WITHDRAWN
WRIGHT STATE UNIVERSITY LIBRARIES

Endocrinology in Clinical Practice

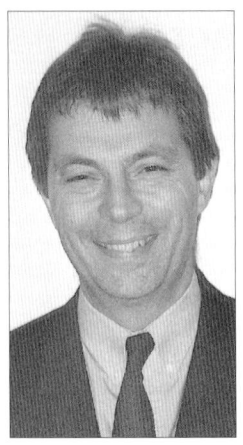

Philip E Harris trained in endocrinology at St Bartholomew's Hospital, London and The University of Newcastle upon Tyne. In 1990-91, Dr Harris worked as an MRC Travelling Fellow at the Endocrine and Reproductive Endocrine Units, Massachusetts General Hospital, Boston, USA. In 1994, he was appointed Senior Lecturer and Consultant Endocrinologist at King's College Hospital, London. His main clinical and research interest is in the field of endocrine oncology, in particular pituitary disease. In April 2001, Dr Harris was appointed Medical Director in Adult Endocrinology Europe, Pharmacia Corporation. He also holds an Honorary Consultant appointment in Endocrinology at St Bartholomew's Hospital, London.

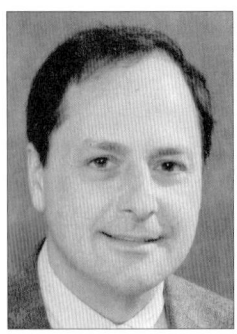

Pierre-Marc G Bouloux is presently Director of the Centre for Neuroendocrinology at the Royal Free and University College of Medicine Schools. He was an MRC Training Fellow under Michael Besser at St Bartholomew's Hospital, London and was subsequently Lecturer in Medicine at the University Department of Medicine at St Bartholomew's. He has held his present post since 1991 and in addition to running a clinical service, he has a special interest in neuroendocrinology. He has published over 150 peer-reviewed publications.

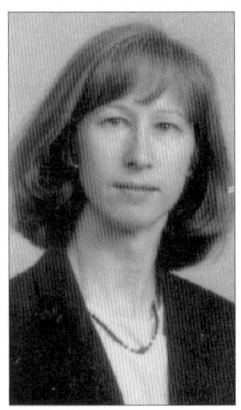

Beverly MK Biller is an associate professor of Medicine at Harvard Medical School, Boston, Massachusetts and on the staff of Massachusetts General Hospital, Boston. She is a supervising physician in the multidisciplinary Neuroendocrine Clinical Center there, and an attending physician on the Endocrinology Consultation Service at Massachusetts General Hospital, where she also serves as Director of the Clinical Fellowship in Endocrinology. Dr. Biller is an associate editor of *Journal of Clinical Endocrinology and Metabolism*. Research interests include neuroendocrine causes of osteoporosis, hormone-secreting pituitary adenomas, and growth hormone deficiency in adults.

Endocrinology in Clinical Practice

Philip E Harris
Honorary Consultant Endocrinologist
St Bartholomew's Hospital
London
UK

Pierre-Marc G Bouloux
Director, Centre for Neuroendocrinology
Royal Free and University College
of Medicine Schools
London
UK
Editors

Beverly MK Biller
Neuroendocrine Unit
Massachusetts General Hospital
Boston MA
USA
Associate Editor

Foreword by Larry Jameson
Chief, Division of Endocrinology,
Metabolism and Molecular Medicine
Northwestern University
Chicago IL
USA

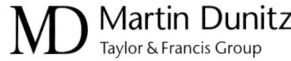

© 2003 Martin Dunitz Ltd, a member of the Taylor & Francis group

First published in the United Kingdom in 2003
by Martin Dunitz Ltd, The Livery House, 7- 9 Pratt Street, London NW1 0AE

Tel.:   +44 (0) 20 74822202
Fax.:   +44 (0) 20 72670159
E-mail: info.dunitz@tandf.co.uk
Website: http://www.dunitz.co.uk

All rights reserved. No part of this publication may be reproduced, stored in a retrieval system, or transmitted, in any form or by any means, electronic, mechanical, photocopying, recording, or otherwise, without the prior permission of the publisher or in accordance with the provisions of the Copyright, Designs and Patents Act 1988 or under the terms of any licence permitting limited copying issued by the Copyright Licensing Agency, 90 Tottenham Court Road, London W1P 0LP.

Although every effort has been made to ensure that drug doses and other information are presented accurately in this publication, the ultimate responsibility rests with the prescribing physician. Neither the publishers nor the authors can be held responsible for errors or for any consequences arising from the use of information contained herein. For detailed prescribing information or instructions on the use of any product or procedure discussed herein, please consult the prescribing information or instructional material issued by the manufacturer.

Although every effort has been made to ensure that all owners of copyright material have been acknowledged in this publication, we would be glad to acknowledge in subsequent reprints or editions any omissions brought to our attention.

A CIP record for this book is available from the British Library.

ISBN 1-84184-186-2

Distributed in the USA by
Fulfilment Center
Taylor & Francis
7625 Empire Drive
Florence, KY 41042, USA
Toll Free Tel.: +1 800 634 7064
E-mail: cserve@routledge_ny.com

Distributed in Canada by
Taylor & Francis
74 Rolark Drive
Scarborough, Ontario M1R 4G2, Canada
Toll Free Tel.: +1 877 226 2237
E-mail: tal_fran@istar.ca

Distributed in the rest of the world by
Thomson Publishing Services
Cheriton House
North Way
Andover, Hampshire SP10 5BE, UK
Tel.: +44 (0)1264 332424
E-mail: salesorder.tandf@thomsonpublishingservices.co.uk

Composition by Tek-Art
Printed and bound in Spain by Grafos S.A. Arte Sobre Papel

Contents

Contributors		*vii*
Foreword		*xi*
Preface		*xii*
1.	Interpretation of biochemical investigations *Joan Butler*	1
2.	Genetic mechanisms of pituitary and thyroid neoplasia *Philip E Harris*	17
3.	Neuroendocrine disease *Philip E Harris*	25
4.	Growth and growth disorders *John Miell, Annice Mukherjee*	83
5.	Carcinoma of the thyroid *Philip E Harris*	107
6.	Multiple endocrine neoplasia *Bin Tean Teh, Catharina Larsson*	115
7.	Amenorrhea and infertility *Beverley Vollenhoven, Henry Burger*	131
8.	Hypogonadism, erectile dysfunction and infertility in men *Shalender Bhasin, Atam B Singh, Charles E Fisher*	147
9.	Hirsutism and virilization *Frances J Hayes, Janet E Hall*	201
10.	Autoimmune disease *Anthony P Weetman*	217
11.	Non-autoimmune thyroid disease *Soo-Mi Park, Luca Persani, Paolo Beck-Peccoz, Krishna Chatterjee*	247
12.	Multinodular goiter, toxic adenoma and thyroiditis *Arie Berghout, Alex F Muller*	269

13. Calcium disorders and bone diseases   287
    Laura Masi, Alberto Falchetti, Luigi Gennari, Maria Luisa Brandi

14. Endocrinology and systemic disease   333
    R Andrew James, Richard Quinton, Steven G Ball

15. Disorders of fluid and electrolytes   367
    Pierre-Marc G Bouloux

16. Endocrine hypertension   387
    Jennifer E Lawrence, Robert G Dluhy

17. Obesity   407
    Pierre-Marc G Bouloux

18. Psychoneuroendocrinology   421
    Salim Janmohamed, Ashley B Grossman

19. Endocrine emergencies   441
    Victor HF Hung, John P Monson

Appendix 1 Pituitary function testing   487
William M Drake, Peter J Trainer

Appendix 2 Pharmacopoeia   499
Pierre-Marc G Bouloux and Jessica M Kubie

Appendix 3 Reference values   543

Index   547

Contributors

Steven G Ball
Senior Lecturer and Honorary Consultant Physician
The Endocrine Unit
Royal Victoria Infirmary
Newcastle-upon-Tyne
UK

Paolo Beck-Peccoz
Institute of Endocrine Sciences
University of Milan
Milan
Italy

Arie Berghout
MCRZ-Zuider
Rotterdam
The Netherlands

Shalender Bhasin
Professor of Medicine
UCLA School of Medicine
Chief, Division of Endocrinology, Metabolism
and Molecular Medicine
Charles R Drew University of Medicine and Science
Los Angeles CA
USA

Maria Luisa Brandi
Full Professor of Endocrinology
Department of Internal Medicine
University of Florence
Florence
Italy

Henry Burger
Director, Prince Henry's Institute of Medical Research
at Monash Medical Centre
Clayton, Victoria
Australia

Joan Butler
Honorary Lecturer
Department of Clinical Biochemistry
Guy's, King's and St Thomas' School of Medicine
London
UK

Krishna Chatterjee
Professor, Department of Medicine
University of Cambridge
Addenbrooke's Hospital
Cambridge
UK

Robert G Dluhy
Professor of Medicine, Harvard Medical School
Brigham and Women's Hospital
Boston MA
USA

William M Drake
Department of Endocrinology
St Bartholomew's and The Royal School of Medicine
and Dentistry
St Bartholomew's Hospital
London
UK

Alberto Falchetti
Endocrinologist and Genetist Assistant in Research
Department of Internal Medicine
University of Florence
Florence
Italy

Charles E Fisher
Charles R Drew University of Medicine and Science
Los Angeles CA
USA

Luigi Gennari
Endocrinologist Assistant in Research
Department of Internal Medicine
University of Florence
Florence
Italy

Ashley B Grossman
Professor of Neuroendocrinology
Department of Endocrinology
St Bartholomew's Hospital
London
UK

CONTRIBUTORS

Janet E Hall
Assistant Professor in Medicine, Harvard Medical School and Reproductive Endocrine Unit
National Center for Infertility Research
Massachusetts General Hospital
Boston MA
USA

Frances J Hayes
Instructor in Medicine, Harvard Medical School and Reproductive Endocrine Unit
National Center for Infertility Research
Massachusetts General Hospital
Boston MA
USA

Victor HF Hung
Department of Endocrinology
St Bartholomew's and The Royal School of Medicine and Dentistry
St Bartholomew's Hospital
London
UK

R Andrew James
Consultant Physician & Senior Lecturer
The Endocrine Unit
Royal Victoria Infirmary
Newcastle-upon-Tyne
UK

Salim Janmohamed
Lecturer in Medicine
Department of Endocrinology
St Bartholomew's Hospital
and Department of Medicine
Salisbury District Hospital
Salisbury
UK

Jessica M Kubie
University of London
London
UK

Catharina Larsson
Department of Molecular Medicine
Karolinska Hospital
Stockholm
Sweden

Jennifer E Lawrence
Brigham and Women's Hospital
Boston MA
USA

Laura Masi
Department of Physiopathology
Endocrine Unit
University of Florence
Florence
Italy

John Miell
Senior Lecturer & Consultant Physician
Guy's, King's and St Thomas' School of Medicine
London
UK

John P Monson
Department of Endocrinology
St Bartholomew's and The Royal School of Medicine and Dentistry
St Bartholomew's Hospital
London
UK

Annice Mukherjee
Registrar in Endocrinology
Christie Hospital
Manchester
UK

Alex F Muller
Hôpital Cantonal Universitaire
Geneva
Switzerland

Soo-Mi Park
Department of Medicine
University of Cambridge
Addenbrooke's Hospital
Cambridge UK

Luca Persani
Institute of Endocrine Sciences
University of Milan
Milan
Italy

Richard Quinton
Consultant Physician and Senior Lecturer
The Endocrine Unit
Royal Victoria Infirmary
Newcastle-upon-Tyne
UK

Atam B Singh
Charles R Drew University of Medicine and Science
Los Angeles CA
USA

Bin Tean Teh
Senior Principal Investigator
Laboratory of Cancer Genetics
Van Andel Research Institute
Grand Rapids MI
USA

Peter J Trainer
Christie Hospital
Manchester
UK

Beverly Vollenhoven
Senior Lecturer
Department of Obstetrics & Gynaecology
Monash Medical Centre
Clayton, Victoria
Australia

Anthony P Weetman
Section of Medicine
Division of Clinical Sciences (North)
Northern General Hospital
Sheffield
UK

Foreword

The practice of endocrinology is based upon a solid foundation of genetics, biochemistry, cell signaling, and physiology. In most cases, the clinical manifestations of hormonal disorders can be explained by understanding the physiologic role of hormones - whether deficient or excessive. The conceptual framework for understanding hormone secretion, hormone action, and principles of feedback control allows the practitioner to design a logical diagnostic approach using appropriate laboratory testing and/or imaging studies. This body of knowledge arms the clinician with abundant evidence for decision-making and makes endocrinology a rewarding field for clinical practice.

Like most fields of medicine, the knowledge base in endocrinology is changing rapidly. In addition to the dramatic advances generated from genetics and molecular biology, the field has benefited from the introduction of an unprecedented number of new drugs, particularly for the management of diabetes and osteoporosis. Common diseases like diabetes, hypertension, obesity, osteoporosis, and polycystic ovarian syndrome have also been the subject of numerous large-scale clinical trials that provide powerful evidence for medical decision-making. These rapid changes in endocrinology mandate that physicians continuously update their knowledge base and clinical skills.

Endocrinology in Clinical Practice is a valuable and practical resource for continuing education and patient management. The chapters are based on common clinical presentations, such as Obesity, Hirsutism and Virilization, Carcinoma of the Thyroid, and Endocrine Emergencies. In addition to consultations for these and other specific endocrine diseases, we are often called upon to provide advice about hormone aberrations or electrolyte management in complex clinical situations. The chapters on Endocrinology and Systemic Disease, Disorders of Fluids and Electrolytes, and Psychoneuroendocrinology exemplify how the book is in synch with clinical practice. The appendices summarizing Pituitary Function Testing and Pharmacopoeia provide a wealth of practical information that should be kept close at hand in the clinic. The book also places special emphasis on how new insights into molecular medicine can enhance our understanding of disease pathogenesis. As examples, the chapters on Genetic Mechanisms of Pituitary and Thyroid Neoplasia, Multiple Endocrine Neoplasia, and several others are timely reviews of these rapidly developing fields.

The authors are a highly select international group of authorities, chosen for their expertise and writing skills. The illustrations are uniformly clear and the book is greatly enriched by numerous photomicrographs of patients and radiologic images using CT and MRI. Endocrinology in Clinical Practice is current, authoritative, and practical. The student, general practitioner, and endocrine specialist will each use this book to improve the care of patients with hormonal disorders.

J. Larry Jameson,
Northwestern University, Chicago, USA

Preface

The aim of this book is to provide cutting edge information on clinical practice in a practical format. The book is aimed primarily at practising endocrinologists and doctors training in endocrinology. A working knowledge of the subject both at the preclinical and clinical levels is assumed. In consequence, there is little in the way of basic physiology and biochemistry. A chapter on the genetic mechanisms of pituitary and thyroid neoplasia is included to provide two models of the way in which oncology is developing in endocrinology. Molecular biology is covered where relevant to disease pathology, such as the multiple endocrine neoplasia syndromes and thyroid hormone resistance.

We have attempted to take a problem-oriented approach to endocrinology. Chapters tend to cover general topics rather than specific disease conditions. In consequence, a number of topics are tackled from varying perspectives in different chapters of the book. Well recognised subjects tend to be covered in a fairly brief manner, the bulk of the emphasis being reserved for new subject areas.

The importance of the laboratory in endocrinology is emphasised by the first chapter, which concentrates on pitfalls in the interpretation of biochemical investigations. We have included normal ranges because we believe that these will provide a useful reference, notwithstanding the fact that these may differ from those of local laboratories. Endocrine investigations are covered in detail in each chapter. Nevertheless, we have provided guidelines for pituitary function testing in Appendix 1, as these tests are central to endocrine practice in most major centres.

Details of pharmacological treatments are included in each chapter. We have, however, included a separate pharmacopoeia as Appendix II, as we feel that this will facilitate the practical use of this book in the clinic.

We are most grateful to the many contributors to this book. We must extend our gratitude to our families for their patience and support whilst the book has been written and edited.

Philip E Harris
Pierre MG Bouloux

1

Interpretation of biochemical investigations
Joan Butler

Introduction

Biochemical data in endocrinology, the results of assays for hormones, offer considerable problems with interpretation. Hormone concentrations must always be considered in context, i.e. with knowledge of the concentrations of the other components of that endocrine system, the state of other endocrine systems and the capabilities of the assays used. In particular, data must be interpreted in the context of the clinical history and examination of the patient. It would be convenient to have strict guidelines and cutoffs for endocrine test results, but these are neither available nor appropriate. The aim of this chapter is to consider the interpretation of data provided by hormone assays, highlighting by example circumstances in which erroneous results might arise or erroneous conclusions be drawn.

The state of the patient

The steady state

Vital to accurate (valid) interpretation of assay results is a knowledge of the state of the patient at the time of blood or urine sampling. If the patient is not in a steady state, then some or all of the components of the feedback system being investigated may fall outside their respective reference ranges for the time being. Obvious examples are: adjustment to thyroxine (T4) replacement therapy, when free T4 and thyroid-stimulating hormone (TSH) may take days or weeks to arrive at their final values for a given dose of T4; recovery from surgical stress, especially cortisol and prolactin; and intercurrent serious non-endocrine illness.

Pulsatile secretion

Although many hormones are secreted in a pulsatile manner, if the half-life in blood is sufficiently long, then a single blood sample may give an adequate estimate of secretion. This is not true for all hormones; for example, for growth hormone (GH), random samples are rarely of any value. If a random sample from a neonate gives a high level, GH deficiency might be ruled out, and similarly an undetectable value from an adult might be considered to exclude acromegaly, but this is generally an expensive and sometimes frankly misleading route to diagnosis. The word 'pituitary' in a possible diagnosis should not generate a list of requests for every pituitary hormone.

Diurnal variation

Diurnal rhythms exist for many hormones, though the change during the day may be small enough to be ignored. Where the change is large, laboratories have reference ranges only for specified times, for example for cortisol only at 0800–1000 hours and at 2300–2400 hours; sampling at other times of day may yield a result which is not interpretable. Diurnal rhythms may be disturbed by admission to hospital and by stress.

It has been known for some time that men show a diurnal rhythm for testosterone, but the size and variability of the diurnal change have generally been ignored in clinical practice. If blood samples are taken in the afternoon, values conspicuously below the morning reference range may be found in the presence of normal gonadotropins (luteinizing hormone (LH); follicle-stimulating hormone (FSH)), possibly leading to the false diagnosis of pituitary insufficiency.[1]

Menstrual cycle

Tests of reproductive hormones in premenopausal women must be done at the appropriate stage of the menstrual cycle. Day 5–7, mid-follicular phase, is chosen for gonadotropin assay, because of the certainty of this date and the clear separation from the time of ovulation and the associated large changes in hormone levels. Day 21, i.e. 7 days after presumed ovulation, is required for progesterone assay for detection of ovulation. If there is doubt about the length of the cycle, then more than one sample should be sent and the timing determined retrospectively, the chosen sample being the nearest to 7 days before the date of onset of the next menstrual period. Results from amenorrheic patients should be compared to ranges for mid-follicular-phase samples.

Medication

It might be considered obvious that medication could invalidate testing for related substances, but requests for cortisol assay to assess residual adrenal function in patients on prednisolone are common. Most antibodies to cortisol show cross-reaction with prednisolone, a closely related steroid. Moreover, generations of doctors, finding steroids a difficult subject, have failed to realize that cortisol the hormone and hydrocortisone the pharmaceutical agent are the same compound, and have attempted to diagnose primary adrenal failure after the patient has received 100 mg of intravenous hydrocortisone.

Apparently unrelated medication is another source of error,[2] e.g. the effect of estrogens, which raise the concentration of cortisol-binding globulin (CBG). A separate reference range for cortisol is required for patients on estrogen therapy, possibly including women on oral replacement therapy, because of the first-pass effect on the liver. Some psychotropic drugs, including some drugs of abuse, cause elevations of prolactin, occasionally to very high levels; medication should be the first possibility considered for the cause of raised prolactin. Heparin in vivo activates lipases, and the resulting increase in free fatty acid concentrations may displace thyroid hormones from albumin and produce a transient increase in free T4.

Table 1.1 gives some examples of commonly occurring interference from medication.

Changes in specific binding protein concentrations

For those hormones which circulate in the blood largely bound to specific serum proteins, disorders

Medication	Hormone	Effect
Hydrocortisone	Cortisol	Grossly raised
Prednisolone	Cortisol	Apparently raised
Estrogens	Cortisol	Raised (CBG raised)
	Testosterone (women)	Raised (SHBG raised)
	Total T4	Raised (TBG raised)
Oral contraceptives	FSH and LH	Suppressed
Dopamine antagonists (many antiemetics, most tranquilizers)	Prolactin	Raised
Some drugs of abuse	Prolactin	Raised
Heparin	Free T4	Raised (transiently)
Salicylates	Free T4	Raised (transiently)

FSH, follicle-stimulating hormone; CBG, cortisol-binding globulin; SHBG, sex hormone-binding globulin; TBG, thyroxine-binding globulin.

Table 1.1
Some commonly occurring effects of medication on hormone levels.

which affect the concentration of the binding protein will affect the total concentration of hormone, even though the free or unbound hormone level (thought to be the biologically active fraction) may be unaffected. The principal hormones in this category are thyroid hormones, cortisol and testosterone. It is difficult to remove the protein-bound fraction, or to assay the free fraction in the presence of the protein-bound fraction, without disturbing the equilibrium, especially if the binding is not tight, and methods for measurement of the free hormone are not available at present for cortisol and testosterone. Although methods for free thyroid hormones are routinely used, they are prone to technical difficulties (see below).

Correction for changes in binding protein by measurement of the concentration of the binding protein and calculation of the hormone/protein ratio has been used for T4 and thyroxine-binding globulin (TBG) and for testosterone and sex hormone-binding globulin (SHBG). For T4, the so-called free thyroxine index can be calculated from the total T4 concentration and the uptake test which measures available protein-binding sites. Such corrections are likely to be invalid when the concentrations of specific binding proteins are very different from normal, and in the case of the T4/TBG ratio, when other binding proteins such as albumin are also abnormal. Opinion is divided on the utility of measuring SHBG and calculation of the testosterone/SHBG ratio, but unsuspected changes in SHBG can be revealed, e.g. low values in patients with pituitary tumors. In women, increased testosterone secretion produces a decrease in SHBG concentration, and these two effects can balance out to give normal total testosterone concentrations. In the absence of methods for free hormone estimation, rigorous validation of these correction techniques is not possible.

Table 1.2 lists some factors which affect the concentrations of serum binding proteins.

Intercurrent illness

Severe intercurrent illness may affect endocrine systems and also the tests used to assess such systems, the most important example of which is the effect of non-thyroidal illness (NTI), otherwise known as the sick euthyroid syndrome, on thyroid function testing. In the absence of pre-existing thyroid dysfunction, major abnormalities of thyroid function tests are seen in serious non-thyroidal illness and in the recovery phase. Some of the difficulties of interpretation of thyroid function tests result from the fact that the patient is not in a steady state, e.g. acute caloric deprivation and increases in serum free fatty acids, introduction of drugs which affect T4 metabolism or displace T4 from its binding sites on serum proteins, a catabolic state and decreases in concentrations of serum proteins. In patients given dopamine or high doses of exogenous corticosteroids, TSH may be suppressed. In some studies, the changes seen in the levels of free thyroid hormones may have been assay-dependent artefacts, and this has tended to hinder understanding of the underlying pathophysiological mechanisms.[3,4]

Immunoassay problems in NTI

The earliest immunoassays for measurement of free T4 were the labeled analog methods. The analog is a molecule closely related to T4 which binds to the reagent antibody but which does not bind to the specific binding protein TBG. The first analogs were found to bind to albumin, and the result obtained was therefore in part a function of the concentration of albumin in the sample, which is likely to be low in NTI. The same problem was present in assays for free triiodothyronine (T3). More recent methods use analogs which do not bind to albumin, notably enzyme-labeled derivatives, or completely different

---

Increased binding protein concentrations
  Genetic
  Estrogen (endogenous or exogenous)
  Pregnancy and hydatidiform mole
  Thyrotoxicosis (SHBG)

Decreased binding protein concentrations
  Genetic
  Androgen
  Liver disease
  Protein-losing states
  Severe illness
  Malnutrition
  Malabsorption
  Acromegaly
  Cushing's disease
  High-dose corticosteroid therapy

Table 1.2
Factors which affect the concentrations of specific binding proteins.

assay designs. Some manufacturers include albumin in the reagents, to take up possible inhibitors of T4 binding in the sample. This and other procedures may in some cases amount to tailoring the result to suit present conceptions of the 'true' values to be found in NTI.

Equilibrium dialysis, considered by many to be the most reliable method available for free thyroid hormones, is also prone to problems in NTI. Incubation of the sample at 37°C during the dialysis procedure, especially after heparin treatment, may release fatty acids from lipids in the sample, which will displace thyroid hormone from serum proteins and artefactually elevate the result. If inhibitors of binding are present, their effect may be diminished if they pass into the dialysate.

Because of the very high affinity of TBG for T4, in theory the free T4 concentration should change very little on dilution of the serum. In practice, the serum has already been diluted manyfold in the assay, but limited further dilution of normal serum should give only a slight drop in free T4. In samples from NTI patients, however, large falls may be seen. This may be a way of assessing whether the free T4 value is a reliable index of thyroid function in a sick patient.

There are many recent reviews of thyroid function in NTI, a sure sign that the problems have not been resolved.[5-7]

Testing for thyroid dysfunction in the presence of NTI or in the short-term recovery phase is not advised unless there are clinical signs of such dysfunction. Thyroid function testing in the sick thyrotoxic patient can be problematic, as the degree of suppression of TSH in thyrotoxicosis is not distinguishable from that in NTI, and total T3 and free T3 may be suppressed into the normal range by NTI, rising sharply when the intercurrent illness has been alleviated.

In patients with chronic renal failure, low albumin and high lipids, assay problems may occur similar to those seen in acute NTI.

The sample
Blood

The taking of a blood sample, the type of anticoagulant used, if any, and the transport and storage of the sample are practical matters which may have considerable effects on assay results, and these factors must not be ignored.

Timing and stress have been considered above. Visible lipid or hemolysis may interfere in the assays. The type of blood collection tube (volume and anticoagulant) to be used will depend on the assay in use in the local laboratory and on the analyte to be measured. Heparin interferes in some immunoassays, and EDTA plasma may be incompatible with enzyme-labeled immunoassays, because of chelation of metal ion cofactors. Fragile analytes like adrenocorticotropic hormone (ACTH) require special handling; EDTA limits in vitro degradation by inhibiting plasma proteases, but rapid separation of the sample and low temperature are also very important. Specific advice about each analyte should be sought from the laboratory before beginning blood sampling.

Urine

Similar considerations apply to urine samples. Preservatives and/or cold storage may be required for some analytes. Duration of collection is an important matter, some hormones being satisfactorily assessed in overnight samples, and some requiring 24 h collections. Completeness of collection is, of course, a major source of error.

Assay methods

The use of antibodies or binding proteins as reagents, stemming from the work of Yalow and Berson and of Ekins in the 1950s,[8,9] is the foundation of biochemical endocrinology. At the present time, almost all endocrine assays are immunoassays, with the exception of methods for small molecules such as steroids and catecholamines. For most clinical purposes, steroids in blood are also measured by immunoassay. Catecholamines and, in some circumstances, steroids are measured by methods involving high-performance liquid chromatography (HPLC) or gas–liquid chromatography (GLC); these techniques are time-consuming and have their own problems of imprecision and interferences. Bioassay is seldom used routinely.

Immunoassay: assay design

There are two basic designs of immunoassay, though many variations exist. In the competitive or limited antibody method, generally termed immunoassay, antigen (the analyte of interest) from the sample (or calibrator) competes with antigen labeled with a tracer or reporter molecule for a limited amount of antibody. The amount of label bound will be inversely related to the amount of antigen in the sample. Separation of the bound and free fractions and quantitation of the label in either (though usually the bound fraction) and comparison with a calibration curve permits quantitation (Figure 1.1). Since binding is maximal in the absence of analyte, anything which inhibits binding will give a falsely high value for the analyte concentration.

In non-competitive or labeled antibody methods, generally termed immunometric assay, the analyte is reacted with an excess of labeled antibody. The bound and free forms are separated, and the bound labeled antibody measured; the amount bound will be directly related to the concentration of analyte (Figure 1.2). For small analytes, the excess labeled antibody may be removed by the addition of analyte coupled to a solid phase; such coupling reduces reactivity, and the coupled analyte does not compete with free analyte from the sample. For larger analytes, another antibody to the analyte may be used, directed against a different epitope. This antibody is termed the capture antibody and is usually coupled to a solid phase. This format is termed the two-site or sandwich assay, and is much used for the assay of polypeptide hormones. Inhibition of binding will result in a falsely low value for the analyte concentration. Only substances capable of crosslinking the two antibodies will give positive interference. Solid phases may be the wall of a tube, the well of a microtiter plate or the surface of a bead or small

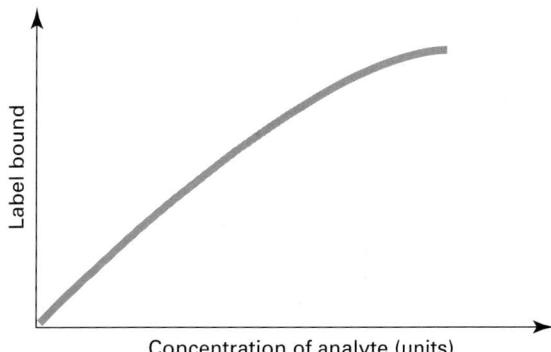

Figure 1.2
Typical standard curve for an immunometric assay.

particles. Polyclonal antisera can be used for immunometric assays, but this type of assay came into general use only with the advent of monoclonal antibodies.

In general, immunometric assays are faster, more sensitive and have a wider working range than competitive immunoassays.

The matrix of the sample, protein content, pH and ionic composition may affect the assay. Assays designed for serum may not be usable for urine or other fluids.

The type of label used has relatively little effect on the quality of the result, though it may affect the speed or convenience of the assay. Radioactive iodine was the first label to be used, and as iodination is relatively simple to do, it is often used in setting up new assays. However, the products are not very stable, and radioisotopes are increasingly regarded as hazardous to health. Some of the alternatives, e.g. time-resolved fluorescence, chemiluminescence or electrochemiluminescence, offer inherently better sensitivity, either because more label can be incorporated or because the label is more easily and quickly measured. Because the equipment required for measurement varies with the label used, changing to alternative methods may involve major capital expenditure, and this will limit the choice of methods.

Immunoassay: specificity and cross-reactivity

Antibodies are highly specific reagents and can recognize short amino acid sequences or clusters, or parts of steroid or thyronine structures, with a specificity largely denied to chemical or physical methods. Depending upon the epitope to which an antibody was

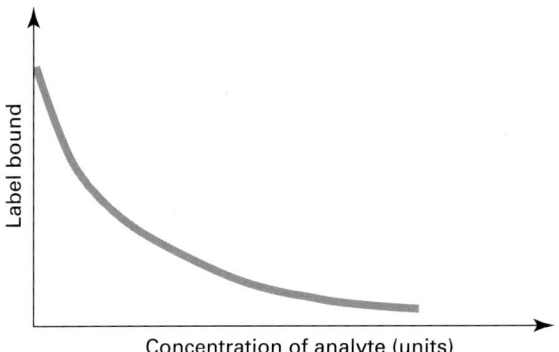

Figure 1.1
Typical standard curve for a competitive immunoassay.

raised, it may or may not be able to distinguish a hormone molecule from its isoforms, precursors, metabolites, fragments and other related molecules. In the case of small molecules such as steroids, which are made antigenic by attachment to a large molecule, the part of the molecule close to the attachment may be 'invisible' and may not contribute to the specificity of the antibodies. A polyclonal antiserum will contain a large number of antibodies of differing affinities and specificities, whereas a monoclonal antibody has a single set of readily characterizable attributes. The two-site assay for large molecules increases the specificity by requiring two connected epitopes, and this can be further modified by the use of several monoclonal antibodies in an oligoclonal system.

Some immunoassays have suffered from serious problems of specificity, due to the antibody being directed to an epitope not unique to the biologically active hormone; for example, early assays for parathyroid hormone measured inactive metabolites together with the active molecule, giving information about the pathophysiology of this hormone which was subsequently found by the use of more specific assays to be incorrect. This kind of difficulty should be borne in mind when reviewing early literature. Structural similarities between hormones cause similar problems, for example: FSH and LH; the inhibins; and LH and chorionic gonadotropin (hCG). Many current assays for LH show some 'cross-reactivity' with hCG, which can be useful in the detection of pregnancy. With such an LH assay, in any patient the combination of undetectable FSH and normal or raised LH should prompt an hCG determination.

The expected problem of hyperspecificity of monoclonal antibodies, i.e. the antibody failing to recognize some of the biologically active forms of a hormone, has rarely been seen. An extreme example is that of an LH genetic variant common in Nordic populations in which a portion of the molecule close to the junction of the subunits is deleted, but biological activity is retained though possibly diminished, subjects with this variant having proven fertility.[10] One commercially available immunoassay, now withdrawn, did not recognize the variant and gave undetectable values for LH in homozygotes. Possibly more misleading was the half-normal value obtained in heterozygotes. In the case of GH, which has two major forms co-secreted in all subjects, the principal 22-kDa form and a 20-kDa splice variant, it is probably not necessary to measure both forms but only the 22-kDa form.[11] Both forms are thought to be biologically active in vivo. There will be marked numerical differences between the results of an immunoassay measuring both forms and the results of one which measures only the 22-kDa form.

Cross-reactivity, unwanted reaction of another molecule in an assay, occurs often, especially in the steroid field. For example, prednisolone is measured in most if not all assays for cortisol. There are several quantitative definitions of cross-reactivity, but they are all arbitrary and are used only to indicate the potential seriousness of such cross-reactivity. The contribution of the cross-reactant to the measured concentration will depend on the concentrations of both the target analyte and the cross-reactant, and calculation of the amount of either the analyte or the cross-reactant in a mixture is not possible.

It will be clear that assays based on different antibodies or antisera may not necessarily give the same results, given the molecular heterogeneity of many polypeptide hormones and the number of potential reactants in body fluids. Since there are no absolute or reference methods for endocrine analytes, with the possible exception of some steroids, thyroid hormones and catecholamines, it is difficult to know which assays are 'right', although there are various tests of validity which can be applied. These include the investigation of potential cross-reactions and interferences and of linearity on dilution. If the calibrant and the analyte are identical, then dilution of the sample should give a (calculated) value the same as that found for the undiluted sample, a situation often described as dilution parallel to the standard. Non-linearity demonstrates a problem of non-identity of some kind, including the presence of cross-reactants or interferents, but the finding of linearity on dilution does not rule out the presence of such substances.

Immunoassay: standardization (calibration)

The preparation of large quantities of pure hormones, especially the polypeptide hormones, is a formidable task. In most cases, it has not been possible to prepare enough pure material by extraction from tissues for measurement by physical methods to provide calibrants for immunoassays. Because of this, the existing International Standards (IS), prepared for use in bioassays, were adopted for use with immunoassays. This did provide a common reference material with internationally accepted, though arbitrary, International Units (IU), but produced a number of problems.

Bioassays measure function, and immunoassays quantitate the amount (of a particular epitope). Where isoforms or variants exist, the estimates by the two types of assay may differ between preparations, as strikingly shown for the IS 83/575 for FSH.[12] This was prepared to have a high content of the more biologically active isoforms, and the bioassay/immunoassay ratio was therefore very much higher than for the previous Standard. This IS has not been adopted for use in immunoassay, as normal values for serum FSH would have gone up by a factor of 4! The existence of isoforms, such as the glycosylation isoforms of FSH, brings into question the whole concept of a pure hormone.

Because the IS are presently calibrated by bioassays in arbitrary IU, and the mass of hormone in the preparation is not accurately known, the IU–mass conversion factors are nominal.[13] Many authorities have ignored this fact and have quoted assay results inappropriately in mass terms, e.g. prolactin or GH in the USA. Unit–mass conversion factors for commercial calibrants will be specific to those calibrants.

It has also been shown, and is evident from UK National External Quality Assessment Schemes data (see below), that the hormone in an IS may not be exactly the same as the form(s) existing in serum. This may be because the material was derived from tissues, e.g. pituitary glands, or because purification induced alterations in the molecule or in the pattern of isoforms or other components. For some important analytes such as ACTH, there is presently no suitable material with which to make an IS.

For the new IS prepared by recombinant technology, the mass of hormone can be measured by physicochemical means, and the content in IU determined by immunoassay to maintain continuity of unitage. A conversion factor or specific activity (IU/mg) can then be set, but this value may still be a compromise because of the differences between immunoassays.[13,14] The ultimate aim is calibration in mass or molar units.

Some of the differences between immunoassays can be ascribed to errors of calibration and some to the fundamental difficulties described above. For a clear and authoritative account of standardization and its current controversies, see Bristow.[12]

Immunoassay: precision

In order that a result be as close as possible to the true value for the sample, laboratories must attempt to minimize all forms of error, from blunders to the imprecision of each step of the assay.

Precision, the reproducibility of the values obtained, is assessed via internal quality control. Because of the complexity of the technique, immunoassay is generally less precise than many of the other methods used in clinical biochemistry. Precision, however, improved sharply with the introduction of automation in the early 1990s. Precision will vary with the concentration of the analyte, the coefficient of variation (CV, the standard deviation (SD) as a percentage of the mean value) usually being highest at very low levels and sometimes increasing again at high levels (Figure 1.3). Inter-assay precision will be worse than intra-assay precision, because of the error of recalibration. The detection limit, sometimes called the sensitivity, of an assay, i.e. the smallest amount which can be reliably distinguished from zero, can be defined in several ways, all of which are dependent on the precision at low levels. Analytical sensitivity is usually defined as the concentration which is 2 (or 2.5) SD above zero, the SD being calculated from 20 replicates of the zero calibrator. Functional sensitivity, a somewhat more realistic parameter, is the concentration at which the CV (ideally between-assay) is 20%, determined using sera with very low analyte content.

Although assays of the immunometric design usually have working ranges of about three orders of magnitude, it is unusual for an assay to be able to measure with adequate precision all concentrations encountered in clinical samples, and many assays are set up for specific clinical purposes. For example, an assay optimized for

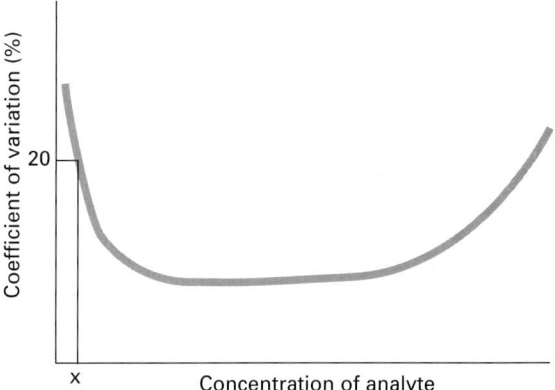

Figure 1.3
A typical precision profile. The concentration at which the CV is 20%, given by x, is the functional sensitivity.

measurement of hCG in pregnancy may not be capable of the precision at very low levels required for the use of hCG as a tumor marker.

When assays with better precision and lower detection limits become available, new clinical information may be revealed. The introduction of immunometric assays for TSH around 1984 revolutionized thyroid function testing,[15] previous assays having been insufficiently sensitive to be able to determine the lower limit of normal and therefore to distinguish low-normal from suppressed values. Using the so-called third-generation or ultrasensitive assays, however, overlap is still seen between the low values found in thyrotoxicosis and those of severe NTI. In the complex field of GH secretion and regulation, considerable advances of understanding have been achieved with recent improvements in assay technology.[16] The improvement in precision associated with automation should be beneficial to clinical studies, conclusions being clearer, with most of the 'noise' due to imprecision removed. Between-laboratory CVs of <5% are now commonly seen over a wide range of concentrations for many hormones.

Immunoassay: accuracy

Accuracy, the closeness of a value to the true value, is difficult to ascertain for endocrine analytes, since the true value is seldom known, given the absence of absolute or reference methods except perhaps for some steroid and thyroid hormones. In the UK, for the validation of immunoassays, laboratories largely rely on external quality assessment schemes (e.g. UK NEQAS), in which the results returned from 'blind' analysis of samples sent out by a central laboratory are considered in terms of laboratory and method precision, adequacy of calibration, consensus of methods, susceptibility of methods to certain interferences, and sometimes interpretation and appropriateness of reference ranges.

Since the characteristics of a method or kit are relatively constant, certainly in the short term, and since the numbers of participants in UK NEQAS may be in the hundreds and the numbers of methods in use 20 or 30, the mean value obtained for a sample will be relatively constant over a period of many months. This mean value (the ALTM or All Laboratory Trimmed Mean, trimmed of gross outliers) can be used as a target value, the only target available for many endocrine analytes. The relationship of each laboratory's result to the ALTM is expressed as percentage bias, and the bias of a method can also be calculated. The 6-month running mean bias is written as BIAS. For some analytes, method BIAS is clearly related to calibration and specificity factors, e.g. GH,[17] but in some cases no explanation is available. The ALTM can be shifted by a highly biased method with a large number of users, and the trend towards automation and fewer methods but larger user groups gives cause for concern. Indicators of consensus of methods are the range of BIAS observed or the overall between-laboratory agreement usually found.

The information provided by UK NEQAS is very valuable and has contributed to the continued improvement of laboratory and method performance, but accuracy can be approached only in terms of consensus, which is not necessarily a reliable index.

Immunoassay: consensus of methods

The consensus of methods is particularly important in the interpretation of the results of dynamic tests, as criteria in use now are in many cases derived from studies carried out some years ago, using assays different from those available today. Clinicians are understandably reluctant to set up studies of dynamic tests in large numbers of normal subjects. Some of the reference ranges in general use for dynamic tests of pituitary–adrenal function were derived in 1969[18] from limited studies using a fluorimetric method for cortisol, a relatively non-specific method no longer in use. Interpretation of results from one assay using criteria derived from a different assay can lead to inappropriate clinical decisions, and this still applies to individual immunoassays. Figure 1.4 is an example of UK NEQAS data comparing the values given by a total of 246 laboratories and 11 current cortisol methods for a single sample in September 1998. Many participant laboratories would have been using the same 'textbook' limit for the response to tetracosactrin (Synacthen), despite the discrepancies between the values produced by their assays.[19] There is evidence from UK NEQAS data that different relationships between assays may be found for unstimulated samples from male and female subjects. Clark et al[20] showed that the value for the 5th centile cutoff for the cortisol response to Synacthen in normal subjects differed not only between assays but also between males and females, and that relationships between the four assays studied differed between basal and post-stimulation samples. The use of a simple factor to derive a new cutoff or a new reference range when

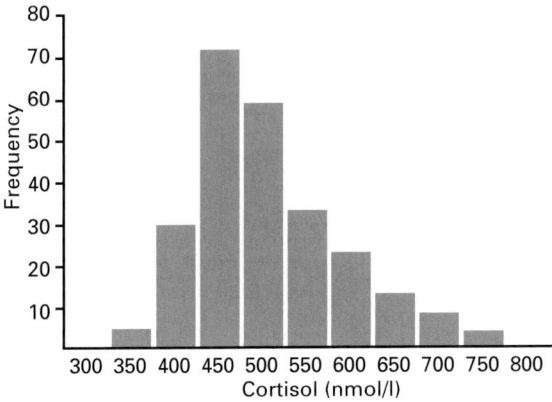

Figure 1.4
Data from UK NEQAS on a single sample showing the spread of results achieved by individual laboratories.

changing assays is unwise; the aim should be to make comparisons in samples taken from all possible types of subject or patient and under all possible conditions.

The difficulties created by poor consensus of assays may occur for any endocrine analyte. Another example is the tradition that in polycystic ovarian syndrome the LH/FSH ratio is around 3. This figure, never diagnostic, cannot be applied to every possible pair of LH and FSH assays, and the characteristics of the assays used to derive the figure of 3 are long forgotten. Even when an individual commercial kit remains on the market for many years, its characteristics may change with time, e.g. errors of calibration being corrected or new antibodies being substituted; such matters are seldom reported in the medical literature.

Consensus is presently good for a few hormones, e.g. TSH and (total) T4, and very poor for free thyroid hormones. It would be very convenient if all assays gave the same values, avoiding errors of interpretation and discontinuities in patients' data, but this situation is unlikely to happen. The alternative, that all laboratories use the same assay, is not a viable option at the present time, and would lead to a loss of scientific information. The differences between assays can be pointers to previously unsuspected problems, as in the case of autoantibodies to prolactin (see below).

When changing from one immunoassay to another, a laboratory will carry out a comparison of the two methods, and the samples analyzed should include some from all types of patients in whom the analyte is to be measured. If the two methods are really measuring the same substance, then the correlation coefficient will be 0.99 or better. If the correlation coefficient is conspicuously less than this, then in one or both assays there are problems of imprecision, cross-reactivity or interference.

Immunoassay: automation

Automated instruments for the performance of immunoassays became available around 1990, with stable reagents permitting random access systems, and the precision of some of these instruments is such that coefficients of variation of 3–4% can be maintained for long periods. Automation does not alter the basic characteristics of immunoassay but only the speed (and effort) with which a result may be obtained and the precision of that result. Laboratories with automated equipment may be unable to change to alternative methods in the short term if problems occur.

Assay failings

Apart from imprecision and blunders such as the incorrect identification of samples, there are certain circumstances when a usually satisfactory immunoassay may give an erroneous result.

The 'high-dose hook' effect

Assays using simultaneous addition of two antibodies (one-step assay) in the two-site immunometric configuration are subject to the 'high-dose hook effect', in which at very high analyte concentrations the value reported is falsely low. When the analyte concentration is very high and the antibodies are no longer in excess, the binding sites of both the capture antibody and the labeled antibody are occupied by separate molecules of analyte. Crosslinking is reduced, diminishing the observed signal. At extremely high concentrations, the signal may be below that of the top calibrator, giving a readable value orders of magnitude lower than the true value (Figure 1.5). The concentration at which this occurs is related to the amounts of the reagent antibodies and therefore varies with the assay used.

Although this effect can occur with a one-step sandwich assay for any analyte, it is of clinical importance only for those analytes for which a concentration range of several orders of magnitude is found in

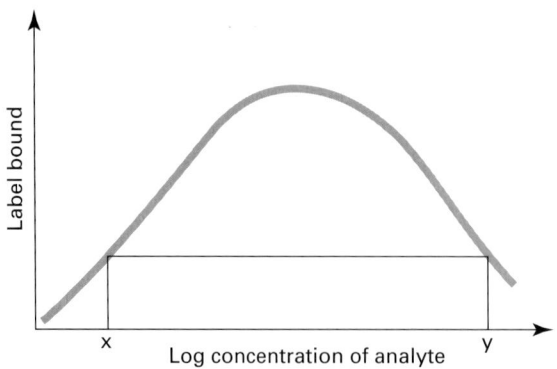

Figure 1.5
The high-dose hook effect. x = concentration of the highest calibrator; y = concentration above which falsely low values will be obtained on samples assayed without dilution. Between x and y, a value of '>x' would be reported.

clinical practice, e.g. prolactin, and must be borne in mind when attempting to determine whether a large pituitary tumor is a prolactinoma. The hook effect has the greatest potential for causing a diagnostic disaster for those analytes whose presence may be 'silent', i.e. some tumor markers. Laboratories try to avoid the hook effect by assaying in dilution samples likely to contain very high concentrations.

The high-dose hook effect does not occur with two-step assays, in which a wash step is included before addition of the labeled antibody. This step, however, introduces further imprecision to the assay.

Interferences

Various substances which interfere in immunoassays are found in blood or urine. Interference may be related to the hormone in question, e.g. cross-reaction of similar molecules (see above) or sequestration of hormone by endogenous binding proteins or auto-antibodies, or it may be general, affecting assays for any hormone in that sample.

Binding proteins

Endogenous binding proteins of high affinity can cause considerable problems in assays for the hormone, as they compete with reagent antibody for the hormone. Prior removal of the binding protein may cause losses of the hormone, and inadequate removal or inactivation may invalidate results, as was the case for insulin-like growth factor 1 (IGF-1) assays using acid–ethanol extraction (a misnomer, actually inactivation) without cryoprecipitation or chromatographic separation.[21] In assays for T4 or steroids, the hormone is released from its binding protein by chemical means. The effect on assays for GH of the high-affinity GH binding protein (GHBP) found in serum was initially discounted[22] and therefore generally ignored, but it is now known that this protein does interfere in some assays.[14,23,24]

In the rare familial condition of dysalbuminemic hyperthyroxinemia, a variant albumin binds T4 much more strongly than does normal albumin, giving raised total T4, but the subject is (usually) euthyroid and TSH will be normal.

Autoantibodies

Autoantibodies to the hormone of interest can produce bizarre results, as seen most obviously in the case of autoantibodies to T4 and/or T3. These antibodies do not of themselves cause a disturbance of the pituitary–thyroid axis, though there may be an increased incidence in patients with thyroid disorders. They may produce high values for total thyroid hormones, if present in sufficiently high titer, but the most marked effect is aberrant values for the free hormones given by some methods, due to participation of the autoantibodies in the assay.[25]

Interferences from autoantibodies to thyroid hormones or from variant albumin can be recognized in the first instance by discrepancies between the various components of the pituitary–thyroid axis and between the biochemistry and the clinical picture.

Autoantibodies to thyroglobulin are present in many patients with autoimmune thyroid dysfunction, and also occur in a substantial proportion of patients with differentiated thyroid cancers. Interference by anti-thyroglobulin antibodies in most current assays for thyroglobulin may prevent the use of this marker in such patients for the detection of residual or recurrent tumor.[26]

Autoantibodies to prolactin are a frequent but less well-recognized source of anomalous results.[27] The major circulating form of prolactin in normal subjects is monomeric prolactin with a molecular mass of 23 kDa. Big prolactin, ~50 kDa, also occurs in blood and may be a dimer. The antibody-bound form is termed macroprolactin or big-big prolactin, with molecular mass 150–170 kDa. Since the antibody-bound form is cleared more slowly from plasma than monomeric prolactin, it tends to become the predominant form in subjects with this condition. Most assays for prolactin presently in use in the UK recognize the antibody-bound form to some extent,[28] though the magnitude of the response varies considerably, and therefore will give high results in patients with macroprolactinemia.

The prevalence of macroprolactinemia has recently been shown to be 15–25% in samples with moderately raised prolactin concentrations,[29–31] and macroprolactinemia may be a major factor in the skewed distribution of total serum prolactin and the difficulty of interpretation of mildly raised prolactin concentrations.

Although many of these patients are fertile, firm evidence for the degree of biological activity in vivo of macroprolactin is difficult to acquire. Most studies have few patients, and the symptoms of hyperprolactinemia are somewhat non-specific. If macroprolactin is not biologically active, then in patients with macroprolactinemia the problem is to assess the level of unbound or monomeric prolactin. Since there is presently no specific assay for either prolactin or macroprolactin, it is necessary to separate the two forms by gel filtration, a cumbersome and expensive procedure, before assay. A simpler alternative is assay after precipitation of the antibody-bound fraction with polyethylene glycol (PEG). This is a useful screening test,[30,31] but it is not very precise and PEG may interfere in some prolactin assays. If the PEG precipitation test is to be used to estimate the monomeric prolactin concentration, the test should first be validated against gel filtration.

The variability of response of different immunoassays when compared on samples from different patients[28,29] suggests that macroprolactin is not a single species. The nature of the variation is presently not known. Occasionally, forms of macroprolactin with very high molecular masses have been found.[32]

Heterophilic antibodies
Human antibodies to immunoglobulins of other species can interfere in all types of immunoassay by binding to reagent antibody and reducing the binding of the analyte, giving increased or decreased results according to assay design, but are most commonly detected in sandwich assays, when crosslinking of capture and signal antibodies gives a spuriously high concentration of analyte.[33] The highest titers of heterophilic antibodies are found in patients who have received murine monoclonal antibodies for diagnostic or therapeutic purposes; these antibodies are termed human anti-mouse antibodies or HAMA. The cause of induction in other subjects is not known, but may be vaccination, handling animals or even the diet. Heterophilic antibodies including HAMA usually react with the immunoglobulins of a number of species (hence their name), and their effects are counteracted by the inclusion in the assay reagents of non-immune serum or polymerized immunoglobulins, usually murine.[34] However, occasionally, the concentration of heterophilic antibodies is sufficiently high to overcome such blockage.

Rheumatoid factor
Rheumatoid factor, human IgM against human IgG, may also react with the immunoglobulins of other species, giving interference similar to that of heterophilic antibodies. Rheumatoid factor is present in the sera of many patients with rheumatoid arthritis or other autoimmune diseases and in the sera of some elderly subjects. Interference is apparently not closely related to the titer of rheumatoid factor as presently measured; it may be that the interference is due in part to other factors commonly found in rheumatoid arthritis patients.

For a review of interference by various types of antibody in thyroid assays see Despres and Grant.[25]

Complement
Complement in vivo is able to destroy immune complexes, and in vitro may interfere with assays using second antibody precipitation or solid-phase separation.[35] Susceptibility to this interference is not a universal feature of immunoassay, and may depend on the immunoglobulin subclass and other factors. Interference will be maximal in fresh serum, as complement itself is labile in vitro. Complement activation depends on calcium ions and can be prevented by the inclusion of a chelating agent, though this may not be feasible for some types of assay.

Detection of interference

The presence of interfering substances is usually detected only by unlikely combinations of results or by discrepancies between the results and the clinical picture. In the case of common problems such as anti-thyroglobulin antibodies, these substances are usually assayed by the laboratory before attempting the assay of thyroglobulin. Discussion of unexpected results with experienced laboratory staff is the first stage in detection of interferences.

Interpretation

Reference ranges

The establishment of reference ranges against which patients' results can be compared is a major undertaking. The numbers of normal subjects required for statistically valid ranges are very large, the minimum number recommended by the International Federation for Clinical Chemistry being 120 for each group of subjects, multiplied up when age or sex differences exist. For most endocrine analytes, this goal is often not attained. In practice, it can be quite difficult to achieve blood or urine samples from even small numbers of apparently normal subjects, e.g. premenopausal women with no menstrual disorder and not on oral contraceptives. Until recently, ethical considerations have prevented the acquisition of data on normal children, especially the results of dynamic tests on which, unfortunately, the diagnosis of GH deficiency has been based (see below). Manufacturers of commercial kits seldom have access to large numbers of appropriate subjects and usually recommend the user to make his own ranges. With the advent of automation and very good between-laboratory precision, it is now possible to make reference ranges by large numbers of laboratories each contributing data on small numbers of subjects. Reference ranges differ not only between assays but also sometimes according to the population under study, for racial, dietary or other reasons.

It is essential to relate results to the reference range for the assay in use, and to request this information if it is not provided. Ranges can be presented as the entire range of results achieved in normal subjects, as the central 95% of those results (the 95% reference interval) or, if the distribution is Gaussian, as the mean ±2 SD. Since both the reference range and a patient's result have some imprecision, intra-personal variation can be considerable, and there will be normal subjects with values just outside the range, however derived and results close to the limits of the range should be interpreted with caution.[36]

Information from the literature

Because of continuing technical advances and also of increasingly high standards of scientific and medical studies, unquestioning acceptance of the findings of published studies is to be avoided. Papers should be scrutinized for the suitability of the assays for the purpose of the study, the comparability of the control and disease groups with respect to age, gender and other relevant variables, the adequacy for statistical reliability of the numbers in these groups, especially if subdivided by age or other characteristics, and the presence of bias in the selection of subjects or the reporting of results. The same matters should be borne in mind when setting up new studies; for example, in some cases it may be exceptionally difficult to find adequate numbers of control subjects, such as normal women not on any type of estrogen treatment. As discussed elsewhere in this chapter, it will be found that accepted wisdom in some fields is based on very slight evidence.

GH as an example

GH provides a good example of many of the problems of assays, tests and interpretation in endocrinology, and despite decades of study it remains a difficult subject. Fortunately, GH is fairly stable in serum, but it is rather less so in urine, partly because the amount of other protein in urine is small, and GH may be lost by adsorption onto the container.

Since secretion of GH is highly pulsatile, serum levels of GH fluctuate enormously. Even present immunometric methods are imprecise at nadir levels, only the new ultrasensitive methods being sufficiently precise to provide values for basal concentrations.[16] Imprecision may have confounded the many attempts to establish determination of GH secretion rate using frequent sampling over 12 h or 24 h as a test for GH deficiency in children. Even in normal subjects, many of the samples would have GH concentrations close to or below the detection limit of a competitive radioimmunoassay. Between-method differences for GH assays can be as large as a factor of 2,[17] and previously may have been even larger.[37] Reactivity of GH immunoassays for the 20-kDa form of GH is a major cause of such differences. As 20-kDa GH is cleared from the blood more slowly than the 22-kDa form, the area under the curve of GH concentration versus time will be greater and the fall in GH concentration after the peak (endogenous or stimulated) apparently delayed if assays recognizing both forms are used. Interference in GH assays from GH-binding protein (the extracellular domain of the GH receptor) has been little appreciated, and agreement on the levels of this protein in blood is poor.[38–40]

There is no absolute method for defining the presence of GH deficiency against which biochemical tests can be assessed, and the insulin stress test has been used for this purpose, despite its known unsuitability.[41,42] Interpretation of the results of a stimulation test requires not only that the test is strictly defined and applied but that sufficient data from normal subjects have been acquired to constitute a proper reference range. Such data were acquired for children in 1996,[43] and demonstrated that as many as 49% of normally growing children might fail such tests. For more than three decades, selection of children for GH therapy has been based on unreliable tests and arbitrary cutoffs. Since the treatment groups will have been markedly heterogeneous, evaluation of the outcome of GH therapy is seriously compromised.[44]

In 1988, Australian pediatricians abandoned GH testing as a criterion in decisions about therapy and used only measurements of height and height velocity.[45]

Precision and specificity will also be factors in the biochemical assessment of acromegalic patients after treatment, and the definition of a cure may be assay-related. The reasons for the lack of relationship between GH levels and disease activity in acromegaly are poorly understood.

Evidence-based medicine

In using the results of the work of others as the basis of diagnostic tests, where possible the quality of the original studies should be taken into account. The trend to evidence-based medicine has been extended to diagnostics, and in many areas the evidence may be found to be insufficient for the uses to which the tests may be put. In the case of pituitary–adrenal function tests, the debate on whether to use the insulin stress test or the short Synacthen test has revealed the paucity and methodological inadequacy of the reference data and the lack of comparability of the study groups.[18,46,47] See above for the problems of diagnosis of GH deficiency in children.

Clinical sensitivity and specificity

Since it is rare for the concentrations of the analyte being measured to be so different in normal and affected subjects that the ranges for the two groups do not overlap at all, few tests provide yes/no answers in all cases. In modern studies of the utility of a test in a given disorder, the concepts of clinical sensitivity and specificity are employed. Sensitivity is the proportion of true positives, i.e. the proportion of patients with a

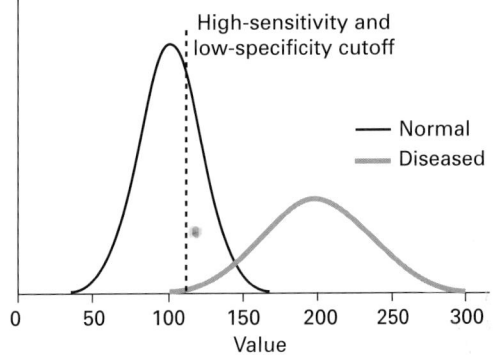

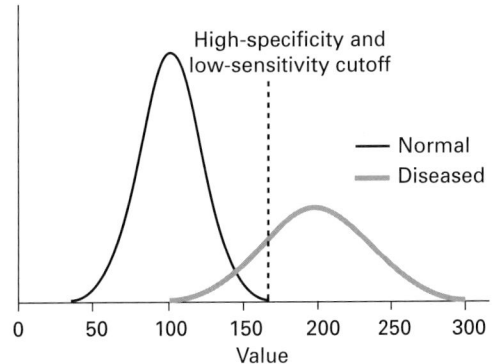

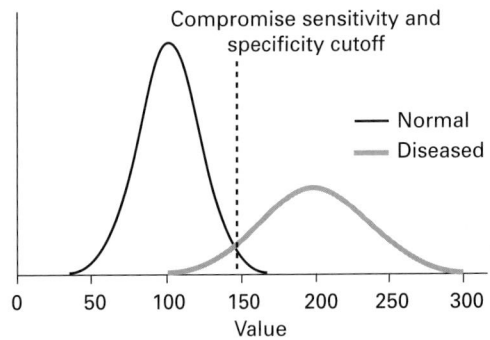

Figure 1.6
The choice of cutoff for a diagnostic test. If the cutoff is moved to a lower value, sensitivity will increase at the expense of specificity. Conversely, moving the cutoff to a higher value will increase specificity but decrease sensitivity. Some compromise is inevitable. Reproduced with permission.[36]

positive result in the disease group, and specificity is the proportion of true negatives, i.e. with a negative result in the control group. Each parameter gives the proportion of subjects in that group correctly identified by the test. These calculations depend on being able to define the disease group by an independent ('gold standard') test, and on the definition of a positive result, i.e. the cutoff value chosen to distinguish between normality and disease. It should be borne in mind that a positive result may mean a low concentration of the analyte. The reliability of the values obtained for sensitivity and specificity will depend on the numbers of patients and normal subjects studied and on the comparability of the patients in the disease group with those encountered in routine clinical practice; that is, the study group should have been selected randomly and not by the severity of their disease.

For virtually all tests, there will be a trade-off between missing some cases of the disease and subjecting some unaffected patients to further inappropriate investigation (Figure 1.6), and the choice of cutoff will depend on the implications, including cost, of these alternatives.

To establish the most appropriate cutoff value for the measured substance, receiver operating characteristic (ROC) curves are used.[48] The name of these curves derives from their origin in the optimization of radar systems. The detection rate (sensitivity) is plotted against the false-positive rate (1-specificity) for various cutoffs (Figure 1.7), and the cutoff giving the best combination of high detection rate with low false-positive rate is obtained. These curves can also be used to compare two or more tests or combinations of tests for the same disorder.

Other useful parameters can be calculated, such as positive and negative predictive values, positive and negative likelihood ratios (Table 1.3) and pre- and

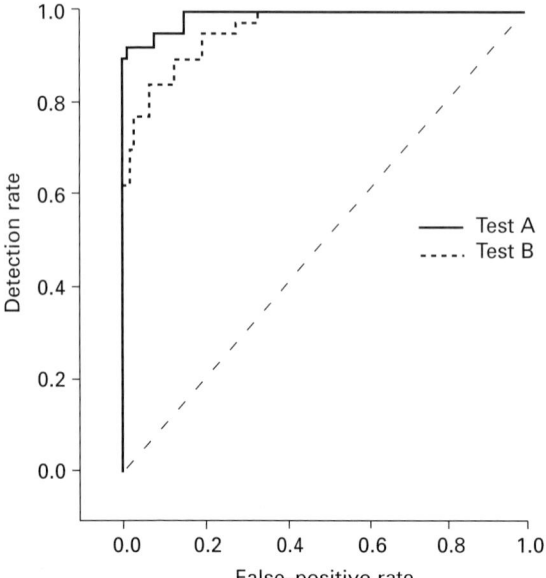

Figure 1.7
Typical ROC curves. Each curve is obtained by changing the cutoff values for a test in the given disease, and plotting the sensitivity and specificity obtained at each cutoff. The test furthest from the diagonal will be the best test, i.e. test A is a better test than test B for this disorder at most cutoffs.

> Sensitivity
>   Detection rate
>   Proportion of patients with the disease who are correctly identified by the test
>   True-positive tests/total patients with the disease
>
> Specificity
>   Proportion of patients without the disease who are correctly identified by the test
>   True-negative tests/total patients without the disease
>
> Positive predictive value
>   Proportion of patients with a positive test who are correctly diagnosed as disease positive
>   True-positive patients/total positive tests
>   Likelihood that a patient with a positive result has the disease
>
> Negative predictive value
>   Proportion of patients with a negative test who are correctly diagnosed as being disease-free
>   True-negative patients/total negative tests
>   Likelihood that a patient with a negative result does not have the disease

Table 1.3
Definitions of performance characteristics of diagnostic tests.

post-test odds. For an exposition of these calculations and their uses in diagnosis, see Jones and Payne.[36] These indices permit the relative utility of various tests in the diagnosis of a given disorder to be systematically assessed, and also allow formal comparison of the results of different studies and the putting together of the results of a number of studies in meta-analysis. The aim of such analysis is the establishment of tests with improved diagnostic capability and the abandonment of less useful tests.

Conclusion

As well as the clinical utility of measurement of the concentrations of hormones, knowledge of the strengths and limitations of the assays available allows the clinician to place an appropriate degree of reliance on the results of biochemical tests. Overinterpretation of results or ignoring them because they do not fit can both lead to errors of diagnosis or management.

Acknowledgments

The author is grateful to UK NEQAS for permission to quote findings, in particular: Dr J. Seth and Mr A. Ellis, UK NEQAS for Peptide Hormones, Edinburgh; Dr J. Middle, UK NEQAS for Steroid Hormones, Birmingham; Mr F. MacKenzie, UK NEQAS for Thyroid Hormones, Birmingham.

Further reading

Price CP, Newman DJ (eds). *Principles and Practice of Immunoassay*, 2nd edn. London: Macmillan Reference, 1997.

Wild DG (ed). *The Immunoassay Handbook*, 2nd edn. London: Macmillan, 2000.

Butler J, In: Crocker J, Burnett D, eds. *The Science of Laboratory Diagnosis*. Oxford: Isis Medical Media, 1998.

Jones RG, Payne RB. *Clinical Investigation and Statistics in Laboratory Medicine*. London: ACB Venture Publications, 1997.

References

1. Diver MJ, Scutt D, Manning JT, Gage AR, Fraser WD. Pituitary insufficiency. *Lancet* 1998; **352**: 816–17.
2. Vanderpump MPJ, Tunbridge WMG. The effects of drugs on endocrine function. *Clin Endocrinol* 1993; **39**: 389–97.
3. Midgley JEM, Sheehan CP, Christofides ND, Fry JE, Browning D, Mardell R. Concentrations of free thyroxin and albumin in serum in severe nonthyroidal illness: assay artefacts and physiological influences. *Clin Chem* 1990; **36**(5): 765–71.
4. Ekins R. The free hormone hypothesis and measurement of free hormones. *Clin Chem* 1992; **38**(7): 1289–93.
5. Docter R, Krenning EP, de Jong M, Henneman G. The sick euthyroid syndrome: changes in thyroid hormone serum parameters and hormone metabolism. *Clin Endocrinol* 1993; **39**: 499–518.
6. Chopra IJ. Euthyroid sick syndrome: is it a misnomer? *J Clin Endocrinol Metab* 1997; **82**(2): 329–34.
7. De Groot LJ. Dangerous dogmas in medicine: the nonthyroidal illness syndrome. *J Clin Endocrinol Metab* 1999; **84**(1): 151–64.
8. Yalow RS, Berson SA. Assay of plasma insulin in human subjects by immunological methods. *Nature* 1959; **184**: 1648–9.
9. Ekins RP. The estimation of thyroxine in human plasma by an electrophoretic technique. *Clin Chim Acta* 1960; **5**: 453–9.
10. Nilsson C, Pettersson K, Millar RP, Coerver KA, Matzuk MM, Huhtaniemi IT. Worldwide frequency of a common genetic variant of luteinizing hormone: an international collaborative research. *Fertil Steril* 1997; **67**(6): 998–1004.
11. Ranke MB, Orskov H, Bristow AF, Seth J, Baumann G. Consensus on how to measure growth hormone in serum. *Hormone Res* 1999; **51**(suppl 1): 27–9.
12. Bristow AF. Standardisation of protein hormone immunoassays: current controversies. *Proc UK NEQAS Meeting* 1998; 66–73.
13. Bristow AF. International Standards for growth hormone. *Hormone Res* 1999; **51**(suppl 1): 7–12.
14. Jansson C, Boguszewski C, Rosberg S, Carlsson L, Albertsson-Wikland K. Growth hormone (GH) assays: influence of standard preparations, GH isoforms, assay characteristics, and GH-binding protein. *Clin Chem* 1997; **43**(6): 950–6.
15. Seth J, Kellett HA, Caldwell G et al. A sensitive immunometric assay for serum thyroid stimulating hormone: a replacement for the thyrotropin-releasing hormone test. *BMJ* 1984; **289**(ii): 1334–6.
16. Veldhuis JD. What have we learned so far from ultrasensitive growth hormone (GH) assays? *Clin Chem* 1996; **42**(11): 1731–2.
17. Seth J, Ellis A, Al-Sadie R. Serum growth hormone measurements in clinical practice: an audit of performance from the UK National External Quality Assessment Scheme. *Hormone Res* 1999; **51**(suppl 1): 13–19.
18. Plumpton FS, Besser GM. The adrenocortical response to surgery and insulin-induced hypoglycaemia in corticosteroid treated and normal subjects. *B J Surg* 1969; **56**: 216–19.

19. Barth JH, Seth J, Howlett TA, Freedman DB. A survey of endocrine function testing by clinical biochemistry laboratories in the UK. *Ann Clin Biochem* 1995; 32(5): 442–9.
20. Clark PMS, Neylon I, Raggatt PR, Sheppard MC, Stewart PM. Defining the normal cortisol response to the short Synacthen test: implications for the investigation of hypothalamic–pituitary disorders. *Clin Endocrinol* 1998; 49: 287–92.
21. Bang P, Baxter RC, Blum WF et al. Valid measurements of total IGF concentrations in biological fluids: recommendations from the 3rd International Symposium on Insulin-like Growth Factors. *Eur J Endocrinol* 1995; 132: 338–9.
22. Jan T, Shaw M, Baumann G. Effects of growth hormone-binding proteins on serum growth hormone measurements. *J Clin Endocrinol Metab* 1991; 72(2): 387–91.
23. Strasburger CJ, Dattani MT. New growth hormone assays: potential benefits. *Acta Paediatr* 1997; Suppl 423: 5–11.
24. Ebdrup L, Fisker S, Sorensen HH, Ranke MB, Orskov H. Variety in growth hormone determinations due to use of different immunoassays and to the interference of growth hormone-binding protein. *Hormone Res* 1999; 51(suppl 1): 20–6.
25. Despres N, Grant AM. Antibody interference in thyroid assays: a potential for clinical misinformation. *Clin Chem* 1998; 44(3): 440–54.
26. Spencer CA, Takeuchi M, Kazarosyan M et al. Serum thyroglobulin autoantibodies: prevalence, influence on serum thyroglobulin measurement, and prognostic significance in patients with differentiated thyroid carcinoma. *J Clin Endocrinol Metab* 1998; 83(4): 1121–7.
27. Lindstedt G. Endogenous antibodies against prolactin – a 'new' cause of hyperprolactinaemia. *Eur J Endocrinol* 1994; 130: 429–32.
28. Fahie-Wilson MN, Ellis AR. Macroprolactin – what should we do about it? *Proc UK NEQAS Meeting* 1998; 121–3.
29. Bjoro T, Morkrid L, Wergeland R et al. Frequency of hyperprolactinaemia due to large molecular weight prolactin (150–170 kD PRL). *Scand J Clin Lab Invest* 1995; 55: 139–47.
30. Fahie-Wilson MN, Soule SG. Macroprolactinaemia: contribution to hyperprolactinaemia in a district general hospital and evaluation of a screening test based on precipitation with polyethylene glycol. *Ann Clin Biochem* 1997; 34(3): 252–8.
31. Olukoga AO, Kane JW. Macroprolactinaemia: validation and application of the polyethylene glycol precipitation test and clinical characterization of the condition. *Clin Endocrinol* 1999; 51: 119–26.
32. Carlson HE, Markoff E, Lee DW. On the nature of serum prolactin in two patients with macroprolactinemia. *Fertil Steril* 1992; 58(1): 78–87.
33. Boscato LM, Stuart MC. Heterophilic antibodies: a problem for all immunoassays. *Clin Chem* 1988; 34(1): 27–33.
34. Kricka LJ. Human anti-animal antibody interferences in immunological assays. *Clin Chem* 1999; 54(7): 942–56.
35. Weber TH, Kapyaho KI, Tanner P. Endogenous interference in immunoassays in clinical chemistry. A review. *Scand J Clin Lab Invest* 1990; 50(suppl 201): 77–82.
36. Jones RG, Payne RB. *Clinical Investigation and Statistics in Laboratory Medicine.* London: ACB Venture Publications, 1997.
37. Celniker AC, Chen AB, Wert RMJ, Sherman BM. Variability in the quantitation of circulating growth hormone using commercial immunoassays. *J Clin Endocrinol Metab* 1989; 68(2): 469–76.
38. Carlsson L, Mercado M, Baumann G et al. Assay systems for the growth hormone-binding protein. *Proc Soc Exp Biol Med* 1994; 206: 312–15.
39. Rajkovic IA, Valiontis E, Ho KKY. Direct quantitation of growth hormone binding protein in human serum by a ligand immunofunctional assay: comparison with immunoprecipitation and chromatographic methods. *J Clin Endocrinol Metab* 1994; 70(3): 772–7.
40. Fisker S, Frystyk J, Skriver L, Vestbo E, Ho KKY, Orskov H. A simple, rapid immunometric assay for determination of functional and growth hormone-occupied growth hormone-binding protein in human serum. *Eur J Clin Invest* 1996; 26: 779–85.
41. Rosenfeld RG, Albertsson-Wikland K, Cassorla F et al. Diagnostic controversy: the diagnosis of childhood growth hormone deficiency revisited. *J Clin Endocrinol Metab* 1995; 80(5): 1532–40.
42. Shalet SM, Toogood A, Rahim A, Brennan BMD. The diagnosis of growth hormone deficiency in children and adults. *Endocrine Rev* 1998; 19(2): 203–23.
43. Ghigo E, Bellone J, Aimaretti G et al. Reliability of provocative tests to assess growth hormone secretory status. Study in 472 normally growing children. *J Clin Endocrinol Metab* 1996; 81: 3323–7.
44. Guyda HJ. Four decades of growth hormone therapy for short children: what have we achieved? *J Clin Endocrinol Metab* 1999; 84(12): 4307–16.
45. Werther GA. Growth hormone measurements versus auxology in treatment decisions: the Australian experience. *J Pediatrics* 1996; 128(5 Pt 2): S47–51.
46. Mukherjee JJ, Jacome de Castro J, Kaltsas G et al. A comparison of the insulin tolerance/glucagon test with the short ACTH stimulation test in the assessment of the hypothalamo–pituitary–adrenal axis in the early post-operative period after hypophysectomy. *Clin Endocrinol* 1997; 47: 51–60.
47. Stewart PM, Clark PMS, Sheppard MC. Comparison of the short ACTH stimulation test with the insulin tolerance/glucagon test. *Clin Endocrinol* 1998; 48: 124–6.
48. Zweig MH, Campbell G. Receiver-operating characteristic (ROC) plots: a fundamental evaluation tool in clinical medicine. *Clin Chem* 1993; 39(4): 561–77.

2

Genetic mechanisms of pituitary and thyroid neoplasia
Philip E Harris

Introduction

The principles of endocrine neoplasia are considered, using pituitary and thyroid tumors as examples. Other forms of endocrine neoplasia are covered as appropriate elsewhere. In keeping with the concept that neoplasia arises as a result of a single mutated somatic cell, most endocrine tumors have been shown to be monoclonal in origin.[1] This implies that they arise from an oncogenic event (gene mutation) in a single cell. Recent evidence, however, suggests that some recurrent pituitary tumors arise from a different clone of cells than the original pituitary tumor.[2] This suggests the possibility that tumors are potentially polyclonal, but that one particular clone develops a growth advantage over the other cells, resulting in the growth of a monoclonal tumor. There are two broad categories of genetic mutations, dominant activating mutations and recessive loss of function mutations.

Oncogenes and growth factors

Protooncogenes control cell proliferation and differentiation in the normal cell. Single-base mutations in a single allele can result in constitutive activation, with loss of the normal control of cell function and growth. One example of this type in endocrine disease is for the stimulatory G protein for adenylyl cyclase (AC), Gs.[3] G proteins are linked to an archetypal receptor consisting of intra- and extracellular domains, linked by seven transmembrane domains. A number of hypothalamic factors act on the anterior pituitary via specific G protein-coupled receptors (GPCRs). Similarly, the trophic hormones thyroid-stimulating hormone (TSH) and adrenocorticotropic hormone (ACTH) also act via GPCRs. Point mutations of Gs at codons 201 (R201C, R201H, R201S) and 227 (Q227R, Q227L) result in loss of the intrinsic GTPase activity of Gs, which normally inactivates Gs by hydrolyzing GTP back to GDP. As a result, Gs becomes constitutively activated (*gsp*), resulting in continuous activation of AC and downstream signaling pathways (Figure 2.1).

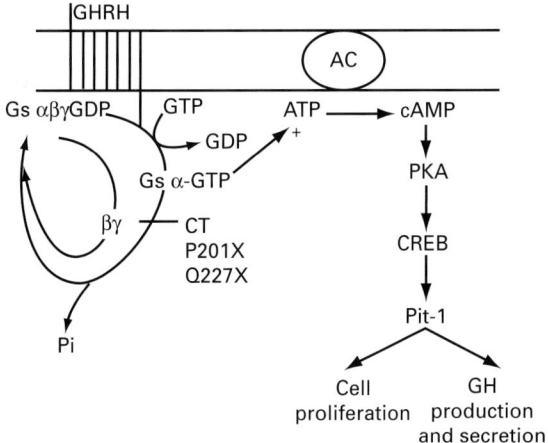

Figure 2.1
G protein cycle. Activation of Gs occurs when growth hormone-releasing factor interacts with its seven-transmembrane domain receptor. This results in the activation of adenylyl cyclase (AC), with consequent stimulation of cAMP production, leading to cell proliferation, stimulation of GH production and secretion. Constitutive activation of Gs by inhibition of intrinsic GTPase results from ADP ribosylation by cholera toxin (CT) or point mutations at codons 210 or 227 of Gsα encoding amino acid X. pKA, protein kinase A.

Gsp mutations have been described in a number of endocrine conditions.[4–6] They have been consistently described in 35–40% of somatotroph adenomas, apart from two Japanese series, which reported prevalences of 4% and 9%.[7] At first sight, this appears to provide a very clear explanation for the development of a large subgroup of somatotroph adenomas. There are, however, no clearcut differences in the clinical phenotypes of *gsp*-positive and *gsp*-negative tumors. There are no sex or age differences, and no clear differences in tumor size or in serum growth hormone (GH) levels.[8] There have been some data to suggest that *gsp*-positive tumors respond less readily to growth hormone-releasing factor (GHRH) and that they are more sensitive to the inhibitory actions of somatostatin.[9] The reported differences have not been great, however, and there is a considerable overlap between the two groups. A possible explanation for the apparent lack of an effect of *gsp* is counterregulation, which could take place by a number of mechanisms (Figure 2.2). A recent report has in fact demonstrated that phosphodiesterase (PDE) activity is increased in the *gsp*-positive tumors.[10] Transgenic animal models with activation of the AC system in somatotrophs develop somatotroph hyperplasia and gigantism, without evidence of tumor formation, except in older animals.[11,12] These data suggest that activation of AC alone is insufficient for tumor formation and that additional oncogenetic effects are also required.

Apart from somatotroph adenomas, *gsp* mutations have also been well documented in autonomously functioning thyroid nodules, where they have been reported to occur with a prevalence of 6–25%.[13–15] More frequently, activating mutations of the TSH receptor has been shown to occur in 60–80% of autonomously functioning thyroid nodules. Point mutations have been described at a number of locations within the seven transmembrane domains, most particularly in the 3rd intracellular loop and 6th transmembrane domain[16] (Figure 2.3). Activating germ-line mutations of the TSHR have also been described as rare, but increasingly recognized, causes of thyrotoxicosis.[17–23] Activating mutations of the inhibitory G protein for AC, Gi2a (*gip*), have also been infrequently identified in endocrine tumors.[4,24]

Ras is a member of the G protein superfamily, and activating mutations similar to those in Gs and Gi have been well described in neoplastic disease. *Ras* mutations have been reported in highly aggressive pituitary tumors or in their metastases.[25] Activating mutations of *ras* have been clearly documented in thyroid neoplasia, in particular follicular adenomas and carcinomas, giving rise to the suggestion that these mutations occur as an early event in the development of malignant thyroid disease.[26]

Protein kinase C (PKC) is a calcium-activated kinase which has a central role in the control of cell function and proliferation. Protein kinase Cα activity has been shown to be increased in invasive pituitary tumors.[27] A point mutation D294G has been demonstrated in these tumors. The same mutation has also been described in thyroid neoplasia.[28] The functional significance is at present unclear.

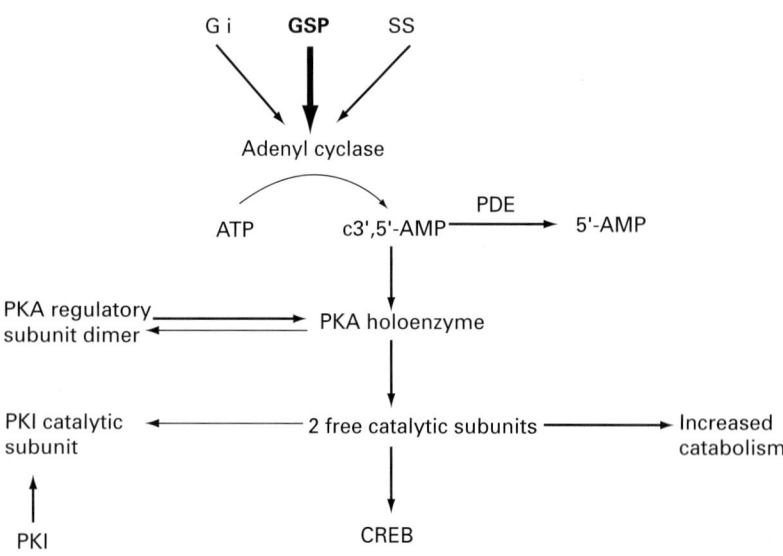

Figure 2.2
Potential counterregulatory mechanisms to gsp in the cell. Gi and somatostatin (SS) both inhibit AC. The activity of phosphodiesterase (PDE) is increased secondary to activation of AC. Activation of PKA results in increased PKA catalytic subunit catabolism, increased production of regulatory subunits, and increased production of protein kinase inhibitor (PKI).

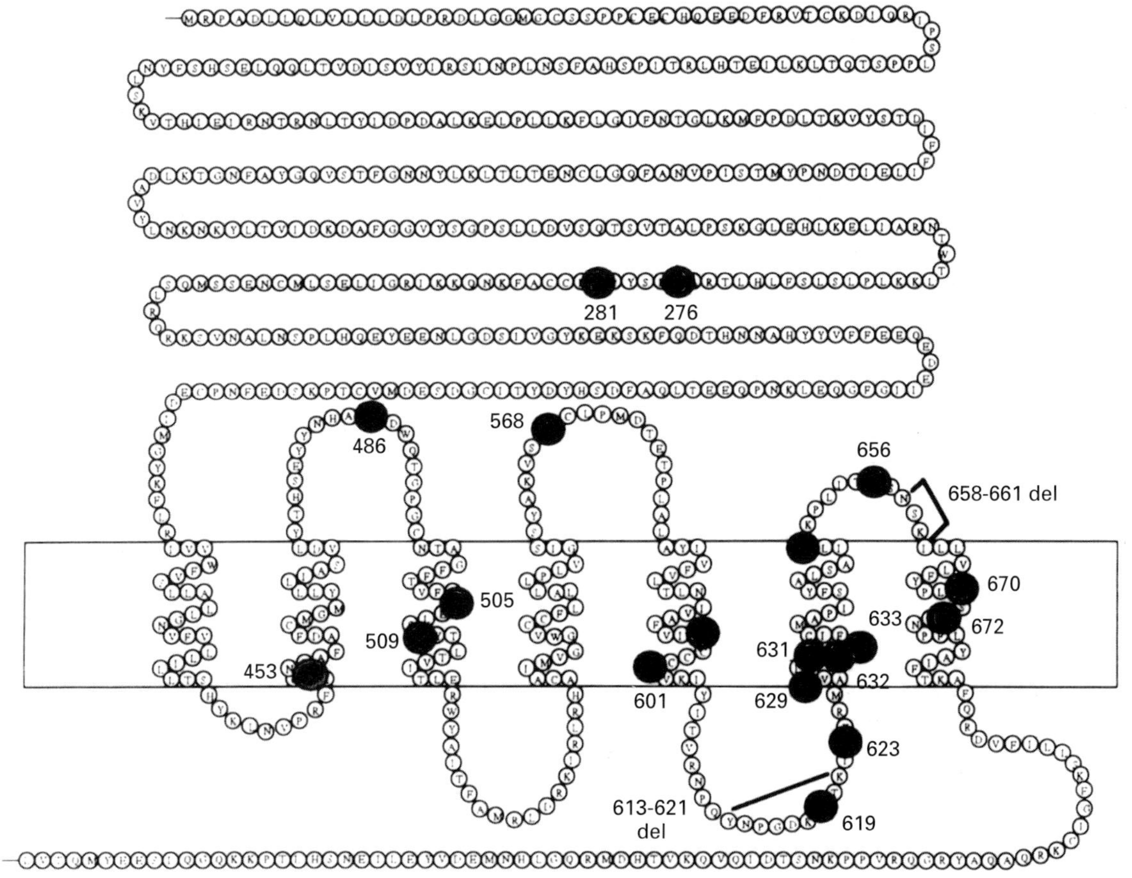

ONCOGENES AND GROWTH FACTORS

Figure 2.3
Activating mutations of the TSHR. This figure illustrates some of the mutations that have been reported in the literature. New mutations are being continually described. The majority of mutations are clustered around the 6th and 7th transmembrane domains.

The human *ret* gene located on chromosome 10q11.2 encodes a transmembrane receptor tyrosine kinase (TK) whose putative ligand is glial cell line-derived neurotropic factor (GDNF). In papillary thyroid carcinoma (PTC), hybrid genes are formed between the TK domain (3′) and the 5′ of highly expressed genes, resulting in constitutive TK activation. Five forms of *ret*/PTC rearrangements have been described in thyroid tumors: *ret*/PTC-1, formed by intrachromosomal inversion, fusing the H4 gene to the TK domain of *ret*; *ret*/PTC-2, formed by fusion of *ret* and the 5′-terminal sequences of R1α (regulatory subunit of protein kinase A (PKA)); and *ret*/PTC-3, formed by intrachromosomal inversion fusing to *ele-1* (Figure 2.4). Two further rearrangements between *ret*

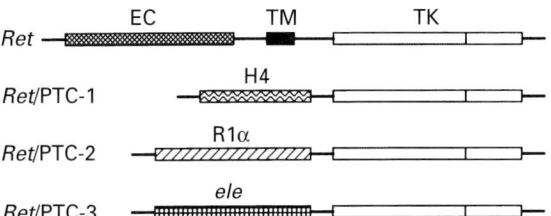

Figure 2.4
Ret/PTC rearrangements in thyroid cancer. See text for details.

and *ele-1* have been described in post-Chernobyl PTC: *ele-1*/PTC-4 and *ele-1*/PTCd.[29,30] Until recently, *ret*/PTC rearrangements were thought to be restricted to papillary carcinomas, with widely reported prevalences of 2.5–34%. A recent study has demonstrated a high prevalence of *ret*/PTC rearrangements in micropapillary carcinomas, raising the possibility that these mutations occur as an early event in thyroid tumor pathogenesis.[31] Another report has demonstrated *ret*/PTC rearrangements in 84% of PTCs and also in 45% of thyroid follicular adenomas in French patients previously exposed to external irradiation.[32] An increased prevalence of *ret*/PTC-3 has been reported in children from contaminated areas following the Chernobyl nuclear accident.[33] In contrast, *ret*/PTC-1 has been reported in papillary carcinomas from adults with a history of external irradiation in childhood.[34] In vivo transgenic studies[35] support an etiological role of *ret*/PTC in the development of papillary carcinomas. Similarly, chromosome rearrangements resulting in activation of *trk*, a transmembrane domain TK receptor for nerve growth factor (NGF),[36] and *met*, a transmembrane TK receptor which binds hepatocyte growth factor, also occur in papillary carcinomas.[37]

A pituitary tumor-transforming gene (*pttg*) has been isolated from pituitary tumors using mRNA differential display PCR. The human *pttg* family consists of at least three homologous genes, of which one, *pttg1*, is located on chromosome 5q33. This gene encodes a 201 amino acid protein, which induces cell transformation in vitro and tumor formation in nude mice.[38] Increased amounts of *pttg1* mRNA have been demonstrated in all types of pituitary tumors. *Pttg1* induces the expression of fibroblast growth factor 2 (FGF-2), which is a mediator of cell growth and angiogenesis. FGF-2 is a potent angiogenic factor regulating vascular endothelial growth factor (VEGF). *Pttg1* has been shown to be induced by estrogen, coincidental with FGF-2 and VEGF induction and angiogenesis.[39] FGF-2 is present in the serum of multiple endocrine neoplasia type 1 (MEN 1) patients with pituitary tumors. Moreover, FGF-2 immunoreactivity disappears following hypophysectomy, suggesting that the pituitary produces this factor. Although FGF-2 does not appear to be mitogenic, it does stimulate prolactin secretion, prolactin being the most commonly produced pituitary hormone in MEN 1.[40] In addition, prolactinomas have been shown to produce FGF-4, a product of the *hst* gene, which is localized on 11q13, close to the MEN 1 locus. FGF-4 is mitogenic to pituitary cells and also stimulates prolactin gene transcription.[41] A recent study reports the identification of a novel pituitary tumour-derived, N-terminally truncated isoform of FGF receptor-4 (ptd-FGFR4). This polypeptide lacks a signal peptide and the first two extracellular Ig-like domains. It is located in the cytoplasm and is constitutively phosphorylated. Immuno-reactivity occurs in about 40% of pituitary tumours of various types, but not in non-tumorous pituitary. It is tumorigenic both in vitro and in vivo and provokes pituitary tumours in transgenic mice.[42]

Another paracrine system, which may be operating in prolactinomas, involves transforming growth factor α (TGF-α) and epidermal growth factor receptor (EGFR). Mice transgenic for TGF-α targeted to lactotrophs develop lactotroph hyperplasia and prolactinomas. TGF-α production appears to be regulated in parallel with prolactin, being stimulated by estradiol and inhibited by bromocriptine.[43] Evidence suggests that galanin has a role as a trophic factor in the development of prolactinomas.[44]

Tumor suppressor genes

Tumor suppressor genes are recessive and need to undergo two mutations on both alleles before function is lost. Usually, one mutation is inherited (germline). The second somatic mutation usually involves the loss of a large amount of chromosome material, the so-called 'loss of heterozygosity' (Figure 2.5).

Multiple endocrine neoplasia type 1 is a dominant inherited syndrome, which includes pituitary tumors in about 50% of cases. The most frequent tumor is the prolactinoma, although any type of tumor can occur. The gene locus has long been known to be at 11q13. Loss of heterozygosity (LOH) at this locus is consistently

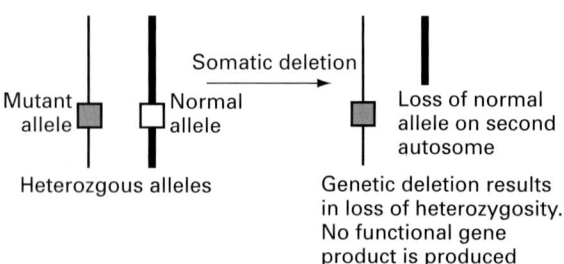

Figure 2.5
Loss of heterozygosity of a putative tumor suppressor gene. Both alleles need to be inactivated before function is lost. In the case of inherited syndromes such as MEN 1, one allele is inactivated as a result of a germline mutation. The second allele is inactivated as a result of a somatic loss of genetic material.

demonstrated in pituitary tumors from patients with MEN 1. Loss of heterozygosity of chromosome 11q13 has also been demonstrated in a number of sporadic pituitary tumors.[45] One large study of 88 pituitary tumors demonstrated LOH in 18% of tumors.[46] Some sporadic follicular adenomas of the thyroid have been reported to demonstrate LOH at 11q13. Whether or not these sporadic tumors have MEN 1 mutations remains to be seen. The MEN 1 gene, termed menin, has recently been cloned.[47] It is ubiquitously expressed and does not have any close identifiable homology to other proteins. It has been shown to regulate transcription of AP-1. The identification of mutations in the menin gene, together with their functional analysis, will provide critical information on the role of menin in the normal organism and in neoplasia.

The retinoblastoma (*Rb*) gene locus is on chromosome 13q14. The Rb protein has a central role in the control of the cell cycle. Proteins called cyclin-dependent kinases (CDKs) phosphorylate Rb, resulting in its inactivation. In its inactivated form, Rb dissociates from a transcription factor E2F, whereupon the cell progresses from the G_1 to the S phase of the cell cycle. Mammalian DNA viral tumor proteins such as T antigen from simian virus 40 and E7 target hypophosphorylated forms of Rb from human papilloma virus. These proteins bind directly to Rb, resulting in its inactivation. Loss of heterozygosity at the *Rb* locus has been found to be associated with a number of different malignancies.[48] There is little evidence, however, to suggest a role of *Rb* gene mutation in thyroid neoplasia.[49] Transgenic mice heterozygous for a disrupted *Rb* gene develop adenocarcinomas of the pituitary.[50] Loss of heterozygosity at 13q14 has been described in invasive pituitary adenomas and in the very rare pituitary carcinomas. *Rb* protein was, however, identifiable by immunocytochemistry.[51] This protein could be non-functional, or there may be loss of function of another unidentified tumor suppressor gene close to the *Rb* gene locus. These data suggest that LOH at 13q14 is a late event in pituitary tumor pathogenesis, possibly predisposing to a change in tumor behavior towards a more aggressive phenotype.

The *p53* gene encodes a nuclear protein that controls the expression of genes important for DNA repair and apoptosis. It is the most commonly mutated gene in malignant disease. The loss of functional p53 protein is particularly associated with poorly differentiated/anaplastic carcinomas.[52] Mutations of the *p53* gene have not been identified in pituitary tumors. Although p53 protein expression may be altered in some cases, there is no evidence that p53 mutations have a role in the pathogenesis of pituitary tumors.[53] In the thyroid, *p53* mutations appear to be restricted to poorly differentiated and anaplastic carcinomas, implicating p53 inactivation as a critical step in the progression of tumors to a clinically aggressive phenotype.[54]

A number of allelic deletions have been detected in pituitary tumors at other loci, apart from 11q13 and 13q14.[55] Allelic loss of 3p occurs in some follicular adenomas.[56] Multiple allelic deletions have been reported in highly aggressive pituitary tumors. Overall, it is difficult to know whether allelic deletions demonstrated in tumors are merely epiphenomena, associated with cellular dedifferentiation, or whether they are true oncogenic mutations, releasing the cells from as yet unidentified tumor suppressor gene control.

CDK inhibitors have a central role in controlling cell cycle progression by binding to and inactivating cyclin–CDK complexes. Disruption of the CDK-inhibitory domain of p27 in mice results in the development of intermediate lobe pituitary tumors.[57] Analysis of pituitary tumors for mutations and expression of the p27 gene, however, has failed to demonstrate any evidence of p27 dysfunction.[58] In contrast, p21 has been found to be truncated or deleted in 10% of thyroid carcinomas.[59] Methylation of CpG islands in p16 have been demonstrated in pituitary tumors, with loss of p16 expression. Methylation has been demonstrated in more than 70% of clinically non-functioning pituitary adenomas, although it appears to occur rarely in somatotroph adenomas. Methylation occurs in both non-invasive and invasive tumors, suggesting that this is an early event in pituitary oncogenesis.[60] Transfection studies of the pituitary AtT20 cell line have demonstrated restoration of growth control following the induction of ectopically expressed p16. These effects were reversed by prior in vitro methylation of the construct's CpG sites within the coding region of the gene.[61]

The *nm23* gene encodes a protein with anti-metastatic properties. High expression of *nm23* has been found in non-invasive pituitary tumors, with reduced expression in invasive tumors.[62] In contrast, high levels of *nm23* gene expression have been demonstrated in advanced metastatic and anaplastic thyroid carcinomas.[63]

Familial non-medullary thyroid cancer is rare and occurs predominantly in papillary carcinomas. About 3% of papillary thyroid carcinomas are familial. There is an increased incidence of papillary carcinoma in Cowden's syndrome, Gardner's syndrome and familial adenomatosis polyposis, the latter being associated with a tumor suppressor gene (FAP) at 5q21.

Conclusions

Overall, data for both thyroid and pituitary neoplasia suggest that single-gene mutations are unlikely to result in the development of a neoplastic phenotype. Knudson originally suggested that tumor development occurs as the result of a stepwise accumulation of a number of oncogenic 'hits'.[64] The identification of multiple-gene mutations, in particular with increasingly aggressive disease, suggests that this is the case. Apart from oncogenic mutations, it is important to realize that circulating growth factors, together with the local production of autocrine/paracrine factors, almost certainly also have significant roles in tumor development. An established monoclonal tumor may grow under the influence of oncogenic mutations, together with the permissive action of growth factors and other local autocrine/paracrine factors.[65] Although understanding of the pathogenesis of thyroid and pituitary tumors is relatively rudimentary, models of tumor development can be put forward (Figures 2.6 and 2.7).

The identification of genetic mutations in thyroid and pituitary disease has had little impact upon clinical practice to date. PCR amplification of genes and microsatellite regions obtained from fine needle aspirates (FNAs) of thyroid nodules may help to classify follicular lesions as being either adenomas or carcinomas preoperatively. Activating Gs mutations can be identified by PCR of FNAs, but the diagnosis of an autonomously functioning nodule can be more easily made by radionuclide scanning. In the future, examination for allelic deletions in pituitary and thyroid tumors may help to predict tumor behavior, with consequent implications for treatment. In spite of these limitations, however, it is important to be aware of the developments of molecular biology in endocrine oncology and in areas of endocrinology that are covered in other chapters of this book. There is no doubt that the applications of molecular biology to clinical practice will continue to expand rapidly over the next few years.

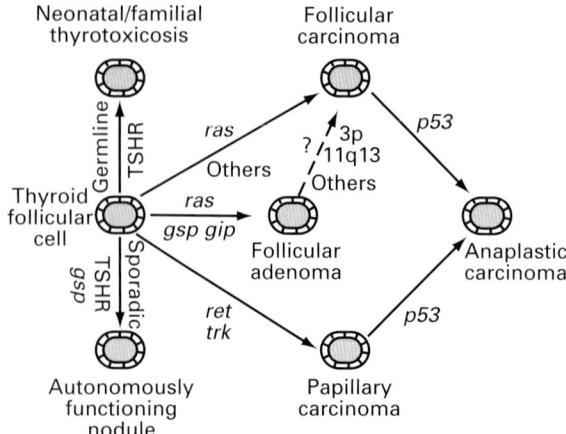

Figure 2.7
Model of the pathogenesis of thyroid cancer.

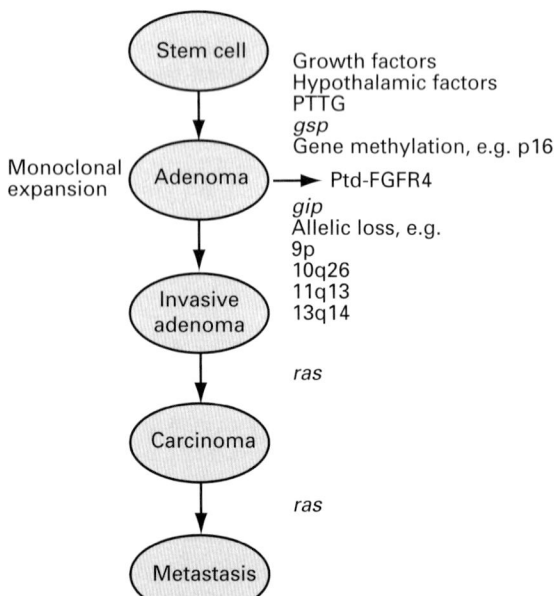

Figure 2.6
Model of pituitary tumor pathogenesis.

References

1. Knudson AG. Mutation and human cancer. *Adv Cancer Res* 1973; **17**: 317–52.
2. Zahedi A, Booth GL, Smyth HS et al. Distinct clonal compositions of primary and metastatic adrenocorticotrophic hormone-producing pituitary carcinoma. *Clin Endocrinol* 2001; **55**: 549–56.
3. Vallar L, Spada A, Giannattasio G. Altered Gs and adenylate cyclase activity in human GH-secreting pituitary adenomas. *Nature* 1987; **330**: 566–8.
4. Lyons J, Landis CA, Harsh G et al. Two G protein oncogenes in human endocrine tumors. *Science* 1990; **249**: 655–9.
5. Weinstein LS, Shenker A, Gejman PV, Merino MJ, Friedman E, Spiegel AM. Activating mutations of the

stimulatory G protein in the McCune–Albright syndrome. *N Engl J Med* 1991; **325**: 1688–95.
6. Williamson EA, Johnson SJ, Foster S, Kendall-Taylor P, Harris PE. G protein gene mutations in patients with multiple endocrinopathies. *J Clin Endocrinol Metab* 1995; **80**: 1702–5.
7. Harris PE. Gs protein mutations and the pathogenesis and function of pituitary tumors. *Metabolism* 1996; **45**(8 suppl 1): 120–2.
8. Harris PE, Alexander JM, Bikkal HA. Glycoprotein hormone α-subunit production in somatotroph adenomas with and without Gs mutations. *J Clin Endocrinol Metab* 1992; **75**: 918–23.
9. Faglia G, Arosio M, Spada A. Gs protein mutations and pituitary tumours: functional correlates and possible therapeutic implications. *Metabolism* 1996; **45**(8 suppl 1): 117–19.
10. Lania A, Persani L, Ballare E, Mantovani S, Losa M, Spada A. Constitutively active Gsα is associated with an increased phosphodiesterase activity in human growth hormone-secreting adenomas. *J Clin Endocrinol Metab* 1998; **83**: 1624–8.
11. Burton FH, Hasel KW, Bloom FE, Sutcliffe JG. Pituitary hyperplasia and giantism in mice caused by a cholera toxin transgene. *Nature* 1991; **350**: 74–7.
12. Asa SL, Kovacs K, Stefaneanu L et al. Pituitary adenomas in mice transgenic for growth hormone releasing hormone. *Endocrinology* 1992; **131**: 2083–9.
13. Russo D, Franko F, Wicker R et al. Genetic alterations in thyroid hyperfunctioning adenomas. *J Clin Endocrinol Metab* 1995; **80**: 1347–51.
14. O'Sullivan CO, Barton CM, Staddon SL et al. Activating point mutations of *gsp* oncogene in human thyroid adenomas. *Mol Carcinog* 1991; **4**: 345–9.
15. Parma J, Duprez L, Van Sande J et al. Diversity and prevalence of somatic mutations in the thyrotropin receptor and Gsα genes as a cause of toxic thyroid adenomas. *J Clin Endocrinol Metab* 1997; **82**: 2695–701.
16. Esapa C, Foster S, Johnson S, Jameson LJ, Kendall-Taylor P, Harris PE. G protein and thyrotropin receptor mutations in thyroid neoplasia. *J Clin Endocrinol Metab* 1997; **82**: 493–6.
17. Kopp P, Van Sande J, Parma J et al. Congenital hyperthyroidism caused by a mutation in the thyrotropin receptor gene. *N Engl J Med* 1995; **332**(3): 150–4.
18. De Roux N, Polak M, Couet J et al. A neomutation of the thyroid-stimulating hormone receptor in a severe neonatal hyperthyroidism. *J Clin Endocrinol Metab* 1996; **81**: 2023–6.
19. Esapa CT, Duprez L, Ludgate M et al. A novel TSH receptor mutation in an infant with severe thyrotoxicosis. *Thyroid* 1999; **9**: 1005–10.
20. Tonacchera M, Van Sande J, Cetani F et al. Functional characteristics of three new germline mutations of the thyrotropin receptor gene causing autosomal dominant toxic thyroid hyperplasia. *J Clin Endocrinol Metab* 1996; **81**: 547–54.
21. Kopp P, Muirhead S, Jourdain N, Gu W-X, Jameson LJ, Rodd C. Congenital hyperthyroidism caused by a solitary toxic adenoma harboring a novel somatic mutation (Serine 281>Isoleucine) in the extracellular domain of the thyrotropin receptor. *J Clin Invest* 1997; **100**: 1634–9.
22. Holzapfel H-P, Wonerow W, Von Petrykowski W, Henschen M, Scherbaum WA, Paschke R. Sporadic congenital hyperthyroidism due to a spontaneous germline mutation in the thyrotropin receptor gene. *J Clin Endocrinol Metab* 1997; **82**: 3879–84.
23. Gruters A, Schoneberg T, Biebermann H et al. Severe congenital hyperthyroidism caused by a germ-line *neo* mutation in the extracellular portion of the thyrotropin receptor. *J Clin Endocrinol Metab* 1998; **83**: 1431–6.
24. Williamson EA, Daniels M, Foster S, Kelly WF, Kendall-Taylor P, Harris PE. Gsα and Gi2α mutations in clinically non-functioning pituitary tumors. *Clin Endocrinol* 1994; **41**: 815–20.
25. Pei L, Melmed S, Scheithauer B, Kovacs K, Prager D. H-*ras* mutations in human pituitary carcinoma metastases. *J Clin Endocrinol* 1994; **78**: 842–6.
26. Esapa CT, Johnson SJ, Kendall-Taylor P, Lennard TWJ, Harris PE. Prevalence of *ras* mutations in thyroid neoplasia. *Clin Endocrinol* 1999, **50**: 529–35.
27. Alvaro V, Levy L, Dubray C et al. Invasive human pituitary tumors express a point-mutated α-protein kinase-C. *J Clin Endocrinol Metab* 1993; **77**: 1125–9.
28. Prevostel C, Alvaro V, de Boisvilliers F, Martin A, Jaffiol C, Joubert D. The natural protein kinase Cα mutant is present in human thyroid neoplasms. *Oncogene* 1995; **11**: 669–74.
29. Fugazzola L, Pierotti MA, Vigano E, Pacini F, Vorontsova TV, Bongarzone I. Molecular and biochemical analysis of RET/PTC4, a novel oncogenic rearrangement between RET and ELE1 genes in post-Chernobyl papillary thyroid cancer. *Oncogene* 1996; **13**: 1093–7.
30. Klugbauer S, Lengfelder E, Demidchik EP, Rabes HM. A new form of RET rearrangement in thyroid carcinomas of children after the Chernobyl reactor accident. *Oncogene* 1996; **13**: 1099–102.
31. Sugg SL, Ezzat S, Rosen IB, Freeman JL, Asa SL. Distinct multiple *RET*/PTC gene rearrangements in multifocal papillary thyroid neoplasia. *J Clin Endocrinol Metab* 1998; **83**: 4116–22.
32. Bounacer A, Wicker R, Caillou B et al. High prevalence of activating ret protooncogene rearrangements in thyroid tumors from patients who had recieved external radiation. *Oncogene* 1997; **15**: 1263–73.
33. Klugbauer S, Lengfelder E, Demidchik EP, Rabes HM. High prevalence of RET rearrangement in thyroid tumors of children from Belarus after the Chernobyl reactor accident. *Oncogene* 1995; **11**: 2459–67.
34. Learoyd DL, Messina M, Zedenius J, Guinea AI, Delbridge LW, Robinson BG. *RET/PTC* and *RET* tyrosine kinase expression in adult papillary thyroid carcinomas. *J Clin Endocrinol Metab* 1998; **83**: 3631–5.

35. Jhiang SM, Sagartz JE, Tong Q et al. Targeted expression of the *ret*/PTC1 oncogene induces papillary thyroid carcinomas. *Endocrinology* 1996; 137: 375–8.
36. Bongarzone I, Pierotti MA, Monzini N et al. High frequency of activation of tyrosine kinase oncogenes in human papillary thyroid carcinoma. *Oncogene* 1989; 4: 1457–62.
37. Di Renzo MF, Olivero M, Ferro S et al. Overexpression of the c-met/HGF receptor gene in human thyroid carcinomas. *Oncogene* 1992; 7: 2549–53.
38. Pei L, Melmed S. Isolation and characterization of a pituitary tumor-transforming gene (PTTG). *Mol Endocrinol* 1997; 11: 433–41.
39. Heaney AP, Horwitz GA, Wang Z, Singson R, Melemd S. Early involvement of estrogen-induced pituitary tumor transforming gene and fibroblast growth factor expression in prolactinoma pathogenesis. *Nature Med* 1999; 5: 1317–21.
40. Zimering MB, Katsumata N, Sato Y et al. Increased FGF in plasma from multiple endocrine neoplasia type 1: relation to pituitary tumor. *J Clin Endocrinol Metab* 1993; 76: 1182–7.
41. Shimon I, Hinton DR, Weiss MH et al. Prolactinomas express human heparin-binding secretory transforming gene (*hst*) protein product: marker of tumor invasiveness. *Clin Endocrinol* 1998; 48: 23–9.
42. Ezzat S, Zheng L, Zhu X-F et al. Targeted expression of a human pituitary tumor-derived isoform of FGF Receptor-4 recapitulates pituitary tumorgenesis. *J Clin Invest* 2002; 109: 69–78.
43. McAndrew J, Kudlow JE. Role of TGFα in pituitary tumorigenesis. *Front Horm Res* 1996; 20: 156–78.
44. Wynick D, Small CJ, Bacon A et al. Galanin regulates prolactin release and lactotroph proliferation. *Proc Natl Acad Sci USA* 1998; 95(21): 12671–6.
45. Thakker RV. Role of chromosome 11 in hereditary and sporadic pituitary tumorigenesis. *Front Horm Res* 1996; 20: 179–93.
46. Boggild MD, Jenkinson S, Pistorello M et al. Molecular genetic studies of sporadic pituitary tumors. *J Clin Endocrinol Metab* 1994; 78: 387–92.
47. Chandrasekharappa SC, Guru SC, Manickam P et al. Positional cloning of the gene for multiple endocrine neoplasia-type 1. *Science* 1997; 276: 404–7.
48. Weinberg RA. Tumor suppressor genes. *Science* 1991; 254: 1138–46.
49. Wynford-Thomas D. Molecular genetics of thyroid cancer. *Current Opin Endocrinol Diabetes* 1995; 2: 429–36.
50. Jacks T, Fazelli A, Schmitt E, Bronson RT, Goodell M, Weinberg RA. Effects of an Rb mutation in the mouse. *Nature* 1992; 359: 295–300.
51. Pei L, Melmed M, Scheithauer B, Kovacs K, Benedict WF, Prager D. Frequent loss of heterozygosity at the retinoblastoma susceptibility gene (RB) locus in aggressive pituitary tumors: evidence for a chromosome 13 tumor suppressor gene other than RB. *Cancer Res* 1995; 55: 1613–16.
52. Harris CC, Hollstein M. Clinical implications of the p53 tumor suppressor gene. *N Engl J Med* 1993; 329: 1318–27.
53. Pei L, Melemd S. Oncogenes and tumor suppressor genes in pituitary tumorigenesis. *Front Horm Res* 1996; 20: 122–36.
54. Fagin JA, Matsuo K, Karmakar A, Chen DL, Tang S-H, Koeffler HP. High prevalence of mutations of the p53 gene in poorly differentiated human thyroid carcinomas. *J Clin Invest* 1993; 91: 179–84.
55. Bates AS, Farrell WE, Bicknell EJ et al. Allelic deletion in pituitary adenomas reflects aggressive biological activity and has potential value as a prognostic marker. *J Clin Endocrinol Metab* 1997; 82: 818–24.
56. Herrmann MA, Hay ID, Bartelt Jr DH et al. Cytogenetic and molecular genetic studies of follicular and papillary thyroid cancers. *J Clin Invest* 1991; 88: 1596–604.
57. Nakayama K, Ishida N, Shirane M et al. Mice lacking p27^{kip1} display increased body size, multiple organ hyperplasia, retinal dysplasia and pituitary tumors. *Cell* 1996; 85: 707–20.
58. Takeuchi S, Koeffler HP, Hinton DR, Miyoshi I, Melmed S, Shimon I. Mutation and expression analysis of the cyclin-dependent kinase inhibitor gene *p27/kip1* in pituitary tumors. *J Endocrinol* 1998; 157: 337–41.
59. Farid NR, Zou M, Shi Y. Genetics of follicular thyroid cancer. *Endocrinol Metab Clin North Am* 1995; 24(4): 865–83.
60. Simpson DJ, Bicknell JE, McNicoll AM, Clayton RN, Farrell WE. Hypermethylation of the p16/CDKN2A/MTS1 gene and loss of protein expression is associated with non-functional pituitary adenomas but not somatotrophinomas. *Genes Chrom Cancer* 1999; 24(4): 328–36.
61. Frost SJ, Simpson DJ, Clayton RN, Farrell WE. Transfection of an inducible p16/CDKN2A construct mediates reversible growth inhibition and G1 arrest in the AtT20 pituitary tumor cell line. *Mol Endocrinol* 1999; 13(11): 1801–10.
62. Takino H, Herman V, Weiss M, Melmed S. Purine-binding factor (*nm23*) gene expression in pituitary tumors: marker of adenoma invasiveness. *J Clin Endocrinol Metab* 1995; 80: 1733–8.
63. Zou M, Shi Y, Al-Sedairy S, Farid NR. High levels of Nm23 gene expression in advanced stage of thyroid carcinomas. *Br J Cancer* 1993; 68: 385–8.
64. Knudson AG, Strong LC, Anderson DE. Heredity and cancer in man. *Prog Med Genet* 1973; 9: 113–58.
65. Spada A. Growth factors and human pituitary adenomas. *Eur J Endocrinol* 1998; 138: 255–7.

3

Neuroendocrine disease
Philip E Harris

The normal hypothalamic–pituitary axis

Normal anterior pituitary function is under the central control of the hypothalamus and higher centers. Hypothalamic releasing and inhibitory factors are secreted into the capillaries of the hypophysial portal circulation at the median eminence. The neurohypophysis consists of neurons arising from the magnocellular and parvocellular neurons of the supraoptic and paraventricular nuclei (Figure 3.1). The anatomical

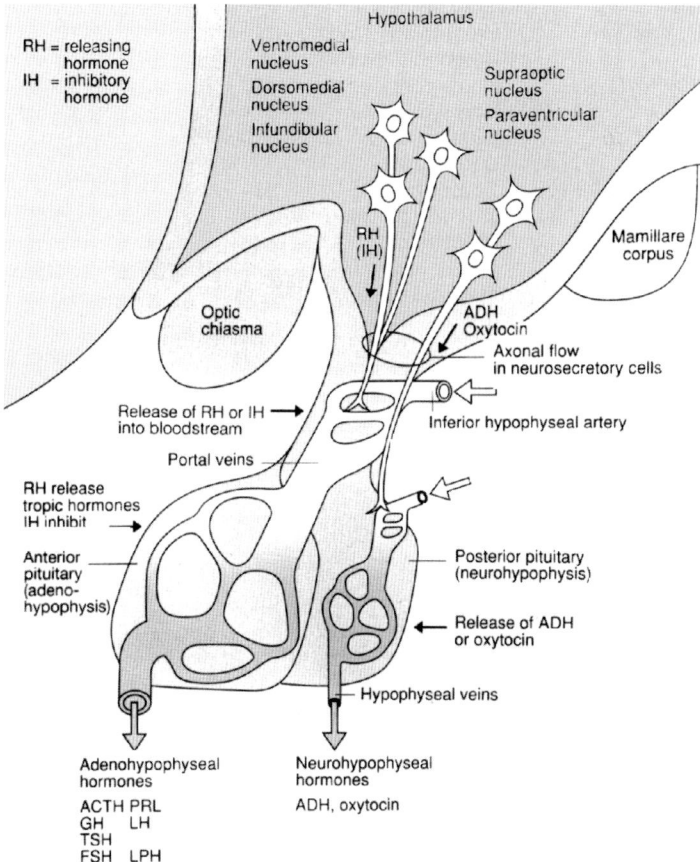

Figure 3.1
The hypothalamic–pituitary axis (from Harris AG. The hypothalamic–pituitary axis. In: Daly AF, ed., Acromegaly and its Management, Lippincott-Raven, 1996; 1–8, with permission.)

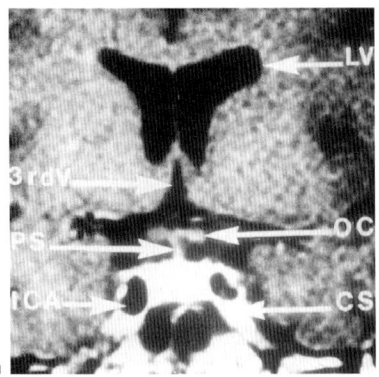 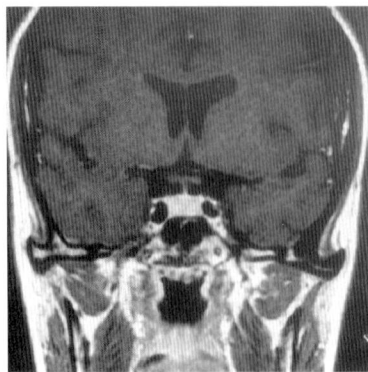

Figure 3.2
(a) and (b) Coronal MRI scan (T1 weighted) of the pituitary gland, hypothalamus and surrounding structures. LV, lateral ventricle; 3rd V, 3rd ventricle; OC, optic chiasm; PS, pituitary stalk; ICA, internal carotid artery; CS, cavernous sinus (includes the third, fourth, first and second divisions of the fifth and sixth cranial nerves).

relationships of the hypothalamus and surrounding brain structures can be clearly demonstrated on magnetic resonance imaging (MRI) scan (Figure 3.2). The posterior pituitary (neurohypophysis) characteristically has a high signal on T1 weighted images, which is lost in cranial diabetes insipidus.

Classification of hypothalamic–pituitary disease

Endocrine dysfunction secondary to hypothalamic disease (Table 3.1) usually results in hypopituitarism. Rarely, activation of the hypothalamic–pituitary axis can occur. A well-recognized but rare example of this is precocious puberty, which may be associated with hypothalamic tumors such as neurofibromas,[1] hamartomas[2] and pinealomas.[3] Very rarely, hypothalamic tumors can produce releasing factors, resulting in pituitary hyperfunction. Acromegaly has been reported to occur as a result of the hypothalamic production of growth hormone-releasing hormone (GHRH) from hypothalamic tumors.[4] Similarly, Cushing's syndrome has been reported in association with the production of corticotropin-releasing hormone (CRH) by hypothalamic gangliocytomas.[5]

Hyperprolactinemia is a frequent accompaniment of hypothalamic disease, secondary to damage of the dopaminergic neurons in the arcuate nucleus. Diabetes insipidus may complicate hypothalamic disease. This is in contrast to primary pituitary disease, where diabetes insipidus is very uncommon. There are certain clinical features that are indicative of hypothalamic rather than of pituitary disease. Obesity and hyperphagia are a

---

Congenital hypophysiotrophic hormone deficiencies
    Isolated GnRH deficiency (olfactory–genital syndrome—Kallman's syndrome)
    Isolated TRH deficiency
    Isolated GHRH deficiency
Hypothalamic tumors
    Craniopharyngioma
    Arachnoid cyst
    Hamartoma
    Gangliocytoma
    Glioma
    Choristoma
    Chordoma
Hypothalamic infiltration
    Sarcoidosis
    Histiocytosis X
    Metastatic disease, e.g. breast
Infection
    Tuberculosis
    Meningitis
    Viral encephalitis
Trauma
    Stalk section, e.g. road traffic accident
    Direct hypothalamic damage, e.g. surgery
    Cranial irradiation
Vascular
    Infarct
    Aneurysm, subarachnoid hemorrhage
    Arteriovenous malformation

GnRH, gonadotropin-releasing hormone; TRH, thyrotropin-releasing hormone; GHRH, growth hormone-releasing hormone. Hypothalamic pathology typically gives rise to hypopituitarism, and/or diabetes insipidus, unless otherwise indicated.

Table 3.1
Classification of hypothalamic diseases.

major problem for some patients. This is almost certainly in part due to the loss of the normal satiety effects of leptin acting upon hypothalamic peptides such as neuropeptide Y, melanocyte-stimulating hormone and CRH.[6] The obesity and hyperphagia of these patients poses a major clinical problem, for which there is, at present, no simple solution. Somnolence is also a characteristic feature, and often occurs in conjunction with hyperphagia and obesity. Thermo-dysregulation and psychiatric disturbance can also occur[7] (Table 3.2).

Pituitary tumors are classified preoperatively in terms of function and size (Figures 3.3–3.6). Functionality depends upon clinical assessment and biochemical investigations. There are a number of ways of classifying pituitary tumor size and invasion.[8] A commonly used practical classification is given in Table 3.3. Postoperatively, tumors can be functionally classified on the basis of electron microscopy, immuno-cytochemistry (Figure 3.7) and in vitro secretory profiles (Table 3.4).[9]

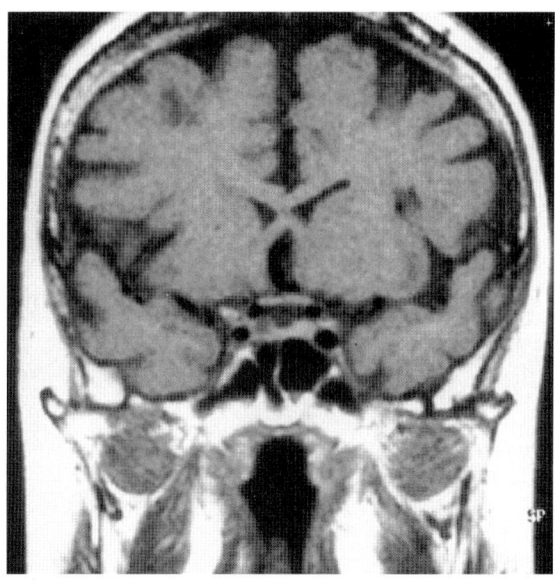

Figure 3.3
Coronal MRI scan (T1 weighted) demonstrating a pituitary microadenoma (hypodense area on the right).

Disorders of food intake
   Hyperphagia
   Anorexia
Disorders of temperature regulation
   Hyperthermia
   Hypothermia
   Poikilothermia
Disorders of drinking
   Adipsia
   Compulsive drinking
Disorders of sleep and consciousness
   Somnolence
   Altered sleeping patterns
Disorders of psychological functioning
   Behavioral changes
   Altered cognition
Disorders of neurological functioning
   Raised intracranial pressure
   Epilepsy
   Impaired motor function
   Impaired sensory function
   Impaired autonomic function

Table 3.2
Non-endocrine manifestations of hypothalamic disease.

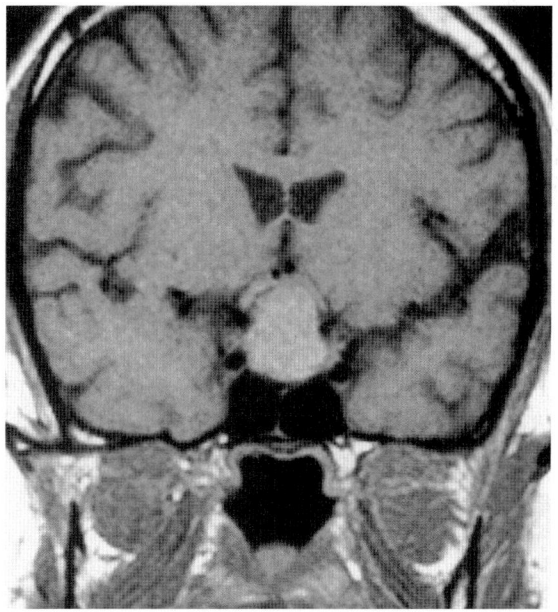

Figure 3.4
Coronal MRI scan (T1 weighted) demonstrating a pituitary macroadenoma with suprasellar extension, compressing the optic chiasm.

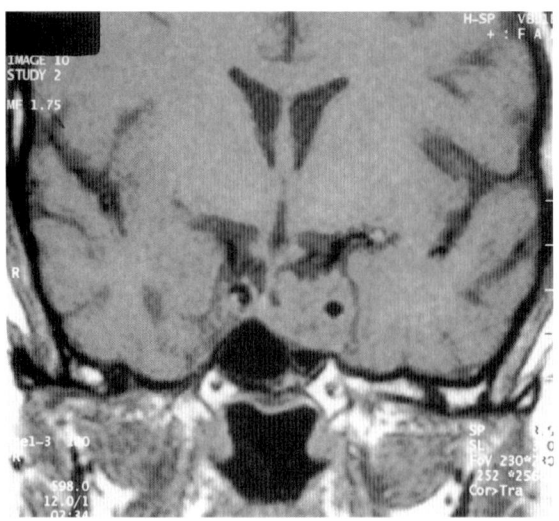

Figure 3.5
Coronal MRI scan (T1 weighted) demonstrating an invasive pituitary macroadenoma extending into the left cavernous sinus, with suprasellar extension.

Tumor grade	Tumor size
1	Microadenoma (<1 cm in diameter)
2	Intrasellar macroadenoma (>1 cm in diameter)
3a	Non-invasive macroadenoma with suprasellar extension
3b	Invasive macroadenoma with suprasellar extension
4	Giant invasive macroadenoma

Table 3.3
Clinical classification of pituitary tumor size (Figures 3.3–3.7).

Unlike hypothalamic disease, which is usually manifest by hormone deficiency syndromes, pituitary tumors can present with a wide variety of different features. In general terms, pituitary tumors can present with local pressure effects (Table 3.5), hypopituitarism and/or syndromes of hormone excess. An increasingly recognized presentation is pituitary apoplexy, which characteristically presents with a sudden onset of severe, debilitating headache, which can last for several days, sometimes in association with cranial nerve lesions and the acute onset of

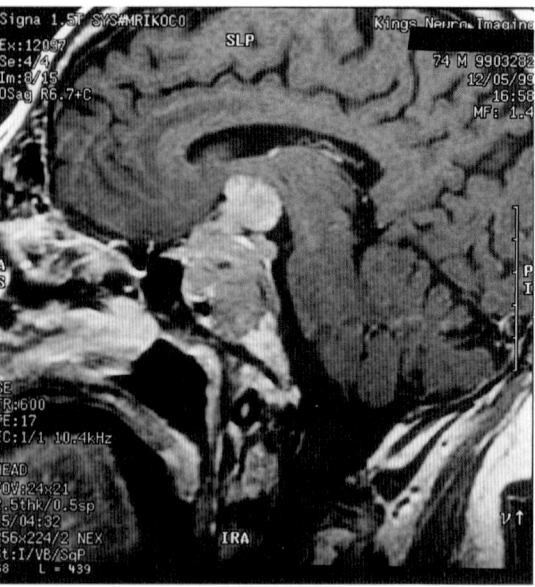

Figure 3.6
MRI scan (T1 weighted) demonstrating a giant invasive pituitary macroadenoma: (a) coronal section; (b) sagittal section.

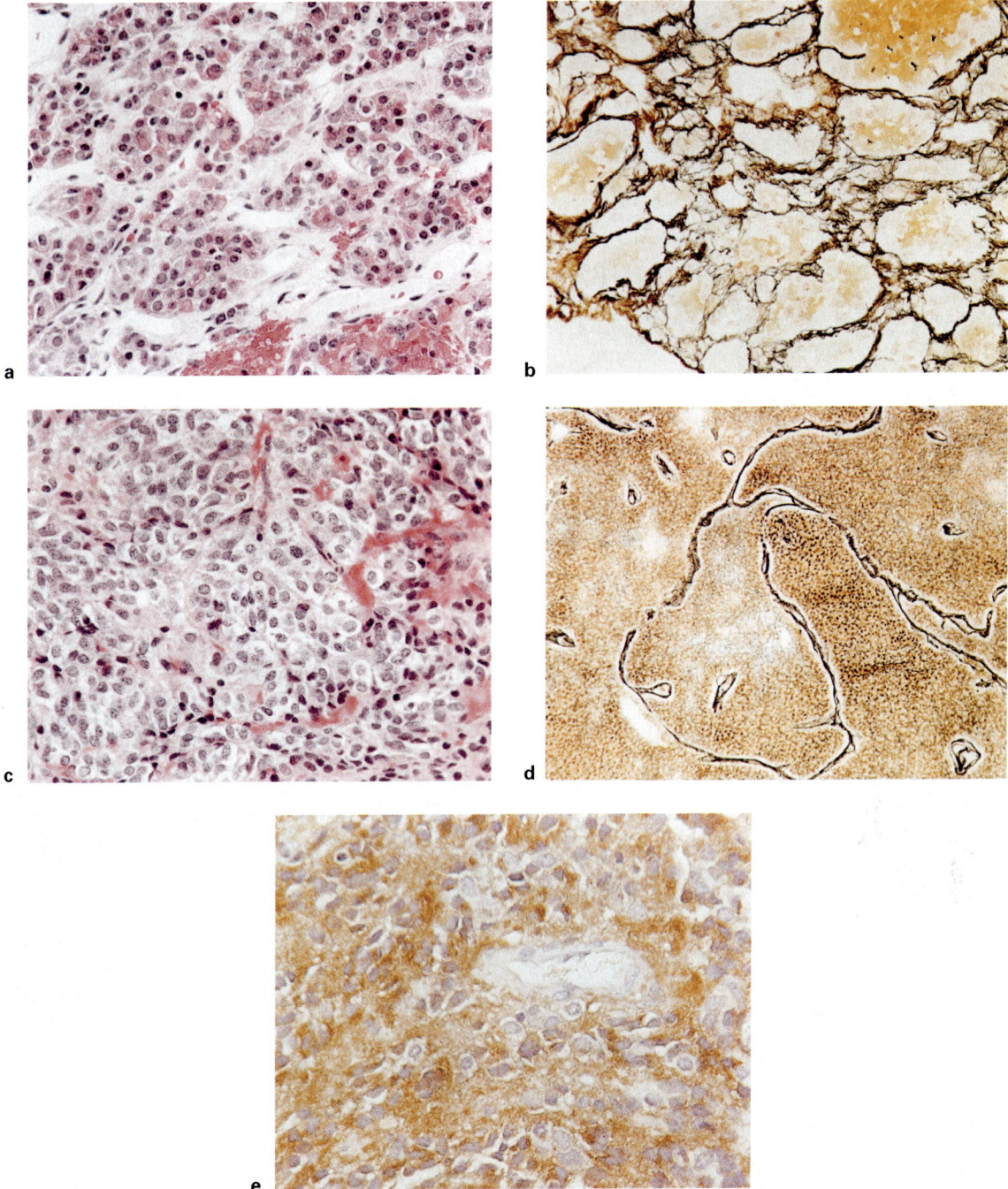

Figure 3.7
Pituitary histology: (a) normal pituitary, H&E stain; (b) normal reticulin pattern; (c) pituitary adenoma, H&E; (d) pituitary adenoma with disruption of normal reticulin pattern; (e) prolactinoma demonstrating immunostaining for prolactin.

Tumor type	Prevalence (%)
Lactotroph adenomas (prolactinomas)	30
Sparsely granulated	
Densely granulated	
Somatotroph adenomas	20
Sparsely granulated	
Densely granulated	
Mixed GH–prolactin cell adenoma	
Mammosomatotroph adenoma	
Acidophil cell adenoma	
Corticotroph adenoma	15
Functioning	
Silent	
Gonadotroph adenoma/non-functioning pituitary adenoma	30
Thyrotroph adenoma	1
Pituitary carcinoma	<1

GH, growth hormone.

Table 3.4
Functional classification of pituitary tumors based on histology, hormone production (immunocytochemistry, mRNA, hormone secretion in vitro) and electron microscopy.

Headache—dural stretching, sudden bleed or infarction

Visual field defect (Figure 3.13)

CSF rhinorrhea

Cavernous sinus invasion—cranial nerve palsies: 3rd, 4th, 5th (ophthalmic and mandibular divisions), 6th

Hydrocephalus

Epilepsy—temporal lobe invasion

Facial pain—invasion of maxillary, sphenoid sinuses

CSF, cerebrospinal fluid.

Table 3.5
Local complications of pituitary tumors.

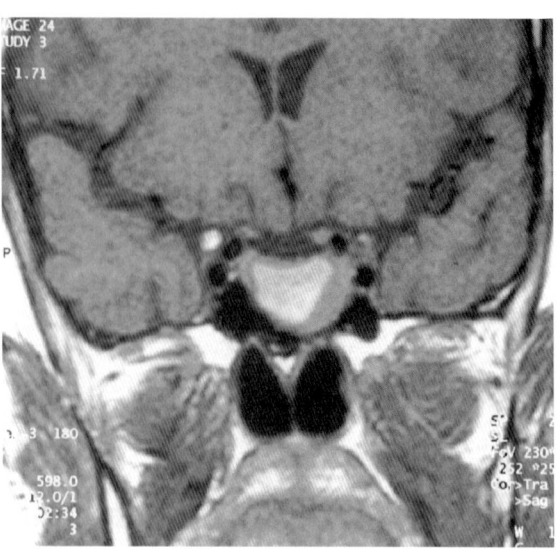

Figure 3.8
Coronal MRI scan (T1 weighted) demonstrating pituitary apoplexy. Note the high signal, indicative of hemorrhage.

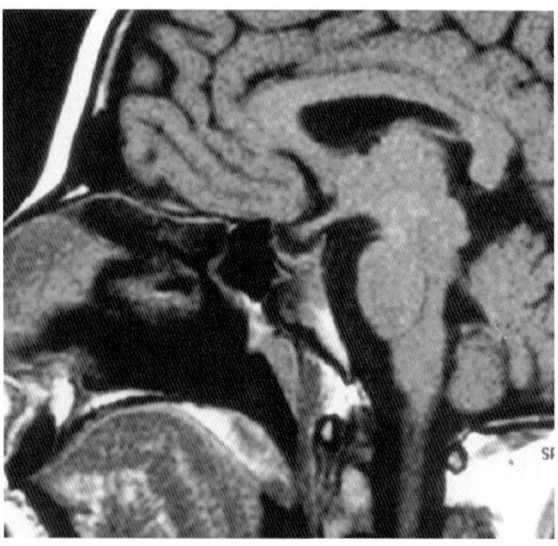

Figure 3.9
Sagittal MRI scan (T1 weighted) demonstrating an empty sella. Note the herniation of cerebrospinal fluid into the fossa.

visual loss (Figure 3.8). Atrophy of the necrotic tumor may result in the development of an 'empty sella' on pituitary imaging (Figure 3.9). The finding of an empty or partially empty sella on pituitary imaging does not necessarily indicate an underlying pathology, since this may represent a normal anatomical variant. Empty sella may also be seen in patients following pituitary surgery or radiotherapy, or in patients with macroprolactinomas, treated with dopamine agonists. Occasionally, patients may develop visual field defects, due to herniation of the optic chiasm into the fossa.[10]

The optic chiasm is normally situated directly over the pituitary gland (80%), pre-fixed (15%) and post-fixed (5%). The characteristic early field defect seen with a symmetrical suprasellar extension impinging on normally located chiasm is a bitemporal superior quadrantopia (Figure 3.10). This is due to the initial involvement of the decussating fibers originating from the inferior and nasal retinas. Further tumor growth involves the upper nasal fibers, with the development of the classical bitemporal hemianopia. Other patterns of visual disturbance, however, are frequently seen, depending upon the position of

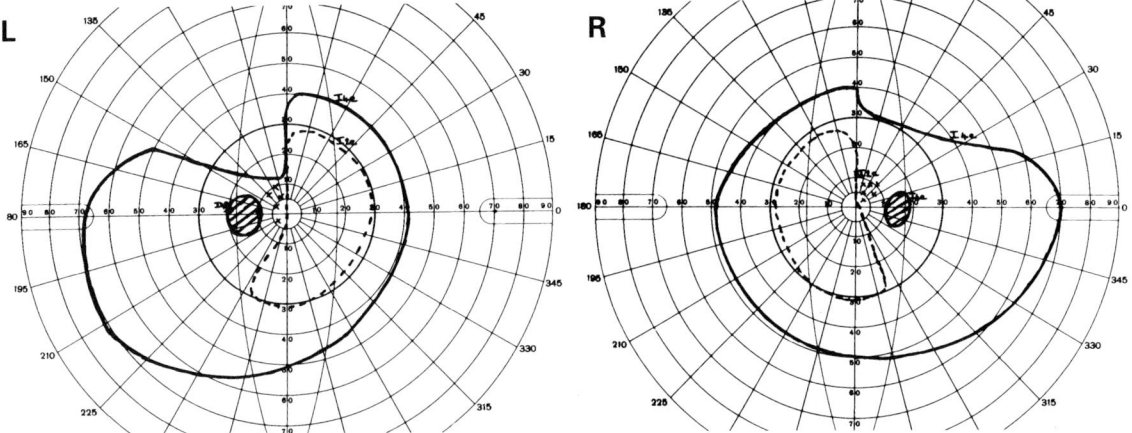

Figure 3.10
Goldman perimetry demonstrating a bitemporal superior quadrantopia.

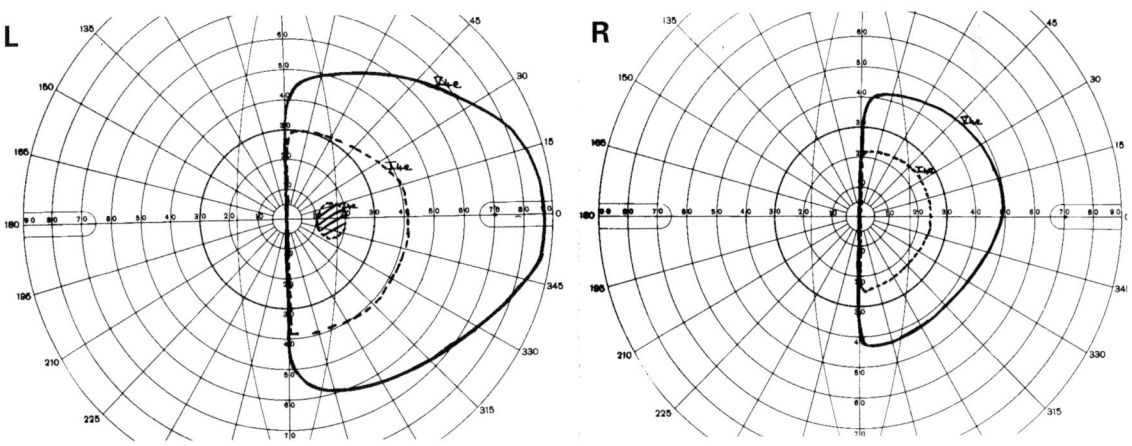

Figure 3.11
Right hononymous hemianopia.

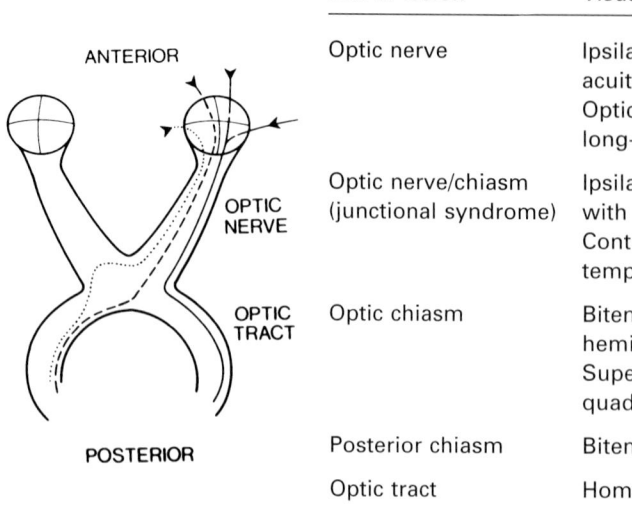

Site of lesion	Visual field/acuity
Optic nerve	Ipsilateral reduced acuity/blindness Optic atrophy with long-standing lesion
Optic nerve/chiasm (junctional syndrome)	Ipsilateral scotoma with reduced acuity Contralateral temporal hemianopia
Optic chiasm	Bitemporal hemianopia Superior bitemporal quadrantopia
Posterior chiasm	Bitemporal scotoma
Optic tract	Homonymous hemianopia

Figure 3.12
Classical visual disturbances produced by pituitary tumors. Solid line, uncrossed temporal fibers; dashed line, superior nasal fibers; dotted line, inferior nasal fibers. (Modified from Melen O. Neuro-ophthalmic features of pituitary tumors. In: Molitch ME, ed., Pituitary Tumors: Diagnosis and Management. Endocrinol Metab Clin North Am 1987; **16**(3): 585–608, with permission.)

the chiasm and the site of suprasellar extension (Figures 3.11 and 3.12).[11]

Principles of treatment

Pituitary surgery

Neuroendocrine tumors should be managed in specialist centers. The management of these tumors requires a multidisciplinary approach involving specialists in endocrinology, neurosurgery, neuroradiology, radiotherapy and neuropathology, who have a particular interest in the subject. The endocrinologist should coordinate the overall management of these patients. Guidelines for the management of pituitary tumors have recently been published by the Royal College of Physicians of London (Figure 3.13).[12] The cure of a pituitary tumor should aim for the complete removal of the tumor, with reversal of associated pressure effects such as visual field defects, the normalization of abnormal hormone secretion and associated metabolic abnormalities, the reversal of abnormal pituitary function or the retention of normal pituitary function.

The advent of MRI imaging is probably the greatest single advance in the management of pituitary tumors over the last decade. Unlike conventional CT scans, which have a safety limit of about six full scans, there is no limit to the frequency with which patients can be safely rescanned with MRI. This has had a profound effect upon the management of pituitary tumors. This is particularly the case for non-functioning pituitary tumors. Some patients who would have previously received surgery can now be safely managed conservatively, with regular monitoring by MRI. Similarly, many patients who in the past would have routinely received radiotherapy following surgery can now also be monitored in a similar fashion.

The standard surgical approach to pituitary tumors is transsphenoidal. This was originally pioneered by Harvey Cushing. Jules Hardy, in particular, has subsequently developed the approach using modern microsurgical techniques.[13] Some surgeons prefer the transethmoidal approach. The sphenoid sinus can be approached either transnasally or through the upper gum. Transsphenoidal surgery is particularly effective in the removal of microadenomas and small non-invasive macroadenomas, where surgical cure can often be obtained without the concomitant effect of rendering the patient hypopituitary. Recently, endoscopic endonasal transsphenoidal surgery has been used in some centers. This is less invasive than conventional transsphenoidal surgery and may be particularly useful in the decompression of cystic lesions. Debulking of larger tumors may be carried out prior to radiotherapy. Intraoperative MRI at the time of surgery enables the extent of tumor resection to be assessed, allowing further resection to be carried out if necessary. Occasionally, with very large tumors, a transcranial approach is necessary.

PRINCIPLES OF TREATMENT

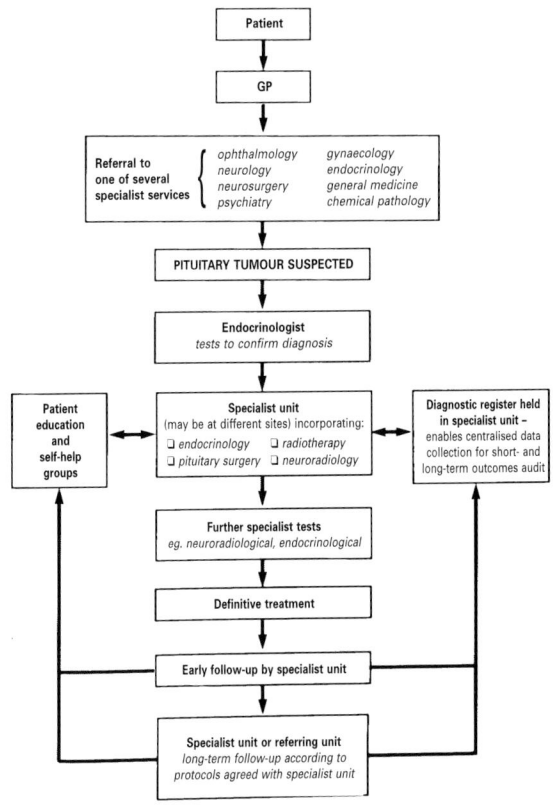

Figure 3.13
Recommended management pathway for patients with pituitary tumors. (From Pituitary Tumours. Recommendations for Service Provision and Guidelines for Management of Patients. Consensus Statement of a Working Party from the Royal College of Physicians Committee on Endocrinology and Diabetes Mellitus and the Society for Endocrinology in conjunction with the Research Unit of the Royal College of Physicians. London: Royal College of Physicians of London, *with permission.)*

Perioperative medical management

Patients undergoing pituitary surgery should be managed jointly by the neurosurgeon and endocrinologist. Although some centers elect not to give glucocorticoid cover to patients with small microadenomas, it is certainly a safe policy to routinely provide all patients with perioperative glucocorticoid cover. Patients are frequently over-treated with glucocorticoids perioperatively, with consequent attendant risks of hypertension, glucose intolerance, poor wound healing, wound infections and electrolyte disturbances. It is quite unnecessary to provide anything more than a modest increase in what would normally be replacement therapy. Patients with Cushing's syndrome should be treated with a higher dose of glucocorticoids than other patients. All patients should receive routine antibiotic prophylaxis as dictated by local neurosurgical preference.

Postoperative diabetes insipidus is not uncommon in the first 2–3 days in patients who have undergone surgery for macroadenomas, but in most cases is transient. This may be masked if the patient is hypoadrenal. A detailed fluid balance chart is mandatory. The diagnosis is confirmed by the demonstration of polyuria (urine output > 200 ml/h), plasma osmolality > 300 mosmol/kg, and inappropriately dilute urine of < 150 mosmol/kg. There may be evidence of intravascular fluid depletion, with high normal plasma sodium and high plasma urea and creatinine. If treatment is required, the patient should be given 1 µg of subcutaneous desmopressin acetate. It is extremely dangerous for the patient to be given desmopressin without clear documentation of diabetes insipidus.

Ideally, patients should undergo a full endocrine assessment before discharge from hospital, or, failing this, within 4–6 weeks of discharge. In the latter event, the patient should be discharged home on glucocorticoid replacement therapy.

Radiotherapy

This subject has recently been reviewed by Plowman.[14] Radiotherapy is generally given as an adjuvant treatment to surgery, usually about 3 months postoperatively. It may also be given as the primary treatment, particularly in elderly patients or in patients with invasive tumors who are receiving medical treatment such as a dopamine agonist as the first-line treatment. Conventional radiotherapy is given via a three-field technique through bitemporal and frontal portals (Figure 3.14). A total treatment of about 4500 cGy is usually given in 25 fractions over 5 weeks. This approach minimizes the irradiation to other brain areas, in particular the optic chiasm.[15] Radiotherapy appears to be very rarely associated with the development of secondary brain tumors, and neuronal and vascular damage.[16]

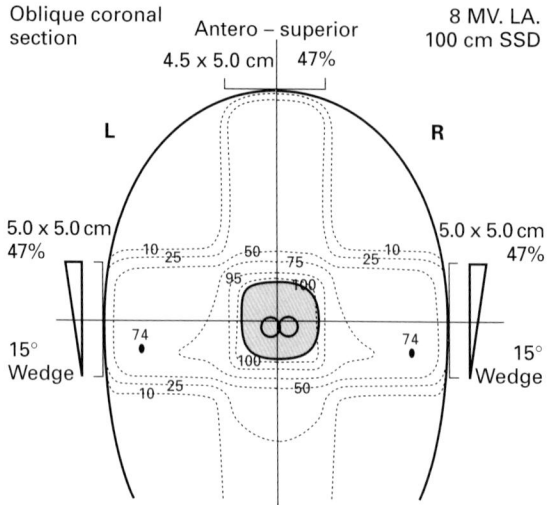

Figure 3.14
Typical isodose plan for irradiation of a pituitary adenoma, using a 6-MV linear accelerator. (From Plowman PN. Radiotherapy in acromegaly. In: Wass JAH, ed. Treating Acromegaly. Bristol: Society for Endocrinology, 1994: 87–94, with permission.)

Headaches—if present, usually mild. Resolve within 2–3 weeks of completion

Tiredness, lethargy—if present, usually mild. Resolves within 2–3 weeks of completion

Hypopituitarism—very frequent. Variable onset, but usually >12 months after treatment. Typical pattern is GH>LH/FSH>ACTH>TSH

Rarely—CNS damage, secondary malignancy

GH, growth hormone; LH, luteinizing hormone; FSH, follicle-stimulating hormone; ACTH; adrenocorticotropic hormone; TSH, thyroid-stimulating hormone.

Table 3.6
Complications of radiotherapy.

Implantation of radioactive sources such as ^{90}Y or ^{198}Au directly into the pituitary fossa has been used in the past, but these techniques have been associated with high complication rates.[17] Stereotactic radiotherapy further minimizes the radiation dose to a given area of the brain and may be used in the rare instances where a tumor recurs despite a conventional course of radiotherapy. Radiotherapy can be delivered in a single dose using a linear accelerator. Stereotactic radiosurgery using ^{60}Co γ-knife has been available for over 30 years. Although this technique has been used in a few centers for the treatment of pituitary tumors, experience is limited.[18,19] The technique does, however, have potential advantages, in that it offers a means of providing a single highly accurately targeted dose of radiation to the pituitary gland, with an accuracy of 0.5 mm. Similar results can be obtained with the x-knife, which uses a modified linear accelerator to deliver a single dose of irradiation.[14] Proton beam radiotherapy delivers a homogenous, high target dose with a minimal exit dose. The Cyclotron machine is extremely expensive and for this reason the technique is unlikely to find widespread use.

A major effect of radiotherapy is hypothalamic–pituitary damage, resulting in hypopituitarism.[20] It appears that the hypothalamus is the major site of damage, as evidenced by the frequent development of hyperprolactinemia and delayed thyroid-stimulating hormone (TSH) and gonadotropin responses to thyrotropin-releasing hormone (TRH) and to gonadotropin-releasing hormone (GnRH) respectively (Appendix 2). The risks of hypopituitarism are minimized by delivering as small an efficacious dose of radiation as possible, in small fractions. By 10 years following radiotherapy, about 50% of patients will be hypogonadal, 30% hypoadrenal and 16% hypothyroid. There is an increased risk of hypopituitarism in patients who have previously undergone pituitary surgery.[21] Growth hormone (GH) deficiency almost invariably occurs first. The implication is that any patient who manifests other evidence of hypopituitarism will almost certainly be GH deficient. This has important implications in terms of treatment with GH replacement therapy (Table 3.6).

Medical treatment

Dopamine agonists

The advent of dopamine agonists in the form of bromocriptine in the early 1970s led to medical treatment being the approach of choice for prolactinomas,[22–25] and, to a lesser extent, acromegaly.[26–28] A major side-effect of bromocriptine is nausea and vomiting. This is a major factor in reducing patient compliance. Postural hypotension is a less frequent problem. Psychiatric complications occur very rarely, but can be

PRINCIPLES OF TREATMENT

Nausea and vomiting ~60%
Postural hypotension ~25%
Constipation ~10%
Dry mouth
Abdominal pain, dyspepsia
Flushing
Nasal congestion
Headache
Leg cramps
Fatigue, weakness
Psychiatric
Pleuropulmonary
Digital vasospasm
Hypertension
Thromboembolic events, particularly postpartum

Table 3.7
Side-effects of dopamine agonists.[22]

extremely serious.[29] In view of this, documented warning of psychiatric side-effects should be given to all patients before starting treatment (Table 3.7). Bromocriptine has been used extensively in pregnancy, with no evidence of teratogenic effects. Most patients can tolerate bromocriptine if it is commenced as a small dose (1–2.5 mg) last thing at night with a snack. The patient should be instructed not to get out of bed on the first night, to minimize the postural effect. After three nights, the bedtime dose can be doubled, and thereafter, the dose can be slowly increased according to tolerance, by starting doses with breakfast and later with lunch. If this is done slowly, the majority of patients will be able to tolerate bromocriptine given in split doses, three times daily. Some patients may be controlled on twice- or once-daily doses. Therapeutic dosages are usually in the region of 2.5–15 mg/day, although some patients, particularly acromegalics, may require doses up to 30 mg/day. If side-effects occur, they will usually disappear if the treatment is continued. There remains, however, a small group of approximately 10–15% of patients who have genuine intolerance to oral bromocriptine. A long-acting depot preparation of bromocriptine, bromocriptine LAR, may be tolerated in some of these patients.[30] A small number of patients are resistant to bromocriptine. Two recently introduced oral dopamine agonists, quinagolide[31,32] and cabergoline,[33] have improved side-effect profiles over bromocriptine. Quinagolide is a non-ergot which selectively binds to the D_2 receptor. Its prolactin-lowering effect is maintained for about 24 h, allowing once-daily administration. The usual starting dose as provided in the manufacturer's 'starting pack' is 25 µg/day for the first 3 days, 50 µg/day for the next 3 days, and then 75 µg/day. The usual maintenance dose is between 75 and 150 µg/day. Cabergoline is a selective D_2 receptor agonist with an extremely long half-life and duration of action. It is usually administered as a once- or twice-weekly dose, although it can be given more frequently, up to daily if necessary. The usual starting dose is 0.25 mg, with the dose being titrated as necessary. Most patients can be controlled on between 0.25 and 0.5 mg twice-weekly. Some patients may require total doses of over 4.5 mg weekly. There is no doubt that most patients who are unable to tolerate bromocriptine can be treated with one of these two preparations. Cabergoline, in particular, appears to be very well tolerated and is more efficacious than both bromocriptine and quinagolide.[34] Other dopamine agonists such as Pergolide[35] and lisuride[36] are also available which are effective in the management of hyperprolactinemia.

One situation where bromocriptine has a clear indication in preference to other dopamine agonists is in pregnancy. There are extensive data available attesting to the safety of bromocriptine in pregnancy which are not available for other dopamine agonists.[37] In view of this, if dopamine agonist therapy is required in pregnancy, preference should be given to bromocriptine. Any patient who is attempting conception on dopamine agonist therapy should be instructed to stop medication as soon as conception has been confirmed.

Somatostatin analogs

Somatostatin analogs provide a means for medically managing somatotroph adenomas. They are also

Somatotroph adenoma
Thyrotroph adenoma
Non-functioning adenoma (rarely)
Medullary carcinoma of thyroid
Carcinoid tumor
Gut hormone tumors

Table 3.8
Endocrine tumors responsive to somatostatin analogs.

efficacious in a number of other endocrine conditions (Table 3.8).[38] Five G protein-linked human somatostatin receptors (SSRs) (types 1–5) have been cloned. Somatostatin analogs bind to the SSR types 2, 3 and 5.[39] SSR2 selectively mediates the inhibition of GH release by somatostatin. The receptor is linked to Gi, activation of which results in the inhibition of adenylyl cyclase activity.[40] In addition to the inhibition of hormone release, somatostatin analogs have been shown to produce a variable degree of pituitary tumor shrinkage. This could occur through a variety of mechanisms, including stimulation of tyrosine phosphatase (SSR2) and the inositol phospholipid/calcium pathway (SSR5).[41]

Pituitary tumors express SSRs 1, 2 and 5.[42] The presence of SSRs in vivo can be demonstrated using SSR scintigraphy with ^{111}In-labeled pentetreotide[43] (Figure 3.15). Positive SSR scintigraphy, however, does not necessarily indicate sensitivity of pituitary tumors to somatostatin analog therapy.[44] Apart from pituitary tumors, SSR scintigraphy has a well-defined role in the anatomical localization of neuroendocrine tumors. In addition, there is the potential for the therapeutic targeting of tumors bearing SSRs with radiolabeled analogs such as ^{90}Y-lanreotide[45] and with cytotoxic drug-coupled somatostatin analogs.

Somatostatin analogs need to be given by injection. Octreotide is a short-acting somatostatin analog which needs to be given by subcutaneous injection three or four times daily.[38] A usual starting dose is 100 μg three times daily, which can be titrated upwards as necessary. Most acromegalic patients can be managed with total daily doses of 600 μg or less. A recent marketing review of 40 UK acromegalic patients on octreotide demonstrated that the mean frequency of injection was 3.23/day and the mean dose per subcutaneous injection was 165 μg. Tachyphylaxis does not occur. This is in contrast to gut hormone and carcinoid tumors, where increasing doses of octreotide are required to control symptoms, until the drug ultimately becomes ineffective.[46] Apart from daily injections, patients can also be managed using continuous subcutaneous infusions of octreotide. Depot preparations of somatostatin analogs are now available, octreotide LAR and lanreotide, which use biodegradable polymer matrices (Figure 3.16). Octreotide LAR is given by intramuscular injection on a monthly basis.[47,48] The starting dose is 20 mg, which may be increased to 30 mg or to 2×20 mg injections monthly (Figure 3.17). Lanreotide is given by a 30-mg intramuscular injection, initially every 2 weeks. The frequency of injection can be increased to every 10 or 7 days if necessary, in order to obtain therapeutic control.[49–51] Octreotide LAR and lanreotide are quite viscous, and care needs to be taken in their preparation and injection. Siliconized wide-bore 20 gauge needles facilitate the injections. A new long-acting aqueous preparation of lanreotide is now available which is administered by deep subcutaneous injection from a small volume, prefilled syringe. The intial dose is 60 mg monthly, increasing to 90 mg or 120 mg monthly. Depot preparations have a number of advantages over conventional short-acting octreotide. Patient compliance problems are eliminated, the clinician assuming overall control of the patient's treatment. From the patient's point of view, infrequent injections

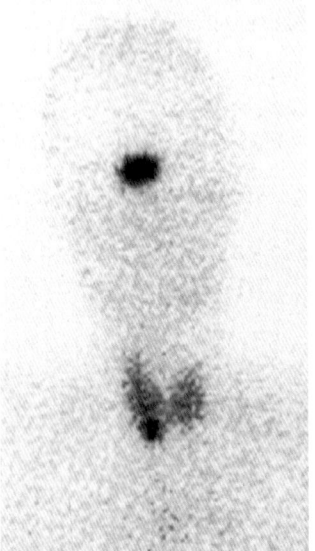

Figure 3.15
Pituitary thyrotroph adenoma (TSHoma) demonstrating binding of ^{111}In pentetreotide. The patient has a goiter and is thyrotoxic, as exemplified by the binding of ^{111}In pentetreotide by the thyroid.

Somatostatin
Ala-Gly-Cys-Lys-Asn-Phe-Phe-Trp-Lys-Thr-Phe-Thr-Ser-Cys

Octreotide
DPhe-Cys-Phe-DTrp-Lys-Thr-Cys-Thr-ol

Lanreotide
DβNal-Cys-Tyr-DTrp-Lys-Val-Cys-Thr-NH$_2$

Figure 3.16
Amino acid sequences of somatostatin-14, octreotide and lanreotide.

PRINCIPLES OF TREATMENT

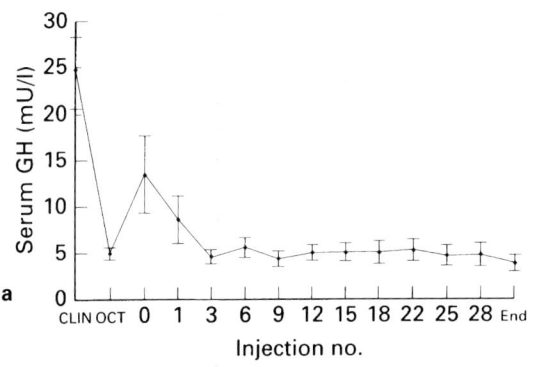 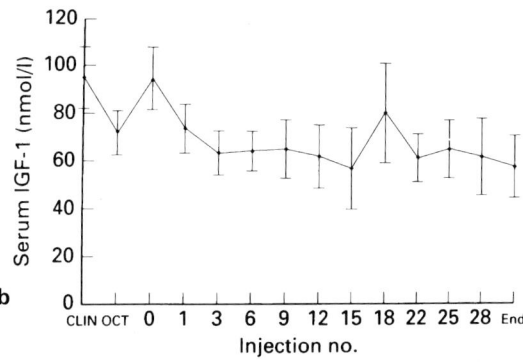

Figure 3.17
(a) Serum GH concentrations following treatment with sandostatin LAR (mean ± SEM; n = 12 until 12 injections, thereafter n = 8). CLIN, pretreatment GH concentration in clinic; OCT, end of 4-week treatment period with subcutaneous octreotide three times daily. (b) Serum insulin-like growth factor-1 (IGF-1) concentrations following treatment with sandostatin LAR (mean ± SEM; n = 12 until 12 injections, thereafter n = 8). CLIN, pretreatment GH concentration in clinic. OCT, end of 4-week treatment period with subcutaneous octreotide, three times daily. (From Davies PH, Stewart SE, Lancranjan I, Sheppard MC, Stewart PM. Long-term therapy with long-acting octreotide (sandostatin LAR) for the management of acromegaly. Clin Endocrinol 1998, 311–16, with permission.)

are preferable to multiple daily injections. In addition, drug administration is simplified for patients who are unable to self-inject. There is evidence that octreotide LAR has increased efficacy compared with the shorter-acting preparation over the long term.[52] From the cost point of view, octreotide, octreotide LAR and lanreotide are closely comparable. Overall, it seems to be appropriate to offer a long-acting formulation to patients.

A major problem with conventional octreotide is patient compliance. Depot preparations have an obvious advantage in this regard. The cost of treatment with the different preparations is comparable. Side-effects occur in about 30% of patients (Table 3.9). The most frequent acute side-effect is abdominal colic, which may occasionally be severe. This may be associated with diarrhea, steatorrhea and flatulence. These symptoms usually disappear after 10–14 days of treatment. Somatostatin inhibits insulin secretion, but this is usually of no clinical relevance in terms of glucose tolerance. Although somatostatin analogs can be effective in the treatment of insulinomas, they may be hazardous in this situation, producing paradoxical worsening of hypoglycemia by the inhibition of glucagon secretion. Stinging at the injection site of the subcutaneous injection may be minimized by warming the injection to room temperature first. A longer-term problem is cholelithiasis, which occurs in 20–30% of patients. This is due to the inhibition of gallbladder and intestinal motility, inhibition of cholecystokinin, and increased production of deoxycholic acid.[38] The development of gallstones is usually asymptomatic. The presence of uncomplicated gallstones or their development during treatment is not a contraindication to therapy. All patients should, however, have an ultrasound scan of the gallbladder carried out before initiating treatment and 6-monthly thereafter. If necessary, patients can be treated with ursodeoxycholic acid.

Intestinal colic
Diarrhea
Steatorrhea
Flatulence
Cholelithiasis

Table 3.9
Frequent side-effects of treatment with somatostatin and analogs.[38]

Miscellaneous medical therapies

A small group of pituitary tumors are relentlessly progressive. Photodynamic therapy using photosensitizing drugs such as photofrin 11 is currently undergoing trials in patients with recurrent pituitary tumors that have failed to respond to conventional therapies. Occasionally, tumors may become frankly malignant and metastasize.[53] Cytotoxic chemotherapy may be of some limited value in delaying disease progression in a small proportion of patients.[54] Adenovirus vectors carrying human pituitary-specific promoters may provide a means of developing gene therapy strategies for the treatment of such tumors in the future.[55]

Hypopituitarism

Hypopituitarism is one of the most frequent clinical problems in neuroendocrinology. It may occur de novo, or as a secondary event, most often as a result of surgery and/or radiotherapy (see above) (Table 3.10). Hypopituitarism is associated with reduced life-expectancy, in part due to vascular disease[56–59]

Hypothalamic
  Craniopharyngioma
  Sarcoidosis
  Histiocytosis X
  Glioma
  Metastatic disease, e.g. breast cancer
  Radiotherapy
  Trauma
  Infection, e.g. tuberculosis, mycoses, syphilis, toxoplasmosis, Whipple's disease
  Genetic, e.g. septo-optic dysplasia
  Infiltrative/invasive, e.g. meningioma, chordoma, dysgerminoma

Pituitary
  Pituitary tumor
  Pituitary apoplexy
  Sheehan's syndrome
  Empty sellar syndrome
  Lymphocytic hypophysitis
  Surgery
  Radiotherapy
  Genetic, e.g. mutations of POU-1 and PROP-1[63], LHX3, LHX4, HESX1,

Table 3.10
Causes of hypopituitarism.

Hypopituitarism classically develops in the sequential fashion GH > luteinizing hormone (LH)/follicle-stimulating hormone (FSH) > adrenocorticotropic hormone (ACTH) > TSH.[60] Prolactin deficiency is usually a late event and does not appear to be of clinical significance, except in women who wish to breastfeed. The developmental sequence of hormone deficiency can vary, although GH is almost invariably affected first. Hypopituitary patients who present de novo often give a preceding history of severe lethargy and weakness, which may have been present over a number of years. Premenopausal women are more likely to present earlier than men, due to the development of secondary amenorrhea. Male patients may or may not volunteer a history of erectile dysfunction and loss of libido, but these symptoms are invariably present on direct questioning. Patients usually describe a loss of axillary and pubic hair. Male patients also lose body hair, and facial hair growth diminishes. In severe cases, patients develop additional symptoms of hypothyroidism such as cold intolerance. Osteoporosis may result in the development of fractures. Ischemic heart disease frequently develops. Often, patients are unable to participate in normal daily activities and work. Many patients become chronic invalids.

Clinical examination may appear to be unremarkable, particularly in women. On closer inspection, however, most patients will have a smooth, sallow facial appearance and thin skin. Male patients, in particular, develop the classical appearance, with loss of facial hair. Most patients will have a diminution or loss of axillary and pubic hair (Figure 3.18). Profoundly hypopituitary patients may be hypotensive with cold skin and delayed tendon jerks. Because of its insidious development, hypopituitarism is frequently missed, often with catastrophic consequences for the patient. Hypopituitarism is particularly likely to be missed in male patients with non-functioning pituitary tumors and prolactinomas (see below). It is important to enquire about the sudden onset of what is often an extremely severe headache, suggesting pituitary apoplexy (Figure 3.8). In these circumstances, the patient will often describe the acute onset of symptoms following the event. Similarly, the onset of a severe headache in the peripartum period, followed by failure of lactation, should suggest the possibility of Sheehan's syndrome.[61]

The most frequent causes of hypopituitarism are pituitary surgery and hypothalamic–pituitary irradiation.[20,21] These causes are predictable and should be detected early with specialist follow-up. It is uncommon for radiotherapy to result in the development of clinically significant hypopituitarism earlier than 1 year after treatment. All patients should have a full pituitary assessment

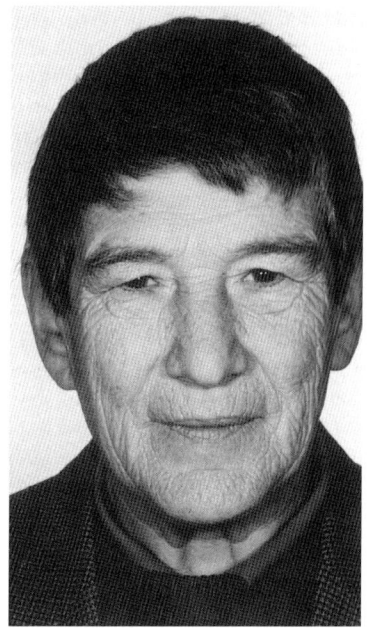 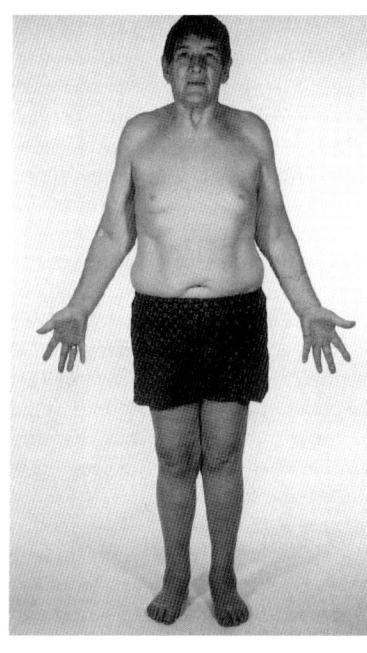

Figure 3.18
(a) and (b) Patient with panhypopituitarism secondary to a macroprolactinoma.

immediately following pituitary surgery. Patients who receive radiotherapy should have baseline endocrinology checked at 6 months post-treatment, followed by a full pituitary assessment at 1 year. It is recommended that patients have annual pituitary assessment for the next 4 years, biannual pituitary assessment over the next 5 years, and 5-yearly pituitary assessment thereafter, unless otherwise clinically indicated. Full baseline testing should be carried out 6–12-monthly in the intervening periods.

Rare causes of hypopituitarism include lymphocytic hypophysitis, granulomatous conditions, infections[62] and congenital causes such as inactivating mutations of the nuclear transcription factors PIT-1 and PROP-1[63] (see below).

Assessment of hypothalamic–pituitary function (see Appendix 1)

Full hypothalamic–pituitary testing should include a baseline screen plus dynamic testing to assess GH and ACTH reserve. The best validated and reproducible test is the insulin tolerance test (ITT). This is a very safe test in adults, provided it is carried out in a specialist endocrine investigation unit with appropriate safeguards.[64] The ITT is contraindicated in patients with a history of ischemic heart disease or epilepsy. In these patients, an alternative test is the glucagon test. This is also a well-validated test, but is less reproducible than the ITT. Some centers use a short tetracosactrin (Synacthen) test to assess adrenal reserve, on the basis that there is adrenal hypofunction in the face of ACTH deficiency. The standard 250-μg dose of tetracosactrin is grossly supraphysiological. In view of this, some centers use a low-dose 1-μg test.[65,66] Although it is simpler than the ITT or glucagon test, some patients will give a normal adrenal response to tetracosactrin, while giving a subnormal response to the ITT.[66,67] A recent study advocates using the low-dose test for the evaluation of the hypothalamic–pituitary–adrenal (HPA) axis, using a cutoff of 600 nmol/l (21.7 mg/δ1).[68] It is important to note that the tetracosactrin test is likely to be unreliable in patients undergoing immediate postoperative assessment and having previously demonstrated a normal ACTH reserve. The ITT and glucagon tests have the added advantage of enabling GH reserve to be assessed at the same time as ACTH reserve. As for the HPA axis, the ITT is regarded as being the test of choice for assessing GH reserve. Other provocative tests of GH reserve include the use of arginine, pyridostigmine, GHRH and hexarelin.[69,70] Serum insulin-like growth factor 1 (IGF-1) provides an integrated profile of GH secretion. Although serum IGF-1 levels may be low in adult GH deficiency, serum IGF-1 levels within the normal range do not exclude a diagnosis of GH deficiency.[71]

The most important deficiency to identify at the start of treatment is ACTH deficiency. This should always be treated first. It is highly dangerous to treat TSH deficiency without adequate glucocorticoid reserve or cover. Most patients will receive adequate replacement therapy with 10 mg hydrocortisone twice daily, although some patients can manage on less than this. The morning dose should be taken immediately on rising. The second dose should normally be taken around 4 pm. Some patients require larger or split doses of hydrocortisone. It is sometimes necessary to carry out a hydrocortisone day curve to optimize dosage and timing. The peak serum cortisol level after the morning dose should be between 700 and 1000 nmol/l (25.3 and 36.2 mg/δ1), and after the evening dose between 500 and 750 nmol/l (18.1 and 27.1 mg/δ1). Patients must be given appropriate advice regarding glucocorticoid cover at times of intercurrent illness. All patients should be given a steroid card and advised to wear a necklace/bracelet such as Medicalert, detailing their treatment.

Testosterone replacement therapy is usually given as a depot injection of testosterone ester(s) or as a patch.[72–74] The usual depot preparations is a mixture of testosterone esters: testosterone propionate, testosterone phenylpropionate, testosterone isocaproate and testosterone decanoate (sustanon). The depot injection is primotesterone or sustanon 250 is usually given every three weeks. Serum testosterone levels are supraphysiological for the first few days following injection, frequently falling to subphysiological levels before the next injection. These fluctuating serum levels are often accompanied by corresponding changes in libido and sense of wellbeing. More stable plasma concentrations of testosterone can be achieved using lower doses of weekly injections, e.g. sustanon 100. Alternatively, testosterone can be administered as a transdermal patch. Scrotal patches and non-genital patches are available. Scrotal patches are associated with supraphysiological serum levels of dihydrotestosterone, due to the high levels of 5-α-reductase in scrotal skin. There is no evidence that this is associated with any short-term deleterious effects, and no long-term problems have been demonstrated with the oral preparation, testosterone undecanoate (see below). Transdermal patches (5 mg) provide a slow release of testosterone over a 24-h period. The serum testosterone remains within the normal range. Some patients find transdermal patches to be esthetically unacceptable. The most common problem with adhesive transdermal patches, however, is local skin irritation. Some patients experience problems with patch adhesion. The recent availability of a 1% testosterone gel which is applied once daily to the skin, avoids these problems. Testosterone can be given orally as testosterone undecanoate. This is a lipophilic compound which is preferentially absorbed into the lymphatics. Testosterone undecanoate is less effective than the parenteral or transdermal preparations, serum testosterone levels rarely rising into the normal range. The usual dose is 80 mg twice daily. As for genital transdermal patches, testosterone undecanoate is associated with high serum dihydrotestosterone levels.[75] Subcutaneous testosterone pellets (600 mg) will provide normal serum testosterone levels for 3 or more months. Technically, this treatment is more complicated than other options. The main problem is pellet extrusion. Implantation of pellets may lead to scarring and occasionally infection. Nonetheless, subcutaneous testosterone pellets are the preferred choice for some patients and practitioners. Patients with prostatic symptoms should have a rectal examination before starting testosterone replacement therapy treatment, and all patients should have annual measurements of prostate-specific antigen (PSA). Testosterone replacement therapy must be started gradually in patients who are profoundly hypogonadal. Serious behavioral problems can be induced if patients are started on a full replacement dose of testosterone. This is particularly the case for patients treated with depot injection preparations, where serum testosterone levels fluctuate widely. Such patients should be commenced on a low dose of depot injection such as sustanon 100 monthly, gradually building the dose up over a period of 3–6 months. Patients treated with transdermal preparations should start with 2.5 mg.

Women may usually be started on conventional hormone replacement therapy (HRT), although patients who have been hypogonadal for many years may need to start on a low dose of estrogen, gradually building up to conventional HRT over a few months.

Thyroxine replacement therapy should only be started after ensuring that the patient has adequate glucocorticoid reserve or is on adequate replacement therapy. Unlike primary hypothyroidism, the serum TSH level is redundant as a means of monitoring replacement. In this situation, reliance has to be placed upon clinical assessment and serum thyroxine levels.

Now that recombinant GH is available, this should be offered to all patients, subject to appropriate inclusion and exclusion criteria. Consensus Guidelines for the Diagnosis and Treatment of Adults with GH Deficiency have been produced.[76]

Central diabetes insipidus is a well-recognized phenomenon in patients with hypothalamic lesions. In contrast, diabetes insipidus is an extremely rare phenomenon in patients presenting with pituitary adenomas.[77] Transient diabetes insipidus is, however, a frequent complication of pituitary surgery for macroadenomas (see above). Extensive surgery may result in permanent diabetes insipidus. In the above situations, the cause of the diabetes insipidus is usually immediately apparent. Patients with established diabetes insipidus usually require medical treatment with desmopressin. Mild disease can occasionally be managed with regular drinking. Desmopressin acetate is usually administered as an intranasal snuff or spray. The dose is adjusted to control the polyuria. Most patients manage with 10–20 μg/day. It is safest to err on the side of undertreatment. Overtreatment will result in fluid overload and hyponatremia, with consequent risk of fits. It is good practise to omit the treatment for one day of the week if possible. Occasionally, the diabetes insipidus may resolve spontaneously, sometimes after many months or even years. Oral desmopressin acetate is available for patients who are unable to take a nasal preparation. This is more expensive than the intranasal preparations and larger doses are required, usually 300–600 μg daily. If there is any doubt about the diagnosis (Table 3.11), the patient should undergo a formal water deprivation test. In some patients, this test is difficult to interpret. This is particularly the case for some patients with psychogenic polydipsia, who may develop variable degrees of nephrogenic diabetes insipidus. In such cases, a hypertonic saline infusion test usually provides the definitive answer.[78]

Differential diagnosis of suprasellar and sellar tumors

There is a large differential diagnosis for both suprasellar and sellar tumors[79] (Table 3.12). In practice, the majority of sellar tumors are pituitary adenomas. Probably the most important pathology to consider in the differential diagnosis of space-occupying lesions in this area is the aneurysm. Aneurysms can mimic large pituitary adenomas. Failure to correctly identify an aneurysm preoperatively can have catastrophic consequences. If there is any doubt about the diagnosis, MR angiography or conventional carotid angiography should be performed. The presence of diabetes insipidus should raise the likelihood of a different pathology to a pituitary adenoma.

Lymphocytic hypophysitis

Lymphocytic hypophysitis is a condition which is now well described (Figure 3.19). This condition has a striking predilection for young females, particularly in late pregnancy or in the postpartum period. Patients usually present with a pituitary mass with suprasellar extension. Visual field defects and hypopituitarism are common. Less frequently, the patient may present with diabetes insipidus. Failure of lactation may occur in the postpartum period.[79–82] Important differential diagnoses are Sheehan's syndrome in the postpartum period and granulomatous conditions such as histiocytosis X and sarcoidosis (Figure 3.20) (see above). The diagnosis can only be made defini-

---

Central (vasopressin-deficient)
  Primary
    Familial (autosomal dominant)
    DIDMOAD syndrome (autosomal recessive)
    Idiopathic
  Secondary
    Hypothalamic disease
    Lymphocytic hypophysitis
    Post-pituitary surgery
    Trauma
    Vascular
    Autoimmune
Nephrogenic (vasopressin insensitive)
  Primary
    Familial (autosomal recessive or X-linked)
    Idiopathic
  Secondary
    Hypercalcemia
    Hypokalemia
    Drug-induced, e.g. lithium, demeclocyline
    Vascular (sickle cell disease)
    Chronic renal disease
    Osmotic, e.g. hyperglycemia
    Psychogenic polydipsia

Table 3.11
Causes of diabetes insipidus.[77]

Embryological cell rests
    Craniopharyngioma
    Rathke's cleft cyst
    Chordoma
Germ cell tumors
    Germinoma
    Dermoid
    Teratoma
    Pinealoma
Gliomas
    Optic nerve glioma
    Oligodendroglioma
    Astrocytoma
    Ependymoma
Meningeal
    Meningioma
Vascular
    Aneurysm
    Angioma
    Arteriovenous malformation
Granulomatous
    Sarcoidosis
    Giant cell granuloma
    Histiocytosis
    Tuberculosis
Inflammatory
    Lymphocytic hypophysitis
    Lymphocytic infundibuloneurohypophysitis
Metastatic
    e.g. Breast, bronchus
Miscellaneous
    Abscess
    Arachnoid cyst

Table 3.12
Differential diagnosis of sellar and suprasellar lesions from pituitary adenomas.

tively by biopsy. If the diagnosis is considered to be a possibility and the patient is not at risk from compressive symptoms, then a conservative approach should be adopted, as in some patients the endocrine dysfunction is only transient. A proportion of patients respond to glucocorticoid treatment, e.g. prednisoline 40 mg daily, titrated as an approximate according to response. Autoantibodies to pituitary cytoplasmic proteins are present in ~70% of patients.[83] Lymphocytic infundibuloneurohypophysitis may initially present with a thickened pituitary stalk together with diabetes insipidus.[84]

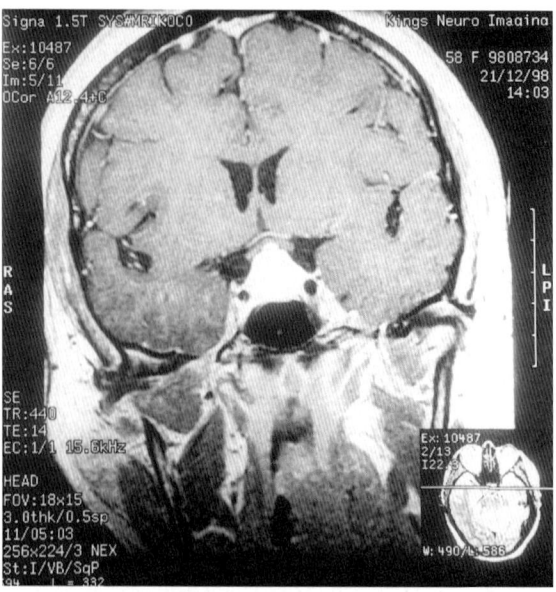

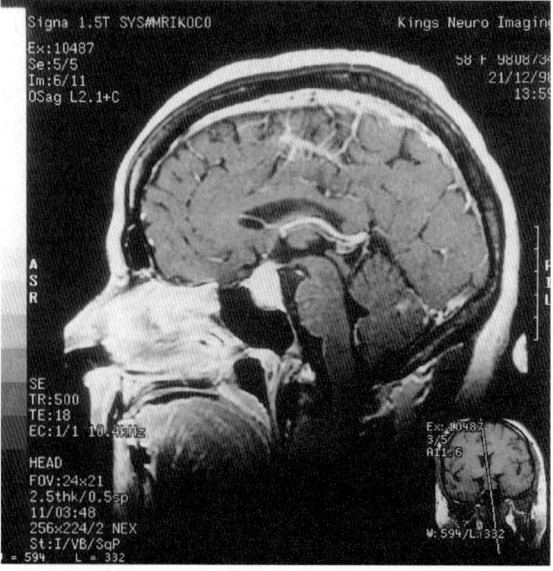

Figure 3.19
MRI scan (T1 weighted) of lymphocytic hypophysitis: (a) coronal section demonstrating homogeneous enhancement of the pituitary mass with gadolinium, with suprasellar extension—note the thickening of the pituitary stalk; (b) sagittal section demonstrating tongue-like extension of the enhancing tissue along the base of the hypothalamus. This is typically seen in granulomatous disease and in lymphocytic hypophysitis.

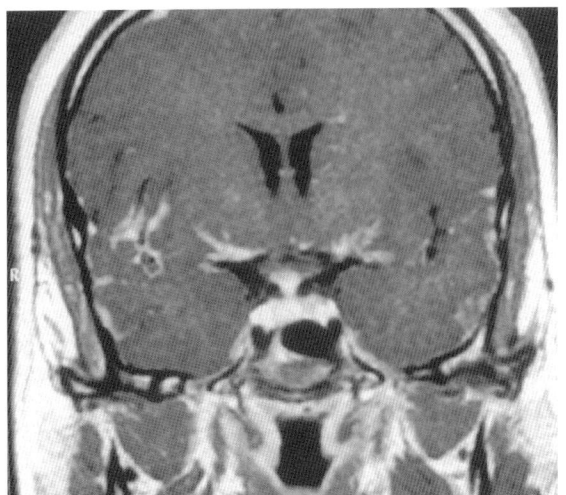

Figure 3.20
Coronal MRI scan (T1 weighted) of pituitary sarcoidosis. Note the thickening of the pituitary stalk, with enhancing tissue extending along the base of the hypothalamus.

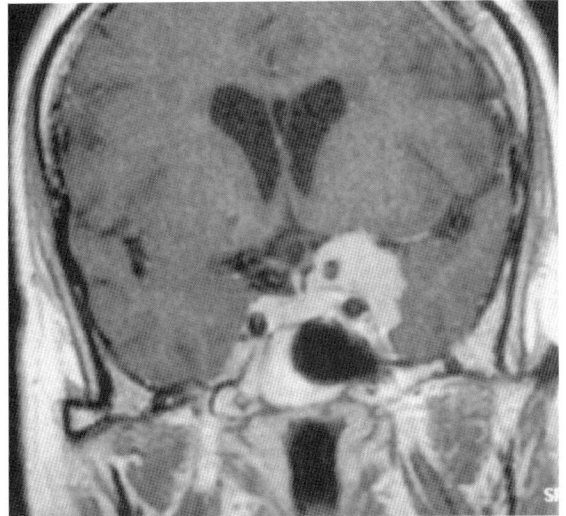

Figure 3.21
Coronal MRI scan (T1 weighted) demonstrating a left-sided suprasellar meningioma.

Apart from aneurysms, there are a number of possible diagnoses to be considered with suprasellar lesions. Craniopharyngiomas, meningiomas (Figure 3.21) and optic gliomas are the most common lesions that are likely to come to the attention of the endocrinologist.

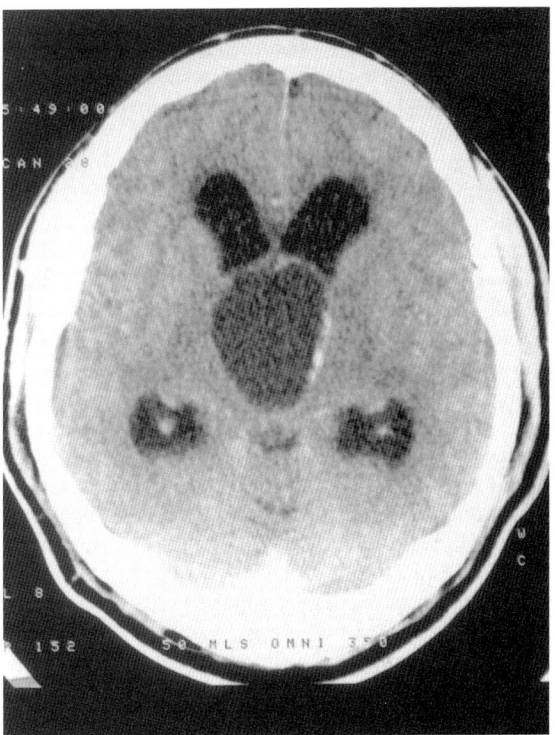

Figure 3.22
Axial CT head scan of a craniopharyngioma. There is a central hypodense mass with a surrounding ring of calcification. There is associated hydrocephalus and effacement of the brain, indicative of raised intracranial pressure.

Craniopharyngioma

Craniopharyngiomas account for 10% of childhood intracranial tumors. Although they present far less commonly in adults, they remain an important cause of neuroendocrine tumors in later life. In contrast to pituitary tumors, craniopharyngiomas are embryological anomalies. They are composed of cystic lesions, lined with squamous epithelium. The cyst fluid tends to be viscous, often described as being like 'engine oil', and cholesterol crystals are frequently present. There is some degree of calcification in the majority of craniopharyngiomas, giving rise to typical appearances on CT scan (Figure 3.22). It should be noted, however, that calcification can also occur in pituitary adenomas. Rathke's cleft cysts are usually small and asymptomatic. They may present with similar features to craniopharyngiomas, although calcification is not a feature.

Craniopharyngiomas are frequently adherent to surrounding structures, which can give rise to problems with surgical removal. They are associated with significant morbidity and mortality. They can have aggressive growth characteristics and tend to recur.[85] Patients usually present with features of hypopituitarism, frequently in association with visual field defects. In children, there is the additional problem of growth failure. Unlike pituitary tumors, diabetes insipidus can also be present. Rarely, patients may also be adipsic, which results in serious management problems. Large craniopharyngiomas may be associated with headaches and raised intracranial pressure. They are usually clearly suprasellar in their localization, but occasionally they can be intrasellar, mimicking pituitary tumors. Craniopharyngiomas elaborate β-human chorionic gonadotrophin (hCG) in the cyst fluid. This is present in high concentrations and provides a useful diagnostic marker. Occasionally, the β-hCG is also measurable in the cerebrospinal fluid (CSF).[86]

The treatment of choice is surgical excision. This often needs to be carried out using a transcranial approach. Incomplete removal is frequent, particularly if the tumor is closely adherent to surrounding structures. Radiotherapy reduces tumor recurrence and should be given as adjuvant treatment in such patients.[87,88] Some tumors continue to grow in spite of surgery and radiotherapy. In addition, cystic fluid reaccumulation can be a recurrent problem. In this situation, a reservoir can be implanted to facilitate repeated cyst aspiration. Persistently raised intracranial pressure may require ventricular shunting. Other approaches to deal with recurrent disease include intracystic implantation of a β-emitting radioactive source[89] and the use of cytotoxic substances such as alcohol during surgery, in an attempt to destroy the cyst lining. In spite of these measures, a small number of craniopharyngiomas continue to grow and are ultimately fatal.

Glycoprotein-producing pituitary tumors

Non-functioning pituitary adenoma/gonadotroph adenomas

Most glycoprotein-producing pituitary tumors are clinically quiescent and are termed non-functioning pituitary adenomas (NFAs). They comprise about 30% of pituitary tumors.[90] They form part of a spectrum of phenotypes, ranging from the truly null cell adenoma to the gonadotroph adenoma, which may be associated with elevated (sometimes markedly) serum gonadotropin levels. As such, NFAs and gonadotroph adenomas are almost certainly derived from the same gonadotroph cell lineage. The majority of NFAs express mRNA and/or immunostain for glycoprotein hormone subunits.[91] Similarly, a majority will secrete one or more of these subunits in vitro.[92] There have been a number of reports describing the measurement of intact gonadotropins and their subunits in patients with NFAs. From the clinical point of view, gonadotroph adenomas can be considered to be tumors that secrete measurable amounts of gonadotropins or their β-subunits in vivo. Gonadotroph adenomas secrete intact FSH more frequently than LH[91] and this may be biologically active.[93] More commonly, tumors secrete biologically inactive β-subunits.[94-96] In addition, paradoxical LH-β and FSH-β responses to TRH are present in a large proportion of these tumors.[94-98] There is often associated hypersecretion of glycoprotein hormone α-subunit. A proportion of NFAs secrete α-subunit alone.[90,99] Unlike other types of pituitary tumor, most NFAs and gonadotroph adenomas present with pressure symptoms and/or hypopituitarism (see above), rather than with clinical syndromes related to hormone hypersecretion.[60] Occasionally, they may be associated with clinical evidence of gonadotropin hypersecretion.[100] Macroadenomas are frequently associated with hyperprolactinemia due to stalk compression.[101] They are frequently mistaken for prolactinomas and vice versa. Any patient presenting as an emergency with visual disturbance must have serum prolactin measured as a matter of urgency (see below). It is essential that the rare but highly aggressive 'silent corticotroph adenoma' is not misdiagnosed as an NFA at this stage. These latter tumors are characteristically large and invasive[102,103] (see below).

Until a few years ago, the standard treatment for NFAs and gonadotroph adenomas was surgery followed by radiotherapy. It is now well recognized that there is a risk of tumor recurrence, even following confident surgical removal and without evidence of residual tumor on postoperative MRI scan. This may in part be due to dural invasion, microscopic evidence of which has been demonstrated in 88% of intrasellar macroadenomas and in 94% of suprasellar tumors.[104] A retrospective audit of patients with NFAs treated without irradiation demonstrated a recurrence rate of around 30% with a mean follow-up time of 76 months.[105] There is no doubt that adjuvant radiotherapy reduces tumor recurrence following surgery.[106] Since the advent of MRI, however, many clinicians have followed patients without automatic recourse to radiotherapy. The author's policy is to refer patients who have surgical and/or MRI evidence of residual tumor for postoperative radiotherapy. Other patients are monitored with annual MRI scans, unless otherwise indicated. Patients are then referred for radiotherapy in the event of tumor recurrence.

The abnormal secretion of gonadotropins or their glycoprotein subunits provides a useful additional means of monitoring individual tumor responses to treatment. Medical therapy of these tumors is largely ineffective. Tumors often express dopamine receptors, and there are case reports of patients who have responded to dopamine analogs.[107] Similarly, tumors frequently express somatostatin receptors, as demonstrated by radiolabeled scintigraphy. As for dopamine analogs, there have been case reports of patients demonstrating variable responses to somatostatin analogs.[108] Ophthalmological responses are sometimes seen in patients without observable effects on tumor size, suggesting that somatostatin analogs may be acting on the optic pathways through different mechanisms.[109] Analogs of GnRH have been found to be unhelpful and may, in fact, stimulate glycoprotein production by tumors.[110]

An important group of 'non-functioning' pituitary tumors was recognized following the advent of MRI. These are incidental pituitary tumors, which are detected coincidentally with MRI scanning. They are small intrasellar microadenomas, which are unassociated with any evidence of endocrine dysfunction or pressure effects. Small pituitary abnormalities are identified in about 30% of pituitary MRI scans. A similar proportion have been found at autopsy. Some of these tumors are microprolactinomas.[111] If such an abnormality is found on scanning, basal endocrine function should be checked. More detailed dynamic testing should be reserved for patients who have clinical or biochemical evidence of endocrine dysfunction. Data for microprolactinomas have demonstrated a cumulative risk of tumor enlargement over a 5-year period of about 5%.[112] The majority, therefore, remain as small microadenomas. Nonetheless, every macroadenoma must have been a microadenoma, so that, as a general rule, patients should be followed up with repeat MRI scans at 1 year, 2–3 years and 5 years. Tumors greater than 1 cm in diameter have a greater propensity to grow.

Thyrotroph adenomas

Thyrotroph adenomas are very rare, accounting for ~1% of pituitary adenomas. It was found that 72% secreted TSH alone, 16% GH and 11% prolactin.[113,114] These tumors are characteristically large and invasive. Patients may present with local pressure effects and/or symptoms of thyrotoxicosis. There may be an associated diffuse goiter. It is essential that these patients are not mistakenly diagnosed as having Graves' disease. Unlike primary hyperthyroidism, thyroid function tests demonstrate elevated levels of thyroid hormones in association with inappropriately normal or elevated serum TSH levels. An important differential diagnosis is the syndrome of thyroid hormone resistance. Such patients may exhibit some clinical features of thyrotoxicosis. A family history must always be sought. Elevated serum total T4 levels together with normal/high serum TSH levels may occur with inherited disorders of thyroid hormone-binding proteins and thyroid hormone autoantibodies. Heterophilic antibodies can produce elevated serum TSH levels, but these effects have now been eliminated in most assay kits. Unlike in the syndrome of thyroid hormone resistance, thyrotroph adenomas characteristically secrete glycoprotein α-subunit, with an elevated molar α-subunit to TSH ratio of >1 (α-subunit μ/l/TSH mU/l × 10).[114] Elevated serum markers of thyroid hormone excess, such as elevated sex hormone-binding globulin, are also useful in the differential diagnosis from the syndrome of thyroid hormone resistance. Dynamic testing with TRH results in a flat or attenuated (<200% of baseline) TSH response in ~70% of patients. In a series of 25 thyrotroph adenomas, the most sensitive test was an elevated α-subunit/TSH ratio (83%), followed by an elevated α-subunit (75%), a flat or attenuated TSH response to TRH (71%), and an elevated TSH (43%). In the differential diagnosis from thyroid hormone resistance, the most specific test was a flat or an attenuated TSH response to TRH (96%), followed by an elevated α-subunit (90%), elevated baseline TSH (88%) and an elevated α-subunit/TSH ratio (65%). In patients who had undergone prior thyroid treatment, the TRH test was less sensitive (64%) but was highly specific (100%).[114]

Pituitary thyrotroph adenomas can often be demonstrated by pentetreotide scintigraphy, and the majority are highly responsive to somatostatin analogs.[43,114]

Surgery is the treatment of choice. Patients should be rendered euthyroid preoperatively using standard antithyroid drug therapy and/or β-blockers. Serum TSH level is likely to rise as a result. If the tumor cannot be fully resected, the patient should be given adjuvant radiotherapy. Approximately one-third of patients can be expected to be cured using this approach. A further one-third will obtain some objective benefit. Patients who are not cured should be offered medical therapy with somatostatin analogs (see above). Most patients will experience a reduction in serum TSH levels, which in the majority of patients will normalize. In addition, approximately 50% of tumors will show variable degrees of shrinkage.[113] Occasionally, patients may demonstrate tachyphylaxis, which responds to an increase in the dose of the somatostatin analog.

Hyperprolactinemia

Hyperprolactinemia is a common clinical problem which is frequently misdiagnosed and mismanaged. A number of different types of clinicians are likely to see patients with hyperprolactinemia, including primary care physicians, urogenital physicians, urologists, obstetricians, gynecologists and endocrinologists. A guiding principle is that any patient with hyperprolactinemia should be fully investigated by a specialist endocrinologist.

There are a number of pitfalls in the investigation of hyperprolactinemia. The first is that prolactin is a stress hormone. As such, a modestly elevated random serum prolactin of up to 2000 mU/l (111 μg/L) can be misleading. It is also important to remember that pregnant women have hyperprolactinemia and secondary amenorrhea Serum prolactin levels correlate with prolactinoma size. A serum prolactin level of >6000 mU/l (333 μg/L) is nearly always indicative of a prolactinoma. Serum prolactin levels below this level may be due to a prolactinoma, but may also be due to a number of other causes (Table 3.13).

Clinical features

The most frequent pathological cause of hyperprolactinemia is the microprolactinoma. Most microprolactinomas remain small. Microprolactinomas typically occur in young women of reproductive age.[115,116] The commonest presentations are oligomenorrhea or amenorrhea. Some patients present with infertility. There may be associated symptoms of estrogen deficiency. Galactorrhea has been reported as having a variable prevalence of 30% upwards, this being largely dependent upon the vigor with which it is sought. It is important to realize, however, that galactorrhea per se is not indicative of hyperprolactinemia.

Although microprolactinomas occur in males, they are less common than in women, most male patients presenting with macroprolactinomas (see below). Hyperprolactinemia in males tends to present more

---

Stress
Pregnancy
Lactation
Hypothyroidism
Drugs
    Major tranquilizers
    Antiemetics
    Tricyclic antidepressants
    Estrogens, e.g. oral contraceptive pill
    Verapamil
    Methyl dopa
    Reserpine
Liver disease
Renal failure
Chest wall trauma
Hypothalamic disease
    Trauma
    Radiotherapy
    Infiltrative diseases, e.g. histiocytosis X, sarcoidosis
    Infection, e.g. tuberculosis
    Metastatic disease, e.g.
        Breast cancer
    Neoplastic disease, e.g.
        Craniopharyngioma
        Glioma
        Meningioma
        Astrocytoma
Stalk section
Pituitary disease
    Microprolactinoma
    Macroprolactinoma
    Mixed lactotroph–somatotroph adenoma
    Mammosomatotroph adenoma
    Acidophil somatotroph adenoma
    Stalk compression from
        Non-functioning adenoma
        Gonadotroph adenoma
        TSHoma
        Corticotroph adenoma
        Lymphocytic hypophysitis
    Miscellaneous causes of pituitary infiltration, e.g. metastatic disease, granulomatous disease
    Empty sellar
Macroprolactin

Table 3.13
Causes of/associations with hyperprolactinemia.

insiduously than in females, with a reduction in libido and associated erectile dysfunction.[117,118] The patient develops clinical features of hypogonadism. Infertility is a presenting problem in about 10% of patients. Galactorrhea occurs occasionally.

Macroprolactinomas behave quite differently from microprolactinomas. These tumors usually grow, and some of them are extremely aggressive in their behavior. A small group are resistant to dopamine agonist therapy. Recent data indicate that many of the tumors resistant to bromocriptine or to quinagolide are sensitive to cabergoline.[34,119] Some tumors which are resistant to dopamine agonists have a reduction in dopamine-2 receptor expression,[120] possibly in association with a decrease in the expression of the inhibitory G protein for adenylyl cyclase, $Gi_2\alpha$.[121] Macroprolactinomas in males, in particular, tend to be aggressive in their growth characteristics. Apart from the effects of hyperprolactinemia, patients may present with symptoms and signs of other hormone deficiencies. Symptoms and signs resulting from local tumor compression occur frequently. A serum prolactin must always be requested as the priority investigation in any patient presenting with signs of chiasmal compression, in association with a pituitary macroadenoma (see above).

Most prolactinomas are sporadic. Familial prolactinomas occur in the MEN 1 syndrome[122] and also rarely as isolated phenomena.[123]

Investigation of hyperprolactinemia

There are a number of causes of hyperprolactinemia which need to be considered in the patient presenting with hyperprolactinemia (Table 3.13). The history and examination of the patient are particularly important. The possibility of pregnancy should be considered in all amenorrheic women of reproductive age. A detailed drug history is essential. Baseline renal, liver, thyroid and gonadal function should be assessed. Stress-induced hyperprolactinemia should be excluded by the measurement of serum prolactin 2 h after intravenous cannulation. Macroprolactin is a recently recognized cause of hyperprolactinemia. This is a high molecular weight 150–175-kDa complex (higher molecular weight complexes occasionally occur) due to immune complex with prolactin molecules. The bioactivity of macroprolactin may be reduced. It occurs in about 15% of patients with serum prolactin < 3500 mU/l.[124,125] It is likely that a number of patients with modest degrees of hyperprolactinemia, associated with otherwise normal endocrinology, have macroprolactinemia. The presence of macroprolactin should be checked in these patients (<194 μg/L). If hyperprolactinemia is confirmed and no cause has been identified, hypothalamic–pituitary disease needs to be considered. All patients should have MRI (T1 weighted) imaging of the hypothalamus and pituitary, with gadolinium enhancement. High-resolution CT scan with contrast may be performed if MRI scan is contraindicated. Dynamic assessment of hypothalamic–pituitary–adrenal reserve (see above) is carried out in patients with identifiable abnormalities. GH reserve is assessed in patients with pituitary macroadenomas. Visual fields are performed where appropriate. The TRH test has been used in many centers, on the basis that it provides discrimination between prolactinomas and other neuroendocrine causes of hyperprolactinemia (see Appendix 1). A normal TRH response in a patient with hyperprolactinemia is at least a doubling of serum prolactin levels following TRH. Prolactinomas have been reported to have a flat prolactin response to TRH, in contrast to other causes of hyperprolactinemia. Recent data,[126] however, demonstrate that the TRH test is of no discriminatory value. Although most prolactinomas have an attenuated or flat prolactin response to TRH, this can also occur with other causes of hyperprolactinemia. A frequent error is to carry out a TRH test, combined with an ITT or glugagon test with measurement of prolactin. This renders the test completely uninterpretable, as prolactin normally rises with ITT or glucagon. Overall, there is no evidence that the TRH test is of diagnostic help, and it may be frankly misleading.

The diagnosis of microprolactinomas and most macroprolactinomas is usually straightforward. There remains, however, a gray area where it is unclear whether the patient has a prolactinoma or non-functioning pituitary adenoma (see above). In most cases, these tumors are small macroadenomas associated with serum prolactin levels in the range of 2000–4500 mU/l (111-250 μg/L). Occasionally, larger tumors may cause diagnostic problems, particularly if the MRI scan demonstrates cystic or hemorrhagic areas in the tumor. In this situation, it is frequently worthwhile giving the patient a trial of a dopamine agonist. If there is no evidence of tumor shrinkage after 3 months of treatment, the diagnosis of prolactinoma can effectively be discounted and other forms of treatment considered (see below).

Management of prolactinomas

The first question to be asked is whether or not the patient requires any treatment. The majority of microprolactinomas are small benign tumors, which will never grow.[112,127] There will, however, be a small group of tumors that are destined to become macroadenomas. With the advent of MRI, it is now possible to closely monitor tumor size without the risk of irradiation. Patients with microprolactinomas that are unassociated with reproductive dysfunction or galactorrhea do not need treatment.

A proportion of the population has small pituitary microadenomas unassociated with any clinical abnormality. Postmortem analysis has demonstrated that these occur in about 30% of the population, and a large proportion of these comprise prolactinomas. More of these 'incidentalomas' are now being detected with MRI scanning[111] (see above).

The first-line treatment of prolactinomas is medical, with dopamine agonist therapy (see above). The majority of microprolactinomas (~90%) and small prolactinomas will rapidly respond, with shrinkage and normalization of serum prolactin, to a small dose of dopamine agonist (Figure 3.23). In most cases, however, hyperprolactinemia will recur after dopamine therapy is stopped, although a small proportion of patients remain normoprolactinemic off treatment.[128,129] Microprolactinomas can also be successfully managed surgically, with remission rates of around 80%.[130–132] Hardy reported that 22% of his patients subsequently relapsed over a 5-year period following surgery.[131] In a summary of the surgical results from a number of studies, Molitch found that initial normalization of prolactin occurred in 71% of microadenomas, with recurrence in 17% and hence long-term normalization of prolactin in 53% of cases.[112] Thomson et al reviewed their surgical results in 61 women with microprolactinomas. Prolactin was normalized in more than 80% of patients following surgery, with an overall success at 10-year follow-up of 73%.[132] In a review of his own results in the management of pituitary tumors, Wilson has concluded that a prolactin level of <400 mU/l (<22μg/L) obtained within 1–2 days after surgery predicts a cure with >90% probability.[133] Personal experience and that of others indicates that, although dopamine agonists are the treatment of choice for microprolactinomas, surgery is a realistic alternative to offer patients with microprolactinomas, in centers where dedicated neuroendocrine surgical expertise is available.

Macroprolactinomas should always be treated medically in the first instance. Children and adolescents have been shown to respond to medical treatment equally as well as adults.[134] In contrast to microprolactinomas, surgical results for macroprolactinomas are poor. Molitch found that initial normalization of prolactin occurred in 32% of macroprolactinomas, with a recurrence rate of 19% and hence long-term normalization of prolactin occurring in only 13% of cases. In addition, as would be expected, surgery on macro-

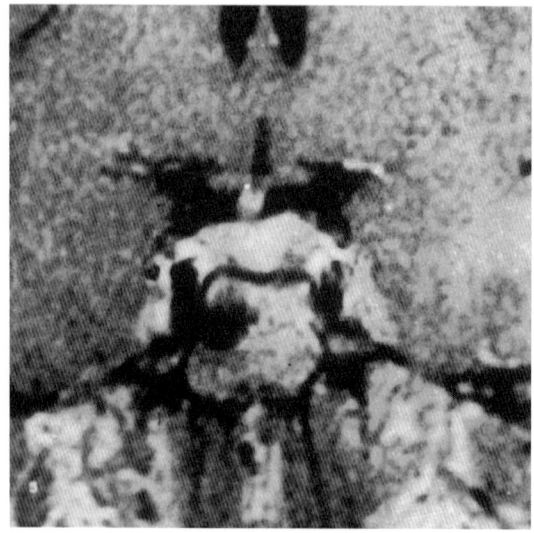
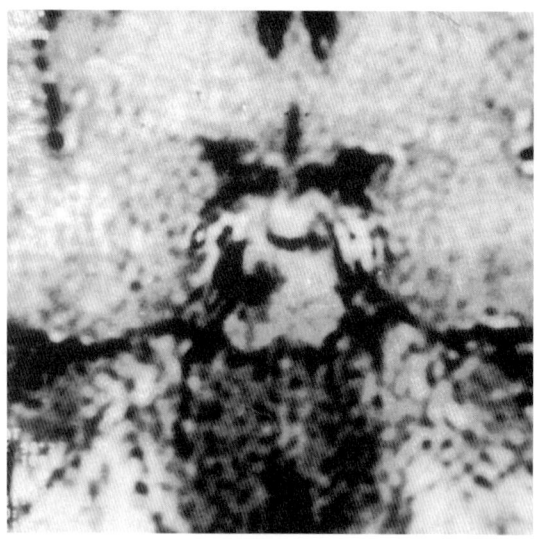

Figure 3.23
Coronal MRI scan (T1 weighted) of an intrasellar macroprolactinoma, (a) before and (b) after dopamine agonist therapy.

prolactinomas is associated with a significant degree of morbidity, quite apart from the risk of long-term damage to pituitary function.[112] Radiotherapy does not have a place as a primary treatment of macroprolactinomas,[112] although it is often given as adjuvant therapy for patients who have failed to respond to medical/surgical treatment. Prolactin can be expected to normalize in about 50% of patients 10 years following radiotherapy. It is essential that an urgent prolactin assay is carried out on any patient presenting with a visual field defect in association with a pituitary macroadenoma. In specialized centers, it should be possible to obtain a result within 2 h. In such circumstances, macroprolactinomas are never cured by surgery and the patients are likely to be rendered permanently hypopituitary. Macroprolactinomas usually demonstrate evidence of tumor shrinkage, with an improvement in visual fields within a few days (see above)[25,119,135–138] (Figure 3.24). Even if patients are hypopituitary at presentation, normal endocrine function may return with dopamine agonist therapy. Continued tumor shrinkage may occur over a number of months,[138,139] so that it is important to continue medical therapy alone, without recourse to other treatment modalities, unless there are specific indications. In spite of this, some large invasive macroprolactinomas may only partially respond to medical treatment in terms of serum prolactin levels, tumor size and invasion of surrounding structures. In these situations, it may be necessary to consider adjuvant surgery and/or radiotherapy.

A subset of macroprolactinomas is particularly aggressive in their behavior, showing only a partial response to dopamine agonist therapy.[140] The tumors frequently have extensive suprasellar extensions, which

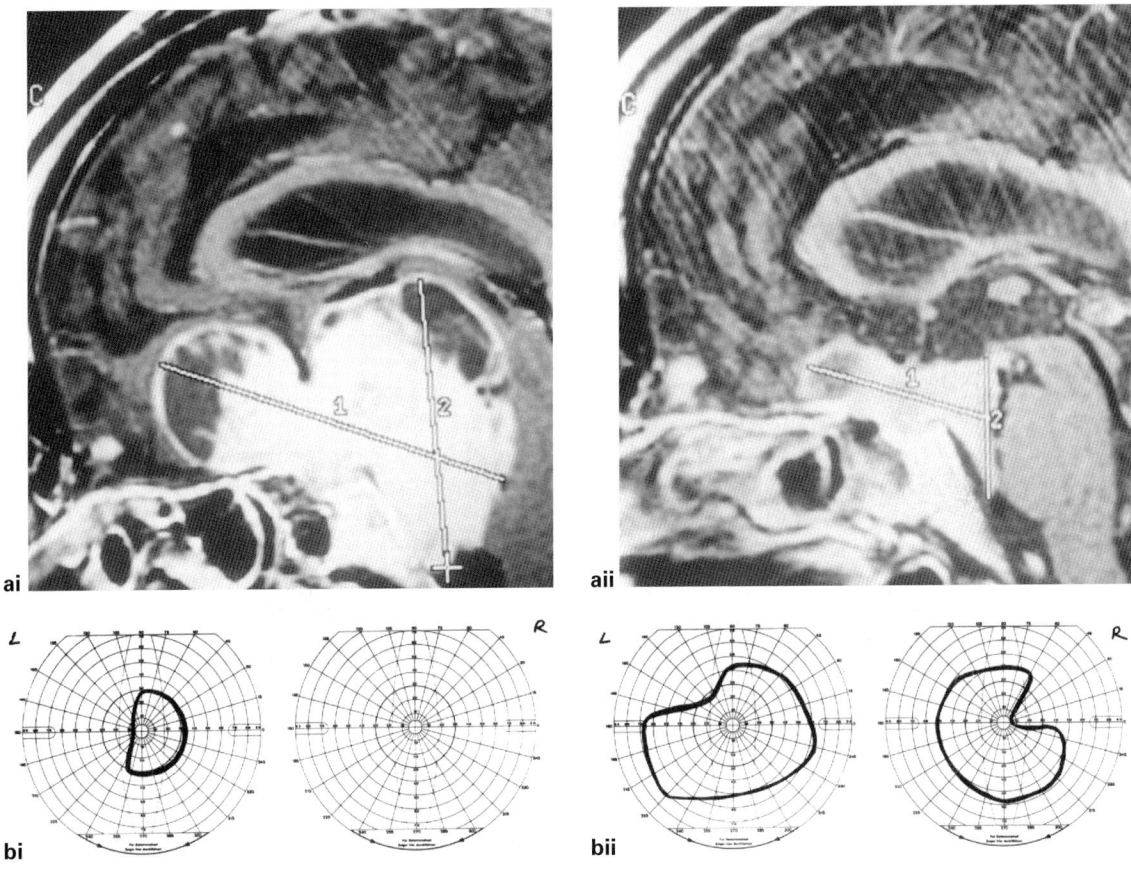

Figure 3.24
(a) Sagittal MRI scan (T1 weighted) of a giant cystic macroprolactinoma, (i) before and (ii) after dopamine agonist therapy. (b) Goldman perimetry, (i) before and (ii) after dopamine agonist therapy.

may produce hydrocephalus. Lateral invasion into the cavernous sinuses is common and may be associated with cranial nerve palsies, most frequently third nerve palsy. The tumors frequently invade downwards into the sphenoid sinus (Figure 3.6). Serum prolactin levels can be greater than a million mU/l. These tumors may continue to grow in spite of high-dose dopamine agonist therapy, radical transcranial surgery and radiotherapy. Rarely, the tumors become frankly malignant and metastasize[53] (Figure 3.25). In this situation, the prognosis is hopeless. Chemotherapy may provide palliation, but the evidence is only anecdotal[54] (see above). If the patient is experiencing severe pain from local tumor invasion, the patient may obtain palliation from octreotide.[53] Molecular biological studies have demonstrated that pituitary tumors that develop increasingly aggressive characteristics of behavior have increasing allelic loss. This is consistent with a 'multiple-hit' theory of tumor development, as has been classically shown to occur in colonic carcinoma.

Prolactinomas in pregnancy

Patients frequently ovulate shortly after starting dopamine agonist therapy. It is essential that they are warned to take appropriate contraceptive precautions.

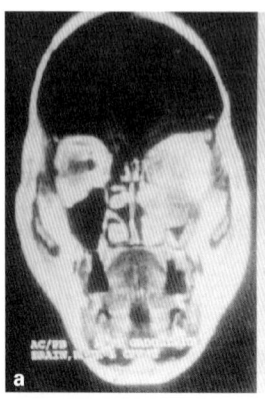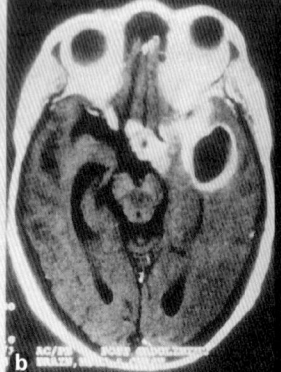

Figure 3.25
MRI scan (T1 weighted) of a malignant prolactinoma: (a) coronal section demonstrating extension of the tumor into the orbit, sphenoid and maxillary sinuses; (b) axial scan demonstrating extension of the tumor into the orbit, together with a cystic cerbral metastasis. The tumor also metastasized to the cervical lymph nodes.

Ideally, this should be a barrier contraceptive method. The oral contraceptive pill has, in the past, been considered to be contraindicated in patients with prolactinomas. This is due to the effects of estrogen in stimulating lactotroph growth and function.[141] The oral contraceptive pill is, however, quite safe in patients who are taking adequate dopamine agonist therapy. Most microadenomas do not in fact grow, even if the patient is treated with the oral contraceptive pill without dopamine agonist therapy. Some practitioners treat amenorrheic patients who do not require fertility with oral contraceptives as a means of providing estrogen replacement and withdrawal bleeds. This is not an approach which is recommended for the routine management of these patients. Conventional HRT, which has a lower estrogen component than the pill, can be a useful alternative to dopamine agonist therapy in certain cases.

There is no evidence that bromocriptine is teratogenic,[37] although data for other dopamine agonists are more limited. Patients should, however, be told to stop treatment immediately following confirmation of conception. The normal pituitary gland approximately doubles in size during pregnancy, largely due to lactotroph hyperplasia. In addition, growth of some macroprolactinomas is stimulated in pregnancy.[142,143]

Conventional microprolactinomas rarely give rise to any cause for concern. Nevertheless, patients with microadenomas should be reviewed at around 4 months and 8 months of gestation, with clinical assessment of visual fields. Patients with macroprolactinomas need to be reviewed more frequently, at least every 3 months. Apart from clinical assessment, patients should also have formalized assessment of visual fields carried out using either Goldmann perimetry or a computerized method. If there is any suspicion of tumor growth, the patient should have an MRI scan carried out. Dopamine agonist therapy should be immediately instituted in any patient with visual field defects or other problems due to tumor growth. In view of its proven safety profile, bromocriptine should be the treatment of choice in pregnancy, although quinagolide or cabergoline may also be used if necessary, particularly if the patient has intolerable side-effects with bromocriptine.

Most patients with microprolactinomas and uncomplicated macroprolactinomas can breastfeed. Patients with clinical evidence of tumor growth in pregnancy should be discouraged from breastfeeding. If the patient started dopamine agonist therapy in pregnancy, this should be continued postpartum.

Acromegaly

Features of acromegaly

Acromegaly is insidious in onset and has often been present for many years at the time of diagnosis. It is, however, a serious condition, which, apart from disfigurement, is associated with significant morbidity and an approximately 2–3-fold increase in mortality.[144,145] European studies have demonstrated an annual incidence of about 3 cases per million or a prevalence of 40–60 per million.[146,147]

Acromegaly is almost invariably caused by a somatotroph adenoma of the pituitary. Most tumors are sporadic. Approximately 40% are associated with activating mutations of Gs (*gsp*) and, as such, they are a feature of the McCune–Albright syndrome (see Cushing's syndrome, below). Somatotroph adenomas occur in MEN 1 and occasionally as isolated familial tumors.[148–150] Occasionally, acromegaly is associated with ectopic GHRH production. Thorner et al[151] and Sassolas et al[152] originally described two acromegalic patients who had endocrine tumors of the pancreas. Subsequently, GHRH was isolated and characterized from these tumors by Rivier et al[153] and Guillemin et al.[154] Ectopic production of GHRH has now been described in a number of cases, most notably in association with carcinoid tumors of the lung and gastrointestinal tract and with islet cell tumors of the pancreas. Occasionally, ectopic production of GHRH has been described in association with intracranial gangliocytomas and other tumors.[155,156]

Key features of the condition relate to the bone and soft tissue swelling. These result in the characteristic symptoms and signs of acromegaly (Tables 3.14 and 3.15). Frequently, the features can best be appreciated by retrospective comparison of the patient's photographs (Figure 3.26). Thickening of the skin is a cardinal physical sign. As a result, venepuncture is often difficult. Skin cuts heal quickly. Patients frequently describe excessive sweating and greasy skin. Skin tags are a common feature, particularly in the axilla and around the nape of the neck. Glossomegaly is also a cardinal sign. This, together with pharyngeal and laryngeal swelling, can result in significant upper airway obstruction. This results in snoring, which is almost always affirmed by partners. Most patients develop a mild myopathy.[157] As a result, acromegalics are often surprisingly weak in comparison to their bulk. Partly because of this and also because of cartilage hypertrophy and laxity of the joint ligaments, degenerative joint disease is common.[158,159] Headaches are a frequent complaint and are usually unrelated to the size of the pituitary adenoma. Characteristically, the headaches in acromegaly are immediately relieved by somatostatin analogs. A cardiomyopathy may develop, which is compounded by cardiac hypertrophy secondary to hypertension.[160] Ischemic heart disease is a common complication. In the longer term, patients can develop sleep apnea and cor pulmonale. Upper airway obstruction can cause problems with intubation at surgery. This is one of the reasons for advocating preoperative medical control. In addition, patients may

---

Thick, greasy skin
Acne
Skin tags
Soft, 'fleshy' hands ('spade-like')
Large feet with thickened heel pads
Thick 'fleshy' lips
Prominent supraorbital ridges
Rhinomegaly
Prognathism
Interdental separation
Glossomegaly
Multinodular goiter (50%)

Table 3.15
Signs of acromegaly.

Increased shoe size
Increased ring size
Increased linear growth before epiphysial fusion (gigantism)
Coarsening of facial features
Headaches
Carpal tunnel syndrome
Arthralgia
Snoring
Sweating
Difficulty with mastication
Tongue biting
Difficulty with phonation
Deepening of voice

Table 3.14
Frequent presenting complaints in acromegalic patients.

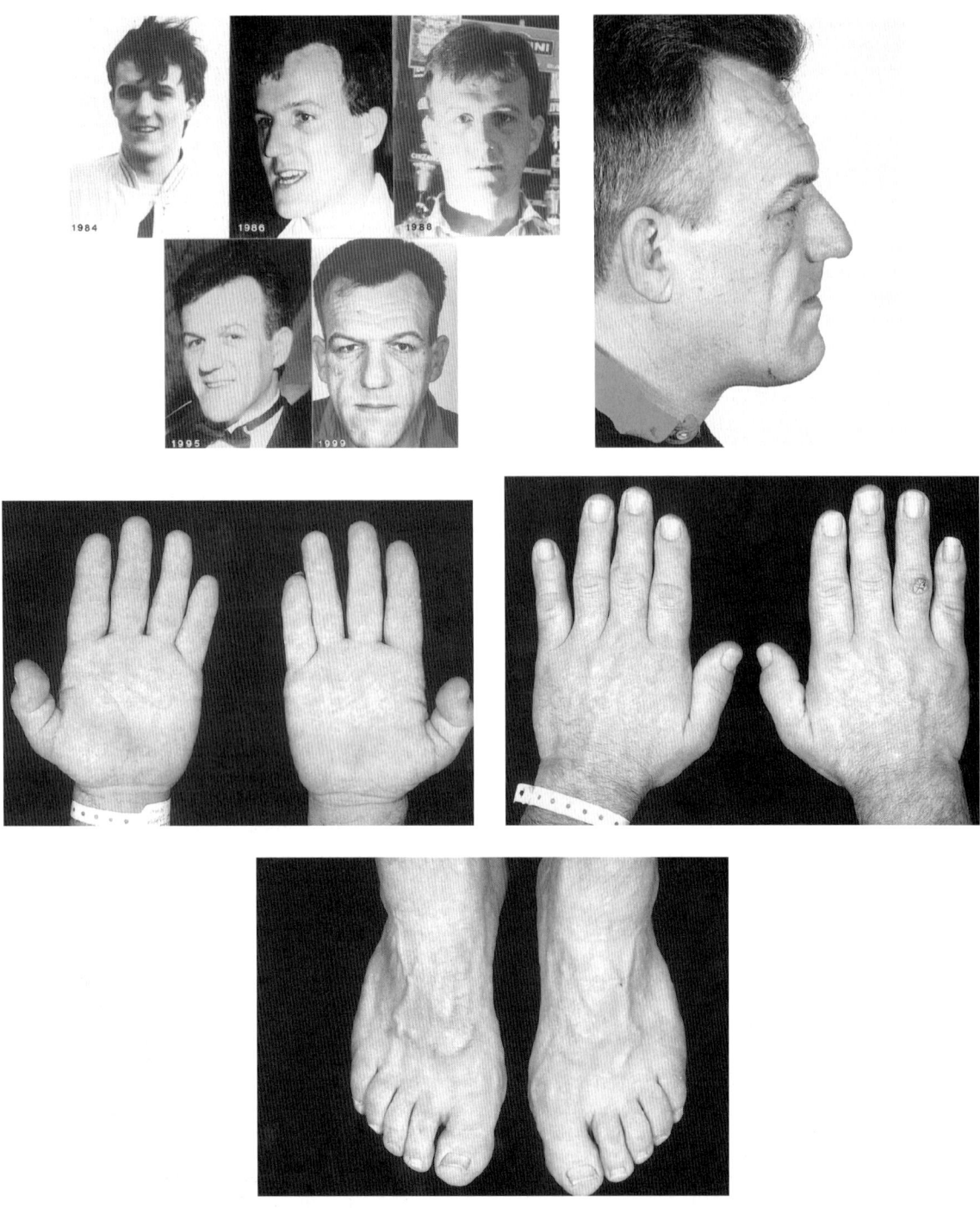

Figure 3.26
Patient with acromegaly in 1999. Sequential photographs over time are useful to assess the duration of disease: 1984; 1986; 1988; 1995; 1999(a).

describe symptoms directly related to the pituitary adenoma, including hypopituitarism (see above). Patients with acromegaly have been reported to have an increased incidence of colonic polyps, predisposing to colonic carcinoma.[144,161] Overall, it seems that acromegali patients have a 2.5-threefold increased risk of colorectal carcinoma. The optimum screening policy for acromegalic patients is still a matter of debate. Some centers routinely carry out colonoscopy at diagnosis and at periodic intervals thereafter. Others advocate a single screening procedure at around age 50–55 years, unless otherwise indicated.[162] A report describing an increased prevalence of prostatic hyperplasia in acromegalics suggests that all male acromegalic patients should undergo prostate screening at diagnosis and follow-up[163] (Table 3.16).

Investigation of acromegaly

Acromegaly is associated with a number of abnormalities which may be apparent on routine laboratory testing. Hyperphosphatemia may be present, due to increased phosphate reabsorption by the renal tubules. Glucose intolerance and frank diabetes mellitus are well recognized, diabetes mellitus occurring in about 20% of patients. GH stimulates the activity of 1-α-hydroxylase activity in the kidney, resulting in elevated levels of 1,25-hydroxyvitamin D levels. Hypercalciuria occurs, and may result in nephrolithiasis.[164]

GH is secreted in a pulsatile fashion. In acromegaly, the GH pulses are increased in frequency about twofold.[165] Random GH levels, therefore, are of little value in either the diagnosis of acromegaly or in the follow-up of patients post-treatment. The oral glucose tolerance test (OGTT) is the 'gold standard' diagnostic test. A normal result is signified by the suppression of plasma GH to <2 mU/l (<1 μg/L), although, in practice, in most normal individuals it will be suppressed to undetectable levels using conventional radioimmunoassay.[166] The OGTT will also enable glucose tolerance to be assessed. False positives may occur in diabetes mellitus, liver disease, renal disease, adolescence and anorexia nervosa. More than 60% of acromegalics demonstrate a paradoxical GH response to TRH,[167] and a proportion also have a paradoxical response to GnRH.[168] Serum IGF-1 is elevated.[169] Unlike GH, which has a half-life of about 22 min and is secreted, albeit abnormally in acromegalics, in a pulsatile fashion, serum IGF-1 has a half-life of 15 h. As a result, it reflects the integrated secretion of GH over the previous few days. Important variables to be aware of are aging and diabetes mellitus, which are associated with reduced serum IGF-1 levels, and pregnancy, in which IGF-1 levels may be increased 2–3-fold. Serum IGFBP-3 is usually elevated in acromegaly, but is less useful in diagnosis and monitoring of treatment than IGF-1.[170,171] Prolactin status must also be assessed. The majority of somatotroph adenomas are macroadenomas.[172] In consequence, a proportion of these will have hyperprolactinemia related to stalk compression. Approximately 20% of patients have tumors, which also produce prolactin. The majority are mixed somatotroph–lactotroph tumors, about 5% being mammosomatotrophs. Acidophil cell adenomas are characteristically associated with hyperprolactinemia, often with relatively low GH production (Table 3.4).[9]

All patients must have a full endocrine assessment, including a dynamic assessment of the hypothalamic–pituitary–adrenal axis, preferably by ITT or glucagon test (see Appendix 1). Ring size provides a simple objective measurement for clinical assessment of the efficacy of treatment. A generalized enlargement of the pituitary without a discrete tumor being demonstrated on MRI scanning should raise the possibility of ectopic GHRH production.

Hypertension
Nephrolithiasis
Glucose intolerance/diabetes mellitus
Cardiomyopathy
Ischemic heart disease
Upper airway obstruction
Cor pulmonale
Chronic airways disease
Malignancy, in particular colon
Prostatic hyperplasia

Table 3.16
Complications of acromegaly.

Management of acromegaly

The first-line treatment of choice is transsphenoidal surgery. The standard approach has been to use adjuvant radiotherapy for patients who still have active disease following surgery. The availability of somatostatin analogs and Pegvisomant, however, has introduced a degree of flexibility in this conventional approach.

The efficacy of treatment is difficult to state, however, as the criteria of remission or cure are constantly changing. Ideally, patients should have normal serum GH and IGF-1 levels, with a return of normal GH pulsatility and control of secretion. The threshold GH level constituting a 'cure' has consistently dropped. Much of the literature in the past has relied upon random rather than mean GH levels to define a cure. This is clearly inappropriate in view of the pulsatile secretion of GH. Nonetheless, mean GH levels <5 mU/l (<2.5 μg/L) are associated with 'normalization' of mortality (see below). Over the last few years, a large proportion of the literature has interpreted a cure as being a mean serum GH level <10 mU/l (<5 μg/l). Using this criterion, however, up to 50% of patients will still have elevated IGF-1 levels.[173] More recently, suppression of GH to less than 4 mU/l (<2 μg/L) after oral glucose has been used as evidence of remission.[174] Studies using highly sensitive immunoradiometric, chemiluminescent and enzyme-linked immunosorbent assays have demonstrated that some patients with elevated IGF-1 levels still had suppressed GH down to less than 2 mU/l (<1 μg/L) following a glucose load. In addition, GH failed to be suppressed normally in 39% of patients who had normal IGF-1 levels.[171] A mean serum level of <5 mU/l (<2.5 μg/l) corresponds to data which suggest that body composition is normalized[175] with the negation of long-term complications.[144,176] Nonetheless, this is clearly not a normal situation. Recent data indicate that mean GH levels should be <0.3 mU/l to consistently achieve normal IGF-1 levels. Normalization of IGF-1 levels has been shown to be associated with 'normalization' of mortality.[176] In practice, it is probably true to say that a large proportion of patients are never truly cured, demonstrating persistent abnormalities of GH secretion, either as pulsatility[165] or in response to agents such as TRH[167] and GnRH.[168] It is still unclear whether or not the retention of abnormal responses in the face of provocative stimuli is associated with increased risk of relapse. In view of these uncertainties, it is probably more accurate to refer to the 'control' of acromegaly rather than to its cure. An international consensus statement on the criteria for cure of acromegaly has recently addressed these issues.[177] A novel GH receptor agonist, Pegvisomant, normalizes serum IGF-1 in more than 90% of cases. This ability will set a new standard in terms of disease control (see below).[178]

In view of the changing criteria, it is difficult to compare the literature in terms of treatment outcomes. Patients may receive somatostatin analog therapy to normalize GH levels for a period of time (~3 months) prior to surgery. Approximately 40–50% of tumors will show a variable, usually modest, reduction in tumor size, which may facilitate surgery.[179] Some surgeons feel that octreotide pretreatment gives the tumor a softer consistency, rendering surgical removal easier. Recent evidence suggests that pretreatment with somatostatin analogs results in improved surgical outcome. Pretreatment may reduce the risks of intubation and anesthesia. In addition, associated problems such as hypertension and diabetes may be ameliorated, resulting in reduced complications and shortened duration of hospitalization.[180]

Overall, following surgery, more than 50% of patients may be expected to suppress GH to <4 mU/l (<2 μg/L) following a glucose load.[176,181] Not surprisingly, the efficacy of surgery is dependent upon tumor size (Figure

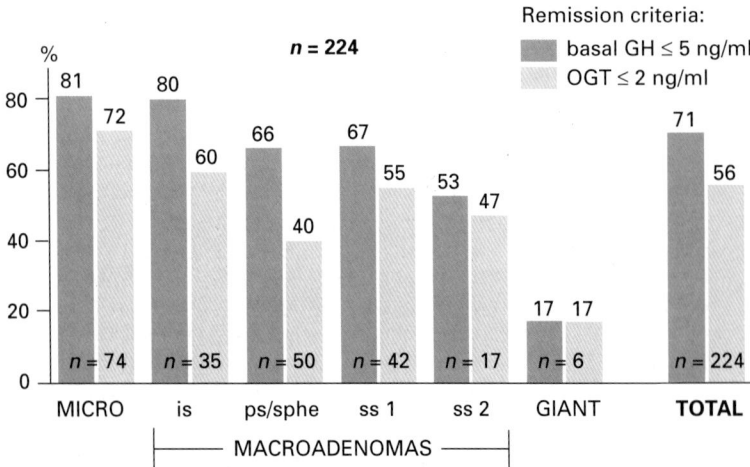

Figure 3.27
Remission rates of primary transsphenoidal operations in acromegaly. 1 ng/ml = 2 mU/l; is, intrasellar; ps, parasellar; sphe, sphenoidal; ss1, suprasellar extension without visual compromise; ss2, suprasellar extension with visual compromise. (From Fahlbusch R, Honegger J, Schott W, Buchfelder M. Results of surgery in acromegaly. In: Wass JAH, ed., Treating Acromegaly, Bristol: Society for Endocrinology, 1994: 49–54, with permission.)

3.27), with remission rates of up to 90% for patients with microadenomas.[181-184] Remission rates for non-invasive macroadenomas range between 48% and 67%.[176,181,184] Recurrence rates were <10% at 10 years.[176,184]

Patients who do not achieve remission by current criteria may be offered adjuvant radiotherapy. Radiotherapy has a rapid effect in controlling tumor growth. Its effects on GH, however, are delayed. In view of this, patients should receive medical treatment for disease control until the radiotherapy becomes effective. The lower the pretreatment GH levels, the more rapid and effective is the treatment. After 2 years, GH levels decrease by about 50% of baseline, falling to about 25% of initial values by 5 years[21,185] (Figure 3.28). The fall in serum GH levels, however, is not necessarily mirrored by a fall in serum IGF-1 levels.[186] This factor, together with the other long-term complications of radiotherapy, brings into question the role of radiotherapy for the routine postoperative management of patients with persisting disease. It can be suggested that with the availability of effective medical therapy, particularly in the form of Pegvisomant with its ability to normalize IGF-1 levels, radiotherapy should now be reserved for patients with large infiltrating tumors, for whom control of tumor growth is a major priority.

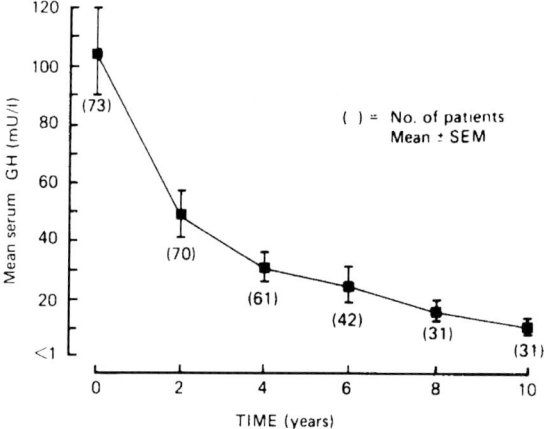

Figure 3.28
GH levels in unoperated acromegaly patients, followed with time after radiotherapy. All data points were taken when patients had been off dopamine agonist therapy for at least 1 month. (From Plowman PN. Radiotherapy in acromegaly. In: Wass JAH, ed., Treating Acromegaly, *Bristol: Society for Endocrinology, 1994; 87–91, with permission.)*

Medical therapy has now assumed a major role in the treatment of acromegaly. Until the advent of somatostatin analogs, dopamine agonists provided the only medical option for acromegaly. Bromocriptine will reduce GH levels in most patients, although only about 20% will show suppression to <10 mU/l (<5μg/L), with IGF-1 levels normalized in 10%. Modest tumor shrinkage occurs in a minority of patients. In spite of this, patients may obtain a subjective improvement in symptoms. Bromocriptine may be required in doses of up to 20 mg to produce a useful effect.[27,28,30,187] Similar results have been obtained with lysuride, pergolide and quinagolide.[188-190] In contrast, cabergoline appears to be more effective than other dopamine agonists, both in terms of GH response and of tumor shrinkage. Normalization of IGF-1 and GH were demonstrated by Abs et al in 39% (25/64) of patients[191] and by Cozzi et al in 27% (5/18) of patients.[192] Remarkably, 61% of the patients in the study of Abs et al demonstrated tumor shrinkage, with more than 50% shrinkage occurring in mixed GH/prolactin-secreting tumors. Previous data have also suggested that overall, mixed GH/prolactin-secreting tumors are more likely to be responsive to dopamine agonists.[187] Unlike with somatostatin analogs, tumor response to dopamine analogs cannot be readily predicted using an acute challenge test. Mixed GH/prolactin-secreting tumors may respond to dopamine agonists, so that these drugs should be considered in patients who have evidence of tumor prolactin production. The only way to assess tumor responsiveness, however, is with a therapeutic trial of dopamine agonist therapy. Effective response to dopamine agonist therapy is most likely in patients who have only modestly elevated levels of GH and IGF-1. Dopamine agonists have been shown to have a synergistic effect with somatostatin analogs in some cases.[193] This effect can be useful when managing aggressive tumors that cannot be medically controlled with somatostatin analogs alone. The main advantage of dopamine agonists is that they are very cheap, particularly when compared with somatostatin analogs. For this reason, they should always be considered as an option in the management of acromegaly.

Somatostatin analogs are more effective than dopamine agonists in the management of acromegaly. Conventionally, tumor responsiveness has been predicted as a >50% reduction in GH levels during hourly sampling for 6 h, following a subcutaneous challenge of octreotide.[194] Another study, however, found that the positive predictive value of a 100-μg subcutaneous injection of octreotide was only 53%, compared with 70% for ^{111}In pentetreotide scintigraphy and 73% for 1 month's octreotide treatment.[195] A number of studies have suggested phenotypic differences, including increased sensitivity to somatostatin analogs in somatotroph adenomas harboring the *gsp* mutation, compared with *gsp* negative tumors.[196] There is, however, a great deal of overlap between the two groups, and from the clinical point of view, there are no useful discriminating features. Recent studies have reported that serum GH levels are suppressed to <10 mU/l (<5 μg/L) in about 65% and to <5 mU/l (<2.5 μg/L) in about 40% of patients. Serum IGF-1 levels have been reported to normalize in ~50% of patients. There is a corresponding improvement in metabolic parameters and in patients' clinical and subjective responses. A European multicenter study with octreotide LAR in acromegalic patients previously treated with octreotide (mean serum GH<20U/L (<10μg/L)), reported a suppression of mean serum GH to <5 mU/l (<2.5 μg/L) in 69.8% of patients over 48 weeks of treatment. This was associated with a commensurate normalization of serum IGF-1 levels.[197] About 40% of patients treated with somatostatin analogs will exhibit some modest reduction of 20–40% in tumor size (Figure 3.29). This may be of benefit in patients with optic nerve compression.[38,43,47–52] Efficacy of treatment should be assessed by a 6-h GH day profile and by normalization of IGF-1. GH levels should be suppressed to <5 mU/l (<2.5 μg/L). On the basis of this, the dose of the somatostatin analog can be titrated as appropriate (see above). An interesting phenomenon is the rapid amelioration of headaches in some acromegalic patients, which can occur within a few minutes of an injection of octreotide. In this situation, the somatostatin analog must be acting on central pathways independent of the effects on GH.

Patients who are unfit for surgery or who decline surgery may be offered treatment with a somatostatin analog as first-line management. Some clinicians suggest that consideration should be given to offering somatostatin analog treatment as primary therapy, particularly in patients with surgically incurable tumors.[198] Another group of patients for whom treatment with a somatostatin analog should be considered are the patients with ectopic production of GHRH.[199] Some patients with ectopic GHRH production also demonstrate an excellent, well-tolerated, long-term response to chemotherapy.[200]

Pegvisomant is a pegylated recombinant 191 amino acid analog of human GH. It has eight mutations at site 1, which increase binding to the GH receptor. It has a further mutation at site 2 (G120R), which inhibits binding to the GH receptor. As a result, the molecule acts as a competitive GH receptor antagonist, by preventing receptor dimerization (Figure 3.30). At the time of writing, Pegvisomant is awaiting regulatory approval. Given its efficacy in disease control, Pegvisomant will have a major role in the future management of acromegaly.[178,202] Pegylation of four or five moieties results in an increased half-life of 72 h, with reduced immunogenicity. The drug is given by subcutaneous injection. Treatment with 10–40 mg daily has resulted in the normalization of IGF-1 in more than 90% of patients treated for 12 months or more. This is mirrored by similar reductions in serum IGFBP-3 and acid-labile subunit. The drug is so effective at lowering IGF-1 levels that the clinician can effectively 'control' the IGF-1 level within the normal range. The fall in

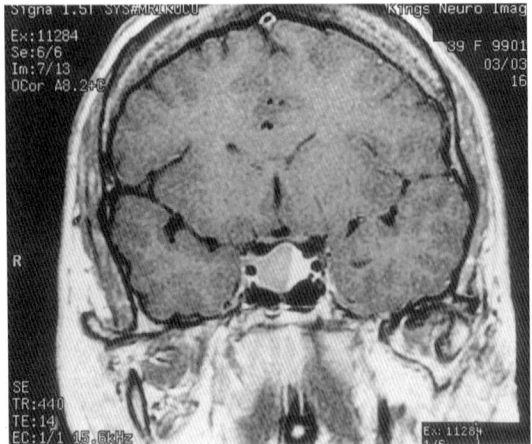
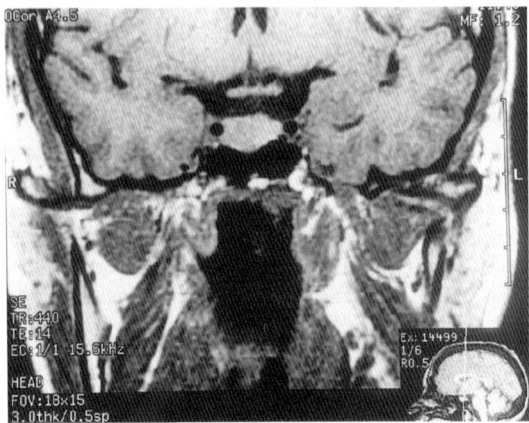

Figure 3.29
Coronal MRI scan (T1 weighted) of a somatotroph adenoma, (a) before and (b) after 9 months of treatment with octreotide LAR. Note the high-signal hemorrhagic component of the tumor.

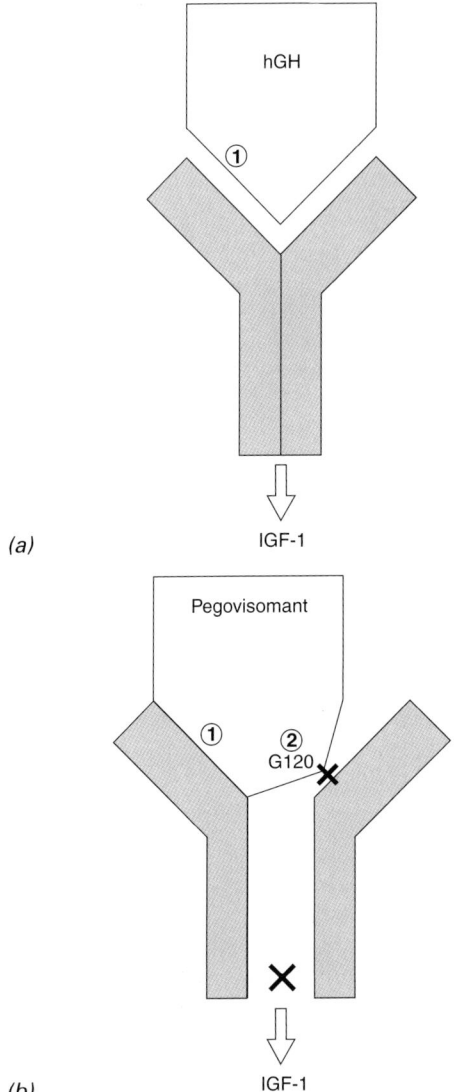

Figure 3.30
Binding of human growth hormone (hGH) and Pegvisomant to the growth hormone eceptor (GHR)

(a) hGH binds to two identical cell surface receptors via binding sites 1 and 2, resulting in receptor dimerization and signal transduction.
(b) Pegvisomant has 8 amino acid mutations at site 1 which result in competitive advantage over GH for GHR. A single point mutation G120R disrupts site 2 binding. Receptor dimerization is prevented, blockingsignal transduction.

serum IGF-1 is mirrored by a rise in serum GH levels which plateau at ~2 weeks. There is no further rise in GH levels and IGF-1 levels remain within the normal range over 18 months' treatment, i.e. there is no tachyphylaxis. Fasting serum insulin levels have been shown to fall, with a concomitant fall in fasting serum glucose levels, although glycated hemoglobin concentrations did not fall significantly. In view of the insulin resistance associated with acromegaly, it is likely that Pegvisomant treatment will result in beneficial changes in glucose metabolism. Two patients have been reported to develop elevated transaminase levels (> 10 times the upper limit of normal) within 12 weeks of starting treatment with pegvisomant, which returned to normal within several months of stopping the drug. There were no other features of hepatic dysfunction. Liver function tests returned to normal within several months after stopping the drug. One patient had a further rise in enzyme levels on rechallenge with the drug. In consequence, liver function tests should be regularly monitored in patients treated with pegvisomant. The drug is well tolerated with dose-related improvements in symptomatic control. Unlike somatostatin and dopamine analogs, the drug does not target the somatotroph adenoma. There is no evidence that treatment with pegvisomant results in tumor growth. Two highly aggressive tumors, which were also refractory to other treatment modalities, have continued to grow with pegvisomant treatment. Concomitant treatment with dopamine and/or somastatin analogues may be effective in controlling disease in such patients.

In conclusion, surgery is unequivocally the treatment of choice for acromegalic patients with microadenomas and non-invasive intrasellar macroadenomas. Surgical remission rates rapidly decline in patients with large macroadenomas and invasive macroadenomas. There is some evidence that pretreatment of patients with somatostatin analogs may improve surgical outcome. Radiotherapy is effective in the management of acromegaly over the long term. Its efficacy is directly related to the pretreatment GH level. This forms part of the rationale behind the surgical debulking of large tumors prior to radiotherapy. The recently recognized disparity between normalization of GH levels and persistently elevated IGF-1 levels, however, remains a concern. In addition, extensive pituitary surgery followed by radiotherapy is inevitably associated with significant morbidity, in particular hypopituitarism (see above). The standard approach to the management of these patients has been surgical debulking, followed by radiotherapy, with adjuvant cover being provided by medical treatment with a somatostatin analog, or, occasionally, a dopamine

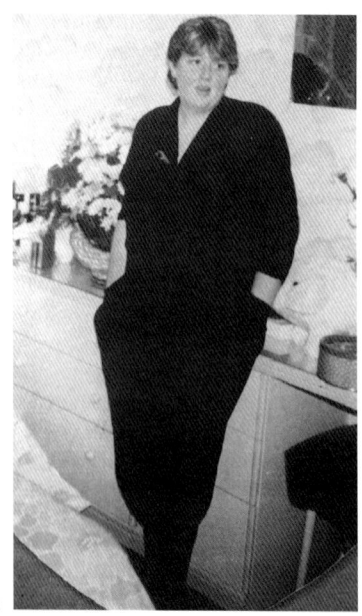
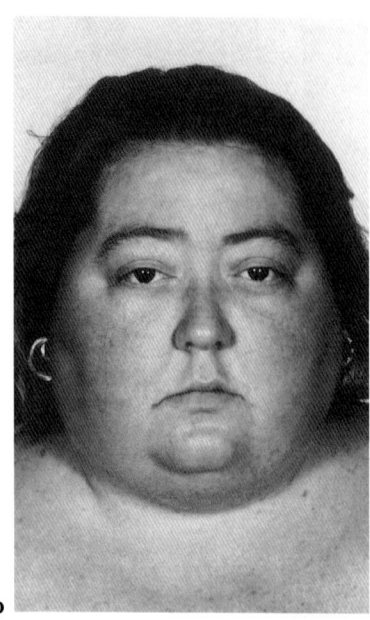
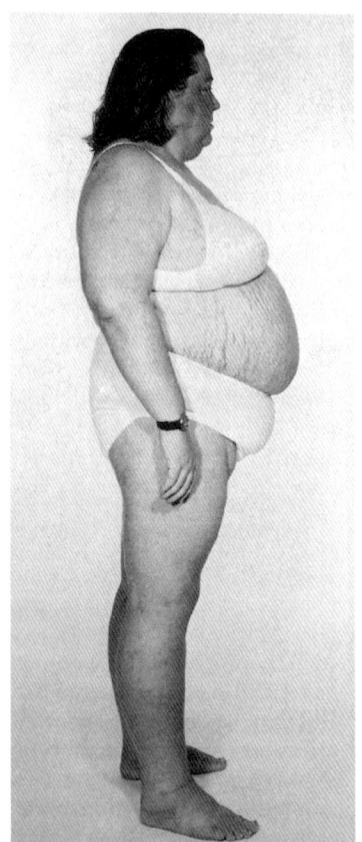
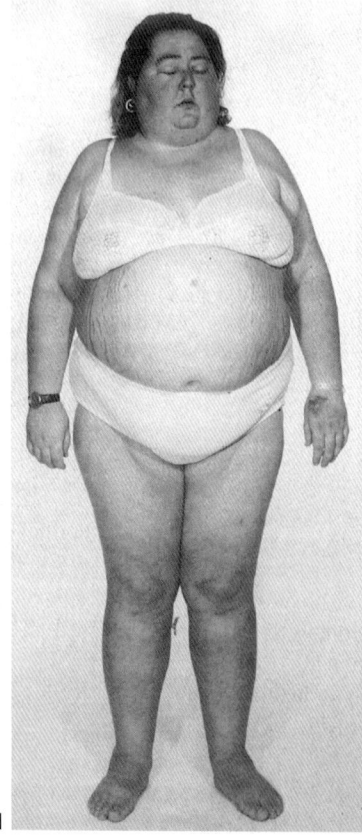

Figure 3.31
Patient with Cushing's disease, (a) 2 years before presentation and (b–d) at presentation.

analog. The availability of effective medical therapy is likely to result in a reduction in the use of post-operative radiotherapy. Medical treatment may offer genuine options as primary therapy in some patients with large tumors and in the patients for whom surgery is not an option. It should, however, be remembered that medical therapy does not offer curative treatment and that the long-term effects of these drugs are unknown. For these reasons, definitive treatment with surgery should always be offered as the treatment of choice to patients with potentially resectable tumors, unless there are clear contraindications.

Cushing's syndrome

The investigation and management of Cushing's syndrome is one of the most challenging areas of endocrinology. Harvey Cushing first described the chromophobe pituitary adenoma as being the underlying cause of some cases of the condition[203] thereafter

Central distribution of body fat, with correspondingly thin arms and legs	90%
Plethoric, rounded face	90%
'Buffalo' hump (cervical fat pad)	50%
Thin skin	76%
Bruising	66%
Poor wound healing, scarring	42%
Livid, purple/red striae	57%
Acne	50%
Alopecia	50%
Hirsuties	76%
Proximal myopathy	66%
Edema	56%

Table 3.17
Clinical signs of Cushing's syndrome.

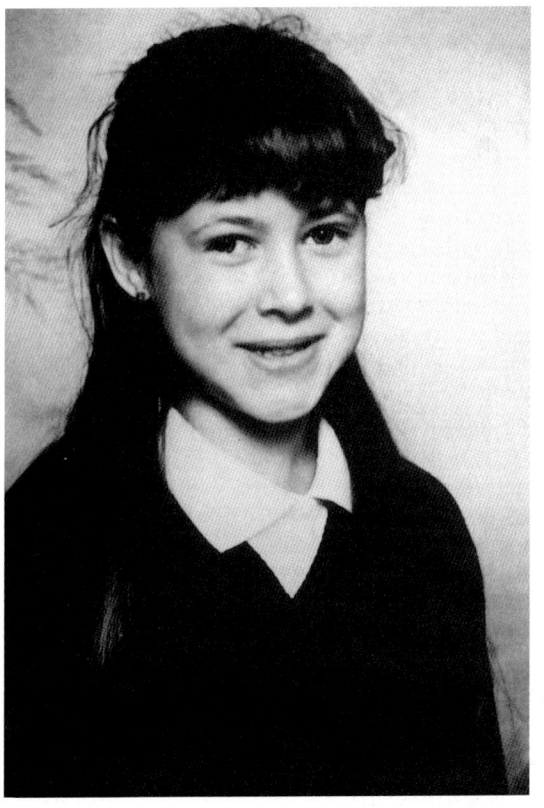
a
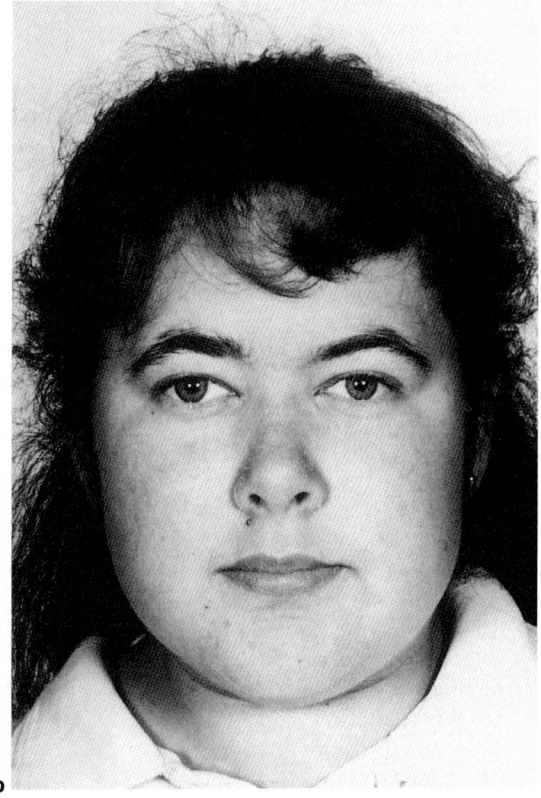
b

Figure 3.32
Teenage patient with Cushing's syndrome secondary to the ectopic production of a CRH-like peptide, (a) 18 months before presentation, and (b) at presentation.

referred to as Cushing's disease. Although florid cases of Cushing's syndrome are easy to diagnose, subtler cases can be extremely difficult. Alcohol abuse, obesity and depression can all give rise to 'pseudo-Cushing's syndrome', which mimics Cushing's syndrome not only clinically, but also, on occasion, biochemically. In addition, some cases of Cushing's syndrome 'cycle' in and out of active disease, with cycles of between a few hours and months.[204,205] Once the diagnosis of Cushing's syndrome has been confirmed, it is necessary to make a specific etiological diagnosis. Although the differentiation of Cushing's syndrome into ACTH-dependent and ACTH-independent disease is straightforward, the identification of the source of ACTH in the former can be very difficult. In addition, very rare Cushing's syndrome secondary to the ectopic expression of various receptors by the adrenal glands have now been recognized.[206–214] Neurosurgery should only be carried out by a dedicated neuroendocrine surgeon. An experienced endocrine surgeon should be available for bilateral adrenalectomy, and there should be ready access to thoracic surgery. The overall management should be coordinated by an endocrinologist.[215]

The clinical features of Cushing's syndrome are well recognized (Figures 3.31 and 3.32) and are summarized in Table 3.17.

Patients most commonly present complaining of rapid weight gain. Growth retardation also occurs in over 80% of children and adolescents.[216] Oligomenorrhea and amenorrhea are common associated presentations in women.[217] Some patients complain of weakness, particularly if their work involves a great deal of physical activity. Recurrent infections are occasionally a presenting problem. The majority of patients will have some form of

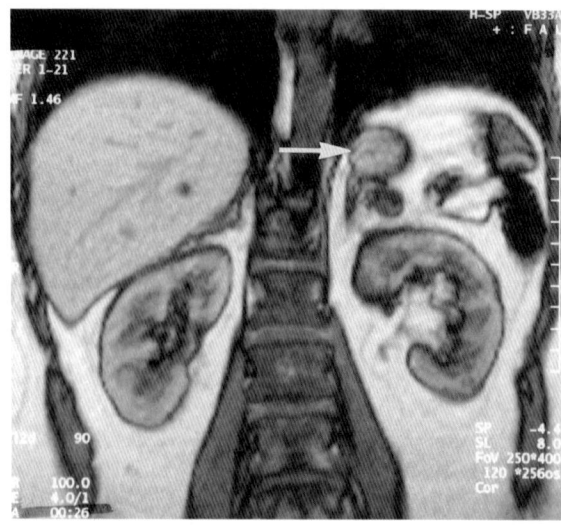

Figure 3.33
Coronal abdominal MRI scan (T1 weighted) of a patient with ACTH-dependent Cushing's syndrome, demonstrating significant retroperitoneal fat and an enlarged nodular left adrenal gland (arrow).

psychological disturbance, ranging from mild symptoms to a severe psychosis (see below).

Patients characteristically have a rounded, plethoric face. There is typically a central distribution of body fat, with contrastingly thin arms and legs, although children tend to have generalized obesity. The skin is thin compared with an individual of comparable age and sex. Bruising is frequently present. Striae, typically violaceous or red, occur most commonly around the axillae and abdomen, but can also occur in the lumbar or gluteal regions, around the thighs, upper arms and breasts. Acne frequently occurs and may be associated with hirsuties and alopecia. Acanthosis nigricans may be present, indicative of hyperinsulinemia. Viral warts, oral candidiasis and cutaneous fungal infections may be present, reflecting immunosuppression. Proximal myopathy should always be sought, and is best assessed by asking the patient to rise from a squat without using a support, with the back kept straight.

Cushing's syndrome has a severe morbidity (Table 3.18) and is associated with a significant mortality, most deaths being from cardiovascular disease, infections or the direct or metastatic effects of the primary tumor. The acquisition of body fat can be rapid, occurring predominantly in the abdomen, both subcutaneously and also intra-abdominally. Intra-abdominal fat is particularly distributed around the viscera and can be clearly demon-

---

Infection
Poor wound healing
Hypertension
Diabetes mellitus
Deep venous thrombosis/pulmonary embolism
Ischemic heart disease
Oligomenorrhea/amenorrhea
Myopathy
Osteoporosis
Glaucoma
Psychiatric

Table 3.18
Clinical associations with Cushing's syndrome.

strated on CT or MRI scans (Figure 3.33). Osteoporosis can be extremely rapid in onset, with serious sequelae. Proximal myopathy can be profound and extremely debilitating. Patients are at increased risk of venous thrombosis and pulmonary embolism, and in consequence it is recommended that patients with uncontrolled disease should receive appropriate thromboembolic prophylaxis.[218,219]

Psychiatric complications occur in more than 60% of patients with Cushing's syndrome, most commonly depression.[220] This can be very severe and may be the presenting symptom. There may be difficulties in differentiating pseudo-Cushing's syndrome secondary to depression from Cushing's syndrome with associated depression. Occasionally, patients may develop psychotic symptoms. Less severe symptoms may also occur, including fatigue, irritability, poor concentration, insomnia, and loss of libido. In particular, many patients have difficulty with work due to tiredness and inability to concentrate. It is essential that all patients with Cushing's syndrome undergo a formal psychiatric assessment both at presentation and following their treatment. It is important to realize that the psychiatric component of the disease is often extremely severe and may take many months to remit following curative treatment. Indeed, patients may actually feel worse rather than better for a prolonged period of time. It is most important that patients are warned of this before treatment is undertaken.

ACTH-dependent	
Corticotroph adenoma (Cushing's disease)	70%
Ectopic ACTH production	10%
ACTH-independent	
Adrenal adenoma	10%
Adrenal carcinoma	5%
Nodular adrenal hyperplasia	5%
Primary pigmented nodular adrenal disease	
Massive macronodular adrenal hyperplasia	
Ectopic receptor expression	

Table 3.19
Causes of Cushing's syndrome.

Causes of Cushing's syndrome

Cushing's syndrome is ACTH dependent in about 85% of cases. About 80% of these cases are caused by a corticotroph adenoma of the pituitary gland (Cushing's disease), the remainder being caused by ectopic ACTH production. Primary adrenal disease accounts for about 20% of cases of Cushing's syndrome[221] (Table 3.19).

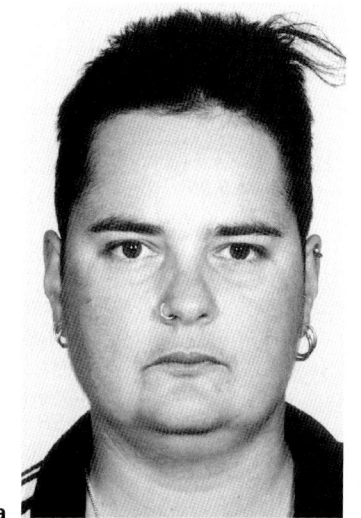 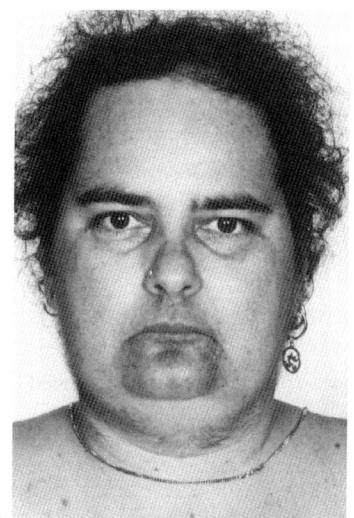 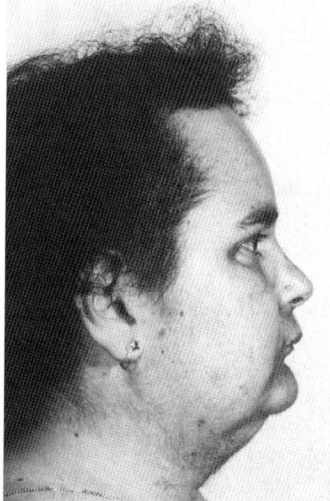

Figure 3.33
Nelson's syndrome: (a) patient at presentation with a recurrent corticotroph adenoma; (b) 2 years later following bilateral adrenalectomy. This patient originally presented with a silent corticotroph adenoma. The patient ultimately died from a pituitary carcinoma.

Cushing's disease

Cushing's disease is very rare, with an estimated prevalence of 10 per million population. It is 4–6 times more common in females.[222] The majority of corticotroph adenomas are microadenomas. Crooke's hyaline change due to corticotroph suppression may be present in surrounding normal corticotrophs and also occasionally within tumor cells themselves.[223] Macroadenomas are often aggressive in their behavior.[224] This is particularly the case for the so-called 'silent' corticotroph adenomas.[102,103,225] These tumors present as clinically non-functioning pituitary adenomas, often with mass effects. Immunostaining of the tumor is positive for ACTH. The tumors tend to be recurrent, increasingly aggressive with their growth characteristics, and associated with increasingly severe clinical disease. Tumors may become frankly malignant. Genetic analysis of one of these tumors has been reported to demonstrate increasing allelic loss with time, presumably representing tumor dedifferentiation.[103,225]

Nelson's syndrome describes the rapid growth of a corticotroph adenoma following medical or surgical adrenalectomy. The reported incidence varies between 40% and 80% over long-term follow-up. This is associated with a rapid increase in serum ACTH levels, manifest by increasing skin pigmentation[226] (Figure 3.34). Nelson's tumors can be highly aggressive, and occasionally can become resistant to treatment. Nelson's syndrome is rarely seen presenting de novo, as bilateral adrenalectomy is now only occasionally performed in patients with Cushing's disease. There is no doubt that pituitary irradiation following bilateral adrenalectomy is the best way of avoiding Nelson's syndrome.[227] Corticotroph hyperplasia rather than adenoma is occasionally seen. Histologically, the differentiation from an adenoma can be difficult to make. The presence of hyperplasia should always raise the possibility of an ectopic source of CRH (see below).[228,229]

Ectopic hormone production

Cushing's syndrome secondary to ectopic production of ACTH is most commonly due to a bronchial or thymic carcinoid tumor.[230–232] These tumors are typically slow-growing and are often difficult to localize. In contrast to Cushing's disease, ectopic ACTH syndrome occurs more commonly in males. Apart from rare cases of Cushing's disease, ectopic ACTH production is often associated with hypokalemic alkalosis. This is a useful diagnostic indicator of ectopic ACTH production.[233,234] Processsing of propiomelanocortin (POMC) is often abnormal, resulting in high circulating levels of ACTH precursors (Figure 3.35).[235,236] Other rare causes include medullary cell carcinoma of the thyroid, pheochromocytoma, paraganglioma, pancreatic islet cell tumors, and malignant gonadal and prostatic disease.[234,237] Ectopic ACTH production by small cell carcinoma of the bronchus is rarely associated with the development of Cushing's syndrome. This is a highly aggressive condition and is usually rapidly fatal. Patients characteristically develop a profound wasting illness, with pigmentation and hypokalemic alkalosis.[234]

Ectopic production of CRH has also been described.[228,229,237] This is very rare, but it is important to recognize. Ectopic production of CRH may produce

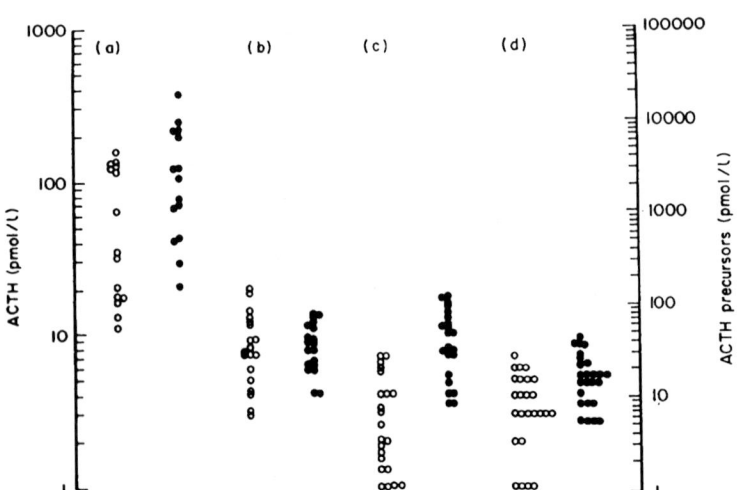

Figure 3.35
ACTH (o), and ACTH precursors (•) plotted on a logarithmic scale in: (a) ectopic ACTH syndrome; (b) Cushing's disease; (c) small cell lung cancer patients; (d) controls. (From Stewart PM, Gibson S, Crosby SR et al. ACTH precursors characterize the ectopic ACTH syndrome. Clin Endocrinol 1994; **40**: 199–204, with permission.)

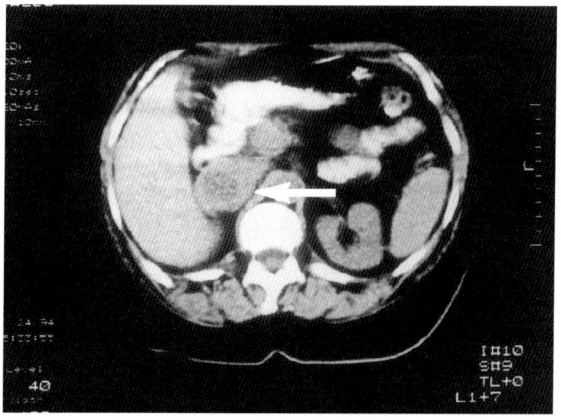

Figure 3.36
CT scan demonstrating an adrenal tumor (arrow) in a patient with pheochromocytoma.

false localization with inferior petrosal sinus sampling (IPSS).[238]

Adrenal disease

Adrenal adenomas account for about 60% of cases of ACTH-independent Cushing's syndrome. The majority of the remainder are accounted for by adrenal carcinomas.[239] Tumors range in size from about 1 cm to 7 cm,[240] overlapping in size with 'non-functioning' adrenal adenomas (see below). These patients often present with a relatively prolonged history, sometimes over a few years. This is in contrast to adrenal carcinomas. These tumors tend to be larger at presentation, often >6 cm. The patients may have typical symptoms of malignant disease, either from the local effects of the tumor or from metastatic disease. The patients may have a short history of rapid onset of Cushing's syndrome, or present with a wasting disease, similar to ACTH-producing small cell carcinoma of the lung. The tumors often produce high levels of steroid precursors, resulting in virilization of females, hypertension, and hypokalemic alkalosis.[241]

Patients are now being identified with incidental adrenal tumors on CT or MRI scanning of the abdomen. Some of these tumors may be functioning, but the majority of them are found to be non-functioning. Metastatic tumor spread to the adrenal gland is an important differential diagnosis of an adrenal mass. Such tumors have been found in up to 4% of abdominal imaging examinations, with an even higher incidence at autopsy. A proportion of clinically non-functioning adrenal adenomas do have autonomous adrenal function, as demonstrated by elevated urinary free cortisol measurement or lack of cortisol suppression by dexamethasone, hyperaldosteronism or medullary hyperfunction (see below).[242,243] Some of these patients may develop clinical features of Cushing's syndrome. It is important that any patient found to have an incidental adrenal mass on abdominal imaging is investigated (Figure 3.36). Any tumor greater than 6 cm in diameter should be removed. A recent study has indicated that mass size of 3 cm or more at diagnosis and exclusive radiocholesterol uptake indicate higher risk of hyperfunction.[244] Tumors can be managed conservatively with periodic observation, once significant underlying pathology has been excluded (Figure 3.37).

Nodular adrenal disease

Primary pigmented nodular adrenal disease

Patients with primary pigmented nodular adrenal disease (PPNAD) present at a younger age than patients with other causes of Cushing's syndrome. The disease ranges from subclinical or mild to severe. About 50% of patients have autosomal dominant disease, as described by Carney and co-workers.[245,246] This is a heterogeneous condition, typically consisting of pigmented/blue naevi and lentigines, in association with a number of different tumors, such as cutaneous myxomas, cardiac myxomas, breast tumors, testicular tumors and peripheral nerve lesions. Imaging of the

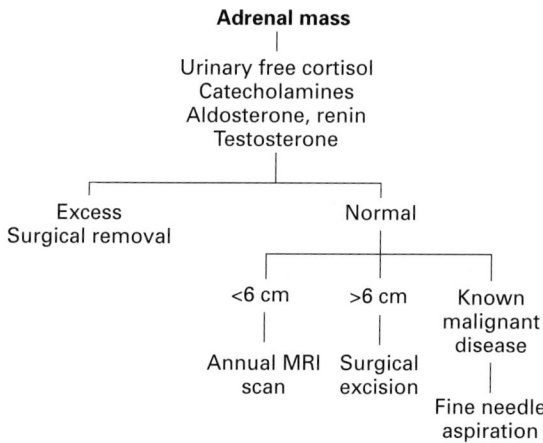

Figure 3.37
Algorithm for the assessment of incidentally identified adrenal tumors.

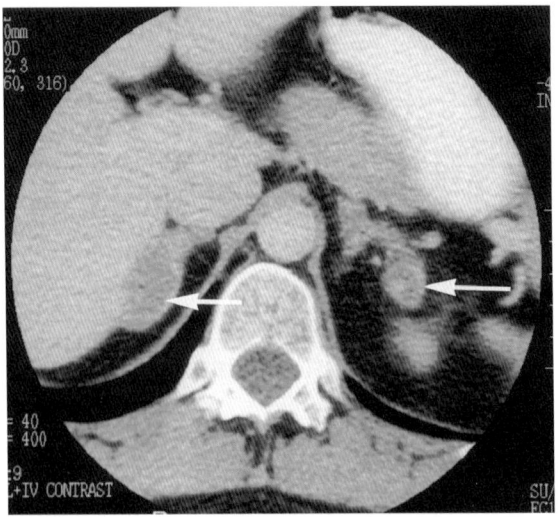

Figure 3.38
Axial CT scan of abdomen of a patient with ACTH-dependent Cushing's syndrome, demonstrating bilateral macronodular adrenal hyperplasia (arrows) together with significant retroperitoneal fat.

adrenal glands can be variable, ranging from apparent normality, to bilateral enlargement or asymmetric nodularity. Pathological examination reveals small, unencapsulated, pigmented adrenal nodules, ranging from 1 cm upwards. There is atrophy of surrounding adrenal tissue, unlike in macronodular adrenal hyperplasia (MAH).

Macronodular adrenal hyperplasia

MAH describes a radiological appearance, rather than a distinct disease entity. The adrenal glands exhibit nodules varying in size from 0.5 to 7 cm. Unlike PPNAD, there is hyperplastic adrenal tissue between the nodules. It is not uncommonly seen in patients with Cushing's syndrome and can give rise to diagnostic confusion. Investigations may demonstrate biochemical evidence of ACTH-dependent disease or adrenal autonomy. Between 20% and 40% of patients with Cushing's disease develop adrenal nodular disease (Figure 3.38). It is likely that some patients with Cushing's disease develop a degree of secondary adrenal autonomy.[247] Occasionally, there may be massive MAH, with both adrenal glands being over 10 times their normal weight. In this situation, adrenal function is ACTH independent.[248]

McCune–Albright syndrome

This is a sporadic condition and is an example of a 'multiple endocrinopathy' syndrome. Patients have been shown to have widespread tissue expression of the *gsp* oncogene, which presumably arises early on in somatic development. The syndrome includes polyostic fibrous dysplasia of bones, pigmented skin lesions,

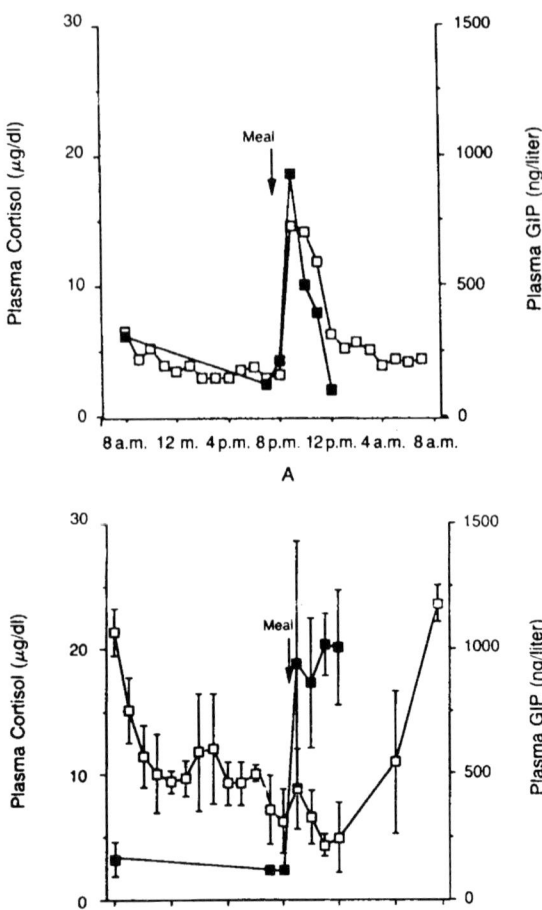

Figure 3.39
*The 24-h profile of plasma cortisol (□) and GIP (■) concentrations in a patient with food-induced Cushing's syndrome (A) and three normal men (B). (From Reznic Y, Allali-Zerah V, Chayvialle JA et al. Food-dependent Cushing's syndrome mediated by aberrant adrenal sensitivity to gastric inhibitory polypeptide. N Engl J Med 1992; **327**: 981–6, with permission.)*

precocious puberty, autonomous functioning thyroid nodules, pituitary somatotroph adenomas and adrenal disease which may be associated with hypercortisolemia. Patients tend to present early on in childhood.

Ectopic adrenal receptor expression
Recently, some cases of Cushing's syndrome have been shown to be associated with ectopic adrenal receptor expression.

Lacroix and Reznik and their respective colleagues both described food-dependent Cushing's syndrome secondary to adrenal expression of gastric inhibitory polypeptide (GIP).[206,207] Their patients only developed biochemical evidence of Cushing's syndrome following

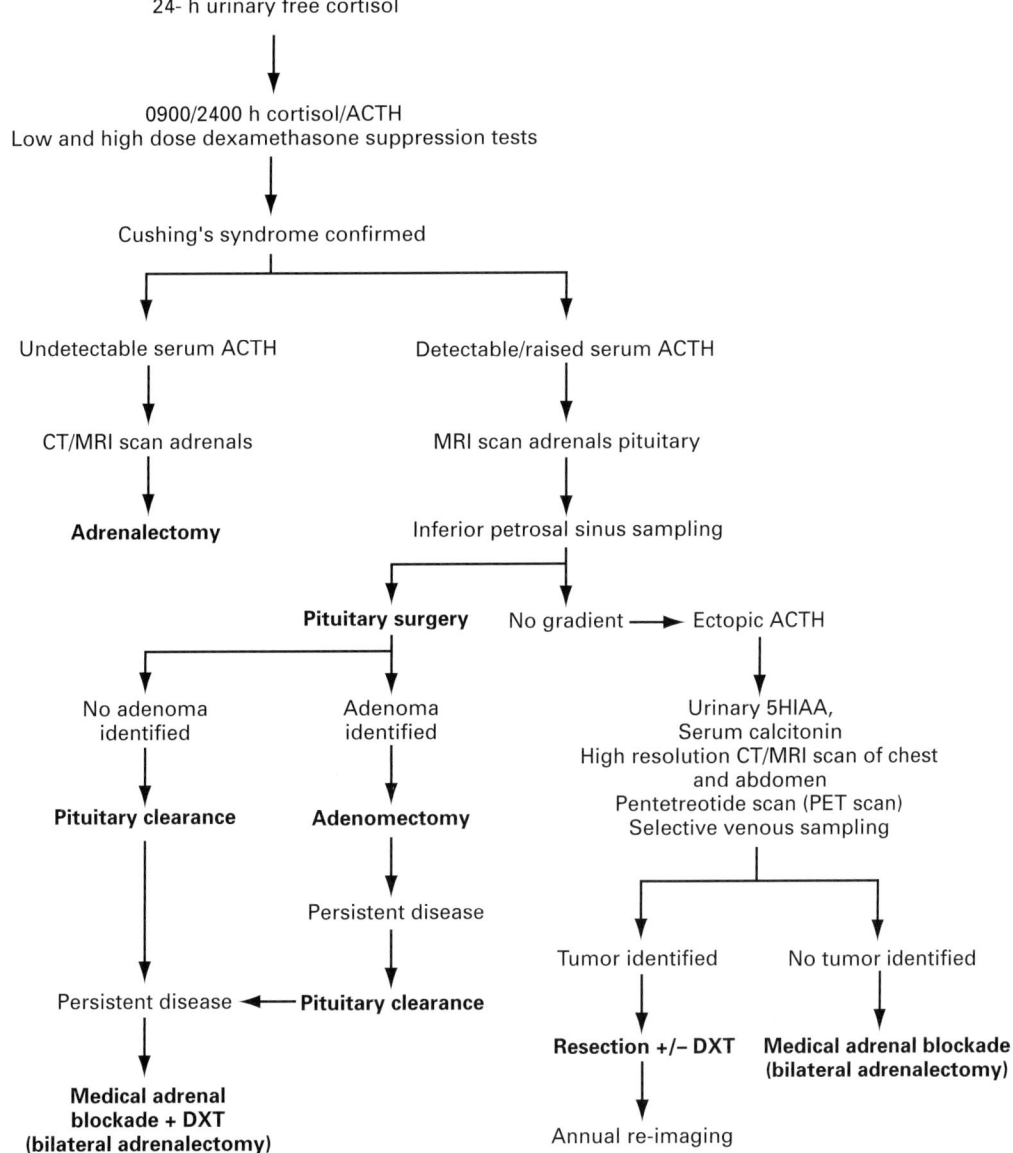

Figure 3.40
Algorithm for the investigation and management of Cushing's syndrome.

a meal (Figure 3.39). These patients and others subsequently identified had MAH.[208] Other patients have been found to have solitary adrenal adenomas.[208,209] One study confirmed that ectopic expression of GIP receptors is the main cause of food-dependent Cushing's syndrome.[210] Similarly, ectopic expression of β-adrenoreceptors, V_1-vasopressin receptors, interleukin-1 receptors and LH receptors, has also been described in association with adrenal disease.[211–214] As more examples of ectopic receptor expression are described, it seems likely that such associations with Cushing's syndrome will be found to be less uncommon than initially thought.

The identification of an adrenal adenoma or of nodular adrenal disease in a patient with Cushing's syndrome does not necessarily denote a primary adrenal cause. The serum ACTH level is of critical importance in the diagnosis (see below). A number of patients with Cushing's disease will have associated 'non-functioning' adrenal adenomas. Patients with ACTH-dependent MAH may have a unilateral dominant nodule on imaging. It is most important that a decision on treatment is only undertaken after a full biochemical evaluation.

Investigation of suspected Cushing's syndrome (Figure 3.40)

A detailed history of alcohol consumption and psychiatric symptomatology and illness needs to be taken.

A useful screen in the clinic is a 24-h urinary free cortisol (UFC) measurement.[247] Two collections should be taken to allow for incomplete samples. UFC excretion on overnight urinary sampling has recently been described, and is more convenient to collect than a 24-h sample.[249] This test will effectively exclude normal patients, with the exception of patients who are in the quiescent phase of cycling. If cyclical Cushing's syndrome is suspected, patients should carry out repeat urine collections at periodic intervals. Cycles may vary from days to months. Rarely, patients may actually cycle between hypercortisolemia and hypocortisolemia.[204,205] It is important to note that UFC measurements may be misleading in patients with renal impairment.[250] Loss of diurnal variation in serum cortisol and ACTH levels are pathognomonic in Cushing's syndrome, although this can also occur in pseudo-Cushing's states.[247] It has been reported that all patients with Cushing's syndrome will have a sleeping midnight serum cortisol level of >50 nmol/l (>1.8 μg/dL).[251] Although this is a useful measurement to make, it should be done while the patient is sleeping and hence can only be done as part of an inpatient assessment. In contrast, salivary late-night cortisol measurement can be carried out as an outpatient procedure, with a reported sensitivity of 92%, rising to 100% if combined with UFC measurement.[252]

Glucocorticoid suppressibility by dexamethasone is frequently used for screening. The original tests described by Liddle used 24-h urinary 17-hydroxycorticosteroids to assess the suppressibility of cortisol production.[253] Dexamethasone suppression tests are now more usually carried out using measurement of serum cortisol. The overnight 1-mg dexamethasone suppression test is a simpler test to perform than the low-dose (0.5 mg dexamethasone, starting at 0900 hours, and thereafter precisely 6-hourly for a total of eight doses) dexamethasone suppression test. Under normal circumstances, serum cortisol at 0900 hours the following day should be <50 nmol/l (<1.8 μg/dL). Both tests have a high sensitivity, approaching 100%. The overnight test, however, has a slightly reduced specificity of 80–90%, compared to reported values of 97–100% for the 48-h test.[254] There are, however, situations where dexamethasone suppression tests may be misleading. Dexamethasone metabolism is enhanced by certain drugs such as phenytoin, rifampicin and phenobarbitone. Estrogens and estrogen analogs such as tamoxifen may cause false-positive results due to increased concentrations of corticosteroid-binding globulin. Pseudo-Cushing's syndrome, associated with excessive alcohol consumption and/or depression, may result in the failure of dexamethasone suppression. Occasionally, it can be difficult to exclude Cushing's syndrome in such patients, particularly as more than 50% of patients with Cushing's syndrome have associated psychiatric features.[220] The ITT is a useful test in this situation, as most patients with pseudo-Cushing's syndrome secondary to depression will show a normal cortisol response, whereas patients with Cushing's syndrome have a flat cortisol response.[255] The abnormal biochemistry associated with alcohol-induced pseudo-Cushing's syndrome is usually reversed following a few days of abstinence in hospital. Stress may also produce failure of dexamethasone suppression and should be interpreted with caution in patients with serious concomitant illnesses. Patients with chronic renal failure may also give false-positive results with dexamethasone testing.

CUSHING'S SYNDROME

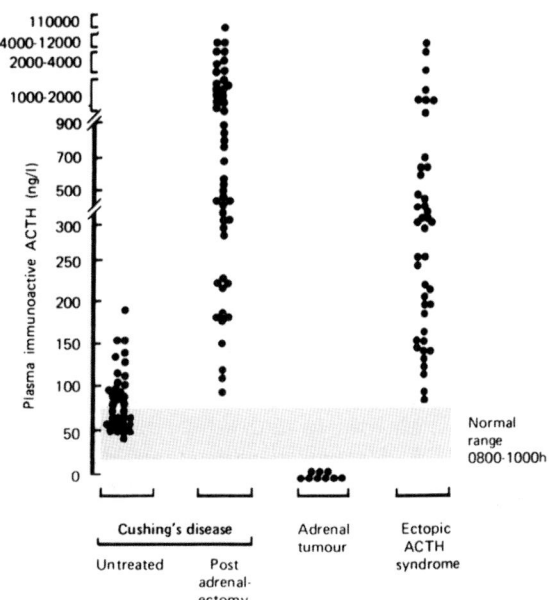

Figure 3.41
Serum ACTH levels in patients with Cushing's syndrome. (From Drury PL, Besser GM. Adrenal cortex. In: Hall R, Besser M, eds. Fundamentals of Clinical Endocrinology, Harcourt Publishers Ltd, 1989; 153–84, with permission.)

The differential diagnosis of Cushing's syndrome

The first determination to be made is whether or not the patient has ACTH-dependent disease. Patients with primary adrenal disease will have suppressed 0900 hours serum ACTH levels, in contrast to patients with ACTH-dependent disease (Figure 3.41). Patients with suppressed serum ACTH levels should proceed directly to adrenal imaging and, if an adrenal tumor is identifiable, to surgery. Patients with ACTH-dependent disease require further investigations. The high-dose (2 mg dexamethasone, starting at 0900 hours, and thereafter precisely 6-hourly, for a total of eight doses) dexamethasone suppression test is used to differentiate Cushing's disease from ectopic ACTH production. In practice, the results of dexamethasone suppression testing can be misleading. In Cushing's disease, the 0900 hours serum cortisol following the last dose of dexamethasone should be suppressed to <50% of baseline values. Dexamethasone suppressibility should be absent in patients with ectopic ACTH

		ACTH (ng/l)	
CRH	Peripheral	LIPS	RIPS
Baseline	64	78	356
CRH + 5'	85	110	482
CRH + 10'	96	260	595

The test demonstrates elevated basal serum ACTH levels, which clearly rise following CRH. In addition, there is a central-to-peripheral gradient, with lateralization to the RIPS. This patient was found to have a right-sided corticotroph adenoma. False lateralization can, however, occur, due to anomalous venous drainage from the contralateral side.[263] LIPS, left inferior petrosal sinus; RIPS, right inferior petrosal sinus.

Table 3.20
Inferior petrosal sinus sampling with CRH (100 μg IV)

production. This test has a sensitivity and a specificity of around 90%.[247] Similar results can be obtained using an overnight 8-mg dexamethasone suppression test[256] or a 7-h intravenous dexamethasone suppression test.[257]

The CRH test (100 μg intravenous CRH; serum cortisol and ACTH at 0 min, 30 min, 60 min, 90 min, 120 min) is a useful, well-validated adjunct in the investigation of Cushing's syndrome. Both ovine and human CRH are available. The response to ovine CRH may be slightly greater, due to its longer half-life. Typically, patients with Cushing's disease demonstrate clear rises in cortisol (peak >800 nmol/l (>30 μg/dL)) of >20% and in ACTH of >35% over basal values, giving sensitivities and specificities of around 90%.[247] Combined testing with high-dose dexamethasone and CRH improves the diagnostic accuracy of the investigation.[247] The conventional CRH test has, however, been superseded by IPSS with CRH.[258] This test is quick and easy to perform in centers having the appropriate expertise and radiological facilities. It must now be regarded as the 'gold standard' test in the investigation of ACTH-dependent Cushing's syndrome. It has a sensitivity and specificity of almost 100%. Anomalous results can rarely be obtained in cases of ectopic CRH production,[238,259] in the early presentation of Cushing's disease, and in patients with hypoplastic or plexiform inferior petrosal sinuses.[260] A central-to-peripheral ACTH gradient of >2, or an ACTH rise of >300% over peripheral ACTH values following CRH, is diagnostic of Cushing's disease (Table 3.20). Lateralization can be misleading, as 40% of pituitaries have venous drainage to the contralateral side. A recent study found that IPSS with CRH had a sensitivity of 83% in correctly lateralizing the pituitary adenoma, compared with a sensitivity of 72% for MRI scanning.[261] It has been suggested that direct cavernous sinus sampling is superior to IPSS for predicting intrapituitary tumor lateralization.[262] Lateralization is unreliable in patients who have had previous pituitary surgery. If lateralization is required in patients undergoing IPSS, venous angiography should be performed to exclude anomalous venous drainage.[263]

Patients with Cushing's disease frequently demonstrate ACTH and cortisol responses to desmopressin, but responses can be variable and the test is unlikely to add much useful information.[264] Patients with ectopic production of ACTH often process proopiomelanocortin (POMC) abnormally. The measurement of serum ACTH precursors can help in the diagnosis of ectopic ACTH production.[235,236]

Imaging

The majority of corticotroph adenomas are microadenomas.[223] Apparently non-functioning microadenomas have been reported in 30% of pituitaries from an unselected population at autopsy.[111] A pituitary abnormality demonstrated on MRI scanning in a patient with Cushing's syndrome cannot, therefore, be inferred to be a corticotroph adenoma. For this reason it is recommended that, as a routine, all patients, apart from those with pituitary macroadenomas, should undergo IPSS with CRH.

Adrenal CT or MRI scanning can be misleading. Patients with ACTH-dependent disease generally demonstrate adrenal hyperplasia, although the adrenal glands may appear to be normal. Nodular adrenal hyperplasia may be seen in more than 20% of patients with Cushing's disease (see above). This may cause diagnostic confusion. The serum ACTH level is essential to avoid the misdiagnosis of primary pituitary disease. Incidental adrenal adenomas have been reported to be present in up to 5% of autopsies. Although these adenomas are said to be non-functioning, subtle abnormalities in adrenal function can often be demonstrated (see above).[242,243]

Patients who have ACTH-dependent disease should undergo MRI scanning of the pituitary. Less than 50% of corticotroph adenomas will be visualized with CT scanning,[265] whereas 50–75% will be visible on MRI scanning.[265–267] Scanning should be carried out both pre- and post-gadolinium.

Patients who have biochemical evidence of ectopic ACTH production should be screened for medullary carcinoma of the thyroid, pheochromocytoma, islet cell tumors and carcinoid tumors.[237] The majority of patients will have a small thymic or bronchial carcinoid tumor, often <1 cm in diameter. Remnant thymic tissue may cause diagnostic confusion.[268] These tumors are notoriously difficult to localize. Spiral CT or MRI are the best imaging modalities. Selective venous sampling for ACTH is frequently carried out in difficult cases, but is often uninformative.[234] The majority of carcinoid tumors express somatostatin receptors 2 and 5. Indium-labeled octreotide has been used for tumor localization (Figure 3.42). In most cases, however, this does not offer any advantages over conventional imaging.[269,270] Positron emission tomography (PET) can be a useful additional localizing tool in some patients.

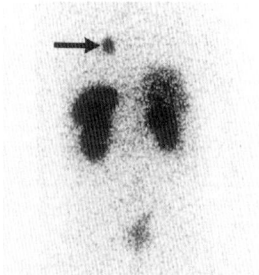

Figure 3.42
^{111}In-pentetreotide scan, demonstrating a bronchial carcinoid tumor in a patient with ectopic ACTH production.

Treatment of Cushing's syndrome

Medical treatment
Medical therapy may be used preoperatively to control disease activity and hence metabolic control. Although there is no evidence that medical pretreatment improves wound healing or reduces infection, it may reduce the postoperative symptoms which almost always accompany the reduction in circulating cortisol levels following successful surgery. Many centers empirically treat patients preoperatively for about 6 weeks. Medical therapy should be given to patients with persisting disease following surgery and/or radiotherapy. Patients with an unidentified source of ectopic

ACTH production should also be treated medically. Efficacy of adrenal blockade is usually assessed by 24-h UFC estimations. Some centers prefer to monitor therapy by taking a mean of a number of serum cortisol measurements through the day, aiming for a value of 150–300 nmol/l.[239]

Metyrapone blocks cortisol production by inhibiting 11-β-hydroxylase, with a consequent rise in serum 11-deoxycortisol levels. This cross-reacts with some cortisol assays and hence may lead to the erroneous impression that cortisol production is not fully blocked. Although serum ACTH levels rise, the block is not overcome.[239] Metyrapone acts rapidly to reduce cortisol levels within 2 h and needs to be given 6–8-hourly with food. Patients should start on 250 mg 8-hourly, increasing as necessary to achieve full blockade. Some patients may need up to 6000 mg daily. It should always be given together with dexamethasone 0.5 mg replacement. The major side-effects are nausea, acne and hirsuties.

Ketoconazole is an imidazole which was originally developed as an antifungal agent. It is, however, also a potent inhibitor at several levels of adrenal steroidogenesis, with its most important action being the 20–22 desmolase step, which catalyzes the conversion of cholesterol to pregnenolone. As a result, the accumulation of androgenic steroid metabolites is avoided.[239] The corollary of this is that ketoconazole is potentially teratogenic to male fetuses. It has a slower onset and a more prolonged duration of action than metyrapone, with the result that it is usually easier to stabilize adrenal blockade, often without the need for concomitant dexamethasone replacement. It may take several weeks for the full effects of ketoconazole to be seen. The most worrying side-effect is hepatotoxicity. Biochemical evidence of abnormal liver function occurs in about 10% of patients and is usually reversible. Clinical evidence of hepatotoxicity is much rarer, but fatalities have been documented.[239] Liver function should be routinely monitored and the drug should be stopped if abnormalities develop. Some patients develop gastrointestinal disturbances with high doses. The absorption of ketoconazole is impaired in the presence of achlorhydria or antacid treatment. Patients should be started on 200 mg daily and the dose adjusted up to 1200 mg daily if necessary, to achieve normal 24-hour UFC excretion.

Aminoglutethimide is a third-line drug after metyrapone and ketoconazole. It inhibits the conversion of cholesterol to pregnenolone, resulting in the inhibition of mineralocorticoid, glucocorticoid and sex hormone production.[239] Skin rashes, sometimes accompanied by fever, are a common side-effect, but will frequently resolve with continuation of the drug. Drowsiness and lethargy are common in the first few weeks of treatment. Gastrointestinal effects occasionally occur. Hypothyroidism due to inhibition of iodine uptake by the thyroid gland and hematological abnormalities occur rarely. Its use should be reserved for patients who cannot be controlled using other agents. Patients should be started on 250 mg daily increasing the dose on a weekly basis until 24-h UFC excretion is normalized.

Mitotane (o,p'-DDD) is useful in the management of Cushing's syndrome[271] and, in particular, adrenal carcinoma.[272] It blocks adrenal cortisol production and, in addition, has a direct cortical adrenolytic action. It has a slow onset of action over several weeks, and similarly has a prolonged action due to its accumulation in adipose tissue. Mitotane increases dexamethasone metabolism. Accordingly, patients taking dexamethasone replacement therapy need to be closely monitored for adrenal insufficiency and the dose of dexamethasone increased as appropriate. Mitotane treatment may be associated with an increase in low-density lipoprotein (LDL) serum cholesterol, as a result of increased HMG-CoA reductase activity. An HMG-CoA reductase inhibitor may be added to the treatment regimen if necessary.[273] Patients with Cushing's syndrome are usually managed with doses up to 4 g/day. Larger doses, up to 12 g/day, may be required for adrenocortical carcinomas, with the attendant development of gastrointestinal (nausea, vomiting, diarrhea) and neurological (weakness, neuropathy) side-effects. It is suggested that low-dose mitotane therapy should be started as adjuvant therapy in all patients with adrenocortical carcinoma following adrenalectomy.[274]

Some patients cannot be controlled using a single agent. Side-effects are frequent with high doses of any of these drugs. In such situations, patients can often be controlled using a combination of drugs at lower doses.

Other preparations that are occasionally useful in individual cases include the glucocorticoid receptor antagonist mifepristone[275] and centrally acting drugs such as sodium valproate, cyproheptadine and dopamine agonists.[276] In emergency situations where oral therapy is not possible, control may be obtained using intravenous etomidate.[277]

Perioperative treatment

All patients with Cushing's syndrome require glucocorticoid cover for surgery. Patients should receive higher doses of glucocorticoids than that recommended for other pituitary patients (see above).

Cushing's disease

The treatment of choice is transsphenoidal surgery. More than 90% of patients with a microadenoma can expect to experience remission after surgery by an experienced operator.[278,279] Macroadenomas, in contrast, have lower overall remission rates of around 60%.[279] Similar results have been obtained for children and adolescents.[280] Failure of surgery at the first attempt may be followed by a repeat procedure with a success rate of about 50%.[281] An important but rare cause of failed surgery is the extrasellar location of a microadenoma. This possibility should always be considered in patients who have negative pituitary MR imaging.[282] An undetectable 0900 hour cortisol following surgery is indicative of remission, but not necessarily of long-term cure. A recent report describes recurrent disease in 11.5% of patients during a mean follow-up period of 36.3 months.[283]. This occurs due to suppression of the normal corticotrophs by the tumor. Patients who have detectable 0900 hour cortisols postoperatively require a full assessment. Patients in remission generally require glucocorticoid supplementation for 6–12 months until the hypothalamic–pituitary–adrenal axis has fully recovered. Between 11.5% and 25% of patients can be expected to relapse, mostly within the first 5 years of surgery.[279,280,283–285]

Patients who experience relapse may be offered further surgery, but in any event will also require radiotherapy. Radiotherapy is an effective adjunct for patients who fail to enter remission or who relapse and for patients with Nelson's syndrome. It may also be used as a primary treatment for patients who, for whatever reason, are not candidates for surgery. Data suggest that a final overall remission rate of approximately 70% may be expected.[286] Such patients should be controlled with medical adrenal blockade until they enter remission. Occasionally, patients require bilateral adrenalectomy to achieve control. A small proportion of corticotroph adenomas are highly aggressive[102,103,225] (see above). These patients may initially enter remission following surgery and radiotherapy and then relapse, or control may never be achieved even with medical adrenal blockade. Further radiotherapy may be required, although in this situation, this will only delay inevitable recurrence. If the tumor is close to the optic chiasm, surgical debulking should be carried out to reduce chiasmal irradiation. Stereotactic radiotherapy is preferred, as this will minimize the irradiation of adjacent structures.[19] Control of hypercortisolemia is best achieved in this situation by bilateral adrenalectomy. Clinicians have always been reluctant to resort to this procedure, except in the most extreme situations, because of the high risk of further stimulating tumor growth.[226,227] These patients are, however, at imminent risk of death from hypercortisolemia. Bilateral adrenalectomy is highly effective and provides immediate remission. In these patients, it can be a life-saving procedure. In view of the immediate benefits of bilateral adrenalectomy, this treatment should be considered early on in the management of these patients, rather than waiting until they are in extremis. The overall prognosis for this group of patients, however, is poor, as the pituitary tumor will inevitably recur.

Adrenal tumors

It is essential that a clear diagnosis of adrenal autonomy is made before a patient is referred for surgery (see above). Adrenal tumors are treated by unilateral adrenalectomy. Massive macronodular hyperplasia requires bilateral adrenalectomy. These conditions are cured by surgery. In contrast, adrenal carcinomas have a poor prognosis, with an overall 5-year survival rate of about 30%.[239] Mitotane is effective in controlling cortisol secretion in about 75% of patients, and some patients may demonstrate regression of tumor mass. Residual or recurrent disease following surgery should be treated with radiotherapy to the tumor bed. Recent evidence suggests that in those patients who enter remission following surgery, the prognosis is improved if mitotane treatment is commenced immediately postoperatively.[274] There is no evidence that chemotherapy is of any benefit.

Ectopic ACTH/CRH-producing tumors

These tumors often remain occult, in spite of strenuous efforts at localization (see above). If a tumor has been unequivocally identified, it should be resected. Bronchial carcinoids frequently metastasize to the hilar lymph nodes. The hilar nodes should be examined both macroscopically and microscopically for evidence of involvement. Prophylactic hilar radiotherapy should be considered. In the event that a tumor cannot be identified, medical adrenal blockade should be carried out (see above). Occasionally, patients will respond to treatment with somatostatin analogs.[237] If adrenal function cannot be readily controlled by medical blockade, the patient should undergo bilateral adrenalectomy. Many patients with occult carcinoid tumors can be managed very successfully either medically or following bilateral adrenalectomy. It frequently takes many years for the tumor to become identifiable. Patients should have annual MR imaging. If and when a tumor is localized, the patient should then undergo definitive surgery.

Postoperative management of patients

It is essential that the patient with Cushing's syndrome understands that full recovery will take many months following successful surgery. Patients should be warned that they may, in fact, feel more unwell for a period of time following surgery than beforehand. The psychological effects such as depression, in particular, are frequently more marked postoperatively. Cognitive functioning may take a considerable period of time to return to premorbid levels. This period of time can be extremely difficult for the patient, and it is most important that the clinician provides particular support and reassurance for the patient and their family.

Regardless of the etiology of the Cushing's syndrome, the patient will require glucocorticoid therapy following successful surgery. The hypothalamic–pituitary axis, and the contralateral adrenal gland in the case of an adrenal tumor, take many months to return to normal functioning. Some clinicians elect to place the patient on a normal replacement dose of glucocorticoid immediately following surgery. Patients may benefit from a higher dose of glucocorticoid therapy, e.g. hydrocortisone 20 mg twice daily, or prednisolone 10 mg daily, in the initial weeks following surgery, tailing the dose down to physiological replacement as quickly as the patient is able to tolerate. Dexamethasone, which does not cross-react with cortisol assays, may be used to monitor endogenous cortisol status in patients deemed to be at risk of relapse. It can take a number of months, occasionally more than a year, before the patient is finally able to stop glucocorticoid therapy. The hypothalamic– pituitary–adrenal axis should be assessed after the patient has been able to tolerate a sub-physiological replacement dose of glucocorticoid, e.g. hydrocortisone 5 mg twice daily or prednisolone 2 mg daily. Initially, the patient should demonstrate a normal cortisol response to depot Synacthen. Thereafter, the patient should undergo an ITT or, if this is contraindicated, a glucagon test (see Appendix 1).

GH reserve recovers in a high proportion of patients with Cushing's disease following surgically induced remission. In view of this, it has been suggested that definitive assessment of GH secretory capacity should be delayed for at least 2 years following surgery.[287]

Finally, a note of caution: a recent report gives rise to some concern regarding the long-term prognosis of patients who have undergone surgical cure of Cushing's disease. Such patients have a high prevalence of atherosclerosis together with increased risk factors for cardiovascular disease. It remains to be seen whether or not this translates into increased morbidity and mortality in these patients.[288]

References

1. Saxena KM. Endocrine manifestations of neurofibromatosis in children. *Am J Dis Child* 1970; **120**: 265–72.
2. Hochman HI, Judge DM, Reichlin S. Precocious puberty and hypothalamic hamartoma. *Pediatrics* 1981; **67**: 236–44.
3. Axelrod L. Endocrine dysfunction in patients with tumors of the pineal region. In: Schmidek HH, ed. *Pineal Tumors*, New York: Masson, 1977: 61–77.
4. Asa SL, Scheithauer BW, Bilbao JM et al. A case for hypothalamic acromegaly: a clinicopathological study of six patients with hypothalamic-gangliocytomas producing growth hormone-releasing factor. *J Clin Endocrinol Metab* 1984; **58**: 796–803.
5. Asa SL, Kovacs K, Tindall GT et al. Cushing's disease associated with an intrasellar gangliocytoma producing corticotrophin-releasing factor. *Ann Intern Med* 1984; **101**: 789–93.
6. Bray GA, York DA. Leptin and clinical medicine: a new piece in the puzzle of obesity. *J Clin Endocrinol Metab* 1997, **82**: 2771–6.
7. Plum FC, Uitert RV. Nonendocrine diseases and disorders of the hypothalamus. In: Reichlin S, Baldessarini RJ, Martin JB, eds. *The Hypothalamus*, New York: Raven, 1978; 415–74.
8. Teasdale G. Surgical management of pituitary adenoma. *Neuroendocrinol/Clin Endocrinol Metab* 1983; **12(3)**: 789–823.
9. Thapar K, Kovacs K, Muller PJ. Clinical-pathological correlations of pituitary tumours. *Baillière's Clin Endocrinol Metab* 1995; **9(2)**: 243–70.
10. James RA, Hall K, Crombie A, Kendall-Taylor P. The chiasmal traction syndrome. *J Endocrinol* 1991; **131(suppl)**: 97.
11. Melen O. Neuro-ophthalmological features of pituitary tumors. *Endocrinol Metab Clin North Am* 1987; **16(3)**: 585–608.

12. *Pituitary Tumours. Recommendations for Service Provision and Guidelines for Management of Patients. Consensus Statement of a Working Party from the Royal College of Physicians Committee on Endocrinology and Diabetes Mellitus and the Society for Endocrinology, in conjunction with the Research Unit of the Royal College of Physicians.* London: Royal College of Physicians of London, 1997.
13. Hardy J. Transsphenoidal microsurgery of the normal and pathological pituitary. *Neurosurgery* 1969; **16**: 185–217.
14. Plowman PN. Pituitary adenoma radiotherapy—when, who and how? *Clin Endocrinol* 1999; **51**: 265–71.
15. Jones A. Complications of radiotherapy for acromegaly. In: Wass JAH, ed. *Treating Acromegaly*, Bristol: Society for Endocrinology, 1994; 115–25.
16. Brada M, Rajan B. The toxicity of radiotherapy in the treatment of pituitary adenoma. In: Wass JAH, ed. *Treating Acromegaly*, Bristol: Society for Endocrinology, 1994; 127–32.
17. Fraser R, Doyle GF, Joplin CW et al. The assessment of endocrine effect and the effectiveness of ablative pituitary treatment by ^{90}Y and ^{198}Au implantation. In: Kohler PO, Ross GT, eds. *Pituitary Tumors*, New York: Elsevier, 1973; 35–47.
18. Landolt AM, Haller D, Lomax N et al. Stereotactic radiosurgery for recurrent treated acromegaly: comparison with fractionated radiotherapy. *J Neurosurg* 1998; **88**: 1002–8.
19. Witt TC, Kondziolka D, Flickinger JC, Lunsford LD. Stereotactic radiosurgery for pituitary tumors. *Radiosurgery* 1996; **1**: 55–65.
20. Littley MD, Shalet SM, Beardwell C et al. Hypopituitarism following external radiotherapy for pituitary tumors in adults. *Q J Med* 1989; **70**: 145–60.
21. Feek CM, McLelland J, Seth S et al. How effective is external pituitary irradiation for growth hormone secreting pituitary tumors? *Clin Endocrinol* 1984; **20**: 401–8.
22. Ho KY, Thorner MO. Therapeutic applications of bromocriptine in endocrine and neurologic diseases. *Drugs* 1988; **36**: 67–82.
23. Crosignani PG, Ferrari C. Dopaminergic treatments for hyperprolactinemia. *Clin Obstet Gynaecol* 1990; **4**: 441–55.
24. Molitch ME. Management of prolactinomas. *Annu Rev Med* 1989; **40**: 225–32.
25. Bevan JS, Webster J, Burke CW, Scanlon MF. Dopamine agonists and pituitary tumor shrinkage. *Endocrine Rev* 1992; **13**: 220–40.
26. Chiodini PG, Liuzzi A, Botalla L et al. Stable reduction of plasma growth hormone (hGH) levels during chronic administration of 2-Br-alpha-ergocryptine (CB-154) in acromegalic patients. *J Clin Endocrinol Metab* 1975; **40**: 705–8.
27. Wass JAH, Williams J, Charlesworth M et al. Long-term treatment of acromegaly with bromocriptine. *BMJ* 1977; **1**: 875–8.
28. Nortier JWR, Croughs RJM, Thijssen JHH, Schwartz F. Bromocriptine therapy in acromegaly: effects on plasma GH levels, somatomedin-C levels and clinical activity. *Clin Endocrinol* 1985; **22**: 209–17.
29. Webster J. A comparative review of the tolerability profiles of dopamine agonists in the treatment of hyperprolactinemia and inhibition of lactation. *Drug Safety* 1996; **14(4)**: 228–38.
30. Tsagarakis S, Tsiganou E, Tzavara I et al. Effectiveness of a long-acting injectable form of bromocriptine in patients with prolactin and growth hormone secreting macroadenomas. *Clin Endocrinol* 1995; **42**: 593–9.
31. Rasmussen C, Bergh T, Wide L et al. CV 205–502: a new long-acting drug for inhibition of prolactin hypersecretion. *Clin Endocrinol* 1987; **26**: 321–6.
32. van der Heijden PFM, de Wit W, Brownell J et al. CV205–502, a new dopamine agonist, versus bromocriptine in the treatment of hyperprolactinemia. *Eur J Obstet Gynaecol Reprod Biol* 1991; **40**: 111–18.
33. Webster J, Piscitelli G, Polli A et al. A comparison of cabergoline and bromocriptine in the treatment of hyperprolactinemic amenorrhea. *N Engl J Med* 1994; **331**: 904–9.
34. Colao A, Di Sarno A, Sarnacchiaro F et al. Prolactinomas resistant to standard dopamine agonists respond to chronic cabergoline treatment. *J Clin Endocrinol Metab* 1997; **82**: 876–83.
35. Freda PU, Andreadis CI, Khandji AG et al. Long-term treatment of prolactin-secreting macroadenomas with pergolide. *J Clin Endocrinol Metab* 2000; **85**: 8–13.
36. Stracke H, Heinlein W, Horowski R et al. Dopamine agonists in the treatment of hyperprolactinemia. Comparison between bromocriptine and lisuride. *Arzneimittel Forschung* 1986; **36**: 1834–6.
37. Krupp P, Monka C. Bromocriptine in pregnancy: safety aspects. *Klin Wochenschr* 1987; **65**: 823–7.
38. Lamberts SWJ, Van der Lely A-J, De Herder WW, Hofland LJ. Octreotide. *N Engl J Med* 1996; **334(4)**: 246–54.
39. Hoyer D, Bell GI, Berelowitz M et al. Classification and nomenclature of somatostatin receptors. *Trends Pharmacol Sci* 1995; **16**: 86–8.
40. Law SF, Woulfe D, Reisine T. Somatostatin receptor activation of cellular effector systems. *Cell Signalling* 1995; **7**: 1–8.
41. Berelowitz M. The somatostatin receptor—a window of therapeutic opportunity? *Endocrinology* 1995; **136**: 3695–7.
42. Virgolini I, Pangerl T, Bischof C et al. Somatostatin receptor subtype expression in human tissues: a prediction for diagnosis and treatment of cancer? *Eur J Clin Invest* 1997; **27**: 645–7.

43. Lamberts SWJ, Krenning EP, Reubi JC. The role of somatostatin and its analogs in the diagnosis and treatment of tumors. *Endocrine Rev* 1991; 12: 450–82.
44. Plockinger U, Bader M, Hopfenmuller W et al. Results of somatostatin receptor scintigraphy do not predict pituitary tumor volume- and hormone-response to octreotide therapy and do not correlate with tumor histology. *Eur J Endocrinol* 1997; 136: 369–76.
45. Smith-Jones PM, Bischof C, Leimer M et al. DOTA-lanreotide: a novel somatostatin analog for tumor diagnosis and therapy. *Endocrinology* 1999; 140: 5136–48.
46. Wynick D, Anderson JV, Williams SJ, Bloom SR. Resistance to metastatic pancreatic endocrine tumors after long-term treatment with the somatostatin analog octreotide (SMS 201–995). *Clin Endocrinol* 1989; 30: 385–8.
47. Davies PH, Stewart SE, Lancranjan I et al. Long-term therapy with long-acting octreotide (sandostatin LAR) for the management of acromegaly. *Clin Endocrinol* 1998; 311–6.
48. Caron P, Beckers A, Cullen DR et al. Efficacy of the new long-acting formulation of lanreotide (lanreotide Artogel) in teh management of acromegaly. *J Clin Endocrinol Metab* 2002; 87: 99–104.
49. Morange I, De Boisvilliers F, Chanson P et al. Slow release lanreotide treatment in acromegalic patients previously normalised by octreotide. *J Clin Endocrinol Metab* 1994; 79: 145–51.
50. Giusti M, Gussoni G, Cuttica CM, Giordano G. Effectiveness and tolerability of slow release lanreotide treatment in active acromegaly: six month report on an Italian multicenter study. *J Clin Endocrinol Metab* 1996; 81: 2089–97.
51. Caron P, Morange-Ramos I, Cogne M, Jaquet P. Three year follow-up of acromegalic patients treated with intramuscular slow-release lanreotide. *J Clin Endocrinol Metab* 1997; 82: 18–22.
52. Lancranjan I, Bruns C, Grass P et al. Sandostatin LAR: a promising therapeutic tool in the management of acromegalic patients. *Metabolism* 1996; 45: 67–71.
53. Hurel SJ, Harris PE, McNicol AM et al. Metastatic prolactinoma: effect of octreotide, cabergoline, carboplatin and etoposide; immunocytochemical analysis of protooncogene expression. *J Clin Endocrinol Metab* 1997; 82: 2962–5.
54. Kaltsas GA, Mukherjee JJ, Plowman PN et al. The role of cytotoxic chemotherapy in the management of aggressive and malignant pituitary tumors. *J Clin Endocrinol* 1998; 83: 4233–8.
55. Lee EJ, Anderson LM, Thimmapaya B, Jameson JL. Targeted expression of toxic genes directed by pituitary hormone promoters: a potential strategy for adenovirus-mediated gene therapy of pituitary tumors. *J Clin Endocrinol Metab* 1999; 84: 786–94.
56. Rosen T, Bengtsson B. Premature mortality due to cardiovascular disease in hypopituitarism. *Lancet* 1990; 336: 285–8.
57. Bates AS, Van't Hoff W, Clayton RN. Life expectancy in hypopituitarism. *J Clin Endocrinol Metab* 1996; 81: 1169–72.
58. Bülow B, Hagmar L, Mikoczy Z et al. Increased cerebrovascular mortality in patients with hypopituitarism. *Clin Endocrinol* 1997; 46: 75–81.
59. Tomlinson JW, Holden N, HIlls RK et al. Association between premature mortality and hypopituitarism. *Lancet* 2001; 357: 425–31.
60. Harris PE, Afshar F, Coates P et al. The effects of transsphenoidal surgery on endocrine function and visual fields in patients with functionless pituitary tumors. *Q J Med* 1989; 71(265): 417–27.
61. Yen SSC. Chronic anovulation due to CNS–hypothalamic–pituitary dysfunction. In: Yen SSC, Jaffe RB, eds. *Reproductive Endocrinology: Physiology, Pathophysiology and Clinical Management*, 2nd ed. Philadelphia: WB Saunders, 1986; 500–45.
62. Brandle M, Ammann P, Giaten A et al. Relapsing Whipple's disease presenting with hypopituitarism. *Clin Endocrinol* 1999; 50: 399–403.
63. Wu W, Cogan JD, Pfaffle RW et al. Mutations in PROP1 cause familial combined pituitary hormone deficiency. *Nature Genet* 1998; 18: 147–9.
64. Erturk E, Jaffe CA, Barkan AL. Evaluation of the integrity of the hypothalamic–pituitary adrenal axis by insulin hypoglycemia test. *J Clin Endocrinol Metab* 1998; 83: 2350–4.
65. Mayenknecht J, Diederich S, Bahr V et al. Comparison of low and high dose corticotropin stimulation tests in patients with pituitary disease. *J Clin Endocrinol Metab* 1998; 83: 1558–62.
66. Oelkers W. The role of high- and low-dose corticotropin tests in the diagnosis of secondary adrenal insufficiency. *Eur J Endocrinol* 1998; 139: 567–70.
67. Harris PE, Kendall-Taylor P. Steroid therapy and surgery. *Current Pract Surg* 1989; 1: 165–9.
68. Abdu TAM, Elhadd TA, Neary R, Clayton RN. Comparison of the low dose short synacthen test (1 μg), the conventional short synacthen test (250 μg) and the insulin tolerance test for the assessment of the hypothalamic–pituitary–adrenal axis in patients with pituitary disease. *J Clin Endocrinol Metab* 1999; 84: 838–43.
69. Hoffman DM, O Sullivan AJ, Baxter RC et al. Diagnosis of growth hormone deficiency in adults. *Lancet* 1994; 343: 1064–8.
70. Korbonits M, Kaltsas G, Perry LA et al. Hexarelin as test of pituitary reserve in patients with pituitary disease. *Clin Endocrinol* 1999; 51: 369–75.
71. Ho KY, Hoffman DM. Diagnosis. In: Johannsson G, Jorgensen JOL, Russell-Jones DL, eds. *Treatment of GH Deficiency in Adults*, Oxford: OCC Ltd, 1998, 2–6.

72. Ghusn HF, Cuningham GR. Evaluation and treatment of androgen deficiency in males. *Endocrinologist* 1991; 1(6): 399–408.
73. Bagatell CJ, Bremner WJ. Androgens in men—uses and abuses. *N Engl J Med* 1996; 334(11): 707–14.
74. Bhasin S, Bremener WJ. Emerging issues in androgen replacement therapy. *J Clin Endocrinol Metab* 1997; 82: 3–8.
75. Gooren LJ. A ten year safety study of the oral androgen testosterone undecanoate. *J Androl* 1994; 15: 212–15.
76. GRS Consensus Guidelines for Diagnosis and Treatment of Adults with GH Deficiency. Port Stevens Workshop, April 1997. Consensus Guidelines for the Diagnosis and Treatment of Adults with Growth Hormone Deficiency: Summary Statement of the Growth Hormone Research Society Workshop on Adult Growth Hormone Deficiency. *J Clin Endocrinol Metab* 1998; 83: 379–81.
77. Baylis PH, Thompson CJ. Osmoregulation of vasopressin secretion and thirst in health and disease. *Clin Endocrinol* 1988; 29: 549–76.
78. Baylis PH, Robertson GL. Plasma vasopressin response to hypertonic saline to assess posterior pituitary function. *J R Soc Med* 1980; 73: 255–60.
79. Post KD, McCormick PC, Bello JA. Differential diagnosis of pituitary tumors. *Endocrinol Metab Clin North Am* 1997; 16(3): 609–45.
80. Thodou E, Asa SL, Kontogeorgos G et al. Lymphocytic hypophysitis: clinicopathological findings. *J Clin Endocrinol Metab* 1995; 80: 2302–11.
81. Jenkins PJ, Chew SL, Lowe DG et al. Lymphocytic hypophysitis: unusual features of a rare disorder. *Clin Endocrinol* 1995; 42: 529–34.
82. Patel MC, Guneratne N, Haq N et al. Peripartum hypopituitarism and lymphocytic hypophysitis. *Q J Med* 1995; 88: 571–80.
83. Stromberg S, Crock P, Lernmark A, Hulting A-L. Pituitary autoantibodies in patients with hypopituitarism and their relatives. *J Endocrinol* 1998; 157: 475–80.
84. Maghnie M, Genovese E, Sommaruga MG et al. Evolution of childhood central diabetes insipidus into panhypopituitarism with a large hypothalamic mass: is 'lymphocytic infundibuloneurohypophysitis' in children a different entity? *Eur J Endocrinol* 1998; 139: 635–40.
85. Bulow B, Attewell R, Hagmar L et al. Postoperative prognosis in craniopharyngioma with respect to cardiovascular mortality, survival and tumor recurrence. *J Clin Endocrinol Metab* 1998; 83: 3897–904.
86. Harris PE, Perry L, Chard T et al. Immunoreactive human chorionic gonadotrophin from the cyst fluid and CSF of patients with craniopharyngioma. *Clin Endocrinol* 1988; 29: 503–8.
87. Nashimoto A, Matsuhisa T, Kunishio K et al. Craniopharyngioma: early and long-term recurrence after partial removal. *J Neurol Neurosurg Psychiatry* 1995; 58(1): 111–12.
88. Van Effenterre R, Boch AL. Craniopharyngiomes de l'adulte et de l'enfant. Etude d'une serie chirurgicale de 106 cas consecutifs. *Neurochirurgie* 1997; 43(4): 187–210.
89. Voges J, Sturm V, Lehrke R et al. Cystic craniopharyngioma: long-term results after intracavitary irradiation with stereotactically applied colloidal beta-emitting radioactive sources. *Neurosurgery* 1997; 40(2): 263–9.
90. Katznelson L, Alexander JM, Klibanski A. Clinically nonfunctioning pituitary adenomas. *J Clin Endocrinol Metab* 1993; 76: 1089–94.
91. Jameson JL, Klibanski A, Black PM et al. Glycoprotein hormone genes are expressed in clinically nonfunctioning pituitary adenomas. *J Clin Invest* 1987; 80: 1472–8.
92. Asa SL, Cheng Z, Raymar L et al. Human pituitary null cell adenomas and oncocytomas *in vitro*: effects of adenohypophysiotropic hormones and gonadal steroids on hormone secretion and tumor cell morphology. *J Clin Endocrinol Metab* 1992; 74: 1128–34.
93. Galway AB, Hsueh AJW, Daneshdoost L, Zhou MH, Paulou SN, Snyder PJ. Gonadotroph adenomas in men produce biologically active follicle-stimulating hormone. *J Clin Endocrinol Metab* 1990; 71: 907–12.
94. Daneshdoost L, Gennarelli TA, Bashey et al. Identification of gonadotroph adenomas in men with clinically nonfunctioning adenomas by the luteinizing hormone β-subunit response to thyrotropin releasing hormone. *J Clin Endocrinol Metab* 1993; 77: 1352–5.
95. Gil-del-Alamo P, Petersson KSI, Saccomanno K et al. Abnormal response of luteinizing hormone beta subunit to thyrotropin-releasing hormone in patients with non-functioning pituitary adenoma. *Clin Endocrinol* 1994; 41: 661–6.
96. Chanson P, Pantel J, Young J et al. Free luteinizing-hormone beta-subunit in normal subjects and patients with pituitary adenomas. *J Clin Endocrinol Metab* 1997; 82: 1397–402.
97. Greenman Y, Tordjman K, Somjen D et al. The use of β-subunits of gonadotropin hormones in the follow-up of clinically non-functioning tumors. *Clin Endocrinol* 1998; 49: 185–90.
98. Harris PE. Biochemical markers for clinically non-functioning pituitary tumors. *Clin Endocrinol* 1998; 49: 163–4.
99. Oppenheim DS, Kana AR, Sangha JS, Klibanski A. Prevalence of α-subunit hypersecretion in patients with pituitary tumors: clinically nonfunctioning and somatotroph adenomas. *J Clin Endocrinol Metab* 1990; 70: 859–64.
100. Heseltine D, White MC, Kendall-Taylor P et al. Testicular enlargement and elevated serum inhibin concentrations in patients with pituitary macroadenomas secreting follicle stimulating hormone. *Clin Endocrinol* 1989; 31: 411–23.

101. Franks S, Nabarro JDN. Prolactin secretion in patients with chromophobe adenomas of the pituitary: incidence and presentation of hyperprolactinemia: results of surgical treatment. *Ann Clin Res* 1978; **10**: 157–63.

102. Vaughan NJA, Laroche CM, Goodman I et al. Pituitary Cushing's disease arising from a previously non-functional corticotrophic chromophobe adenoma. *Clin Endocrinol* 1985; **22**: 147–53.

103. Harris PE. Clinical and genetic changes in a case of a Cushing's carcinoma. *Clin Endocrinol* 1995; **42**: 671–2.

104. Selman WR, Laws ER, Scheithauer BW, Carpenter SM. The occurrence of dural invasion in pituitary adenomas. *J Neurosurg* 1986; **64**: 402–7.

105. Turner HE, Stratton IM, Byrne JV et al. Audit of selected patients with non functioning pituitary adenomas treated without irradiation—a follow-up study. *Clin Endocrinol* 1999; **51**: 281–4.

106. Brada M, Rajan B, Traish D et al. The long-term efficacy of conservative surgery and radiotherapy in the control of pituitary adenomas. *Clin Endocrinol* 1993; **38**: 571–8.

107. Kwekkeboom DJ, Lamberts SWJ. Long-term treatment with the dopamine agonist CV205–502 of patients with a clinically non-functioning gonadotroph, or a α-subunit secreting pituitary adenoma. *Clin Endocrinol* 1992; **36**: 171–6.

108. Borson-Chazot F, Houzard C, Ajzenberg C et al. Somatostatin receptor imaging in somatotroph and non-functioning pituitary adenomas: correlation with hormonal and visual responses to octreotide. *Clin Endocrinol* 1997; **47**: 589–98.

109. De Bruin TWA, Kwekkeboom DJ, Vant Verlaat JW et al. Clinically non-functioning pituitary adenoma and octreotide response to long term high dose treatment and studies *in vitro*. *J Clin Endocrinol Metab* 1992; **75**: 1310–17.

110. Klibanski A, Jameson JL, Biller BMK et al. Gonadotropin and α-subunit responses to chronic LHRH analog administration in patients with pituitary tumors. *J Clin Endocrinol Metab* 1989; **68**: 81–6.

111. Molitch ME. Pituitary incidentalomas. *Endocrinol Metab Clin North Am* 1997; **26**(4): 725–40.

112. Molitch ME. Pathological hyperprolactinemia. *Endocrinol Metab Clin North Am* 1992; **21**(4): 877–901.

113. Beck-Peccoz P, Brucker-Davis F, Persani L et al. Thyrotropin-secreting pituitary tumors. *Endocrine Rev* 1996; **17**(6): 610–38.

114. Brucker-Davis F, Oldfield EH, Skarulis MC et al. Thyrotropin-secreting pituitary tumors: diagnostic criteria, thyroid hormone sensitivity and treatment outcome in 25 patients followed at the National Institutes of Health. *J Clin Endocrinol Metab* 1999; **84**: 476–86.

115. Franks S, Murray MAF, Jequier AM et al. Incidence and significance of hyperprolactinemia in women with amenorrhoea. *Clin Endocrinol* 1975, **4**: 597–607.

116. Bachman GA, Kemmann E. Prevalence of oligomenorrhea and amenorrhea in a college population. *Am J Obstet Gynecol* 1982; **144**: 98–102.

117. Carter JN, Tyson JE, Tolis G. Prolactin-secreting tumors and hypogonadism in 22 men. *N Engl J Med* 1978; **299**: 847–52.

118. Schwartz MF, Baumann JE, Masters WH. Hyperprolactinemia and sexual disorders in men. *Biol Psychiatry* 1982; **17**: 861–76.

119. Verhelst J, Abs R, Maiter D et al. Cabergoline in the treatment of hyperprolactinemia: a study of 455 patients. *J Clin Endocrinol Metab* 1999; **84**: 2518–22.

120. Pellegrini I, Rasolonjanahary R, Gunz G et al. Resistance to bromocriptine in prolactinomas. *J Clin Endocrinol Metab* 1989; **69**: 500–9.

121. Caccavelli L, Morange-Ramos I, Kordon C et al. Alteration of Gα mRNA levels in bromocriptine resistant prolactinomas. *J Neuroendocrinol* 1996; **8**: 737–46.

122. Flanagan DEH, Armitage M, Clein GP, Thakker RV. Prolactinoma presenting in identical twins with multiple endocrine neoplasia type 1. *Clin Endocrinol* 1996; **45**: 117–120.

123. Berezin M, Karasik A. Familial prolactinoma. *Clin Endocrinol* 1995; **42**: 483–6.

124. Alquist JAO, Fahie-Wilson MN. Macroprolactin: incidence and prevalence in moderate and marked hyperprolactinemia. *J Endocrinol* 1998; **156**(suppl): OC32.

125. Olukoga AO, Kane JW. Macroprolactinemia: validation and application of the polyethylene glycol precipitation test and clinical characterization of the condition. *Clin Endocrinol* 1999; **51**: 119–26.

126. Smith A, Harris PE. A comparison of prolactin responses to TRH and high resolution MRI in the assessment of patients with hyperprolactinemia. *J Endocrinol* 2000; **164**(suppl): 29.

127. Martin TL, Kim M, Malarkey WB. The natural history of idiopathic hyperprolactinemia. *J Clin Endocrinol Metab* 1985; **60**: 855–8.

128. Wang C, Lam KSL, Ma JTC et al. Long-term treatment of hyperprolactinemia with bromocriptine: effect of drug withdrawal. *Clin Endocrinol* 1987; **27**: 363–71.

129. Ferrari C, Paracchi A, Mattei AM et al. Cabergoline in the long-term therapy of hyperprolactinemic disorders. *Acta Endocrinol* 1992; **126**: 489–94.

130. Randall RV, Laws ER Jr, Abboud CF et al. Transsphenoidal microsurgical treatment of prolactin-producing pituitary adenomas: results in 100 patients. *Mayo Clin Proc* 1983; **58**: 108–21.

131. Hardy J. Transsphenoidal microsurgery of microprolactinomas. In: Black P, Zervas NT, Ridgeway EC et al, eds. *Secretory Tumors of the Pituitary Gland*. New York: Raven Press, 1984: 73–81.

132. Thomson JA, Davies DL, McLaren EH, Teasdale GM. Ten year follow up of microprolactinoma treated by transsphenoidal surgery. *BMJ* 1994; 1409–10.

133. Wilson CB. Surgical management of pituitary tumors. *J Clin Endocrinol Metab* 1997; **82**: 2381–5.
134. Colao A, Loche S, Cappa M et al. Prolactinomas in children and adolescents. Clinical presentation and long-term follow-up. *J Clin Endocrinol Metab* 1998; **83**: 2777–80.
135. Barnett PS, Dawson JM, Butler J et al. CV 205–502, a new non-ergot dopamine agonist reduces prolactinoma size in man. *Clin Endocrinol* 1990; **33**: 307–16.
136. van der Lely AJ, Brownell J, Lamberts SWJ. The efficacy and tolerability of CV 205-502 (a non-ergot dopaminergic drug) in macroprolactinoma patients and in prolactinoma patients intolerant to bromocriptine. *J Clin Endocrinol Metab* 1991; **72**: 1136–41.
137. Mbanya JCN, Mendelow AD, Crawford PJ et al. Rapid resolution of visual abnormalities with medical therapy alone in patients with large prolactinomas. *Br J Neurosurg* 1993; **7**: 519–27.
138. Biller BMK, Molitch ME, Vance ML et al. Treatment of prolactin-secreting macroadenomas with the once-weekly dopamine agonist cabergoline. *J Clin Endocrinol Metab* 1996; **81**: 2338–43.
139. Colao A, Sarno AD, Landi ML et al. Long-term and low-dose treatment with cabergoline induces macroprolactinoma shrinkage. *J Clin Endocrinol Metab* 1997; **82**: 3574–9.
140. Davis JR, Sheppard MC, Heath DA. Giant invasive prolactinoma: a case report and review of nine further cases. *Q J Med* 1990; **74**: 227–38.
141. Lloyd RV. Estrogen-induced hyperplasia and neoplasia in the rat anterior pituitary gland: an immunohistochemical study. *Am J Pathol* 1983; **113**: 198–206.
142. Gemzell C, Wang CF. Outcome of pregnancy in women with pituitary adenoma. *Fertil Steril* 1979; **31**: 363–72.
143. Molitch ME. Pregnancy and the hyperprolactinemic woman. *N Engl J Med* 1985; **312**: 1364–70.
144. Orme SM, McNally RJQ, Cartwright RA, Belchetz PE. Mortality and cancer incidence in acromegaly: a retrospective cohort study. *J Clin Endocrinol Metab* 1998; **83**: 2730–4.
145. Tremble JM, McGregor AM. Epidemiology, complications and mortality. In: Wass JAH, ed. *Treating Acromegaly*, Bristol: Society for Endocrinology, 1994: 5–12.
146. Alexander L, Appleton D, Hall R et al. Epidemiology of acromegaly in the Newcastle region. *Clin Endocrinol* 1980; **12**: 71–9.
147. Etxabe J, Gaztambide P, Latorre P et al. Acromegaly: an epidemiological study. *J Endocrinol Invest* 1993; **16**: 181–7.
148. Pestell RG, Alford FP, Best JD. Familial acromegaly. *Acta Endocrinol* 1989; **121**: 286–9.
149. McCarthy MI, Noonan K, Wass JAH, Monson JP. Familial acromegaly: studies in three families. *Clin Endocrinol* 1990; **32**: 719–28.
150. Yamada S, Yoshimoto K, Sano T et al. Inactivation of the tumor suppressor gene on 11q13 in brothers with familial acrogigantism without multiple endocrine neoplasia type 1. *J Clin Endocrinol Metab* 1997; **82**: 239–42.
151. Thorner MO, Perryman RL, Cronin MJ et al. Somatotroph hyperplasia. Successful treatment of acromegaly by removal of a pancreatic islet tumor secreting a growth hormone-releasing factor. *J Clin Invest* 1982; **70**: 965–77.
152. Sassolas G, Chayvialle JA, Partensky C et al. Acromegalie, expression clinique de la production de facteurs de liberations de l'hormone de croissance (G.R.F.) par une tumeur pacreatique. *Ann Endocrinol* 1983; **44**: 347–54.
153. Rivier J, Speiss J, Thorner M, Vale W. Characterisation of a growth hormone releasing factor from a human pancreatic tumor. *Nature* 1982; **300**: 276–8.
154. Guillemin R, Brazeau P, Bohlen P et al. Growth hormone releasing factor from a human pancreatic tumor that caused acromegaly. *Science* 1982; **218**: 585–7.
155. Sano T, Asa SL, Kovacs K. Growth hormone-releasing hormone-producing tumors: clinical, biochemical and morphological manifestations. *Endocrine Rev* 1988; **9**: 357–73.
156. Faglia G, Arosio M, Bazzoni N. Ectopic acromegaly. *Endocrinol Metab Clin North Am* 1992; 575–95.
157. Pickett JBE, Layzer RB, Levin SR et al. Neuromuscular complications of acromegaly. *Neurology* 1975; **25**: 638–45.
158. Lieberman SA, Bjorkengren AG, Hoffman AR. Rheumatologic and skeletal changes in acromegaly. *Endocrinol Metab Clin North Am* 1992; **21**(3): 615–31.
159. Colao A, Marzullo P, Vallone G et al. Reversibility of joint thickening in acromegalic patients: an ultrasonography study. *J Clin Endocrinol* 1998; **83**: 2121–5.
160. Minniti G, Jaffrain-Rea ML, Moroni C et al. Echocardiographic evidence for a direct effect of GH/IGF-1 hypersecretion on cardiac mass and function in young acromegalics. *Clin Endocrinol* 1998; **49**: 101–6.
161. Jenkins PJ, Fairclough PD. Colorectal neoplasia in acromegaly. *Clin Endocrinol*, 2001; **55**: 727–9.
162. Atkin WS. Risk of colorectal neoplasia in acromegaly: An independant view. *Clin Endocrinol* 2001; **55**: 723–5.
163. Colao A, Marzullo P, Ferone D et al. Prostatic hyperplasia: an unknown feature of acromegaly. *J Clin Endocrinol Metab* 1998; **83**: 775–9.
164. Hennessey JV, Jackson IMD. Clinical features and differential diagnosis of pituitary tumors with emphasis on acromegaly. *Baillière's Clin Endocrinol Metab* 1995; **9**(2): 271–314.
165. Hartman ML, Veldhuis JD, Vance ML et al. Somatotropin pulse frequency and basal concentrations

are increased in acromegaly and are reduced by successful therapy. *J Clin Endocrinol Metab* 1990; **70**: 1375–84.
166. Hattori N, Shimatsu A, Kato Y et al. Growth hormone responses to oral glucose loading measured by highly sensitive enzyme imunoassay in normal subjects and patients with glucose intolerance and acromegaly. *J Clin Endocrinol Metab* 1990; **70**: 771–6.
167. De Marinis L, Mancini A, Zuppi P et al. Paradoxical growth hormone response to thyrotropin releasing hormone in active acromegaly: clinical correlations and prognostic value. *Acta Endocrinol* 1990; **122**: 433–49.
168. Ishibashi M, Yamaji T, Kosaka K. Induction of growth hormone and prolactin secretion by luteinizing-hormone-releasing hormone and its blockade by bromoergocriptine in acromegalic patients. *J Clin Endocrinol Metab* 1978; **47**: 418–21.
169. Roelfsema F, Van Dulken H, Frolich M. Long-term results of transsphenoidal pituitary microsurgery in 60 acromegalic patients. *Clin Endocrinol* 1985; **23**: 555–65.
170. Grinspoon S, Clemmons D, Swearomgem B et al. Serum insulin-like growth factor-binding protein-3 levels in the diagnosis of acromegaly. *J Clin Endocrinol Metab* 1995; **80**: 927–32.
171. Freda PU, Post KD, Powell JS, Wardlaw SL. Evaluation of disease status with sensitive measures of growth hormone secretion in 60 postoperative patients with acromegaly. *J Clin Endocrinol Metab* 1998; **83**: 3808–16.
172. Nabarro JDN. Acromegaly. *Clin Endocrinol* 1987, **26**: 481–512.
173. Sheppard MC. Aims of treatment and definition of cure. In: Wass JAH, ed. *Treating Acromegaly*, Bristol: Society for Endocrinology, 1994: 17–23.
174. Melmed S. Acromegaly. *N Engl J Med* 1990; **322**: 966–77.
175. McLellan AR, Connell JMC, Beastall GH et al. Growth hormone, body composition and somatomedin C after treatment of acromegaly. *Q J Med* 1988; **260**: 997–1008.
176. Swearingen B, Barker FG, Katznelson L et al. Long-term mortality after transsphenoidal surgery and adjunctive therapy for acromegaly. *J Clin Endocrinol Metab* 1998; **83**: 3419–26.
177. Giustina A, Barkan A, Casanueva FF et al. Criteria for cure of acromegaly: a consensus statement. *J Clin Endocrinol Metab* 2000; **85**: 526–9.
178. van der Lely AJ, Hutson RK, Trainer PJ et al. Long-term treatment of acromegaly with Pegvisomant, a growth hormone receptor agonist. *Lancet* 2001; **358**: 1754–9.
179. Newman CB, Melmed S, George A et al. Octeoride as primary therapy for acromegaly. *J Clin Endocrinol Metab* 1998; **83**: 3034–40.
180. Colao A, Ferone D, Cappabianca P et al. Effect of octreotide pretreatment on surgical outcome in acromegaly. *J Clin Endocrinol Metab* 1997; **82**: 3308–14
181. Fahlbusch R, Honegger J, Schott W, Buchfelder M. Results of surgery in acromegaly. In: Wass JAH, ed. *Treating Acromegaly*, Bristol: Society for Endocrinology, 1994: 49–54.
182. Laws ER. Results of transsphenoidal microsurgical management of acromegaly. In: Wass JAH, ed. *Treating Acromegaly*, Bristol: Society for Endocrinology, 1994: 59–63.
183. Kendall-Taylor P, Osman IA, James RA et al. Outcome of surgery for acromegaly. In: Wass JAH, ed. *Treating Acromegaly*, Bristol: Society for Endocrinology, 1994: 65–8.
184. Abosch A, Tyrrell JB, Lamborn KR et al. Transsphenoidal microsurgery for growth hormone secreting pituitary adenomas: initial outcome and long-term results. *J Clin Endocrinol Metab* 1998; **83**: 3411–8.
185. Plowman PN. Radiotherapy in acromegaly. In: Wass JAH, ed. *Treating Acromegaly*, Bristol: Society for Endocrinology, 1994: 87–91.
186. Barkan AL, Halasz I, Dornfeld KJ et al. Pituitary irradiation is ineffective in normalizing plasma insulin-like growth factor 1 in patients with acromegaly. *J Clin Endocrinol Metab* 1997; **82**: 3187–91.
187. Jaffe CA, Barkan AL. Treatment of acromegaly with dopamine agonists. *Endocrinol Metab Clin North Am* 1992; **21**: 713–35.
188. Verde G, Chiodini PG, Liuzzi A et al. Effectiveness of the dopamine agonist lysuride in the treatment of acromegaly and pathological hyperprolactinemic states. *J Endocrinol Invest* 1980; **4**: 405–410.
189. Kleinberg DL, Boyd AE, Wardlaw S et al. Pergolide for the treatment of pituitary tumors secreting prolactin or growth hormone. *N Engl J Med* 1983; **309**: 704–9.
190. Chiodini PG, Attanasio R, Cozzi R et al. CV 205–502 in acromegaly. *Acta Endocrinol* 1993, **128**: 389–93.
191. Abs R, Verhelst J, Maiter D et al. Cabergoline in the treatment of acromegaly: a study in 64 patients. *J Clin Endocrinol Metab* 1998, **83**: 374–8.
192. Cozzi R, Attanasio R, Barausse M et al. Cabergoline in acromegaly: a renewed role for dopamine agonist treatment? *Eur J Endocrinol* 1998; **139**: 516–21.
193. Lamberts SWJ, Verleun T, Hofland L, Del Pozo E. A comparison between the effects of SMS 201–995, bromocriptine and a combination of both drugs on hormone release by the cultured pituitary tumor cells of acromegalic patients. *Clin Endocrinol* 1987; **27**: 11–23.
194. Lamberts SWJ, Uitterlinden P, Schuijff PC, Klijn JG. Therapy of acromegaly with sandostatin: the predictive value of an acute test, the value of serum somatomedin-C measurements in dose adjustment and

the definition of a biochemical 'cure'. *Clin Endocrinol* 1988; **29**: 411–20.
195. Colao A, Ferone D, Lastoria S et al. Prediction of efficacy of octreotide therapy in patients with acromegaly. *J Clin Endocrinol Metab* 1996; **81**: 2356–62.
196. Barlier A, Gunz G, Zamora AJ et al. Prognostic and therapeutic consequences of Gsα mutations in somatotroph adenomas. *J Clin Endocrinol Metab* 1998; **83**: 1604–10.
197. Lancranjan I, Atkinson BA. Results of a European multicenter study with sandostatin LAR in acromegalic patients. *Pituitary* 1999; **1**: 105–14.
198. Newman CB, Melmed S, George A et al. Octreotide as primary therapy for acromegaly. *J Clin Endocrinol Metab* 1998; **83**: 3034–40.
199. Drange MR, Melmed S. Long-acting lanreotide induces clinical and biochemical remission of acromegaly caused by disseminated growth hormone-releasing hormone-secreting carcinoid. *J Clin Endocrinol Metab* 1998; **83**: 3104–9.
200. Harris PE, Bouloux PMG, Wass JAH, Besser GM. Succesful treatment by chemotherapy for acromegaly associated with ectopic growth hormone releasing hormone secretion from a carcinoid tumor. *Clin Endocrinol* 1990; **32**: 315–21.
201. van der Lely AJ, Muller AF, Janssen JA et al. Control of tumor size and disease activity during co-treatment with octreotide and the growth hormone receptor agonist Pegvisomant in an acromegalic patient. *J Clin Endocrinol Metab* 2001; **86**: 478–81.
202 Trainer PJ, Drake WM, Katznelson L et al. Treatment of acromegaly with the growth hormone-receptor antagonist pegvisomant. *N Engl J Med* 2000; **342**: 1171–7.
203. Cushing H. The basophil adenomas of the pituitary body and their clinical manifestations (pituitary basophilism). *Bull John Hopkins Hosp* 1932; **50**: 137–95.
204. Sakiyama R, Ashcraft MW, Van Herle AJ. Cyclic Cushing's syndrome. *Am J Med* 1984; **77**: 944–6.
205. Vagnucci AH, Evans E. Cushing's disease with intermittent hypercortisolism. *Am J Med* 1986; **80**: 83–8.
206. Lacroix AL, Bolte E, Tremblay J et al. Gastric inhibitory polypeptide-dependent cortisol hypersecretion—a new cause of Cushing's syndrome. *N Engl J Med* 1992; **327**: 974–80.
207. Reznik Y, Allali-Zerah V, Chayvialle JA et al. Food-dependent Cushing's syndrome mediated by aberrant adrenal sensitivity to gastric inhibitory polypeptide. *N Engl J Med* 1992; **327**: 981–6.
208. N'Diaye N, Tremblay J, Hamet P et al. Adrenocortical overexpression of gastric inhibitory polypeptide receptor underlies food-dependent Cushing's syndrome. *J Clin Endocrinol Metab* 1998; **83**: 2781–5.
209. de Herder WW, Hofland LJ, Usdin TB et al. Food-dependent Cushing's syndrome resulting from abundant expression of gastric inhibitory polypeptide receptors in adrenal adenoma glands. *J Clin Endocrinol Metab* 1996; **81**: 3168–72.
210. Lebrethon MC, Avallet O, Reznik Y et al. Food-dependent Cushing's syndrome: characterisation and functional role of gastric inhibitory polypeptide receptor in the adrenals of three patients. *J Clin Endocrinol Metab* 1998; **83**: 4514–19.
211. Lacroix A, Tremblay J, Rousseau G et al. Propranolol therapy for ectopic β-adrenergic receptors in adrenal Cushing's syndrome. *N Engl J Med* 1997; **337**: 1429–34.
212. Lacroix A, Tremblay J, Touyz RM et al. Abnormal adrenal and vascular responses to vasopressin mediated by a V_1-vasopressin receptor in a patient with adrenocorticotropin-independent macronodular adrenal hyperplasia, Cushing's syndrome and orthostatic hypotension. *J Clin Endocrinol Metab* 1997; **82**: 2414–22.
213. Willenberg HS, Stratakis CA, Marx C et al. Aberrant interleukin-1 receptors in a cortisol-secreting adrenal adenoma causing Cushing's syndrome. *N Engl J Med* 1998; **339**: 27–31.
214. Lacroix A, Hamet P, Boutin J-M. Leuprolide acetate therapy in luteinizing hormone-dependent Cushing's syndrome. *N Engl J Med* 1999; **341**: 1577–81.
215. Boscaro M, Barzon L, Fallo F, Sonino N. Cushing's Syndrome. *Lancet* 2001; **357**: 783–91.
216. Styne DM, Grumbach MM, Kaplan SL et al. Treatment of Cushing's disease in childhood and adolescence by transsphenoidal microadenomectomy. *N Engl J Med* 1984; **310**: 889–94.
217. Lado-Abeal J, Rodriguez-Arnao J, Newell-Price JDC et al. Menstrual abnormalities in women with Cushing's disease are correlated with hypercortisolemia rather than raised circulating androgen levels. *J Clin Endocrinol Metab* 1998; **83**: 3083–8.
218. Small M, Lowe GD, Forbes CD et al. Thromboembolic complications in Cushing's syndrome. *Clin Endocrinol* 1983; **19**: 503–11.
219. Soberg HE, Blomback M, Granberg PO. Thromboembolic complications, heparin treatment and increase in coagulation factors in Cushing's syndrome. *Acta Med Scand* 1976; **199**: 95–8.
220. Haskett RF. Diagnostic characterization of psychiatric disturbance in Cushing's syndrome. *Am J Psychiatry* 1985; **142**: 911–16.
221. Trainer PJ, Grossman A. The diagnosis and differential diagnosis of Cushing's syndrome. *Clin Endocrinol* 1991; **34**: 317–30.
222. Neiman LK, Cutler GB. Cushing's syndrome. In: De Groot LJ, ed. *Endocrinology*. WB Saunders, 1995: 1741–69.
223. Thapar K, Kovacs K, Muller PJ. Clinical–pathological correlations of pituitary tumors. *Baillière's Clin Endocrinol Metab* 1995; **9**(2): 243–70.
224. Scheithauer BW, Kovacs K, Laws ER et al. Pathology of invasive pituitary adenomas with special reference

to functional classification. *J Neurosurg* 1986; **65**: 733–44.
225. Bates AS, Buckley N, Boggild MD et al. Clinical and genetic changes in a case of a Cushing's carcinoma. *Clin Endocrinol* 1995; **42**: 663–70.
226. Nelson DH, Meakin JW, Thorn GW. ACTH-producing pituitary tumors following adrenalectomy for Cushing's syndrome. *Ann Intern Med* 1960; **52**: 560–9.
227. Orth DN, Liddle GW. Results of treatment in 108 patients with Cushing's syndrome. *N Engl J Med* 1971; **285**: 243–7.
228. Carey RM, Varna SK, Drake CR et al. Ectopic secretion of corticotropin-releasing factor as a cause of Cushing's syndrome. *N Engl J Med* 1984; **311**: 13–20.
229. Muller OA, Von Werder K. Ectopic production of ACTH and corticotropin-releasing hormone. *J Steroid Biochem Mol Biol* 1992; **43**: 403–8.
230. Leinung MC, Young WF Jr, Whitaker MD et al. Diagnosis of corticotropin-producing bronchial carcinoid tumors causing Cushing's syndrome. *Mayo Clin Proc* 1990; **65**: 1314–21.
231. Limper AH, Carpenter PC, Scheithauer B et al. The Cushing syndrome induced by bronchial carcinoid tumors. *Ann Intern Med* 1992; **117**: 209–14.
232. Wollensak G, Herbst EW, Beck A et al. Primary thymic carcinoid with Cushing's syndrome. *Virchows Arch A Pathol Anat* 1992; **420**: 191–5.
233. Blunt SB, Sandler LM, Burrin JM et al. An evaluation of the distinction of ectopic and pituitary ACTH dependent Cushing's syndrome by clinical features, biochemical tests and radiological findings. *Q J Med* 1990, **77**: 1113–33.
234. Howlett TA, Drury PL, Perry L et al. Diagnosis and management of ACTH-dependent Cushing's syndrome: comparison of the features in ectopic and pituitary ACTH production. *Clin Endocrinol* 1986, **24**: 699–713.
235. Stewart PM, Gibson S, Crosby SR et al. ACTH precursors characterize the ectopic ACTH syndrome. *Clin Endocrinol* 1994; **40**: 199–204.
236. Gibson S, Ray DW, Crosby SR et al. Impaired processing of proopiomelanocortin in corticotroph macroadenomas. *J Clin Endocrinol Metab* 1996; **81**: 497–502.
237. Becker M, Aron DC. Ectopic ACTH syndrome and CRH-mediated Cushing's syndrome. *Endocrinol Metab Clin North Am* 1994; **23**(3): 585–606.
238. Harris PE, Buxton-Thomas M, Kane P et al. Cushing's syndrome associated with a circulating CRF-like peptide. *J Endocrinol* 1998; **156**(suppl): P37.
239. Trainer PJ, Besser M. Cushing's syndrome. Therapy directed at the adrenal glands. *Endocrinol Metab Clin North Am* 1994; **23**(3): 571–84.
240. Bertagna C, Orth DN. Clinical and laboratory findings and results of therapy in 58 patients with adrenocortical tumors admitted at a single medical center (1951–1978). *Am J Med* 1981; **71**: 855.
241. Samuels MH, Loriaux DL. Cushing's syndrome and the nodular adrenal gland. *Endocrinol Metab Clin North Am* 1994; **23**(3): 555–69.
242. Osella G, Terzolo M, Borretta G et al. Endocrine evaluation of incidentally discovered adrenal masses (incidentalomas). *J Clin Endocrinol Metab* 1994; **79**: 1532–9.
243. Barzon L, Scaroni C, Sonino N et al. Incidentally discovered adrenal tumors: endocrine and scintigraphic correlates. *J Clin Endocrinol Metab* 1998; **83**: 55–62.
244. Barzon L, Scaroni C, Nicoletta S et al. Risk factors and long-term follow-up of adrenal incidentalomas. *J Clin Endocrinol Metab* 1999; **84**: 520–6.
245. Carney JA, Young WF. Primary pigmented nodular adrenocortical disease and its associated conditions. *Endocrinologist* 1992; **2**: 6.
246. Sarlis NJ, Chrousos GP, Doppman JL et al. Primary pigmented nodular adrenocortical disease: reevaluation of a patient with Carney complex 27 years after unilateral adrenalectomy. *J Clin Endocrinol Metab* 1997; **82**: 1274–8.
247. Trainer PJ, Grossman A. The diagnosis and differential diagnosis of Cushing's syndrome. *Clin Endocrinol* 1991; **34**: 317–30.
248. Malchoff CD, Rosa J, DeBold CR et al. Adrenocorticotropin-independent bilateral macronodular adrenal hyperplasia: an unusual cause of Cushing's syndrome. *J Clin Endocrinol Metab* 1989; **68**: 855–60.
249. Corcuff J-B, Tabarin A, Rashedi M et al. Overnight urinary free cortisol determination: a screening test for the diagnosis of Cushing's syndrome. *Clin Endocrinol* 1998; **48**: 503–8.
250. Issa BG, Page MD, Read G et al. Undetectable urinary free cortisol concentrations in a case of Cushing's disease. *Eur J Endocrinol* 1999; **140**: 148–51.
251. Newell-Price J, Trainer P, Perry L et al. A single sleeping midnight cortisol has 100% sensitivity for the diagnosis of Cushing's syndrome. *Clin Endocrinol* 1995; **43**: 545–50.
252. Raff H, Raff JL, Findling JW. Late-night salivary cortisol as a screening test for Cushing's syndrome. *J Clin Endocrinol Metab* 1998; **83**: 2681–6.
253. Liddle GW. Tests of pituitary–adrenal suppressibility in the diagnosis of Cushing's syndrome. *J Clin Endocrinol Metab* 1960; **20**: 1539–61.
254. Wood PJ, Barth JH, Freedman DB et al. Evidence for the low dose dexamethasone suppression test to screen for Cushing's syndrome—recommendations for a protocol for biochemistry laboratories. *Ann Clin Biochem* 1997; **34**: 222–9.
255. Lampe TH, Fariss BL, Risse SC et al. Laboratory evaluation for Cushing's syndrome in psychiatric patients with cortisol non-suppression following the

overnight dexamethasone suppression test. *Biol Psychiatry* 1987; 22: 1264–70.
256. Dichek HL, Nieman LK, Oldfield EH et al. A comparison of the standard high dose dexamethasone suppression test and the overnight 8-mg dexamethasone suppression test for the differential diagnosis of adrenocorticotropin-dependent Cushing's syndrome. *J Clin Endocrinol Metab* 1994; 78: 418–22.
257. van den Bogaert DPM, de Herder WW, de Jong FH et al. The continuous 7-hour intravenous dexamethasone suppression test in the differential diagnosis of ACTH-dependent Cushing's syndrome. *Clin Endocrinol* 1999; 51: 193–8.
258. Oldfield EH, Doppman JL, Nieman LK et al. Petrosal sinus sampling with and without corticotropin-releasing hormone for the differential diagnosis of Cushing's syndrome. *N Engl J Med* 1991; 325: 897–905.
259. Young J, Deneux C, Grino M et al. Pitfall of petrosal sinus sampling in a Cushing's syndrome secondary to ectopic adrenocorticotropin–corticotropin releasing hormone (ACTH-CRH) secretion. *J Clin Endocrinol Metab* 1998; 83: 305–8.
260. Doppman JL, Chang R, Oldfield EH et al. The hypoplastic inferior petrosal sinus: a potential source of false-negative results in petrosal sampling for Cushing's disease. *J Clin Endocrinol Metab* 1999; 84: 533–40.
261. Kaltsas GA, Giannulis MG, Newell-Price JDC et al. A critical analysis of the value of simultaneous inferior petrosal sinus sampling in Cushing's disease and the occult ectopic adrenocorticotropin syndrome. *J Clin Endocrinol Metab* 1999; 84: 487–92.
262. Graham KE, Samuels MH, Nesbit GM et al. Cavernous sinus sampling is highly accurate in distinguishing Cushing's disease from the ectopic adrenocorticotropin syndrome and in predicting intrapituitary tumor location. *J Clin Endocrinol Metab* 1999; 84: 1602–10.
263. Namelak AN, Dowd CF, Tyrrell JB et al. Venous angiography is needed to interpret inferior petrosal sinus and cavernous sinus sampling data for lateralising adrenocorticotropin-secreting adenomas. *J Clin Endocrinol Metab* 1996; 81: 475–81.
264. Newell-Price J. The desmopressin test and Cushing's syndrome: current state of play. *Clin Endocrinol* 1997; 47: 173–4.
265. Buchfelder M, Nistor R, Fahlbusch R, Huk WJ. The accuracy of CT and MR evaluation of the sella turcica for detection of adrenocorticotropic hormone-secreting adenomas in Cushing disease. *Am J Neuroradiol* 1993; 14: 1183–90.
266. Colombo N, Loli P, Vignati F, Scialfa G. MR of corticotropin-secreting pituitary microadenomas. *Am J Neuroradiol* 1994; 15: 1591–5.
267. de Herder WW, Uitterlinden P, Pieterman H et al. Pituitary tumor localization in patients with Cushing's disease by magnetic resonance imaging. Is there a place for petrosal sinus sampling? *Clin Endocrinol* 1994; 40: 87–92.
268. Hanson JA, Sohaib SA, Newell-Price J et al. Computed tomography appearance of the thymus and anterior mediastinum in active Cushing's syndrome. *J Clin Endocrinol Metab* 1999; 84: 602–5.
269. Torpy DJ, Chen CC, Mullen N et al. Lack of utility of ^{111}In-pentetreotide scintigraphy in localizing ectopic ACTH producing tumors: follow-up of 18 patients. *J Clin Endocrinol Metab* 1999; 84: 1186–92.
270. Tabarin A, Valli N, Chanson P et al. Usefulness of somatostatin scintigraphy in patients with occult ectopic adrenocorticotropin syndrome. *J Clin Endocrinol Metab* 1999; 84: 1193–202.
271. Scheingart DE, Tsao HS, Taylor CI. Sustained remission in Cushing's disease with mitotane and pituitary irradiation. *Ann Intern Med* 1980; 92: 613–18.
272. Luton J, Cerdas S, Billaud L et al. Clinical features of adrenocortical carcinoma, prognostic factors and the effect of mitotane therapy. *N Engl J Med* 1990; 322: 1195–201.
273. Maher VMG, Trainer PJ, Scoppola A et al. Possible mechanisms and treatment of o,p'DDD-induced hypercholesterolemia. *Q J Med* 1992; 84: 671–9.
274. Dickstein G, Shechner C, Arad E et al. Is there a role for low doses of mitotane (o,p'-DDD) as adjuvant therapy in adrenocortical carcinoma? *J Clin Endocrinol Metab* 1998; 83: 3100–3.
275. Nieman LK, Chroususm GP, Kellner CH et al. Successful treatment of Cushing's syndrome with the glucocorticoid antagonist RU 486. *J Clin Endocrinol Metab* 1985; 61: 536–40.
276. Mercado-Asis LB, Yanovski JA, Tracer HL et al. Acute effects of bromocriptine, cyproheptadine and valproic acid on plasma adrenocorticotropin secretion in Nelson's syndrome. *J Clin Endocrinol Metab* 1997; 82: 514–17.
277. Drake WM, Perry LA, Hinds CJ et al. Emergency and prolonged use of intravenous etomidate to control hypercortisolemia in a patient with Cushing's syndrome and peritonitis. *J Clin Endocrinol Metab* 1998; 83: 3542–4.
278. Mampalam TJ, Tyrrell JB, Wilson CB. Transsphenoidal microsurgery for Cushing's disease. A report of 216 cases. *Ann Intern Med* 1988; 109: 487–93.
279. Blevins LS, Christy JH, Khajavi M, Tindall GT. Outcomes of therapy for Cushing's disease due to adrenocorticotropin-secreting pituitary macroadenomas. *J Clin Endocrinol Metab* 1998; 83: 63–7.
280. Devoe DJ, Miller WL, Conte FA et al. Long-term outcome in children and adolescents after transsphenoidal surgery for Cushing's disease. *J Clin Endocrinol Metab* 1997; 82: 3196–202.
281. Friedman RB, Oldfield EH, Nieman LK et al. Repeat transsphenoidal surgery for Cushing's disease. *J Neurosurg* 1989; 71: 520–7.

282. Pluta RM, Nieman L, Doppman JL et al. Extrapituitary parasellar microadenoma in Cushing's disease. *J Clin Endocrinol Metab* 1999; **84**: 2912–23.
283. Yap LB, Turner HE, Adams CBT, Wass JAH. Undetectable postoperative cortisol does not always predict long-term remission in Cushing's disease: a single centre audit. *Clin Endocrinol* 2002; **56**: 25–31.
284. Bochicchio D, Losa M, Buchfelder M, the European Cushing's Disease Survey Study Group. Factors influencing the immediate and late outcome of Cushing's disease treated by transsphenoidal surgery: a retrospective study by the European Cushing's Disease Survey Group. *J Clin Endocrinol Metab* 1995; **80**: 3114–20.
285. Sonino N, Zielezny M, Fava GA et al. Risk factors and long-term outcome in pituitary-dependent Cushing's disease. *J Clin Endocrinol Metab* 1996; **81**: 2647–52.
286. Howlett TA, Plowman PN, Wass JAH et al. Megavoltage pituitary irradiation in the management of Cushing's disease and Nelson's syndrome: long-term follow-up. *Clin Endocrinol* 1989; **31**: 309–32.
287. Hughes NR, Lissett CA, Shalet SM. Growth hormone status following treatment for Cushing's syndrome. *Clin Endocrinol* 1999; **51**: 61–6.
288. Colao A, Pivonello R, Spiezia S et al. Persistence of increased cardiovascular risk in patients with Cushing's disease after five years of successful cure. *J Clin Endocrinol Metab* 1999; **84**: 2664–72.

4

Growth and growth disorders
John Miell, Annice Mukherjee

Physiology of growth hormone secretion

Growth hormone (GH) is a single-chain protein consisting of 191 amino acid residues and two disulfide bridges. It is a somatomammotropic hormone, along with prolactin and placental lactogen, and has growth-promoting and lactogenic properties. The GH gene complex is situated on chromosome 17. It consists of five related genes, only one of which is expressed in the pituitary (hGH-N), and is responsible for directing GH synthesis. A human GH variant (GHV) is secreted by the placenta during pregnancy.[1,2] GH is synthesized in the somatotroph cells of the anterior pituitary as a preprohormone, which is spliced to form the precursor hormone, cleavage then takes place to produce the final secretory form. This is predominantly a 22-kDa molecule which is stored in cytoplasmic granules prior to pulsatile release into the bloodstream by exocytosis. A 20-kDa form of GH is also secreted by the somatotroph cells and constitutes only about 5–10% of secreted pituitary GH. A third monomeric form of GH is incompletely characterized. In addition to monomeric forms of the hormone, much larger immunoreactive species can be detected in pituitary extracts and plasma, and this 'big' GH is thought to represent a dimer attached by interchain disulfide linkages. It has been shown to be secreted directly by the somatotroph cells, and its amino acid composition may differ from that of monomeric GH. 'Big' GH can bind to and displace monomeric GH from hepatic membrane receptors; however, it has less biological activity and its physiological significance is uncertain.

Approximately 70% of circulating GH is transported bound, and the major binding protein involved in transport is a 61-kDa glycoprotein which is identical to the extracellular domain of the GH receptor and is generated by enzymatic cleavage of the receptor. Growth hormone-binding protein (GHBP) prolongs the half-life of GH, allowing it to persist in the circulation for 10 times as long.[3] The GH receptor itself is located in the peripheral tissues, and its activation results in a cascade of events which lead to growth-promoting effects in target tissues (see below). Its absence through genetic defects results in GH resistance syndromes (see below).

GH secretogogs

Under physiological conditions, GH secretion is tightly regulated by an integral system of neural, metabolic and hormonal factors, which have inhibitory and stimulatory effects. Growth hormone-releasing hormone (GHRH) and growth hormone release-inhibiting hormone (somatostatin) are both of hypothalamic origin and act as the mediators for control of GH secretion.

GHRH

GHRH is the major physiological stimulus for GH synthesis and secretion. It is a peptide hormone and circulates in two major biologically active forms, one with 40 and the other with 44 amino acids. It is structurally similar to the family of gut–brain peptides. It was first completely characterized in 1982.[4] The human GHRH gene is located on chromosome 20. GHRH cell bodies are situated in the perifornical and infundibular nuclei of the hypothalamus. GHRH neuronal axons project to the median eminence and terminate on the capillaries of the portal circulation. GHRH release is pulsatile, contributing to the pulsatility of GH release.

In the pituitary, GHRH binds to specific G protein-coupled receptors on somatotroph cell membranes and, via a process involving generation of cyclic AMP and free cytosolic calcium, acts as a powerful GH secretagog. It is also thought to induce somatotroph proliferation.

Somatostatin

Somatostatin is the other major hypothalamic hormone contributing to the control of GH release. It has two major biologically active forms, of 14 and 28 amino acid residues.[5] Like GHRH, it is released episodically. However, unlike GHRH, it is widely distributed in the central nervous system and in tissues of neuroectodermal origin. Hypothalamic somatostatin binds to five different membrane receptor subtypes which are tissue specific and differ in their mechanisms of intracellular action and bind to somatostatin analogs differently. Only two of these are found in the pituitary, and mediate the inhibitory effects on basal and stimulated pituitary GH release.[6] These receptors are G protein-coupled systems with seven transmembrane spanning sequences, which inhibit intracellular cAMP formation and indirectly inhibit calcium channels in the somatotroph cell membrane. This process lowers free cytosolic calcium within the somatotroph cell, which inhibits somatotrophin secretion. Unlike GHRH, somatostatin is not thought to modulate GH synthesis. Somatostatin actions appear to be generally inhibitory, as it also suppresses pituitary release of thyrotropin and, under certain conditions, corticotropin and prolactin secretion. Multiple physiological and pathological stimuli contribute to the relative secretions of GHRH and somatostatin and therefore GH secretion (Figure 4.1).

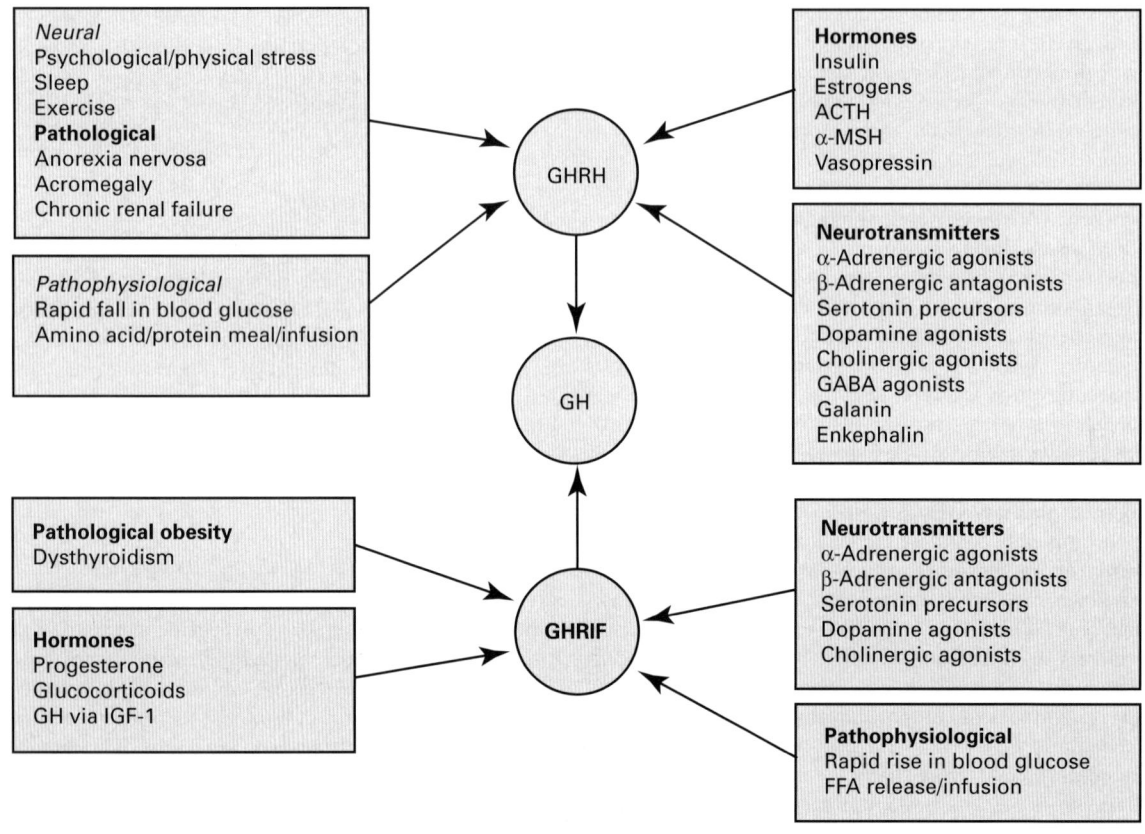

Figure 4.1
Control of growth hormone secretion. FFA, free fatty acid; ACTH, adrenocorticotropic hormone; IGF-1, insulin-like growth factor-1; GHRH, growth hormone-releasing hormone.

Growth hormone-releasing peptides (GHRPs)

GHRPs are synthetic GH secretagogs which have potent, reproducible and dose-related GH-releasing activity in humans.[7]

GHRPs, like endogenous GH secretagogs stimulate GH secretion by acting on receptors, which are present in the pituitary, in the hypothalamus, elsewhere in the central nervous system (CNS) and in the peripheral tissues.

Hexarelin is a potent GHRP which has been shown to produce profound GH release in normal human subjects after oral, intravenous and subcutaneous administration.[8] Its oral availability and its ability to produce pulsatile GH release make it a promising future therapeutic GH secretagog with obvious benefits over subcutaneous GH and GHRH analogs. The success of hexarelin as a therapeutic entity will be determined by its ability to induce GH release with chronic administration, and there is a suggestion that chronic subcutaneous administration may result in an attenuated GH response.[9] Further research in this area is awaited.

Physiology of GH action

The first step in the process of GH action occurs when GH binds to its receptor in the peripheral tissues. The GH receptor consists of two adjacent receptor molecules on the target cell membrane, and receptor binding results in the formation of a dimeric unit. A tyrosine kinase, JAK2, is associated with the receptor and is activated by receptor binding. This activates pathways that result in intracellular protein phosphorylation, which ultimately results in intracellular expression of

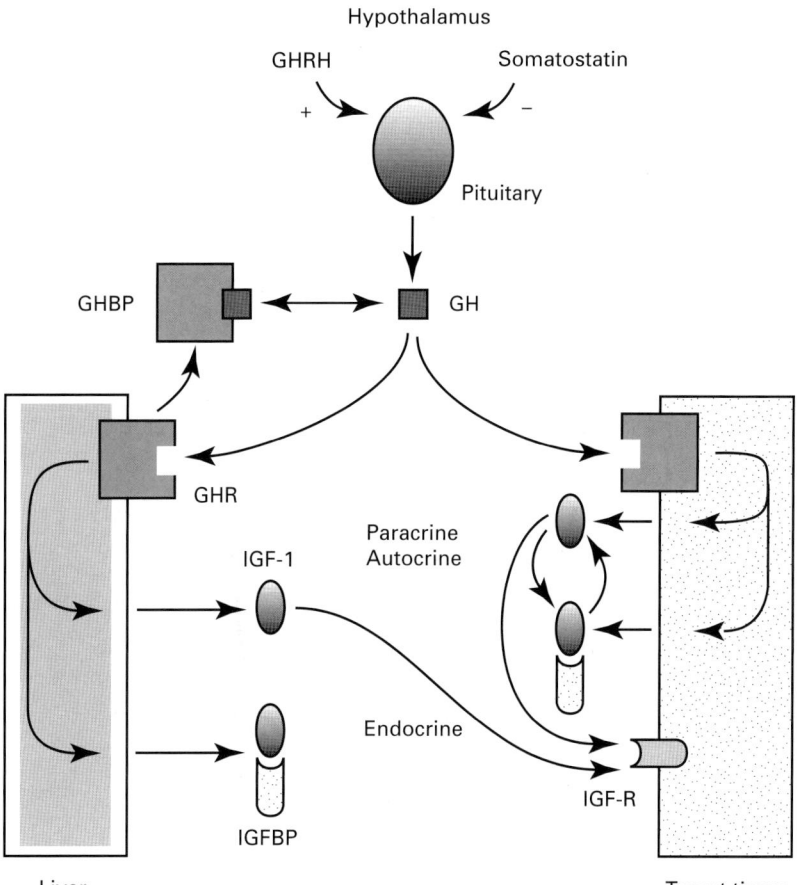

Figure 4.2
GH–IGF–IGF binding protein axis. GHRH, growth hormone-releasing hormone; GHBP, growth hormone-binding protein; GHR, growth hormone receptor; IGF-1, insulin-like growth factor-1; IGFBP, insulin-like growth factor-binding protein; IGF-R, insulin-like growth factor receptor.

GH action. GH receptor binding also activates a membrane-bound phospholipase C via activation of a G protein system. This results in an increase in free intracellular calcium and activation of protein kinase C, which can activate other intracellular proteins such as transcription factors. In the liver, GH stimulates hepatic production of insulin-like growth factor-1 (IGF-1), which has 10–13% of the activity of insulin. The GH–IGF axis interaction is summarized in Figure 4.2.

Insulin-like growth factor physiology

The existence of the insulin-like growth factors was first recognized in 1957, and since then considerable information on and understanding of these blood-borne growth factors has accumulated. IGFs are mitogenic, and their actions are determined by the availability of free IGF to interact with the IGF receptors. IGF-2 exerts tissue growth-promoting activity, particularly in the fetus, but its GH dependence is less well established than that of IGF-1. One of the major mediators of GH in peripheral tissues is IGF-1.

IGF-1

IGF-1 is a 70 amino acid peptide and is similar in structure to proinsulin, with domains analogous to the A and B domains of insulin and the C peptide of proinsulin. It is the product of a single gene, which is on the long arm of chromosome 12. It is a blood-borne molecule released predominantly by the liver in response to GH, and is present in the circulation in readily detectable concentrations, the majority circulating bound to its binding proteins (IGFBPs). IGF-1 predominantly circulates bound to IGFBP-3 and an acid-labile glycoprotein subunit. The bound form is known as a ternary complex and comprises approximately 95% of circulating IGF-1.[10] The advantages of the ternary complex are that it prolongs the half-life of both IGF-1 and IGFBP-3. The half-life of unbound IGFBP-3 is between 30 and 90 min, the half-life of free IGF-1 is less than 10 min, and the half-life of the 150-kDa complex is approximately 12 h.[11] This enables IGF-1 to remain in the intravascular space for steady delivery to the tissues, in contrast to the pulsatility of GH. The latter enables its distribution to many tissues, and enables maintenance of higher blood levels. IGF-1 is not stored but secreted shortly after synthesis. IGF-1 can stimulate proliferation of many cell types, and in others promotes cellular differentiation and specialized function.[10]

IGF-1 regulation of expression and action

The level of free circulating IGF-1 is in part determined by the degree of binding to IGFBPs. Other contributory factors are rates of IGF-1 production and clearance. GH and nutritional status are major regulators of IGF-1 by stimulating its transcription in the liver as well as other tissues.[12] Severe GH deficiency and nutritional deprivation therefore markedly reduce hepatic IGF-1 mRNA transcription. IGF-1 can be regulated by other factors or hormones, depending on the specific target issue of IGF-1 expression; for example, thyroid-stimulating hormone (TSH) stimulates IGF-1 mRNA expression in the thyroid. IGF-1 levels vary with age, as illustrated in Table 4.1.

IGF-1 receptors

IGF-1 actions are mediated by activation of the type I IGF receptor.[13] This receptor possesses tyrosine kinase domains, is the product of a single gene and shares structural homology with the insulin receptor. As well as mediating growth-promoting activity, it also mediates the mitogenic activity of IGF-1. A further IGF receptor—the type II receptor—which is identical to the mannose 6-phosphate receptor, has also been discovered, but its signaling function is thus far unknown. Disruption of the type II IGF receptor in type II IGF receptor-knockout mice does not result in growth retardation, suggesting that this receptor is not part of the IGF growth-signaling system.

Interaction of IGF-1 with the type I IGF receptor results in a conformational change in the receptor with autophosphorylation and a series of intracellular events, which ultimately result in transcription of early-response genes. These generally encode transcription factors, which stimulate the transcription of late-response genes that produce the effectors of growth

Age (years)	Normal range Mean (+/− 2 SDs)
25–29	257 (127–387) ng/ml
30–54	212 (128–296) ng/ml
55+	196 (98–294) ng/ml

Data are from reference range provided by Diagnostic Services Laboratories Inc.

Table 4.1
Changes in serum IGF-1 with age.

factor stimulation, such as progression through the cell cycle and differentiation.

IGF-1 actions

In vitro studies have shown IGF-1 to have anabolic effects analogous to insulin, with amino acid and glucose uptake and synthesis of extracellular matrix proteins. It exhibits direct negative feedback of GH secretion and can act synergistically with other hormones to stimulate specialized cell function.[14]

In vivo, IGF-1 infusion stimulates tissue glucose uptake, leading to hypoglycemia and protein synthesis.[10] Detailed experiments in transgenic mice with ablation or overexpression of genes encoding the various key proteins in the pathway of GH and IGF-1 action mediation have established vital information regarding their individual roles in health and disease. IGF-1 knockout mice exhibit marked in utero and postnatal growth retardation and are subsequently infertile. IGF-1-overexpressing mice become larger than their non-transgenic siblings at about 6 weeks of age. As adults, they weigh about 30% more than normals.

IGF-2

IGF-2 is an anabolic peptide of 67 amino acids. It shares structural homology with proinsulin and IGF-1, and a summary of similarities between insulin, IGF-1 and IGF-2 is given in Table 4.2. IGF-2 is the product of a single large, complex gene located on the short arm of chromosome 11, just downstream from the insulin gene. The IGF-2 gene is an imprinted gene, imprinting being a type of gene regulation in which only one of the parental alleles is expressed in a tissue- and developmental stage-specific manner.

IGF-2 does not behave in a classical endocrine fashion. Levels in humans are detectably high but not highly regulated, as is the case for IGF-1. IGF-2, like IGF-1 and in contrast to peptide hormones, is secreted soon after synthesis, with no storage phase. Its expression is influenced to a lesser extent by GH and nutritional status than IGF-1, and transcription is much more abundant in embryonic and fetal tissues, where it acts as a local growth factor to provide growth signals in a tissue-specific manner.

IGF-2-knockout mice have growth retardation confined to the in utero period, predominantly during

	IGF-1	IGF-2	Insulin
Molecular mass	7649 Da	7471 Da	5734 Da
Structure	One chain E-peptide cleaved	One chain E-peptide cleaved	Two chains C-peptide cleaved
Origin	Liver, ubiquitous	Liver, ubiquitous	β-cells of the pancreas
Secretion	Constant Slow-release	Constant Slow-release	Pulsatile
Production rate	10 mg/day$l$	13 mg/day$l$	2 mg/day$l$
Adult serum concentration	200 µg/l	700 µg/l	0.5–5 µg/l
Binding proteins	Yes µ	Yes µ	No µ
Daily variation	Little or none	Little or none	Yes
Half-life	12–15 h	15 h	10 min
Receptor affinity	Type 1>2>insulin	Type 2>1>insulin	Insulin>type 1
Action	Endocrine and local	Endocrine and local	Endocrine
GH dependence	++++	+	–

Table 4.2
Comparison between serum IGF-1, IGF-2 and insulin.

a brief period of early gestation. Postnatally, growth velocities are normal, but catch-up growth does not occur. IGF-2 overexpressing transgenic mice show no enhancement of somatic growth, even with markedly elevated circulating levels of IGF-2, the only abnormality to note being evident in tissues expressing the transgenes; for example, thymic enlargement occurs. However, these mice seem to develop multiple types of cancer with advancing age.[15]

The mechanism by which IGFs induce tumorigenesis is still not fully understood and may be mediated through overexpression of IGFs and the type I IGF receptor, although an etiological role has not been confirmed. Gene mutations occur spontaneously throughout life, resulting in damaged cells which are usually deleted by apoptosis, and the latter can be prevented by a number of external signals, of which IGF-1 is the most abundant and potent for many cell types. IGFBP-3 is the main carrier protein for IGF-1 and has independent apoptosis-promoting actions. The IGF-1–IGFBP-3 interaction, which is widespread throughout the body, may therefore play an important role in the balance of signals for cell survival and death, and therefore in whether damaged cells can survive to accumulate mutations and undergo malignant transformation.

IGFBP physiology

IGFBPs are a family of proteins which bind to IGFs with high affinity and specificity. Six proteins have been identified to date. IGFBPs potentially modulate IGF actions by prolonging their half-life, limiting free IGF and thus reducing IGF receptor binding, augmenting IGF actions by delivering IGFs to the cell surface as a steady stream, protecting them from degradation and regulating IGF passage into the extravascular space. In addition, IGFBPs have IGF-independent functions, which are mediated via their own receptors. Several enzymes capable of degrading IGFBPs by proteolytic cleavage have been identified, and these appear to have effects on IGF levels and actions. IGFBP-3 is primarily involved in growth, and it is the most abundant IGFBP in postnatal serum; its levels do not change acutely.

IGFBP-3

IGFBP-3 is the most abundant IGFBP in postnatal serum. Its gene is located on chromosome 7, adjacent to the *HoxA* gene, which encodes a DNA-binding protein.

IGFBP-3 is predominantly synthesized in the liver.[16] It is the major binding protein responsible for transporting IGF-1 in the circulation, and plays an important role in the regulation of IGF-1 action. Circulating levels of IGFBP-3, like those of IGF-1, are age dependent, being low at birth, increasing during childhood and peaking at puberty, and decreasing thereafter, but the postpubertal decline in IGFBP-3 precedes that of IGF-1. The serum levels of IGFBP-3 do not change acutely and are less affected by nutritional status than those of IGF-1.[17] The exact mechanism by which GH stimulates IGFBP-3 production is still under investigation. In vitro studies show that IGFBP-3 can decrease the stimulatory effects of IGF-1, generally by inhibiting receptor binding, because the affinity of IGF-1 for IGFBP-3 is higher than that for the IGF-1 receptor. In vitro studies have also shown that, in small amounts, IGFBP-3 can potentiate the effects of IGF-1, possibly by acting as a reservoir for IGF-1, providing a sustained release of IGF-1 for interaction with its receptor, and therefore preventing receptor downregulation.[18]

IGFBP-3 proteolysis is important in the regulation of IGF-1 action. Cleavage of IGFBP-3 decreases its affinity for IGF-1, leading to release of free IGF-1, allowing it to be transported to the extravascular space.

IGFBP proteases

The IGFBP proteases were first described in 1994 in pregnancy serum as proteolytic activity against IGFBP-3. Since then they have been described in many other circumstances and have been shown to cleave IGFBP-2–6 with varying degrees of affinity. At least three classes of proteases have been identified, including kallikreins, cathepsins and matrix metalloproteinases. The proteolysis of the IGFBPs is thought to play an integral part in the regulation of IGF action.[19] Fragmentation of IGFBPs decreases their affinity for IGFs, allowing release of free mitogenic IGF, which can be transported to the extra-vascular space. Further binding to IGFBPs occurs in the extravascular space, where again specific proteases can promote release of IGF at the tissue level.

IGF-independent actions of IGFBPs

IGFBP-I and IGFBP-3 have been shown to have IGF-independent functions, and these are also postulated for the other IGFBPs, several studies having drawn similar conclusions.[19]

IGFBP-3 has been shown to have an inhibitory action on synthesis of DNA by embryonic fibroblasts, even in the presence of high concentrations of insulin, which should provoke effects mediated through the type I IGF receptor. This suggests an inhibitory action independent of IGFs. It has also been shown, using a cell transfection system, that IGFBP-3 has independent inhibitory effects on cell growth.

> Congenital
>   Isolated GHD
>   Genetically inherited; usually recovers in adulthood; reassessment necessary
>   Genetically inherited; combined with other pituitary hormone deficiencies
>   Primary GH resistance syndromes
>   Normal or elevated levels of circulating GH (discussed below)
> Acquired
> Tumors
>   Pituitary
>   Craniopharyngioma
>   Meningiomas
>   Optic nerve gliomas
>   Secondary deposits, particularly breast, lung, reticuloses
> Infection
>   Tuberculous meningitis
>   Syphilis
>   Viral encephalitis
> Granulomas
>   Sarcoidosis
>   Histiocytosis X
> Vascular disease
>   Temporal arteritis
>   Carotid aneurysms
>   Vascular malformations
> Trauma
>   Basal skull fracture
> Iatrogenic
>   Surgery to the pituitary or surrounding structures
>   Radiotherapy
> Functional
>   Anorexia nervosa
>   Malnutrition
> Autoimmune
>   Lymphocytic hypophysitis
>   Lymphocytic infundibuloneuronitis

Table 4.3
Causes of adult GH deficiency/growth failure.

IGF-1 measurement

Historically, there were several problems with assay methodologies for IGFs, due to interference by IGFBPs. These have been largely addressed and are, at least in the majority of circumstances, no longer an issue. There has been a huge increase in the availability of commercial assays, though there remain standardization problems, making it difficult to compare studies carried out with different assays. There is still incomplete use of standard international reference preparations (IRPs). Binding protein assays are also more readily available, IGFBP-3 being used diagnostically and the others still largely as research tools. Recent exciting developments include the technology for measuring IGF/IGFBPs using blood spots immobilized on filter paper.[20] These will be much easier to take and transport for epidemiological studies, and will allow rapid assessment of adequate GH replacement in adult GH-deficient subjects (see below).

GH deficiency in adulthood
Causes

The major causes of GH deficiency (GHD) in adulthood include primary tumors (predominantly benign) in the region of the pituitary gland, parasellar and suprasellar regions, and treatments thereof, including surgery and radiotherapy.[21] Other, rarer, causes include granulomas, metastatic deposits and lymphocytic hypophysitis. Any cause of generalized pituitary disease will lead to GH deficiency relatively early in the disease. The true incidence of adult-onset GHD is not known, but estimates based on the incidence of pituitary tumors suggest an annual incidence of 10 people per million. Table 4.3 provides a list of causes of GHD/growth failure seen in adulthood, including those of childhood onset, many of which cause generalized pituitary disease.

Clinical characteristics

The recognition of adult-onset GHD as a specific clinical syndrome has resulted from a growing body of evidence describing its characteristics after detailed investigation of subjects with long-standing and severe deficiency of GH. Further evidence supporting the existence of this clinical syndrome has been obtained from placebo-controlled

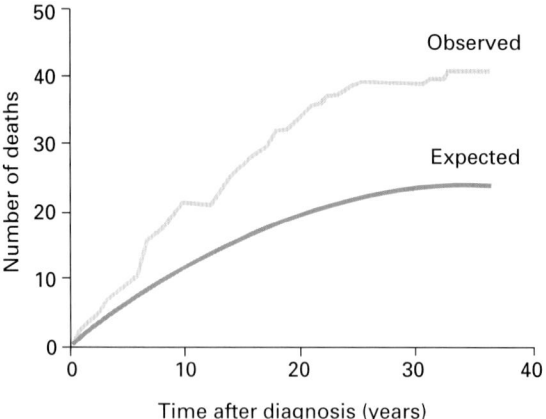

Figure 4.3
Cardiovascular mortality rate is increased in patients with GHD. (From Rosén and Bengtsson.[23])

4.3.[23-25] The syndrome is characterized by specific symptoms and signs, as well as biochemical and radiological abnormalities.

Psychological characteristics

Psychological health as assessed by validated general health questionnaires has been found to be impaired in subjects with adult-onset GHD as compared with age-, sex- and socio-economic class-matched controls.[26,27] Quality of life in these subjects has been shown to improve as assessed by such questionnaires after treatment with GH.[28-30] The benefits of treatment are illustrated in Figures 4.4 and 4.5. In addition to the general health questionnaires, a disease-specific questionnaire has been developed which has been found to be reliable and robust, particularly for assessment of response to treatment with GH replacement.[31] However, the symptom bias of subjects choosing to take part in randomized GH replacement studies[34] and the technical difficulties of enforcing a double-blind protocol in subjects who may exhibit obvious side-effects of an active treatment produces flaws in interpretation and validity of the results of such trials.

trials and open studies of the effects of replacement GH in these subjects which have recently been comprehensively reviewed by Carroll et al.[22] Furthermore, additional interest in adult onset GHD has arisen from studies suggesting that hypopituitary subjects, including those who have had all pituitary hormones except GH replaced, have a reduced life-expectancy, as illustrated in Figure

Body composition

The body composition of adults with GHD has been investigated in detail and, despite the widely varying methods used, a consistent finding has been that of a reduction in lean body mass of around 7%[35-39] and an increase in fat mass of a similar magnitude.[40-46] The

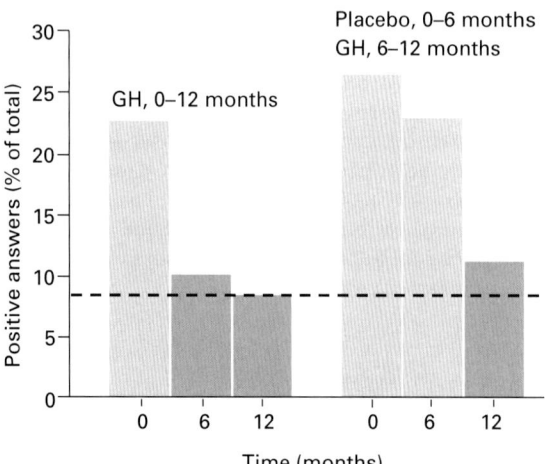

Figure 4.4
GH replacement therapy improves energy scores of the Nottingham Health Profile.

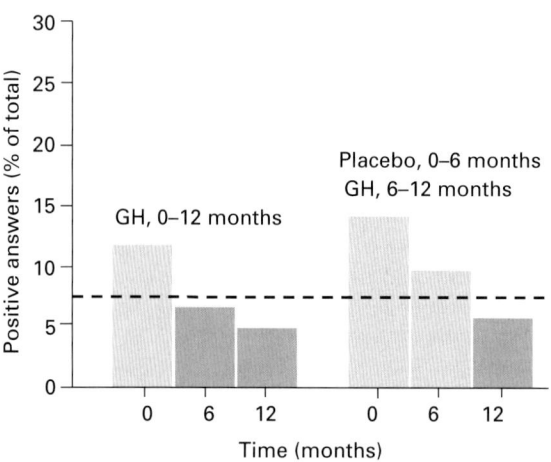

Figure 4.5
GH replacement improves emotional reaction scores of the Nottingham Health Profile.

GH DEFICIENCY IN ADULTHOOD

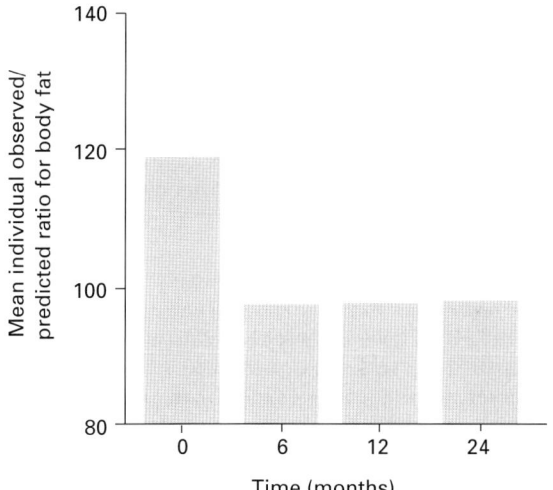

Figure 4.6
Two years of GH replacement therapy reduces body fat.

generally to significant levels.[36-39,41,45-53] The beneficial effects on fat mass are illustrated in Figure 4.6. Additionally, an increase in total body water, predominantly due to an increase in extracellular fluid volume, generally occurs in 3–5 days[40,47] and does not lead to a concurrent rise in blood pressure.[45,54]

Bone mineral density

Epidemiological studies have suggested an increased risk for osteoporotic fracture in subjects with both adult-onset and childhood-onset GHD. Further studies assessing bone mineral density have supported these findings by consistently demonstrating, despite the use of different techniques, reduced bone mass at different skeletal sites in subjects with adult-onset GHD when compared with matched control subjects.[55-57] These findings are reproduced on assessment of subjects with isolated GHD of childhood origin and deficiencies of mixed origin.

distribution of the excess adipose tissue in these individuals is predominantly abdominal and visceral, a finding which has been shown to be associated with premature mortality from cardiovascular disease.

The effects of GH treatment on body composition are unequivocal, with universal results showing an increased lean body mass, and a reduced fat mass,

The effects of GH replacement on bone mass in subjects with GHD seem to depend on length of administration as well as dose, and are reviewed in detail by Carroll et al.[22] Those studies investigating the effect of GH replacement over a 3–6-month period have shown no overall change in bone mass. Studies assessing GH effects over 6–12 months have shown a reduction in bone mass. An increase in bone density with GH treatment is only evident after 12 months of treatment, as demonstrated in Figures 4.7 and 4.8.

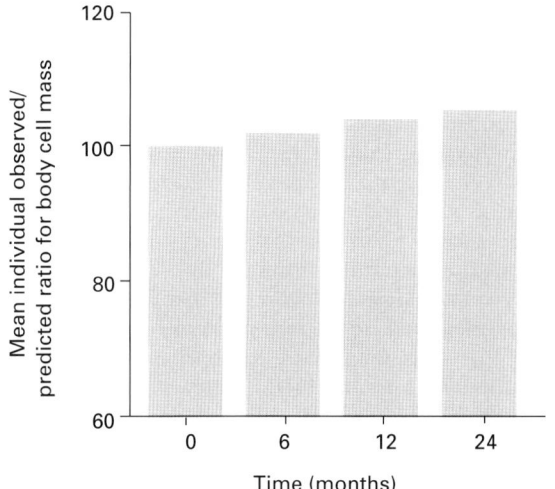

Figure 4.7
Two years of GH replacement therapy increases bone mineral density in the lumbar spine (L2–L4).

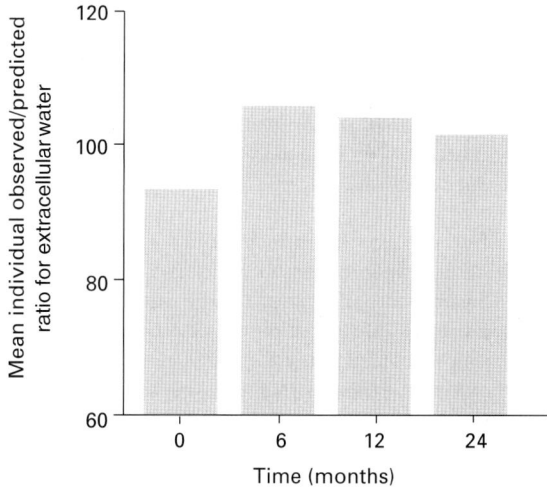

Figure 4.8
Two years of GH replacement therapy increases bone mineral density in the femoral neck.

91

These beneficial effects appear to continue with prolonged treatment, being most marked in subjects with the lowest initial bone mass.[58] The early transient reduction in bone mass in GH-treated subjects may be explained by an expansion of the 'remodeling space' resulting from the increased bone turnover.[59]

Muscle strength and exercise performance

The reduction in lean body mass, which appears to be universal in adult GHD, results in a reduction in muscle strength of a mild to moderate degree. This effect has been demonstrated by comparing isometric quadriceps force in adult GHD subjects with that of age- and sex-matched normal controls.[60,61] The effects of GH replacement in GHD subjects have been documented in several studies.[22] Thigh muscle cross-sectional area increases and limb girdle force has been shown to increase after 6 months of GH replacement; however, isometric quadriceps force and quadriceps torque have not been shown to increase until at least 12 months of GH replacement, but after 3 years of GH replacement these characteristics have been shown to normalize.[50]

Exercise performance is reduced in adults with GHD, even allowing for a reduction in muscle mass as confirmed by increased shoulder fatigability and reduced quadriceps force.[60] Several studies have assessed maximal exercise performance using cycle ergometry before and after GH replacement. Exercise performance improves significantly after 6 months of GH replacement, but this improvement appears to be solely the result of the increased muscle mass rather than any improvement in cardiovascular performance.[62]

Cardiovascular performance

The association of long-standing severe GHD with premature cardiovascular mortality is well documented in the epidemiological setting. Recent studies have supported this association by showing an increased risk of death in hypopituitary subjects as compared with their healthy neighbors, with the excess mortality predominantly due to cardiovascular disease.[25] GHD has been proposed as being the prime contributor to the excess mortality in these subjects. However, the exact mechanism of excess cardiovascular mortality is unknown. It is associated with a higher body mass index, higher plasma triglycerides, lower high-density lipoprotein cholesterol fractions and higher blood pressure when compared with normal subjects.[63] GHD is also associated with a reduced left ventricular mass with impaired systolic function compared with matched control subjects which is fully reversible with 6 months of GH replacement, although recurrence of these abnormalities occurs within 6 months of stopping replacement therapy.[41,64] With prolonged GH replacement (up to 3 years), the beneficial effects of therapy appear to continue.[65] However, the long-term effects of GH replacement on these subjects are unknown.

Metabolism

Resting energy expenditure is largely dependent on lean body mass and has been shown to be reduced in adult GHD. However, once the reduction in lean body mass in these subjects is controlled for, it is unclear whether resting energy expenditure is affected by GHD, as the results of published studies are conflicting.[39,66] GH replacement in GHD subjects results in an increased level of circulating triiodothyronine (T3) in euthyroid subjects and those receiving thyroxine replacement.[36] This suggests that GH is a physiological regulator of thyroid function, with a specific role in the peripheral conversion of thyroxine to T3.

Adult GHD subjects have altered protein metabolism, with reduced protein flux and synthesis. The effect of GH replacement is transient; protein synthesis is increased during the first 6 months, and thereafter returns to baseline rates.[22]

Adult GHD appears to induce a state of hyperinsulinemia and insulin resistance.[68] These characteristics produce the classic central obesity associated with adult GHD. GH replacement in the first few weeks of therapy appears to exacerbate insulin resistance. Carbohydrate metabolism, however, normalizes after 3 months of therapy.[68]

Studies investigating the effects of adult GHD on lipoprotein metabolism and the effects of GH replacement in these subjects have confirmed that GH is involved in hepatic lipoprotein metabolism and may influence the lipoprotein profiles seen in subjects with adult GHD.[22] Further long-term studies will be required to determine whether the restoration of a more physiological lipoprotein profile with GH replacement will prevent the premature atherosclerosis and therefore the excess cardiovascular mortality associated with adult GHD.

Skin

The skin in GHD adults is described as dry and thin. The capacity to secrete sweat is reduced, particularly during exercise or heat stress.[69] This feature may contribute to the impaired exercise performance in these subjects.

Immune system

Animal studies suggest a role for IGF-1 in the regulation of cell-mediated and humoral immunity. There is, however, no evidence that adults with GHD have impaired immunity.

Diagnosis

With evidence demonstrating the probable increased morbidity and mortality associated with adult GHD and an increasing body of evidence demonstrating reversal of many of the detrimental features of adult GHD with treatment with human GH, there has been an increasing consensus to treat all such subjects. However, a major setback in the management of these subjects has been confirmation of the deficiency by laboratory methods. This problem is primarily due to the fact that varying degrees of deficiency exist and that assays vary considerably between laboratories.

Because of the diagnostic dilemmas faced by clinicians managing adult subjects with possible GHD, a GH research society workshop was set up in 1997 in order to provide a consensus statement for the diagnosis and treatment of adult GHD.[70] The workshop report suggested that an appropriate definition of adult GHD should include biochemical and clinical characteristics and should only be made in subjects with predisposing risk factors. These include subjects with evidence of hypothalamo–pituitary disease, those who have previously received cranial irradiation, and those with childhood-onset GHD who require reassessment.

In generalized hypothalamo–pituitary disease, the likelihood of GHD increases with the number of other pituitary hormone deficiencies (Figure 4.9). Subjects without appropriate risk factors should not be evaluated for GHD, to prevent false-positive results.

A biochemical diagnosis should be confirmed by provocative testing in a subject who has had other hormone deficits fully replaced. Currently, the provocative test of choice is the insulin stress test (IST), which, provided that adequate hypoglycemia is achieved, is able to distinguish between true GHD and the reduced GH secretion which accompanies certain conditions, including aging (Figure 4.10). A normal response to IST involves inducing hypoglycemia to a laboratory glucose level of less than 2.0 mmol/l, and results in a peak GH of greater than 15 mU/l (5 mg/l) using polyclonal competitive radioimmunoassay. Severe GHD is defined as a peak GH of less than 9 mU/l (3 mg/l). Inter-laboratory variation in methodology will give rise to variation in diagnostic thresholds. The IST is contraindicated in certain circumstances, including a history of epilepsy, known ischemic heart disease, an abnormal electrocardiogram, untreated hypothyroidism and hypocortisolism, and it should be used with caution in the elderly. Various alternative stimulatory tests are available; however, their diagnostic value is less well established. All second-line tests work on the principle of stimulating GH release, and include glucagon, arginine, L-DOPA, clonidine, pyridostigmine and GHRH tests. Clonidine is less useful in adults than in children. Adults with hypothalamo–pituitary disease

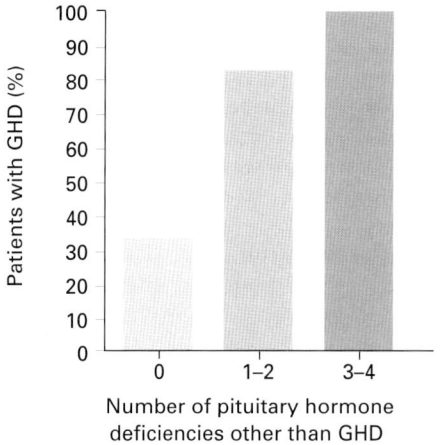

Figure 4.9
Patients with other pituitary hormone deficiencies are more likely to be GH deficient. (From Sönksen et al.[110])

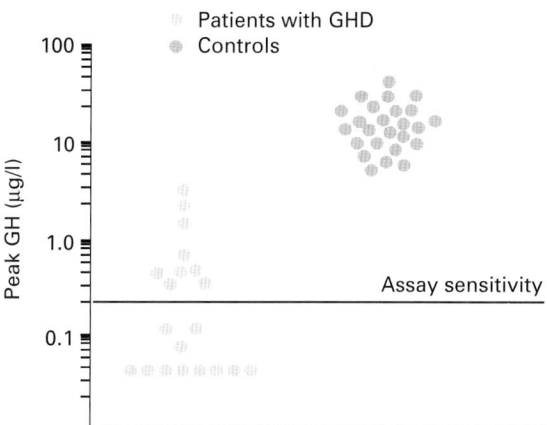

Figure 4.10
The insulin tolerance test is the test of choice in the diagnosis of adult GHD. (From Hoffman et al.[71])

and one or more other pituitary hormone deficiencies require only one positive provocation test of GH secretion for the diagnosis of GHD. Childhood-onset GHD requires reconfirmation in adulthood. Other biochemical markers of GH action such as IGF-1, although useful as supportive evidence of GHD and in assessing response to treatment, do vary with age and are not of proven benefit in establishing a diagnosis of adult GHD (Figures 4.11 and 4.12). They should therefore be used in this context with caution.[71]

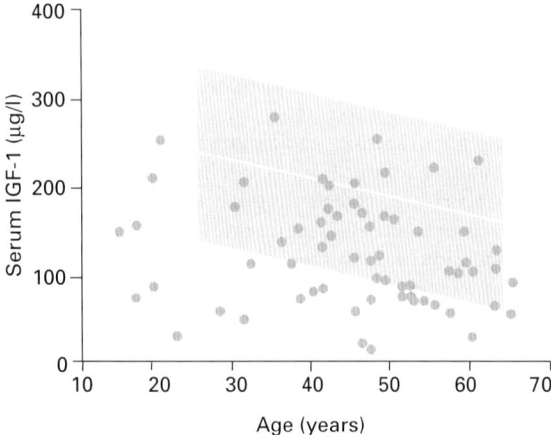

Figure 4.11
Serum IGF-I concentrations in women with GHD. (From Svensson et al.[111])

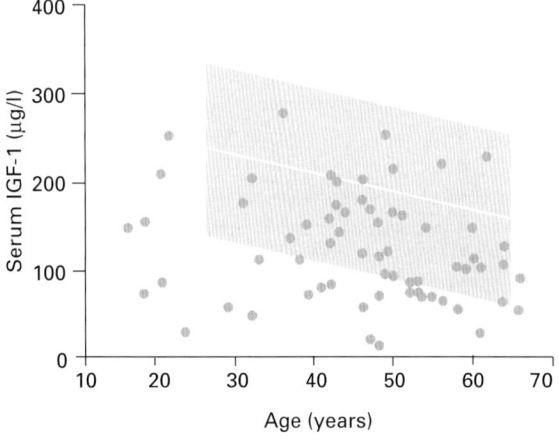

Figure 4.12
Serum IGF-1 concentrations in men with GHD. (From Svensson et al.[111])

Treatment

Subjects who fulfill the criteria for severe GHD on dynamic testing should receive GH replacement therapy as a single subcutaneous injection daily. In order to minimize side-effects while obtaining maximum benefit of treatment, a low initial dose of 1.0 iu or 0.3 mg/day should be used, and thereafter the dose may be titrated up at monthly intervals, depending on clinical and biochemical response. The dose rarely needs to exceed 0.6 mg/day. The response to GH therapy in adults with GHD varies considerably. Generally, the response with regard to serum IGF-1 concentrations is significantly lower in females than in males with GHD, which could at least partly be explained by the use of estrogen replacement therapy. The mechanism is not well understood, but higher concentrations of estrogen in the liver after oral ingestion of estrogen might inhibit IGF-1 secretion and alter exogenous GH requirements. Women on oral hormone replacement therapy have been shown to require higher doses of GH than women using transdermal preparations, which is an important financial consideration.[72] In a recent study, serum estrone levels significantly decreased, serum sex hormone-binding globulin levels significantly decreased, and serum estradiol levels also decreased, albeit non-significantly, whereas serum IGF-1 levels significantly increased, after a switch from oral to transdermal estrogen therapy.[73] Further investigation is necessary to answer the question of whether the increase in serum IGF-1 levels with transdermal estrogen therapy is due to lower serum levels of estradiol or to differences in the mode of administration of estradiol.

An initial assessment for consideration of GH replacement should include physical examination, including blood pressure, and blood should be analyzed for glucose, glycated hemoglobin, lipid, liver and renal profiles. Other baseline tests include ECG and bone mineral density scan. Treatment should be monitored by regular medical assessment, including full physical examination. Follow-up by an endocrinologist with an interest in pituitary disease is desirable. Quality-of-life questionnaires are often used. Biochemical markers of success of treatment are of value, particularly in assessing over-replacement, the most robust marker being IGF-1. IGFBP-3 is also used. These markers of treatment are particularly useful in assessing initial dose titration and can be checked monthly during this period. Once a steady dose is achieved, these markers should be measured at annual or biannual review, as dose requirements may change (usually reduce) with time and the treatment is usually lifelong.

The benefit of GH replacement therapy in GHD subjects is now unequivocal, and its widespread use is only limited by cost.

Side-effect profile

Recombinant human GH should only result in side-effects in supraphysiological doses, as it is identical to natural human GH. The most common side-effect noted by treated subjects is attributable to salt and water retention, including dependent edema, tightness of the hands, carpal tunnel syndrome and weight gain. Also reported are arthralgia and myopathy. All these side-effects appear to improve with dose reduction and are usually attributable to excess dosage. Other side-effects reported in adults treated with GH are hypertension and atrial fibrillation, but these are extremely rare.[36] There is no evidence that GH therapy exacerbates tumor growth in adulthood, and data for tumors in childhood show no increased risk of recurrence. However, absolute contraindications to therapy include active malignancy, intracranial hypertension, and preproliferative and proliferative diabetic retinopathy. GH therapy should be discontinued in the second trimester of pregnancy, as a GHV is produced by the placenta.

Data regarding the long-term safety of GH replacement therapy are accumulating in the Pharmacia and Upjohn international database (KIMS) and the Eli Lilly database (HYPOCCS), which have thus far provided reassurance, with no unexpected adverse events observed to date and low discontinuation rates.

GH—other potential therapeutic uses

GH treatment of critical illness

In the acute phases of critical illness, circulating levels of GH are elevated, with high basal levels and attenuated peak levels, with low concomitant levels of serum IGF-1.[74] This picture may be interpreted as indicating a state of GH resistance. In the chronic phase of critical illness the pattern of GH secretion changes with reduced amplitude but increased frequency of pulses, with basal levels that are not undetectable but with resulting low mean GH levels. This diverse pathophysiological response to critical illness may explain the so far lack of demonstrable response of subjects with acute critical illness to treatment with GH and, in contrast, the promising results of initial studies of treatment of subjects in the chronic phase of critical illness with GH secretagogs. Outcome studies are awaited. However, intercurrent acute illness such as intercurrent sepsis may complicate the chronic phase of critical illness, giving rise to a paradoxical GH response, and the inevitability of this mixed picture in some critically ill patients may be responsible for discrepancies in results of previously published and forthcoming interventional studies.[75] One particular concern is that a large (unpublished) European multicenter trial of GH therapy in intensive-care patients had to be terminated early because of an increased mortality in the GH-treated patients as compared with the placebo-treated subjects. This rather dramatic finding has led to a great deal of reflection on the role of GH in the treatment of catabolic states. However, this study was criticized on several counts, including the large, non-physiological doses of GH used, which may well have been relevant to the adverse outcomes.

GH treatment of chronic fatigue syndrome (CFS)

CFS is a common condition with an unknown etiology, and disturbed neuroendocrine function is one possible hypothesis for its pathogenesis. A small number of studies have assessed GH secretion in subjects with CFS, and only one study has demonstrated a statistically significantly reduced peak GH response to insulin-induced hypoglycemia.[76] Impaired GH secretory function may therefore be associated with CFS, but the results of further studies are awaited. GH treatment as a therapeutic option has been attempted in a 12-week study of CFS patients with low peak GH levels during stage-controlled sleep. In this study, quality of life did not improve significantly.[77]

GH neurosecretory dysfunction

This is the descriptive term used to describe a spectrum of individuals who have poor growth and short stature, and who have normal GH responses to stimulatory testing but low IGF-1 levels and low 24-h serum GH levels. It has therefore been assumed that these subjects have insufficiency of spontaneous GH secretion due to neuroendocrine abnormalities in spite of a normal releasable pool of GH. There is an association with prior cranial irradiation. A subgroup of these subjects may benefit from treatment with recombinant human GH.[78] There is no association with idiopathic short stature, where 24-h serum GH levels as well as stimulatory tests of GH secretion are normal.

GH resistance syndromes

The GH resistance syndromes comprise a group of conditions in which failure of GH action occurs despite normal or high circulating levels of immunoreactive GH of endogenous or exogenous origin. Primary causes of this GH resistance or insensitivity (GHI) are due to GH receptor deficiency (GHRD), GH–GH-receptor signal transduction defects, IGF-1 gene defect, or deficiency or defective IGF-1–IGF-receptor signal transduction. An example of a rare cause of primary GHI has been described in a family with normal GH and IGFBP-3 levels but very low IGF-1 levels, thought to be due to a post-receptor defect.[79] This family possessed the clinical characteristics of severe GHD. However, another recently described defect of the IGF-1 gene was associated with severe intra-uterine growth retardation and mental retardation.[80]

Improved understanding of these disorders is allowing increasing understanding of the physiology and pathophysiology of GH action. Secondary causes of GHI include GH-inhibiting antibodies, malnutrition, diabetes and uremia. GHI due to GHRD only will be discussed here.

Laron syndrome

The commonest cause of primary GHI is GH receptor deficiency or Laron syndrome, first described by Laron and co-workers in 1966. There are now over 200 cases reported worldwide. Ninety per cent of reported cases are of Middle-East, Mediterranean or Indian subcontinent extraction, and there is a high frequency of consanguinity in the families of the probands.

The underlying molecular defects giving rise to the clinical phenotype of GHI are markedly heterogeneous. Homozygosity or compound heterozygosity for point mutations or major deletions of the extracellular domain of the GH receptor gene have been identified in subjects with the characteristic phenotype of Laron syndrome.[81–83] Because of the involvement of the extracellular domain of the GH receptor, these subjects, as expected, have reduced serum GHBP activity.[84] There are also reports of a mutation involving exons usually encoding the transmembrane and intracellular domains of the GH receptor.[85] In this situation, the mutant GH receptor is unable to anchor in the cell membrane, and serum concentrations of GHBP are therefore elevated in these individuals.

The majority of reports suggest an equal sex distribution, an exception being a report of 20 subjects from Loja province in southern Ecuador with a strongly female preponderance.[86] Overall, GHRD is thought to be an autosomal, fully penetrant recessive condition, the explanation for the Lojanean female predominance of probands being an association between GHRD and a trait lethal for the male fetus in this population.

The birthweight and length of the probands are normal, and as IGF-1 is essential for intrauterine growth, this indicates that intrauterine IGF-1 synthesis is not GH dependent.

At birth, although the overall size is normal, distinctive phenotypic characteristics can be identified by the informed eye. The nasal bridge is hypoplastic, the orbits are shallow and the vertical dimensions of the face are reduced. The hands and feet are small and the fingernails hypoplastic. There is an association with blue sclera, unilateral ptosis and facial asymmetry.

Growth velocity is reduced from birth and is 50% of normal, indicating that growth from birth is GH dependent. Poor longitudinal growth is associated with low serum IGF-1, IGF-2 and IGFBP-3, and there is no correlation with non-affected first-degree relatives, indicating that the heterozygous state does not confer any partial resistance to GH.

There is sparse hair in early childhood, with frontotemporal recession later in all probands. Bone age is delayed, but advanced for height. Reduced muscle mass leading to delayed motor milestones occurs in 70%, although cognition is normal. There is an increased incidence of avascular necrosis of the femoral head and congenital hip dislocation (25% and 5% respectively). Limited elbow extension occurs in the majority. Children tend to be underweight for height. High random GH levels with exaggerated response to stimulation tests are found in childhood.

Puberty is delayed by 3–7 years in about 50% of probands, but normal secondary sexual characteristics and normal reproductive capacity are expected.

In males, the penis is small in childhood but becomes normal for body size in adulthood. In adulthood, there is a prominent forehead and a large head size, out of proportion with the short stature. There is reduced upper and lower arm span and small hands and feet in the majority. Adults are usually overweight for height, with a reduced lean body mass. There is osteopenia despite normal sex hormone status. There is a tendency towards hypoglycemia in all ages, an increase in total cholesterol due to an increase in the LDL subfraction, and decreased sweating. In adulthood, the GH levels are normal but there is an exaggerated response to stimulation tests. Characteristically reduced levels of IGF-1, IGF-2 and IGFBP-3 occur, with higher levels in adults than in children, and markedly elevated levels of IGFBP-1 and IGFBP-2 occur, with lower levels in adults than in children. GHBP is markedly reduced in most cases, although GHBP-positive GHRD has been reported.[87]

IGF-1 treatment

Studies are underway assessing the short- and long-term effects of recombinant human IGF-1 (rhIGF-1) treatment. A major pitfall of its administration in these subjects has been the incidence of hypoglycemia after intravenous administration, which is likely to be due to the coexisting deficiency of IGFBP-3 allowing rapid delivery of IGF-1 to the tissues in the absence of its major carrier protein. The absence of IBFBP-3 also theoretically means more rapid clearance of the rhIGF-1, leading to a blunted therapeutic effect. Hypoglycemia is much less likely to occur with treatment with rhIGF-1 in normal subjects. However, treatment of children with GHRD with subcutaneous rhIGF-1 has been assessed with double-blind placebo-controlled trials and has shown some promising results.[88] However, IGFBP-3 levels have not been shown to rise with rhIGF-1 therapy, either in the short or long term, and it is possible that the improvements in growth in the actively treated subjects may simply represent improved nutrition. Side-effects of rhIGF-1 treatment include parotid swelling, lymphoid hyperplasia, papilledema and benign intracranial hypertension as well as pain at the injection site.

IGF and cancer epidemiology

Gene mutations occur spontaneously throughout life; however, the resulting damaged cells are usually deleted by apoptosis, one of the body's sophisticated protective mechanisms. Apoptosis can be prevented by a number of external signals, of which IGF-1 is the most abundant and potent for many cell types. IGFBP-3, the main carrier protein for IGF-1, has independent apoptosis-promoting actions on breast and prostate epithelial cells.[89,90] The IGF-1–IGFBP-3 interaction, which is widespread throughout the body, may therefore play an important role in the balance of signals for cell survival and death and, moreover, in whether damaged cells can survive to accumulate mutations and undergo malignant transformation.

Therapeutic manipulation of the IGF system by administration of exogenous GH or IGF-1 has previously been argued to be safe, as, historically, acromegaly has not been thought to be associated with an increase in cancer incidence. There is now a consensus opinion that the colonic cancer mortality rate is increased in acromegaly. A recent large survey has shown a non-significant increase in colonic cancer incidence but a significant increase in colonic cancer mortality rate in acromegaly.[91]

The perturbation of the IGF system in subjects with cancer has previously been attributed to the cancer itself. There is now emerging evidence from prospective studies of an association between the plasma concentration of IGF-1 and prostate and breast cancer incidence.[92,93] Early data suggest a possible etiological association between circulating IGF-2 and IGFBP-2 levels and colorectal tumors.[94] There is growing evidence that the IGF system is critical in maintaining neoplastic growth. The reports linking IGF-1 with breast and prostate cancer incidence also indicate a negative association between cancer risk and IGFBP-3 concentrations, so that those at greatest cancer risk appear to be those with high IGF-1 and low IGFBP-3.

Many subjects with adult GHD do not have low IGF-1 concentrations, and treatment with GH often raises these levels to the upper end of the normal range or above. However, in this situation, the IGFBP-3 levels are also elevated, as is the case in acromegaly. IGFBP-3 may therefore play a protective role, and this may explain why high IGF-1 concentrations in acromegaly do not appear to be associated with a markedly increased risk of development of cancers and why there has so far been no evidence of any association between GH replacement and cancer incidence.

The effect of drugs which alter the balance between IGF-1 and IGFBP-3 could therefore be used therapeutically in the treatment and prevention of cancers. Certain estrogen antagonists appear to work in this way, and are already used in the treatment of breast cancers.[95] Their preventative use in subjects at high risk is currently being studied.

The emerging association between IGF concentrations and cancer incidence remains, despite theoretical mechanisms, largely unexplained, and further research into this area is ongoing and imperative to enable future strategies for cancer treatment and prevention.

Missed childhood growth disorders leading to adult short stature (Table 4.4)

Turner syndrome (syndrome of gonadal dysgenesis)

First described by Turner in 1938, this clinical syndrome is now a well-recognized clinical entity. However, the classical features may be subtle, due to the presence of lesser degrees of sex chromosome deficiency, so that the syndrome of gonadal dysgenesis is viewed as a continuum ranging from the classical Turner phenotype to that of a normal female or male. The diagnosis may therefore be delayed, and the affected subject may present with primary amenorrhea in early adulthood.

The growth disorder associated with the Turner phenotype will be discussed here, as adult short stature is inevitable without intervention, and therapeutic treatment is now available to enhance final adult height. Growth failure begins in utero. The growth retardation is evident by the middle of the second trimester of gestation and affects all the long bones.[96] The average birthweight and length are one standard deviation below the mean for normal infants of comparable gestational age. For the first 3 years of life, growth velocity is usually within the normal range. Thereafter, growth velocities decelerate, so that by a bone age of 9 years, the difference in mean height between affected and non-affected individuals is close to the difference at maturity.[97] The mean final height correlates with birthweight and target height and ranges from 142 to 147 cm.[98]

Although overt deficiency of GH is not associated with Turner syndrome, decreased amplitude and frequency of GH pulses have been reported after 8 years of age, IGF-1 levels being normal up to the age of ten years, but low thereafter. Administration of estrogen or GH will induce a rise in plasma IGF-1 level. The changes in GH secretory dynamics and IGF-1 concentrations after the age of 8–10 years are thought to be secondary to the absence of the estrogen-induced rise in plasma GH concentration and IGF-1 levels at puberty. However, the progressive growth failure seen in Turner syndrome is not specifically attributable to a deficiency of any hormone. The cause is incompletely understood, but is thought to be attributable at least in part to the missing *PARI*, *PHOG* or *SHOX* genes on the absent or structurally abnormal second sex chromosome.[97]

Although specific hormonal deficiencies are not causal for the growth failure associated with Turner syndrome, there are clearly characterized abnormalities of growth axis hormonal dynamics. This observation has resulted in extensive manipulation of the growth axis in therapeutic trials in an attempt to enhance final adult height. Treatment with oxandrolone has given rise to conflicting reports, and although short-term improvements in growth velocity have been reported, final adult height has been found to be either

---

Hypothyroidism
Hypogonadism
Isolated gonadotropin deficiency (Kallmann's syndrome)
Male primary hypogonadism (Kleinfelter's syndrome)
Cushing's syndrome
Pseudohypoparathyroidism
Rickets
Osteochondrodysplasias
Down's syndrome
CAH
Laron syndrome
Precocious puberty
Pseudoprecocious puberty
Chronic disease
Secondary causes of GHI include GH-inhibiting antibodies, malnutrition, diabetes and uremia
Turner syndrome
Noonan syndrome

CAH. congenital adrenal hyperplasia.

Table 4.4
Childhood growth disorders resulting in adult short stature.

unchanged or to show a very modest gain. Therapeutic trials of low-dose estrogens have generally been unsuccessful, with unchanged or reduced final adult height. Treatment with recombinant human GH (rhGH) accelerates growth in Turner syndrome, and beneficial effects on final adult height have been found in several studies.[98–104] Some of these trials showed a specific benefit of combined therapy with oxandrolone.[101,104] As an example of benefit quantification, in one study six girls with Turner syndrome would need to be treated with GH starting at 12 or 13 years of age for a period of 3–4 years in order for one girl's final adult height to improve by at least 5 cm.[105]

In summary, early commencement of treatment with rhGH gives rise to the best results in terms of final adult height achieved in Turner syndrome, possibly in combination with oxandrolone. The addition of estrogens to treat the primary gonadal failure should be left as late as possible, as these are associated with cessation of growth.

Noonan syndrome

Noonan syndrome is a common form of familial short stature; the phenotypic characteristics are similar to those of Turner syndrome, but the chromosomes are normal. Features include short stature in 70%, micrognathia, and cardiac defects; the most notable cardiac defect is pulmonary stenosis, but any cardiac defect may occur, and hypertrophic cardiomyopathy (HOCM) is well recognized. Postnatal growth in Noonan syndrome is reviewed in detail elsewhere.[105] Birthweight is normal, and thereafter the growth curve follows the 3rd to 5th centile through childhood. Late puberty is a persistent feature in both sexes; however, gonadotropin deficiency has not been recognized. The final adult height achieved in both sexes is close to the 3rd centile. The pathogenesis of short stature is not well understood. Skeletal and growth plate abnormalities have been hypothesized, and there may be growth plate resistance to the effects of GH. Few studies of GH treatment in Noonan syndrome have been undertaken, and none have been randomized or controlled. These are reviewed in detail by Dunger and Mohn.[106] Low-dose GH regimens are unsuccessful, possibly due to relative GH resistance, and higher-dose regimens have given more promising results; however, these studies are relatively short term, and results on final adult height are predominantly still awaited. A major concern in this group is the GH effect on left ventricular wall thickness, in view of the association of Noonan syndrome with HOCM. No adverse cardiac events have been reported thus far; however, the effects of GH treatment in patients with early evidence of HOCM have not been specifically studied.

Hypothyroidism

The development of newborn screening programs for the detection of congenital hypothyroidism has resulted in prompt diagnosis and treatment of these subjects, and growth in appropriately treated subjects is normal. The features of hypothyroidism in older children can be subtle, and the typical symptoms seen in adulthood are often absent. Moreover, the cardinal feature seen in childhood is growth failure. However, this may take several years to become clinically evident, not least because the poor growth is more apparent in height than weight, and the affected children tend to be overweight in relation to height. Body proportions are immature, with an increased upper/lower body segment ratio. Skeletal age is usually markedly reduced. Failure to make a diagnosis results in delayed puberty, and primary amenorrhea may be a presenting feature. Loss of height may be permanent if the diagnosis is delayed, even though growth may continue for a longer period with thyroxine treatment.[107] Catch-up growth may be particularly compromised when therapy is initiated near puberty.[108] In these circumstances, it may be more appropriate to use lower than usual replacement doses of thyroxine or to consider a pharmacological delay of puberty and epiphyseal fusion, or both.

Congenital adrenal hyperplasia (CAH)

Non-classical forms of CAH due to 21-hydroxylase deficiency include asymptomatic as well as 'late-onset' symptomatic forms. The latter may present in females with precocious puberty and symptoms of androgen excess in early childhood. Accelerated linear growth and bone maturation usually lead to short stature unless the diagnosis is made promptly. In adult females, the late-onset variant may be difficult clinically to differentiate from polycystic ovarian syndrome, and in males the late-onset variant may result in oligospermia and decreased fertility.

Overgrowth syndromes (Table 4.5)

The commonest syndrome of overgrowth is acromegaly due to an excess production of pituitary GH, usually by a somatotrope tumor of the pituitary gland. A number of overgrowth syndromes have now been identified which arise from genetic defects due to a putative imbalance between the relative contributions of growth-promoting genes and growth-inhibiting genes in specific tissues at critical developmental stages.

Beckwith–Wiedemann syndrome (BWS) is a human overgrowth syndrome with a complex genetic etiology. It is caused by abnormal variations in chromosome 11p15, which is a region subject to genomic imprinting. The abnormal changes at this site result in increased expression of IGF-2. Genomic imprinting is a type of gene regulation in which only one of the two parental alleles is expressed in a tissue- and developmental stage-specific manner. There are six known imprinted genes on chromosome 11p15, and these include the IGF-2 gene and the H19 gene. H19 is a non-translated mRNA, which may be a tumor suppressor gene and can function as an imprintor of IGF-2. BWS is characterized by fetal macrosomia with omphalocele. There is also renal medullary hyperplasia, neonatal hypoglycemia with islet cell hyperplasia, and excess fetal, neonatal and childhood growth. Early epiphyseal fusion occurs, leading to no increase in adult height. There is an increased risk of embryonal tumors.[109]

Simpson–Golabi–Behmel syndrome is an x-linked overgrowth syndrome phenotypically similar to BWS but genetically distinct. It is caused by alterations in glypican-3 (GPC3), which is a molecule which may interact with IGF-2 and also p57KIP2, which is another gene product on chromosome 11p15 identified as being important in the BWS phenotype.[109]

Insulin resistance syndromes

These will be mentioned briefly here, in view of the fact that they represent a group of disorders comprising hyperinsulinism, and as such represent a type of growth disorder encountered in adulthood. However, detailed description of these syndromes is out of the scope of this chapter. The association of hyperandrogenism, severe insulin resistance and acanthosis nigricans constitutes a specific subset of polycystic ovarian syndrome (PCOS). A number of syndromes are associated with this triad.

Type A insulin resistance syndrome is characterized by the clinical features of PCOS in the absence of obesity or lipoatrophy and incorporates a heterogeneous group of disorders due to different mutations in the insulin receptor gene. It is distinguished from type B insulin resistance by a lack of antibodies to the insulin receptor or other evidence of autoimmune disease.

Type B insulin resistance syndrome is an autoimmune condition characterized by moderate to severe hyperandrogenism, very high insulin levels and detectable insulin antibodies. Other insulin resistance syndromes include Leprechaunism, Rabson–Mendenhall syndrome and lipoatrophic diabetes mellitus.

Perspective

It was previously thought that GH was functionally useful only in childhood growth, becoming superfluous in adulthood.

Over the last two decades, a wealth of information has emerged regarding the role of GH and growth factors in adult health and disease. Evidence has been produced indicating negative health effects in adult subjects with GH deficiency and associated abnormalities of the IGF system. Furthermore, GH and IGF functional abnormalities in childhood and adulthood may also have deleterious effects on physical and psychiatric health, which could be reversed by correction or treatment of the underlying defect.

Treatment of growth disorders, as with any therapeutic treatment, is not without risks, and careful study of treatment regimens and patient follow-up are still ongoing to investigate long-term effects.

Acromegaly
Simpson–Golabi–Behmel syndrome
Klippel–Trenaunay–Weber syndrome
Nevo syndrome
Beckwith–Wiedemann syndrome
Perlman syndrome
Proteus syndrome

Table 4.5
Overgrowth syndromes

The area of GH and growth factor research in adulthood is a contemporary field, and the important evidence emerging needs to be followed by evidence-based practice with appropriate investigation, treatment and follow-up of adult patients affected by growth disorders.

References

1. Frankenna F, Closset J, Gomez F et al. The physiology of growth hormones (GHs) in pregnant women and partial characterisation of the placental GH variant. *JCE&M* 1988; 66: 1171–80.
2. Martinez-Rodriguez HG, Guerra-Rodriguez NE, Iturbe-Cantu MA, Martinez-Torres A, Barrera-Saldana HA. Expression of human placental lactogen and variant growth hormone genes in placentas. *Arch Med Res* 1997; 28(4): 507–12.
3. Baumann G, Amburn KD, Buchanan TA. The effect of circulating growth hormone-binding protein on metabolic clearance, distribution, and degradation of human growth hormone. *JCE&M* 1987; 64: 657–60.
4. Frohman LA, Jansson J-O. Growth hormone-releasing hormone. *Endocrine Rev* 1986; 7: 223–53.
5. Shen LP, Picket RL, Rutter WJ. Human somatostatin I: sequence of the cDNA. *Proc Natl Acad Sci USA* 1982; 79: 4575–9.
6. Patel YC, Greenwood MT, Panetta R et al. The somatostatin receptor family: a mini review. *Life Sci* 1995; 57: 1249–65.
7. Ghogo E, Arvat E, Muccioli G, Camanni F. Growth hormone-releasing peptides. *Eur J Endocrinol* 1997; 136: 445–60.
8. Ghogo E, Arvat E, Gianotti L et al. Growth hormone-releasing activity of hexarelin, a new synthetic hexapeptide, after intravenous, subcutaneous, intranasal and oral administration in man. *JCE&M* 1994; 78: 693–8.
9. Rahim A, Shalet SM. Does desensitization to hexarelin occur? *Growth Horm IGF Res* 1998; 8: 141–3.
10. Jones JL, Clemmons DR. Insulin-like growth factors and their binding proteins: biological actions. *Endocrine Rev* 1995; 16(1): 3–34.
11. Hasegawa T, Cohen P, Rosenfeld RG. Characterisation of the insulin-like growth factor axis in TM Leydig cells. *Growth Regul* 1995; 5: 151–9.
12. Rotwein P, Bichell DP, Kilkuchi K. Multifactorial regulation of IGF-1 gene expression. *Mol Reprod Dev* 1993; 35(4): 358–63.
13. LeRoith D, Werner H, Beitner-Johnson D, Roberts CT Jr. Molecular and cellular aspects of the insulin-like growth factor I receptor. *Endocrine Rev* 1995; 16(2): 143–63.
14. Auernhammer CJ, Strasburger CJ. Effects of growth hormone and insulin-like growth factor I on the immune system. *Eur J Endocrinol* 1995; 133(6): 635–45.
15. Rogler CE, Yang D, Rosetti L et al. Altered body composition and increased frequency of diverse malignancies in insulin-like growth factor-II transgenic mice. *J Biol Chem* 1994; 269(19): 13779–84.
16. Arany E, Afford S, Strain AJ, Winwood PJ, Arthur MJ, Hill DJ. Differential cellular synthesis of insulin-like growth factor binding protein I and IGFBP-3 within the human liver. *JCE&M* 1994; 79(6): 1871–6.
17. Underwood LE, Thissen JP, Lemozy S, Ketelslegers JM, Clemmons DR. Hormonal and nutritional regulation of IGF-1 and its binding proteins. *Horm Res* 1994; 42(4-5): 145–51.
18. Conover CA, Powell DR. Insulin-like growth factor (IGF)-binding protein-3 blocks IGF-1-induced receptor down regulation and cell desensitization in cultured bovine fibroblasts. *Endocrinol* 1991; 129(2): 710–16.
19. Collett-Solberg PF, Cohen P. The role of the insulin-like growth factor binding proteins and IGFBP proteases in modulating IGF action. *Endocrinol Metab Clin North Am* 1996; 25: 591–614.
20. Diamandi A, Khosravi MJ, Mistry J, Martinez V, Guevara-Aguirre J. Filter paper blood spot assay of human insulin-like growth factor I (IGF-I) and IGF-binding protein-3 and preliminary application in the evaluation of growth hormone status. *JCE&M* 1998; 83(7): 2296–301.
21. Sonksen PH. Replacement therapy in hypothalamo–pituitary insufficiency after childhood: management in the adult. *Horm Res* 1990; 33(4): 45–51.
22. Carroll PV, Christ ER, the members of the Growth Hormone Research Society Scientific Committee. Growth hormone deficiency in adulthood and the effects of growth hormone replacement: a review. *JCE&M* 1998; 83(2): 382–95.
23. Rosen T, Bengtsson B-A. Premature mortality due to cardiovascular disease in hypopituitarism. *Lancet* 1990; 336: 285–8.
24. Shahi M, Beshyah SA, Hackett D, Sharp PS, Johnston DG, Foale RA. Myocardial dysfunction treated adult hypopituitarism: a possible explanation for increased cardiovascular mortality. *Br Heart J* 1992; 67: 92–6.
25. Bates, Van't Hoff W, Jones PJ, Clayton RN. The effects of hypopituitarism on life expectancy. *JCE&M* 1996, 81: 1169–72.
26. Stabler B, Turner JR, Girdler SS, Light KC, Underwood LE. Reactivity to stress and psychological adjustment in adults with pituitary insufficiency. *Clin Endocrinol* 1992; 6: 467–73.
27. Rosen T, Wiren L, Wilhelmsen L, Wiklund I, Bengtsson BA. Decreased psychological well-being in adult patients with growth hormone deficiency. *Clin Endocrinol* 1994; 40: 111–16.
28. Mardh G, Lindeberg A. Growth hormone replacement therapy in adult hypopituitary patients with growth hormone deficiency: combined clinical safety data

from clinical trials in 685 patients. *Endocrinol Metab Suppl* 1995; **2**(B): 11–16.
29. Burman P, Broman JE, Hetta J. Quality of life in adults with growth hormone (GH) deficiency: response to treatment with recombinant GH in a placebo controlled 21 month trial. *JCE&M* 1995; **80**: 3585–90.
30. Giusti M, Meineri I, Malagamba D et al. Impact of recombinant human growth hormone treatment on psychological profiles in hypopituitary patients with adult-onset growth hormone deficiency. *Eur J Clin Invest* 1998; **28**(1): 13–19.
31. Holmes SJ, McKenna SP, Doward LC, Shalet SM. Development of a questionnaire to assess the quality of life of adults with growth hormone deficiency. *Endocrine Metab* 1995; **2**: 63–9.
32. Hunt SM, McKenna SP, Doward LC. Preliminary report on the development of a disease specific instrument for assessing quality of life of adults with growth hormone deficiency. *Acta Endocrinol* 1993; **128**(suppl 2): 37–40.
33. Wallymahmed ME, Baker GA, Humphrist G, Dewey M, McFarlane IA. The development, reliability and validity of a disease-specific quality of life model for adults with growth hormone deficiency. *Clin Endocrinol* 1996; **44**: 403–11.
34. Holmes SJ, Shalet SM. Characteristics of adults who wish to enter a trial of growth hormone replacement. *Clin Endocrinol* 1995; **43**(6): 613–18.
35. Beshyah SA, Freemantle C, Shahi M et al. Replacement therapy with biosynthetic human growth hormone in growth hormone-deficient hypopituitary adults. *Clin Endocrinol* 1995; **42**: 73–81.
36. Salomon F, Cuneo RD, Hesp R, Sonkson PH. The effects of treatment with recombinant human growth hormone on body composition and metabolism in adults with growth hormone deficiency. *N Engl J Med* 1989; **321**: 1797–803.
37. Binnerts A, Swart GR, Wilson JHP et al. The effects of growth hormone administration in growth hormone deficient adults on bone, protein, carbohydrate and lipid homeostasis, as well as body composition. *Clin Endocrinol* 1992; **37**(1): 79–87.
38. Johansson G, Rosen T, Lindstedt G, Bosaeus I, Bentsson BA. Effects of 2 years of growth hormone treatment on body composition and cardiovascular risk factors in adults with growth hormone deficiency. *Endocrinol Metab* 1995; **4**(3A): 3–12.
39. Chong PKK, Jung RT, Scrimegeour CM, Rennie MJ, Paterson CR. Energy expenditure and body composition in growth hormone deficient adults on exogenous growth hormone. *Clin Endocrinol* 1994; **40**: 103–10.
40. De Boer H, Blok GJ, Voerman HJ, De Vries PM, Van der Veen EA. Body composition in adult growth hormone deficient men assessed by anthropometry and bioimpedance analysis. *Clin Endocrinol Metab* 1992; **75**: 833–7.
41. Amato G, Carella C, Fazio S et al. Body composition, bone metabolism, and heart structure and function in growth hormone-deficient adults before and after replacement therapy at low doses. *JCE&M* 1993; **77**(6): 1671–6.
42. Rosen T, Bosaeus I, Tolli J, Lindstedt G, Bengtsson BA. Increased body fat mass and decreased extracellular fluid volume in adults with growth hormone deficiency. *Clin Endocrinol* 1993; **38**: 63–71.
43. Hoffman DM, O'Sullivan AJ, Freud J, Ho KK. Adults with growth hormone deficiency have abnormal body composition but normal energy metabolism. *JCE&M* 1995; **80**: 72–7.
44. Beshyah SA, Freemantle C, Thomas E et al. Abnormal body composition and reduced bone mass in growth hormone deficient hypopituitary adults. *Clin Endocrinol* 1995; **42**(2): 179–89.
45. Snel YE, Doerga ME, Brummer RJ, Zelissen PM, Zonderland ML, Koppeschaar HP. Resting metabolic rate, body composition and related hormonal parameters in growth hormone-deficient adults before and after growth hormone replacement therapy. *Eur J Endocrinol* 1995; **133**: 445–50.
46. Snel YE, Doerga ME, Brummer RM, Zelissen PM, Koppeschaar HP. Magnetic resonance imaging-assessed adipose tissue and serum lipid and insulin concentrations in growth hormone-deficient adults. Effects of growth hormone replacement. *Arterioscler Thromb Vasc Biol* 1995; **15**: 1543–8.
47. Moller J, Frandsen E, Frisker S, Jorgensen JOL, Christiansen JS. Decreased plasma and extracellular volume in growth hormone-deficient adults and the acute and prolonged effects of GH administration: a controlled experimental study. *Clin Endocrinol* 1996; **44**: 533–9.
48. Jorgensen JOL, Pendersen SA, Thuesen L et al. Beneficial effects of growth hormone treatment in growth hormone-deficient adults. *Lancet* 1989; **1**: 1221–5.
49. Orme SM, Sebastian JP, Oldroyd B et al. Comparison of measures of body composition in a trial of low dose growth hormone replacement therapy. *Clin Endocrinol* 1992; **37**: 453–9.
50. Jorgensen JO, Thuesen L, Muller J, Ovesen P, Skakkebaek NE, Christiansen JS. Three years of growth hormone treatment in growth hormone-deficient adults: near normalization of body composition and physical performance. *Eur J Endocrinol* 1994; **130**(3): 224–8.
51. Lonn L, Johansson G, Sjostrom L, Kvist H, Oden A, Bengtsson BA. Body composition and tissue distributions in growth hormone deficient adults before and after growth hormone treatment. *Obes Res* 1996; **4**: 45–54.
52. Hansen TB, Vahl N, Jorgsen JO, Christiansen JS, Hagen C. Whole body and regional soft tissue changes in growth hormone deficient adults after one year of growth hormone treatment: a double blind, random-

ized, placebo-controlled study. *Clin Endocrinol* 1995; 43: 689–96.
53. Baum HB, Biller BM, Finkelstein JS et al. Effects of physiologic growth hormone therapy on bone density and body composition in patients with adult-onset of growth hormone deficiency. A randomized, placebo-controlled trial. *Ann Intern Med* 1996; 125(11): 883–90.
54. Hoffman DM, Crampton L, Sernia C, Nguyen TV, Ho KKY. Short term growth hormone (GH) treatment of GH-deficient adults increases body sodium and extracellular water, but not blood pressure. *JCE&M* 1996; 81: 1123–8.
55. Johannsson AG, Burman P, Westmark K, Ljunghall S. The bone mineral density in acquired growth hormone deficiency correlates with circulating insulin-like growth factor I. *J Intern Med* 1992; 232: 447–52.
56. Bing-Yo RG, Denis MC, Rosen CJ. Low bone mineral density in adults with previous hypothalamic–pituitary tumors; correlation with growth hormone response to GHRH, IGF-1 and IGFBP-3. *Calcif Tissue Int* 1993; 53: 183–7.
57. Holmes SJ, Economou G, Whitehouse RW, Adam JE, Shalet SM. Reduced bone mineral density in adults with adult onset growth hormone deficiency. *JCE&M* 1994; 78: 669–74.
58. Johannsson G, Rosen T, Bosaeus I, Sjostrom L, Bengtsson BA. Two years of growth hormone (GH) treatment increases bone mineral content and density in hypopituitary patients with adult-onset GH deficiency. *JCE&M* 1996; 81: 2865–73.
59. Bravenboer N, Holzmann P, De Boer H et al. The effects of growth hormone (GH) on histomorphometric indices of bone structure and bone turnover in GH-deficient men. *JCE&M* 1997; 82: 1818–22.
60. Cuneo RC, Salomon F, Wiles CM, Sonksen PH. Skeletal muscle performance in adults with growth hormone deficiency. *Horm Res* 1990; 33(suppl 4): 50–60.
61. Rutherford OM, Beshyah SA, Johnson DG. Quadriceps strength before and after growth hormone replacement in hypopituitary adults: relationship to change in lean body mass and IGF-1. *Endocrinol Metab* 1994; 1: 41–7.
62. Cuneo RC, Salomon F, Wiles CM, Hesp K, Sonksen PH. Growth hormone treatment in growth hormone-deficient adults. II. Effects on exercise performance. *J Appl Physiol* 1991; 70(2): 695–700.
63. Rosen T, Eden S, Larson G, Wilhelmsen L, Bengtsson B-A. Cardiovascular risk factors in adult patients with growth hormone deficiency. *Acta Endocrinol (Coppenh)* 1993; 129: 195–200.
64. Merola B, Cittadini A, Colao A et al. Cardiac structural and functional abnormalities in adult patients with growth hormone deficiency. *JCE&M* 1993; 77(6): 1658–61.
65. Thuesen L, Jorgensen JOL, Muller JR et al. Short and long-term cardiovascular effects of growth hormone therapy in growth hormone deficient adults. *Clin Endocrinol* 1994; 41: 615–20.
66. Salomon F, Cuneo RC, Umpleby AM, Sonksen PH. Interactions of body fat and muscle mass with substrate concentrations and fasting insulin levels in adults with growth hormone deficiency. *Clin Sci* 1994; 87(2): 201–6.
67. Karnieli E, Laron Z, Richer N. Insulin resistance in GH-deficient adult patients treated with growth hormone: evidence for a postbinding defect in vivo. In: Laron Z, Butenandt O, eds. *Growth Hormone Replacement Therapy in Adults: Pros and Cons*. London, Tel Aviv: Freund, 41–9.
68. Fowelin J, Attvall S, Larger I, Bengtsson BA. Effects of treatment with recombinant human growth hormone on insulin sensitivity and glucose metabolism in adults with growth hormone deficiency. *Metab Clin Exp* 1993; 42: 1443–7.
69. Juul A, Behrenscheer A, Timms T, Nielsen B, Halkjaer-Kristensen J, Skakkebaek NE. Impaired thermoregulation in adults with growth hormone deficiency during heat exposure and exercise. *Clin Endocrinol* 1993; 38(3): 237–44.
70. Invited Report of a Workshop. Consensus Guidelines for the diagnosis and treatment of adults with growth hormone deficiency. *JCE&M* 1998; 83(2): 379–81.
71. Hoffman DM, O'Sullivan AJ, Baxter RC, Ho KKY. Diagnosis of growth-hormone deficiency in adults *Lancet* 1994; 343: 1064–8.
72. Cook DM, Ludlam WH, Cook MB. Route of estrogen administration helps to determine growth hormone (GH) replacement dose in GH-deficient adults. *J Clin Endocrinol Metab* 1999; 84(11): 3956–60.
73. Janssen YJ, Helmerhorst F, Frolich M, Roelfsema F. A switch from oral (2 mg/day) to transdermal (50 microg/day) 17beta-estradiol therapy increases serum insulin-like growth factor-I levels in recombinant human growth hormone (GH)-substituted women with GH deficiency. *J Clin Endocrinol Metab* 2000; 85(1): 464–7.
74. Ross R, Miell J, Freeman E et al. Critically ill patients have high basal growth hormone levels with attenuated oscillatory activity associated with low levels of insulin-like growth factor-I. *Clin Endocrinol* 1991; 35: 47–54.
75. Van den Berghe G, De Zegher F, Bouillon R. Acute and prolonged critical illness as different neuroendocrine paradigms. *JCE&M* 1998; 83(6): 1827–34.
76. Allain TJ, Bearn JA, Coskeran P et al. Changes in growth hormone, insulin-like growth factors (IGFs), and IGF-binding protein-1 in chronic fatigue syndrome. *Biol Psychiatry* 1997; 41: 567–73.
77. Moorkens G, Wynants H, Abs R. Effect of growth hormone treatment in patients with chronic fatigue syndrome: a preliminary study. *Growth Horm IGF Res* 1998; 8: 131–3.

78. Spiliotis BE, August GP, Hung W, Sonis W, Mendelson W, Bercu BB. Growth hormone neurosecretory dysfunction. A treatable cause of short stature. *JAMA* 1984; 251(17): 2223–30.
79. Laron Z, Klinger B, Eshet R, Kaneti H, Karasik A, Silbergeld A. Laron syndrome due to a post-receptor defect: response to IGF-1 treatment. *Isr J Med Sci* 1993; 29(12): 757–63.
80. Woods KA, Camacho-Hubner C, Savage MO, Clark AJ. Intrauterine growth retardation and postnatal growth failure associated with deletion of the insulin-like growth factor-1 gene. *N Engl J Med* 1996; 335(18): 1363–7.
81. Amselem S, Duquesnoy P, Attree O et al. Laron dwarfism and mutations of the growth hormone-receptor gene. *N Engl J Med* 1989; 321: 989.
82. Amselem S, Sobrier ML, Duquesnoy P et al. Recurrent nonsense mutations in the growth hormone receptor from patients with Laron type dwarfism. *J Clin Invest* 1991; 87: 1098.
83. Sobrier M-L, Dastot F, Duquesnoy P et al. Nine novel growth hormone receptor gene mutations in patients with Laron syndrome. *JCE&M* 1997; 82: 435.
84. Baumann G, Shaw MA, Winter RJ. Absence of plasma growth hormone-binding protein in Laron-type dwarfism. *JCE&M* 1987; 65: 814.
85. Woods KA, Fraser NC, Postel-Vinay MC et al. A homozygous splice site mutation affecting the intracellular domain of the growth hormone (GH) receptor resulting in Laron syndrome with elevated GH-binding activity. *JCE&M* 1996; 8: 1686.
86. Rosenbloom AL, Guevara-Aguirre J, Rosenfeld RG, Fielder PJ. The little women of Loja—growth hormone receptor deficiency in an inbred population of southern Ecuador. *N Engl J Med* 1990; 323: 1367–74.
87. Buchanan CR, Maheshwari HG, Norman MR, Morrell DJ, Preece MA. Laron-type dwarfism with apparently normal high affinity serum growth hormone-binding protein. *Clin Endocrinol* 1991; 35(2): 179–85.
88. Rosenbloom AL, Rosenfeld RG, Guevara-Aguirre J. Growth hormone insensitivity. *Pediatr Clin North Am* 199; 44(2): 423–42.
89. Gill ZP, Perks CM, Newcomb PVN, Holly JMP. Insulin-like growth factor binding protein-3 (IGFBP-3) predisposes breast cancer cells to programmed cell death in a non-IGF dependent manner. *J Biol Chem* 1997; 272: 25602–6.
90. Rajah R, Valentinis B, Cohen P. Insulin-like growth factor (IGF)-binding protein-3 induces apoptosis and mediates the effects of transforming growth factor-β1 on programmed cell death through a p53- and IGF-independent mechanism. *J Biol Chem* 1997; 272: 11281–8.
91. Orme SM, McNally R, Cartwright RA, Belchetz PE. Mortality and cancer incidence in acromegaly: a retrospective cohort study. *JCE&M* 1998; 83: 2730–4.
92. Chan JM, Stampfer MJ, Giovanucci E et al. Plasma insulin-like growth factor-1 and prostate cancer risk: a prospective study. *Science* 1998; 279(5350): 563–6.
93. Rowe PM. Unravelling the complexities of environmental effects on breast cancer risk. *Lancet* 1998; 351(9118): 1791.
94. Renehan A, Painter J, Potten CS, O'Dwyer ST, Shalet SM. Altered levels of serum insulin-like growth factors in patients with colorectal tumors. *Clin Endocrinol* 1999; P113.
95. Helle SI, Holly JMP, Tally M, Hall K, Vander-Stappen J, Lonning PE. Influence of treatment with tamoxifen and change in tumor burden on the IGF-system in breast cancer patients. *Int J Cancer* 1996; 69(4): 335–9.
96. Fitzsimmons J, Fantel A, Shepard TH. Growth parameters in mid-trimester fetal Turner syndrome. *Early Hum Dev* 1994; 38: 121–9.
97. Ranke MB. Growth in Turner's syndrome. *Acta Pediatr Scand* 1994; 83(3): 343–4.
98. Grumbach MM, Conte FA. Disorders of sex differentiation. In: *Williams Textbook of Endocrinology*, 9th edn. WB Saunders Company, 1339.
99. Ranke MB, Price DA, Maes M, et al. Factors influencing the final height in Turner syndrome following GH treatment: results of the Kabi International Growth study (KIGS). In: Albertsson-Wikland K, Ranke MB, eds. *Turner Syndrome in a Life-span Perspective: Research and Clinical Aspects*. Amsterdam: Elsevier Scientific Publications BV, 1995: 161–6.
100. Nilsson KO, Wikland KA, Alm J et al. Improved final height in girls with Turner's syndrome treated with growth hormone and oxandrolene. *JCE&M* 1996; 81: 635–40.
101. Takano K, Shizume K, Hibi I et al. Long-term effects of growth hormone treatment on height in Turner syndrome: results of a six-year multi-centre study in Japan. *Horm Res* 1995; 43(4): 141–3.
102. Massa G, Otten BJ, De Muinck Keizer-Schrama SM et al. Treatment with two growth hormone regimens in girls with Turner syndrome: final height results. *Horm Res* 1995; 43: 144–6.
103. Rocchicciolo P, Battin J, Bertrand AM et al. Final stature in cases of Turner's syndrome treated with growth hormone. *Arch Pediatrics* 1994; 1: 359–62.
104. Rosenfeld RG, Frane J, Attie KM et al. Six year results of a randomized, prospective trial of human growth hormone and oxandrolone in Turner syndrome. *J Pediatrics* 1992; 121: 49–55.
105. Taback SP, Collu R, Deal CL et al. Does growth-hormone supplementation affect adult height in Turner syndrome? *Lancet* 1996; 348: 25–7.
106. Dunger DB, Mohn A. Is there a role for growth hormone therapy in Noonan syndrome? In: Monson JP, ed. *Challenges in Growth Hormone Therapy*. Blackwell Science, 36–53.

107. Pantsiouou S, Stanhope R, Uruena M et al. Growth prognosis and growth after menarche in primary hypothyroidism. *Arch Dis Child* 1991; 66: 838–40.
108. Boersma B, Otten BJ, Stoelings GBA et al. Catch-up growth after prolonged hypothyroidism. *Eur J Pediatr* 1996; 155: 362–7.
109. Li M, Squire JA, Weksberg R. Molecular genetics of Beckwith–Wiedemann Syndrome. *Curr Opin Paediatrics* 1997; 9: 623–9.
110. Sonksen PH et al. In: Adashi EY, Thorner MO, eds. *The Somatotrophic Axis of the Reproductive Process in Health and Disease.* New York: Springer-Verlag, 1995.
111. Svensson J, Johannsson G, Bengtsson B-A. Insulin-like growth factor-I in growth hormone-deficient adults: relationship to population-based normal values, body composition and insulin tolerance test. *Clin Endocrinol* 1997; 46: 579–86.

5

Carcinoma of the thyroid
Philip E Harris

Thyroid nodules occur in about 5–10% of adults. Thyroid carcinoma, however, is rare, accounting for <1% of all cancers. The incidence shows a geographical variation and is higher in females (2.4/100 000 UK; 5.2/100 000 USA) than in males (0.9/100 000 UK; 2.1/100 000 USA).[1,2] The median age at diagnosis is 45–50 years. Neoplasms of the thyroid follicular cell encompass a wide spectrum of phenotypes, from benign follicular adenomas to follicular carcinomas, papillary carcinomas and anaplastic carcinomas. The prevalences of follicular carcinoma and anaplastic cancers are partly dependent upon the iodine intake in particular geographical areas, being more common in areas of iodine deficiency.[3,4] In iodine-sufficient areas, papillary carcinomas account for about 80% of tumors. In areas of iodine deficiency, as the prevalence of follicular carcinoma rises, the prevalence of papillary carcinoma falls to 35–55%.

Benign thyroid nodules frequently occur in autoimmune disease. There is, however, an increased risk of lymphoma in patients with Hashimoto's thyroiditis. Most patients presenting with thyroid nodules are asymptomatic. A history of exposure to external ionizing radiation should always be sought. Familial disease occasionally occurs (see below). Thyroid nodules in patients presenting over the age of 60 years or in childhood should always be viewed with suspicion. A fixed thyroid nodule, in the presence of lymphadenopathy, is highly suggestive of malignancy.

Apart from clinical examination, thyroid nodules should have thyroid scintigraphy together with fine needle aspiration (FNA) for histology.[5] Ultrasound may be helpful, particularly if the nodule(s) is large and possibly cystic. Occasionally, FNA needs to be carried out under ultrasound control. FNA requires a skilled operator together with an experienced cytologist and, as such, has a high degree of diagnostic accuracy.[6] Patients who have symptoms and/or signs suggesting upper airway obstruction or superior vena cava obstruction should have CT or MRI imaging performed. Objective evidence of upper airway obstruction should be obtained with flow-loop analysis.[7] Approximately 1% of thyroid nodules are medullary carcinomas. For this reason, basal calcitonin is routinely measured in a number of centers.[8] UK guidelines for the management of thyroid cancer in adults have recenlty been published.[9,10]

Papillary thyroid carcinoma

Papillary carcinoma is an unencapsulated tumor with both papillary and follicular structures. The papillae have a fibrovascular core covered by a single layer of tumor cells (Figure 5.1). The nuclei are typically pale-staining 'ground-glass' in appearance, with longitudinal grooves. Cytoplasmic inclusion vacuoles may be present within the nuclei. Psammoma bodies are calcified degenerative changes that occur in the papillae. They are characteristic of papillary carcinomas, occurring in 40–50% of tumors.

Tumor type	Relative proportion (%)
Classical papillary carcinoma	70
Encapsulated	10
Follicular	10
Tall cell	4
Diffuse sclerosing	3
Hurtle cell (oncocytic)	2
Other	1

Table 5.1
Subtypes of papillary carcinoma.[5]

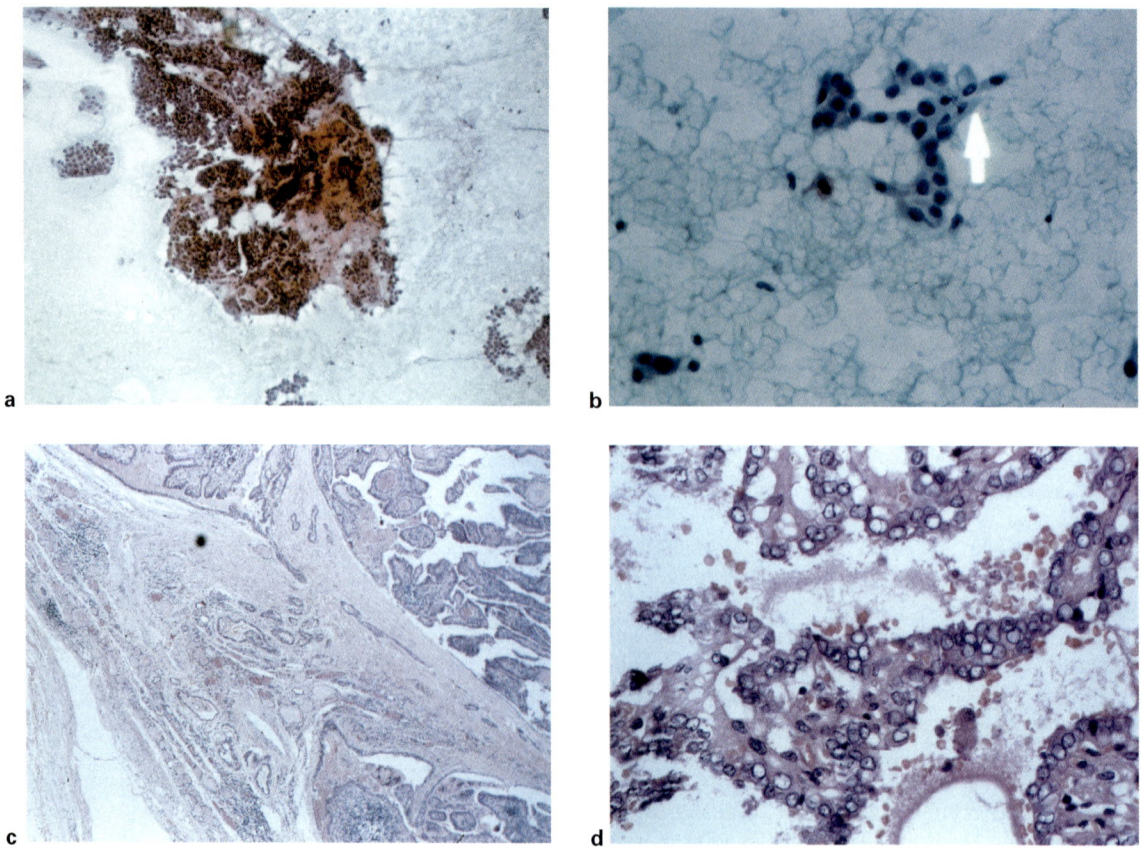

Figure 5.1
Papillary thyroid carcinoma: (a) low-power (×40) fine needle aspirate (FNA) demonstrating papillary structures; (b) high-power (×400) FNA demonstrating intranuclear cytoplasmic inclusion (arrow); (c) low-power (×40) demonstrating papillary tumor surrounded by normal, compressed thyroid tissue; (d) high-power (×400) demonstrating ground glass nuclei.

Multifocality is present in 20–80% of cases, 30% being bilateral.[11] A number of subtypes or variants of papillary carcinoma have been identified (Table 5.1).[11] Recent evidence suggests that patients with lymphocytic thyroiditis have lower pathological tumor node metastasis (pTNM) staging (see below), a lower recurrence rate and a lower mortality rate than patients without lymphocytic thyroiditis.[12] About 3% of papillary carcinomas are familial.[13] There is an association with familial adenomatosis coli[14] and Cowden's disease.[15] There is a clear relationship between papillary carcinoma and exposure to external ionizing radiation.[16] Although the use of ^{131}I in the treatment of thyroid disease is not associated with an increase in thyroid cancer, radioactive isotopes of iodine do have a tumorigenic effect on the thyroid gland.[16,17]

This has been particularly well exemplified by an approximately 50-fold increase in the incidence of childhood papillary carcinoma following the Chernobyl nuclear disaster. Children, particularly those under the age of 5 at the time of the accident, account for the majority of cases to date. Forty-five per cent of these tumors are atypical solid papillary carcinomas. The tumors tend to behave more aggressively than papillary carcinomas presenting in children from other geographical areas.[18]

The overall mortality for treated papillary carcinoma is in the region of 8%. Although there is a 2–3-fold increased incidence in women, the risks of recurrence and death appear to be higher in males. Age is a critical factor. The mortality from papillary carcinoma increases dramatically after the age of 45 years.[19,20] More than

40% of papillary carcinomas are found to be multifocal.[11,19] A primary tumor larger than 3 cm in diameter correlates with an increased probability of recurrence and death.[11,19,20] Papillary carcinomas frequently exhibit local metastatic spread to lymph nodes.[19] Local lymph node metastases are more common in children than in adults, being seen in 50–89% of cases.[11] The relevance of cervical lymph node involvement is controversial. Some studies have reported an increase in disease-specific mortality, whereas other studies have reported an increase in local disease recurrence without an effect on mortality.[11,19,20] Extra-thyroidal invasion is associated with an increased risk of disease recurrence and a 5–10-fold increase in mortality.[11,19,20] Distant metastatic spread is uncommon, occurring in less than 10% of patients. It is a powerful predictor of death, being associated with a more than 50-fold increase in mortality.[11,19,20]

Follicular carcinoma

Follicular carcinomas are encapsulated tumors with follicular differentiation but without the nuclear changes characteristic of papillary carcinoma. Capsular invasion is the key feature which distinguishes follicular carcinomas from follicular adenomas.[21] It is for this reason that follicular carcinomas cannot be differentiated from benign follicular adenomas on FNA. Two main types are recognized; minimally invasive, infiltrating the tumor capsule; and widely invasive, with involvement of the surrounding blood vessels (Figure 5.2). Follicular

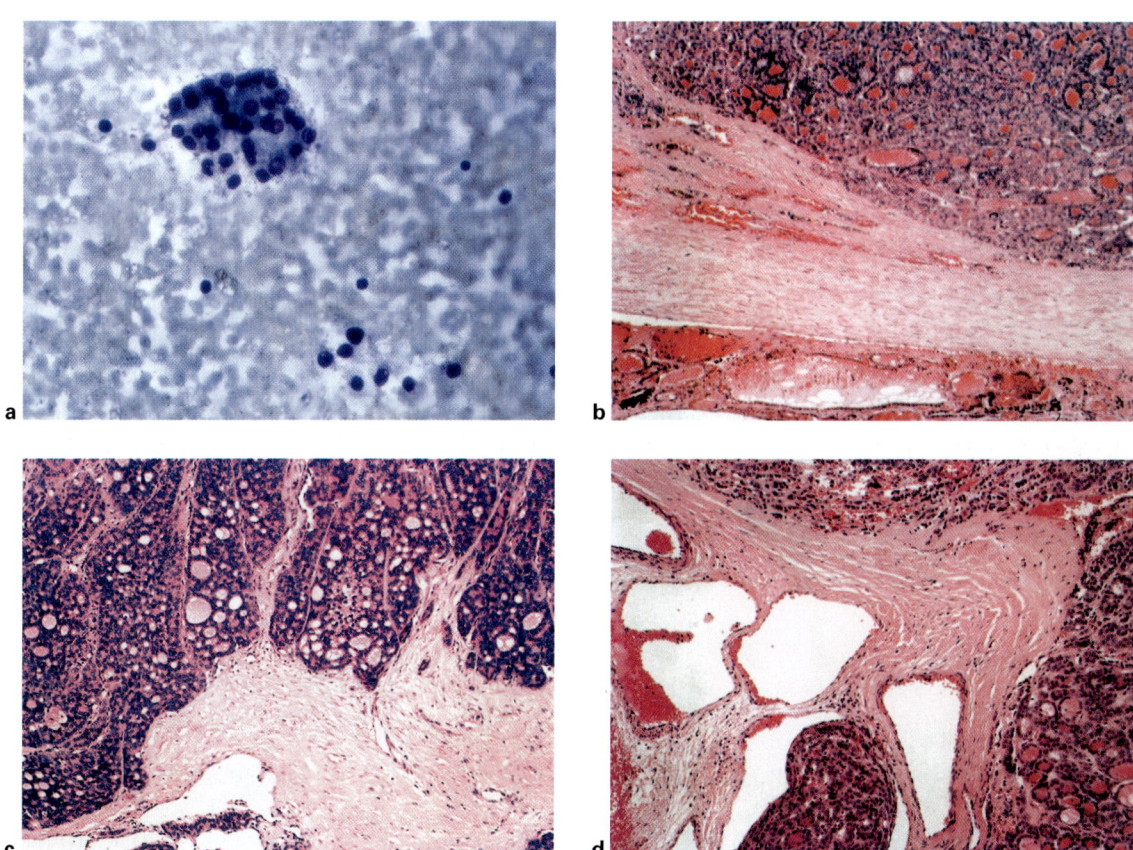

Figure 5.2
Follicular neoplasm: (a) FNA (×200) demonstrating microfollicles, follicular neoplasm; (b) follicular carcinoma demonstrating minimal invasion of the tumor capsule (arrow) (×100); (c) follicular carcinoma demonstrating capsular invasion (×100); (d) follicular carcinoma demonstrating vascular invasion (×100).

tumors, unlike papillary carcinomas, characteristically metastasize by hematogenous spread, most commonly to lung and bone. Metastatic disease may occur in up to 40% of patients[21] (Figure 5.3). Variable 10-year survival figures for follicular carcinoma have been published, ranging from 40% to 95%.[21] One report found that the average age at diagnosis for follicular carcinoma was 44 years, compared to 36 years for papillary carcinoma, although the age at death was younger in the patients with the follicular tumors. The final incidence of deaths was double that for papillary carcinoma (16% follicular versus 8% papillary).[22] Another study has reported a 3.4-fold higher cancer mortality in follicular than in papillary cancer.[23] As with papillary carcinoma, there is a higher mortality rate for patients >45 years age and with tumors >2.5 cm in size.[20–22] The Hurtle cell carcinomas (oncocytic variant) are more often multifocal, frequently involving regional nodes. They appear to have a greater tendency for tumor recurrence and possibly increased mortality.[21,22] The insular form has a poor prognosis. Uniquely, an insular carcinoma has recently been described, presenting with thyrotoxicosis secondary to an activating TSHR mutation.[21]

Prognostic classification of thyroid cancer

There have been several prognostic scoring schemes described for thyroid cancer. A simple system has been used which is based solely on the extent of tumor.[19,22] The pTNM staging for papillary and follicular carcinomas has wide international use[23] (Table 5.2). Other classification schemes include: the European Organization for Research and Treatment of Cancer (EORTC),[25] age, metastasis and extent of primary tumor and size of primary tumor (AMES),[26] and metastasis, age at the time of surgery, completeness of surgery, invasion of extrathyroidal tissues and primary tumor size (MACIS).[27] Although these systems are of use in auditing clinical data, they do not at present have a clear role in the everyday clinical management of individual patients.

Treatment of thyroid cancer (Figure 5.4)

The most important point to make at the outset is that thyroid cancer should only be managed in centers where there is specialist expertise in endocrinology, nuclear medicine and thyroid surgery. It is entirely

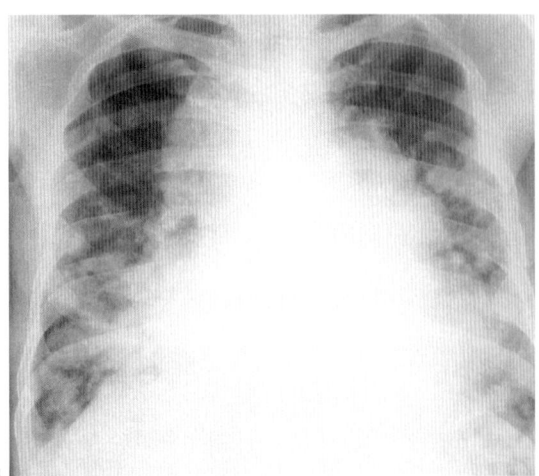

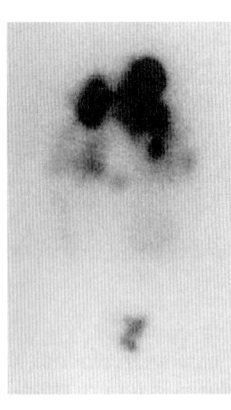

Figure 5.3
Metastatic thyroid follicular carcinoma: (a) chest X-ray; and (b) ^{131}I scan, demonstrating multiple pulmonary metastases.

Stage	Age <45 years	Age >45 years	Anaplastic (any age)
I	M0	T1	
II	M1	T2–3	
III		T4 or N1	
IV		M1	Any T, N or M

T (tumor): T1, <10 mm; T2, 10–40 mm; T3, >40 mm; T4, extra-thyroidal. N (node): N0, node negative; N1, node positive. M (metastasis): M0, no distant metastasis; M1, distant metastasis.

Table 5.2
Pathological pTNM staging for papillary and follicular thyroid cancers.[23]

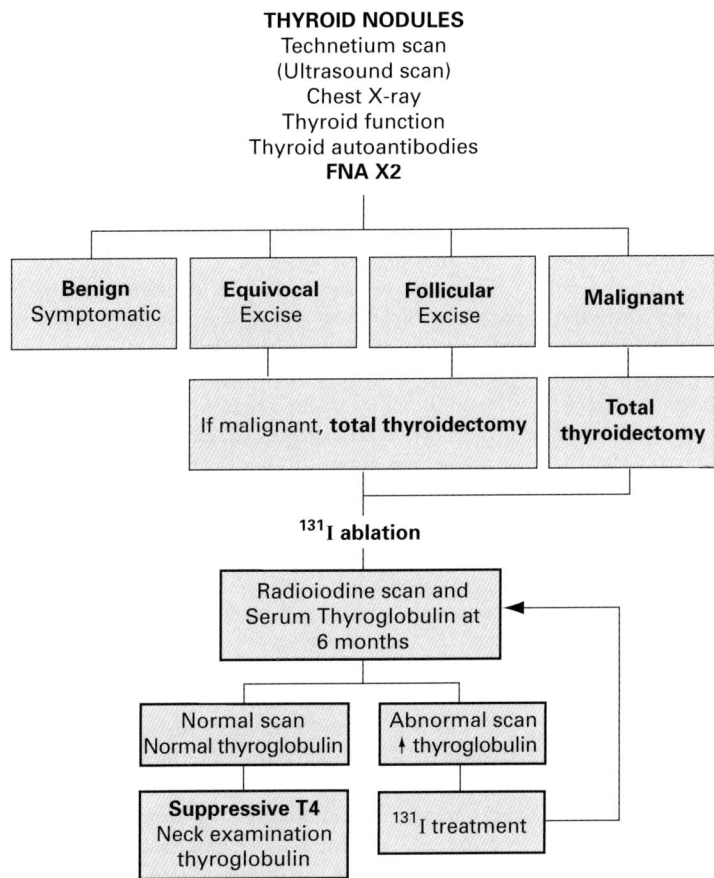

Figure 5.4
Algorithm for the management of thyroid cancer. All patients have thyroid scintigraphy carried out, together with FNA for cytology. Ultrasound may be helpful, particularly if the nodule(s) is large and possibly cystic. Some centers measure serum calcitonin to screen for medullary cancer. Chest X-ray is performed in the event of surgical resection. Further imaging and flow-loops are required in patients with evidence of venous or upper airway obstruction. T4, thyroxine.

inappropriate for thyroid cancer to be treated on an occasional basis by different surgeons.[9,10]

One standard policy is to manage all patients, regardless of age, tumor type or size, with a near-total thyroidectomy. Patients who have cervical lymphadenopathy demonstrated prior to surgery or in whom lymph node involvement is identified at the time of surgery have cervical lymph node dissection carried out. Some thyroid cancer specialists would argue that such extensive treatment is unnecessary, particularly in young patients (<45 years) who have a localized papillary carcinoma <1 cm in diameter.[19] Such patients may be managed with a more limited resection, such as a lobectomy. Balanced against this is the evidence that even in the good prognostic group detailed above, less extensive resections may be associated with an increased risk of recurrence and mortality, this clearly becoming significant with tumors of >1 cm in diameter.[19,20] The management of micropapillary tumors found incidentally during surgery for benign thyroid disease remains a subject of debate. Some cases are carefully followed up, without resorting to further thyroid surgery. Follicular carcinoma is diagnosed by careful histological examination of an excised tumor. In the first instance, a patient with a follicular neoplasm on FNA is subjected to a thyroid lobectomy. Histological confirmation of follicular carcinoma is followed by a near-total thyroidectomy.

Near-total thyroidectomy has a number of advantages in the management of thyroid cancer. Apart from maximizing the likelihood of tumor resection, it enables postoperative ^{131}I thyroid ablation to be performed. Long-term monitoring can then be carried out by the measurement of serum thyroglobulin. The disadvantages are the postoperative complications of thyroid surgery, particularly recurrent laryngeal nerve damage and hypoparathyroidism. These risks are minimized if the operation is performed by a dedicated endocrine surgeon. In addition, patients need to remain on lifelong thyroxine replacement therapy. The dose of thyroxine should be adjusted to ensure that the serum thyroid-stimulating hormone (TSH) level is suppressed to <0.15 mU/l. The risk of recurrent disease increases with higher serum TSH levels.[28] In the period between surgery and ablative treatment, patients are usually treated with triiodothyronine (T3) (~20 μg three times daily), which has a shorter half-life than thyroxine. Some centers do not attempt to give ablative treatment to the low-risk groups of patients. As such, their protocols for the management of these patients will differ from that detailed below.[3]

Thyroid ablation is carried out using ^{131}I following surgery. Radioiodine treatment is contraindicated in pregnant women. Conception should be avoided for the following year.[3] An administered dose of ~3.7 GBq will usually be given. This treatment is not associated with serious side-effects in the majority of patients. Patients may experience some nausea and indigestion secondary to a transient gastritis and are treated with an antiemetic such as metoclopramide and an H_2 receptor blocker such as ranitidine. Transient sialadenitis is treated with mucaine lozenges. Dexamethasone is given to minimize the effects of radiation-induced thyroiditis or inflammation of metastatic tumor. Patients with extensive metastatic pulmonary disease may develop lung fibrosis. Long-term marrow toxicity or secondary malignancy is only seen in patients who have received high cumulative doses of ^{131}I.

T3 is stopped 10 days before treatment. By the end of this time, serum TSH should be in the hypothyroid range (>30 mU/l), facilitating ^{131}I ablation. If thyroxine is used instead of T3, patients need to stop treatment for 4 weeks. There is a theoretical risk of tumor stimulation when thyroid hormone replacement is stopped, as a result of increased serum TSH. This may be deleterious, particularly in patients known to have extensive metastatic disease. Recombinant human TSH (rhTSH) (Genzyme Corporation, Cambridge MA, USA) is now available. This preparation is presently licensed in the UK for ^{131}I tracer studies. This preparation enables ^{131}I to be given without the need to stop thyroid hormone replacement. There are, necessarily, cost implications with this, but it is undoubtedly of value for certain patients. It should be used for patients with hypopituitarism who lack endogenous TSH drive. It is also useful in patients with severe ischaemic heart disease in whom thyroid hormone withdrawal may cause difficulties.

Four to five days after ^{131}I ablation, most patients are scanned to assess whether or not there is any residual thyroid uptake either in the thyroid bed or elsewhere. They are then commenced on suppressive thyroxine replacement therapy. The UK guidelines recommend that a diagnostic radio-iodine scan should be carried out about six months following ^{131}I ablation. As for the first scan, thyroid hormone replacement is stopped, or the patient is treated with rhTSH. Uptake of radio-iodone and/or elevated serum thyroglobulin are indications for a further treatment dose of ^{131}I. A whole body scan is carried out three days after treatment. If there is evidence of residual disease, the patient is scanned again six months later. Patients with abnormal scans receive further ablation doses of 5.5–7.4 GBq 6-monthly, until ablation is complete. Thereafter, the patients are monitored in the clinic by means of clinical examination and serum thyroglobulin measurements. Radioiodine has limited use in some tumors, such as Hurtle cell carcinomas, due to poor ^{131}I uptake. Anaplastic carcinomas do not take up radioiodine. They are associated with an extremely poor prognosis and should be managed by palliation (see below).

Serum thyroglobulin is an excellent predictor of relapse and indicator of residual disease.[3] Serum thyroglobulin should be undetectable in patients who have undergone total thyroid ablation. A measurable serum thyroglobulin indicates the presence of thyroid tissue or recurrent disease. Circulating anti-thyroglobulin antibodies can interfere with thyroglobulin assays. This interference can be minimized using an immunometric assay, with monoclonal antibodies against antigenic determinants on the thyroglobulin molecule, which are not recognized by the majority of circulating antibodies. A recovery estimation of added thyroglobulin to the patient's serum is normally used to detect antibody interference. Thyroxine therapy suppresses serum thyroglobulin to undetectable levels in a small number of patients with metastatic disease. For this reason, some centers measure serum thyroglobulin off suppressive therapy. Recent evidence suggests that rhTSH-stimulated thyroglobulin testing is as sensitive as measuring serum thyroglobulin after thyroxine withdrawal.[31]

Radiotherapy should be considered in patients with evidence of rapidly progressive disease or in whom there is no radioiodine uptake in known tumor sites. Radiotherapy is particularly effective as palliation in patients with painful bone metastases. It should also be considered in patients with extensive inoperable residual disease and in patients with anaplastic tumors.

Chemotherapy has no proven role in patients with differentiated follicular or papillary thyroid cancer. Its palliative use may be considered in patients with dedifferentiating or anaplastic tumors.

References

1. Office of Population Censuses and Surveys. *Cancer Statistics Registrations for 1982*, Series MB1, England and Wales, 1985.
2. Biometry Branch Division of Cancer Cause and Prevention. Third National Cancer Survey Incidence Data. In: Cutler SJ, Young JL, eds. *DHEW Publications* No. 75–789, NCI Monograph No. 41. Washington DC, 1975: 25.
3. Schlumberger MJ. Papillary and follicular thyroid carcinoma. *N Engl J Med* 1998; 297–306.
4. Schneider AB, Ron E. Pathogenesis. In: Braverman LE, Utiger RD, eds. *Werner and Ingbar's The Thyroid: A Fundamental and Clinical Text*, 7th edn. Lippincott-Raven, Philadelphia: 1996: 902–9.
5. Jones MK. Management of nodular thyroid disease. *Br Med J* 2001; 323: 293–4.
6. Oertel YC. Fine-needle aspiration and the diagnosis of thyroid cancer. *Endocrinol Metab Clin North Am* 1996; 25(1): 69–91.
7. Miller MR, Pincock AC, Oates GD, Wilkinson R, Skene-Smith H. Upper airways obstruction due to goitre: detection, prevalence and results of surgical management. *Q J Med* 1990; 74: 177–88.
8. Mayr B, Brabant G, von zur Mühlen A. Incidental detection of familial medullary thyroid carcinoma by calcitonin screening for nodular thyroid disease. *Eur J Endocrinol* 1999; 141: 286–9.
9. Guidelines for the management of thyroid cancer in adults. Royal College of Physicians, London 2002.
10. Harris PE. The management of thyroid cancer in adults: A review of new guidelines. *Clin Med* 2002, in press.
11. Ain KB. Papillary thyroid carcinoma. *Endocrinol Metab Clin North Am* 1995; 24(4): 711–60.
12. Loh K-C, Greenspan FS, Dong F, Miller TR, Yeo PPB. Influence of lymphocytic thyroiditis on the prognostic outcome of patients with papillary thyroid carcinoma. *J Clin Endocrinol Metab* 1999; 84: 458–63.
13. Goldgar DE, Easton DF, Cannon-Albright LA, Skolnick MH. Systematic population-based assessment of cancer risk in first-degree relatives of cancer probands. *J Natl Cancer Inst* 1994; 86: 1600–8.
14. Bell B, Mazzaferri EL. Familial adenomatous polyposis (Gardner's syndrome) and thyroid carcinoma. A case report and review of the literature. *Dig Dis Sci* 1993; 38: 185.
15. Thyresson HN, Doyle JA. Cowden's disease (multiple hamartoma syndrome). *Mayo Clin Proc* 1981; 56: 179.
16. Dobyns BM, Hyrmer BA. The surgical management of benign and malignant thyroid neoplasms in Marshall Islanders exposed to hydrogen bomb fallout. *World J Surg* 1992; 16: 126–40.
17. Kazakov VS, Demidchik EP, Astskhova LN. Thyroid cancer after Chernobyl. *Nature* 1992; 359: 21.
18. Becker DV, Robbins J, Beebe GW, Bouville AC, Wachholz BW. Childhood thyroid cancer following the Chernobyl accident. *Endocrinol Metab Clin North Am* 1996; 25(1): 197–211.
19. DeGroot LJ, Kaplan EL, McCormick M, Straus FH. Natural history, treatment and course of papillary thyroid carcinoma. *J Clin Endocrinol Metab* 1990; 71: 414–24.
20. Mazzferri EL, Kloos RT. Current approaches to primary therapy for papillary and follicular thyroid cancer. *J Clin Endocrinol* 2001; 86:1441–630.
21. Grebe SKG, Hay I. Follicular thyroid cancer. *Endocrinol Metab Clin North Am* 1995; 24(4): 761–801.
22. DeGroot LJ, Kaplan EL, Shulka MS, Salti G, Straus FH. Morbidity and mortality in follicular thyroid cancer. *J Clin Endocrinol Metab* 1995; 80: 2946–53.
23. Loh K-C, Greenspan FS, Gee L, Miller TR, Yeo PPB. Pathological tumor-node-metastasis (pTNM) staging for papillary and follicular thyroid carcinomas: a retrospective analysis of 700 patients. *J Clin Endocrinol Metab* 1997; 82: 3553–62.
24. Russo D, Tumino S, Arturi F et al. Detection of an activating mutation of the thyrotropin receptor in a case of an autonomously hyperfunctioning thyroid insular carcinoma. *J Clin Endocrinol Metab* 1997; 82: 735–8.
25. Byar DP, Green SB, Dor P et al. A prognostic index for thyroid carcinoma: a study of the EORTC Thyroid Cancer Cooperative Group. *Eur J Cancer* 1979; 15: 1033.
26. Cady B, Rossi R. An expanded view of risk-group definition in differentiated thyroid carcinoma. *Surgery* 1988; 104: 947.
27. Hay ID, Bergstralh EJ, Goellner JR et al. Predicting outcome in papillary thyroid carcinoma: development of a reliable prognostic scoring system in a cohort of 1779

patients surgically treated at one institution during 1940 through 1989. *Surgery* 1993; 114: 1050.
28. Pujol P, Daures J-P, Nsakala N, Baldet L, Bringer J, Jaffiol C. Degree of thyrotropin suppression as a prognostic determinant in differentiated thyroid cancer. *J Clin Endocrinol Metab* 1996; 81: 4318–23.
29. Park HM. Stunned thyroid after high dose ^{131}I imaging. *Clin Nucl Med* 1992; 17: 501–2.
30. Ladenson PW, Braverman LE, Mazzaferri EL et al. Comparison of administration of recombinant human thyrotropin with withdrawal of thyroid hormone for radioactive iodine scanning in patients with thyroid carcinoma. *N Engl J Med* 1997; 337: 888–96.
31. Pacini F, Lippi F. Clinical experience with recombinant human thyroid-stimulating hormone (rhTSH): serum thyroglobulin measurement. *J Endocrinol Invest* 1999; 22: 25–9.

6

Multiple endocrine neoplasia
Bin Tean Teh, Catharina Larsson

Introduction

The findings of multiple endocrine tumors in a patient and their usual clusterings in families have long fascinated clinicians. Not only do they pose challenges to definite diagnosis and optimal management, but their underlying etiologies have remained puzzling for decades. Now, thanks to new advances in molecular genetics, these questions are being solved, leading to improved diagnosis and management. In this chapter, we review these recent developments in the multiple endocrine neoplasia type 1 and 2 syndromes as well as the two closely related syndromes hyperparathyroidism–jaw tumor syndrome and familial isolated hyperparathyroidism.

Multiple endocrine neoplasia type 1 (MEN 1)

Clinical manifestations

In 1954, Wermer described adenomatosis of endocrine glands affecting several members of a family which spanned two consecutive generations.[1] This hereditary disease, also called Wermer syndrome and now called multiple endocrine neoplasia type 1, or MEN 1 for short, is transmitted as an autosomal dominant trait with over 95% penetrance and an equal sex distribution.[2] Its prevalence is estimated to be 0.02–0.2/1000. While the majority of MEN 1 families are of Caucasian origin, MEN 1 has also been described in families from a variety of ethnic backgrounds.[3,4] The syndrome is classically characterized by a triad of neoplasia affecting the parathyroid glands (90–97% of the patients), the enteropancreatic endocrine tissues (30–80%), and the anterior pituitary gland (15–50%). The age of diagnosis is dependent on two factors: (1) if the patient is symptomatic or asymptomatic and diagnosed by biochemial screening; and (2) the type of tumor that the patient develops.[5-7] The asymptomatic patients are diagnosed at an earlier age by biochemical screening than are those who are symptomatic. For example, Trump et al showed that in the symptomatic group, the cumulative percentages of patients who had developed MEN 1 are 18%, 52% and 78% at the ages of 20, 35 and 50 years. In the asymptomatic group who were diagnosed by biochemical screening, however, the cumulative percentages increased to 43%, 85% and 94% in the same age groups. In a study of the largest MEN 1 kindred, it was shown that by the age of 20 years two-thirds of patients were found to have primary hyperparathyroidism, and by age 30 years, the rate increased to 95%.[6] Both studies showed that endocrine pancreatic tumors have two patterns: gastrinomas occur commonly in the older group of patients (i.e. above 30 or 40), whereas insulinomas tend to occur in the young patients (i.e. below 30 or 40). For anterior pituitary tumors, most patients were diagnosed between their 20s and 40s.[5-7]

The MEN 1 patients may have only one type of endocrine gland involved or any combination, but, in addition, may also develop tumors in a range of endocrine and non-endocrine tissues (Table 6.1). This spectrum of MEN 1-related tumors is still expanding. They vary in frequency, and include lipomas, foregut and midgut carcinoids, thyroid neoplasms, adrenocortical neoplasia, spinal ependymoma, renal angiomyolipoma and leiomyoma of the esophagus.[8] Adrenocortical tumors, which were originally thought to be uncommon in MEN 1, have been found in up to one-third of patients.[6,9] A number of cutaneous manifestations of MEN 1 have also been described.[10] Facial angiofibroma

Syndrome symbol	Chromosomal location	Gene name	Gene function	Main lesions	Associated features
MEN 1	11q13	MEN 1	TSG	Parathyroid hyperplasia Endocrine pancreatic tumors Anterior pituitary tumors	Adrenocortical tumors, ependymoma, carcinoids, thyroid neoplasms, skin angiofibroma/collagenoma, renal angiomyolipoma, gastrointestinal leiomyoma
FIHP	11q13	MEN 1	TSG	Parathyroid hyperplasia	None
MEN 2A	10q11	RET	Oncogene	Medullary thyroid carcinoma Pheochromocytoma	Parathyroid hyperplasia/adenoma
MEN 2B	10q11	RET	Oncogene	Medullary thyroid carcinoma Pheochromocytoma	Marfanoid facies, mucosal neuromas, intestinal ganglioneuromatosis, neurological disturbances, musculoskeletal abnormalities
FMTC	10q11	RET	Oncogene	Medullary thyroid carcinoma	None

TSG, tumor suppressor gene; FIHP, familial isolated hyperparathyroidism; FMTC, familial medullary thyroid carcinoma.

Table 6.1
Characteristics of the MEN 1 and MEN 2 syndromes.

and collagenoma were identified in up to 75% of MEN 1 patients. Other cutaneous lesions, including confetti-like hypopigmented macules and multiple gingival papules, have been reported. It is not known at present if other tumors, such as breast carcinoma and melanoma, occur more frequently in patients with MEN 1 than in the general population, although a number of these cases have been noted in MEN 1 patients.[11]

Treatment of MEN 1

MEN 1-related hyperparathyroidism (Table 6.2) is invariably a multiglandular disease, and recurrence after parathyroidectomy is well known.[12,13] Hence, the surgery of choice is either total parathyroidectomy with autotransplantation or subtotal resection of three and a half parathyroid glands. The choice is dependent on the preference of the surgeon, since to date there are no conclusive long-term studies comparing the two strategies. With either approach, however, concurrent thymectomy is highly recommended, for two reasons. First, it will remove any supernumerary parathyroid gland in the thymus. Second, MEN 1 patients, particularly males, have a higher risk of developing thymic carcinoid, which has a poor prognosis with no known effective treatment.[14,15]

Syndrome	Syndrome symbol	Chromosomal location	Gene product	Function	Parathyroid finding	S-Ca preop.	S-Ca postop.	U-Ca preop.	S-PTH preop.	Parathyroid surgery
Familial hyperparathyroidism–jaw tumor syndrome	HPT-JT	1q21-q32	NI	Suggested TSG	Adenoma/cystic/ carcinoma	>ref	Normal	>ref	>ref	Curative
Multiple endocrine neoplasia type 1	MEN 1	11q13	MEN 1 menin	TSG	Hyperplasia	>ref	Normal	>ref	>ref	Curative
Familial isolated hyperparathyroidism	FIHP	1q21-q32	N.I.	Suggested TSG	Adenoma/cystic	>ref	Normal	>ref	>ref	Curative
		11q13	MEN 1 menin	TSG	Hyperplasia/ adenoma	>ref	Normal	>ref	>ref	Curative
Familial hypercalcemia and hypercalciuria		3q13.3-q21	CaR	Calcium-sensing receptor	Hyperplasia/ adenoma	>ref	Normal	>ref	Inappropriate within ref	Mostly curative
Familial hypercalcemic hypocalciuria	FHH	3q13.3-q21	CaR	Calcium-sensing receptor	Normal/ hyperplasia	>ref	>ref	Normal	Inappropriate within ref	Not curative
		19p13.3 and 19q13	NI			>ref	>ref	Normal	Inappropriate within ref	Not curative

TSG, tumor suppressor gene; ref, normal reference values; NI, not identified.

Table 6.2
Familial disorders predisposing to hypercalcemia as a major feature.

Pancreatic tumors are a main cause of morbidity and mortality in MEN 1.[16-18] The most frequently encountered are gastrinomas, which are symptomatic secretory enteropancreatic tumors giving rise to the Zollinger–Ellison syndrome.[19,20] These tumors are typically multicentric microgastrinomas (<6 mm), which are often not detectable by conventional preoperative imaging techniques. A number of studies have shown that control of the hyperparathyroidism can ameliorate hypergastrinemia, and parathyroidectomy together with medical management of the gastric hyperacidity produces a satisfactory symptomatic response.[21-23] However, as this strategy does not 'cure' the gastrinoma, which has a predilection for recurrence and metastasis, some authors advocate a more rigorous procedure.[20,24] Strategies which include percutaneous transhepatic selective venous sampling for gastrin, distal pancreatectomy, duodenotomy, enucleation of pancreatic tumors and peripancreatic lymph node dissection, have all been described. Total pancreatectomy has also been proposed, but this approach is not widely practiced, due to the high level of morbidity associated with total pancreatectomy. The forms of medical treatment include symptomatic treatment such as omeprazole and H_2 receptor blockers, but recently the somatostatin analog octreotide has been used to treat hypergastrinemic patients.[25] This agent suppresses gastrin secretion, and it may also have the added benefit of inhibiting gastrin-induced neuroendocrine cell hyperplasia and carcinoidosis in gastric mucosa. Surgical resection is generally recommended for all other species of symptomatic enteropancreatic tumor as well as for lesions that are larger than 3 cm in diameter.[23] Tumor resection is particularly important in the case of insulinoma. Resection is generally curative and disease recurrence uncommon.[26] In tumor localization, conventional radiological imaging can be augmented by somatostatin receptor scintigraphy and intraoperative ultrasonography.[27]

The treatment for MEN 1-related pituitary tumors depends on its type and severity, but all patients should have close follow-up. Small and asymptomatic 'non-functioning' tumors do not require specific therapy. For prolactinomas, bromocriptine is the choice of treatment, but occasionally surgery is indicated when intolerance is a problem. For non-functioning tumors, growth hormone (GH) and adrenocorticotropic hormone (ACTH)-secreting tumors, surgery and/or radiotherapy are usually indicated. Somatostatin has also been shown to be effective in treating GH-secreting tumors.

Molecular genetics of MEN 1

The *MEN1* gene was first assigned to chromosomal region 11q13, based on the study of loss of heterozygosity in MEN 1-related tumors and linkage analysis in affected families.[28] The results from this tumor study were consistent with Knudson's two-hit mutation theory pointing towards the involvement of a tumor suppressor gene in the development of these tumors.[29] Worldwide linkage studies in MEN 1 families which allowed correlation of the inheritance of phenotypes with the inheritance of genotypes have failed to find a second MEN 1 gene locus.[30] The *MEN1* gene was identified in 1997, based on positional cloning. The *MEN1* gene contains 10 exons (only exons 2–9 were transcribed) which encode a 610 amino acid protein product (Figure 6.1). So far, two transcripts have been identified, most likely as the result of alternative splicing: a 2.9-kb transcript expressed in all tissues, and a 4.2-kb transcript in pancreas and thymus.[31,32] The significance of the two transcripts is yet to be established.

The *MEN1* protein product, menin, has no homology to any other known protein, and the first clue of its function came from studies of yeast two-hybrid systems to identify its interacting protein(s). Its first interacting protein turns out to be the AP1 transcription factor JunD.[33] The AP1 transcription factors have basic leucine zipper (bZip) domains that pair to bind DNA as a Y-shaped heterodimer. Menin has been found to specifically bind to JunD via its N-terminus

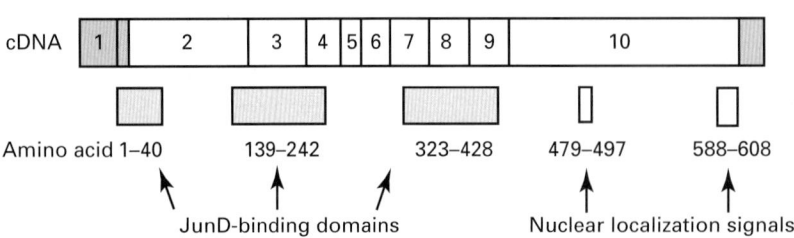

Figure 6.1
Schematic illustration of the MEN1 *gene and the regions coding for the amino acids interacting with JunD as well as encoding the nuclear localization signal.*

but not to the other members of the Jun or Fos families (Figure 6.1). Disruption of this binding activity by *MEN1* mutations leads to inhibition of JunD-activated transcription; however, not all *MEN1* mutations have this property. Based on the binding effects of *MEN1* mutations from different locations, three binding domains have been identified: amino acids 1–40, 139–242 and 323–428. Obviously, more studies are needed to explain the pathophysiological effects of those mutations found in between these domains. The identification of other interacting proteins, which may constitute parts of the menin–JunD complex or be separate functional entities, may contribute to its elucidation.

To date, mutation analysis of MEN 1 patients has identified over 250 different mutations spread over the translated exons 2–9.[34] Approximately 80% of these mutations result in truncated proteins which are likely to eliminate their functions, and further support its TSG role. Several mutations, such as 357del4, have been found more frequently in patients of different origin, and represent 'warm spots'. Some groups have reported a reasonably high rate of mutation detection in so-called 'sporadic MEN 1',[35–37] i.e. patients with two or more MEN 1-related endocrine tumors without clear family history, therefore making it worthwhile to screen for mutations in this group of patients. In the largest MEN 1 family, found in Tasmania, Australia, a high rate of phenocopies has been found, most likely due to diligent screening and the detection of common endocrinopathies such as hyperparathyroidism in non-gene carriers.[38]

Genotype–phenotype correlation in MEN 1 has so far been difficult. First, its clinical presentation, age of onset and natural history are known to vary extensively, even among members of the same family. Second, the wide spectrum of mutations found throughout the gene make any correlation formidable. Still, our findings of two missense mutations in close proximity in exon 4 (Figure 6.2) in two large families with isolated hyperparathyroidism—considered a milder form of MEN 1—may be an exception.[39,40] Interestingly, these two mutations, E255K and Q260P, fall outside the sites for the nuclear localization signals and JunD binding, suggesting a correlation of functionally 'milder' mutations with a milder form of disease. In another study, we looked at the mutations in MEN 1 families with one or more thymic carcinoids, a very malignant form of the disease (Teh, unpublished). There is no correlation with any specific mutation, but all mutations in these families result in a truncated protein, the truncation involving the functionally important regions. In this cohort, there is not one missense mutation, which would otherwise constitute about 20% of all mutations in regular MEN 1 families. However, more studies are needed to test whether functionally important mutations may predispose to more severe phenotypes.

Molecular diagnosis of MEN1

With the identification of the *MEN1* gene, mutation analysis is now the standard tool for diagnosis. Various approaches, including single-strand conformation polymorphism (SSCP), dideoxyfingerprinting (DDF), and denaturing gradient gel electrophoresis (DGGE), have been used with various degreee of success in mutation detection. However, due to the wide spectrum of mutations found throughout the gene, direct sequencing of all coding exons is considered the most effective approach.

To date, in approximately 10–20% of MEN 1 families, a mutation could not be found. It is likely that these families still harbor a *MEN1* mutation that may lie in the regulatory or untranslated regions or constitute large deletions which could not be identified by sequencing alone. In these families, linkage analysis using

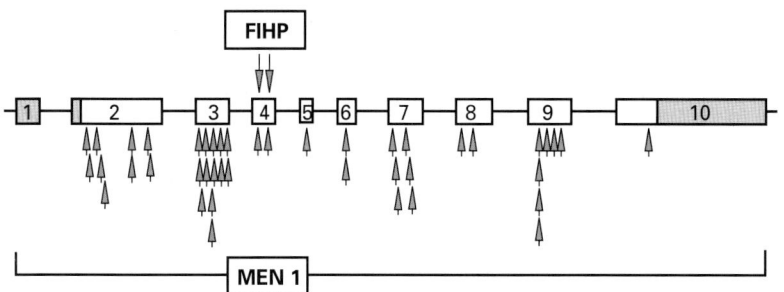

Figure 6.2
Diagrammatic representation of constitutional MEN1 missense mutations reported in families with MEN 1, as well as in two large families with familial isolated hyperparathyroidism (FIHP).

chromosome 11q13 polymorphic markers is still informative and useful. In this process, blood samples from at least two affected relatives and those seeking presymptomatic diagnosis are needed. The analysis involves PCR-based detection of polymorphic microsatellite loci.

The hyperparathyroidism–jaw tumor syndrome (HPT-JT)

In 1958, Jackson described a family with hereditary hyperparathyroidism in which four of the five affected members were found to have jaw tumors also.[41] It was first thought to be a variant of MEN 1, but subsequent identification of more family members with both entities and the exclusion of its linkage to the *MEN1* locus suggested that it is a clinically and genetically distinct syndrome (McKusick number 145001).

Clinically, the hyperparathyroidism in the HPT-JT syndrome is characterized by solitary adenoma, but some patients may have more than one adenoma (Table 6.2). Histologically, they are mainly chief cell tumors, although in one family both chief cell and oncocytic cells were described. In contrast with MEN 1-related hyperparathyroidism, which invariably consists of benign multiglandular parathyroid hyperplasia, the HPT-JT syndrome is associated with an increased risk of carcinoma.[42,43] In addition, cystic structures were found to be prominent in these tumors, but their significance in relation to pathophysiology is not known. Another interesting observation is the reduced penetrance of hyperparathyroidism in female gene carriers, but again the reason behind this phenomenon is unknown.[42]

The fibro-osseous jaw tumors which occur in the maxilla and the mandible usually consist of dense fibrocellular connective tissue with osteoid and bone formation. They are histopathologically distinct from classical primary HPT-related brown tumors, which are characterized by the abundance of multinucleated osteoclasts. Clinically, they are not responsive to the correction of hyperparathyroidism, and although some of these tumors may be fast growing, they are never found to be malignant.

Besides hyperparathyroidism and jaw tumors, the HPT-JT syndrome is associated with a whole spectrum of renal lesions. The most common is cystic kidney disease, which may be very severe, requiring renal transplantation.[42] Other renal lesions reported include Wilm's tumor, renal hamartoma and papillary carcinoma.[42–44]

Molecular genetics of HPT-JT

The putative HPT-JT gene was first designated *HRPT2*, in contrast to *HRPT1*, which refers to an unidentified FIHP gene implicated from studies of a large FIHP family.[45] However, this family has recently been confirmed to be a true HPT-JT family, as cases of jaw tumors and polycystic kidney disease have been found, and it has been genetically linked to the HPT-JT locus.[46] The HPT-JT gene was first mapped to a 60-cM region in 1q21-q32, which has since been narrowed to 15-cM.[42,45] The nature of the HPT-JT gene is still unresolved. It has been considered to be a tumor suppressor gene based on the findings of LOH involving the wild-type alleles in 1q-related renal and parathyroid tumors. However, these findings are not as frequent as in MEN 1-related tumors, where a high percentage of cases show loss of the *MEN1* locus. An alternative and yet unknown mechanism for tumorigenesis may be operating in HPT-JT.

Molecular diagnosis of HPT-JT

As the gene is not yet identified, linkage analysis using chromosome 1q polymorphic markers is still the only tool for genetic diagnosis.

Familial isolated hyperparathyroidism

FIHP (HRPT1, OMIM 145000) is a rare disorder manifesting in the adult, and is typically inherited as an autosomal dominant trait with a reduced penetrance. In the classical case, FIHP is clinically characterized by hypercalcemia, elevated parathyroid hormone levels, and uni- or multiglandular parathyroid tumors (Table 6.2). The diagnosis involves the exclusion of other familial disorders characterized by primary hyperparathyroidism, mainly MEN 1 and HPT-JT. To date, more than 100 FIHP families have been reported. It has been considered a separate entity, based on a previous study of an FIHP family that was not linked to the MEN 1 locus. However, this particular family has been re-analyzed and found to be an HPT-JT family, since linkage to the HPT-JT locus has been confirmed, and additional features, including jaw tumors and polycystic kidney disease, found.[46]

Molecular genetics of FIHP

Two main histopathological entities are found in FIHP. One is characterized by benign multiglandular disease or hyperplasia, and the other by solitary parathyroid adenoma, which in some cases is associated with parathyroid carcinomas. The former is consistent with the primary hyperparathyroidism found in MEN 1 patients, whereas the latter is comparable with that of the HPT-JT syndrome. Subsequent genetic analyses of these types of families confirmed such a phenotype–genotype correlation. FIHP families can be divided into the following subgroups: (1) true MEN 1 variants with demonstrated *MEN1* mutations;[39,40] (2) variants of the HPT-JT syndrome mapped to 1q21–q32;[45–47] (3) variants of familial benign hypercalciuric hypercalcemia (FBHH)—one family had all the features of hyperparathyroidism, including hypercalciuria, but, as for FBHH, the underlying etiology was associated with a mutated calcium-sensing receptor;[48] and (4) genetically undefined families—most of these families are small with two or three affected cases. They are neither associated with *MEN1* mutations nor are they linked to 1q. It is possible that some of these families may represent chance clusterings of sporadic hyperparathyroidism.

Molecular diagnosis of FIHP

The histopathology of the parathyroid tumors should guide the form of genetic testing. If a family is characterized by multiple cases with multiglandular disease, *MEN1* mutation analysis or linkage analysis (if the family is large enough) should be the priority. On the other hand, if parathyroid adenoma or even carcinoma is the main feature, then, until the gene is cloned, linkage analysis using 1q-linked polymorphic markers should be performed. Once the molecular diagnosis is established, it is important to follow up the patients with an understanding of the disease and their associated features. For small FIHP families (two or three affected members), one should realize that there is a high possibility that neither will yield any results. One should also be aware of other differential diagnoses, such as FBHH or, more rarely, the variant of FBHH characterized by hypercalciuria and mildly hyperplastic glands (Table 6.2). If these are suspected, linkage analysis and mutation analysis of the calcium-sensing receptor should be performed.

Case 1

A healthy 33-year-old man (II-2) was found to have hypercalcemia on routine medical check-up by his general practitioner. He was subsequently confirmed to have hyperparathyroidism. Neck exploration revealed four mildly enlarged glands. The enlarged gland was removed, and after a period of hypocalcemia, the calcium level was restored to normal. A few months later, the patient's brother was admitted acutely to the hospital for renal calculi and later was found to have hyperparathyroidism. A detailed family history (Figure 6.3) revealed that his mother (I-2) had died from a perforated ulcer, one paternal cousin (II-4) had been

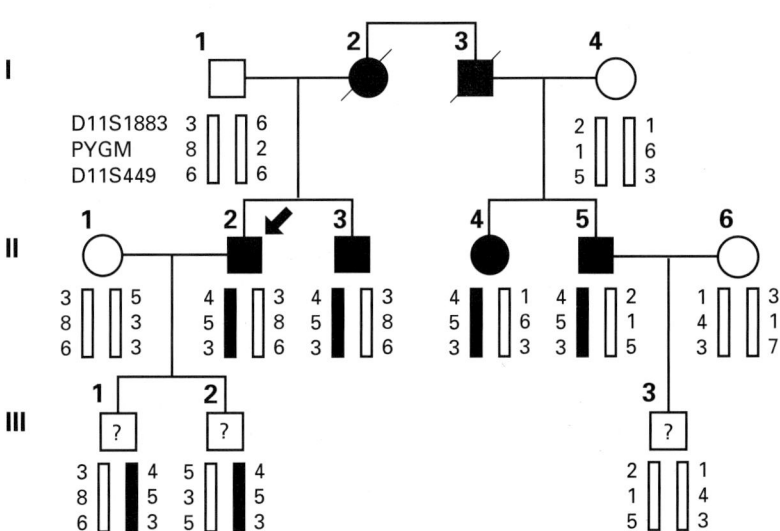

Figure 6.3

Pedigree of case 1, showing DNA-based predictive testing for MEN 1. Filled symbols indicate affected family members, and the arrow the proband. Numbers alongside the two lines below each individual indicate the genotypes for the informative marker systems, listed next to the symbol of I-1. The inferred mutant chromosome is indicated by a thick line with genotypes 4, 5 and 3. Of the individuals in generation III, both III-1 and III-2 carry the disease gene.

treated for prolactinoma, and another paternal cousin (II-5) had been treated for hyperparathyroidism and thymic carcinoid. The proband has two teenage children (III-1, III-2) and one teenage nephew (III-3). All of them have been healthy and asymptomatic.

Considerations

1. What is the management for the family?
2. If MEN 1 is confirmed, what is the optimum management for the patient and his brother?
3. What constitutes the biochemical and radiological screening for MEN 1?

Discussion of case 1

1. The case could not stress more the importance of careful family history. All family members should be contacted for consent for genetic testing. If such facilities are not available, blood samples can be sent to centers that have a special interest in this area. Genetic testing will help to establish the diagnosis of MEN 1 in this family, besides determining who the gene carriers are. In this case, no mutation could be identified by full sequencing of the *MEN 1* gene, and linkage analysis using MEN 1-linked markers was performed (Figure 6.3). Those who test negative can be exempted from further routine biochemical and radiological screening (III-2, III-3). Those who are positive (II-2, -3, -4, -5; III-1) should be followed up carefully by biochemical and radiological investigations, but no surgical interventions should be performed until hyperfunction or neoplasia is proven. It is very important to explain the condition in detail to all family members. A simple information sheet or booklet is very valuable, and psychological counseling should be made available.
2. Irrespective of the findings during neck exploration, $3\frac{1}{2}$ gland removal or total parathyroidectomy followed by autotransplantation should be performed together with thymectomy in MEN 1 patients. The likelihood that this patient will develop recurrence is high, and there is also a risk of developing thymic carcinoid. This patient should be carefully followed up, with the intent of re-exploration and thymectomy. Similar operations should be performed on his brother.
3. MEN 1 is a complex disease, and hence the patients and their families should be under the care of specialists. We recommend initial screening with: (1) for parathyroid involvement—serum intact PTH, total and ionized calcium, albumin and phosphate; (2) for endocrine pancreatic or adrenal involvement—chromogranin, fasting gastrin, glucose, C-peptide, abdominal ultrasound, CT scan or MRI; (3) for pituitary involvement—serum prolactin, and MRI or CT of the pituitary; (4) for foregut carcinoid—CT of the chest; and (5) for gastroduodenal carcinoid—upper gastrointestinal endoscopy. All blood tests and the abdominal ultrasound are performed yearly, and the rest or other special tests should be considered according to the history, signs and symptoms, and clinical examination of an individual.

Conclusion for case 1

Genetic testing for MEN 1 using mutation analysis or linkage analysis has allowed identification of gene carriers, for whom closer surveillance and follow-up should be carried out. This will allow early detection of any hyperfunctioning glands. In fact, these days most MEN 1-related hyperparathyroidism is detected by biochemical screening, as most patients are asymptomatic. This is also the case for non-functioning endocrine pancreatic tumors and anterior pituitary tumors. Before hyperfunction or tumor can be demonstrated, no prophylactic operation is indicated in MEN 1 patients, except concurrent thymectomy with parathyroidectomy when treating primary hyperparathyroidism.

Multiple endocrine neoplasia type 2 (MEN 2)
Clinical manifestations of MEN 2

Multiple endocrine neoplasia type 2A (Sipple's syndrome) is an autosomal dominantly inherited disease with a high degree of penetrance and variable expression (Table 6.2). It is characterized by the association of medullary thyroid carcinoma (MTC) with pheochromocytoma and, in some cases, hyperparathyroidism (HPT). MTC originates from the thyroid parafollicular C-cells, which secrete calcitonin. Virtually all patients with MTC have elevated serum levels of calcitonin, either basally or after stimulation by intravenous administration of pentagastrin.[49] Hence, serum levels serve as a good marker for MTC, and can be used both at the initial diagnosis and for the postoperative evaluation as a sign of persistent or recurrent disease.

Despite elevated serum calcitonin levels, patients with MTC usually present only with a mass in the neck region, and only rarely with general symptoms such as diarrhea and weight loss. MTC can usually be diagnosed by preoperative fine needle biopsy. The familial form constitutes about 25% of all cases of MTC. It is seen in almost all MEN 2A patients, and usually differs from the sporadic counterparts in that the tumors occur bilaterally and are preceded by general C-cell hyperplasia.[50] Thus, if MTC occurs in both lobes at fine needle biopsy, familial disease should be suspected.

Pheochromocytoma is seen in half of all MEN 2A patients. Like MTC, it occurs bilaterally and multicentrically and is preceded by diffuse and nodular hyperplasia.[51] Extra-adrenal tumors, especially in accessory adrenal glands, are described in nearly 50% of cases.[52] The delay in onset between MTC and pheochromocytoma can be more than 25 years.

MEN 2B (Froboese's syndrome or MEN 3) is characterized by the association of MTC and pheochromocytoma with a distinct phenotype: mucosal neuromas, intestinal ganglioneuromatosis and neurological disturbances.[53] A few hundred patients with this condition have been reported so far. About half of the cases appear to be new mutations, i.e. they have no family history of the disease but their children have a 50% risk of developing the disease.[54] Not uncommonly, the MTC in these patients is very aggressive and shows an early age of onset.[55]

Familial medullary thyroid carcinoma (FMTC) is a variant of MEN 2 in which C-cell tumors of the thyroid are the only lesions. FMTC is less common than MEN 2A, tends to present later and appears to be less aggressive than MEN 2A.[56] FMTC is only recognizable in large families where there is no sign of the associated MEN 2A lesions. In fact, it is more likely that a small family with only MTC is instead a MEN 2A family where pheochromocytoma or hyperparathyroidism has not yet been diagnosed.

Molecular genetics of MEN 2

The gene for MEN 2 was assigned in 1987 to the pericentromeric region of chromosome 10, and subsequent studies confirmed that MEN 2B and FMTC were also linked to the same region.[57,58] One of the candidate genes in this region, the *RET* protooncogene, had previously been shown to be expressed in the neuroectodermal tissues involved in MEN 2.[59] *RET* was subsequently shown to be the gene responsible for

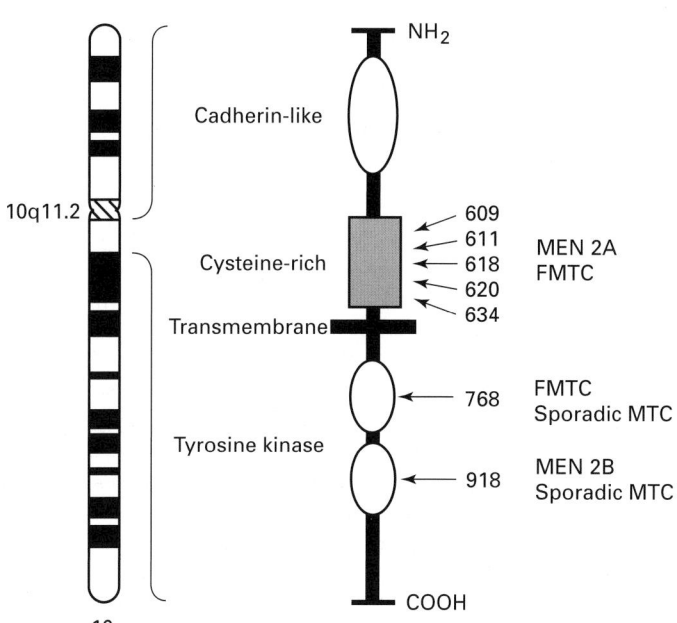

Figure 6.4
An idiogram of chromosome 10 and the RET protooncogene which is located in chromosome 10q11.2. The gene contains a cadherin-like, a cysteine-rich and two intracellular tyrosine kinase regions. The arrows indicate the number for each codon where the common germline mutations for each disease are found.

MEN 2A, MEN 2B, and FMTC when germline mutations were identified in affected patients but not in their unaffected relatives (Figure 6.4). The *RET* protooncogene encodes for a tyrosine kinase receptor, and both its upstream and downstream partners in RET signaling have been elucidated. The RET-mediated cell-transforming effect is most likely mediated by the activation of the phophatidylinositol-3-kinase/AKT pathway.[60] On the upstream side, the ligand glial cell line-derived neurotrophic factor (GDNF) and neurturin (NTN), and their membrane-bound receptors GFR-α_1 and GFR-α_2, form a complex with RET. This results in the dimerization of RET, leading to the activation of its tyrosine kinase function, and allowing it to transduce downstream signaling to the nucleus by phosphorylation of tyrosine residues in signaling proteins.[61] In vitro and in vivo studies have shown that GDNF and NTN can enhance the survival of various neurons by preventing apoptosis.[62,63] NTN and GFR-α_2 are structurally highly homologous to GDNF and GFR-α_1 respectively.[64,65] Recently, two additional ligand complexes have been described for RET. These are artemin and persephin, which activate RET by binding to the membrane-bound receptors designated GFR-α_3 and GFR-α_4 respectively.[66,67]

Nearly all mutations related to FMTC and MEN 2A involve the alteration of one of five cysteine residues within exons 10 and 11.[68,69] MEN 2B patients show instead a mutation altering a methionine to a threonine in codon 918 in exon 16 of *RET*.[70–72] To some extent, the type of mutation seems to correlate with the type of disease; that is, there seems to be a correlation between the phenotype and genotype.[73,74] Interestingly, the *RET* protooncogene was also found to be responsible for a subset of Hirschprung's disease.[75,76] The difference is that mutations in MEN 2A, MEN 2B and FMTC abnormally increase the function of the gene, whereas the mutations in Hirschprung's disease remove its normal function. MEN 2 has now clearly been shown to be an inherited mutation of a protooncogene.[77]

Management of MEN 2

Biochemical screening for C-cell hyperplasia and pheochromocytoma is an effective method to identify early stages of MEN 2. Family registers have been established in many countries and have helped to reduce morbidity and mortality for the disease.[78] However, these screenings are not only unpleasant for the patient but also costly, especially since the program has to be repeated many times. In non-carriers, biochemical screening will be negative, but has to be repeated year after year, due to the risk of late-presenting disease. Furthermore, this screening leads to false-positive results, and we now know that in some instances this has led to unnecessary thyroidectomy. In some of these cases, elevated calcitonin levels appear to have other causes than C-cell hyperplasia caused by MEN 2.[79,80]

Using DNA testing, it is now possible to exclude the non-carriers from screening and also to perform thyroidectomy on gene carriers before they have developed MTC.[79,81] This is important, since in a few cases metastatic MTC has developed before surgery in small children. Family mutational screenings are relatively simple to perform, but rely on the identification of the individual mutation in each family by DNA sequencing. Depending on the mutation, a simple restriction enzyme-based test might be developed in order to screen the family members at risk. By amplification of the mutated exon by PCR, and digestion with the appropriate restriction enzyme, the risk of MEN 2A can easily be confirmed or excluded.

At the 5th International Workshop on Multiple Endocrine Neoplasia in the summer of 1994, a consensus was reached concerning DNA testing for MEN 2. It is important to determine the individual mutation segregating in each MEN 2 kindred. One affected individual should be subjected to either DNA sequencing of exon 10 and/or 11 of the *RET* gene or a restriction enzyme-based test which will identify the mutation. Then, each at-risk individual should be offered a DNA test, which may be based on sequencing or on a restriction enzyme digest. If an at-risk individual tests negative (non-carrier), the test should be repeated on a newly drawn blood sample to avoid the risk of sample mix-up. After two negative DNA tests, the individual and her/his offspring can be taken off the screening program.

In patients who have (twice) tested positive for a MEN 2-associated mutation, total thyroidectomy should be performed. The time for the operation is subject to some controversy. Metastatic MTC has been reported as early as 6 years of age.[82] Therefore, the consensus at the Workshop was that, since the risk of operating on children is small, and considering the risk for metastatic disease, total thyroidectomy should be performed upon children at the age of 5–6 years. It should be emphasized that prophylactic thyroidectomies should be preferably performed at surgical centers with such experience and that proper genetic counseling should be made available to the patients and the family. Prophylactic thyroidectomy would cure at least 95% of MEN 2 gene carriers for MTC. The patients should then continue to be screened for early detection of pheochromocytoma.

The only effective treatment for MTC is surgery. When an MTC has been diagnosed, the treatment of choice is total thyroidectomy (risk of bilateral disease) with central lymph node resection.[83,84] Even persistent disease and recurrences can be successfully treated by surgery in selected cases.[85] So far, radiotherapy and chemotherapy have had little success in MTC treatment. In contrast to surgery for MTC, the surgical approach for MEN 2-related pheochromocytoma remains controversial. For a seemingly normal tumor, some advocate unilateral adrenalectomy,[86] while others prefer bilateral adrenalectomy, to lower the risk for recurrence, but at the cost of complicated hormone replacement.[87,88] However, even subtotal adrenalectomy has been performed with satisfactory results.[89,90] Whatever operative approach is employed, today the preoperative risk for the patient is acceptable.[91] The recent introduction of laparoscopic adrenalectomy will probably also be of benefit for this group of patients.[92,93]

Case 2

A 32-year-old woman was operated on for a single thyroid nodule which was clinically considered as sporadic, since no history of familial disease could be established. Histopathology of the tumor showed a medullary thyroid carcinoma with multifocal growth pattern and C-cell hyperplasia in the surrounding tissue. Owing to these findings, she was examined for MEN 2, but no evidence of other follow-up glandular involvement could be found. Six years of follow-up did not reveal signs of recurrence of MTC. Genetic analysis of the *RET* gene was performed on the patient's blood. This analysis revealed that she was indeed a carrier of a germline MEN 2-causing mutation. Subsequently, her offspring were tested, and two sons aged 11 and 5, were found to carry the same mutation. This 32-year-old patient is now pregnant.

Considerations for case 2

1. What are the future implications for the patient?
2. What should be done for her sons, who have known germline mutations, but are asymptomatic?
3. Should genetic testing be performed on her neonate, and, if so, when?

Discussion of case 2

1. As this patient has a mutation (codon 634 of *RET*) known to be associated with pheochromocytoma (and occasionally hyperparathyroidism) in addition to MTC, it is most important to investigate for this before delivery. As she was considered a 'sporadic' MTC, we may have overlooked this important feature. The patient should be followed-up lifelong for early detection of pheochromocytoma and hyperparathyroidism. In addition, it is important to investigate the patient's other family members, regardless of their age. The benefit of identifying other MEN 2 gene carriers is obvious.[94,95]

2. As in all situations concerning hereditary disease, it is most important to provide the family with detailed information both verbally and in written form and to explain that the boys are at risk of developing MTC. Current opinion would be to perform prophylactic thyroidectomies on both. Possible complications and the fact that the patients will need to be on lifelong thyroid hormone replacement therapy should be considered and discussed. Again, we emphasize that these patients should be referred to a highly specialized surgical center.

3. When to perform *RET* mutation analysis on a neonate remains an ethical dilemma. It seems most rational to withhold the genetic analysis until treatment can be offered. However, if the child turns out to be negative, the psychological relief to the family can be very rewarding. Obviously, this delicate issue has to be carefully discussed and considered by both the parents and clinicians.

Conclusions for case 2

Genetic testing now constitutes a part of the management plan for MEN 2 and FMTC. Besides its predictive value, it should be sought and the mutations confirmed for all patients from these families who have elevated calcitonin prior to total thyroidectomy. Prophylactic thyroidectomy can be considered in gene carriers as young as 5 years old without evidence of calcitonin elevation. Histopathological findings of C-cell hyperplasia and multifocal growth pattern of sporadic MTCs should lead to suspicion of MEN 2 disease. In our opinion, all patients with MTC displaying such phenomena should undergo molecular analysis for mutations in *RET*. Since approximately 30% of all MTC patients belong to an FMTC or MEN 2A family, perhaps all patients with MTC should be subjected to such analysis.

Familial cancer clinic

In the last decade, the molecular bases of hereditary cancer, including MEN, have been elucidated, and this large amount of genetic information has been transferred to clinical medicine. This rapid development has led to better management of cancer families, which has allowed identification of gene carriers, genetic counseling, surveillance programs to detect tumors, and prophylactic operations. In many countries, these multidisciplinary approaches have been integrated and organized into what is known as the familial cancer clinic (Figure 6.5).[96]

A typical familial cancer clinic usually consists of a genetic counselor and a clinical geneticist who have a special interest in hereditary cancer. Their roles are to explain to patients and their family members the nature of the disease, and the genetic issues such as transmission mode, penetrance and probability of inheritance, and to inform the patients of the cost of genetic testing and whether it is covered by health insurance. Besides providing genetic counseling, they may have to touch on psychosocial issues associated with the disease. Finally, they have to consent to the patients' genetic testing and organize the genetic tests. The clinical geneticist is usually in charge of or involved in the operation of a DNA diagnostic laboratory, and he or she has to validate the genetic test results. In most centers, the treating physicians or surgeons also participate in running the clinic, and this is especially important when dealing with complex diseases such MEN or when the management of patients is dependent on genetic results. It may be an enormous psychological burden for both patients and their family members to be aware of the diagnosis of a hereditary cancer, and therefore it is also important not to ignore their psychological wellbeing. If necessary, the geneticists and treating clinicians should refer them for psychological counseling.

In places where the luxury of such an organized clinic is not available, the treating clinician should be aware of the latest developments in hereditary cancer and know where to get assistance either for genetic testing or for clinical management.

Summary

In MEN, the appropriate application of genetic tools will permit early detection of the diseases and offer relief for the non-gene carriers. For those who carry the mutated gene, close surveillance, early intervention and even prophylactic operation (in the case of MEN 2) will be possible, with the intention of reducing its morbidity and mortality. It is expected that further genetic studies will continue to influence the development of its management.

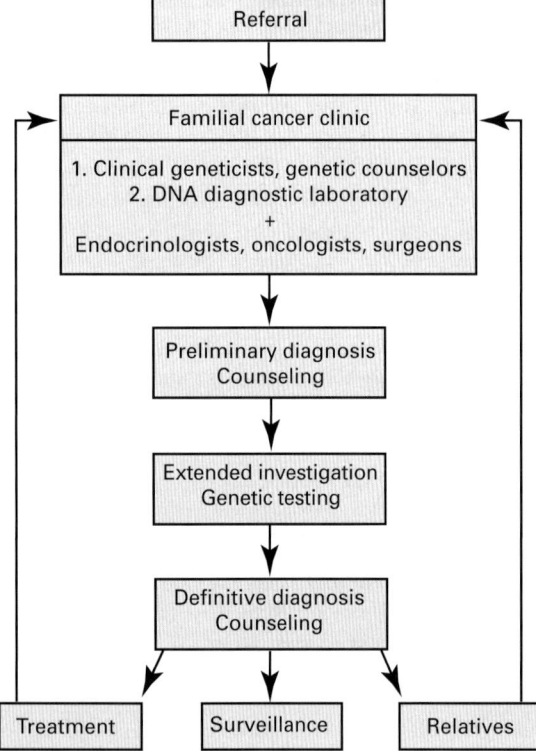

Figure 6.5
The flow chart of the organization and operation of a familial cancer clinic.

References

1. Werner P. Genetic aspects of adenomatosis of endocrine glands. *Am J Med* 1954; 16: 363–71.
2. Brandi ML, Marx SJ, Aurbach GD, Fitzpatrick LA. Familial multiple endocrine neoplasia type 1: a new

look at pathophysiology. *Endocrine Rev* 1987; **8**: 391–405.
3. Teh BT, Hii S, David R et al. Multiple endocrine neoplasia type 1 in two Asian families. *Hum Genet* 1994; **94**: 468–72.
4. Sakurai A, Katai M, Itakura Y, Nakajima K, Baba K, Hashizume K. Genetic screening in hereditary multiple endocrine neoplasia type 1: absence of a founder effect among Japanese families. *Jpn J Cancer Res* 1996; **87**: 985–94.
5. Trump D, Farren B, Wooding C et al. Clinical studies of multiple endocrine neoplasia type 1 (MEN1). *QJ Med* 1996; **89**: 653–69.
6. Burgess JR, Greenaway TM, Shepherd JJ. Expression of the MEN1 gene in a large kindred with multiple endocrine neoplasia type 1. *J Intern Med* 1998; **243**: 465–70.
7. Marx SJ, Spiegel AM, Skarulis MC, Doppman JL, Collins FS, Liotta LA. Multiple endocrine neoplasia type 1: clinical and genetic topics. *Ann Intern Med* 1998; **129**: 484–94.
8. Teh BT. Recent advances in multiple endocrine neoplasia type 1. *Curr Opin Diabetes Endocrinol* 1998; **5**: 35–9.
9. Skogseid B, Larsson C, Lindgren PG et al. Clinical and genetic features of adrenocortical lesions in multiple endocrine neoplasia type 1. *J Clin Endocrinol Metab* 1992; **75**: 76–81.
10. Darling TN, Skarulis MC, Steinberg SM, Marx SJ, Spiegel AM, Turner M. Multiple facial angiofibromas and collagenomas in patients with multiple endocrine neoplasia type 1. *Arch Dermatol* 1997; **133**: 853–7.
11. Nord B, Platz A, Smoczynski K et al. Malignant melanoma in patients with multiple endocrine neoplasia type 1 and the involvement of the MEN1 gene in sporadic melanoma. *Int J Cancer* 2000; **15**: 463–7.
12. Mallete L. Management of hyperparathyroidism in the multiple endocrine neoplasia syndromes and other familial endocrinopathies. *Endocrinol Metab Clin North Am* 1994; **1**:19–36.
13. Teh BT, McArdle J, Parameswaran V et al. Sporadic primary hyperparathyroidism in the setting of multiple endocrine neoplasia type 1. *Arch Surg* 1996; **131**: 1230–2.
14. Teh BT, McArdle J, Chan SP et al. Clinicopathologic studies of thymic carcinoids in multiple endocrine neoplasia type 1. *Medicine* 1997; **76**: 21–9.
15. Teh BT, Zedenius J, Kytölä S et al. Thymic carcinoids in multiple endocrine neoplasia type 1. *Ann Surg* 1998; **228**: 99–105.
16. Ballard HS, Frame B, Hartsock RJ. Familial multiple endocrine adenoma peptic ulcer complex. *Medicine* 1964; **43**: 481–516.
17. Skogseid B, Eriksson B, Lundqvist G et al. Multiple endocrine neoplasia type 1: a ten-year prospective screening study in four kindreds. *J Clin Endocrinol Metab* 1991; **73**: 281–7.
18. Wilkinson S, Teh BT, Davey KR, McArdle JP, Young M, Shepherd JJ. Cause of death in MEN1. *Arch Surg* 1993; **128**: 683–90.
19. Pipeleers-Marichal M, Somers G, Willems G et al. Gastrinomas in the duodenums of patients with multiple endocrine neoplasia type 1 and the Zollinger–Ellison syndrome. *N Engl J Med* 1990; **322**: 723–7.
20. Thompson NW. Management of pancreatic endocrine tumours in patients with multiple endocrine neoplasia type 1. *Surg Oncol Clin North Am* 1998; **7**: 881–91.
21. Grama D, Skogseid B, Wilander E et al. Pancreatic tumors in multiple endocrine neoplasia type 1: clinical presentation and surgical treatment. *World J Surg* 1992; **16**: 611–18.
22. Shepherd JJ, Challis DR, Davies PF, McArdle JP, Teh BT, Wilkinson S. Multiple endocrine neoplasms, microcarcinoids, the Zollinger–Ellison syndrome, lymph nodes and hepatic metastases. *Arch Surg* 1993; **128**: 1133–42.
23. Burgess JR, Greenaway TM, Parameswaran V, Challis DR, David R, Shepherd JJ. Enteropancreatic malignancy in MEN1-risk factors and pathogenesis. *Cancer* 1998; **83**: 428–34.
24. Lairmore TC, Chen VY, Debenedetti MK, Gillanders WE, Norton JA, Doherty GM. Duodenopancreatic resections in patients with multiple endocrine neoplasia type 1. *Ann Surg* 2000; **231**: 909–18.
25. Burgess JR, Greenaway TM, Parameswaran V, Shepherd JJ. Octreotide improves biochemical, radiological and symptomatic indices of gastroenteropancreatic neoplasia in patients with multiple endocrine neoplasia type 1 (MEN 1)—implications for an integrated model of MEN1 tumorigenesis. *Cancer* 1999; **86**: 2154–9.
26. O'Riordan D, O'Brien T, van Heerden J, Service F, Grant C. Surgical management of insulinoma associated with multiple endocrine neoplasia type 1. *World J Surg* 1994; **18**: 488–94.
27. Skogseid B, Öberg K, Åkerström G et al. Limited tumour involvement found at multiple endocrine neoplasia type 1 pancreatic exploration: can it be predicted by pre-operative tumour localisation? *World J Surg* 1998; **22**: 673–7.
28. Larsson C, Skogseid B, Oberg K, Nakamura Y, Nordenskjöld M. Multiple endocrine neoplasia type 1 gene maps to chromosome 11 and is lost in insulinoma. *Nature* 1988; **332**: 85–7.
29. Knudson AG. Mutation and cancer—statistical study of retinoblastoma. *Proc Natl Acad Sci USA* 1971; **68**: 820–3.
30. Larsson C, Calender A, Grimmond S et al. Molecular tools for presymptomatic testing in multiple endocrine neoplasia type 1. *J Intern Med* 1995; **238**: 239–44.
31. Chandrasekharappa SC, Guru SC, Manickam P et al. Positional cloning of the gene for multiple endocrine neoplasia type 1. *Science* 1997; **276**: 404–7.
32. European Consortium on MEN1. Identification of the multiple endocrine neoplasia type 1 (MEN1) gene. *Hum Mol Genet* 1997; **6**: 1177–83.

33. Agarwal SK, Guru SC, Heppner C et al. Menin interacts with the AP1 transcription factor JunD and represses JunD-activated transcription. *Cell* 1999; **96**: 143–52.
34. Wong FK, Burgess J, Nordenskjöld, Larsson C, Teh BT. Multiple endocrine neoplasia type 1. *Semin Cancer Biol* (in press).
35. Agarwal SK, Kester MB, Debelenko LV et al. Germline mutations of the MEN1 gene in familial multiple endocrine neoplasia type 1 and related states. *Hum Mol Genet* 1997; **6**: 1169–75.
36. Bassett JH, Forbes SA, Pannett AA et al. Characterization of mutations in patients with multiple endocrine neoplasia type 1. *Am J Hum Genet* 1998; **62**: 232–44.
37. Teh BT, Kytölä S, Farnebo F et al. Mutation analysis of the MEN1 gene in multiple endocrine neoplasia type 1, familial acromegaly and familial isolated hyperparathyroidism. *J Clin Endocrinol Metab* 1998; **83**: 2621–6.
38. Burgess JR, Nord B, Greenaway TM et al. Clinical and genetic correlates in multiple endocrine neoplasia type 1 (MEN1). *Clin Endocrinol* (in press).
39. Teh BT, Esapa CT, Grandell U et al. Familial isolated hyperparathyroidism associated with a constitutional MEN1 mutation. *Am J Hum Genet* 1998; **63**: 1544–9.
40. Kassem M, Kruse TA, Wong FK, Larsson C, Teh BT. Familial isolated hyperparathyroidism—a variant of MEN1. *J Clin Endocrinol Metab* 2000; **85**: 165–7.
41. Jackson CE. Hereditary hyperparathyroidism associated with recurrent pancreatitis. *Ann Intern Med* 1958; **49**: 829–36.
42. Teh BT, Farnebo F, Kristoffersson U et al. Autosomal dominant primary hyperparathyroidism–jaw tumour syndrome associated with renal hamartomas and cystic kidney disease: linkage to 1q21–q32 and loss of the wild-type allele in renal hamartomas. *J Clin Endocrinol Metab* 1996; **81**: 4204–11.
43. Szabo J, Heath B, Hill VM et al. Hereditary hyperparathyroidism–jaw-tumor syndrome: the endocrine-tumor gene HRPT2 maps to chromosome 1q21–q31. *Am J Hum Genet* 1995; **59**: 944–50.
44. Haven CJ, Wong FK, van Dam E et al. A genotypic and histological study of a large Dutch kindred with hyperparathyroidism–jaw tumor syndrome. *J Clin Endocrinol Metab* 2000; **85**: 1449–54.
45. Wassif WS, Moniz CF, Friedman E et al. Familial isolated hyperparathyroidism: a distinct genetic entity with an increased risk of parathyroid cancer. *J Clin Endocrinol Metab* 1993; **77**: 1485–9.
46. Wassif W, Farnebo F, Teh BT et al. Follow-up studies of a well-known FIHP family. *Clin Endocrinol* 1999; **50**: 191–6.
47. Teh BT, Farnebo F, Twigg S et al. Familial isolated hyperparathyroidism maps to the hyperparathyroidism–jaw tumor locus in 1q21–q32 in a subset of families. *J Clin Endocrinol Metab* 1998; **83** 2114–20.
48. Carling T, Szabo E, Bai M et al. Familial hypercalcemia and hypercalciuria caused by a novel mutation in the cytoplasmic tail of the calcium receptor. *J Clin Endocrinol Metab* 2000; **85**: 2042–7.
49. Wells SA. Multiple endocrine neoplasia type II. *Recent Results Cancer Res* 1990; **118**: 70–8.
50. Block MA, Jackson CE, Greenawald KA, Yott JB, Tashjian AH. Clinical characteristics distinguishing hereditary from sporadic medullary thyroid carcinoma. *Arch Surg* 1980; **115**: 142–8.
51. Carney JA, Sizemore GW, Sheps SG. Adrenal medullary disease in multiple endocrine neoplasia type 2. Pheochromocytoma and its precursors. *Am J Clin Pathol* 1976; **83**: 177–96.
52. Lips CJM, Lamers CBHW, Vasen HFA. Multiple endocrine neoplasia syndromes. *Critic Rev Oncol* 1984; **2**: 117–84.
53. Khairi MRA, Dexter RN, Burzynski NJ, Johnston CC. Mucosal neuroma, pheochromocytoma, and medullary thyroid carcinoma: multiple endocrine neoplasia type 3. *Medicine* 1975; **54**: 85–112.
54. Fryns JP, Chryzanowska K. Mucosal neuromata syndrome (MEN type IIb (III)). *J Med Genet* 1988; **25**: 703–6.
55. Norton JA, Froome LC, Farrell RE, Wells SA Jr. Multiple endocrine neoplasia type IIb—the most aggressive form of medullary thyroid carcinoma. *Surg Clin North Am* 1979; **59**: 109–18.
56. Farndon JR, Leight GS, Dilley WG et al. Familial medullary thyroid carcinoma without associated endocrinopathies: a distinct clinical entity. *Br J Surg* 1986; **73**: 278–81.
57. Mathew CG, Chin KS, Easton DF et al. A linked genetic marker for multiple endocrine neoplasia type 2A on chromosome 10. *Nature* 1987; **328**: 527–8.
58. Simpson NE, Kidd KK, Goodfellow PJ et al. Assignment of multiple endocrine neoplasia type 2A to chromosome 10 by linkage. *Nature* 1987; **328**: 528–30.
59. Santoro M, Rosati R, Grieco M et al. The *ret* proto-oncogene is consistently expressed in human pheochromocytomas and thyroid medullary carcinomas. *Oncogene* 1990; **5**: 1595–8.
60. Segouffin-Cariou C, Billaud M. Transforming ability of MEN2A-RET requires activation of the phosphatidylinositol 3–kinase/AKT signaling pathway. *J Biol Chem* 2000; **275**: 3568–76.
61. Jing S, Wen D, Yu Y et al. GDNF-induced activation of the RET protein tyrosine kinase is mediated by GDNFR-α, a novel receptor for GDNF. *Cell* 1996; **85**: 1113–24.
62. Lin LF, Doherty DH, Lile D, Bektesh S, Collins F. GDNF: a glial cell line-derived neurotrophic factor for midbrain dopaminergic neurons. *Science* 1993; **260**: 1130–2.
63. Oppenheim RW, Houenou LJ, Johnson JE, Lin LF, Li L, Lo AC. Developing motor neurons rescued from programmed and axotomy-induced cell death by GDNF. *Nature* 1995; **373**: 344–6.

REFERENCES

64. Kotzbauer PT, Lampe PA, Heuckeroth RO et al. Neurturin, a relative of glial cell-line-derived neurotrophic factor. *Nature* 1996; **384**: 467–70.
65. Buj-Bello A, Adu J, Pinon LG et al. Neurturin responsiveness requires a GPI-linked receptor and the RET receptor tyrosine kinase. *Nature* 1997; **387**: 721–4.
66. Baloh RH, Tansey MG, Lampe PA et al. Artemin, a novel member of the GDNF ligand family, supports peripheral and central neurons and signals through the GFRalpha3-RET receptor complex. *Neuron* 1998; **21**: 1291–302.
67. Milbrandt J, de Sauvage FJ, Fahrner TJ et al. Persephin, a novel neurotrophic factor related to GDNF and neurturin. *Neuron* 1998; **20**: 245–53.
68. Mulligan LM, Kwok JB, Healey CS et al. Germ-line mutations of the RET proto-oncogene in multiple endocrine neoplasia type 2A. *Nature* 1993; **363**: 458–60.
69. Donis-Keller H, Dou S, Chi D et al. Mutations in the RET proto-oncogene are associated with MEN2A and FMTC. *Hum Mol Genet* 1993; **2**: 851–6.
70. Hofstra RM, Landsvater RM, Ceccherini I et al. A mutation in the RET proto-oncogene associated with multiple endocrine neoplasia type 2B and sporadic medullary thyroid carcinoma. *Nature* 1994; **367**: 375–6.
71. Carlson KM, Dou S, Chi D et al. Single missense mutation in the tyrosine kinase catalytic domain of the RET protooncogene is associated with multiple endocrine neoplasia type 2B. *Proc Natl Acad Sci USA* 1994; **91**: 1579–83.
72. Eng C, Smith DP, Mulligan LM et al. Point mutation within the tyrosine kinase domain of the RET proto-oncogene in multiple endocrine neoplasia type 2B and related sporadic tumours. *Hum Mol Genet* 1994; **3**: 237–41.
73. Mulligan LM, Eng C, Healey CS et al. Specific mutations of the RET proto-oncogene are related to disease phenotype in MEN2A and FMTC. *Nature Genet* 1994; **6**: 70–4.
74. Mulligan LM, Eng C, Attie T et al. Diverse phenotypes associated with exon 10 mutations of the RET proto-oncogene. *Hum Mol Genet* 1994; **3**: 2163–7.
75. Edery P, Lyonnet S, Mulligan LM et al. Mutations of the ret proto-oncogene in Hirschsprung's disease. *Nature* 1994; **367**: 378–80.
76. Romeo G, Ronchetto P, Luo Y et al. Point mutations affecting the tyrosine kinase domain of the ret proto-oncogene in Hirschsprung's disease. *Nature* 1994; **367**: 377–8.
77. Santoro M, Carlomagno F, Romano A et al. Activation of RET as a dominant transforming gene by germline mutations of MEN2A and MEN2B. *Science* 1995; **267**: 381–3.
78. Gagel RF, Tashjian AH Jr, Cummings T et al. The clinical outcome of prospective screening for multiple endocrine neoplasia type 2a. *N Engl J Med* 1988; **318**: 478–84.
79. Lips CJ, Landsvater RM, Hoppener JW et al. Clinical screening as compared with DNA analysis in families with multiple endocrine neoplasia type 2A. *N Engl J Med* 1994; **331**: 828–35.
80. Gagel RF, Cote GJ, Martins Bugalho MJ et al. Clinical use of molecular information in the management of multiple endocrine neoplasia type 2A. *J Intern Med* 1995; **238**: 333–41.
81. Wells SA Jr, Chi DD, Toshima K et al. Predictive DNA testing and prophylactic thyroidectomy in patients at risk for multiple endocrine neoplasia type 2A. *Ann Surg* 1994; **220**: 237–50.
82. Graham SM, Genel M, Touloukian RJ, Barwick KW, Gertner JM, Torony C. Provocative testing for occult medullary carcinoma of the thyroid: findings in seven children with multiple endocrine neoplasia type IIA. *J Pediatr Surg* 1987; **22**: 501–3.
83. Cance WG, Wells SA Jr. Multiple endocrine neoplasia type IIa. *Current Problems Surg* 1985; **22**: 1–56.
84. Russell CF, Van Heerden JA, Sizemore GW et al. The surgical management of medullary thyroid carcinoma. *Ann Surg* 1983; **197**: 42–8.
85. Moley JF, Wells SA Jr, Dilley WG, Tisell LE. Reoperation for recurrent or persistent medullary thyroid cancer. *Surgery* 1993; **114**: 1090–6.
86. Lairmore TC, Ball DW, Baylin SB, Wells SA Jr. Management of pheochromocytomas in patients with multiple endocrine neoplasia type 2 syndromes. *Ann Surg* 1993; **217**: 595–601.
87. Freier DT, Thompsson NW, Sisson JC, Nishiyama RH, Freitas JE. Dilemmas in the early diagnosis and treatment of multiple endocrine adenomatosis, type II. *Surgery* 1977; **82**: 407–13.
88. Van Heerden JA, Sizemore GW, Carney JA, Grant CS, ReMine WH, Sheps SG. Surgical management of the adrenal glands in the multiple endocrine neoplasia type II syndrome. *World J Surg* 1984; **8**: 612–21.
89. Hamberger B, Telenius-Berg M, Cedermark B, Grondal S, Hansson BG, Werner S. Subtotal adrenalectomy in multiple endocrine neoplasia type 2. *Henry Ford Hosp Med J* 1987; **35**: 127–8.
90. Klempa I, Menzel J, Baca I. Subtotal adrenalectomy versus autotransplantation of the adrenal cortex—an alternative procedure in bilateral adrenalectomy in MENII? *Chirurgie* 1989; **60**: 266–71.
91. Gröndal S, Bindslev L, Sollevi A, Hamberger B. Adenosine: a new antihypertensive agent during pheochromocytoma removal. *World J Surg* 1988; **12**: 581–5.
92. Gagner M, Lacroix A, Bolte E. Laparoscopic adrenalectomy in Cushing's syndrome and pheochromocytoma. *N Engl J Med* 1992; **327**: 1033.
93. Evans DB, Lee JE, Merrell RC, Hickey RC. Adrenal medullary disease in multiple endocrine neoplasia type 2. Appropriate management. *Endocrinol Metabol Clin North Am* 1994; **23**: 167–76.

94. Telenius-Berg M, Berg B, Hamberger B, Tibblin S. Impact of screening on prognosis in the multiple endocrine neoplasia type 2 syndromes: natural history and treatment results in 105 patients. *Henry Ford Hosp Med J* 1984; **32**: 225–31.

95. Ponder BA, Ponder MA, Coffey R et al. Risk estimation and screening in families of patients with medullary thyroid carcinoma. *Lancet* 1988; **1**: 397–401.

96. Lindblom A, Nordenskjold M. Hereditary cancer. *Acta Oncol* 1999; **38**: 439–47.

7

Amenorrhea and infertility
Beverley Vollenhoven, Henry Burger

Definitions

Normal menstrual cyclicity is the result of ovarian follicular maturation, ovulation, and the formation of a corpus luteum and its subsequent demise, with falling concentrations of estradiol and progesterone leading to endometrial shedding and menstrual bleeding. Such cyclicity depends on intact mechanisms governing the secretion of the gonadotropins, follicle-stimulating hormone (FSH) and luteinizing hormone (LH). These mechanisms include pulsatile secretion of gonadotropin-releasing hormone (GnRH) and an intact ovarian feedback system, in which estradiol, progesterone and the inhibins influence gonadotropin secretion. Amenorrhea can thus result from disordered gonadotropin secretion, disordered ovarian function, an absent or abnormal endometrium, or anatomical abnormalities of the lower genital tract.

Primary amenorrhea is defined as the absence of menstruation by the age of 14 years in the absence of growth or secondary sexual characteristics, or the absence of menstruation by the age of 16 years regardless of the presence of secondary sexual characteristics.[1]

Secondary amenorrhea is defined as the absence of menstruation for 6 months in a woman who has previously menstruated.[1–3] Obviously, one of the most common reasons for secondary amenorrhea is pregnancy, so this must be ruled out.

Oligomenorrhea is the occurrence of irregular menstrual bleeding at intervals varying between 6 weeks and 6 months, and frequently represents a menstrual cycle disorder less severe than that leading to secondary amenorrhea.

Etiology

Causes of amenorrhea can be divided as follows:

1. Disorders of the hypothalamus
   (a) Functional
   (b) Organic
2. Disorders of the anterior pituitary
   (a) Hyperprolactinemia
   (b) Other anterior pituitary failure
3. Disorders of the ovary
   (a) Polycystic ovary syndrome
   (b) Premature ovarian failure
       (i) Iatrogenic
       (ii) Non-iatrogenic
4. Disorders of the outflow tract
   (a) Congenital
   (b) Acquired
5. Idiopathic delay of menstruation.

Disorders of the hypothalamus (hypogonadotropic amenorrhea)

The amenorrhea of hypothalamic dysfunction results from alterations in the normal pulsatile pattern of GnRH secretion, due to changes in the frequency, amplitude or both of the GnRH pulse generator.[4] This in turn leads to an abnormal pattern, particularly in the secretion of LH, with failure of normal follicular maturation and absence of the mid-cycle LH surge.

Functional

Hypothalamic amenorrhea is the most common cause of hypogonadotropic amenorrhea and is usually a diagnosis of exclusion; that is, pituitary, ovarian and outflow disorders must be excluded. It frequently involves problems such as stress, chronic illness, loss of weight and/or excessive physical exercise. Affected women may have normal or low concentrations of gonadotropins, particularly LH, with concentrations <3 IU/l. FSH is often in the normal follicular phase range. Prolactin concentrations are normal, CT scan or MRI shows no organic abnormalities, and there is a negative progestagen challenge test.[1]

In the past, women who had been on the oral contraceptive pill (OCP) and had ceased taking it with no return of their periods were said to have post-pill amenorrhea. It is now recognized that many of these women may have lost weight while on the OCP, and this is the reason for their amenorrhea. In others, the OCP may have been prescribed for a menstrual cycle disturbance, with failure of menses to occur after OCP cessation.

In general, fertility in women with functional hypogonadotropic hypogonadism is best achieved by reversing the cause for the hypothalamic disorder. If this is not possible, alternatives include administration of GnRH (subcutaneous or intravenous) or induction of ovulation with gonadotropins. Clomiphene citrate (CC) does not work in these women. In the absence of fertility concerns, hormone replacement therapy (HRT) should be administered, even in those who exercise, to prevent the development of osteoporosis and the long-term adverse cardiovascular consequences.[5,6] If contraception is a concern, the OCP should be administered.

Weight loss, anorexia nervosa and bulimia

Of women in Western cultures, 2.5% have an eating disorder. Two per cent suffer from bulimia nervosa, and 0.5% from anorexia nervosa.[7] Acute weight loss leads to a reduction in the pulsatility of GnRH secretion. The weight loss may be due to crash dieting or life-threatening anorexia nervosa.

Anorexia nervosa generally occurs in young, white middle-class females under the age of 25 years who often have an obsessive-compulsive disorder, prior history of depression or family history of psychiatric problems. There is a refusal to maintain the minimal body mass index (BMI), leading to a body weight less than 85% of that expected.[8]

The clinical signs include obvious thinness or emaciation, lanugo-type hair on the buttocks and back, rough dry skin, excessive sensitivity to cold, bradycardia, hypotension, hypothermia, edema, overactivity, hypercarotenemia due to a defect in vitamin A utilization, and hypokalemia due to laxative and diuretic abuse. Excessive exercise may be the first sign of incipient anorexia nervosa.[4,9] In reproductive terms, there is severe estrogen deficiency with the associated features due to hypoestrogenism. Pubertal delay may occur if the disorder begins prior to this cascade of events.

Gonadotropin concentrations are often undetectable, serum cortisol concentration is elevated due to a decrease in clearance with normal production, and there is relative hypothyroidism due to an increase in the formation of rT3 with a low T3. Thyroid-stimulating hormone (TSH) and thyroxine (T4) concentrations remain normal, as does the prolactin concentration. Thirty per cent of these women may remain amenorrheic despite normal gonadotropin concentrations which occur with weight gain.[4,8,10]

Bulimia is a less severe condition and is characterized by episodes of secretive binge eating followed by self-induced vomiting, fasting or laxative and diuretic abuse to combat weight increase. Weight changes are not as dramatic, and these women only rarely stop menstruating. In comparison to women with anorexia nervosa, depression is more likely to be present.[8]

Exercise

Exercise-induced amenorrhea may be present in athletes, in those involved in strenuous recreational activity, i.e. 'fitness fanatics', and in ballet dancers. Menarche may be delayed and, if menstrual cycles have been established, there is a higher incidence of short luteal phases, anovulation, oligomenorrhea and secondary amenorrhea.[6]

The etiological factors involved may include not only the exercise itself, but also poor nutritional intake, low body fat and low body weight. There is abnormal activation of the hypothalamic–pituitary–adrenal axis, with elevated concentrations of cortisol and an abnormal respose to CRH.[11]

Generalized osteoporosis may not occur as a result of the hypogonadal state in this condition, and cortical weight-bearing sites have been shown to have normal bone density in some studies; however, non-weight-bearing sites and weight-bearing sites with predominantly trabecular bone have been shown to have a reduced bone density.[5,6,12]

Organic

Organic causes of hypothalamic amenorrhea make up the minority of these conditions. There may be the rare syndrome of anosmia and amenorrhea, or alternatively a brain tumor may lead to hypothalamic dysfunction. These causes interfere with the normal pattern of GnRH synthesis, secretion or connection with the pituitary.[13]

Idiopathic hypogonadotropic hypogonadism and Kallmann's syndrome

These conditions are rare, more common in males and due to an isolated defect in GnRH secretion.[13] Kallmann's syndrome also includes absent olfactory bulbs clinically presenting as anosmia, though this is not universally the case.[14] Other anomalies present in Kallmann's syndrome include craniofacial defects of the midline (cleft palate and lip), sensorineural deafness, synkinesia, cerebellar ataxia and renal agenesis.[15] In reproductive terms, women present with primary amenorrhea, a lack of secondary sexual characteristics, low gonadotropin concentrations, normal karyotype and anosmia.

The genetics of these conditions is complicated and heterogeneous. Inheritance may be as an autosomal dominant, autosomal recessive or X-linked trait. There is variable expression of Kallmann's syndrome within families.[13]

Brain tumors and other conditions

In the presence of such a lesion, neurological symptoms and signs may be present, and areas of the hypothalamus controlling appetite, sleep, temperature and mood may be affected.[4] There may also be multiple pituitary hormone deficiencies, including a lack of gonadotropins.[13] Such tumors include craniopharyngiomas, gliomas and meningiomas, and other conditions include infiltrative disorders such as sarcoidosis and hemochromatosis, brain trauma and radiation therapy.[13] In the presence of infiltrative disorders, there are often systemic signs of the disease.

Disorders of the anterior pituitary (hypogonadotropic amenorrhea)

Hyperprolactinemia

Prolactin secretion is normally under tonic inhibition by hypothalamic dopamine. Hyperprolactinemia leads to altered GnRH pulsatility and hence amenorrhea by causing increased hypothalamic dopamine levels via an ultra-short feedback mechanism.

A variety of pharmacological agents cause hyperprolactinemia, and a number of pathological states also lead to this condition.

Pharmacological agents include:

1. Psychotropic drugs such as phenothiazines, butyrophenones, imipramine, amitryptyline and monoamine oxidase inhibitors.
2. Antihypertensives such as methyldopa and rauwolfia derivatives.
3. Hormones such as thyrotopin-releasing hormone (TRH) and OCP.
4. Opiates such as morphine.
5. Antiemetics such as metoclopramide.
6. Antihistamines such as meclazine.
7. Histamine (H_2) receptor antagonists such as cimetidine.[16]

Pathological states include:

1. Structural lesions of the central nervous system.
2. Structural lesions of the hypothalamus.
3. Pituitary tumors such as prolactinomas or mixed tumors.
4. Empty sella syndrome.
5. Lymphocytic adenohypophysitis.
6. Primary hypothyroidism.
7. Chronic renal failure.
8. Prolonged postpartum state.
9. Polycystic ovary syndrome (PCOS).
10. Chest wall disease.
11. Stress.
12. Ectopic sources.
13. Idiopathic.[16]

Pharmacological agents

These medications either decrease dopamine concentrations or block dopamine receptors and so cause hyperprolactinemia. If hyperprolactinemia is due solely to the use of a psychotropic drug for a psychiatric condition, the hyperprolactinemia should not be treated with a dopamine agonist until consultation with the treating psychiatrist. There is, however, some controversy as to whether dopamine agonists given in this situation will worsen the patient's psychiatric condition. There should still be protection against the development of osteoporosis by the administration of estrogen (see below).

Structural lesions of the central nervous system and hypothalamus

Such lesions generally cause hyperprolactinemia due to stalk compression. This leads to loss of tonic inhibition by dopamine. Such lesions include tumors such as craniopharyngiomas or Rathke's pouch cysts. Head injuries may cause similar problems.

Prolactinoma

Ten per cent (9–27%) of the population, on autopsy, have an asymptomatic prolactinoma.[10] These are the most common pituitary tumors. The sex distribution is equal; however, women present more often than men because of a disruption in reproduction or menstrual cycles. In men, the only symptoms are usually decreased libido or impotence. Prolactinomas are usually laterally placed in the pituitary and, if central, the possibility exists of a mixed tumor. One-third of patients who present with hyperprolactinemia have a pituitary tumor. The majority of these tumors are microadenomas (<1 cm) and are confined to the pituitary fossa, with a minority being macroadenomas (>1 cm), which may extend into the 3rd ventricle and cause optic nerve compression. They may also extend laterally and compress the cavernous sinus. Visual field assessment must be performed but will rarely show abnormalities in the presence of a microadenoma. Other pituitary hormone concentrations are usually normal.

Significant growth of a microadenoma is rare, hemorrhage is also rare, and both are more likely to occur during pregnancy.[17]

Mixed tumors
The presence of mixed tumors involving adrenocorticotropic hormone (ACTH), growth hormone (GH) or TSH is rare.[4]

Empty sella syndrome
This is a relatively rare condition mostly present in women (4–16% of women who present with amenorrhea and galactorrhea) and due to either congenital incompleteness of the sella diaphragm or secondary to surgery or radiotherapy. The subarachnoid space extends into the pituitary fossa, and the cerebrospinal fluid (CSF) exerts pressure on the sella floor. The pituitary gland becomes separated from the hypothalamus, and the control by dopamine of prolactin secretion is lost. It is a benign condition and does not lead to pituitary failure.[2,16]

Lymphocytic adenohypophysitis
This is a rare condition usually recognized in pregnancy or postpartum. It may present with the clinical features either of hypopituitarism or of a pituitary mass lesion. Mild hyperprolactinemia and diabetes insipidus may occur. CT scanning or MRI show a homogeneously enhancing pituitary mass with suprasellar extension. It should be suspected as the cause of pituitary enlargement in a woman presenting in pregnancy or postpartum. The definitive diagnosis requires pituitary biopsy, which will show lymphocytic infiltration. Spontaneous regression may occur, particularly with pituitary hormone replacement therapy.[18]

Primary hypothyroidism
In women with long-standing primary hypothyroidism, a pituitary adenoma or acidophilic hyperplasia may develop due to long-standing stimulation by TRH. Two per cent of women with hyperprolactinemia will be found to have primary hypothyroidism.[19]

Chronic renal failure
Chronic renal failure may cause hyperprolactinemia due to stress as well as a decrease in glomerular filtration rate. There is also an altered release mechanism and a decrease in the clearance and metabolism of prolactin.

Polycystic ovary syndrome
Hyperprolactinemia may coexist with anovulatory conditions such as PCOS. There is no conclusive support for one condition causing the other or vice versa.[20] Nevertheless, the practitioner is faced with a difficult clinical situation when a woman presents with obvious PCOS and has a mildly elevated prolactin concentration. Concentrations >1000 mU/l require exclusion of a pituitary adenoma.

Chest wall disease
This problem causes hyperprolactinemia by the same reflex that leads to prolactin secretion in response to suckling.

Ectopic sources
Rarely, prolactin may be produced by lung, renal or fibroid tumors.[2]

Idiopathic
This probably represents very small adenomas that are not detectable by MRI scanning, or lactotroph hyperplasia.

The clinical features of hyperprolactinemia include those of the underlying cause of the problem as well as specific symptoms related to the hyperprolactinemia itself. These symptoms and signs include the following:

1. Amenorrhea—30% of women who present with secondary amenorrhea have hyperprolactinemia, and not all will have galactorrhea. If amenorrhea and galactorrhea are both present, half of these women will have a pituitary adenoma.

2. Intermittent anovulation and oligomenorrhea.
3. Infertility.
4. Inadequate luteal phase and early miscarriage.
5. Galactorrhea—one-third of women with hyperprolactinemia present with galactorrhea. Not all women will develop galactorrhea, however, because the low-estrogen environment may prevent the normal action of prolactin on the breast. A minority of women with galactorrhea will have normal prolactin concentrations.
6. Estrogen-deficiency symptoms including hot flushes. Osteoporosis is the major concern of hypoestrogenism.
7. Headaches—a rare presentation. The headaches are usually bifrontal, retro-orbital or bitemporal.
8. Hirsutism.[2,16,21–24]

The physical examination may be normal, except for the presence of galactorrhea. Visual field examination is usually likewise normal, and need only be consistently performed if a macroadenoma is present. If optic nerve compression has occurred, bitemporal hemianopia will be found. There may rarely also be signs of acromegaly or Cushing's syndrome.

The diagnosis of hyperprolactinemia and its causes involves various diagnostic tests, including the following:

1. Prolactin concentration—hyperprolactinemia is defined based on an individual laboratory's standard in its radioimmunoassay (RIA). This usually varies from 100 to 600 mU/ml, most women having serum concentrations less than 400 mU/ml.[25] An elevated concentration should be present on two separate occasions for the diagnosis to be made.
2. TSH to exclude primary hypothyroidism as the cause.
3. MRI represents the gold standard for the detection of a pituitary tumor. In many centers this may not be available, and therefore a CT scan with intravenous contrast enhancement remains adequate, as, if an adenoma is present, it is only important to differentiate a microadenoma from a macroadenoma. In the presence of a tumor, there may also be enlargement of the sella or demineralization of bone.

If the concentration of prolactin is ≥1000 mU/ml, 25% of patients will have a pituitary microadenoma; if the level is ≥2000 mU/ml, 50% of women will have a tumor, and if the level is ≥4000 mU/ml, then almost 100% of women will have a tumor.[25,26]

FSH and LH concentrations are generally normal, but they may also be low (<3 IU/l).

The aims of treatment are four-fold: to treat infertility, reduce tumor size, treat galactorrhea if causing discomfort, and prevent osteoporosis and treat hypoestrogenic symptoms.

The major class of drugs used to treat hyperprolactinemia are the dopamine agonists. These drugs include bromocriptine (Parlodel), cabergoline and pergolide.

Bromocriptine is a semisynthetic ergot alkaloid which binds to dopamine receptors and mimics the dopamine inhibition of prolactin secretion. It also blocks TRH stimulation of prolactin and decreases DNA synthesis and reduces mitotic activity in the pituitary. Peak blood levels occur 2–3 h after an oral dose, but suppression is maintained for 8 h, so only twice-daily dosage is required. During treatment, tumors usually decrease in size, fibrosis may occur and visual defects will also be reversed. Once treatment is stopped, the prolactin concentration will usually return to the pretreatment level.[2,10] The side-effects of bromocriptine are postural hypotension, headaches, nausea and vomiting, constipation, hallucinations (<1%), nasal stuffiness and lethargy. The excretion of bromocriptine is via the biliary tract (90%), with 6–7% being excreted in the urine.

Bromocriptine is commenced at a dose of 1.25 mg (half a tablet) at night for 3–4 days, increasing to 2.5 mg at night. The initial dose should be given with the patient in bed, and with food. The drug is normally ingested in the middle of a meal. After 3–4 weeks, the prolactin concentration should be measured and the dose can be incrementally increased (doubled) until the concentration is in the normal range and the patient commences regular menstruation. It is rare to require greater than 20 mg twice daily, and most women will respond to a dose of 2.5–5 mg twice daily. If side-effects are not tolerated, the medication can be self-administered vaginally. The most common cause of treatment failure is non-compliance.

Eighty per cent of women will develop regular menstrual cycles. The resolution of galactorrhea is much slower. If the woman is being treated for infertility, conception usually occurs within six ovulatory cycles. The mean number of ovulatory cycles for conception is 1.9. There is an 80% pregnancy rate, with no increase in the multiple pregnancy rate. In some women (5%), adequate prolactin suppression is not associated with a return of ovarian function, and these women will also require CC. In a further 5% of women, despite high doses of bromocriptine, the prolactin level may not be suppressed. In this situation, the bromocriptine should be decreased to 20 mg/day and T4 can also be administered, even though thyroid function may be normal. If ovulation still does not occur, CC can be added.[2,10] Alternatively, cabergoline may be tried (see below).

In the woman with a macroadenoma, bromocriptine works less predictably. These tumors may decrease by about 50% in size, with a corresponding reduction in the prolactin level.

Once pregnancy does occur, bromocriptine can be ceased. However, if the patient has a macroadenoma, and particularly if the floor or the walls of the sella turcica are destroyed, the medication should be continued because of the risk of growth and hemorrhage. There are no known teratogenic effects of bromocriptine.[27,28] During pregnancy, it is mandatory that formal visual field testing is carried out once in each trimester. Five per cent of women with a microadenoma will have asymptomatic tumor growth during pregnancy, and 2% will have symptomatic growth. In women with a macroadenoma, 15% will have symptomatic growth of their tumors. Headaches occur before visual symptoms in most cases. If tumor growth does occur or if symptoms are present, bromocriptine treatment will be effective in resolving the situation with no adverse fetal effects. Breastfeeding can take place with no risk of tumor growth. In some women, there is no recurrence of the tumor or hyperprolactinemia after pregnancy. This may be due to infarction of the tumors during pregnancy.[10]

Cabergoline is an ergoline-selective D_2 dopamine agonist that has a longer duration of action than bromocriptine. It inhibits prolactin secretion in women with and without hyperprolactinemia. A single dose of 0.3–1 mg may last for 21 days.[29] As with bromocriptine, there is shrinkage of prolactinomas and the drug can also be used to inhibit postpartum lactation.[30] The European Cabergoline study group has reported that this drug, compared to bromocriptine, achieves ovulatory cycles or pregnancy in more women (72% versus 52%) as well as stable prolactin concentrations in more women (83% versus 58%).[29] Cabergoline is likely to be safe in pregnancy.[31] As far as side-effects are concerned, the drug appears to be better tolerated than bromocriptine, with fewer women stopping the drug because of side-effects (3% versus 12%).[29,30] The side-effects are similar to those experienced with bromocriptine. The starting dose of cabergoline is 0.5 mg weekly, with dosage increments occurring no more frequently than monthly. Most women are controlled on doses of 0.5 mg weekly to 1 mg twice weekly. Because of its efficacy and long half-life, allowing weekly administration in most patients, cabergoline is becoming the drug of first choice for the management of hyperprolactinemia.

Pergolide (50–100 μg/day) is also more potent and longer-lasting than bromocriptine. Pergolide may be administered as a single daily dose. Its major application is in patients intolerant of bromocriptine or cabergoline.

Surgery and radiotherapy are also options for a woman with a pituitary adenoma. Surgery is best reserved for women who are unresponsive to medical therapy. Surgery is carried out through the sphenoid sinus via a sublabial incision. Once the adenoma extends beyond the sella, total removal is impossible. Therefore, there is a high rate of recurrence (50% overall, 90% for macroadenomas, and 10% for microadenomas) and also a high postoperative morbidity rate in terms of panhypopituitarism (10–52% for macroadenomas).[32] Short-term morbidity includes CSF leaks, meningitis and diabetes insipidus. The results with radiotherapy are poor. The response of the tumor is slow (it may take years to decrease in size), and panhypopituitarism may develop up to 10 years later.[10]

A common management problem is that of the patient with hyperprolactinemia and secondary amenorrhea who is not desirous of fertility. Because the dopaminergic agonists are expensive drugs with side-effects, a safe and effective strategy is to give such patients the OCP only, with 6–12-monthly monitoring of serum prolactin concentrations. Only persistently rising levels would lead to a reassessment of the need for dopaminergic agonists in addition, or further neuroradiology to assess the state of an underlying pituitary adenoma.[33] The OCP will relieve the hypoestrogenic side-effects as well as prevent osteoporosis. It has been shown that women with hyperprolactinemic amenorrhea develop significant osteoporosis and that the osteoporosis may be worse than in naturally menopausal women.[34,35]

Other anterior pituitary failure

Anterior pituitary failure may also occur due to other pituitary tumors which, due to their size, may cause compression and stop secretion of other hormones, including gonadotropins. Other conditions include craniopharyngiomas, malignant cerebral tumors, tuberculomas, gummas, internal carotid artery aneurysms, and hydrocephalus, all of which may cause amenorrhea due to pituitary compression and disruption of the hypothalamic–pituitary axis.

Pituitary insufficiency may also occur due to Sheehan's or Simmonds' syndrome or after severe head injury, as well as after cranial irradiation.[2]

Disorders of the ovary

Polycystic ovary syndrome

PCOS was first described in 1935 by Stein and Leventhal.[36] They reported the triad of amenorrhea, infertility and hirsutism with characteristic ovarian morphological changes, including ovarian enlargement, thickened sclerotic ovarian capsule, multiple peripheral follicles and stromal hyperplasia. It is now recognized that this syndrome displays a spectrum of disease severity, with Stein–Leventhal syndrome being at the severe end of the spectrum.

The terms polycystic ovaries and polycystic ovary syndrome (PCOS) are a source of considerable confusion to many clinicians. It is important to distinguish the two. The term polycystic ovaries refers primarily to appearances seen at high-resolution transvaginal pelvic ultrasonography. Principal features include the presence of more than 10 ovarian follicles, 2–8 mm in diameter, peripherally arrayed around each ovary, with increased stromal echogenicity and, usually, an increase in ovarian volume. These ultrasonographic appearances have been described in approximately one-quarter of normal subjects with regular menstrual cycles.[37] The significance of incidentally discovered polycystic ovaries in an otherwise normal subject is not known, although it could be postulated that she may be at increased risk of the development of menstrual cycle abnormalities and/or hirsutism, should she gain weight.

The term PCOS is used to describe a clinical disorder which may have one or more of several different features. A National Institutes of Health Conference on the disorder proposed that three minimal criteria should be used: chronic anovulation leading to menstrual irregularity, evidence of hyperandrogenism, and the exclusion of other diseases.[38] This, too, is not a completely satisfactory definition. A not uncommon clinical situation is that of a young woman who describes menstrual irregularity from the time of menarche but who has no other evidence of any disorders, including no evidence of hyperandrogenism, either clinical or biochemical. The present authors would classify her as having PCOS if her ovaries had the typical appearance on ultrasonography, although she would not fit the NIH guidelines precisely. The authors are unaware of a satisfactory resolution to this dilemma.

It should also be noted that great confusion can be planted in the mind of a patient who is told that she has polycystic ovaries or PCOS. This is frequently interpreted as meaning that she has significant ovarian cysts and that she is likely to require one or more pelvic operations to deal with them. It is most important for the clinician to describe carefully the meaning of a term which does not imply the presence of ovarian cysts in the normal sense of that term.

The genetics of polycystic ovary syndrome

There is considerable evidence that PCOS clusters in families, with most studies suggesting an autosomal dominant pattern of inheritance, perhaps modified by environmental factors. Several genetic loci have been proposed as being linked to the syndrome, including the gene coding for the cholesterol side-chain cleavage enzyme (CYP 11a), the insulin gene and the follistatin gene, but the situation remains unresolved. The topic has been reviewed recently.[39]

Clinical presentation and clinical assessment

Patients fitting the definition of PCOS can present in several different ways:

1. A lifelong history of oligomenorrhea, i.e. menses occurring at intervals of more than 6 weeks but less than 6 months, since the time of menarche without features of hyperandrogenism. Such patients typically give a history of the occurrence of 2–4 menstrual bleeds per annum, often without any preceding features suggestive of the occurrence of an ovulatory cycle, such as premenstrual irritability, mastalgia or bloating. Such patients may present to the clinician primarily because of their concern about menstrual irregularity or because of their concerns regarding fertility.
2. Hirsutism with or without menstrual irregularity.
3. Obesity with or without menstrual disturbance.
4. Type II diabetes or gestational diabetes mellitus: the recognition that insulin resistance is a major component of PCOS raises the possibility that the disorder may be present in patients presenting with type II diabetes or with gestational diabetes mellitus, and recent investigations in particular suggest the possibility that the latter is an important presentation requiring subsequent management.[40]

The clinical assessment of the patient will depend on her reasons for presentation. If she presents with a history of oligomenorrhea, then a careful menstrual history is required. Inquiry about excessive hair growth or the treatment of it will assist in the clinical definition. A history of weight changes since menarche may also be important. Patients with PCOS often give a history of childhood obesity continuing after the menarche. Weight gain after menarche may also induce oligomenorrhea in patients with PCOS who may previously have had regular cycles. The clinical assessment of the patient presenting with infertility will clearly require the normal assessment of sexual function, timing of intercourse, possibility of infertility in the male partner, and exclusion of other disorders such as hypothyroidism or hyperprolactinemia with a history of galactorrhea.

In the clinical examination, the presence of obesity should be recorded, with particular reference to measurements of both height and weight and the calculation of a BMI. The presence of hirsutism should be sought carefully. Patients with PCOS which includes significant obesity and hirsutism sometimes have the clinical sign of acanthosis nigricans, characterized by brown prominent verrucous lesions at the base of the neck, in the axillae or under the breasts. Acanthosis nigricans is a clinical sign of marked insulin resistance. Pelvic examination is mandatory for the patient presenting with infertility, but in these authors' views is not mandatory for the patient presenting primarily with oligomenorrhea, particularly if she has not been previously sexually active.

Investigations
The patient who presents with infertility
Investigations are appropriate for the patient in whom a clinical diagnosis of PCOS has been made as part of the overall assessment of an infertile couple. Other reversible causes of oligomenorrhea should be excluded such as significant hyperprolactinemia and primary hypothyroidism. Hyperprolactinemia in the patient presenting with oligomenorrhea and the clinical diagnosis of PCOS can be a problem, as it may occur in up to a quarter of patients with this condition. If hyperprolactinemia is confirmed, radiological assessment is necessary (see above).

Because of the presence of insulin resistance and hyperlipidemia in patients with PCOS, baseline estimates of serum cholesterol and its subfractions and serum triglycerides is important, and increasingly a baseline fasting blood glucose with concomitant insulin measurement and calculation of ratio is recommended to screen for insulin resistance or a glucose tolerance test should be performed.[41] Pelvic ultrasonography should be done before ovulation induction is attempted, and routine steps such as semen analysis in the partner and the checking of rubella immunity status should be the standard infertility investigations.

The question of whether tubal patency needs to be established prior to ovulation induction in a patient with PCOS is controversial. The authors' practice is to wait until at least three ovulatory cycles have been induced by CC before checking tubal status, ideally by laparoscopy. If the patient requires gonadotropin ovulation induction, it is mandatory that tubal status is checked prior to treatment commencement.

The patient who presents with abnormal bleeding
For the patient presenting with oligomenorrhea, the assessment of prolactin and thyroid status is similar to that described above, as is the assessment of serum lipids and insulin resistance status. In such patients, ultrasonography is helpful to assess whether endometrial abnormalities are present.

Management of the the patient with oligomenorrhea
The major clinical problems requiring management in the patient with oligomenorrhea include the unexpected and inconvenient occurrence of spontaneous menses, the possibility of unwanted pregnancy in the woman who is sexually active, and the protection of the endometrium, as women with PCOS are classically anovulatory, their endometrium thus being exposed to unopposed estrogen.

For the woman who is not sexually active, it is the authors' practice to prescribe the OCP, or recommend the intermittent cyclic use of a progestin only if contraindications to estrogen are present. A typical regimen for the latter would be the use of medroxyprogesterone acetate 10 mg daily or norethisterone 1.25–2.5 mg daily for the first 12 days of every calendar month or every second calendar month. These doses are adequate to provide endometrial protection.

For the woman who is sexually active, the most convenient therapy is a routine combined OCP. If the oligomenorrhea is accompanied by excessive weight, and/or lipid abnormalities, then weight control and a prescription of an adequate exercise regimen are appropriate. Whether the use of drugs to treat the underlying insulin resistance is appropriate for women presenting only because of oligomenorrhea is unresolved at the time of writing.

Management of the patient with infertility

Infertility management requires first the management of any other potentially reversible disorders and the exclusion of a significant male factor. If the patient is overweight, attempts at weight reduction are particularly appropriate.

If such measures are either inappropriate or unsuccessful, conventional initial therapy for anovulatory infertility due to PCOS is the use of the ovulatory stimulant CC. Given in the form of 50-mg tablets, it is conventional to use CC beginning between the 2nd and 5th day of a spontaneous cycle or after the induction of a withdrawal bleed using cyclic progestagen as described above. Preceding pelvic ultrasonography is mandatory to exclude other lesions, in particular to exclude the unlikely but important possibility of an ovarian tumor. CC therapy can be monitored using a basal body temperature chart or using hormone measurements. It is the authors' practice to advise the use of a temperature chart and the obtaining of a blood sample a week or so after a temperature rise, if such can be demonstrated. An alternative is simply to take the sample on day 21 or day 22 to confirm whether or not ovulation has occurred. If facilities are readily available, monitoring pelvic ultrasonography to detect the presence of an ovulatory follicle and to assist in the timing of sexual intercourse can be very helpful. However, it is generally recommended that couples have intercourse on alternate days from days 10–20 of the CC cycle. If ovulation is not induced by the use of 50 mg daily of CC, the dose can be increased to 100 mg and up to 150 mg per day.

For the patient who does not ovulate in response to adequate doses of CC or who ovulates but fails to conceive, the next step in infertility management has currently become quite controversial. The possibilities include the use of gonadotropins for ovulation induction, the use of ovarian cautery to attempt to restore spontaneous cyclic menses, or the use of drugs which decrease insulin resistance in an attempt to reverse the underlying pathogenesis of the disorder. Such drugs include metformin and troglitazone. Practice in regard to the choice of these possibilities varies in different parts of the world and will be dictated by what is available to the managing clinician.

In the authors' practice, the usual next step after failed CC therapy is the use of gonadotropins. The details of gonadotropin therapy are beyond the scope of the present text—such patients require referral to units specializing in ovulation induction therapy. A useful account of such therapy is that by Vollenhoven and Healy.[42]

The use of ovarian cautery is again generally regarded as a specialist procedure for the reproductive endocrine surgeon. This topic has been reviewed by Donesky and Adashi.[43]

The use of antidiabetic drugs has been described recently in a small number of publications. In general, these women have been treated in small numbers and have been obese. No larger detailed studies are available to evaluate long-term effectiveness in significant numbers of women, especially those who are not obese.

Both metformin and troglitazone are insulin-sensitizing drugs and may reduce ovarian androgen secretion. Some reports indicate that they may restore normal menstrual cyclicity.[44–49]

It seems likely that the use of such agents will become increasingly popular, particularly as they represent a non-invasive approach to the restoration of spontaneous ovulatory function and hence a much more desirable approach to the management of infertility, particularly when a theoretically underlying abnormality is dealt with.

Premature ovarian failure (hypergonadotropic amenorrhea)

The term hypergonadotropic amenorrhea is perhaps more accurate a term than premature ovarian failure (POF), as, if serum FSH concentrations are measured on a daily basis, they are not elevated at all times. Some patients may even ovulate and become pregnant, although this is rare.[50]

POF has significant long-term consequences, both psychosocial and physical. These women have twice the age-specific mortality rate compared to women without this problem. All causes of death are increased.[51]

By the age of 40 years, 1% of women have undergone POF, and by the age of 30 years, 0.1% have this diagnosis.[52]

The diagnosis is made in a woman who is aged <40 years, has primary or secondary amenorrhea, has hypoestrogenic symptoms, and has gonadotropin concentrations in the postmenopausal range.[50,53]

The etiology of POF can be divided into iatrogenic and non-iatrogenic causes.

Iatrogenic
Surgical removal of the ovaries
This may occur for a number of reasons, including removal because of endometriosis as well as gynecological cancer, including childhood cancer.

Radiotherapy or chemotherapy

The adverse effects of radiotherapy and chemotherapy on the ovary may be temporary and short-lived, but the recovery is often unpredictable and there may be permanent damage to ovarian function.[54] The effect of radiotherapy depends on the age at treatment and the dose (Table 7.1). Dose for dose, the younger the woman, the less likely it is that she will be permanently affected. If the effect is temporary and ovarian function returns and she becomes pregnant, there is no higher incidence of congenital abnormalities.[2,54]

An attempt to preserve ovarian function prior to radiotherapy has been made by transposing the ovaries. This has been shown to decrease ovarian dysfunction, but its routine use prior to radiotherapy for Hodgkin's lymphoma remains controversial.[55] The excision of ovarian tissue prior to treatment (both radiotherapy and chemotherapy), its freezing and subsequent replacement after remission have recently become an option.

Similar to radiotherapy, the effects of chemotherapeutic agents on the ovary depend on the woman's age and the type of agent and the dose. Alkylating agents, including cyclophosphamide, are particularly toxic and, similarly to radiotherapy, if the adverse ovarian effect is short-lived and the woman becomes pregnant, there is no increase in congenital abnormalities.[54] The combination of radiotherapy and chemotherapy is worse than each individually.[10]

Non-iatrogenic
Autoimmunity

Some of these patients may have been classified as having idiopathic POF in the past. Histologically, the ovaries contain normal-appearing primordial follicles, but developing follicles contain lymphocytes and plasma cells. It may present as a component of autoimmune polyglandular syndrome, which encompasses Hashimoto's thyroiditis, hypoparathyroidism, Addison's disease and mucocutaneous candidiasis.[56,57] Other autoimmune disorders which are associated with POF are myasthenia gravis, idiopathic thrombocytopenic purpura, rheumatoid arthritis, vitiligo, and autoimmune hemolytic anemia.[58] Antibodies against thyroglobulin, nuclear antigen, heart and tissue gluten and increased concentrations of immunoglobulin (IgM) or decreased concentrations of complement, C2 and C4, have been reported in women with POF compared to the normal population.[59] There is also some evidence for the presence of ovarian antibodies,[60] although, in practice, testing for such antibodies is not useful diagnostically.

Chromosomal abnormalities

Disorders of gonadal development (gonadal dygenesis) may present as primary or secondary amenorrhea with 40–50% of cases of primary amenorrhea being due to gonadal dysgenesis.[61] The most common chromosomal abnormality is 45,XO (Turner's syndrome), followed by a variety of mosaicisms (45,XO/46,XX: 46,XX/47,XXX) and Xp or Xq deletions.[62] If the woman has a mosaicism with a Y chromosome present, it is important that all gonadal tissue is excised, because of the 1 in 4 risk of gonadal malignancies such as gonadoblastomas, dysgerminomas and yolk sac tumors.[4,63] The presence of an XX component (XX/XO) yields a variety of responses with often some degree of feminization, menstruation and fertility. Such women may have normal or, more usually, short stature.[4] Premature ovarian failure in the presence of a chromosomal abnormality occurs because the functioning follicles undergo atresia at a faster rate.[2]

Infections

Rarely, infections such as mumps or chicken pox may cause irreversible ovarian damage and POF.[10] Other infections implicated, with no definite cause–effect relationship established, are *Shigella* and malaria.[64]

Gonadotropin and gonadotropin receptor abnormalities

These conditions are rare. Mutations of the β-subunit of FSH, mutations in the gene for the FSH receptor and mutations in the gene for the LH receptor have all been described (reviewed by Kalantaridon et al[62]).

Galactosemia

Galactosemia, an inborn error of galactose metabolism, is a rare autosomal recessive condition where

Ovarian dose	Sterilization effect
60 rads	No effect
150 rads	Some risk >40 years
250–500 rads	Ages 15–40: 60% sterilized
500–800 rads	Ages 15–40: 60–70% sterilized
>800 rads	100% permanently sterilized

Table 7.1
Sterilization effects of radiotherapy.[2]

high gonadotropin concentrations are present with normal ovarian follicles. In women with galactosemia, there is a deficiency of galactose-1-phosphate uridyl transferase, and an abnormal carbohydrate component of the gonadotropin molecule renders both FSH and LH inactive. The problem may also be present within the ovary. The accumulation of galactose and/or galactose 1-phosphate may cause damage to the oocytes as well as to the ovarian stroma. Fewer eggs may be present, as a result of galactose affecting the migration of germ cells from the genital ridge. These are hypotheses, and the actual cause of POF in these women remains unknown. They may be mentally retarded and suffer hepatic, renal, lenticular and neurological abnormalities. Early diagnosis and the institution of the appropriate diet permits normal health and survival.[10]

Enzyme deficiences

These include cholesterol desmolase, 17α-hydroxylase and 17–20 desmolase. In affected women, there is impairment of estrogen synthesis, and therefore primary amenorrhea and absence of secondary sex characteristics, despite the presence of normal ovarian follicles (reviewed by Kalantaridou et al[62]). Individuals with the first condition rarely survive to maturity. 17α-Hydroxylase deficiency affects both ovaries and adrenals and, as well as having POF, the woman is also hypertensive and hypokalemic. In 17–20 desmolase deficiency, there is normal adrenal function[10] (reviewed by Kalantaridon et al[62]).

Idiopathic or true POF

In most cases, no cause for the POF can be found.[65] There is persistent elevation of gonadotropin concentrations, normal karyotype and no detectable autoantibodies. Ovarian biopsy may show either the type of ovary seen in a menopausal woman or an ovary of the 'streak' type.[2,10]

The clinical features include amenorrhea either primary or secondary, symptoms of estrogen deficiency, incomplete sexual development, depending on the time of onset of the estrogen deficiency, stigmata of chromosomal abnormalities, and possible immunological abnormalities. As far as immunological abnormalities are concerned, it is most important that symptoms of adrenal failure are elicited, as this process tends to have a long and insidious course.

The diagnosis of POF is made by evaluating the following:

1. FSH concentration in the menopausal range on more than one occasion at least 1 month apart.
2. Karyotype if the woman is less than 35 years of age. Gonadal tumors in the presence of a Y chromosomal mosaicism do not present after this age.
3. Diagnosis of other autoimmune conditions. Investigations include TSH, antimicrosomal antibodies, anti-thyroglobulin antibodies, anti-adrenal antibodies, random blood glucose, serum calcium, and serum electrolytes, to screen for a polyendocrinopathy. Pernicious anemia ia another possible association.
4. The accuracy of testing for anti-ovarian antibodies is not known,[50] and ovarian biopsy is not required.

Rarely, gonadotropin concentrations are in the postmenopausal range because of ectopic production of gonadotropins by a tumor, usually a lung tumor. A high FSH level and a low LH level may indicate a gonadotropin-secreting pituitary adenoma, which is very rare and usually occurs in men.[2]

The treatment of POF includes both medical and psychological components. Not only do these women require emotional support and sometimes formal psychological counseling, but often their families require the same considerations. The medical treatment of POF depends on the onset of the disease. If loss of follicles is rapid, primary amenorrhea and lack of sexual development will occur. In this case, the initial aim is to cause development of secondary sexual characteristics, most importantly breast formation. Low-dose unopposed conjugated equine estrogen (CEE) (0.3 mg) will accomplish this with incremental doses at 6-monthly intervals until the ideal dose is found. Cyclical progestagen therapy can be added after 2 years of treatment.[62]

HRT to protect against the development of osteoporosis and cardiovascular disease needs to be administered. Often, these women require a higher dose (CEE 1.25 mg) than the standard given to postmenopausal women, in order to prevent bone loss.[62] A cyclical regimen of progestagen must be used as endometrial protection, e.g. norethisterone 1.25–2.5 mg or medroxyprogesterone acetate 10 mg for convenience given on days 1–12 of each calendar month. Testosterone may also be required, especially in those women who have had their ovaries surgically removed.

Spontaneous pregnancies are rare in this condition, but if this would be an unwanted occurrence, the OCP should be used. Spontaneous pregnancies have mostly occurred after treatment with HRT, which suggests that the estrogen component may activate receptor formation on the follicles. This is more likely to occur with gonadotropin receptor abnormalities or in those women with autoimmune POF. Success with ovulation induction using human menopausal gonadotropin (hMG)/human chorionic gonadotropin and/or gonadotropin hormone-releasing hormone agonists (GnRHa) and immunosuppressant doses of glucocorticoids in women with autoimmune POF was investigated by Blumenfeld et al.[59] They reported a conception rate of 40% in three cycles. However, they advocated that if the patient did not become pregnant within three cycles, HRT and donor eggs be used. Others have not shown any success with GnRHa downregulation and hMG ovulation induction compared with hMG alone.[66] The agonists have been used in order to cause suppression of the high FSH concentrations. There also appears to be no value in using high doses of estrogen to decrease the gonadotropin concentrations and then using hMG. CC definitely does not work. Most would advocate that the best chances of conception in women with POF is through the use of donor eggs (reviewed by Kalantaridou et al[62]).

The use of steroids to treat the autoimmune component of this disease has not been successful.

Disorders of the outflow tract (eugonadotropic amenorrhea)

Congenital
Mullerian agenesis
Mayer–Rokitansky–Kuster–Hauser syndrome presents as primary amenorrhea in a woman with an absent vagina. This is the second most common cause of primary amenorrhea after gonadal dysgenesis. In this condition, there may be an absent or markedly hypoplastic vagina, the uterus may be normal but may lack a path to the introitus or may only have rudimentary bicornuate cords, the fimbriated ends of both tubes may be present, or, rarely, the entire mullerian system may be absent. If there is some functioning endometrium in a uterine rudiment, monthly cyclical abdominal pain may occur. Ovarian function, growth and development and karyotype are normal. The ovaries may be high in the pelvis or may be present in the abdomen.[67]

In association with mullerian agenesis, one-third of cases may have a urinary tract abnormality, which most often is unilateral renal agenesis or a solitary pelvic kidney. Twelve per cent of cases will have a skeletal abnormality, usually involving the spine.[10,67,68]

The most widely used operative procedure for the construction of a neovagina is a McIndoe procedure, which involves the creation of the vaginal space lined by a skin graft, often from the buttock. Alternatively, the use of progressively larger dilators (Frank procedure) for 20 min daily can create a functional vagina within 12 weeks. If mullerian structures are present, especially a uterus without a cervix, it is recommended that these structures be removed at the time of vaginal reconstructive surgery.[2,68]

Other mullerian abnormalities
Such abnormalities, which cause primary amenorrhea, include imperforate hymen and transverse vaginal septum, which is usually in the upper third of the vagina.[68] These problems are often complicated by the presence of a hematocolpos and/or hematometra and/or hematoperitoneum due to obstruction of the outflow. This may lead to endometriosis and future infertility. The problem of imperforate hymen is resolved easily by simple drainage after cruciate incisions are made in the hymen. A transverse vaginal septum is treated by establishing continuity of the mullerian duct and this should be undertaken from below. An imperforate hymen can be differentiated from a transverse vaginal septum by the presence of distention at the introitus with a Valsalva maneuver.[2,10,68]

Complete androgen insensitivity syndrome (testicular feminization)
This diagnosis should be suspected in a female who presents with primary amenorrhea, a blind-ending vagina with no uterus, normal-appearing breasts, sparse or absent pubic and axillary hair, and normal or tall stature. There is a failure of virilization in a genetic male, whose testes may be abdominal or within the inguinal canal. Incomplete forms may exist. Transmission is by an X-linked recessive gene responsible for the androgen intracellular receptor. Once full development is attained after puberty, the gonads should be removed because of the risk of neoplasia, and the patient should be started on HRT.[2] The gonads can be removed after puberty is completed rather than before, because development is better with endogenous hormones, and gonadal tumors in these patients rarely occur before the age of 18 years.[62] Testosterone concentrations are in the normal to high range for males (greater than 6 nmol/l), so the condition represents an

insensitivity to androgen (endogenous or exogenous) because of the abnormality rendering the androgen receptor inactive.

Incomplete testicular feminization represents forms with some testosterone action. There may be clitoromegaly, the presence of a phallus, axillary and pubic hair and breast growth. Gonadectomy should be performed as soon as the condition is diagnosed, to prevent further virilization.

Differences between mullerian agenesis and complete androgen insensitivity syndrome are shown in Table 7.2.

Acquired
Asherman's syndrome (amenorrhea traumatica)
This diagnosis is present in 7% of women who present with secondary amenorrhea. Such women are normal hormonally. This condition was first described by Asherman in 1948[69] as being due to obliteration of the endometrial cavity following curettage. The condition is now known to be caused by destruction of the basal layer of the endometrium after a currettage is performed in a postpartum setting, in the setting of an infected miscarriage; rarely after a termination of pregnancy, or after a routine but overvigorous curettage. It may also occur as a result of uterine surgery (cesarian section, myomectomy, or metroplasty) or as a result of infection (tuberculosis, schistosomiasis). Adhesions may partially or fully obliterate the endometrial cavity and/or the internal cervical os and/or the cervical canal.[70] These women may also present with infertility, recurrent miscarriage, dysmenorrhea or a decrease in menstrual flow. Intrauterine adhesions are seen on hysterosalpingogram or hysteroscopy. The treatment is to perform a hysteroscopic adhesionolysis and stimulate endometrial growth using high doses of estrogen (CEE 2.5 mg twice daily).[4] Subsequently, 70–80% of women will have a successful pregnancy, although it may be complicated by premature labor, placenta accreta, placenta previa or postpartum hemorrhage.

Idiopathic delay of menstruation

This is a diagnosis of exclusion in a female who presents with primary amenorrhea, normal secondary sexual characteristics, normal gonadotropin concentrations, a normal mullerian system, and no evidence of virilization. It may represent a delay in hypothalamic maturation. Spontaneous menstruation usually occurs by the age of 21 years.[10]

Management
History

When a woman presents with either primary or secondary amenorrhea, it is mandatory that a meticulous history is taken, as this often leads to a high suspicion of the diagnosis. Important factors to elicit in the history include:

- evidence of stress or psychiatric dysfunction
- changes in weight or obsession with weight
- standard and amount of exercise
- central nervous system (CNS) disease, including headaches and past history of problems
- sense of smell
- symptoms of hypothyroidism
- galactorrhea
- symptoms of hypoestrogenism
- symptoms of hirsutism and virilism

	Mullerian agenesis	Testicular feminization
Karyotype	46XX	46XY
Heredity	Unknown	Maternal X linked recessive
Sexual hair	Normal female	Absent to sparse
Testosterone level	Normal female	Normal to elevated male
Other anomalies	Renal and skeletal	Rare
Gonadal neoplasia	Normal incidence	25% malignant tumors

Table 7.2
Differences between mullerian agenesis and complete androgen insensitivity syndrome.[2]

- prior menstrual history
- gynecological or obstetrical operations
- family history of genetic abnormalities.

Examination

The examination should concentrate on the following features:

- diagnosis of normal growth and development
- secondary sexual characteristics—a female of 15–16 years who has no secondary sexual characteristics has not been exposed to any form of stimulation from gonadal hormones
- signs of hypothyroidism
- galactorrhea
- abnormalities of the reproductive tract
- signs of current estrogen secretion, including moist, pink vagina and presence of cervical mucus.

Investigations

- Exclude pregnancy.
- Serum concentration of FSH, LH, prolactin, estradiol, testosterone, dehydroepiandrosterone sulfate (DHEAS) and TSH as elicited by history and examination (see above).
- Progestagen challenge test can be performed at the first visit to assess the level of endogenous estrogen and the competence of the outflow tract. This test is performed by administering 10 mg medroxyprogesterone acetate for 5 days. A positive test is diagnosed in the presence of any bleeding occurring within 2–7 days after the completion of medication. However, in some anovulatory women, the progestagen may cause ovulation, and a bleed will then occur 14 days after the medication has finished. A negative challenge test, once pregnancy has been excluded, occurs if the outflow tract is non-functional, there is inadequate estrogen or if there is adequate endogenous estrogen but the endometrium is decidualized due to high concentrations of androgens.
- Karyotype in a woman less than 35 years of age who presents with hypergonadotropic amenorrhea.
- MRI if the serum prolactin concentration is elevated. If MRI is unavailable, CT scanning is more than adequate (see above).
- Ultrasound or hysteroscopy if a mullerian abnormality is suspected. If such an abnormality is present, investigation of the renal tract by IVU and/or skeletal X-ray is required.
- Dynamic pituitary function testing may occasionally be necessary.

References

1. Doody KM, Carr BR. Amenorrhea. *Obstet Gynecol Clin North Am* 1990; 17: 361–72.
2. Speroff L, Glass RH, Kase NG. *Clinical Gynecologic Endocrinology and Infertility*, 4th edn. Baltimore: Williams and Wilkins, 1989.
3. Ferrin M, Jewelewicz R, Warren MP. *The Menstrual Cycle*. New York: Oxford University Press, 1993.
4. Warren MP. Evaluation of secondary amenorrhea. *J Clin Endocrinol Metab* 1996; 81: 437–42.
5. Young N, Formica C, Szmukler G et al. Bone density at weight-bearing and nonweight-bearing sites in ballet dancers: the effects of exercise, hypogonadism, and body weight. *J Clin Endocrinol Metab* 1994; 78: 449–54.
6. RACOG Education. Resource Units 121–124. *Women, Sport and Menstruation,* 1995.
7. Hsu LKG. Epidemiology of the eating disorders. *Psychiatr Clin North Am* 1996; 19: 681–700.
8. Wilhelm KA, Clarke SD. Eating disorders from a primary care perspective. *Med J Aust* 1998; 168: 458–63.
9. Warren MP, Vande Wiele RL. Clinical and metabolic features of anorexia nervosa. *Am J Obstet Gynecol* 1973; 117: 435–8.
10. Shearman RP (ed.). *Clinical Reproductive Endocrinology,* Melbourne: Churchill Livingstone, 1985.
11. Warren MP. Amenorrhea in endurance runners. *J Clin Endocrinol Metab* 1992; 75: 1393–7.
12. Rencken ML, Chestnut III CH, Drinkwater BL. Bone density at multiple sites in amenorrheic athletes. *JAMA* 1996; 276: 238–40.
13. Hayes FJ, Seminara SB, Crowley WF. Hypogonadotrophic hypogonadism. *Endocrinol Metab Clin North Am* 1998; 27: 739–63.
14. Quinton R, Duke VM, de Zoysa PA et al. The neuroradiology of Kallman's syndrome: a genotypic and phenotypic analysis. *J Clin Endocrinol Metab* 1996; 81: 3010–17.
15. Waldstreicher J, Seminara SB, Jameson JL et al. The genetic and clinical heterogeneity of gonadotropin-releasing hormone deficiency in the human. *J Clin Endocrinol Metab* 1996; 81: 4388–95.
16. Yazigi RA, Quintero CH, Salameh WA. Prolactin disorders. *Fertil Steril* 1997; 67: 215–25.
17. Weiss MH, Teal J, Gott P et al. Natural history of microprolactinomas: six year follow up. *Neurosurgery* 1983; 12: 180–90.

18. Cosman F, Post KD, Holub DA et al. Lymphocytic adenohypophisitis: report of 3 new cases and review of the literature. *Medicine* 1989; **68**: 240–56.
19. Honbo KS, van Herle AJ, Kellet KA. Serum prolactin levels in untreated primary hypothyroidism. *Am J Med* 1978; **64**: 782–7.
20. Murdoch AP, Dunlop W, Kendall-Taylor P. Studies of prolactin secretion in polycystic ovary syndrome. *Clin Endocrinol (Oxf)* 1986; **24**: 165–75.
21. Schlechte JA, Sherman B, Martin R. Bone density in amenorrheic women with and without hyperprolactinemia. *J Clin Endocrinol Metab* 1983; **56**: 1120–3.
22. Klibanski A, Biller BMK, Resenthal DI, Schoenfeld DA, Saxe V. Effects of prolactin and estrogen deficiency in amenorrheic bone loss. *J Clin Endocrinol Metab* 1988; **67**: 124–30.
23. Katz E, Adashi EY. Hyperprolactinaemic disorders. *Clin Obstet Gynecol* 1990; **33**: 622–39.
24. Ho YB. Etiology and treatment of hyperprolactinemia. *Semin Reprod Endocrinol* 1992; **10**: 228–35.
25. Batrinos ML, Panitsa-Faflia C, Tsinganou E et al. Contribution to the problem of hyperprolactinaemia: experience with 4199 prolactin assays and 117 prolactinomas. *Int J Fertil* 1994; **39**: 120–5.
26. Blackwell RE, Boots LR, Goldenberg RL et al. Assessment of pituitary function in patients with serum prolactin levels greater than 100 ng/mL. *Fertil Steril* 1979; **32**: 177–80.
27. Kurachi K, Aono T, Koike K et al. A follow-up survey of infants born to mothers treated with bromocriptine. *Sanka to Fujinka* 1983; **50**: 126–9.
28. Raymond JP, Goldstein E, Konopka R et al. Follow-up of children born of bromocriptine treated mothers. *Horm Res* 1985; **22**: 239–43.
29. Webster J, Piscitelli G, Polli A et al. A comparison of cabergoline and bromocriptine in the treatment of hyperprolactinaemic amenorrhea. *N Engl J Med* 1994; **331**: 904–9.
30. Bevan JS, Davis JRE. Cabergoline: an advance in dopaminergic therapy. *Clin Endocrinol* 1994; **41**: 709–12.
31. Robert E, Musatti L, Piscitelli C, Ferrara CL. Pregnancy outcome after treatment with the ergo derivative, cabergoline. *Reprod Toxicol* 1996; **10**: 333–7.
32. Kane LA, Leinung MC, Scheithauer BW et al. Pituitary adenomas in childhood and adolescence. *J Clin Endocrinol Metab* 1994; **79**: 1135–40.
33. Corenblum B, Donovan L. The safety of physiological estrogen plus progestin replacement therapy and with oral contraceptive therapy in women with pathological hyperprolactinemia. *Fertil Steril* 1993; **59**: 671–3.
34. Pahuja DN, DeLuca HF. Stimulation of intestinal calcium transport and bone calcium mobilization by prolactin in vitamin-D deficient rats. *Science* 1981; **214**: 1038–40.
35. Koppelman MCS, Kurtz DW, Morrison KA et al. Vertebral body bone mineral content in hyperprolactinemic women. *J Clin Endocrinol Metab* 1984; **59**: 1050–4.
36. Stein IF, Leventhal ML. Amenorrhea associated with bilateral polycystic ovaries. *Am J Obstet Gynecol* 1935; **29**: 181–91.
37. Polson DW, Wadsworth J, Adams J et al. Polycystic ovaries—a common finding in normal women. *Lancet* 1988; **i**: 870–2.
38. Zawadzki JK, Dunaif A. Diagnostic criteria for polycystic ovary syndrome: towards a rational approach. In: Dunaif A, Givens JR, Haseltine FP, Merriam GR, eds. *Polycystic Ovary Syndrome. Current Issues in Endocrinology and Metabolism*, Vol. 4. Boston: Blackwell Scientific, 1992.
39. Kovacs GT ed. *Polycystic Ovary Syndrome*. Cambridge: Cambridge University Press, 2000: 23, 35.
40. Anttila L, Kartala K, Penttila TA, Ruutiainen K, Ekblad U. Polycystic ovaries in women with gestational diabetes. *Obstet Gynecol* 1998; **92**: 13–16.
41. Legro RS, Finegood D, Dunaif A. A fasting insulin ratio is a useful measure of insulin sensitivity in women with polycystic ovary syndrome. *J Clin Endocrinol Metab* 1998; **83**: 2694–8.
42. Vollenhoven BJ, Healy DL. Short- and long-term effects of ovulation induction. *Endocrinol Metab Clin North Am* 1998; **27**: 903–14.
43. Donesky BW, Adashi EY. Surgically induced ovulation in the polycystic ovary syndrome: wedge resection revisited in the age of laparoscopy. *Fertil Steril* 1995; **63**: 439–63.
44. Dunaif A, Scott D, Finegood D et al. The insulin-sensitizing agent troglitazone improves metabolic and reproductive abnormalities in the polycystic ovary syndrome. *J Clin Endocrinol Metab* 1996; **81**: 3299–306.
45. Ehrmann DA, Cavaghan MK, Imperial J et al. Effects of metformin on insulin secretion, insulin action and steroidogenesis. *J Clin Endocrinol Metab* 1997; **82**: 524–30.
46. Ehrmann DA, Schneider DJ, Sobel BE et al. Troglitazone improves defects in insulin action, insulin secretion, ovarian steroidogenesis, and fibrinolysis in women with polycystic ovary syndrome. *J Clin Endocrinol Metab* 1997; **82**: 2108–16.
47. Nestler JE, Jakubowicz DJ. Decreases in ovarian cytochrome P450c17-alpha activity and serum free testosterone after reduction of insulin secretion in polycystic ovary syndrome. *N Engl J Med* 1996; **335**: 617–23.
48. Nestler JE, Jakubowicz DJ. Lean women with polycystic ovary syndrome respond to insulin reduction with decreases in ovarian P450c17α activity and serum androgens. *J Clin Endocrinol Metab* 1997; **81**: 4075–9.
49. Velazquez EM, Mendoza S, Hamer T et al. Metformin therapy in polycystic ovary syndrome reduces hyper insulinemia, insulin resistance, hyperandrogenemia, and systolic blood pressure, while facilitating normal menses and pregnancy. *Metab* 1994; **43**: 647–54.

50. La Barbara AR, Miller MM, Ober C et al. Autoimmune etiology in premature ovarian failure. *Am J Reprod Immunol* 1988; **16**: 115–222.
51. Snowden DA, Kane RL, Beeson WL et al. Is early natural menopause a biologic marker of health and aging? *Am J Public Health* 1989; **79**: 709–14.
52. Coulam CB, Adamson SC, Annegers JF. Incidence of premature ovarian failure. *Obstet Gynecol* 1986; **67**: 604–6.
53. de Morales-Ruehsen M, Jones GS. Premature ovarian failure. *Fertil Steril* 1967; **18**: 440–61.
54. Howell S, Shalet S. Gonadal damage from chemotherapy and radiotherapy. *Endocrinol Metab Clin North Am* 1998; **27**: 927–43.
55. Ray GR, Trueblood HW, Enright LP et al. Oophoropexy: a means of preserving ovarian function following pelvic megavoltage radiotherapy for Hodgkin's disease. *Radiology* 1970; **96**: 175–8.
56. Neufeld M, Maclaren NK, Blizzard RM. Two types of autoimmune Addison's disease associated with different polyglandular autoimmune (PGA) syndromes. *Medicine* 1981; **60**: 355–9.
57. Wheatcroft N, Weetman AP. Is premature ovarian failure an autoimmune disease? *Autoimmunity* 1997; **25**: 157–61.
58. Alper MM, Garner PR. Premature ovarian failure: its relationship to autoimmune disease. *Obstet Gynecol* 1985; **66**: 27–30.
59. Blumenfeld Z, Halachmi S, Peretz BA et al. Premature ovarian failure—the prognostic application of autoimmunity on conception after ovulation induction. *Fertil Steril* 1993; **59**: 750–5.
60. Coulam CB, Ryan RJ. Premature menopause. I. Etiology. *Am J Obstet Gynecol* 1979; **133**: 639–43.
61. Sarto GE. Cytogenetics of fifty patients with primary amenorrhea. *Am J Obstet Gynecol* 1974, **119**: 14–23.
62. Kalantaridou SN, Davis SR, Nelson LM. Premature ovarian failure. *Endocrinol Metab Clin North Am* 1998; **27**: 989–1006.
63. Manuel M, Katayama KP, Jones HW Jr. The age of occurrence of gonadal tumors in intersex patients with a Y chromosome. *Am J Obstet Gynecol* 1976; **124**: 293–6.
64. Rebar RW, Connolly HV. Clinical features of young women with hypergonadotrophic amenorrhea. *Fertil Steril* 1990; **53**: 804–10.
65. Rebar RW, Cedars MI. Hypergonadotrophic forms of amenorrhea in young women. *Endocrinol Metab Clin North Am* 1992; **21**: 173–91.
66. Van Kasteren YM, Hoek A, Schoemaker J. Ovulation induction in premature ovarian failure: a placebo controlled randomized trial combining pituitary suppression with gonadotropin stimulation. *Fertil Steril* 1995; **64**: 273–8.
67. Jones Jr HW. Mullerian abnormalities. *Hum Reprod* 1998; **13**: 789–91.
68. Golan A, Langer R, Bukovsky I, Caspi E. Congenital anomalies of the mullerian system. *Fertil Steril* 1989; **51**: 747–55.
69. Asherman JG. Amenorrhea traumatica (atretica). *J Obstet Gynaecol Br Emp* 1948; **55**: 23–7.
70. Klein SM, Garcia CF. Asherman's syndrome: a critique and current review. *Fertil Steril* 1973; **24**: 722–30.

8

Hypogonadism, erectile dysfunction and infertility in men

Shalender Bhasin, Atam B Singh, Charles E Fisher

Hypogonadism in men

Hypogonadism is a multisystem syndrome associated with impaired androgen production or action. Androgen deficiency can result from abnormalities of testicular function (primary hypogonadism), or hypothalamic or pituitary regulation of testicular function (secondary hypogonadism), or from impairment of androgen action at the target tissue (androgen resistance).

Failure to diagnose and treat androgen deficiency can have serious health consequences. It is important to screen for androgen deficiency, because hypogonadism may be a manifestation of a serious underlying disease such as a pituitary tumor or HIV infection. If left untreated, androgen deficiency may contribute to osteoporosis and increased risk of fracture,[1–6] loss of muscle mass and function,[2,7–9] impaired sexual function,[10–15] lowered mood and energy level,[7] increased fat mass, particularly in the visceral fat compartment,[16–20] and insulin resistance.[16–20]

Who should be screened for androgen deficiency?

Androgen deficiency is a common disorder that frequently remains undetected because the symptoms of androgen deficiency in adult men are often non-specific.[21,22] For instance, in the Massachusetts Male Aging Study,[21,22] 4% of men, 40–70 years of age, who were asymptomatic, had serum testosterone levels less than 150 ng/dl in association with increased luteinizing hormone (LH) levels. The symptoms commonly attributed to androgen deficiency, such as decreased sexual desire and activity and low energy, do not have a high correlation with low testosterone levels.[21,22] Therefore, a high index of suspicion is the key to its diagnosis.

While men presenting with loss of sexual desire and function and diminished secondary sex characteristics should undoubtedly be screened for androgen deficiency, the Massachusetts Male Aging Study[21,22] demonstrated that these symptoms are uncommon in middle-aged men with androgen deficiency. If screening were triggered only by the presence of these symptoms, a majority of hypogonadal men would remain undiagnosed. Since the following patient groups have a high prevalence of low testosterone levels, they should be screened for androgen deficiency (Table 8.1):

1. Patients presenting with delayed sexual development may have constitutional delay of puberty, primary or secondary hypogonadism, or one of a variety of other causes; testosterone levels should be measured in all such patients.
2. Men presenting with infertility. Approximately 10% of men presenting with infertility have Klinefelter's syndrome,[23,24] and an additional 1–3% have hypogonadotropic hypogonadism.
3. Men below the age of 50 presenting with minimal trauma fractures. Minimal trauma fractures are uncommon in men below age 50,[6,7] but when they do occur in younger men, impaired androgen secretion or action is often a contributory cause.
4. Men with chronic illness. There is a high prevalence of low testosterone levels in chronic illness[25–34] such as that associated with HIV infection,[25–30] end-stage renal disease[31–33] and chronic obstructive lung disease.[34] Testosterone replacement increases lean body mass and muscle strength in HIV-infected men with weight loss and low testosterone levels.[35–37]
5. Men being treated with medications that impair testosterone secretion, alter its metabolism, or

> The following groups of men have high prevalence of androgen deficiency and warrant measurement of serum testosterone levels:
> 1. Men with loss of sexual desire and function
> 2. Men with loss of secondary sex characteristics
> 3. Men with delayed pubertal development
> 4. Men being evaluated for infertility
> 5. Men with erectile dysfunction
> 6. Men presenting with minimal trauma fracture before the age of 50
> 7. Men with chronic illness such as that associated with HIV infection, chronic obstructive lung disease, and end-stage renal disease
> 8. Men being treated with medications that impair testosterone production or action
> 9. Men over the age of 60

Table 8.1
Clinical states that are associated with high prevalence of androgen deficiency and warrant screening.

attenuate its action. Particular attention should be paid to the use of glucocorticoids,[38,39] ketoconazole,[40,41] megesterol acetate,[42,43] gonadotropin-releasing hormone agonists,[44,45] neuropsychiatric drugs,[46–48] cancer chemotherapeutic drugs and long-term opiate use.

6. Men over the age of 60. Serum testosterone levels progressively decrease with advancing age,[1,49–55] so that by age 60, approximately 25% of men have serum testosterone levels in the hypogonadal range. Testosterone replacement in older men with low normal testosterone levels is associated with gains in lean body mass, muscle strength and bone mineral density.[54,56–61]

7. Men presenting with erectile dysfunction. Eight per cent of men presenting with erectile dysfunction have low testosterone levels.[51,62–69] Androgen deficiency and erectile dysfunction are two common, but independently distributed, clinical disorders in middle-aged and older men.[51,62–69]

Morley has developed and validated a 10-question ADAM (Androgen Deficiency in Aging Males) questionnaire to detect older male candidates for testosterone testing.[70,71]

Evaluation

History

The diagnostic work-up of androgen deficiency is initiated by an assessment of the general health of the patient, because systemic illness is frequently associated with low testosterone levels (Figure 8.1). Twenty to thirty per cent of men infected with the human immunodeficiency virus have low testosterone levels.[25–30] Similarly, a substantial proportion of patients with chronic obstructive lung disease,[34] diabetes mellitus, end-stage renal disease[31–33] and many types of cancer have low testosterone levels.

It is important to evaluate lifestyle factors and substance abuse, because they can be associated with androgen deficiency. Eating disorders, excessive exercise and recreational drug abuse are often associated with delayed pubertal development and hypogonadism.[72–74] The energy balance and the hypothalamic control of the reproductive axis are intimately linked (Figure 8.2). Excessive exercise is associated with hypogonadotropic hypogonadism; the degree of gonadotropin deficiency is correlated with the magnitude of energy drain.[73] Weight loss in patients with anorexia nervosa is associated with functional gonadotropin-releasing hormone (GnRH) deficiency and hypogonadotropic hypogonadism.[73,74] Leptin is believed to be one of the biochemical links between energy stores and the central regulation of reproduction.[75]

Use of recreational drugs such as alcohol, marijuana, opiates and cocaine can be associated with hypogonadotropic hypogonadism.[76,77] Alcohol has inhibitory effects at all levels of the hypothalamic–pituitary–testicular axis. The physician should ask about the use of glucocorticoids,[38,39] ketoconazole,[40,41] cancer chemotherapeutic agents, GnRH agonists and antagonists[44,45] and neuroleptic agents,[47,48] or a previous

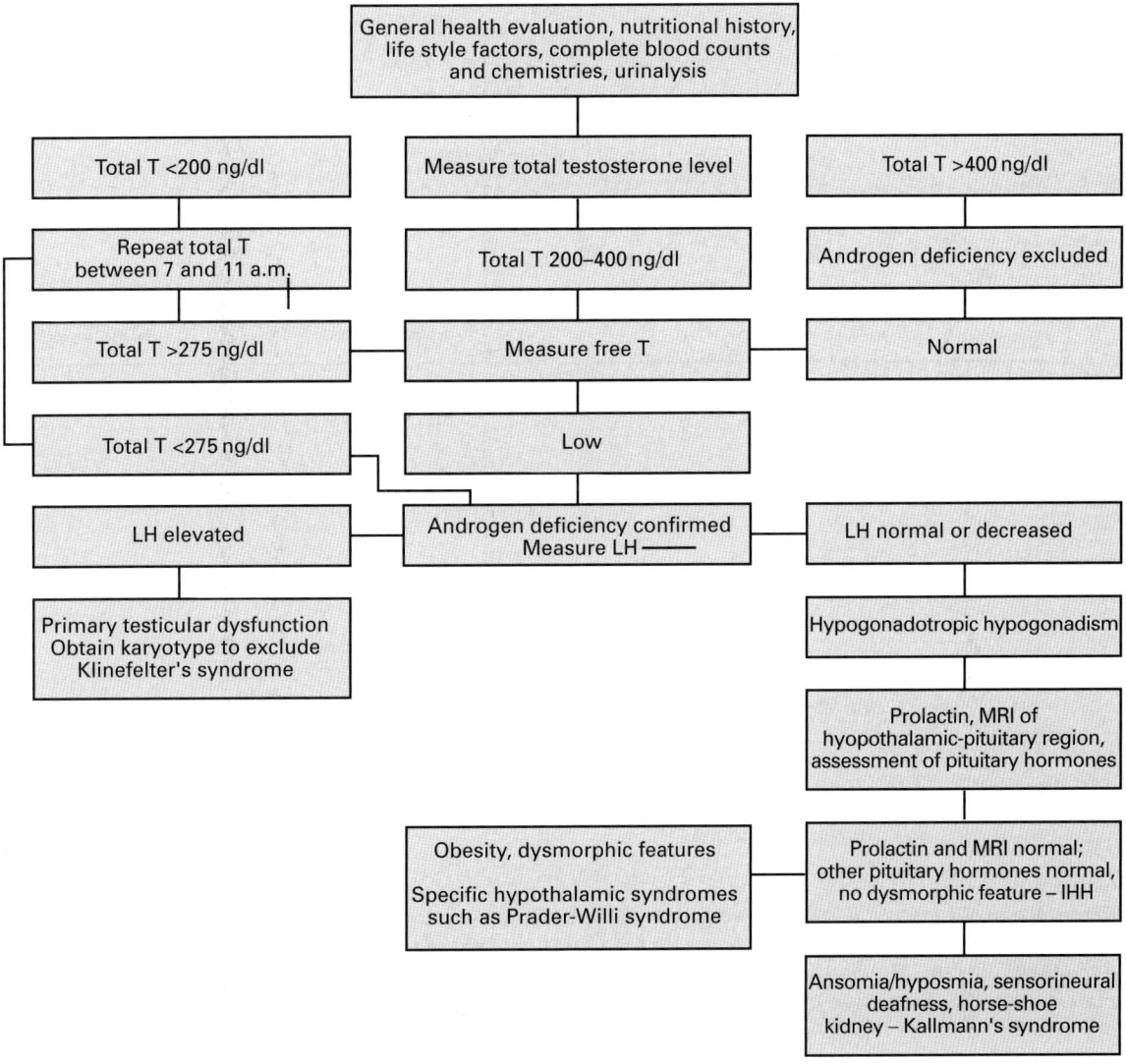

Figure 8.1
An algorithmic approach to the diagnosis of androgen deficiency. T, testosterone; IHH, idiopathic hypogonadotrophic hypogonadism.

history of pelvic irradiation. Glucocorticoids inhibit LH and follicle-stimulating hormone (FSH) secretion by multiple mechanisms and also directly inhibit testicular function.[38,39] Ketoconazole is an inhibitor of several P450-linked steroidogenic enzymes in the testosterone biosynthetic pathway, including CyP450scc.[40,41] Androgen deficiency and subfertility are well-known, frequent, long-term complications of cancer chemotherapy. Many antipsychotic and antidepressant drugs are associated with hyperprolactinemia that can cause hypogonadotropic hypogonadism.[47,48]

The physician should enquire about early-morning erections, frequency of sexual thoughts, intensity of sexual feelings, and frequency of sexual acts such as masturbation and intercourse. Overall frequency of sexual acts and libido is decreased in androgen-deficient men.[7,10–15] However, young, hypogonadal men are able to achieve erections in response to visual erotic

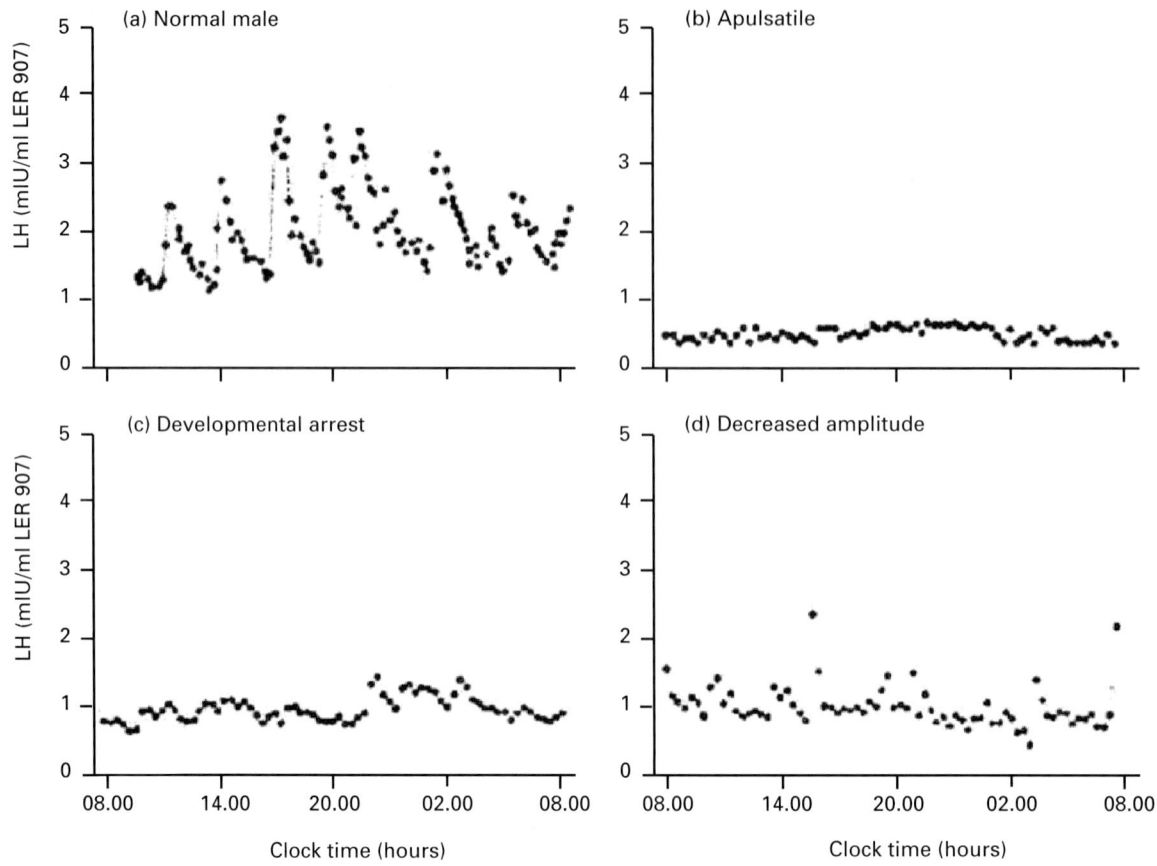

Figure 8.2
*Heterogeneity in the profiles of LH and follicle-stimulating hormone (FSH) secretion in patients with IHH. The pulsatile LH secretion in a healthy young man (a) is contrasted with complete absence of LH pulses in a man with IHH (b). The patient in (c) has a few low-amplitude, night-time, LH pulses, reminiscent of early puberty, while the patient in (d) has a normal frequency of LH pulses, all of which have low amplitude. We do not know whether this clinical heterogeneity in LH pulsatile secretion is due to different degrees of gonadotropin-releasing hormone (GnRH) deficiency, or reflects genetic heterogeneity in the pathophysiology of this syndrome. (Adapted from: Crowley WF Jr, Filicori M, Spratt DI, Santoro NF. The physiology of gonadotropin-releasing hormone (GnRH) secretion in men and women. Recent Prog Horm Res 1985; **41**:473–531.)*

stimuli.[13] Mood and energy level should be ascertained; men with acquired androgen deficiency often report decreased energy and increased irritability.[78] Androgen replacement improves positive aspects of mood and reduces irritability in androgen-deficient men.[78]

Physical examination

In addition to general physical examination, attention should be focused on assessing secondary sex characteristics such as hair growth, testicular volume, breast enlargement, prostate, height and span and body proportions. Hair growth in the beard, chest and pubic regions is androgen dependent. There are ethnic differences in the intensity of hair growth.

Testicular volume can be measured by using a Prader orchidometer. Patients with Klinefelter's syndrome have markedly reduced testicular volumes (1–2 ml).[23,24] In men with congenital hypogonadotropic hypogonadism, testicular volumes are a good marker for the degree of gonadotropin deficiency and the likelihood of response to therapy.[79,80] In general, men with idiopathic hypogonadotropic hypogonadism whose testicular volume is less than 4 ml have more severe gonadotropin deficiency and are less likely to respond to hCG alone than those with testicular volumes greater than 8 ml.

Androgen deficiency can be associated with breast enlargement in men, although gynecomastia is more often due to other causes such as liver and kidney disease, medication, or physiological hormonal changes during the neonatal period, puberty and old age. Breast enlargement may also occur after institution of androgen replacement therapy.

Laboratory evaluation

Complete blood counts, including hemoglobin level, BUN and creatinine, fasting blood glucose, aspartate aminotransferase (AST), alanine aminotransferase (ALT), bilirubin, alkaline phosphatase and urinalysis, should be performed as part of general health evaluation.

The measurement of total serum testosterone level, preferably in an early-morning sample obtained between 8 and 11 a.m., remains the best biochemical test for the diagnosis of androgen deficiency. A total serum testosterone level of less than 200 ng/dl (7 nmol/l) in an early-morning serum sample in association with consistent symptoms is evidence of testosterone deficiency. An early-morning serum testosterone level greater than 350 ng/dl (12 nmol/l) makes the diagnosis of androgen deficiency unlikely. In men with serum testosterone levels between 200 and 350 ng/dl (7–12 nmol/l), the measurement of total testosterone level should be repeated, and free testosterone level should be measured. In older men, patients with Klinefelter's syndrome and in other clinical states that are associated with increased sex hormone-binding globulin (SHBG) levels, measurements of total testosterone level may underestimate the degree of testosterone deficiency. In these patients, a direct measurement of free testosterone level can be useful in unmasking testosterone deficiency.

Serum LH levels should be measured in men with low testosterone levels, because it can help in defining whether the site of lesion is in the testis or at the hypothalamic–pituitary site. The men with androgen deficiency can be classified into hypergonadotropic (high LH) or hypogonadotropic (low or inappropriately normal LH) based on their LH levels.

An elevated LH level indicates that the defect is at the testicular level. Common causes of primary testicular failure include Klinefelter's syndrome, HIV infection, uncorrected cryptorchidism, cancer chemotherapeutic agents, radiation, surgical orchiectomy and prior infectious orchitis. A karyotype should be determined to exclude Klinefelter's syndrome in men with low testosterone and elevated LH level.

The men who have low testosterone levels but 'inappropriately normal' or low LH levels have hypogonadotropic hypogonadism; their defect resides at the hypothalamic–pituitary site.[81] The causes of hypogonadotropic hypogonadism include space-occupying lesions of the hypothalamic–pituitary site, hyperprolactinemia, eating disorders, excessive exercise, substance abuse, chronic illness and a number of hypothalamic syndromes characterized by hypogonadotropic hypogonadism.[81]

In men with hypogonadotropic hypogonadism, the physician should verify or exclude the presence of systemic illness, eating disorders, excessive exercise and substance abuse. Serum prolactin level should be measured, and a CT or MRI scan of the hypothalamic–pituitary region with a contrast agent should be obtained. Measurement of serum prolactin and MRI scan of the hypothalamic–pituitary region can help exclude the presence of a space-occupying lesion. Patients in whom all other detectable causes of hypogonadotropic hypogonadism have been excluded are classified as having idiopathic hypogonadotropic hypogonadism (IHH). Some men with IHH have hyposmia or anosmia, horse-shoe shaped kidney and sensorineural deafness; these patients have Kallmann's syndrome. Several hypothalamic syndromes are associated with hypogonadotropic hypogonadism; these syndromes are recognized by the pattern of associated dysmorphic features.

When should free testosterone levels be measured?

Measurement of free testosterone levels can be useful in diagnosing androgen deficiency in men with alterations in SHBG levels.[82–85] Most of the circulating testosterone is bound to SHBG and albumin; only 0.5–2.0% of circulating testosterone is unbound or 'free'. Total testosterone levels are affected by the prevalent SHBG concentrations. Alterations in SHBG levels due to normal aging,[82,83] obesity,[86,87] some types of medications, chronic illness, or on a congenital basis, can confound interpretation of total testosterone levels. Therefore, measurement of free testosterone levels, presumably reflecting the biologically active fraction, can be useful in the following conditions, particularly if the total testosterone levels are in the borderline zone.

Obesity

Obese men have decreased SHBG levels. Most obese men with mild to moderate obesity have lower serum total testosterone levels due to decreased SHBG concentrations;[86,87] their free testosterone concentrations are normal. Severely obese men may have hypogonadotropic hypogonadism due, in part, to the increased estradiol levels that suppress LH and FSH secretion.[87]

Older men

Serum SHBG concentrations are increased in older men.[82,83] Therefore, total testosterone levels underestimate the degree of age-related decline in serum testosterone levels.

Chronic illness

Serum SHBG concentrations are increased in HIV-infected men[25] and in some types of liver disease, but may be decreased in men with nephrotic syndrome.

Hyperthyroidism

SHBG concentrations are increased in hyperthyroidism.

The methods for free testosterone measurement (Table 8.2)

The measurements of serum free testosterone levels are fraught with difficulty and are not recommended as a general screening test. Serum free testosterone levels should only be measured in specific clinical situations, as described above, and measurements should be obtained from a reliable laboratory that has experience with the assay, by using an appropriate assay that is not affected by the SHBG concentration.

The tracer analog methods are relatively inexpensive and convenient but are dependent on SHBG concentrations and, therefore, do not provide a true index of 'free' testosterone.[88] They should not be used, because of concerns about validity.

Method	Potential merits and demerits	Utility
Tracer analog methods	These methods are affected by SHBG concentrations and therefore do not provide a true index of 'free' testosterone	They are convenient to perform, but should not be used, because of concerns about validity
Equilibrium dialysis using tracer or direct measurement of dialyzed testosterone	Free testosterone levels measured by equilibrium dialysis have good clinical correlation. The equilibrium dialysis methods are techically demanding, affected by dialysis conditions, and available only from a few commercial laboratories	They are clinically useful if performed in a reliable laboratory
Bioavailable testosterone level (unbound plus albumin-bound testosterone fraction)	Measurement of bioavailable testosterone levels by ammonium sulfate precipitation has good clinical correlation	Clinically useful if performed in a reliable laboratory. The method is available only from a few commercial laboratories
Calculation of free testosterone levels by measurement of total testosterone and SHBG levels	Total testosterone and SHBG levels can be measured accurately and precisely by direct immunoassays. The validity of the algorithms used to calculate free testosterone from total testosterone and SHBG concentrations in men with chronic illness has not been established	Useful in healthy, young men, but validity not established in different illnesses that might affect SHBG concentrations and binding

Table 8.2
Methods for the measurement of serum-free testosterone levels.

Free testosterone levels measured by equilibrium dialysis have good clinical correlation.[84,85] The equilibrium dialysis methods are technically demanding, affected by dialysis conditions and available only from a few commercial laboratories.

Measurement of bioavailable testosterone levels by the ammonium sulfate precipitation method has good clinical correlation.[83]

Free testosterone concentrations can also be calculated from total testosterone and SHBG concentrations using previously published algorithms. Total testosterone and SHBG levels can be measured accurately and precisely by direct immunoassays. The validity of the algorithms used to calculate free testosterone from total testosterone and SHBG concentrations in men with chronic illness has not been established; this method may be useful in healthy, young men, but its validity has not been established in different illnesses that might affect SHBG concentrations and binding.

Genetic syndromes associated with hypogonadism

In men with hypogonadotropic hypogonadism, in whom detectable causes of gonadotropin deficiency have been excluded, specific hypothalamic syndromes can be recognized by the associated somatic stigmata.[89] A number of hypothalamic syndromes are characterized by the presence of hypogonadotropic hypogonadism in association with a constellation of dysmorphic somatic features such as horse-shoe kidney, sensorineural deafness, marked obesity, hyperphagia, polydactyly, retinitis pigmentosa and mental retardation.[89–91] A diagnosis of these hypothalamic syndromes is made by pattern recognition.[89–91]

Idiopathic hypogonadotropic hypogonadism
Men who have hypogonadotropic hypogonadism in the absence of a detectable cause have IHH.[81] This is a heterogeneous group of disorders. These patients have selective gonadotropin deficiency resulting from an isolated defect in GnRH secretion. The primary pathogenic defect in these patients is hypothalamic, and the impaired gonadotropin secretion is secondary to the hypothalamic abnormality in GnRH secretion.

Associations
Although anosmia and hyposmia are the most well-known and the first associations described in this syndrome, a number of other somatic abnormalities have been recorded.[81,92] The more common associations include color blindness, cleft lip and palate, cranial nerve defects (including eighth nerve deafness), horse-shoe-shaped kidneys, cryptorchidism and optic atrophy.

Heterogeneity of pulsatile gonadotropin secretion in patients with idiopathic hypogonadotropic hypogonadism
There is considerable heterogeneity in the clinical presentation of IHH (Figure 8.3).[93,94] Those with the most severe deficiency may present with complete absence of pubertal development, sexual infantilism and, in some cases, varying degrees of hypospadias and undescended testes. Male patients may have complete absence of secondary sex characteristics, infantile testes and azoospermia. Female patients may present with primary amenorrhea. Patients with partial GnRH deficiency may have varying degrees of delay in sexual development in proportion to the severity of gonadotropin deficiency.

The patients with IHH are quite heterogeneous in their LH-secretory profiles (Figure 8.3).[94] The largest subset comprises patients who display no pulsatile LH secretion at all; these men have the most severe GnRH deficiency. A smaller subset displays low-amplitude pulses. Another subset of patients has LH pulses at a markedly reduced frequency. A fourth subset is characterized by sleep-entrained pulses reminiscent of the pattern seen in early stages of puberty; these patients can be considered to suffer from a 'developmental arrest.'

Two variants of IHH are particularly interesting. The term 'fertile eunuch syndrome' has been used to describe patients with eunuchoidal proportions and delayed sexual development but who have normal-sized testes. Such individuals appear to have sufficient gonadotropins to stimulate high intratesticular testosterone levels and to initiate spermatogenesis, but not enough testosterone secretion into the blood to adequately virilize the peripheral tissues; they are, in fact, partially gonadotropin deficient. Another variant with predominantly FSH deficiency has also been described,[95] although these patients are rare.

Genetics of IHH
One-third of IHH patients have a positive family history.[92] Of those with a positive family history, approximately 20% have an X-linked pattern of inheritance, one-third have an autosomal recessive mode of

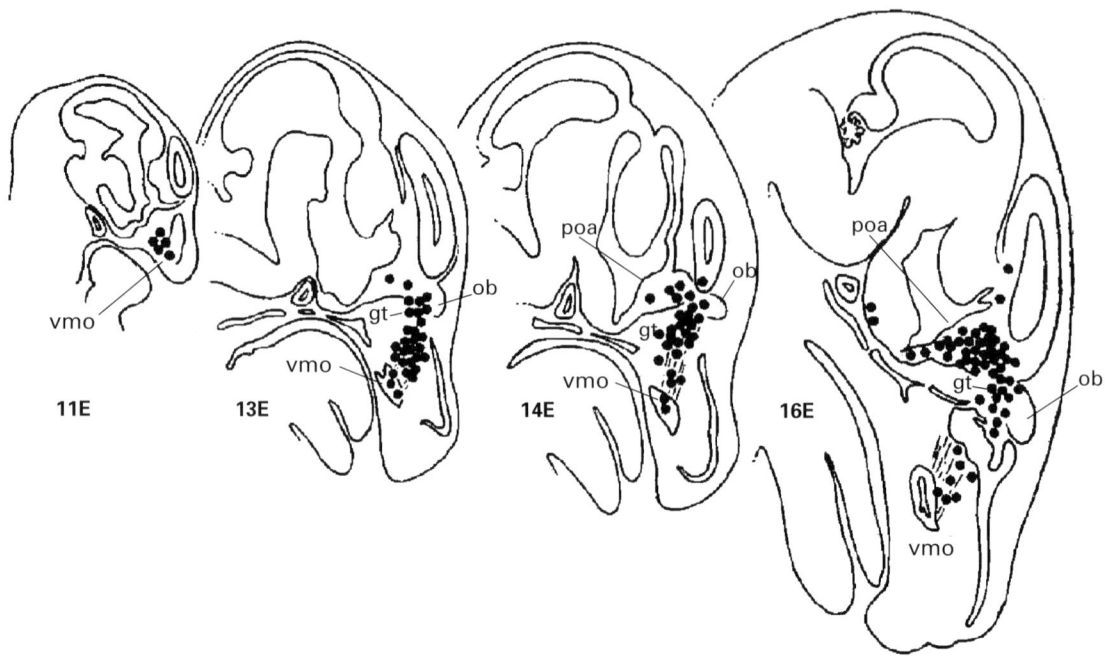

Figure 8.3
Migration of the GnRH neurons in the mouse brain. The numbers below each section indicate the embryonic day on which the section was obtained. Abbreviations: vmo, vomeronasal organ; poa, preoptic area; ob, olfactory bulb; gt, ganglion terminalis. Immunohistochemical staining for GnRH has revealed that GnRH-secreting neurons first appear in the region of the olfactory placode, and start migrating along the vomeronasal and olfactory nerves around embryonic day 11 (11E). These neurons find their way through the forebrain and finally into the supraoptic region of the hypothalamus by day 16. The precise developmental migration of these neurons requires the coordinated action of direction-finding molecules, tissue proteases, and adhesion molecules. (From Schwanzel-Fukuda M, Pfaff DW. Origin of luteinizing hormone-releasing hormone neurons. Nature 1989; 338(6211):161–4.)

inheritance, and one-half an autosomal dominant mode of inheritance.[90,93,96] The locus for the X-linked form of Kallmann's syndrome has been assigned to chromosomal region Xp22.3.[76,77] Two groups[97,98] independently cloned an adhesion molecule-like protein from this region encoded by the *KALIG-1* (Kallmann's syndrome interval-1) gene. The protein product of the *KALIG-1* gene presumably regulates migration of the GnRH and olfactory neurons and their morphogenesis. Mutations in *KALIG-1* have been found in some patients with the X-linked form of IHH, but can account for only a small fraction of patients with the X-linked form of IHH;[99–104] additional as yet unidentified X-linked genes are probably implicated in other subsets of Kallmann's syndrome.[92]

The GnRH neurons first appear in the epithelium of the olfactory placode in the mouse embryo (Figure 8.4A)[105] and then migrate to the forebrain and finally to their ultimate hypothalamic location. Such observations suggest that IHH may be a developmental defect resulting from an abnormal migration of the LH-releasing hormone (LHRH) neurons. MRI studies show that the olfactory bulbs and sulci are poorly developed in patients with IHH who have anosmia or hyposmia (Figure 8.4B).[106]

Mutations of the DAX-1 gene are associated with hypogonadotropic hypogonadism

The product of the *DAX-1* gene is an orphan nuclear receptor.[107–118] The mutations in the C-terminal end of

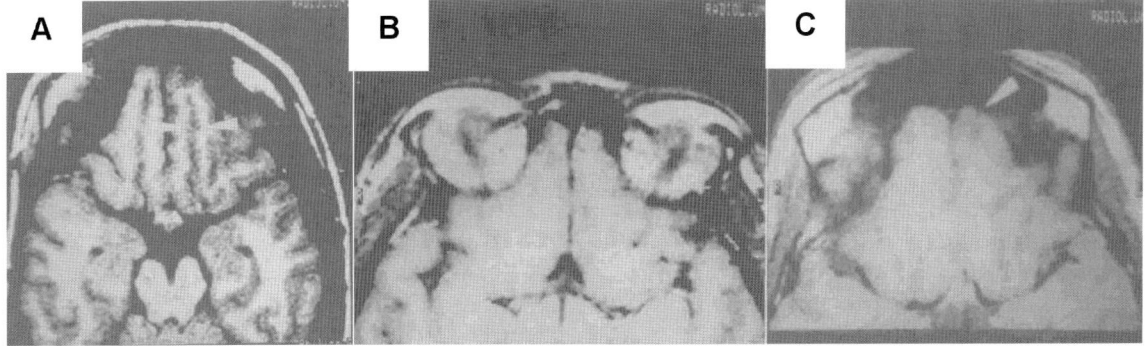

Figure 8.4
MRI scans of a normal person, and two patients with pallmann's syndrome. (A) MRI section of a normal brain, with well-developed rhinencephalon and olfactory sulcus (arrows). (B), (C) Sections of the rhinencephalon from patients with idiopathic hypogonadotropic hypogonadism and anosmia, showing poorly developed olfactory bulbs and absence of olfactory sulci. (From Klingmuller D, Dewes W, Krahe T, Brecht G, Schweikert HU. Magnetic resonance imaging of the brain in patients with anosmia and hypothalamic hypogonadism (Kallmann's syndrome). J Clin Endocrinol Metab 1987; **65**(3): 581–4.)

the *DAX-1* gene have been associated with X-linked hypogonadotropic hypogonadism and adrenal insufficiency (adrenal hypoplasia congenita). However, mutations in the *DAX-1* gene are an unusual cause of idiopathic hypogonadotropic hypogonadism, accounting for less than 1% of the cases. These patients typically have normal testosterone response to human chorionic gonadotropin (hCG), indicating normal Leydig cell function.

Mutations of the GnRH receptor gene are associated with hypogonadotropic hypogonadism

Several families with hypogonadotropic hypogonadism due to mutations of the GnRH receptor have been reported.[88,119] The GnRH receptor is a G protein-coupled receptor with an extracellular N-terminus, seven transmembrane regions and an intracellular C-terminus.[88] De Roux et al[88] described a family with a compound heterozygous mutation of the GnRH receptor. One mutation was in the first extracellular loop of the GnRH receptor and was associated with decreased GnRH binding to its receptor.[88] The second mutation, which was located in the third intracellular loop, did not alter GnRH binding to the receptor but decreased the activation of phospholipase C.[88]

The patients with GnRH receptor mutations have a normal sense of smell. In these families, the pattern of inheritance of idiopathic hypogonadotropic hypogonadism is autosomal recessive. Consanguinity is often present in these families. The male/female distribution among affected individuals is equal. GnRH receptor mutations account for almost 40% of cases in families with autosomal recessive patterns of inheritance and for 10% of sporadic cases.

Major deletions or rearrangements of the GnRH gene have not been found in patients with IHH by Southern blot analysis or sequencing of PCR products. However, more subtle defects within the GnRH gene have not been completely excluded.

Known mutations of the *KALIG-1*, GnRH receptor and *DAX-1* gene can account for only 25–30% of cases of hypogonadotropic hypogonadism (10–15% *KALIG-1*, 15% GnRH receptor, and <1% *DAX-1*). Therefore, additional autosomal and X-linked genes will probably be implicated in other cases of IHH.

Mutations in the genes encoding LH β and FSH β subunits

Hypogonadism caused by mutations in the FSH β subunit gene

Inherited mutations of the FSH β genes are uncommon,[120,121] but have been reported to produce male hypogonadism and delayed puberty in boys.[120,121] FSH-deficient male mice are fertile, although they have small testes and subnormal spermatogenesis.[122] Female mice deficient in the FSH β subunit, produced by the embryonic stem cell technology, are infertile, with a block in folliculogenesis prior to antral follicle formation.[122]

A 46,XX patient, homozygous for an FSH β point mutation, presented with primary amenorrhea, infertility and low serum FSH levels.[120] Analysis of the FSH β gene revealed a two-nucleotide deletion that resulted in a frame shift of subsequent codons and premature termination.[120] A relative of the index case was postmenopausal and had subnormal FSH levels. The two point mutations in the FSH β gene observed in this family were both located in exon 3 at codons 51 and 61.[120]

Hypogonadism associated with inactivating mutations of the LH β gene

A single patient with mutation of the LH β subunit gene has been reported;[123] this individual presented with delayed pubertal development. He had increased serum immunoreactive LH levels but decreased bioactive LH concentrations. The mutant LH in this patient had decreased receptor-binding activity, due to homozygous substitution of glycine in position 54 with arginine (G54R). The male individuals in the family who were heterozygous for this mutation had lower testosterone levels.

A polymorphic variant of LH has been reported in Finland and Japan.[124,125] The variant LH has two amino acid substitutions, W8R and I15T, that are associated with increased bio-activity and a reduced serum half-life. The clinical significance of this polymorphism is not known.

Activating mutations of the LH and FSH receptor genes

Activating or gain-of-function mutations of the LH receptor are associated with gonadotropin-independent sexual precocity in boys, but do not produce a discernible phenotype in females.[126] Analysis of the LH receptor in this patient showed a C to T substitution in exon 11 that resulted in an Ala to Val change. When the COS-7 cells were transiently transfected with the wild-type or Ala373Val mutant LH receptor cDNA, the mutant cDNA construct had higher basal and hCG-stimulated cAMP accumulation.

Only a single case of activating mutation of the FSH receptor is on record; this patient was fertile even after surgical hypophysectomy that had lowered his FSH immunoreactivity to undetectable levels.[127–129]

Prader–Willi syndrome

Patients with this syndrome have been well described. They typically have obesity, hypotonic musculature, mental retardation, hypogonadism, short stature and small hands and feet.[90,91] Hypogonadism, cryptorchidism and micropenis are common.[90] The LH response to a single bolus of GnRH is subnormal in comparison to obese controls.[90] The degree of gonadotropin deficiency in these patients is variable. A few patients with hypergonadotropic hypogonadism have also been described.

Prader–Willi syndrome is a disorder of genomic imprinting that commonly results from deletions of the proximal portion of paternally derived chromosome 15q.[91] The maternally derived copies of genes responsible for the Prader–Willi syndrome in proximal 15q are normally silent.[91] Therefore, the deletion of the paternally derived copy of the normally active genes produces the disease. Prader–Willi syndrome can also result if both copies of the gene are derived from the mother, because the maternal copies are inactivated, presumably by DNA methylation; this condition is known as uniparental disomy. Structural abnormalities of the imprinting center can also produce the Prader–Willi syndrome. The genes responsible for the Prader–Willi syndrome have not been identified. Allele-specific methylation at locus D15S63 can be detected by a PCR-based diagnostic test for this syndrome.

Developmental disorders of the pituitary due to mutations of the homeodomain transcription factors (Table 8.3)

A number of homeodomain transcription factors are involved in the development and differentiation of the different hormone-producing cells within the pituitary gland; mutations in these transcription factors have been associated with deficiencies of pituitary hormones.[116,130–138]

Pit-1

Mutations in the *Pit-1* homeodomain transcription factor have been associated with failure of several differentiated cell types to develop within the pituitary gland and deficiencies of GH, prolactin and thyroid-stimulating hormone (TSH).[130,133–136] These patients have either small or normal-sized pituitary glands. Both autosomal dominant and recessive forms of inheritance have been described, depending on the DNA-binding properties of the mutant protein.

Prop1

Patients with mutations of *Prop1* have deficiencies of LH and FSH in addition to the deficiencies of GH, prolactin and TSH.[130,133] Adrenocorticotropic hormone (ACTH) secretion is normal at birth, but corticotrophs may degenerate secondarily.[134,138] These patients have normal, small or sometimes large pituitary glands.

Gsx1

Gsx1, an orphan homeobox gene, is required for normal pituitary development. Homozygous mutations of the *Gsx1* gene are associated with extreme dwarfism, sexual infantilism and increased perinatal mortality.[134] The pituitary gland in affected individuals is small and hypocellular, and has reduced numbers of GH- and prolactin-producing cells.[134]

Hesx1

Another homeobox gene, *Hesx1*, encodes a pituitary transcription factor whose mutations are associated with septo-optic dysplasia.[132]

Rieger syndrome

A homeodomain gene that is transcribed as two alternately spliced mRNAs that encode for two separate proteins, *Ptx2a* and *Ptx2b*, is a candidate gene for Rieger syndrome, an autosomal dominant disorder with variable craniofacial, dental, eye and pituitary anomalies.[133,137,139]

Lhx3

Combined pituitary hormone deficiency has been linked to missense mutations in the *Lhx3* gene, which encodes a member of the LIM class of homeodomain proteins.[134] Homozygous mutations in *Lhx3* in members of two unrelated consanguineous families were associated with deficiencies of multiple pituitary hormones, except ACTH, and a rigid cervical spine.

Hypergonadotropic disorders

Inactivating mutations of the LH receptor gene

Inactivating mutations of the LH receptor gene are associated with hypogonadism and Leydig cell hypoplasia. A number of families with resistance to LH action due to inactivating mutations of the LH receptor have been reported.[140-143] Men with LH receptor mutations present with a spectrum of phenotypic abnormalities ranging from feminization of external genitalia in 46,XY males to Leydig cell hypoplasia, primary hypogonadism and delayed sexual development. In a patient with Leydig cell hypoplasia and hypogonadism, a T to A mutation in position 1874 of the LH receptor gene was found.[140] Testicular histology in this man revealed the absence of mature Leydig cells; the seminiferous tubules had thickened basal lamina and spermatogenic arrest at the elongated spermatid stage. Female members of the kindred with LH receptor mutation revealed normal development of secondary sex characteristics, increased LH levels and amenorrhea.

Gene mutation	Pit1	Prop1	Hesx1
GH	Absent	Low	Low
Prolactin	Absent	Low	?
TSH	Low	Low	?
LH, FSH	Normal	Absent	?
ACTH	Normal	Low in one-third	?
ADH	Normal	Normal	Normal/Low
Pituitary size	Small/medium	S/M/L/XL/XXL	Small
Complex phenotype	No	No	Septo-optic dysplasia

From: Parks, JS. Commentary: heritable disorders of pituitary development. *J Clin Endocrinol Metab* 1999; **84**(12): 4362-70.

Table 8.3
Mutations of homeodomain transcription factors are associated with heritable disorders of pituitary development.

Inactivating mutations of the FSH receptor gene

It would be expected that a loss-of-function mutation of the gene for the human FSH receptor (2p21) would be associated with hypergonadotropic ovarian dysgenesis. In 1995, a search for linkage in multiple affected Finnish families reported finding a C566T transition predicting an Ala189Val substitution.[144] This mutation segregated perfectly with the disease phenotype of primary amenorrhea, arrest of follicular development and infertility. Expression of the gene in transfected cells showed almost no signal transduction. Compared with similar patients with ovarian dysgenesis who did not have the mutation, patients with the mutation were shorter and had more ovarian follicles.[145] In contrast to females, males with this mutation were fertile but had reduced sperm counts. Population studies have shown this mutation in about 1% of Finns, with geographical enrichment suggestive of a founder effect.

To date, five additional inactivating mutations have been described, including cases with double heterozygosity of mutations. The clinical features are slightly different, apparently due to differences in residual activity in the mutated proteins.

Treatment of androgen deficiency

Testosterone replacement therapy can be administered by using one of several available formulations with appropriate attention to its pharmacokinetics (Table 8.4). The benefits of testosterone replacement therapy have only been demonstrated in men who have androgen deficiency, as indicated by serum testosterone levels that are distinctly below the lower limit of the normal male range.

We do not know what dose of testosterone is optimum for replacement, because we do not know the dose dependency of various androgen-dependent physiological processes. Although serum testosterone concentrations that are at the lower end of the normal male range can normalize sexual function in men, it is not clear whether low normal testosterone levels can maintain bone mineral density and muscle mass. We also do not know whether serum testosterone concentrations in the high normal range that might restore bone mineral density will adversely affect insulin sensitivity or plasma lipids. In light of these uncertainties, the current recommendation is to restore serum testosterone levels into the mid-normal range.

Clinical pharmacology of the available androgen formulations and key points about testosterone replacement therapy (Table 8.4).

Testosterone replacement therapy should be guided in part by an understanding of the clinical pharmacology of the formulation used. Testosterone serves as a prohormone, and is converted in the body to 17-b-estradiol by the enzyme CyP450 aromatase and to 5-a-dihydrotestosterone by the enzyme 5-a-reductase. The effects of testosterone on bone resorption, plasma lipids, gonadotropin inhibition and certain organizational effects on the brain require its conversion to estradiol. Similarly, 5-a-reduction of testosterone to 5-a-dihydrotestosterone is obligatory for mediating its effects on the skin and the prostate. It is generally believed that testosterone may have direct effects on the muscle and bone formation. Therefore, while evaluating testosterone formulations, it is important to ascertain that the formulation being used can achieve physiological estradiol and dihydrotestosterone concentrations in addition to mid-normal testosterone concentrations.

Orally administered, 17-α-alkylated derivatives of testosterone (17-α-methyltestosterone)

Testosterone is well absorbed after its oral administration, but is quickly degraded during its passage through the liver. Therefore, it is not possible to achieve sustained blood levels of testosterone after oral administration of crystalline testosterone. 17-α-alkylated derivatives of testosterone are relatively resistant to hepatic degradation and can be given orally; however, because of the potential for hepatotoxicity, these formulations should not be used for testosterone replacement.[146,147] Hereditary angioedema due to C1 esterase deficiency is the only exception to this general recommendation; in this condition, oral, 17-α-alkylated androgens are useful because they stimulate hepatic synthesis of the C1 esterase inhibitor.

Injectable testosterone esters

The esterification of testosterone at the 17-β-hydroxy position makes the molecule hydrophobic and extends its duration of action.[148–150] De-esterification of testosterone esters occurs quickly in plasma, is not limiting and cannot account for the long duration of action. It is the slow release of testosterone ester from its oily depot in the muscle that accounts for its extended duration. The longer the side-chain, the greater the

Formulation	Regimen	Pharmacokinetic profile	DHT and estradiol	Advantages	Disadvantages
Testosterone enanthate or cypionate[128–130]	100 mg IM weekly or 200 mg IM every 2 weeks	After a single IM injection, serum testosterone levels rise into the supraphysiological range and then decline gradually into the hypogonadal range by the end of the dosing interval[128–130]	DHT and estradiol levels rise in proportion to the increase in testosterone levels. T/DHT and T/E2 ratios do not change	Corrects symptoms of androgen deficiency Relatively inexpensive, if self-administered Flexibility of dosing	Requires IM injection Peaks and valleys in serum testosterone levels
Scrotal testosterone patch[131,132]	One scrotal patch designed to nominally deliver 6 mg over 24 h, applied daily	Normalizes serum testosterone levels in many but not all androgen-deficient men	Serum estradiol levels are in the physiological male range, but DHT levels rise into the suprahysiological range. T/DHT ratio is significantly lower than in healthy men[131–133]	Corrects symptoms of androgen deficiency	To promote optimum adherence of the patch, scrotal skin needs to be shaved High DHT levels
Non-genital transdermal system[134,135]	One or two patches, designed to nominally deliver 5–10 mg testosterone over 24 h, applied daily on non-pressure areas	Restores serum testosterone, DHT and estradiol levels into the physiological male range	T/DHT and T/estradiol levels are in the physiological male range	Ease of application, corrects symptoms of androgen deficiency, and mimics the normal diurnal rhythm of testosterone secretion. Lesser increase in hemoglobin than injectable esters	Serum testosterone levels in some androgen-deficient men may be in the low normal range; these men may need application of two patches daily Skin irritation at the application site may be a problem for some patients
Testosterone gel	Testosterone gel containing 50–100 mg testosterone should be applied daily	Restores serum testosterone and estradiol levels into the physiological male range	Serum DHT levels are higher and T/DHT ratios are lower in hypogonadal men treated with the testosterone gel than in healthy eugonadal men	Corrects symptoms of androgen deficiency, provides flexibility of dosing, ease of application, good skin tolerability	Potential of transfer to a female partner or child by direct skin-to-skin contact; moderately high DHT levels
17-α-methyl testosterone[136]	Orally active, 17-α-alkylated compound that should not be used because of potential for liver toxicity	Orally active			Clinical responses variable; potential for liver toxicity Should not be used for treatment of androgen deficiency

T, testosterone.

Table 8.4
Clinical pharmacology of the testosterone formulations available in the USA.

hydrophobicity of the ester and greater the duration of action. Thus testosterone enanthate and cypionate, with longer side-chains, have longer durations of action than testosterone propionate.

Within 24 h after intramuscular administration of 200 mg testosterone enanthate or cypionate, serum testosterone levels rise into the high normal or supraphysiological range and then gradually decline into the hypogonadal range over the next 2 weeks.[149,150] A bimonthly regimen of testosterone enanthate or cypionate results in 'highs' and 'lows' in serum testosterone levels that are attended by changes in the patient's mood, sexual desire and activity and energy level.

The kinetics of testosterone enanthate and cypionate are identical.

Serum levels of estradiol and dihydrotestosterone (metabolites that are derived by conversion from testosterone) are normal if testosterone replacement is physiological.

Testosterone transdermal systems

Three transdermal testosterone patches are now commercially available: a scrotal testosterone patch (Testoderm, ALZA Corporation, Palo Alto, CA, USA) and two non-genital patches (Androderm, Watson-TheraTech, Salt Lake City, UT, USA, and Testoderm TTS, ALZA Corporation, Menlo Park, CA, USA) (Table 8.4).

The scrotal transdermal system

The scrotal transdermal system, when applied daily on the scrotal skin, can produce mid-normal serum testosterone levels in hypogonadal men 4–8 h after application of the patch followed by a gradual decrease in serum testosterone levels over the next 24 h.[151] Serum estradiol levels are normal, but dihydrotestosterone levels are high in hypogonadal men treated with the scrotal testosterone patch, presumably due to the high rates of 5-α reduction of testosterone to dihydrotestosterone during its passage through the scrotal skin. Because testosterone effects on the prostate are mediated through its metabolite, dihydrotestosterone, there was initial concern that long-term exposure to high serum dihydrotestosterone levels might have deleterious effects on the prostate. However, long-term follow-up of men treated with the scrotal patch has not revealed an unusual increase in prostate problems.[152]

Non-genital patches

One or two non-genital patches can be applied on the non-scrotal skin. Serum testosterone and estradiol levels are in the mid-normal range 4–12 h after application of the patch.[148,153] Unlike the scrotal patch, the non-genital patch produces physiological levels of serum dihydrotestosterone. Sexual function and sense of well-being is restored in androgen-deficient men treated with the non-genital patch.

The transdermal systems are more expensive than testosterone esters. The expense of testosterone esters is increased if injections are given in a medical office; however, nearly all patients or their close family members can be taught to administer the injections. The use of non-genital patches may be associated with skin irritation in some individuals; the frequency of local skin reactions is greater with the Androderm patch than with the Testoderm patch.

Testosterone gel

The Food and Drug Administration of the USA recently approved a testosterone hydroalcoholic gel for the treatment of classical hypogonadism in men. The testosterone gel is available in 2.5- and 5-g unit doses that nominally deliver 25 and 50 mg of testosterone to the application site. Initial pharmacokinetic studies[154] have demonstrated that 50-, 75- and 100-mg doses applied daily to the skin can raise and maintain serum total and free testosterone concentrations into the middle to high normal range in healthy, hypogonadal men. Serum total and free testosterone concentrations are uniform throughout the 24-h application period. The current recommendations are to start with a 75-mg dose and adjust the dose based on the measurement of serum testosterone levels. If steady-state total testosterone concentrations are in excess of 800 ng/dl on this dose, the dose should be reduced to 50 mg daily. Conversely, if the serum testosterone concentrations are less than 500 ng/dl, the dose should be increased to 100 mg daily.

The relative advantages of the testosterone gel are the ease of application, its invisibility after application and the flexibility of dosing. The major concern about the use of the gel is the potential for transfer to sexual partner and to children, who may come in close contact with the patient. Initial studies have shown that significant transfer can occur to the female partner after vigorous and direct skin-to-skin contact. Less than 5% of treated individuals reported skin irritation at the application site.

Testosterone undecanoate

This testosterone ester, when administered orally in oleic acid, is absorbed preferentially through the lymphatics into the systemic circulation and is spared the first-pass degradation through the liver. Doses of 40–80 mg given two or three times daily are typically used. However, the clinical responses are variable in different individuals and on different days in the same individual. Serum dihydrotestosterone-to-testosterone ratios are higher in hypogonadal men treated with oral testosterone undecanoate, as compared to healthy eugonadal men.

Testosterone implants

Implants of crystalline testosterone have been used for androgen replacement in men and women for over 40 years. The implants are inserted in the subcutaneous tissue by means of a trocar through a small skin incision. Testosterone is released by surface erosion from the implant and absorbed into the systemic circulation. Four to six 200-mg implants can maintain serum testosterone concentrations in the middle to high normal range for up to 6 months. The need for skin incision for insertion and removal, spontaneous extrusions and fibrosis at the site of implant insertion are potential drawbacks of this formulation.

Novel androgen formulations

A number of novel androgen formulations with better pharmacokinetics or more selective activity profiles are under development. These novel delivery systems may provide greater convenience, more physiological testosterone profile, or longer duration of action.

A biodegradable testosterone microsphere formulation has been shown to provide physiological testosterone levels for 10–11 weeks.

Two long-acting esters, testosterone buciclate and testosterone undecanoate, when injected intramuscularly, can maintain circulating testosterone concentrations in the male range for 7–12 weeks.

Initial clinical trials have demonstrated the feasibility of administering testosterone by the sublingual route using a cyclodextrin-complexed formulation, and by the buccal route.

7-α-Methyl-19-nortestosterone is an androgen that cannot be 5-α-reduced; therefore, compared to testosterone, it has relatively greater agonist activity on the muscle and gonadotropin suppression, but is less potent in supporting prostate growth that requires 5-α-reduction.

The efforts to develop non-steroidal, selective androgen receptor modulators (SARMs) with defined properties represent a most exciting development. In a manner analogous to the selective estrogen receptor modulators such as raloxifene, it may be possible to administer androgen agonists that exert the desired physiological effects on the muscle, bone and sexual function, but do not adversely affect the prostate and the cardiovascular system.

Contraindications for androgen administration in men

Testosterone replacement is contraindicated or should be administered with caution in men with certain androgen-sensitive clinical disorders.

Prostate cancer

Prostate cancer is an androgen-dependent tumor, and androgen administration may promote tumor growth. Testosterone administration is absolutely contraindicated in men with a history of prostate cancer.

Benign prostatic hypertrophy with severe symptoms

Testosterone replacement can be administered safely to men with benign prostatic hypertrophy who have mild to moderate symptom scores. Androgen deficiency is associated with decreased prostate volume, and androgen replacement increases prostate volumes to those in age-matched controls.[95,155–157] In patients with pre-existing, severe symptoms of benign prostatic hypertrophy, even small increases in prostate volume during testosterone administration may exacerbate obstructive symptoms. In these men, testosterone should either not be administered or administered with caution, with careful and frequent monitoring of obstructive symptoms.

Erythrocytosis

Testosterone replacement is associated with increase in red cell mass, presumably through its effects on erythropoietin and stem cell proliferation.[158–161] Therefore, testosterone replacement should not be administered to men with baseline hematocrit of 52% or greater without appropriate evaluation and treatment of erythrocytosis.

Sleep apnea

Testosterone can induce sleep apnea or exacerbate pre-existing sleep apnea because of its neuromuscular effects on the upper airway,[162–167] and should not be given to men with severe obstructive sleep apnea without appropriate evaluation and treatment of sleep apnea.

Breast cancer

Because testosterone is converted to estrogen, it is contraindicated in patients with breast cancer.

> Restoration and maintenance of sexual function
> Induction and maintenance of secondary sex characteristics such as hair growth
> Restoration of energy and sense of wellbeing
> Restoration of serum testosterone level in the mid-normal range for healthy, eugonadal men

Table 8.5
Assessment of treatment efficacy.

Monitoring androgen replacement therapy

Tables 8.5 and 8.6 list the clinical outcomes and laboratory tests that should be monitored in order to assess the adequacy and safety of testosterone replacement therapy.

Frequency of monitoring

The evaluation for clinical effectiveness and safety of testosterone replacement therapy should be performed 3 and 6 months after initiating testosterone therapy and annually thereafter.

Establishing efficacy of testosterone replacement therapy (Table 8.5)

Target testosterone levels

We do not have a clinically useful biological marker of androgen action. The complexities of the diurnal, pulsatile and circannual rhythms of testosterone make it difficult to mimic the endogenous pattern of testosterone secretion. Therefore, restoration of serum testosterone levels into the mid-normal range remains the goal of therapy.[153] Serum testosterone level should be measured 3 months after initiating therapy, to assess adequacy of therapy. In patients being treated with testosterone enanthate or cypionate, serum testosterone levels should be 400–700 ng/dl 1 week after the injection. If nadir levels 14 days after the injection are low, the interval between injections may be shortened; a less preferred option is to increase the dose.

In men on chronic transdermal therapy, serum testosterone levels 4–12 h after the patch application should be mid-normal. If serum testosterone levels are less than 450 ng/dl 4–8 h after patch application, the dose should be increased to two patches daily.

In men being treated with the testosterone gel, serum testosterone levels should be 450–800 ng/dl. If serum testosterone levels are outside this range, the dose should be appropriately adjusted.

Clinical evidence of efficacy

Restoration of sexual function, secondary sex characteristics, energy level and sense of wellbeing are important objectives of testosterone replacement therapy. Therefore, it is important to ask the patient about sexual desire and activity, whether the patient has early-morning erections, and whether he is able to achieve and maintain erections that are adequate for sexual intercourse.

Some hypogonadal men continue to complain of sexual dysfunction even after testosterone replacement has been instituted; these patients can benefit from counseling. Hypogonadal men with prepubertal onset of androgen deficiency who are started on testosterone in their late 20s or 30s may find it difficult to cope with their new-found sexuality and need counseling. If the patient has a sexual partner, it is crucial to include the partner in counseling because of the dramatic physical and sexual changes that occur with androgen treatment.

The facial hair growth in response to androgen replacement is variable and dependent on the ethnic background.

LH and FSH levels

The usefulness of LH and FSH levels to assess the adequacy of testosterone replacement remains questionable. In men with hypergonadotropic hypogonadism, particularly those with Klinefelter's syndrome, it is uncommon for serum LH and FSH levels to be normalized by physiological replacement doses of

> Clinical
>   Clinical evaluation should focus on ascertaining the presence of:
>   Breast tenderness or enlargement
>   Acne and oiliness of skin
>   Symptoms of sleep apnea
>   Symptoms of benign prostatic hypertrophy
>   Digital rectal examination for prostatic enlargement or nodules
> Biochemical
>   Hemoglobin level
>   Serum PSA

Table 8.6
Monitoring of adverse effects.

testosterone that restore sexual function. Similarly, measurements of LH and FSH levels are not useful in men with hypogonadotropic hypogonadism, because in these men the feedback relationship between serum testosterone and LH secretion is perturbed because of the underlying hypothalamic–pituitary disorder.

Bone mineral density
Institution of testosterone replacement therapy is associated with an increase in bone mineral density in androgen-deficient men. Men with idiopathic hypogonadotropic hypogonadism who have closed epiphyses experience an increase in cortical bone density, while those with open epiphyses demonstrate increases in both cortical and trabecular bone density after testosterone treatment. In adult men with androgen deficiency that is acquired after the completion of pubertal development, testosterone replacement induces an improvement primarily in the trabecular bone density. The bone density is, however, not normalized in most hypogonadal men by physiological testosterone replacement. The clinical utility of following bone mineral density in androgen-deficient men has not been demonstrated.

Body composition assessment
Testosterone treatment is associated with an increase in lean body mass and muscle strength;[168–171] however, measurements of body composition are not clinically indicated at this time.

Monitoring potential adverse experiences (Table 8.6)
The men receiving androgen replacement therapy should be monitored for potential adverse effects.

Hemoglobin levels
Administration of testosterone to androgen-deficient men is typically associated with a 3–5% increase in hemoglobin levels. Clinically significant polycythemia is uncommon in young hypogonadal men, but can occur in men with sleep apnea, significant smoking history, or chronic obstructive lung disease; in such patients, hemoglobin levels should be closely monitored after institution of testosterone replacement. Testosterone administration in older men is associated with greater increments in hemoglobin than observed in young, hypogonadal men. The magnitude of hemoglobin increase during testosterone therapy appears to be related to the magnitude of the peak serum testosterone levels. Testosterone replacement by means of a transdermal system has been reported to produce a lesser increase in hemoglobin levels than that associated with testosterone esters.

Digital examination of the prostate and serum PSA levels (Table 8.7)
Testosterone replacement therapy increases prostate volumes and PSA levels to those seen in age-matched controls, but continued androgen treatment does not further increase prostate volume beyond that expected for age.[95,152,155–157,172,173] There is no evidence that testosterone replacement causes prostate cancer. However, androgen can exacerbate pre-existing prostate cancer and should not be administered to men with a history of prostate cancer. Many older men harbor microscopic foci of cancer in their prostates. In addition, older men with prostate cancer may have low testosterone levels.[174] We do not know whether long-term testosterone administration to older men will unmask microscopic foci of prostate cancer. This uncertainty is the main reason for periodic PSA measurements in men receiving testosterone replacement therapy.

Serum PSA levels are lower in testosterone-deficient men and are restored to normal following testosterone replacement;[152,155,172,173,175] however, serum PSA levels do not increase progressively in healthy hypogonadal men with replacement doses of testosterone. In two recent placebo-controlled trials of testosterone administration in older men, the change in serum PSA levels over a 3-year treatment period was not significantly different between placebo- and testosterone-treated men.

Serum PSA levels tend to fluctuate when measured repeatedly in the same individual over time. Therefore, when serum PSA levels in androgen-deficient men on testosterone replacement therapy show a change from a previously measured value, the clinician has to decide whether the change warrants detailed evaluation of the patient for prostate cancer, or whether it is simply due to test-to-test variability in PSA measurement. The data from the Finasteride Study for Benign Prostatic Hypertrophy demonstrated that the 95% confidence interval for the change in PSA values measured 3–6 months apart is 1.4 ng/ml. Therefore, a change in PSA of >1.5 ng/ml between any two values measured 3–6 months apart in the same patient should be verified by a repeat PSA measurement. If the repeated measurement confirms a change of >1.5 ng/ml from the previous value, then that patient should be referred for urological evaluation. In addition, in patients in whom sequential PSA measurements are available for more

> 1. Enquire about symptoms of benign prostatic hypertrophy using an American Urologic Association (AUA) symptom questionnaire, perform a digital rectal examination, and obtain a baseline PSA measurement before initiating androgen replacement therapy
> 2. Testosterone should not be administered to men with baseline PSA greater than 4 ng/ml, AUA symptom score >14, or a palpable abnormality on digital rectal examination without a urological evaluation
> 3. The presence of benign prostatic hypertrophy by itself is not a contraindication for testosterone replacement therapy. However, testosterone should not be prescribed to men with AUA symptom score greater than 14 without a thorough urological evaluation
> 4. After institution of testosterone replacement therapy, serum PSA measurement and digital rectal examination should be performed at 3 months, 9 months, and annually thereafter. In addition, at these points, an assessment of the symptoms of benign prostatic hypertrophy should be made by using the AUA symptom score
> 5. There is considerable test-to-test variability in PSA measurements. A change in serum PSA level of greater than 1.5 ng/ml between two measurements 3–6 months apart should be verified by retesting. A persistent increase of 1.5 ng/ml or greater should warrant a urological evaluation to exclude prostate cancer.
> 6. In men in whom sequential PSA levels are available over a period of greater than 2 years, PSA velocity can be calculated as the change from baseline in PSA levels divided by the elapsed time in years; PSA velocity is expressed as ng/ml/year. A PSA velocity of greater than 0.75 ng/ml/year should warrant a urological evaluation to exclude prostate cancer. However, PSA velocity criteria must not be applied to follow-up data of less than 2 years' duration.

Table 8.7
Guidelines for prostate follow-up in hypogonadal men receiving androgen replacement.

than 2 years, the PSA velocity criterion can be used; a change of greater than 0.75 ng/ml/year in PSA velocity is unusual in men with benign prostatic disease and should warrant evaluation for prostate cancer. However, Carter has emphasized that the PSA velocity criterion should not be used for time periods of less than 2 years.

Sleep apnea
Testosterone can induce or exacerbate sleep apnea in some individuals, particularly those with obesity or chronic obstructive lung disease.[162–166] This appears to be due to direct effects of testosterone on laryngeal muscles.

Evaluation of the local application site in men treated with the transdermal patches and gel
In patients being treated with the testosterone patch or the testosterone gel, the application site should be inspected for local skin reactions, including erythema and induration, that can occur in 5–10% of patients receiving the non-genital patch. Blister formation is relatively rare. Local skin reactions are less common with the Testoderm patch than with the Androderm patch.

Cardiovascular risk assessment
The long-term effects of testosterone supplementation on cardiovascular risk are unknown. Testosterone effects on plasma lipids depend on the dose (physiological or supraphysiological), the route of administration (oral or parenteral) and the formulation (whether aromatizable or not). Physiological testosterone replacement by an aromatizable androgen has a modest or no effect on plasma high-density lipoprotein (HDL). In middle-aged men with low testosterone levels, physiological testosterone replacement has been shown to improve insulin sensitivity and reduce visceral obesity. In epidemiological studies, serum testosterone concentrations are inversely related to waist-to-hip ratio and plasma HDL levels, which are surrogate markers for the risk of heart disease. These data suggest that physiological testos-

terone replacement may reduce cardiovascular risk in androgen-deficient men. While no specific recommendations can be made at this time, men receiving androgen replacement therapy should undergo cardiovascular risk assessment as part of their general health evaluation.

Breast enlargement

Testosterone administration can induce breast enlargement due to testosterone conversion to estradiol, although this is an uncommon complication. Even with administration of supraphysiological doses of testosterone enanthate, less than 4% of men in a contraceptive trial developed detectable breast enlargement. Breast cancer is listed as a contraindication for testosterone replacement therapy, primarily because of concern that increased estrogen levels during testosterone treatment might exacerbate breast cancer growth. There are, however, few case reports of breast cancer occurring as a complication of testosterone treatment. Men with Klinefelter's syndrome have a higher risk of breast cancer than the general population.

Erectile dysfunction in men

Erectile dysfunction is the inability of the male to attain and/or maintain an erection sufficient to allow sexual intercourse.[62,176,177] Impotence is a more general term that also includes libidinal, orgasmic and ejaculatory dysfunction in addition to the inability to attain or maintain penile erection.[62]

Prevalence

Erectile dysfunction is a common problem, affecting 10 million to 30 million men in the USA alone.[14,62,176–179] The prevalence of erectile dysfunction increases with age; it affects less than 3% of men younger than 45 years of age, but 75% of men over 80 years of age.[14,179] Men suffering from other medical problems such as hypertension, diabetes, cardiovascular disease and end-stage renal disease have a significantly higher prevalence of erectile dysfunction than healthy men.[14,62,179]

The regulation of sexual function and the physiology of penile erection

Sexual function is a complex, multicomponent system that comprises central mechanisms for regulation of libido and arousability, and local mechanisms for the generation of penile tumescence, rigidity, orgasm and ejaculation. Androgen-deficient men have decreased overall sexual activity but can achieve normal erections in response to visual erotic stimuli.[11–13,15] These observations have led to the prevalent dogma that libido is testosterone dependent and that the local mechanisms for penile erection are androgen independent. There is emerging evidence that testosterone is a regulator of

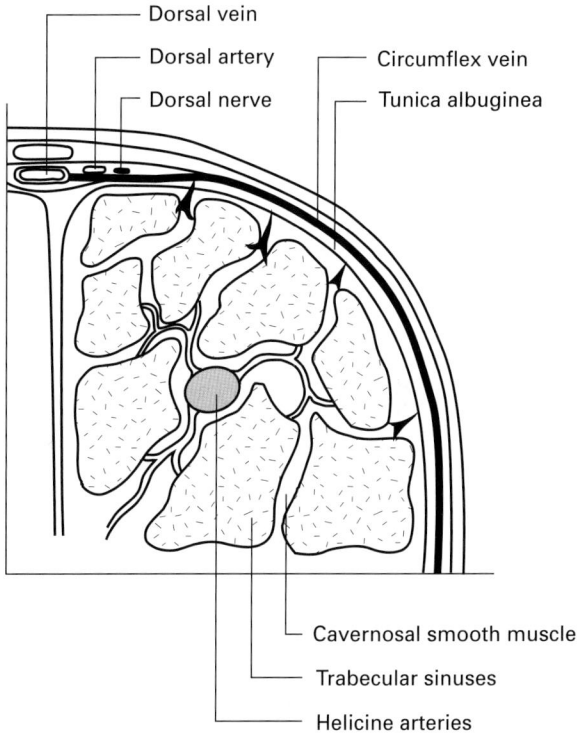

Figure 8.5

*Anatomy of penile erection. Corpora cavernosa are made up of trabecular spaces that are surrounded by cavernosal smooth muscle. Helicine arteries provide the arterial supply to the cavernosal spaces. The dorsal nerve provides the sensory innervation to the penis. During erection, the relaxation of the trabecular smooth muscle and increased bloodflow result in engorgement of the sinusoidal spaces in the corpora cavernosa. The expansion of the sinusoids compresses the venous return against the tunica albuginea, resulting in entrapment of blood. This imparts rigidity to the tumescent penis. (Adapted from Lue TF. Erectile dysfunction. N Engl J Med 2000; **342**(24): 1802–13.)*

nitric oxide synthase activity in the cavernosal smooth muscle.[180] Therefore, it is possible that physiologically normal testosterone concentrations might be required for optimum penile rigidity. Orgasm and ejaculation are not androgen dependent and can occur without a full penile erection.

Normal penile erection requires coordinated involvement of intact central and peripheral nervous systems, corpora cavernosa and spongiosa, as well as a normal arterial blood supply and venous drainage (Figure 8.6).[181–184] The cavernosal arteries and their branches, the helicine arteries, provide bloodflow to the penis.[184] Helicine arteries drain blood into the cavernosal sinuses.[181,182] Dilatation of the helicine arteries increases the bloodflow and pressure in the cavernosal sinuses.[181,182] Relaxation of the cavernosal smooth muscle that surrounds the cavernosal sinuses along with increased bloodflow results in pooling of blood in the cavernosal spaces and penile engorgement. The expanding corpora cavernosa compress the venules against the rigid tunica albuginea, restricting the venous outflow from the cavernosal spaces. This facilitates entrapment of blood in the cavernosal sinuses and achievement of a rigid erection.[181]

The relaxation of the cavernosal smooth muscle trabeculae is under the regulation of the autonomic nervous system.[181–186] Although cholinergic, adrenergic and noradrenergic non-cholinergic (NANC) mediators all play a role, the principal biochemical regulator of cavernosal smooth muscle relaxation is nitric oxide derived from the nerve terminals innervating the corpora cavernosa, endothelial lining of penile arteries and cavernosal sinuses.[181–186] Nitric oxide also induces arterial dilatation. The actions of nitric oxide on the cavernosal smooth muscle and the arterial bloodflow are mediated through the activation of guanyl cyclase and production of cyclic

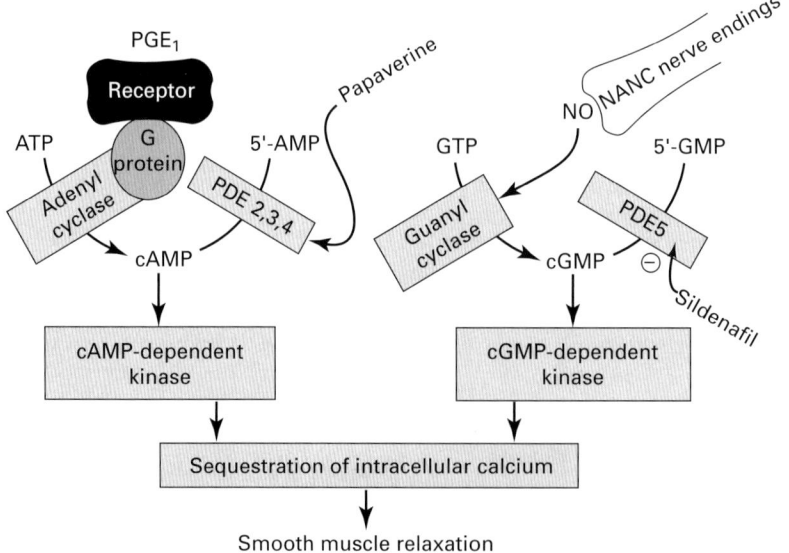

Figure 8.6
Biochemical mechanisms of penile smooth muscle relaxation. The relaxation of the cavernosal smooth muscle is regulated by intracellular cAMP and cGMP. These intracellular second messengers, by activation of specific protein kinases, cause sequestration of intracellular calcium and closure of calcium channels. This results in a net decrease in intracellular calcium, causing smooth muscle relaxation. Nitric oxide, released by noradrenergic, non-cholinergic nerve endings, stimulates guanyl cyclase. Sildenafil, by inhibiting phosphodiesterase type 5 (PDE5), increases the amount of intracellular cGMP. Prostaglandin E_1 stimulates cAMP generation. Papaverine inhibits phosphodiesterases 2, 3 and 4, and thereby increases the amount of intracellular cAMP. cAMP, 3',5'-cyclic adenosine monophosphate; cGMP, 3',5'-guanyl monophosphate; ATP, adenosine triphosphate; NANC, noradrenergic, non-cholinergic nerve endings; NO, nitric oxide; PGE_1, prostaglandin E_1.

GMP.[181–187] The latter acts as an intracellular second messenger and causes smooth muscle relaxation by lowering intracellular calcium.[184]

A class of enzymes called cyclic nucleotide phosphodiesterases degrade cGMP into an inactive form, GMP. There are many isoforms of cyclic nucleotide phosphodiesterases, and these isoforms are widely distributed throughout the body; the predominant isoform of this enzyme in the cavernosal smooth muscle is cyclic nucleotide phosphodiesterase 5 (PDE5).[177,181,184] Hydrolysis of cGMP by this enzyme results in reversal of the smooth muscle relaxation and relief of penile erection. Sildenafil, a potent and selective inhibitor of the activity of PDE5, prevents breakdown of cGMP and enhances penile erection.[96]

Additional cGMP-independent pathways, some of which proceed through cyclic adenosine monophosphate (cAMP)-dependent mechanisms, also contribute to trabecular smooth muscle relaxation. For instance, prostaglandin E1, normally synthesized by corpus cavernosum smooth muscle, can increase intracellular cAMP concentration and potentiate smooth muscle relaxation.[181–187]

Evaluation of patients with erectile dysfunction (Table 8.8)

History
The diagnostic work-up of the patient with erectile dysfunction should start with an evaluation of general health.[176,177] General medical history should be directed at identifying etiological factors as well as factors that might affect the selection and response to therapy. The presence of diabetes mellitus, coronary artery disease, peripheral vascular disease and hypertension may suggest a vascular cause. History of stroke, spinal cord or back injury, multiple sclerosis or dementia may point to a neurological disorder. Also relevant are a history of pelvic trauma, prostate surgery, or priapism. Social history should include ascertainment of recreational drug abuse—particularly alcohol, cocaine, marijuana and tobacco. Information about medications, particularly antihypertensives, antiandrogens, anti-depressants and antipsychotic drugs is important, because almost a quarter of all cases of impotence can be attributed to medications. Psychiatric illnesses such as depression or psychosis, or drugs used to treat these disorders, might be associated with sexual dysfunction.

A detailed sexual history, including the nature of relationships, partner expectations, situational erectile failure, performance anxiety and marital discord, should be elicited (Table 8.8).[176,177] It is important to distinguish between inability to achieve erection, changes in sexual desire, failure to achieve orgasm and ejaculation, and dissatisfaction with a sexual relationship. The physician should inquire about the onset, duration, quality and duration of erections and the presence of nocturnal and early-morning erections.

Physical examination
A directed physical examination should assess secondary sex characteristics, the presence or absence of breast enlargement and testicular volume. An evaluation of femoral and pedal pulses can provide clues to the presence of peripheral vascular disease (Table 8.8). The neurological examination should focus on the presence of motor weakness, perineal sensation, rectal sphincter tone and bulbocavernosus reflex. The examination of the penis should ascertain any unusual curvature or palpable cordae.

Laboratory tests
The work-up of the man with erectile dysfunction should start with general health evaluation.[176,177] Measurements of hemoglobin, white blood count, AST, ALT, bilirubin, alkaline phosphatase, BUN and creatinine can provide useful information about general health and the presence of liver and kidney disease.

Evaluation of penile vasculature and blood flow
There are several tests that can evaluate the integrity of penile vasculature and bloodflow.[176,177] Of these, the penile brachial blood pressure index is the simplest. For computation of this index, brachial and penile blood pressure measurements are taken on either side in the supine position before and after leg exercise.[188–191] The ratio of the penile to brachial systolic blood pressure is calculated on both sides under these conditions. An abnormal response is defined as any penile to brachial systolic blood pressure ratio of <0.65 or a decrease in the index of >0.15 after exercise. The penile brachial blood pressure index is a relatively specific but not very sensitive marker of vascular insufficiency.[188–191] This index can provide a useful clue to the presence of vascular insufficiency, which should then be further investigated by duplex sonography or angiography. Recent publications have raised questions about the reproducibility and accuracy of this index.[190]

Intracavernosal injection of a vasoactive amine such as prostaglandin E_1 can be helpful in men for whom this mode of therapy is being considered.[176,177] This procedure can show whether the patient will respond to this therapeutic modality and facilitate patient education about the procedure and its potential side-effects. Failure to respond to intracavernosal injection can raise the suspicion of vascular insufficiency or a venous leak that might need further evaluation and treatment. The penile brachial blood pressure index and the response to intracavernosal injection may diverge in about 20% of men with vascular problems. A venous leak should be suspected in these individuals.

Most men with erectile dysfunction do not need duplex color sonography, cavernosography, or pelvic angiography.[176,177] These procedures should be performed only in patients where the results of these tests would alter the management or prognosis, and only by those with considerable experience with their use. For instance, angiography could be useful in a young man

---

History
A. Ascertain psychosexual history of:
  1. The strength of marital relationship and marital discord
  2. Depression
  3. Stress
  4. Performance anxiety
B. Ascertain etiological factors, such as:
  1. The presence of diabetes mellitus, hypertension, end-stage renal disease, peripheral vascular disease
  2. History of spinal cord injury, stroke, or Alzheimer's disease
  3. Prostate or pelvic surgery
  4. Pelvic injury
  5. Concomitant medications such as antihypertensive, antidepressant, antipsychotic, anti-androgens such as flutamide, casadex, cyproterone acetate, and cimetidine, inhibitors of androgen production such as ketoconazole and GnRH agonists
  6. The use of recreational drugs such as alcohol, cocaine, opiates, and tobacco
C. Ascertain factors that might affect choice of therapy and the patient's response to it, such as:
  1. Coexisting coronary artery disease and its symptoms and severity
  2. The use of nitrates for angina
  3. Exercise tolerance
  4. The use of vasodilators for hypertension or congestive heart failure

Physical examination
  1. Ascertain signs of androgen deficiency such as loss of secondary sex characteristics, eunuchoidal proportions, small testicular volume, or breast enlargement
  2. Neurological findings of spinal cord lesion, previous stroke, or peripheral neuropathy; genital and perineal sensation
  3. Palpation of femoral and pedal pulses, and evidence of lower extremity ischemia
  4. Penile examination to exclude Peyronie's disease

Laboratory evaluation
  1. Brachial penile blood pressure index
  2. Intracavernosal injection of vasodilator
  3. Duplex ultrasonography
  4. Pelvic arteriography
  5. Cavernosography

Table 8.8
Diagnostic evaluation of erectile dysfunction.

with arterial insufficiency associated with pelvic trauma. Similarly, suspicion of congenital or traumatic venous leak in a young man presenting with erectile dysfunction would justify a cavernosography. In each instance, confirmation of the vascular lesion might lead to consideration of surgery. Duplex ultrasonography can provide a non-invasive evaluation of vascular function.[177]

Nocturnal penile tumescence

Although recording of nocturnal penile tumescence (NPT) can help differentiate organic from psychogenic impotence, this test is expensive, labor-intensive and not required in most men with erectile dysfunction. A history of night-time or early-morning erections, or a stamp test, have a high correlation with erections recorded by an NPT device.

Diagnostic tests to exclude androgen deficiency and hypothalamic–pituitary lesions

There is considerable debate about the usefulness and cost-effectiveness of hormonal evaluation and the extent to which androgen deficiency should be investigated in men presenting with erectile dysfunction. Eight to ten per cent of men with erectile dysfunction have low testosterone levels; the prevalence of androgen deficiency increases with advancing age.[51,63–65,67,69] The prevalence of low testosterone levels is not significantly different among men who present with erectile dysfunction and in an age-matched population.[51] These data are consistent with the proposal that erectile dysfunction and androgen deficiency are two common but independently distributed disorders.[51]

It is important to exclude androgen deficiency in this patient population, for several reasons.[66] Androgen deficiency is a correctable cause of sexual dysfunction and many, though not all, men with erectile dysfunction and low testosterone levels would respond to testosterone replacement. Second, hypogonadism might have additional deleterious effects on the individual's health; for instance, hypogonadism might contribute to osteoporosis, loss of muscle mass and function, increased risk of disability, falls and fracture, insulin resistance and cardiovascular disease. Therefore, regardless of the presence of sexual dysfunction, androgen deficiency should be corrected by appropriate hormone replacement therapy. Further, androgen deficiency might be a manifestation of a serious underlying disease, such as HIV infection or a hypothalamic–pituitary space-occupying lesion, and needs evaluation.

In large studies,[51,63,65] only a small fraction of men with erectile dysfunction and low testosterone levels have been found to have space-occupying lesions of the hypothalamic–pituitary region. In one large survey, all of the hypothalamic–pituitary lesions were found in men with serum testosterone levels less than 150 ng/dl.[65] Therefore, the cost-effectiveness of the diagnostic work-up to rule out an underlying lesion of the hypothalamic–pituitary region can be increased by limiting the work-up to men with serum testosterone levels less than 150 ng/dl.

Treatment of erectile dysfunction

The selection of the therapeutic modality should be based on the underlying etiology, patient preference, the nature and strength of the relationship with the sexual partner, and the absence or presence of underlying cardiovascular disease and other comorbid conditions.[176,177] A step approach that first utilizes non-invasive therapies that are easier to use and have fewer adverse effects and progresses to therapies that require injections or surgical interventions only after the first-line choices have been exhausted can minimize risk and increase patient acceptance (Table 8.9). The physician should discuss the risks and benefits of all the diagnostic procedures and therapies with the couple. The treatment of associated medical disorders should be optimized. In men with diabetes mellitus, efforts to optimize glycemic control should be instituted, although improving glycemic control may not improve sexual function. In men with hypertension, control of blood pressure should

---

1. All patients and their sexual partners can benefit from and should receive psychosexual counseling
2. First-line therapies:
   (a) Sildenafil citrate
   (b) Vacuum constriction devices
3. Second-line therapies:
   (a) Intracavernosal injection of alprostadil
   (b) Intracavernosal injections of other vasoactive amines
4. Third-line therapies:
   (a) Penile prosthesis
   (b) Vascular surgery

Table 8.9
A stepwise approach to treatment of erectile dysfunction.

be optimized and, if possible, the therapeutic regimen should be modified to remove antihypertensive drugs that impair sexual function. This strategy is not always possible, because almost all antihypertensive agents have been associated with sexual dysfunction; the frequency of this adverse event is less with converting enzyme inhibitors than with other agents.

All patients with erectile dysfunction can benefit from and should receive psychosexual counseling.

First line therapies

Psychosexual counseling

Counseling is always indicated in both psychogenic and organic impotence. It can help decrease performance anxiety and increase the patient's ability to cope with the problem.[176,177] Involving the partner in the counseling can help dispel misperceptions about the problem, decrease stress, enhance intimacy and ability to talk about sex, and increase the chances of successful outcome of therapy. Counseling sessions are also helpful in uncovering conflicts in relationships, psychiatric problems, alcohol and drug abuse, and significant misperceptions about sex. Although psychobehavioral therapy has been claimed to relieve depression and anxiety, there is a striking paucity of outcome data on the effectiveness of this therapeutic modality.

Sildenafil

Sildenafil is a selective type 5 phosphodiesterase inhibitor that is a safe and effective first-line oral treatment for erectile dysfunction.[95,192–197]

Mechanism of action

Sildenafil blocks the hydrolysis of cGMP induced by nitric oxide.[95,192,193] Therefore, sildenafil action requires an intact nitric oxide response, as well as constitutive synthesis of cGMP by the cells. By selectively inhibiting cGMP catabolism in the cavernosal smooth muscle cells, sildenafil restores the natural erectile response to sexual stimulation, but does not produce an erection in the absence of such stimulation. The intactness of the nitric oxide production pathway and sexual stimulation are both necessary for sildenafil to successfully induce an erection.

Efficacy

The efficacy of sildenafil was demonstrated in a randomized dose–response study[187] in which 532 men with organic, psychogenic or mixed erectile dysfunction were randomized to receive placebo or 25, 50, or 100 mg sildenafil for 24 weeks. In this dose–response study,[187] patients on sildenafil performed better in terms of increased rigidity, frequency of vaginal penetration and maintenance of erection. Increasing doses of sildenafil were associated with higher mean scores for the questions assessing frequency of penetration and maintenance of erections after sexual penetration. In a follow-up dose escalation study,[187] 329 men were randomly assigned to receive placebo or 50 mg sildenafil for 12 weeks. At each follow-up, the dose of sildenafil was increased or decreased by 50%, depending upon the therapeutic response or side-effects. Sixty-four per cent of attempts at intercourse were successful for the men receiving sildenafil, as compared to 22% for men receiving placebo. The mean numbers of successful attempts per month were 5.9 for men receiving sildenafil and 1.5 for those receiving placebo. The mean scores for orgasms, intercourse satisfaction and overall satisfaction were also significantly higher in the sildenafil group than in the placebo group.[187]

Sildenafil has been shown to be effective in men with diabetes mellitus in a separate clinical trial.[66] In this randomized clinical trial, 268 men with diabetes mellitus and erectile dysfunction received either placebo or sildenafil for 12 weeks. Fifty-six per cent of men receiving sildenafil reported improved erections, compared with 10% of those receiving placebo ($P < 0.001$). The percentage of men reporting at least one successful attempt at intercourse was 61% for the sildenafil versus 22% for the placebo group. This study[66] demonstrated that sildenafil is an effective treatment for erectile dysfunction in patients with diabetes mellitus.

Sildenafil is also effective in men with erectile dysfunction due to a variety of other causes, including spinal cord injury and prostatectomy.[194,195] In general, baseline sexual function and the etiology of sexual dysfunction are good predictors of response to therapy;[194] however, there is no baseline characteristic that predicts absolute failure to respond to sildenafil therapy. Therefore, a therapeutic trial of sildenafil is warranted in all patients except in those in whom it is contraindicated.[194]

Adverse effects associated with sildenafil therapy (Table 8.11)

In clinical trials, the adverse effects that have been reported with greater frequency in sildenafil-treated men than placebo-treated men include headaches, flushing, dyspepsia, respiratory tract disorders and visual disturbances.[196] Sildenafil does not affect semen characteristics.[197–204] No cases of priapism were noted in any of the pivotal clinical trials.

1. Sildenafil is absolutely contraindicated in men taking long-acting or short-acting nitrate drugs on a regular basis.
2. If the patient has stable coronary artery disease, is not taking long-acting nitrates, and uses short-acting nitrates only infrequently, the use of sildenafil should be guided by careful consideration of risks.
3. All men taking nitrates should be warned about the risks of the potential interaction between nitrates and sildenafil. The patients should also be warned that concurrent recreational use of inhaled nitrates or poppers could result in marked hypotension that could be serious or even fatal.
4. Sildenafil is contraindicated within 24 h of the ingestion of any form of nitrate.
5. In men with pre-existing coronary artery disease, the risks of inducing cardiac ischemia during sexual activity should be assessed before prescribing sildenafil. This assessment may include a stress test.
6. Men who are taking a combination antihypertensive medication should be warned about the possibility of sildenafil-induced hypotension. This is of particular concern in men with congestive heart failure who have low blood volume or who are receiving complex regimens that include vasodilators or diuretics.

Table 8.10
American College of Cardiology and American Heart Association recommendations for the use of sildenafil by men with cardiac disease.[44]

Hemodynamic effects of sildenafil citrate

In post-marketing surveillance, several instances of myocardial infarction and sudden death were reported[198–204] in men using sildenafil. Forty-four of the 130 deaths reported by the US Food and Drug Administration during March to November 1998 occurred in temporal relation to the ingestion of sildenafil;[198–204] 16 of these deaths occurred in individuals who were taking nitrates. Because most men presenting with erectile dysfunction also have a high prevalence of cardiovascular risk factors, it is unclear whether these events were causally related to the ingestion of sildenafil, underlying heart disease, or both.[204] In a rigorously controlled study,[205] oral administration of 100 mg sildenafil to men with severe coronary artery disease produced only small decreases in systemic blood pressure and no significant changes in cardiac output, heart rate, coronary bloodflow and coronary artery diameter. This led the American Heart Association to conclude that the pre-existence of coronary artery disease by itself does not constitute a contraindication for the use of sildenafil.[204]

Guidelines for the use of sildenafil in men with coronary artery disease (Table 8.10)[204]

Before prescribing sildenafil, it is crucial to assess cardiovascular risk factors. If the patient has hypertension or symptomatic coronary artery disease, the treatment of those clinical disorders should be optimized.[177,204] The physician must enquire about the use of nitrates, because sildenafil is absolutely contraindicated in individuals taking any form of nitrates or nitrites on a daily basis.

Adverse event	Sildenafil (%)	Placebo (%)
Headache	16	4
Flushing	10	1
Dyspepsia	7	2
Rate of discontinuation	2.5	2.3

Morales et al[38] reviewed the safety and tolerability data on 4274 men with erectile dysfunction from a series of placebo-controlled and open-label studies of sildenafil. Most adverse effects were reported to be mild to moderate in intensity and transient.[38] In other studies, visual disturbances resulting in blue–green color-tinged vision, increased light perception, and blurred vision, and myalgias have also been reported in association with the use of sildenafil.[44]

Table 8.11
Common adverse events associated with the use of sildenafil in men with erectile dysfunction.

Sildenafil can be used in men who use nitrates infrequently. However, sildenafil should not be used within 24 h of the use of nitrates.[204]

In men with pre-existing coronary artery disease, sexual activity can induce coronary ischemia;[203] these individuals should undergo assessment of their exercise tolerance. One practical way to assess exercise tolerance is to have the patient climb one or two flights of stairs. If the individual can safely climb one or two flights of stairs without angina or excessive shortness of breath, he can probably engage in sexual intercourse with a stable partner without similar symptoms. Exercise testing before prescribing sildenafil may be indicated in some men with significant heart disease to assess the risk of inducing cardiac ischemia during sexual activity.[204]

In men with congestive heart failure, receiving vasodilator drugs, or on complex regimens of antihypertensive drugs, it is advisable to monitor blood pressure after initial administration of sildenafil.[204]

There have been extensive reviews published on the safety of sildenafil therapy.[206–213]

Drug–drug interactions

Sildenafil is metabolized mostly by the P450 2C9 and the P450 3A4 pathways.[204] Cimetidine and erythromycin, inhibitors of P450 3A4, increase the plasma concentrations of sildenafil. Protease inhibitors may also alter the activity of the P450 3A4 pathway and affect the clearance of sildenafil.[204]

Conversely, sildenafil is an inhibitor of the P450 2C9 metabolic pathway, and its administration could potentially affect the metabolism of drugs metabolized by this system, such as warfarin and tolbutamide.[204]

The most serious interactions of sildenafil are with the nitrates. The vasodilator effects of nitrates are augmented by sildenafil; this also applies to inhaled forms of nitrates such as amyl nitrate or nitrite, which are sold under the street name 'poppers'. Concomitant administration of the two drugs can cause a potentially fatal decrease in blood pressure.[204]

Therapeutic regimens

In most men with erectile dysfunction, sildenafil should be started at an initial dose of 25 mg. If this dose does not produce any adverse effects, then the dose should be increased to 50 mg.[95,204] Further dose adjustment should be guided by the therapeutic response to therapy and occurrence of adverse effects. Increments in unit dose should be limited to 25 mg at one time. Typically, unit doses higher than 100 mg are not recommended. To minimize the risk of hypotension and adverse cardiovascular events in association with the use of sildenafil, the American Heart Association has prepared a list of recommendations (Table 8.10), which should be followed rigorously.[204]

Sildenafil should be taken at least 1 hour before sexual intercourse. It should not be taken more than once in any 24-h period.

Cost-effectiveness of sildenafil use for erectile dysfunction

A number of studies have evaluated the economic cost of treating erectile dysfunction in men in managed-care organizations.[214–216] These analyses, using a prevalence-based cost of illness approach, have concluded that sildenafil and vacuum constriction devices are the most cost-effective of all the available therapeutic options in the managed-care setting and should be considered as first-line strategies.[214–216]

Vacuum devices for inducing erection

Commercially available vacuum devices consist of a plastic cylinder, a vacuum pump and an elastic constriction band.[176,177] The plastic cylinder fits over the penis and is connected to a vacuum pump. The vacuum within the cylinder draws blood into the penis, producing an erection. An elastic band slipped around the base of the penis traps the blood in the penis, maintaining an erection as long as the rubber band is retained around the base. The constriction band should not be left in place for more than 30 min.

These devices are safe, relatively inexpensive and reasonably effective. These devices impair ejaculation, resulting in entrapment of semen. They are difficult and awkward for some patients to use. Some couples dislike the lack of spontaneity engendered by the use of these devices. Partner cooperation is usually important for successful use of these devices.[217–224]

Testosterone replacement in androgen-deficient men presenting with erectile dysfunction

Testosterone replacement in healthy, young, androgen-deficient men restores sexual function.[10,13,14,225–232] In healthy young men, relatively low normal levels of serum testosterone can maintain sexual function.[10,229,232] In male rats,[230,231] a decrease in serum testosterone concentrations to castration levels is associated with marked impairment of all measures of mating behavior, and testosterone replacement to levels that are at the lower end of the adult male range normalizes all measures of mating behavior. In general, supraphysiological doses of testosterone do not further improve sexual function. It is possible that increasing testosterone levels above the physiological range might increase arousability; however, this has not been conclusively demonstrated.

Androgen deficiency and erectile dysfunction are two common but independently distributed clinical disorders in middle-aged and older men that often coexist in the same patient. Eight to ten per cent of men presenting with erectile dysfunction have low testosterone levels.[51,63–65,67] The prevalence of low testosterone levels is not significantly different between middle-aged and older men with impotence and those without impotence.[51] Testosterone administration is unlikely to improve sexual function in men with normal testosterone levels. Therefore, indiscriminate use of testosterone replacement in all older men with erectile dysfunction is not warranted. However, it is important to exclude testosterone deficiency in older men presenting with erectile dysfunction. Androgen deficiency may be a manifestation of an underlying disease such as a pituitary tumor. Additionally, therapies directed just at erectile dysfunction in men will not correct androgen deficiency, which, if left uncorrected, will have deleterious effects on bone, muscle, energy level and sense of wellbeing.

Many, but not all, of the impotent men with low testosterone levels experience improvements in their libido and overall sexual activity with androgen replacement therapy.[66,233] The response to testosterone supplementation even in this group of men is variable,[51,63–65,67] because of the coexistence of other disorders such as diabetes mellitus, hypertension, cardiovascular disease and psychogenic factors.[51] A meta-analysis[233] of the usefulness of androgen replacement therapy concluded that testosterone administration is associated with greater improvements in sexual function than those associated with placebo in men with erectile dysfunction and low testosterone levels.[233]

Erectile dysfunction in middle-aged and older men is often a multifactorial disorder. Common causes of erectile dysfunction in men include diabetes mellitus, hypertension, medication, peripheral vascular disease, psychogenic factors and end-stage renal disease. These factors often coexist in the same patient. Therefore, it is not surprising that testosterone treatment might not improve sexual function in all men with androgen deficiency.

Testosterone treatment does not improve sexual function in impotent men who have normal testosterone levels.[64] We do not know whether testosterone replacement improves sexual function in impotent men with borderline serum testosterone levels.

Second-line therapies
Intraurethral therapies
Intrauretheral prostadil
Mechanism of action
Alprostadil is a stable, synthetic form of prostaglandin E_1 which causes an increase in cAMP levels and thereby promotes cavernosal smooth muscle relaxation.

Efficacy
Alprostadil, when applied into the urethra, has been shown to improve erectile function in approximately 43% of patients with organic impotence in placebo-controlled, double-blind clinical trials.[234–236] Use of a constriction device after application of transurethral alprostadil can increase the efficacy of this form of therapy.

Treatment regimen
Typically, the initial dose of 500 μg is applied in the doctor's office. The patient should be observed for clinical response and adverse effects such as decrease in blood pressure and local bleeding. The dose of alprostadil can be increased to 1000 μg per application or decreased to 250 μg, depending upon the clinical response and the adverse effects.

Potential complications of transurethral aprostadil
Common side-effects of transurethral alprostadil therapy are penile pain and urethral burning.[234–236] Urethral bleeding and priapism are unusual side-effects of transurethral aprostadil.

Relative merits and demerits of transurethral therapy
The major shortcomings of the transurethral alprostadil are its relatively low and inconsistent response rates and penile pain. The advantages include local application and low incidence of systemic complications.

Intracavernosal injection of vasoactive amines (Table 8.12)
Several formulations of alprostadil are commercially available (Caverject, Pharmacia and Upjohn; Prostin VR, Pharmacia and Upjohn; and Edex, Schwarz Pharma). In addition, a combination of phentolamine, papaverine and alprostadil is also available (Trimix).

Intracavernosal alprostadil

Mechanism of action
Alprostadil increases cAMP generation and thereby causes cavernosal smooth muscle relaxation.

Efficacy
Intracavernosal injections of alprostadil can result in successful erection in almost 75% of treated men. It is more effective than papaverine and phentolamine.

1. The patient should be instructed on how to inject the medication, and should be educated about the risks of this form of therapy.
2. Physicians who wish to prescribe intracavernosal injections must have contingency plans and a designated urologist to handle emergencies related to complications of intracavernosal injections, such as priapism.
3. It is advisable to administer the first injection in the physician's office and observe the blood pressure and heart rate response. This provides an excellent opportunity for educating the patient, observing adverse effects, and determining whether the patient will respond to this form of therapy.
4. The dose of the vasoactive substance should be adjusted to achieve an erection that is sufficient for sexual intercourse, but that does not last for more than 30 min.
5. The patient should be advised that priapism and fibrosis are potential complications of intracavernosal therapy.
6. After the injection, the patient should compress the injection site to minimize the risk of hematoma formation and subsequent fibrosis.
7. If the erection does not abate in 30 min, the patient should be instructed to take a tablet of pseudoephedrine or an intracavernosal injection of phenylephrine. If this is not effective, the patient should either call a designated urologist or come to the emergency room.
8. Intracavernosal therapy is not suitable for patients with psychiatric disorders, hypercoagulable states, or sickle cell disease, and for those who are receiving anticoagulant therapy.

Table 8.12
Checklist before administering intracavernosal therapy.

Regimens
The usual dose range is 5–20 μg. The first injection should be administered in the physician's office; this can help determine whether the patient will respond to this form of therapy. This can also be useful in educating the patient about the technique and potential adverse effects.

Potential side-effects
The common-side effects of intracavernosal alprostadil injections are painful erections, hyperalgesia, priapism and fibrosis. The incidence of priapism and fibrosis is lower than that observed with papaverine.

Relative merits and demerits
High rates of efficacy and low incidence of priapism are the main advantages of alprostadil over other forms of intracavernosal therapies. However, the need for intracavernosal injection, painful erections and the need for urological backup in the event of priapism are its relative drawbacks.

Papaverine

Mechanism of action
Papaverine is an antispasmodic agent and exerts its action as a non-selective phosphodiesterase inhibitor. As such, it would be expected to increase both cAMP and cGMP levels within the trabecular smooth muscle cell, resulting in an increase in penile blood inflow and cavernous artery diameter and cavernosal smooth muscle relaxation.

Efficacy
Intracavernous injection of vasoactive substances has been shown to be an effective treatment of organic erectile dysfunction in 50–80% of treated patients.

Dose regimen
The usual dose regimen is 15–60 mg.

Potential complications
Up to 50% of men discontinue this kind of therapy due to the inconvenience of injections, needle phobia and side-effects such as plaque or nodule formation, hematoma and infection. The incidence of priapism and corporal fibrosis (up to a third of treated men) is high.

Relative merits and demerits
Papaverine is not commercially available in the USA. A topical preparation of papaverine has been studied and is not as effective as intracavernosal injection.[14] High rates of priapism and fibrosis make it an unacceptable

choice in an internist's practice without adequate urological backup.

α-adrenergic receptor blockers
The sympathetic α-adrenergic receptors are thought to mediate and maintain corpus cavernosum tone in a detumescent state. All three subtypes of α-adrenergic receptors are expressed in human corpus cavernosum. Phentolamine, an α_1- and α_2-adrenergic antagonist, has been used alone and in combination with other agents for the treatment of erectile dysfunction.

Efficacy
When given alone, phentolamine is not very effective in producing rigid erections. However, in combination with papaverine, it is highly effective in producing successful erections in over 75% of treated men.

Dose regimen
One-half to one milligram of phentolamine is usually given in combination with 30 mg papaverine.

Potential complications
Major side-effects of phentolamine are hypotension and palpitations due to reflex tachycardia. When given in combination with papaverine, it can induce priapism and fibrosis.

Third-line therapies
Penile prosthesis
Insertion of penile prostheses should be limited to men who have failed other forms of therapy. The available prosthetic devices are of three types: inflatable, semirigid and malleable. The major complications of prosthetic devices include infections, erosions and the risk of mechanical failure. Penile prostheses have a finite lifespan and need replacement in 5–10 years. They produce an unnatural erection. Because of the concern about silicone implants, their use has decreased significantly in recent years. Migration of silicone particles to regional lymph nodes has been reported, although we do not know whether this migration has any adverse health consequences.

Newer therapeutic approaches under development
A number of novel selective phosphodiesterase inhibitors are under development. Milrinone is a selective type 3 phosphodiesterase inhibitor in human corpus cavernosum. Rolipram is a selective type 4 phosphodiesterase inhibitor.

Doxazocin, an α-adrenergic blocker, was evaluated for its potential in enhancing the effects of intracavernosal therapy; results showed limited efficacy. Chlorpromazine, deliquamine, moxysylate, prazosin and yohimbine have not been shown to be efficacious in large-scale, placebo-controlled, randomized clinical trials. Trazodone has been shown to cause priapism and induce erection when injected intracavernosally. Oral trazodone has been used to treat psychogenic erectile dysfunction.

Apomorphine, a dopamine receptor agonist, is known to induce erection when administered orally. Side-effects, including nausea and vomiting, may be unacceptable.

Endothelin is a potent vasoconstrictor and is synthesized by trabecular smooth muscle cells. Therefore, endothelin receptor antagonists may be useful in the treatment of erectile dysfunction. Most of the studies to date have been in animal models.

Infertility and subfertility in men

Infertility, defined as the inability of a couple to achieve pregnancy despite unprotected intercourse for a period of greater than 12 months, affects 10–15% of couples.[237–242] In a third of infertile couples, the primary problem resides in the male partner, in a third in the female partner, and in the remaining third in both the male and the female partner.[238–242]

Germ cell development in the testis

The process of spermatogenesis takes place in the seminiferous tubules of the testis, and is divided into three major stages[242] (Figure 8.7): spermatogonial replication, meiosis, and spermiogenesis. During the first stage, the spermatogonial stem cells divide mitotically several times to give rise to successive generations of spermatogonia, of which there are at least three main types in the human tubules, the dark type A, pale type A, and type B.[242] The type B spermatogonia proliferate to give rise to primary spermatocytes at the preleptotene stage of meiosis, in which DNA is actively synthesized. The second stage is the process of meiosis, which consists of two successive divisions of the spermatocyte accompanied by only one duplication of chromosomes. (Figure 8.7) At the completion of meiosis, four spermatids are produced, each containing a single, or haploid, set of

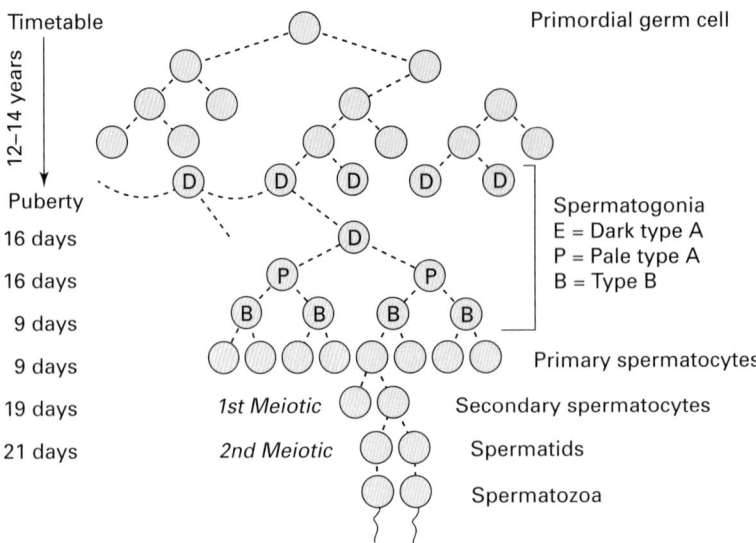

Figure 8.7
Stages of spermatogenesis in the human testis. After the migration of germ cells into the gonadal ridges is complete during embryogenesis, there are approximately 300 000 germ cells per gonad. The primordial germ cells differentiate and undergo mitotic divisions, so that at the time of puberty there are approximately 6 million germ cells in each testis. The germ cell development is arrested at the stage of spermatogonia dark type A. With sexual maturation, each spermatogonium differentiates and gives rise to 16 primary spermatocytes. Each primary spermatocyte enters meiosis and gives rise to four haploid spermatids. The spermatids are initially round and undergo a series of differentiation steps that include the reorganization of the nucleus and cytoplasm and development of a flagellum, resulting in the formation of spermatozoa. Each spermatogonium gives rise to 64 spermatozoa. (Adapted from Griffin JE, Wilson JD. In: Wilson JD, Foster DW, eds. Williams Textbook of Endocrinology, 8th edn. Philadelphia: Saunders, 1992: 810.

chromosomes. The final stage of spermatogenesis is called spermiogenesis, which involves a complex process of structural transformation and differentiation of the spermatid. During spermiogenesis, the chromatin of the spermatid condenses into a compact mass of dense granules, and the nucleus becomes invested by a membranous derivative of the Golgi apparatus, the acrosome, which contains enzymes that will digest a path for the sperm to penetrate the outer vestments of the egg. The cytoplasm elongates and surrounds the flagellum, which sprouts from a centriole. At the time of sperm formation, most of the cytoplasm is cast off in the form of a residual body. The spermatid completes its metamorphosis into a spermatozoon by forming a complex tail by the axonemal complex of two inner singlet and nine outer doublet microtubules. In man, the total duration of spermatogenesis is 74 days.[242]

Normal spermatogenesis requires complex interactions between germ cells and various somatic cells, such as Sertoli and Leydig cells, and the synergistic actions of the pituitary gonadotropins LH and FSH. LH, after binding to its G protein-coupled receptor, stimulates the production of testosterone by the Leydig cells; high intratesticular testosterone concentrations are essential for the initiation and maintenance of spermatogenesis within the testis. FSH initiates function in immature Sertoli cells by stimulating the formation of the blood–testis barrier and the secretion of a wide range of proteins and growth factors, such as androgen-binding protein, inhibin, activin, stem cell factor, plasminogen activator, transferrin, sulfated glycoproteins, and lactate.[243] Once spermatogenesis is established in the adult testis, Sertoli cells become less responsive to FSH.

Failure of spermatogenesis can result from impaired secretion or action of LH and FSH or from intrinsic defects in spermatogenesis within the testis. While a multitude of acquired causes can impair spermatogenesis, there is reason to believe that a genetic basis exists in a majority of infertile men. It is worth emphasizing that the molecular defects that result in infertility in a majority of infertile men remain unknown. Although the number of human genes known to be implicated in the pathophysiology of infertility is small, a significantly larger database exists for the mouse and *Drosophila*. For instance, 2400 *Drosophila* loci have been implicated in male sterility! It is certain that additional autosomal and X- and Y-specific candidate genes that are associated with defects of germ cell replication, meioisis or spermiogenesis will be discovered in man.

Pathogenesis of infertility

Common causes of infertility are listed in Table 8.13. Several large surveys of infertile men have been published.[237–242,244] Although differences exist in the frequency of various etiological factors in surveys from different centers, based in part on patient referral patterns, the nature and extent of investigation, and geography, these surveys are in agreement that subfertility and infertility in men form a heterogeneous group of disorders.[244] A specific cause of infertility is not determinable in most men. Most infertile men have idiopathic oligozoospermia or male factor infertility.

Of infertile men, 15–20% are azoospermic. An additional 10% have severe oligozoospermia (sperm density less than 1 million/ml). Correctable or treatable causes of infertility, such as gonadotropin deficiency and obstruction, are present in only a small number of men.

Although varicoceles are present in 10–30% of men with infertility, their role, if any, in the pathophysiology of male infertility remains controversial.

Diagnosis

History

In the diagnostic work-up of infertility, it is important to evaluate both the male and the female partner simultaneously (Figure 8.8).[245] The history should focus on duration of infertility, previous evidence of fertility in the man or the woman, contraceptive use, sexual function, and frequency and timing of intercourse in relation to the menstrual cycle. The inquiry should also be directed at ascertaining the timing of pubertal development, shaving frequency, hair loss, and hair distribution. A history of scrotal trauma, genitourinary infection, sexually transmitted disease, and scrotal or inguinal surgery may also be pertinent. Details of other medical problems such as erectile dysfunction, diabetes mellitus and autonomic neuropathy that might be associated with retrograde ejaculation should be obtained.

Physical examination

Physical examination should focus on determining whether patient has evidence of androgen deficiency. The measurements of body proportions (height to span and upper segment to lower segment ratio), voice

Diagnosis	Incidence (%)
Idiopathic infertility	60–80
Primary testicular failure (chromosomal disorders including Klinefelter's syndrome, undescended testis, irradiation, orchitis, drugs)	8–10
Genital tract obstruction (congenital absence of vas, vasectomy, epididymal obstruction)	5
Coital disorders	<1
Hypogonadotropic hypogonadism (pituitary adenomas, panhypopituitarism, idiopathic hypogonadotropic hypogonadism, hyperprolactinema)	3–4
Varicocele[a]	15–35
Other (sperm autoimmunity, drugs, toxins, systemic illness)	5

[a]Although the prevalence of varicocele in infertile men is higher than in the general population, it is not known whether the presence of varicocele causes or contributes to infertility. Adapted from Baker et al[4] with permission.

Table 8.13
Major etiologic diagnoses in infertile men.

HYPOGONADISM, ERECTILE DYSFUNCTION AND INFERTILITY IN MEN

(high pitched or not), hair distribution, including escutcheon, muscle mass and body habitus, and the absence or presence of gynecomastia can point to hypogonadism. Measurement of testicular volume by Prader orchidometer is an important part of the evaluation. The presence of cryptorchidism, varicocele or nodularity of vas deferens should be recorded. A digital rectal examination for assessment of prostate size should be performed.

Laboratory evaluation

An algorithm for the evaluation is provided in Figure 8.8. Initial evaluation should focus on assessment of general health and include a complete blood count, blood chemistries, and urinalysis.[245]

Semen analysis

Three or more semen samples should be obtained by masturbation after a 48-h abstinence period. Semen should be assessed for volume, sperm density and count, sperm motility, and sperm morphology.[246,247] According to the World Health Organization,[246,247] a normal semen specimen should have a volume of more than 2 ml, sperm density of greater than 20 million/ml, and a total sperm count of 40 million per ejaculate. More than 50% of sperm should show forward motility, and more than 30% of cells should have normal morphology.

The significance of leukocytes in the semen is not clear. The presence of leukocytes in the semen does not necessarily indicate accessory gland infection.

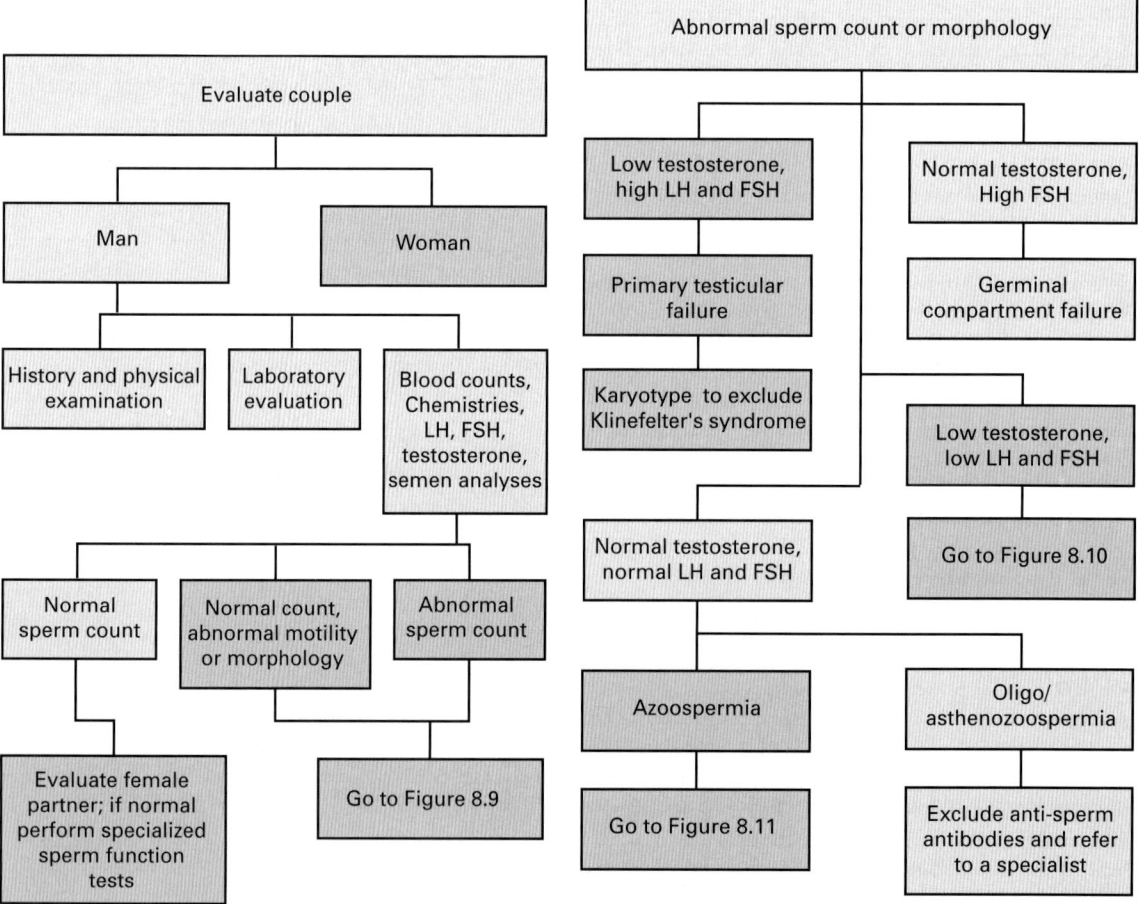

Figure 8.8
Evaluation of an infertile couple.

Figure 8.9
Evaluation of an infertile man with abnormal sperm count and morphology.

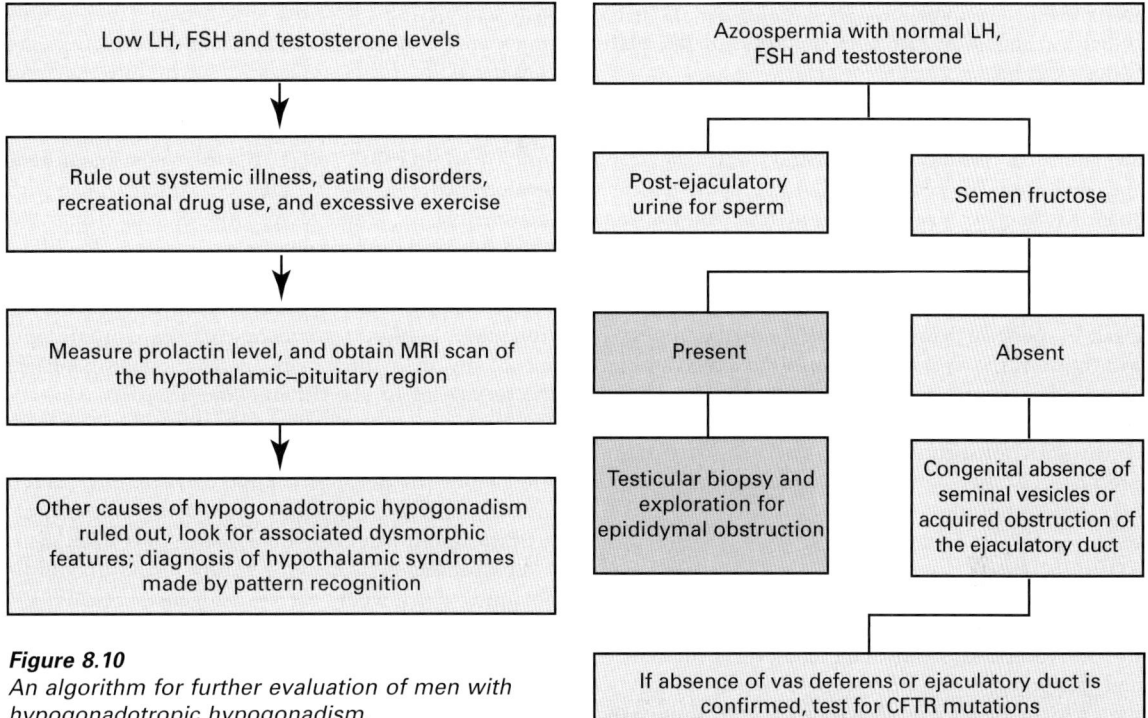

Figure 8.10
An algorithm for further evaluation of men with hypogonadotropic hypogonadism.

Figure 8.11
Evaluation of azoospermic men with normal LH, FSH and testosterone levels. CFTR, cystic fibrosis transmembrane conductance regulator.

Hormonal evaluation

Measurement of testosterone, LH and FSH can help in the diagnosis of hypogonadism and determine whether hypogonadism is hypogonadotropic or hypergonadotropic[245] (Figures 8.9–8.11).

High LH and FSH levels in the presence of low testosterone concentrations suggest primary testicular failure. In these men, a karyotype should be performed to exclude the presence of Klinefelter's syndrome (47,XXY) or its variants. A normal karyotype, however, does not exclude the possibility of mosaicism (46,XY/47,XXY).

Elevated testosterone and elevated LH levels in a man who appears hypogonadal suggest androgen insensitivity. Analysis of skin fibroblasts for androgen binding or analysis of peripheral lymphocyte DNA can help to confirm mutations in androgen receptor or 5-α-reductase genes. An isolated increase in serum FSH levels with normal LH and testosterone levels suggests failure of the germ cell compartment.

If the patient has hypogonadotropic hypogonadism, a history of eating disorders, excessive exercise, and systemic illness should be looked for (Figure 8.10). Serum prolactin levels should be measured, and an MRI scan of the hypothalamic–pituitary region should be obtained to exclude a space-occupying lesion. In older men with mild hypogonadotropic hypogonadism, the search for additional causes of hypogonadotropism is often unrewarding, and the cost-effectiveness of extensive pituitary evaluation has not been established. Older men with severe hypogonadotropic hypogonadism with serum testosterone levels less than 150 ng/dl (5.2 nmol/l) should be evaluated for the presence of a pituitary pathology by obtaining prolactin measurements and an MRI scan.

Men with azoospermia and normal LH and testosterone levels may have an obstructive lesion, such as congenital absence of vas or epididymis or an acquired obstruction (Figure 8.11). In such patients, post-ejaculatory urine should be checked to exclude retrograde ejaculation, and seminal fructose should be measured. Very low fructose concentrations suggest the absence of seminal vesicles or obstruction. In such patients, exploration and testicular biopsy should be performed to rule out obstruction or germ cell failure. If absence of vas deferens or seminal vesicles is confirmed, then the individual should be tested for mutations in the cystic fibrosis conductance regulator gene.

In men who have normal hormone levels and low or normal sperm count, specialized sperm function tests are indicated. Various sperm function tests, including the cervical mucus penetration test, acrosome reaction, zona-free hamster egg penetration test, human zona pellucida binding test, and specialized sperm biochemistry, are used in specialized andrology laboratories. The clinical utility of the acrosome reaction is not clear. A positive hamster oocyte penetration test is indicative of the ability of sperm to undergo capacitation and acrosome reaction, and penetrate and fuse with the hamster egg. This reaction has good concordance with fertilization in an in vitro fertilization procedure. It has, however, a significant number of false-negative results.

Testicular biopsy

Although testicular biopsy can provide information about the spermatogenic defect, there are very few instances where this procedure alters the management and prognosis. For instance, testicular biopsy is indicated in an infertile man who is azoospermic, and has normal testosterone and LH concentrations. This individual should undergo further work-up to exclude the presence of obstruction, including examination of post-ejaculatory urine for sperm and seminal fructose. If seminal fructose is present, testicular biopsy and exploration should be performed to rule out obstruction and establish the presence of spermatogenesis in the testis. Testicular biopsy has also been used to retrieve sperm or spermatids for intracytoplasmic sperm injection in men with azoospermia in whom sperm cannot be obtained from the semen. Fertility has been achieved by intracytoplasmic injection of sperm obtained from testicular biopsy in men with azoospermia associated with Klinefelter's syndrome or other causes.

Computer-aided sperm analysis

Many computer-aided sperm analysis systems are commercially available. These systems are convenient, but offer no real advantage over manual methods for assessment of sperm morphology. These automated systems are susceptible to error in the estimation of sperm concentration.

Genetic testing

Because genetic disorders account for a significant fraction of infertile men, genetic testing of the infertile man and of the offspring will become increasingly important, especially in those couples who are being considered for intracytoplasmic sperm injection. For instance, infertile men with congenital absence of vas deferens or seminal vesicles should be screened for mutations in the cystic fibrosis transmembrane conductance regulator (CFTR) gene. Infertile men with azoospermia or severe oligozoospermia in whom the cause of infertility cannot be ascertained should be screened for Y chromosome microdeletions. Offspring born through the use of intracytoplasmic sperm injection have a higher frequency of sex chromosome aneuploidy than the general population; in addition, the prevalence of sex chromosome disorders is 6–10-fold higher among infertile men, especially those with azoospermia. This has led some to conclude that infertile men with non-obstructive azoospermia should undergo karyotype analysis. Men with post-meiotic germ cell arrest may have mutations in the *CREM* gene.

In all instances, a detailed family history should be obtained, which would then guide genetic testing.

Genetic disorders associated with infertility in man (Table 8.14)

Genetic disorders associated with impaired gonadotropin secretion or action

These disorders were discussed earlier. This section will focus only on the genetic disorders of germ cell development.

Primary defects of spermatogenesis
Sex chromosome disorders

Approximately 5% of infertile men carry chromosome abnormalities; of these, a majority involve sex chromosomes (4% on average), and 1% involve the autosomes.[248–251] The prevalence of sex chromosomal and autosomal abnormalities in infertile men is 15 and 6 times higher respectively than in the general population.[252,253]

Klinefelter's syndrome

Klinefelter's syndrome is the most common chromosomal disorder associated with male infertility and is found in 1:500 to 1:1000 live-born males.[252,253] The most frequent karyotype in men with Klinefelter's syndrome is 47,XXY (93%), but 46,XY/47,XXY, 48,XXXY, 48,XXYY and 49,XXXXY karyotypes have also been reported.[24,254,255]

The XXY chromosomal constitution has been described in other mammals such as mouse, Chinese hamster, cat, dog, sheep, ox, and pig, and is associated with sterility. The testes of 47,XXY animals are devoid of germ cells.[24,255]

Azoospermia is the rule in men with Klinefelter's syndrome who have the 47,XXY karyotype. Men with mosaicism may have germ cells in their testes, especially at a younger age.

Testicular histology in men with Klinefelter's

Genetic or chromosomal disorder	Genotype	Hormonal profile	Histology	Semen
Klinefelter's syndrome	47,XXY, 46,XY/47,XXY	Low or low normal testosterone, increased LH and FSH	Hyalinization of seminiferous tubules, absence of germ cells, normal or hyperplastic Leydig cells	Azoospermia
Y chromosome microdeletions	46,XY, microdeletions of AZFa, AZFb, AZFc, AZFd regions	Usually normal or low normal testosterone, normal LH, and normal or increased FSH	Variable. Some men may have Sertoli cell-only phenotype, others have germ cell arrest	Azoospermia or severe oligozoospermia
Bilateral congenital absence of vas deferens	Mutations of the CFTR gene	Usually normal testosterone, LH and FSH	Testicular histology tends to be normal, but patients have obstructive azoospermia	Azoospermia. May or may not have clinical features of cystic fibrosis
CREM mutations	Mutations of the CREM gene	Normal testosterone and LH, normal or elevated FSH	Germ cell arrest at the spermatid stage early in spermiogenesis	Azoospermia
Thalessemia	Mutations of one or more β-globin gene/s	Typically, have hypogonadotropic hypogonadism with low testosterone, and low LH and FSH; occasionally primary testicular failure may also occur		Azoospermic, depending on degree of gonadotropin deficiency
Sickle cell disease	Mutations of the globin gene	May have primary testicular failure due to testicular infarcts resulting in low testosterone and high LH and FSH. Some patients may have iron overload and hypogonadotropic hypogonadism	Testicular infarcts	May have oligozoospermia, depending on the severity of the disease and the degree of LH and FSH deficiency

Table 8.14
Relatively common chromosomal and genetic disorders in infertile men in which genetic testing is possible.

syndrome shows hyalinization of seminiferous tubules and absence of spermatogenesis.[23,24] Patients with mosaicism may have normal-sized testes and spermatogenesis at puberty. However, progressive degeneration and hyalinization of seminiferous tubules takes place after puberty. In some men, the tubular dysgenesis is patchy; degenerating tubules are interspersed with apparently normal tubules. The Leydig cells appear to be increased, although their function is impaired.

The 47,XXY karyotype in patients with Klinefelter's syndrome results from non-dysjunction during the first meiotic division in one of the parents. Non-dysjunction of maternal chromosomes is the cause of the 47,XXY karyotype in two-thirds of affected men. Advanced maternal age is a risk factor for non-dysjunction. The mechanism by which an extra X chromosome renders patients infertile is not known. In male germ cells, inactivation of the single X chromosome in primary spermatocytes of heterogametic males is necessary for spermatogenesis to proceed through meiosis. The necessity for X inactivation in male germ cell differentiation in heterogametic species is not clearly understood; however, inactivation of the single X may be necessary for normal sex chromosome pairing or to prevent expression of some X-linked genes that are detrimental to spermatogenesis.

Noonan's syndrome, the male Turner's syndrome
These patients have 46,XY karyotype, male external genitalia, and clinical stigmata of Turner's syndrome.[256] The testis size is reduced, and the Leydig cell function is impaired. Sterility and cryptorchidism are common.

XYY syndrome
There is a higher frequency of the 47,XYY karyotype in men with tall stature and nodular cystic acne, among prisoners and among mental hospital patients.[257] The mean intelligence quotient and educational level are lower in 47,XYY individuals than healthy controls.

Mixed gonadal dysgenesis (45,X/46,XY)
The patients with mixed gonadal dysgenesis usually have a 45,X/46,XY karyotype, and a testis on one side and a streak gonad on the other.[258] Some degree of ambiguity in the genitalia is usual. The phenotypic males with mixed gonadal dysgenesis often have abdominal testes with normal Leydig cells but without any germ cells.[258] The dysgenetic gonad is at high risk for neoplastic degeneration.

XX males
These patients have a male phenotype and normal-looking testes, but are azoospermic and have high LH and FSH levels.[259,260] The portion of the Y chromosome that contains the Sry may be translocated onto the X chromosome or an autosome; a few patients may be mosaics and carry some 46,XY cell lines. However, because they lack other Y-specific genes required for spermatogenesis, they are sterile.

The Y chromosome microdeletion syndrome
Large deletions of the Y chromosome that can be seen under the microscope in late prophase and hence are detectable on routine karyotype are uncommon in infertile men. However, submicroscopic deletions of the long arm of the Y chromosome, which are not detectable on karyotype and hence are called microdeletions, are present in 5–10% of azoospermic men.[261–273] These microdeletions can be detected by PCR-based sequence-tagged site mapping or by Southern hybridization. The initial studies had focused on infertile men with severe defects of spermatogenesis, i.e. those with azoospermia. However, more recent studies have shown that Y deletions are also present in oligozoospermic men.[274,275] (Bhasin, Ma, Mallidis, and De Kretser, unpublished data). Most infertile men with Y deletions have severe defects of spermatogenesis, i.e. they have either azoospermia or severe oligozoospermia.[276–278] Although the total number of infertile men with Y deletions that have been studied in detail is small, most of these patients have had testicular volumes of less than 15 ml and elevated FSH levels. The testicular histologies in the small number of reported cases of Y deletions have revealed either Sertoli cell only or germ cell arrest phenotypes. The limited number of patients in whom testicular histology has been examined has not allowed a correlation between the location and size of the deletion and the histological phenotype. However, Vogt et al[279] have reported that three loci can be identified in Yq, termed AZFa, AZFb, and AZFc, wherein deletions are associated with specific testicular histopathology.

Two Y-specific candidate gene families have been cloned by deletion mapping of infertile men with Yq deletions and proposed as candidates for the putative AZF locus, the *RBM* (RNA binding motif containing) gene family,[274,280] and the *DAZ* (deleted in azoospermia) gene family.[277,281–283] Both are multiple-copy gene families[283,284] that contain the RNA binding motif. The *RBM* gene family has more than

30 copies spread throughout the Y chromosome, most of the copies being located in deletion intervals 6A and 6B. At least two members of the *RBM* gene family, *RBM-1* and *RBM-2*, are expressed in the testis.[284] The presence of the RNA-binding motif in the predicted protein sequence suggests that these genes play a role in RNA processing; however, the precise role of the RBM protein/s in germ cell development remains unclear.

The *DAZ* gene family is also a multiple-copy gene family.[283] The mouse and *Drosophila* homologs of *DAZ* have been mapped to chromosomes 17 and 3, respectively.[281,285] An autosomal homolog of *DAZ* has also been identified in the human and mapped to chromosome 3.[261,286] The homologs of the autosomal *DAZ*-like gene, *DAZL1*, are present in all mammalian species; *DAZ* homologs are present only on the Y chromosomes of great apes and Old World monkeys. Mutations of the *DAZL1* gene in *Drosophila*, *boule*, are associated with meiotic arrest and azoospermia.[281] Similarly, *DAZL1* mutations in knockout mice are associated with sterility, providing further evidence for the role of this gene product in germ cell development.[262]

In infertile men with *DAZ* deletions, both meiotic arrest and Sertoli cell only phenotypes have been described; it is possible that germ cell degeneration may occur secondarily.

The precise physiological function and role of the *RBM* and *DAZ* gene families in human spermatogenesis remain unclear. The RNA molecules that are the targets of these RNA-binding proteins have not been identified. Using DAZ as bait in a two-hybrid system, Tsui et al[287] identified two novel proteins, *DAZ*-associated proteins (DAZAP) 1 and 2, that interact with *DAZ* and *DAZL1*. The *DAZAP* genes have been mapped to chromosomal regions 19p13.3, and 2q33–q34.

Although deletions involving the *DAZ* genes appear to be the most frequent, a large proportion of Y deletions are outside the *DAZ* region; some of these involve the *RBM* gene. Additional candidate gene families, including *BPY2*, *CDY1*, *PRY*, and *TTY2*, have been identified in the AZFc region of the Y chromosome.[263] The role of these additional Y-specific gene families in germ cell development and infertility is not understood. It is also not clear how deletions of one or two copies of the *RBM* or *DAZ* genes could explain infertility when there are multiple copies of these genes elsewhere on the Y chromosome. A significant proportion of infertile men with *DAZ* deletions are oligozoospermic and not azoospermic. Furthermore, only 5–10% of infertile men have Y deletions. These data suggest that additional Y-specific and autosomal genes may be involved in other infertility phenotypes.[263]

The length of the polyglutamine tract in the androgen receptor protein and infertility[264–267]

The length of the CAG trinucleotide repeat in exon 1 of the androgen receptor gene that encodes for the polyglutamine tract in the androgen receptor protein is polymorphic in humans.[264–267] In vitro studies have demonstrated that the transactivational activity of the androgen receptor protein is related inversely to the length of the polyglutamine tract. Individuals with very long tracts have spinobulbal muscular atrophy (Kennedy's disease), a degenerative disease of the spinal cord neurons. However, several reports indicate that men with idiopathic oligozoospermia have a higher likelihood of having longer polyglutamine tracts than fertile men.[264–266] For instance, in one study of 153 infertile men and 72 healthy controls, Yong et al[266] reported that 20% of infertile men have reduced androgenicity because of long CAG repeat length in exon 1 of the androgen receptor gene. These authors have proposed that long polyglutamine tracts are associated with increased risk of infertility and reduced risk of prostate cancer. Conversely, these authors assert that short polyglutamine tracts are associated with increased transactivational activity, increased risk of prostate cancer and reduced risk for infertility. Dadze et al,[267] on the other hand, found no relationship between the CAG repeat length and impaired spermatogenesis in a sample of infertile men of German origin. Therefore, the validity of this hypothesis remains to be verified.

Autosomal gene defects and male infertility
Cyclic adenosine 3´,5´-monophosphate-response element modulator gene expression and spermatogenic arrest[268–272]

The cyclic AMP-response element modulator gene codes for a transcription factor that is expressed in post-meiotic germ cells and is important for physiological regulation of the balance between differentiation and apoptosis during normal germ cell development.[268–272] Mice that are null for CREM protein are sterile and reveal spermatogenic arrest at the first step of spermiogenesis.[272] Late spermatids are absent, and there is an increase in the number of apoptotic germ cells in the seminiferous tubules of *CREM*-mutant mice.[272] Normal spermatogenesis in fertile men is characterized by a switch from CREM repressors to CREM activator isoforms in post-meiotic germ cells. In situ hybridization studies on testicular biopsies obtained from infertile men with germ cell arrest have demonstrated the absence of activator isoforms of CREM in postmeiotic germ cells and increased apoptosis.[268–271] These data suggest that germ cell arrest could result from failure of this normal transition from repressor to activator isoforms of CREM in the seminiferous tubule.

Bilateral congenital absence of vas deferens and the CFTR mutations
Mutations in the coding region of the *CFTR* gene may result in congenital absence of vas without causing the classical pulmonary disease.[273] Fifty to seventy per cent of men with congenital absence of the vas deferens harbor mutations of the *CFTR* gene. About 50% are homozygous for the common cystic fibrosis gene abnormality such as F508, and some have compound heterozygosity.

Gonadal dysfunction associated with sickle cell disease and thalessemia
A significant proportion of men with sickle cell disease have low testosterone levels. The majority of men with sickle cell disease and low testosterone levels suffer from primary testicular dysfunction.[288] It is assumed that testicular dysfunction results from microinfarcts in the testis because of the vaso-occlusive disease. However, hypogonadotropic hypogonadism due to hypothalamic–pituitary dysfunction has also been reported in men with sickle cell disease.

The pituitary and gonadal dysfunction occurs in thalessemia due to iron deposition in these tissues.[289] Hypogonadotropic hypogonadism is the predominant form of androgen deficiency syndrome in men with thalessemia and can be treated effectively with gonadotropin replacement therapy. Pituitary and testicular overload and the resulting hypogonadism can be prevented by prophylactic iron-chelating therapy.

Testicular dysfunction in myotonic dystrophy
Myotonic dystrophy is an autosomal dominant disorder associated with CTG repeats in the dystrophin gene. Testicular atrophy occurs in 75% of these men, primarily due to degeneration of the seminiferous tubules. Although Leydig cells are preserved, serum testosterone levels are low in many patients due to primary testicular failure.[290]

Subfertility associated with diabetes
Men with diabetes mellitus may experience infertility if they have retrograde ejaculation due to autonomic neuropathy or if they have poor glycemic control. Impotence is common in men who have had diabetes for more than 10 years.

Treatment

The role of the internist in the management of the infertile couple
The internist can play an important role in the treatment of infertile men by initiating a rational diagnostic evaluation and referring those who require more specialized care.[291] The internist should focus on ascertaining a specific treatable cause of infertility, even though specific treatment modalities may be applicable to only a fraction of infertile men. In this regard, it is particularly important to identify and treat gonadotropin deficiency, because hormone replacement therapy in this disorder is highly effective. Similarly, it is also useful to quickly ascertain whether the patient has untreatable sterility, in which case the couple should be appropriately counseled about adoption or artificial insemination with donor sperm. One of the most useful roles that an internist can play is to present to the couple a realistic prognosis, the pros and cons of different treatment options, and estimates of costs, and guide the couple away from interventions that have not been shown to be effective (Table 8.15).

Gonadotropin treatment of men with hypogonadotropic hypogonadism
Preparations
Human chorionic gonadotropin (hCG) and human menopausal gonadotropin (hMG) preparations have been commercially available for over three decades.[292–296] hCG is purified from the urine of pregnant women, being secreted primarily by the human placenta during pregnancy. hMG is derived from the urine of postmenopausal women. While hCG primarily stimulates Leydig cell testosterone production by interacting with LH/hCG receptors, hMG contains LH and FSH activities in almost equal proportions.

> Clomiphene and anti-estrogens
> Varicocelectomy
> LH and FSH
> Testosterone rebound
> Antibiotics
> Vitamins and minerals
> Artificial insemination by husband's sperm
> Low-dose glucocorticoid therapy
>
> Adapted from Burger and Baker[1] with permission.

Table 8.15
Treatment modalities whose beneficial effects have not been demonstrated in male factor infertility.

Highly purified preparations of hLH and hFSH, derived from human cadaver pituitaries, had become available for research studies from the National Pituitary Agency of the NIDDK. However, occurrence of a slow virus degenerative disease (Creutzfeldt–Jakob disease) in a few patients treated with earlier preparations of human GH[287] led to the withdrawal and cessation of the use of all human pituitary hormones for therapeutic purposes. A highly purified hFSH preparation is commercially available and is being used extensively in gynecological applications.[297] Recombinant LH is not commercially available at this time, but recombinant hFSH, expressed in Chinese hamster ovary cell lines and purified to homogeneity, is now available and has received recent FDA approval for induction of spermatogenesis in men with idiopathic hypogonadotropic hypogonadism.[298–300] The mature β subunit of rhFSH has seven fewer amino acids than reported in the literature, but has similar oligosaccharide structures as purified urinary hFSH preparation.[298] Recombinant hFSH is also indistinguishable from purified urinary hFSH in its biological activity in vitro and in vivo. rhFSH is available in ampoules containing 75 IU (approximately 7.5 μg FSH), which accounts for >99% of protein content. The pharmacokinetics of urinary hFSH and recombinant hFSH are similar.

Biological effects of gonadotropin therapy

Pharmacological doses of hCG, when administered to normal men, lead to biphasic testosterone and estradiol responses.[301–304] When 1500–6000 units of hCG are given intramuscularly to normal adult men, an initial peak in serum testosterone levels can be observed 2 h after the injection, followed by a second larger and more sustained peak at 72–96 h. Serum testosterone levels may remain elevated for as long as 6 days after a single hCG injection. Serum estradiol levels also exhibit a similar biphasic response. It should be noted that the biphasic testosterone and estradiol responses are characteristic only of the postpubertal, normally virilized men.[301–306] In prepubertal boys or hypogonadotropic men, not previously primed with gonadotropins, only a monophasic increase in serum testosterone, peaking 72–96 h after hCG injection, can be seen, and there is significant latency before testosterone levels begin to rise. Smals et al[301] have suggested that an early testosterone response in normally virilized postpubertal men results from testosterone release from a readily releasable pool of preformed hormone and/or rapid induction of mature enzymatic machinery. Wang et al[304] demonstrated that hypogonadotropic men, previously primed with hCG treatment, also exhibit a biphasic testosterone response to LH infusion, consistent with the proposal that maturation of the biphasic adult pattern is a function of prior gonadotropin priming of the testis.

Multiple injections of pharmacological doses of hCG lead to diminished testosterone response to subsequent hCG injections, a phenomenon referred to as desensitization.[301–303] Desensitization to hCG can be seen under several different clinical and experimental circumstances: first, multiple daily hCG injections do not result in higher serum testosterone levels than single daily injections; second, men with hCG-secreting neoplasia do not usually have elevated serum testosterone levels.[301]

It has long been known that in prepubertal males, hCG, given alone, widens the seminiferous tubules and increases the number of primary spermatocytes.[309,310] However, spermatogenesis does not progress to completion, and germ cell development remains arrested. Addition of hMG to patients on hCG results in an increase in testis size, progression of germ cell development, completion of spermiogenesis, and appearance of sperm in the ejaculate.

Therapeutic aspects

The two best predictors of success of gonadotropin therapy in hypogonadotropic men are testicular volume at presentation and the time of onset of hypogonadotropism (prepubertally or postpubertally).

In general, the larger the testis size, the greater the likelihood of success; best responses are seen in men with initial testicular volume greater than 8 ml.[80,311] Similarly, patients who became hypogonadotropic after puberty (e.g. because of a pituitary tumor, surgery, or irradiation) experience higher overall success rates than those who have never undergone pubertal changes.[80,311] The presence of a coincidental or associated primary testicular abnormality will, of course, attenuate the testicular response to gonadotropin therapy. Some patients with IHH may also have cryptorchidism; earlier studies[312,313] indicated that these patients did not respond well to hCG therapy, leading to an erroneous speculation that there may be dual defects in IHH, the first hypothalamic and the second testicular.

Although a variety of treatment regimens are being used, there is no consensus on what constitutes the optimum dose and schedule of gonadotropin administration. Published data and empirical clinical experience indicate that a reasonable starting dose is 1000–1500 IU[80,311–313] given intramuscularly three times weekly. Serum testosterone levels should be measured 6–8 weeks later, 48–72 h after the hCG injection, in order to adjust and optimize the regimen. The goal should be to adjust the dose to achieve serum testosterone levels in the mid-normal range. Sperm counts should be monitored on a monthly basis. It may take several[80,311–313] months for spermatogenesis to be restored, and patients often get very impatient and prematurely disappointed. Therefore, it is very important to forewarn patients about the potential length and expense of the treatment, and to provide conservative estimates of success rates.

If, after 6 months of therapy with hCG alone, serum testosterone levels are in the mid-normal range but the sperm concentrations are low, it is time to add FSH. This can be done by using hMG, highly purified FSH, or recombinant FSH. The selection of FSH dose is empirical. A common practice is to start with the addition of a $\frac{1}{2}$–1 ampoule of hMG (1 ampoule = 75 IU LH plus 75 IU FSH) three times each week in conjunction with the hCG injections. If, after 3 months of combined treatment, sperm densities are still low, the dose of hMG should be increased to one or two ampoules. It may occasionally take 18–24 months or longer for spermatogenesis to be restored.

The therapy is expensive but is otherwise well tolerated. Development of antibodies to hCG is not a common event.[314–317] Braunstein et al[314] found no evidence of antibodies in 41 people treated with hCG for weight reduction. Another study found antibodies in less than 1% of men treated with short courses of hCG.[315] There are only a handful of case reports of treatment failure due to development of anti-hCG antibodies.[314–317]

In men with postpubertal onset of hypogonadotropism, spermatogenesis can usually be reinitiated by hCG alone, and the success rates are high.[80] On the other hand, men in whom hypogonadotropic hypogonadism developed prior to completion of the pubertal maturation usually do not respond to hCG alone, but require combined treatment with hCG and hMG for longer duration, and the overall success rates are lower. Prior androgen therapy appears not to affect subsequent responsiveness to gonadotropin therapy.[318]

The degree of gonadotropin deficiency, as reflected by the pretreatment testicular volume, is an important determinant of the response to gonadotropin therapy. In general, men with testicular volumes greater than 8 ml have higher response rates than those with testicular volumes less than 4 ml.[311]

An open-label clinical trial by the Spanish Collaborative Group on Male Hypogonadotropic Hypogonadism[297] evaluated the efficacy of self-administered highly purified hFSH (150 IU three times a week) and hCG (2500 IU twice a week) in men with idiopathic hypogonadotropic hypogonadism. Serum testosterone concentrations normalized in all but one patient. Testicular volume increased three-fold during treatment, and 80% of men who were initially azoospermic achieved a positive sperm count. The maximum sperm density during treatment was 25 ± 8 million/ml. Three men developed gynecomastia.

Pulsatile GnRH therapy

Pioneering studies by Knobil's group[319–321] had predicted that pulsatile administration of GnRH would be required to maintain normal LH and FSH output from the pituitary. Continuous infusion of GnRH in monkeys, made hypogonadotropic by radiofrequency lesions of the hypothalamic GnRH-secreting nuclei, downregulates LH and FSH secretion.

Synthetic GnRH is commercially available for therapy of patients with hypogonadotropism due to GnRH deficiency.[322] However, success of GnRH therapy assumes normal pituitary and gonadal function. The agonist analogs of GnRH are not useful for restoring gonadotropin secretion, because after an initial short-lived stimulatory phase, GnRH agonists downregulate pituitary LH and FSH output.[323–325]

A large number of clinical studies utilizing GnRH in a variety of treatment regimens have demonstrated successful induction of puberty by pulsatile administration of low doses of GnRH. Therapy is usually started with an initial dose of 25 ng/kg per pulse, administered subcutaneously every 2 h by a portable infusion pump.[305,306,311–313,326] Serum testosterone, LH and FSH levels need to be monitored. The dose of GnRH may need to be increased until serum testosterone levels in the mid-normal range are reached. There is considerable variability in GnRH dose requirement among different subjects, and doses ranging from 25 to 200 ng/kg may be required to induce virilization.[305] Once pubertal changes have been initiated, the dose of GnRH can be reduced without any adverse effects on serum testosterone, LH and FSH levels.

The gonadotropin secretion and gonadal function can be maintained for extended periods of time (months to years) in a majority of carefully selected patients with IHH by pulsatile GnRH therapy.[305,306,326] Development of anti-GnRH antibodies is an uncommon occurrence, but can be a cause of treatment failure. Increase in sperm counts and testicular volume have been reported in over 70% of treated men, and improvements in sexual function and virilization can be induced in over 90% of subjects. Some of the patients with IHH have associated cryptorchidism, and these men might have an additional testicular defect. Local cutaneous infections do occur but are infrequent and minor. While induction of virilization by pulsatile GnRH administration in patients with IHH has provided important insights into the mechanisms of puberty and regulation of gonadotropin secretion by GnRH, this approach has no particular advantage over the traditional gonadotropin therapy.[312,313] Carrying a portable infusion device can be cumbersome, and follow-up of these patients often requires considerable physician supervision and laboratory monitoring.

Liu et al[311] compared an hCG/hMG regimen with pulsatile GnRH therapy in its efficacy in inducing spermatogenesis. After 2 years of therapy, 40% of GnRH-treated men and 80% of the hCG/hMG-treated men produced sperm. The sperm concentrations in all men were below 5×10^6/ml and were comparable in the two groups.

In another retrospective review,[312,313] hCG/hMG and pulsatile GnRH therapy were found to be equally effective in inducing spermatogenesis. Spermatogenesis was induced in 54 of 57 courses of therapy, and pregnancies occurred in 26 of 36 courses. The two therapies did not significantly differ in terms of the time to first appearance of sperm or pregnancy rates. These and other data[311–313] demonstrate that both pulsatile GnRH therapy and traditional gonadotropin replacement therapy are equally effective in inducing spermatogenesis in men with IHH.

Treatment options for patients with azoospermia

The presence of azoospermia, total teratozoospermia and primary testicular failure with azoospermia indicates a poor prognosis.[307] In these instances, adoption or artificial insemination using donor sperm are reasonable options.[237,307]

With the advent of intracytoplasmic sperm injection, the prognosis for these men has improved. There are several case reports of successful pregnancies in partners of men with Klinefelter's syndrome using intracytoplasmic injection of the sperm retrieved from testicular biopsy into the oocyte.[308,327,328] Palermo et al[327] have reported high success rates with the use of intracytoplasmic sperm injection using spermatozoa surgically retrieved from azoospermic men. These investigators report clinical pregnancy rates of 49% for non-obstructive cases, and 57% for testicular spermatozoa obtained from men with obstructive azoospermia.[327] Success rates vary considerably among centers, depending upon patient selection and experience with the procedure.

Couples who are undergoing intracytoplasmic sperm injection using testicular spermatozoa should be counseled about the risk of sex chromosome aneuploidy and other genetic disorders being transmitted to the offspring through intracytoplasmic sperm injection. Also, it is best to present a realistic prognosis and dampen expectations at the very outset.

Should varicoceles be treated surgically or left alone in infertile men?

Varicoceles are present in 10–30% of infertile men; however, they are also common in men of known fertility.[329] Therefore, the role of varicoceles in the pathophysiology of male infertility remains unclear.[329–334] Although many uncontrolled studies have reported improvements in sperm density and sperm motility after varicocele resection, these data are difficult to interpret because of the lack of appropriate control groups. Most varicocele studies have lacked scientific rigor and are uninterpretable. Only a few controlled clinical trials have been performed, and these trials have failed to show significantly greater improvements in fertility after surgical resection of varicocele than after counseling alone.[331] Therefore, there are insufficient data to support a recommendation for surgical resection of varicoceles in most infertile men.

The expert opinion among urologists favors surgical correction of varicoceles in adolescent boys; the rationale is that there is catch-up growth of the testes after varicocelectomy which might not occur without the surgical correction. However, prospective data from controlled clinical trials are lacking.

Intracytoplasmic sperm injection for male factor infertility

Intracytoplasmic sperm injection (ICSI), first used successfully in 1992 for the treatment of infertility, has become a widely used treatment modality worldwide.[335] Tens of thousands of infertile couples have undergone this procedure since then, at hundreds of centers around the world.[291,335–337] A recent survey convened by the European Society of Human Reproduction and Embryology[335] has reported that the fertilization rates obtained with ejaculated, epididymal, and testicular spermatozoa for 1995 were 64%, 62% and 52%, respectively. Eighty to ninety per cent of couples had embryo transfer, and the viable pregnancy rates were 21% for ejaculated, 22% for epididymal, and 19% for testicular sperm. The incidence of multiple gestation was 30–40%. The pregnancy rates were similar for obstructive and non-obstructive azoospermia.[335]

There has been considerable concern about the possibility of transmitting genetic disorders from the parents to the offspring born through the use of ICSI. Reassuringly, the perinatal outcome of children born after ICSI was not significantly different from that after in vitro fertilization or natural conception.[290,335–337] A small increase in frequency of congenital malformations has been explained on the basis of the higher prevalence of multiple births. When multiplicity is taken into account, the incidence of major or minor malformations is not increased.[291,335–337] There is, however, a small but significant increase in the frequency of chromosome aneuploidy, especially sex chromosome aneuploidy, among the offspring of ICSI. The data from the Swedish Medical Birth Registry[291,338] have also demonstrated an increase in relative risk of hypospadias. Long-term data on the mental and physical wellbeing of children born through the use of ICSI are not available.

Therefore, a large body of carefully collected data indicates that ICSI is a safe treatment modality that can be effective in many cases of male factor infertility.[338] However, ICSI is an expensive and complicated procedure. The couples should undergo extensive counseling before they are referred for ICSI. They should also be advised to undergo genetic counseling and testing.

References

1. Finkelstein JS, Klibanski A, Neer RM, Greenspan SL, Rosenthal DI, Crowley WF, Jr. Osteoporosis in men with idiopathic hypogonadotropic hypogonadism. *Ann Intern Med* 1987; 106(3): 354–61.
2. Katznelson L, Finkelstein JS, Schoenfeld DA, Rosenthal DI, Anderson EJ, Klibanski A. Increase in bone density and lean body mass during testosterone administration in men with acquired hypogonadism. *J Clin Endocrinol Metab* 1996; 81(12): 4358–65.
3. Stepan JJ, Lachman M, Zverina J, Pacovsky V, Baylink DJ. Castrated men exhibit bone loss: effect of calcitonin treatment on biochemical indices of bone remodeling. *J Clin Endocrinol Metab* 1989; 69(3): 523–7.
4. Boonen S, Vanderschueren D, Cheng XG et al. Age-related (type II) femoral neck osteoporosis in men: biochemical evidence for both hypovitaminos. *J Bone Miner Res* 1997; 12(12): 2119–26.
5. Kenny AM, Gallagher JC, Prestwood KM, Gruman CA, Raisz LG. Bone density, bone turnover, and hormone levels in men over age 75. *J Gerontol A Biol Sci Med Sci* 1998; 53(6): M419–M425.
6. Stanley HL, Schmitt BP, Poses RM, Deiss WP. Does hypogonadism contribute to the occurrence of a minimal trauma hip fracture in elderly men? *J Am Geriatr Soc* 1991; 39(8): 766–71.
7. Bhasin S, Bremner WJ. Clinical review 85: emerging issues in androgen replacement therapy. *J Clin Endocrinol Metab* 1997; 82(1): 3–8.
8. Katznelson L, Rosenthal DI, Rosol MS et al. Using quantitative CT to assess adipose distribution in adult men with acquired hypogonadism. *Am J Roentgenol* 1998; 170(2): 423–7.
9. Mauras N, Hayes V, Welch S et al. Testosterone deficiency in young men: marked alterations in whole body protein kinetics, strength, and adiposity. *J Clin Endocrinol Metab* 1998; 83(6): 1886–92.
10. Bagatell CJ, Heiman JR, Rivier JE, Bremner WJ. Effects of endogenous testosterone and estradiol on sexual behavior in normal young men [published erratum appears in *J Clin Endocrinol Metab* 1994; 78(6): 1520]. *J Clin Endocrinol Metab* 1994; 78(3): 711–16.
11. Carani C, Granata AR, Bancroft J, Marrama P. The effects of testosterone replacement on nocturnal penile tumescence and rigidity and erectile response to visual erotic stimuli in hypogonadal men. *Psychoneuroendocrinology* 1995; 20(7): 743–53.
12. Cunningham GR, Hirshkowitz M, Korenman SG, Karacan I. Testosterone replacement therapy and sleep-related erections in hypogonadal men. *J Clin Endocrinol Metab* 1990; 70(3): 792–7.
13. Davidson JM, Camargo CA, Smith ER. Effects of androgen on sexual behavior in hypogonadal men. *J Clin Endocrinol Metab* 1979; 48(6): 955–8.

14. Kwan M, Greenleaf WJ, Mann J, Crapo L, Davidson JM. The nature of androgen action on male sexuality: a combined laboratory–self-report study on hypogonadal men. *J Clin Endocrinol Metab* 1983; **57**(3): 557–62.
15. Salmimies P, Kockott G, Pirke KM, Vogt HJ, Schill WB. Effects of testosterone replacement on sexual behavior in hypogonadal men. *Arch Sex Behav* 1982; **11**(4): 345–53.
16. Barrett-Connor E, Khaw KT. Endogenous sex hormones and cardiovascular disease in men. A prospective population-based study. *Circulation* 1988; **78**(3): 539–45.
17. Marin P, Holmang S, Jonsson L et al. The effects of testosterone treatment on body composition and metabolism in middle-aged obese men. *Int J Obes Relat Metab Disord* 1992; **16**(12): 991–7.
18. Marin P. Testosterone and regional fat distribution. *Obes Res* 1995; **3**(suppl 4): 609S–12S.
19. Marin P, Oden B, Bjorntorp P. Assimilation and mobilization of triglycerides in subcutaneous abdominal and femoral adipose tissue in vivo in men: effects of androgens. *J Clin Endocrinol Metab* 1995; **80**(1): 239–43.
20. Seidell JC, Bjorntorp P, Sjostrom L, Kvist H, Sannerstedt R. Visceral fat accumulation in men is positively associated with insulin, glucose, and C-peptide levels, but negatively with testosterone levels. *Metabolism* 1990; **39**(9): 897–901.
21. Gray A, Feldman HA, McKinlay JB, Longcope C. Age, disease, and changing sex hormone levels in middle-aged men: results of the Massachusetts Male Aging Study. *J Clin Endocrinol Metab* 1991; **73**(5): 1016–25.
22. Gray A, Berlin JA, McKinlay JB, Longcope C. An examination of research design effects on the association of testosterone and male aging: results of a meta-analysis. *J Clin Epidemiol* 1991; **44**(7): 671–84.
23. Bandmann HJ, Breit R, Perwein E. *Klinefelter's Syndrome.* Berlin: Springer-Verlag, 1984.
24. Paulsen CA, Gordon DL, Carpenter RW, Gandy HM, Drucker WD. Klinefelter's syndrome and its variants: a hormonal and chromosomal study. *Recent Prog Horm Res* 1968; **24**: 321–63.
25. Arver S, Sinha-Hikim I, Beall G, Guerrero M, Shen R, Bhasin S. Serum dihydrotestosterone and testosterone concentrations in human immunodeficiency virus-infected men with and without weight loss. *J Androl* 1999; **20**(5): 611–18.
26. Coodley GO, Loveless MO, Nelson HD, Coodley MK. Endocrine function in the HIV wasting syndrome. *J AIDS* 1994; **7**(1): 46–51.
27. Dobs AS, Dempsey MA, Ladenson PW, Polk BF. Endocrine disorders in men infected with human immunodeficiency virus. *Am J Med* 1988; **84**(3 Pt 2): 611–16.
28. Dobs AS, Few WL III, Blackman MR, Harman SM, Hoover DR, Graham NM. Serum hormones in men with human immunodeficiency virus-associated wasting. *J Clin Endocrinol Metab* 1996; **81**(11): 4108–12.
29. Grinspoon S, Corcoran C, Lee K et al. Loss of lean body and muscle mass correlates with androgen levels in hypogonadal men with acquired immunodeficiency syndrome and wasting. *J Clin Endocrinol Metab* 1996; **81**(11): 4051–8.
30. Laudat A, Blum L, Guechot J et al. Changes in systemic gonadal and adrenal steroids in asymptomatic human immunodeficiency virus-infected men: relationship with the CD4 cell counts. *Eur J Endocrinol* 1995; **133**(4): 418–24.
31. Berns JS, Rudnick MR, Cohen RM. A controlled trial of recombinant human erythropoietin and nandrolone decanoate in the treatment of anemia in patients on chronic hemodialysis. *Clin Nephrol* 1992; **37**(5): 264–7.
32. Chopp RT, Mendez R. Sexual function and hormonal abnormalities in uremic men on chronic dialysis and after renal transplantation. *Fertil Steril* 1978; **29**(6): 661–6.
33. Handelsman DJ, Dong Q. Hypothalamo–pituitary gonadal axis in chronic renal failure. *Endocrinol Metab Clin North Am* 1993; **22**(1): 145–61.
34. Casaburi R. Rationale for anabolic therapy to facilitate rehabilitation in chronic obstructive pulmonary disease. *Baillières Clin Endocrinol Metab* 1998; **12**(3): 407–18.
35. Bhasin S, Storer TW, Asbel-Sethi N et al. Effects of testosterone replacement with a nongenital, transdermal system, Androderm, in human immunodeficiency virus-infected men with low testosterone levels. *J Clin Endocrinol Metab* 1998; **83**(9): 3155–62.
36. Bhasin S, Storer TW, Javanbakht M et al. Testosterone replacement and resistance exercise in HIV-infected men with weight loss and low testosterone levels. *JAMA* 2000; **283**(6): 763–70.
37. Grinspoon S, Corcoran C, Askari H et al. Effects of androgen administration in men with the AIDS wasting syndrome. A randomized, double-blind, placebo-controlled trial. *Ann Intern Med* 1998; **129**(1): 18–26.
38. MacAdams MR, White RH, Chipps BE. Reduction of serum testosterone levels during chronic glucocorticoid therapy. *Ann Intern Med* 1986; **104**(5): 648–51.
39. Reid IR, Ibbertson HK, France JT, Pybus J. Plasma testosterone concentrations in asthmatic men treated with glucocorticoids. *BMJ (Clin Res Ed)* 1985; **291**(6495): 574.
40. Trachtenberg J, Halpern N, Pont A. Ketoconazole: a novel and rapid treatment for advanced prostatic cancer. *J Urol* 1983; **130**(1): 152–3.
41. Pont A, Williams PL, Azhar S et al. Ketoconazole blocks testosterone synthesis. *Arch Intern Med* 1982; **142**(12): 2137–40.

42. Johnson DE, Babaian RJ, Swanson DA, von Eschenbach AC, Wishnow KI, Tenney D. Medical castration using megestrol acetate and minidose estrogen. *Urology* 1988; **31**(5): 371–4.
43. Venner P. Megestrol acetate in the treatment of metastatic carcinoma of the prostate. *Oncology* 1992; **49**(suppl 2): 22–7.
44. Bhasin S, Swerdloff RS. Mechanisms of gonadotropin-releasing hormone agonist action in the human male. *Endocrine Rev* 1986; **7**(1): 106–14.
45. Kim WH, Swerdloff RS, Bhasin S. Regulation of alpha and rat luteinizing hormone-beta messenger ribonucleic acids during gonadotropin-releasing hormone agonist treatment in vivo in the male rat. *Endocrinology* 1988; **123**(4): 2111–16.
46. Okonmah AD, Bradshaw WG, Couceyro P, Soliman KF. The effect of neuroleptic drugs on serum testosterone level in the male rat. *Gen Pharmacol* 1986; **17**(2): 235–8.
47. Rinieris P, Hatzimanolis J, Markianos M, Stefanis C. Effects of treatment with various doses of haloperidol on the pituitary–gonadal axis in male schizophrenic patients. *Neuropsychobiology* 1989; **22**(3): 146–9.
48. Halbreich U, Palter S. Accelerated osteoporosis in psychiatric patients: possible pathophysiological processes. *Schizophr Bull* 1996; **22**(3): 447–54.
49. Carter HB, Pearson JD, Metter EJ et al. Longitudinal evaluation of serum androgen levels in men with and without prostate cancer. *Prostate* 1995; **27**(1): 25–31.
50. Ferrini RL, Barrett-Connor E. Sex hormones and age: a cross-sectional study of testosterone and estradiol and their bioavailable fractions in community-dwelling men. *Am J Epidemiol* 1998; **147**(8): 750–4.
51. Korenman SG, Morley JE, Mooradian AD et al. Secondary hypogonadism in older men: its relation to impotence. *J Clin Endocrinol Metab* 1990; **71**(4): 963–9.
52. Morley JE, Kaiser FE, Perry HM III et al. Longitudinal changes in testosterone, luteinizing hormone, and follicle-stimulating hormone in healthy older men. *Metabolism* 1997; **46**(4): 410–13.
53. Simon D, Preziosi P, Barrett-Connor E et al. The influence of aging on plasma sex hormones in men: the Telecom Study. *Am J Epidemiol* 1992; **135**(7): 783–91.
54. Tenover JS. Effects of testosterone supplementation in the aging male. *J Clin Endocrinol Metab* 1992; **75**(4): 1092–8.
55. Tsitouras PD, Martin CE, Harman SM. Relationship of serum testosterone to sexual activity in healthy elderly men. *J Gerontol* 1982; **37**(3): 288–93.
56. Morley JE, Perry HM III, Kaiser FE et al. Effects of testosterone replacement therapy in old hypogonadal males: a preliminary study. *J Am Geriatr Soc* 1993; **41**(2): 149–52.
57. Sih R, Morley JE, Kaiser FE, Perry HM, III, Patrick P, Ross C. Testosterone replacement in older hypogonadal men: a 12-month randomized controlled trial. *J Clin Endocrinol Metab* 1997; **82**(6): 1661–7.
58. Snyder PJ, Peachey H, Hannoush P et al. Effect of testosterone treatment on body composition and muscle strength in men over 65 years of age. *J Clin Endocrinol Metab* 1999; **84**(8): 2647–53.
59. Snyder PJ, Peachey H, Hannoush P et al. Effect of testosterone treatment on bone mineral density in men over 65 years of age. *J Clin Endocrinol Metab* 1999; **84**(6): 1966–72.
60. Urban RJ, Bodenburg YH, Gilkison C et al. Testosterone administration to elderly men increases skeletal muscle strength and protein synthesis. *Am J Physiol* 1995; **269**(5 Pt 1): E820–6.
61. Tenover JL. Testosterone for all? The 80th Endocrine Society Meetings, New Orleans. S8-1, 1998.
62. Benet AE, Melman A. The epidemiology of erectile dysfunction. *Urol Clin North Am* 1995; **22**(4): 699–709.
63. Buvat J, Lemaire A. Endocrine screening in 1,022 men with erectile dysfunction: clinical significance and cost-effective strategy. *J Urol* 1997; **158**(5): 1764–7.
64. Carani C, Zini D, Baldini A, Della CL, Ghizzani A, Marrama P. Effects of androgen treatment in impotent men with normal and low levels of free testosterone. *Arch Sex Behav* 1990; **19**(3): 223–34.
65. Citron JT, Ettinger B, Rubinoff H et al. Prevalence of hypothalamic–pituitary imaging abnormalities in impotent men with secondary hypogonadism. *J Urol* 1996; **155**(2): 529–33.
66. Hajjar RR, Kaiser FE, Morley JE. Outcomes of long-term testosterone replacement in older hypogonadal males: a retrospective analysis. *J Clin Endocrinol Metab* 1997; **82**(11): 3793–6.
67. Kaiser FE, Viosca SP, Morley JE, Mooradian AD, Davis SS, Korenman SG. Impotence and aging: clinical and hormonal factors. *J Am Geriatr Soc* 1988; **36**(6): 511–19.
68. Morales A, Johnston B, Heaton JP, Lundie M. Testosterone supplementation for hypogonadal impotence: assessment of biochemical measures and therapeutic outcomes. *J Urol* 1997; **157**(3): 849–54.
69. Lugg JA, Rajfer J. Drug therapy for erectile dysfunction. *AUA Update* 1996; **15**: 290.
70. Morley JE. Sex hormones and diabetes. *Diabetes Metab Rev* 1998; **6**: 6–15.
71. Morley JE and Perry HM III. Androgen deficiency in aging men. *Med Clin North Am* 1999; **83**(5): 1279–89, vii.
72. van der Walt LA, Wilmsen EN, Jenkins T. Unusual sex hormone patterns among desert-dwelling hunter-gatherers. *J Clin Endocrinol Metab* 1978; **46**(4): 658–63.
73. Sherman BM, Halmi KA, Zamudio R. LH and FSH response to gonadotropin-releasing hormone in anorexia nervosa: effect of nutritional rehabilitation. *J Clin Endocrinol Metab* 1975; **41**(1): 135–42.

74. Comerci GD. Medical complications of anorexia nervosa and bulimia nervosa. *Med Clin North Am* 1990; 74(5): 1293–310.
75. Mozaffarian GA, Higley M, Paulsen CA. Clinical studies in an adult male patient with 'isolated follicle stimulating hormone (FSH) deficiency'. *J Androl* 1983; 4(6): 393–8.
76. Ballabio A, Bardoni B, Carrozzo R et al. Contiguous gene syndromes due to deletions in the distal short arm of the human X chromosome. *Proc Natl Acad Sci USA* 1989; 86(24): 10001–5.
77. Hardelin JP, Levilliers J, Young J et al. Xp22.3 deletions in isolated familial Kallmann's syndrome. *J Clin Endocrinol Metab* 1993; 76(4): 827–31.
78. Rebuffe-Scrive M, Marin P, Bjorntorp P. Effect of testosterone on abdominal adipose tissue in men. *Int J Obes* 1991; 15(11): 791–5.
79. Burris AS, Rodbard HW, Winters SJ, Sherins RJ. Gonadotropin therapy in men with isolated hypogonadotropic hypogonadism: the response to human chorionic gonadotropin is predicted by initial testicular size. *J Clin Endocrinol Metab* 1988; 66(6): 1144–51.
80. Finkel DM, Phillips JL, Snyder PJ. Stimulation of spermatogenesis by gonadotropins in men with hypogonadotropic hypogonadism. *N Engl J Med* 1985; 313(11): 651–5.
81. Whitcomb RW, Crowley WF Jr. Clinical review 4: diagnosis and treatment of isolated gonadotropin-releasing hormone deficiency in men. *J Clin Endocrinol Metab* 1990; 70(1): 3–7.
82. Longcope C, Goldfield SR, Brambilla DJ, McKinlay J. Androgens, estrogens, and sex hormone-binding globulin in middle-aged men. *J Clin Endocrinol Metab* 1990; 71(6): 1442–6.
83. Nankin HR, Calkins JH. Decreased bioavailable testosterone in aging normal and impotent men. *J Clin Endocrinol Metab* 1986; 63(6): 1418–20.
84. Rosner W. Errors in the measurement of plasma free testosterone. *J Clin Endocrinol Metab* 1997; 82(6): 2014–15.
85. Sinha-Hikim I, Arver S, Beall G et al. The use of a sensitive equilibrium dialysis method for the measurement of free testosterone levels in healthy, cycling women and in human immunodeficiency virus-infected women [published erratum appears in *J Clin Endocrinol Metab* 1998; 83(8): 2959]. *J Clin Endocrinol Metab* 1998; 83(4): 1312–18.
86. Glass AR, Swerdloff RS, Bray GA, Dahms WT, Atkinson RL. Low serum testosterone and sex-hormone-binding-globulin in massively obese men. *J Clin Endocrinol Metab* 1977; 45(6): 1211–19.
87. Zumoff B, Strain GW, Miller LK et al. Plasma free and non-sex-hormone-binding-globulin-bound testosterone are decreased in obese men in proportion to their degree of obesity. *J Clin Endocrinol Metab* 1990; 71(4): 929–31.
88. de Roux N, Young J, Misrahi M et al. A family with hypogonadotropic hypogonadism and mutations in the gonadotropin-releasing hormone receptor. *N Engl J Med* 1997; 337(22): 1597–602.
89. Rimoin DL, Schimke RN. Mechanisms of gene action in disorders of the endocrine glands. *Birth Defects Orig Artic Ser* 1971; 7(6): 5–11.
90. Gunay-Aygun M, Cassidy SB, Nicholls RD. Prader–Willi and other syndromes associated with obesity and mental retardation. *Behav Genet* 1997; 27(4): 307–24.
91. LaSalle JM, Ritchie RJ, Glatt H, Lalande M. Clonal heterogeneity at allelic methylation sites diagnostic for Prader–Willi and Angelman syndromes. *Proc Natl Acad Sci USA* 1998; 95(4): 1675–80.
92. Waldstreicher J, Seminara SB, Jameson JL et al. The genetic and clinical heterogeneity of gonadotropin-releasing hormone deficiency in the human. *J Clin Endocrinol Metab* 1996; 81(12): 4388–95.
93. Crowley WF Jr, Whitcomb RW, Jameson JL, Weiss J, Finkelstein JS, O'Dea LS. Neuroendocrine control of human reproduction in the male. *Recent Prog Horm Res* 1991; 47: 27–62.
94. Spratt DI, Carr DB, Merriam GR, Scully RE, Rao PN, Crowley WF Jr. The spectrum of abnormal patterns of gonadotropin-releasing hormone secretion in men with idiopathic hypogonadotropic hypogonadism: clinical and laboratory correlations. *J Clin Endocrinol Metab* 1987; 64(2): 283–91.
95. Behre HM, Bohmeyer J, Nieschlag E. Prostate volume in testosterone-treated and untreated hypogonadal men in comparison to age-matched normal controls. *Clin Endocrinol (Oxf)* 1994; 40(3): 341–9.
96. Goldstein I, Lue TF, Padma-Nathan H, Rosen RC, Steers WD, Wicker PA. Oral sildenafil in the treatment of erectile dysfunction. Sildenafil Study Group [published erratum appears in *N Engl J Med* 1998; 339(1): 59]. *N Engl J Med* 1998; 338(20): 1397–404.
97. Franco B, Guioli S, Pragliola A et al. A gene deleted in Kallmann's syndrome shares homology with neural cell adhesion and axonal path-finding molecules. *Nature* 1991; 353(6344): 529–36.
98. Legouis R, Hardelin JP, Levilliers J et al. The candidate gene for the X-linked Kallmann syndrome encodes a protein related to adhesion molecules. *Cell* 1991; 67(2): 423–35.
99. Seminara SB, Hayes FJ, Crowley WF Jr. Gonadotropin-releasing hormone deficiency in the human (idiopathic hypogonadotropic hypogonadism and Kallmann's syndrome): pathophysiological and genetic considerations. *Endocrine Rev* 1998; 19(5): 521–39.
100. O'Neill MJ, Tridjaja B, Smith MJ, Bell KM, Warne GL, Sinclair AH. Familial Kallmann syndrome: a novel splice acceptor mutation in the KAL gene. *Hum Mutat* 1998; 11(4): 340–2.

101. Maya-Nunez G, Zenteno JC, Ulloa-Aguirre A, Kofman-Alfaro S, Mendez JP. A recurrent missense mutation in the KAL gene in patients with X-linked Kallmann's syndrome. *J Clin Endocrinol Metab* 1998; **83**(5): 1650–3.

102. Duke V, Quinton R, Gordon I, Bouloux PM, Woolf AS. Proteinuria, hypertension and chronic renal failure in X-linked Kallmann's syndrome, a defined genetic cause of solitary functioning kidney. *Nephrol Dial Transplant* 1998; **13**(8): 1998–2003.

103. Weissortel R, Strom TM, Dorr HG, Rauch A, Meitinger T. Analysis of an interstitial deletion in a patient with Kallmann syndrome, X-linked ichthyosis and mental retardation. *Clin Genet* 1998; **54**(1): 45–51.

104. Georgopoulos NA, Pralong FP, Seidman CE, Seidman JG, Crowley WF Jr, Vallejo M. Genetic heterogeneity evidenced by low incidence of KAL-1 gene mutations in sporadic cases of gonadotropin-releasing hormone deficiency. *J Clin Endocrinol Metab* 1997; **82**(1): 213–17.

105. Schwanzel-Fukuda M, Pfaff DW. Origin of luteinizing hormone-releasing hormone neurons. *Nature* 1989; **338**(6211): 161–4.

106. Klingmuller D, Dewes W, Krahe T, Brecht G, Schweikert HU. Magnetic resonance imaging of the brain in patients with anosmia and hypothalamic hypogonadism (Kallmann's syndrome). *J Clin Endocrinol Metab* 1987; **65**(3): 581–4.

107. Muscatelli F, Strom TM, Walker AP et al. Mutations in the DAX-1 gene give rise to both X-linked adrenal hypoplasia congenita and hypogonadotropic hypogonadism. *Nature* 1994; **372**(6507): 672–6.

108. Guo W, Mason JS, Stone CG Jr et al. Diagnosis of X-linked adrenal hypoplasia congenita by mutation analysis of the DAX1 gene. *JAMA* 1995; **274**(4): 324–30.

109. Burris TP, Guo W, McCabe ER. The gene responsible for adrenal hypoplasia congenita, DAX-1, encodes a nuclear hormone receptor that defines a new class within the superfamily. *Recent Prog Horm Res* 1996; **51**: 241–59.

110. Habiby RL, Boepple P, Nachtigall L, Sluss PM, Crowley WF Jr, Jameson JL. Adrenal hypoplasia congenita with hypogonadotropic hypogonadism: evidence that DAX-1 mutations lead to combined hypothalamic and pituitary defects in gonadotropin production. *J Clin Invest* 1996; **98**(4): 1055–62.

111. Tamai KT, Monaco L, Alastalo TP, Lalli E, Parvinen M, Sassone-Corsi P. Hormonal and developmental regulation of DAX-1 expression in Sertoli cells. *Mol Endocrinol* 1996; **10**(12): 1561–9.

112. Wang J, Killinger DW, Hegele RA. A microdeletion within DAX-1 in X-linked adrenal hypoplasia congenita and hypogonadotrophic hypogonadism. *J Invest Med* 1999; **47**(5): 232–5.

113. Caron P, Imbeaud S, Bennet A, Plantavid M, Camerino G, Rochiccioli P. Combined hypothalamic–pituitary–gonadal defect in a hypogonadic man with a novel mutation in the DAX-1 gene. *J Clin Endocrinol Metab* 1999; **84**(10): 3563–9.

114. Achermann JC, Gu WX, Kotlar TJ et al. Mutational analysis of DAX1 in patients with hypogonadotropic hypogonadism or pubertal delay. *J Clin Endocrinol Metab* 1999; **84**(12): 4497–500.

115. Seminara SB, Achermann JC, Genel M, Jameson JL, Crowley WF Jr. X-linked adrenal hypoplasia congenita: a mutation in DAX1 expands the phenotypic spectrum in males and females. *J Clin Endocrinol Metab* 1999; **84**(12): 4501–9.

116. Layman LC. Genetics of human hypogonadotropic hypogonadism. *Am J Med Genet* 1999; **89**(4): 240–8.

117. Tabarin A, Achermann JC, Recan D et al. A novel mutation in DAX1 causes delayed-onset adrenal insufficiency and incomplete hypogonadotropic hypogonadism. *J Clin Invest* 2000; **105**(3): 321–8.

118. Lalli E, Ohe K, Hindelang C, Sassone-Corsi P. Orphan receptor DAX-1 is a shuttling RNA binding protein associated with polyribosomes via mRNA. *Mol Cell Biol* 2000; **20**(13): 4910–21.

119. Pralong FP, Gomez F, Castillo E et al. Complete hypogonadotropic hypogonadism associated with a novel inactivating mutation of the gonadotropin-releasing hormone receptor. *J Clin Endocrinol Metab* 1999; **84**(10): 3811–16.

120. Layman LC, Lee EJ, Peak DB et al. Delayed puberty and hypogonadism caused by mutations in the follicle-stimulating hormone beta-subunit gene. *N Engl J Med* 1997; **337**(9): 607–11.

121. Phillip M, Arbelle JE, Segev Y, Parvari R. Male hypogonadism due to a mutation in the gene for the beta-subunit of follicle-stimulating hormone. *N Engl J Med* 1998; **338**(24): 1729–32.

122. Kumar TR, Wang Y, Lu N, Matzuk MM. Follicle stimulating hormone is required for ovarian follicle maturation but not male fertility. *Nat Genet* 1997; **15**(2): 201–4.

123. Weiss J, Axelrod L, Whitcomb RW, Harris PE, Crowley WF, Jameson JL. Hypogonadism caused by a single amino acid substitution in the beta subunit of luteinizing hormone. *N Engl J Med* 1992; **326**(3): 179–83.

124. Raivio T, Huhtaniemi I, Anttila R et al. The role of luteinizing hormone-beta gene polymorphism in the onset and progression of puberty in healthy boys. *J Clin Endocrinol Metab* 1996; **81**(9): 3278–82.

125. Nilsson C, Pettersson K, Millar RP, Coerver KA, Matzuk MM, Huhtaniemi IT. Worldwide frequency of a common genetic variant of luteinizing hormone: an international collaborative research. International Collaborative Research Group. *Fertil Steril* 1997; **67**(6): 998–1004.

126. Gromoll J, Partsch CJ, Simoni M et al. A mutation in the first transmembrane domain of the lutropin receptor causes male precocious puberty. *J Clin Endocrinol Metab* 1998; **83**(2): 476–80.
127. Conway GS. Clinical manifestations of genetic defects affecting gonadotrophins and their receptors. *Clin Endocrinol (Oxf)* 1996; **45**(6): 657–63.
128. DiMeglio LA, Pescovitz OH. Disorders of puberty: inactivating and activating molecular mutations. *J Pediatr* 1997; **131**(1 Pt 2): S8–12.
129. Gromoll J, Simoni M, Nordhoff V, Behre HM, De Geyter C, Nieschlag E. Functional and clinical consequences of mutations in the FSH receptor. *Mol Cell Endocrinol* 1996; **125**(1–2): 177–82.
130. Pfaffle RW, Blankenstein O, Wuller S, Kentrup H. Combined pituitary hormone deficiency: role of Pit-1 and Prop-1. *Acta Paediatr Suppl* 1999; **88**(433): 33–41.
131. Castrillo JL, Theill LE, Karin M. Function of the homeodomain protein GHF1 in pituitary cell proliferation. *Science* 1991; **253**(5016): 197–9.
132. Dattani MT, Martinez-Barbera JP, Thomas PQ et al. Mutations in the homeobox gene HESX1/Hesx1 associated with septo-optic dysplasia in human and mouse. *Nat Genet* 1998; **19**(2): 125–33.
133. Parks JS, Brown MR. Transcription factors regulating pituitary development. *Growth Horm IGF Res* 1999; **9**(suppl B): 2–8.
134. Parks JS, Brown MR, Hurley DL, Phelps CJ, Wajnrajch MP. Heritable disorders of pituitary development. *J Clin Endocrinol Metab* 1999; **84**(12): 4362–70.
135. Pfaffle RW, DiMattia GE, Parks JS et al. Mutation of the POU-specific domain of Pit-1 and hypopituitarism without pituitary hypoplasia. *Science* 1992; **257**(5073): 1118–21.
136. Radovick S, Nations M, Du Y, Berg LA, Weintraub BD, Wondisford FE. A mutation in the POU-homeodomain of Pit-1 responsible for combined pituitary hormone deficiency. *Science* 1992; **257**(5073): 1115–18.
137. Semina EV, Reiter R, Leysens NJ et al. Cloning and characterization of a novel bicoid-related homeobox transcription factor gene, RIEG, involved in Rieger syndrome. *Nat Genet* 1996; **14**(4): 392–9.
138. Wu W, Cogan JD, Pfaffle RW et al. Mutations in PROP1 cause familial combined pituitary hormone deficiency. *Nat Genet* 1998; **18**(2): 147–9.
139. Sadeghi-Nejad A, Senior B. Autosomal dominant transmission of isolated growth hormone deficiency in iris-dental dysplasia (Rieger's syndrome). *J Pediatr* 1974; **85**(5): 644–8.
140. Themmen AP, Martens JW, Brunner HG. Gonadotropin receptor mutations. *J Endocrinol* 1997; **153**(2): 179–83.
141. Latronico AC, Anasti J, Arnhold IJ et al. Brief report: testicular and ovarian resistance to luteinizing hormone caused by inactivating mutations of the luteinizing hormone-receptor gene. *N Engl J Med* 1996; **334**(8): 507–12.
142. Laue L, Wu SM, Kudo M et al. A nonsense mutation of the human luteinizing hormone receptor gene in Leydig cell hypoplasia. *Hum Mol Genet* 1995; **4**(8): 1429–33.
143. Laue LL, Wu SM, Kudo M et al. Compound heterozygous mutations of the luteinizing hormone receptor gene in Leydig cell hypoplasia. *Mol Endocrinol* 1996; **10**(8): 987–97.
144. Aittomaki K, Lucena JL, Pakarinen P et al. Mutation in the follicle-stimulating hormone receptor gene causes hereditary hypergonadotropic ovarian failure. *Cell* 1995; **82**(6): 959–68.
145. Aittomaki K, Herva R, Stenman UH et al. Clinical features of primary ovarian failure caused by a point mutation in the follicle-stimulating hormone receptor gene. *J Clin Endocrinol Metab* 1996; **81**(10): 3722–6.
146. Bagheri SA, Boyer JL. Peliosis hepatis associated with androgenic-anabolic steroid therapy. A severe form of hepatic injury. *Ann Intern Med* 1974; **81**(5): 610–18.
147. Yoshida EM, Erb SR, Scudamore CH, Owen DA. Severe cholestasis and jaundice secondary to an esterified testosterone, a non-C17 alkylated anabolic steroid. *J Clin Gastroenterol* 1994; **18**(3): 268–70.
148. Dobs AS, Meikle AW, Arver S, Sanders SW, Caramelli KE, Mazer NA. Pharmacokinetics, efficacy, and safety of a permeation-enhanced testosterone transdermal system in comparison with bi-weekly injections of testosterone enanthate for the treatment of hypogonadal men. *J Clin Endocrinol Metab* 1999; **84**(10): 3469–78.
149. Snyder PJ, Lawrence DA. Treatment of male hypogonadism with testosterone enanthate. *J Clin Endocrinol Metab* 1980; **51**(6): 1335–9.
150. Sokol RZ, Palacios A, Campfield LA, Saul C, Swerdloff RS. Comparison of the kinetics of injectable testosterone in eugonadal and hypogonadal men. *Fertil Steril* 1982; **37**(3): 425–30.
151. Cunningham GR, Cordero E, Thornby JI. Testosterone replacement with transdermal therapeutic systems. Physiological serum testosterone and elevated dihydrotestosterone levels. *JAMA* 1989; **261**(17): 2525–30.
152. Behre HM, Von Eckardstein S, Kliesch S, Nieschlag E. Long-term substitution therapy of hypogonadal men with transscrotal testosterone over 7–10 years. *Clin Endocrinol (Oxf)* 1999; **50**(5): 629–35.
153. Meikle AW, Mazer NA, Moellmer JF et al. Enhanced transdermal delivery of testosterone across nonscrotal skin produces physiological concentrations of testosterone and its metabolites in hypogonadal men. *J Clin Endocrinol Metab* 1992; **74**(3): 623–8.
154. Wang C, Berman N, Longstreth JA et al. Pharmacokinetics of transdermal testosterone gel in hypogonadal men: application of gel at one site versus

four sites: a General Clinical Research Center Study. *J Clin Endocrinol Metab* 2000; **85**(3): 964–9.
155. Cooper CS, Perry PJ, Sparks AE, MacIndoe JH, Yates WR, Williams RD. Effect of exogenous testosterone on prostate volume, serum and semen prostate specific antigen levels in healthy young men. *J Urol* 1998; **159**(2): 441–3.
156. Meikle AW, Arver S, Dobs AS et al. Prostate size in hypogonadal men treated with a nonscrotal permeation-enhanced testosterone transdermal system. *Urology* 1997; **49**(2): 191–6.
157. Sasagawa I, Nakada T, Kazama T, Satomi S, Terada T, Katayama T. Volume change of the prostate and seminal vesicles in male hypogonadism after androgen replacement therapy. *Int Urol Nephrol* 1990; **22**(3): 279–84.
158. Rencricca NJ, Solomon J, Fimian WJ Jr, Howard D, Rizzoli V, Stohlman F Jr. The effect of testosterone on erythropoiesis. *Scand J Haematol* 1969; **6**(6): 431–6.
159. Naets JP, Wittek M. The mechanism of action of androgens on erythropoiesis. *Ann NY Acad Sci* 1968; **149**(1): 366–76.
160. Fried W, Marver D, Lange RD, Gurney CW. Studies on the erythropoietic stimulating factor in the plasma of mice after receiving testosterone. *J Lab Clin Med* 1966; **68**(6): 947–51.
161. Dexter DD, Dovre EJ. Obstructive sleep apnea due to endogenous testosterone production in a woman. *Mayo Clin Proc* 1998; **73**(3): 246–8.
162. Cistulli PA, Grunstein RR, Sullivan CE. Effect of testosterone administration on upper airway collapsibility during sleep. *Am J Respir Crit Care Med* 1994; **149**(2 Pt 1): 530–2.
163. Emery MJ, Hlastala MP, Matsumoto AM. Depression of hypercapnic ventilatory drive by testosterone in the sleeping infant primate. *J Appl Physiol* 1994; **76**(4): 1786–93.
164. Grunstein RR. Metabolic aspects of sleep apnea. *Sleep* 1996; **19**(10 suppl): S218–20.
165. Matsumoto AM, Sandblom RE, Schoene RB et al. Testosterone replacement in hypogonadal men: effects on obstructive sleep apnoea, respiratory drives, and sleep. *Clin Endocrinol (Oxf)* 1985; **22**(6): 713–21.
166. Schneider BK, Pickett CK, Zwillich CW et al. Influence of testosterone on breathing during sleep. *J Appl Physiol* 1986; **61**(2): 618–23.
167. Tripathy D, Shah P, Lakshmy R, Reddy KS. Effect of testosterone replacement on whole body glucose utilisation and other cardiovascular risk factors in males with idiopathic hypogonadotrophic hypogonadism. *Horm Metab Res* 1998; **30**(10): 642–5.
168. Bhasin S, Storer TW, Berman N et al. Testosterone replacement increases fat-free mass and muscle size in hypogonadal men. *J Clin Endocrinol Metab* 1997; **82**(2): 407–13.
169. Brodsky IG, Balagopal P, Nair KS. Effects of testosterone replacement on muscle mass and muscle protein synthesis in hypogonadal men—a clinical research center study. *J Clin Endocrinol Metab* 1996; **81**(10): 3469–75.
170. Wang C, Eyre DR, Clark R et al. Sublingual testosterone replacement improves muscle mass and strength, decreases bone resorption, and increases bone formation markers in hypogonadal men—a clinical research center study. *J Clin Endocrinol Metab* 1996; **81**(10): 3654–62.
171. Bhasin S, Tenover JS. Age-associated sarcopenia—issues in the use of testosterone as an anabolic agent in older men. *J Clin Endocrinol Metab* 1997; **82**(6): 1659–60.
172. Hanash KA, Mostofi KF. Androgen effect on prostate specific antigen secretion. *J Surg Oncol* 1992; **49**(3): 202–4.
173. Svetec DA, Canby ED, Thompson IM, Sabanegh ES Jr. The effect of parenteral testosterone replacement on prostate specific antigen in hypogonadal men with erectile dysfunction. *J Urol* 1997; **158**(5): 1775–7.
174. Morgentaler A, Bruning CO III, DeWolf WC. Occult prostate cancer in men with low serum testosterone levels. *JAMA* 1996; **276**(23): 1904–6.
175. Winters SJ, Atkinson L. Serum LH concentrations in hypogonadal men during transdermal testosterone replacement through scrotal skin: further evidence that ageing enhances testosterone negative feedback. The Testoderm Study Group. *Clin Endocrinol (Oxf)* 1997; **47**(3): 317–22.
176. NIH Consensus Conference. Impotence. NIH Consensus Development Panel on Impotence. *JAMA* 1993; **270**(1): 83–90.
177. Lue TF. Erectile dysfunction. *N Engl J Med* 2000; **342**(24): 1802–13.
178. Furlow WL. Prevalence of impotence in the United States. *Med Aspects Hum Sex* 1985; **19**: 13–16.
179. Feldman HA, Goldstein I, Hatzichristou DG, Krane RJ, McKinlay JB. Impotence and its medical and psychosocial correlates: results of the Massachusetts Male Aging Study. *J Urol* 1994; **151**(1): 54–61.
180. Lugg JA, Rajfer J, Gonzalez-Cadavid NF. Dihydrotestosterone is the active androgen in the maintenance of nitric oxide-mediated penile erection in the rat. *Endocrinology* 1995; **136**(4): 1495–501.
181. Andersson KE, Wagner G. Physiology of penile erection. *Physiol Rev* 1995; **75**(1): 191–236.
182. Christ GJ. The penis as a vascular organ. The importance of corporal smooth muscle tone in the control of erection. *Urol Clin North Am* 1995; **22**(4): 727–45.
183. Lue TF, Tanagho EA. Hemodynamics of erection. In: Tanagho EA, Lue TF, McClure RD, eds. *Contemporary Management of Impotence and Infertility*. Baltimore: Williams and Wilkins, 1988: 28–38.
184. Naylor AM. Endogenous neurotransmitters mediating penile erection. *Br J Urol* 1998; **81**(3): 424–31.

185. Rajfer J, Aronson WJ, Bush PA, Dorey FJ, Ignarro LJ. Nitric oxide as a mediator of relaxation of the corpus cavernosum in response to nonadrenergic, noncholinergic neurotransmission. *N Engl J Med* 1992; 326(2): 90–4.
186. McDonald LJ, Murad F. Nitric oxide and cyclic GMP signaling. *Proc Soc Exp Biol Med* 1996; 211(1): 1–6.
187. Nehra A, Barrett DM, Moreland RB. Pharmacotherapeutic advances in the treatment of erectile dysfunction. *Mayo Clin Proc* 1999; 74(7): 709–21.
188. Ruutu ML, Virtanen JM, Lindstrom BL, Alfthan OS. The value of basic investigations in the diagnosis of impotence. *Scand J Urol Nephrol* 1987; 21(4): 261–5.
189. Takasaki N, Kotani T, Miyazaki S, Saitou S. [Measurement of penile brachial index (PBI) in patients with impotence]. *Hinyokika Kiyo* 1989; 35(8): 1365–8.
190. Aitchison M, Aitchison J, Carter R. Is the penile brachial index a reproducible and useful measurement? *Br J Urol* 1990; 66(2): 202–4.
191. Mueller SC, Wallenberg-Pachaly H, Voges GE, Schild HH. Comparison of selective internal iliac pharmacoangiography, penile brachial index and duplex sonography with pulsed Doppler analysis for the evaluation of vasculogenic (arteriogenic) impotence. *J Urol* 1990; 143(5): 928–32.
192. Rendell MS, Rajfer J, Wicker PA, Smith MD. Sildenafil for treatment of erectile dysfunction in men with diabetes: a randomized controlled trial. Sildenafil Diabetes Study Group. *JAMA* 1999; 281(5): 421–6.
193. Boolell M, Allen MJ, Ballard SA et al. Sildenafil: an orally active type 5 cyclic GMP-specific phosphodiesterase inhibitor for the treatment of penile erectile dysfunction. *Int J Impot Res* 1996; 8(2): 47–52.
194. Moreland RB, Goldstein I, Traish A. Sildenafil, a novel inhibitor of phosphodiesterase type 5 in human corpus cavernosum smooth muscle cells. *Life Sci* 1998; 62(20): PL309–18.
195. Giuliano F, Hultling C, el Masry WS et al. Randomized trial of sildenafil for the treatment of erectile dysfunction in spinal cord injury. Sildenafil Study Group. *Ann Neurol* 1999; 46(1): 15–21.
196. Jarow JP, Burnett AL, Geringer AM. Clinical efficacy of sildenafil citrate based on etiology and response to prior treatment. *J Urol* 1999; 162(3 Pt 1): 722–5.
197. Dinsmore WW, Hodges M, Hargreaves C, Osterloh IH, Smith MD, Rosen RC. Sildenafil citrate (Viagra) in erectile dysfunction: near normalization in men with broad-spectrum erectile dysfunction compared with age-matched healthy control subjects [published erratum appears in *Urology* 1999; 53(5): 1072]. *Urology* 1999; 53(4): 800–5.
198. Morales A, Gingell C, Collins M, Wicker PA, Osterloh IH. Clinical safety of oral sildenafil citrate (VIAGRA) in the treatment of erectile dysfunction. *Int J Impot Res* 1998; 10(2): 69–73.
199. Aversa A, Mazzilli F, Rossi T, Delfino M, Isidori AM, Fabbri A. Effects of sildenafil (Viagra) administration on seminal parameters and post-ejaculatory refractory time in normal males. *Hum Reprod* 2000; 15(1): 131–4.
200. Feenstra J, Drie-Pierik RJ, Lacle CF, Stricker BH. Acute myocardial infarction associated with sildenafil. *Lancet* 1998; 352(9132): 957–8.
201. Zusman RM, Morales A, Glasser DB, Osterloh IH. Overall cardiovascular profile of sildenafil citrate. *Am J Cardiol* 1999; 83(5A): 35C–44C.
202. Arora RR, Timoney M, Melilli L. Acute myocardial infarction after the use of sildenafil. *N Engl J Med* 1999; 341(9): 700.
203. Muller JE, Mittleman A, Maclure M, Sherwood JB, Tofler GH. Triggering myocardial infarction by sexual activity. Low absolute risk and prevention by regular physical exertion. Determinants of Myocardial Infarction Onset Study Investigators. *JAMA* 1996; 275(18): 1405–9.
204. Cheitlin MD, Hutter AM Jr, Brindis RG et al. Use of sildenafil (Viagra) in patients with cardiovascular disease. Technology and Practice Executive Committee [published erratum appears in *Circulation* 1999; 100(23): 2389]. *Circulation* 1999; 99(1): 168–77.
205. Herrmann HC, Chang G, Klugherz BD, Mahoney PD. Hemodynamic effects of sildenafil in men with severe coronary artery disease. *N Engl J Med* 2000; 342(22): 1622–6.
206. Padma-Nathan H, Steers WD, Wicker PA. Efficacy and safety of oral sildenafil in the treatment of erectile dysfunction: a double-blind, placebo-controlled study of 329 patients. Sildenafil Study Group. *Int J Clin Pract* 1998; 52(6): 375–9.
207. Goldenberg MM. Safety and efficacy of sildenafil citrate in the treatment of male erectile dysfunction. *Clin Ther* 1998; 20(6): 1033–48.
208. Conti CR, Pepine CJ, Sweeney M. Efficacy and safety of sildenafil citrate in the treatment of erectile dysfunction in patients with ischemic heart disease. *Am J Cardiol* 1999; 83(5A): 29C–34C.
209. Osterloh IH, Collins M, Wicker P, Wagner G. Sildenafil citrate (VIAGRA): overall safety profile in 18 double-blind, placebo controlled, clinical trials. *Int J Clin Pract Suppl* 1999; 102: 3–5.
210. Young J. Sildenafil citrate (VIAGRA) in the treatment of erectile dysfunction: a 12-week, flexible-dose study to assess efficacy and safety. *Int J Clin Pract Suppl* 1999; 102: 6–7.
211. Goldstein I. A 36-week, open label, non-comparative study to assess the long-term safety of sildenafil citrate (VIAGRA) in patients with erectile dysfunction. *Int J Clin Pract Suppl* 1999; 102: 8–9.
212. Kloner RA. Cardiovascular risk and sildenafil. *Am J Cardiol* 2000; 86(2A): 57F–61F.

213. McMahon CG, Samali R, Johnson H. Efficacy, safety and patient acceptance of sildenafil citrate as treatment for erectile dysfunction. *J Urol* 2000; 164(4): 1192–6.
214. McGarvey MR. Tough choices: the cost-effectiveness of sildenafil. *Ann Intern Med* 2000; 132(12): 994–5.
215. Smith KJ, Roberts MS. The cost-effectiveness of sildenafil. *Ann Intern Med* 2000; 132(12): 933–7.
216. Tan HL. Economic cost of male erectile dysfunction using a decision analytic model: for a hypothetical managed-care plan of 100,000 members. *Pharmacoeconomics* 2000; 17(1): 77–107.
217. Witherington R. Vacuum devices for the impotent. *J Sex Marital Ther* 1991; 17(2): 69–80.
218. Lewis JH, Sidi AA, Reddy PK. A way to help your patients who use vacuum devices. *Contemp Urol* 1991; 3(12): 15–21.
219. Morley JE. Management of impotence. Diagnostic considerations and therapeutic options. *Postgrad Med* 1993; 93(3): 65–72.
220. Morales A. Nonsurgical management options in impotence. *Hosp Pract (Off Ed)* 1993; 28(3A): 15–20, 23.
221. Lewis RW, Witherington R. External vacuum therapy for erectile dysfunction: use and results. *World J Urol* 1997; 15(1): 78–82.
222. Ganem JP, Lucey DT, Janosko EO, Carson CC. Unusual complications of the vacuum erection device. *Urology* 1998; 51(4): 627–31.
223. Finelli A, Hirshberg ED, Radomski SB. The treatment choice of elderly patients with erectile dysfunction. *Geriatr Nephrol Urol* 1998; 8(1): 15–19.
224. Oakley N, Moore KT. Vacuum devices in erectile dysfunction: indications and efficacy. *Br J Urol* 1998; 82(5): 673–81.
225. Skakkebaek NE, Bancroft J, Davidson DW, Warner P. Androgen replacement with oral testosterone undecanoate in hypogonadal men: a double blind controlled study. *Clin Endocrinol (Oxf)* 1981; 14(1): 49–61.
226. McClure RD, Oses R, Ernest ML. Hypogonadal impotence treated by transdermal testosterone. *Urology* 1991; 37(3): 224–8.
227. Nankin HR, Lin T, Osterman J. Chronic testosterone cypionate therapy in men with secondary impotence. *Fertil Steril* 1986; 46(2): 300–7.
228. Arver S, Dobs AS, Meikle AW, Allen RP, Sanders SW, Mazer NA. Improvement of sexual function in testosterone deficient men treated for 1 year with a permeation enhanced testosterone transdermal system. *J Urol* 1996; 155(5): 1604–8.
229. Buena F, Swerdloff RS, Steiner BS et al. Sexual function does not change when serum testosterone levels are pharmacologically varied within the normal male range. *Fertil Steril* 1993; 59(5): 1118–23.
230. Bhasin S, Fielder T, Peacock N, Sod-Moriah UA, Swerdloff RS. Dissociating antifertility effects of GnRH-antagonist from its adverse effects on mating behavior in male rats. *Am J Physiol* 1988; 254(1 Pt 1): E84–91.
231. Fielder TJ, Peacock NR, McGivern RF, Swerdloff RS, Bhasin S. Testosterone dose-dependency of sexual and nonsexual behaviors in the gonadotropin-releasing hormone antagonist-treated male rat. *J Androl* 1989; 10(3): 167–73.
232. Bhasin S. The dose-dependent effects of testosterone on sexual function and on muscle mass and function. *Mayo Clin Proc* 2000; 75(suppl): S70–5.
233. Jain P, Rademaker AW, McVary KT. Testosterone supplementation for erectile dysfunction: results of a meta-analysis. *J Urol* 2000; 164(2): 371–5.
234. Engelhardt PF, Plas E, Hubner WA, Pfluger H. Comparison of intraurethral liposomal and intracavernosal prostaglandin-E1 in the management of erectile dysfunction. *Br J Urol* 1998; 81(3): 441–4.
235. Kim ED, McVary KT. Topical prostaglandin-E1 for the treatment of erectile dysfunction. *J Urol* 1995; 153(6): 1828–30.
236. Peterson CA, Bennett AH, Hellstrom WJ et al. Erectile response to transurethral alprostadil, prazosin and alprostadil–prazosin combinations. *J Urol* 1998; 159(5): 1523–7.
237. Bhasin S, de Kretser DM, Baker HW. Clinical review 64: pathophysiology and natural history of male infertility. *J Clin Endocrinol Metab* 1994; 79(6): 1525–9.
238. de Kretser DM, Burger HG, Fortune D et al. Hormonal, histological and chromosomal studies in adult males with testicular disorders. *J Clin Endocrinol Metab* 1972; 35(3): 392–401.
239. Lamb DJ, Niederberger CS. Animal models that mimic human male reproductive defects. *Urol Clin North Am* 1994; 21(3): 377–87.
240. Jaffe T, Oates RD. Genetic abnormalities and reproductive failure. *Urol Clin North Am* 1994; 21(3): 389–408.
241. Skakkebaek NE, Giwercman A, de Kretser D. Pathogenesis and management of male infertility. *Lancet* 1994; 343(8911): 1473–9.
242. Heller CG, Clermont Y. Kinetics of the germinal epithelium in man. *Recent Prog Horm Res* 1964; 20: 545–75.
243. Griswold MD. Protein secretions of Sertoli cells. *Int Rev Cytol* 1988; 110: 133–56.
244. Baker HW, Burger HG, de Kretser DM, Hudson B. Relative incidence of etiologic factors in male infertility. In: Santen RJ, Swedloff RS, eds. *Reproductive Dysfunction: Diagnosis and Management of Hypogonadism.* New York: Marcel Dekker, 1986: 341–72.
245. Swerdloff RS, Boyers SP. Evaluation of the male partner of an infertile couple. An algorithmic approach. *JAMA* 1982; 247(17): 2418–22.
246. World Health Organization: *Laboratory Manual for the Examination of Human Semen and Semen–Cervical Mucus Interaction.* Cambridge: Cambridge University Press, 1987.

247. Wang C, Chan SY, Ng M et al. Diagnostic value of sperm function tests and routine semen analyses in fertile and infertile men. *J Androl* 1988; 9(6): 384–9.
248. Zuffardi O, Tiepolo L. Frequencies and types of chromosome abnormalities associated with human male infertility. In: Crosignani PG, Rubin BL, eds. *Genetic Control of Gametic Production and Function.* Academic Press, 1982: 261–73.
249. Kjessler B. *Karyotype, Meiosis and Spermatogenesis in a Sample of Men Attending an Infertility Clinic.* Basel and New York: S. Karger, 1966.
250. Chandley AC. The chromosomal basis of human infertility. *Br Med Bull* 1979; 35(2): 181–6.
251. Koulischer L, Schoysman R. Studies of the mitotic and meiotic chromosomes in infertile males. *J Genet Hum* 1975; 23(suppl): 58–70.
252. Jacobs PA, Melville M, Ratcliffe S, Keay AJ, Syme J. A cytogenetic survey of 11,680 newborn infants. *Ann Hum Genet* 1974; 37(4): 359–376.
253. Hamerton JL, Canning N, Ray M, Smith S. A cytogenetic survey of 14,069 newborn infants. I. Incidence of chromosome abnormalities. *Clin Genet* 1975; 8(4): 223–43.
254. Bryns JP, Kleckowska A, van den Berghe H. *The X Chromosome and Sexual Development: Clinical Aspects.* New York: Alan R. Liss, Inc., 1983.
255. Huckins C, Bullock LP, Long JL. Morphological profiles of cryptorchid XXY mouse testes. *Anat Rec* 1981; 199(4): 507–11.
256. Sharland M, Burch M, McKenna WM, Paton MA. A clinical study of Noonan syndrome. *Arch Dis Child* 1992; 67(2): 178–83.
257. Santen RJ, DeKretser DM, Paulsen CA, Vorhees J. Gonadotrophins and testosterone in the XYY syndrome. *Lancet* 1970; 2(7668): 371.
258. Davidoff F, Federman DD. Mixed gonadal dysgenesis. *Pediatrics* 1973; 52(5): 725–42.
259. Page DC, Brown LG, de la Chapelle A. Exchange of terminal portions of X- and Y-chromosomal short arms in human XX males. *Nature* 1987; 328(6129): 437–40.
260. Page DC, de la CA, Weissenbach J. Chromosome Y-specific DNA in related human XX males. *Nature* 1985; 315(6016): 224–6.
261. Chai NN, Phillips A, Fernandez A, Yen PH. A putative human male infertility gene DAZLA: genomic structure and methylation status. *Mol Hum Reprod* 1997; 3(8): 705–8.
262. Ruggiu M, Speed R, Taggart M et al. The mouse Dazla gene encodes a cytoplasmic protein essential for gametogenesis. *Nature* 1997; 389(6646): 73–7.
263. Saut N, Terriou P, Navarro A, Levy N, Mitchell MJ. The human Y chromosome genes BPY2, CDY1 and DAZ are not essential for sustained fertility. *Mol Hum Reprod* 2000; 6(9): 789–93.
264. Lim HN, Chen H, McBride S et al. Longer polyglutamine tracts in the androgen receptor are associated with moderate to severe undermasculinized genitalia in XY males. *Hum Mol Genet* 2000; 9(5): 829–34.
265. Tut TG, Ghadessy FJ, Trifiro MA, Pinsky L, Yong EL. Long polyglutamine tracts in the androgen receptor are associated with reduced trans-activation, impaired sperm production, and male infertility. *J Clin Endocrinol Metab* 1997; 82(11): 3777–82.
266. Yong EL, Ghadessy F, Wang Q, Mifsud A, Ng SC. Androgen receptor transactivation domain and control of spermatogenesis. *Rev Reprod* 1998; 3(3): 141–4.
267. Dadze S, Wieland C, Jakubiczka S et al. The size of the CAG repeat in exon 1 of the androgen receptor gene shows no significant relationship to impaired spermatogenesis in an infertile Caucasoid sample of German origin. *Mol Hum Reprod* 2000; 6(3): 207–14.
268. Tamai KT, Monaco L, Nantel F, Zazopoulos E, Sassone-Corsi P. Coupling signalling pathways to transcriptional control: nuclear factors responsive to cAMP. *Recent Prog Horm Res* 1997; 52: 121–39.
269. Peri A, Krausz C, Cioppi F et al. Cyclic adenosine 3`,5`-monophosphate-responsive element modulator gene expression in germ cells of normo- and oligo-azoospermic men. *J Clin Endocrinol Metab* 1998; 83(10): 3722–6.
270. Lin WW, Lamb DJ, Lipshultz LI, Kim ED. Absence of cyclic adenosine 3`:5` monophosphate responsive element modulator expression at the spermatocyte arrest stage. *Fertil Steril* 1998; 69(3): 533–8.
271. Weinbauer GF, Behr R, Bergmann M, Nieschlag E. Testicular cAMP responsive element modulator (CREM) protein is expressed in round spermatids but is absent or reduced in men with round spermatid maturation arrest. *Mol Hum Reprod* 1998; 4(1): 9–15.
272. Blendy JA, Kaestner KH, Weinbauer GF, Nieschlag E, Schutz G. Severe impairment of spermatogenesis in mice lacking the CREM gene. *Nature* 1996; 380(6570): 162–5.
273. Anguiano A, Oates RD, Amos JA et al. Congenital bilateral absence of the vas deferens. A primarily genital form of cystic fibrosis. *JAMA* 1992; 267(13): 1794–7.
274. Reijo R, Alagappan RK, Patrizio P, Page DC. Severe oligozoospermia resulting from deletions of azoospermia factor gene on Y chromosome. *Lancet* 1996; 347(9011): 1290–3.
275. Pryor JL, Kent-First M, Muallem A et al. Microdeletions in the Y chromosome of infertile men. *N Engl J Med* 1997; 336(8): 534–9.
276. Nagafuchi S, Namiki M, Nakahori Y, Kondoh N, Okuyama A, Nakagome Y. A minute deletion of the Y chromosome in men with azoospermia. *J Urol* 1993; 150(4): 1155–7.
277. Najmabadi H, Huang V, Yen P et al. Substantial prevalence of microdeletions of the Y-chromosome in

infertile men with idiopathic azoospermia and oligozoospermia detected using a sequence-tagged site-based mapping strategy. *J Clin Endocrinol Metab* 1996; **81**(4): 1347–52.

278. Henegariu O, Hirschmann P, Kilian K et al. Rapid screening of the Y chromosome in idiopathic sterile men, diagnostic for deletions in AZF, a genetic Y factor expressed during spermatogenesis. *Andrologia* 1994; **26**(2): 97–106.

279. Vogt P, Chandley AC, Hargreave TB, Keil R, Ma K, Sharkey A. Microdeletions in interval 6 of the Y chromosome of males with idiopathic sterility point to disruption of AZF, a human spermatogenesis gene. *Hum Genet* 1992; **89**(5): 491–6.

280. Martinez MC, Bernabe MJ, Gomez E et al. Screening for AZF deletion in a large series of severely impaired spermatogenesis patients. *J Androl* 2000; **21**(5): 651–5.

281. Eberhart CG, Maines JZ, Wasserman SA. Meiotic cell cycle requirement for a fly homologue of human deleted in azoospermia. *Nature* 1996; **381**(6585): 783–5.

282. Reijo R, Seligman J, Dinulos MB et al. Mouse autosomal homolog of DAZ, a candidate male sterility gene in humans, is expressed in male germ cells before and after puberty. *Genomics* 1996; **35**(2): 346–52.

283. Saxena R, Brown LG, Hawkins T et al. The DAZ gene cluster on the human Y chromosome arose from an autosomal gene that was transposed, repeatedly amplified and pruned. *Nat Genet* 1996; **14**(3): 292–9.

284. Najmabadi H, Chai N, Kapali A et al. Genomic structure of a Y-specific ribonucleic acid binding motif-containing gene: a putative candidate for a subset of male infertility. *J Clin Endocrinol Metab* 1996; **81**(6): 2159–64.

285. Cooke HJ, Lee M, Kerr S, Ruggiu M. A murine homologue of the human DAZ gene is autosomal and expressed only in male and female gonads. *Hum Mol Genet* 1996; **5**(4): 513–16.

286. Yen PH, Chai NN, Salido EC. The human autosomal gene DAZLA: testis specificity and a candidate for male infertility. *Hum Mol Genet* 1996; **5**(12): 2013–17.

287. Fradkin JE, Schonberger LB, Mills JL et al. Creutzfeldt–Jakob disease in pituitary growth hormone recipients in the United States. *JAMA* 1991; **265**(7): 880–4.

288. Abbasi AA, Prasad AS, Ortega J, Congco E, Oberleas D. Gonadal function abnormalities in sickle cell anemia. Studies in adult male patients. *Ann Intern Med* 1976; **85**(5): 601–5.

289. Kletzky OA, Costin G, Marrs RP. Gonadotropin insufficiency in patients with thalassemia major. *J Clin Endocrinol Metab* 1979; **48**(6): 901–5.

290. Takeda R, Ueda M. Pituitary–gonadal function in male patients with myotonic dystrophy—serum luteinizing hormone, follicle stimulating hormone and testosterone levels and histological damage of the testis. *Acta Endocrinol (Copenh)* 1977; **84**(2): 382–9.

291. Wennerholm UB, Bergh C, Hamberger L, Westlander G, Wikland M, Wood M. Obstetric outcome of pregnancies following ICSI, classified according to sperm origin and quality. *Hum Reprod* 2000; **15**(5): 1189–94.

292. Heller CG, Elson WO. Classification of male hypogonadism and discussion of the pathologic physiology, diagnosis and treatment. *J Clin Endocrinol Metab* 1948; **8**: 345–66.

293. MacLeod J. Restoration of human spermatogenesis by menopausal gonadotropins. *Lancet* 1964; **i**: 1196–7.

294. Santen RJ, Paulsen CA. Hypogonadotropic eunuchoidism. II. Gonadal responsiveness to exogenous gonadotropins. *J Clin Endocrinol Metab* 1973; **36**(1): 55–63.

295. Gemzell C, Kiessler G. Treatment of infertility after partial hypophysectomy with human pituitary gonadotrophins. *Lancet* 1964; **i**: 44–7.

296. Johnson SG. A study of human testicular function by the use of human menopausal gonadotropin and human chorionic gonadotropin in male hypogonadotropic eunuchoidism and infantilism. *Acta Endocrinol (Copenh)* 1966; **53**: 315–41.

297. Burgues S, Calderon MD. Subcutaneous self-administration of highly purified follicle stimulating hormone and human chorionic gonadotrophin for the treatment of male hypogonadotrophic hypogonadism. Spanish Collaborative Group on Male Hypogonadotropic Hypogonadism. *Hum Reprod* 1997; **12**(5): 980–6.

298. Recombinant Human FSH Product Development Group. Recombinant follicle stimulating hormone: development of the first biotechnology product for the treatment of infertility. *Hum Reprod Update* 1998; **4**(6): 862–81.

299. Liu PY, Turner L, Rushford D et al. Efficacy and safety of recombinant human follicle stimulating hormone (Gonal-F) with urinary human chorionic gonadotrophin for induction of spermatogenesis and fertility in gonadotrophin-deficient men. *Hum Reprod* 1999; **14**(6): 1540–5.

300. Zitzmann M, Nieschlag E. Hormone substitution in male hypogonadism. *Mol Cell Endocrinol* 2000; **161**(1–2): 73–88.

301. Smals AG, Pieters GF, Drayer JI, Benraad TJ, Kloppenborg PW. Leydig cell responsiveness to single and repeated human chorionic gonadotropin administration. *J Clin Endocrinol Metab* 1979; **49**(1): 12–14.

302. Padron RS, Wischusen J, Hudson B, Burger HG, de Kretser DM. Prolonged biphasic response of plasma testosterone to single intramuscular injections of human chorionic gonadotropin. *J Clin Endocrinol Metab* 1980; **50**(6): 1100–4.

303. Saez JM, Forest MG. Kinetics of human chorionic gonadotropin-induced steroidogenic response of the human testis. I. Plasma testosterone: implications for human chorionic gonadotropin stimulation test. *J Clin Endocrinol Metab* 1979; 49(2): 278–83.

304. Wang C, Paulsen CA, Hopper BR. Acute steroidogenic responsiveness to human luteinizing hormone in hypogonadotropic hypogonadism. *J Clin Endocrinol Metab* 1980; 51(6): 1269–73.

305. Hoffman AR, Crowley WF Jr. Induction of puberty in men by long-term pulsatile administration of low-dose gonadotropin-releasing hormone. *N Engl J Med* 1982; 307(20): 1237–41.

306. Whitcomb RW, Crowley WF Jr. Male hypogonadotropic hypogonadism. *Endocrinol Metab Clin North Am* 1993; 22(1): 125–43.

307. Burger HG, Baker HW. The treatment of infertility. *Annu Rev Med* 1987; 38: 29–40.

308. Bourne H, Stern K, Clarke G, Pertile M, Speirs A, Baker HW. Delivery of normal twins following the intracytoplasmic injection of spermatozoa from a patient with 47,XXY Klinefelter's syndrome. *Hum Reprod* 1997; 12(11): 2447–50.

309. Bergada C, Mancini RE. Effect of gonadotropins on the induction of spermatogenesis in human prepubertal testis. *J Clin Endocrinol Metab* 1973; 37(6): 935–43.

310. Mancini RE, Seiguer AC, Lloret AP. Effect of gonadotropins on the recovery of spermatogenesis in hypophysectomized patients. *J Clin Endocrinol Metab* 1969; 29(4): 467–78.

311. Liu L, Banks SM, Barnes KM, Sherins RJ. Two-year comparison of testicular responses to pulsatile gonadotropin-releasing hormone and exogenous gonadotropins from the inception of therapy in men with isolated hypogonadotropic hypogonadism. *J Clin Endocrinol Metab* 1988; 67(6): 1140–5.

312. Buchter D, Behre HM, Kliesch S, Nieschlag E. Pulsatile GnRH or human chorionic gonadotropin/human menopausal gonadotropin as effective treatment for men with hypogonadotropic hypogonadism: a review of 42 cases. *Eur J Endocrinol* 1998; 139(3): 298–303.

313. Kliesch S, Behre HM, Nieschlag E. High efficacy of gonadotropin or pulsatile gonadotropin-releasing hormone treatment in hypogonadotropic hypogonadal men. *Eur J Endocrinol* 1994; 131(4): 347–54.

314. Braunstein GD, Bloch SK, Rasor JL, Winikoff J. Characterization of antihuman chorionic gonadotropin serum antibody appearing after ovulation induction. *J Clin Endocrinol Metab* 1983; 57(6): 1164–72.

315. Nieschlag E, Bernitz S, Topert M. Antigenicity of human chorionic gonadotrophin preparations in men. *Clin Endocrinol (Oxf)* 1982; 16(5): 483–8.

316. Sokol RZ, McClure RD, Peterson M, Swerdloff RS. Gonadotropin therapy failure secondary to human chorionic gonadotropin-induced antibodies. *J Clin Endocrinol Metab* 1981; 52(5): 929–32.

317. Claustrat B, David L, Faure A, Francois R. Development of anti-human chorionic gonadotropin antibodies in patients with hypogonadotropic hypogonadism. A study of four patients. *J Clin Endocrinol Metab* 1983; 57(5): 1041–7.

318. Burger HG, de Kretser DM, Hudson B, Wilson JD. Effects of preceding androgen therapy on testicular response to human pituitary gonadotropin in hypogonadotropic hypogonadism: a study of three patients. *Fertil Steril* 1981; 35(1): 64–8.

319. Belchetz PE, Plant TM, Nakai Y, Keogh EJ, Knobil E. Hypophysial responses to continuous and intermittent delivery of hypothalamic gonadotropin-releasing hormone. *Science* 1978; 202(4368): 631–3.

320. Knobil E. The neuroendocrine control of the menstrual cycle. *Recent Prog Horm Res* 1980; 36: 53–88.

321. Wildt L, Hausler A, Marshall G et al. Frequency and amplitude of gonadotropin-releasing hormone stimulation and gonadotropin secretion in the rhesus monkey. *Endocrinology* 1981; 109(2): 376–85.

322. Spratt DI, Hoffman AR, Crowley WF Jr. Hypogonadotropic hypogonadism. In: Santen RJ, Swerdloff RS, eds. *Male Reproductive Dysfunction*. New York: Marcel Dekker, Inc, 1986: 227–49.

323. Moore MP, Smith R, Donald RA, Espiner EA, Stronach S. The effects of different dose regimes of D-SER(TBU)6-LHRH-EA10 (HOE 766) in subjects with hypogonadotrophic hypogonadism. *Clin Endocrinol (Oxf)* 1981; 14(1): 93–7.

324. Laron Z, Dickerman Z, Ben Zeev Z, Prager-Lewin R, Comaru-Schally AM, Schally AV. Long-term effect of D-Trp6-luteinizing hormone-releasing hormone on testicular size and luteinizing hormone, follicle-stimulating hormone, and testosterone levels in hypothalamic hypogonadotropic males. *Fertil Steril* 1981; 35(3): 328–31.

325. Vickery BH. Comparison of the potential for therapeutic utilities with gonadotropin-releasing hormone agonists and antagonists. *Endocrine Rev* 1986; 7(1): 115–24.

326. Spratt DI, Finkelstein JS, O'Dea LS et al. Long-term administration of gonadotropin-releasing hormone in men with idiopathic hypogonadotropic hypogonadism. A model for studies of the hormone's physiologic effects. *Ann Intern Med* 1986; 105(6): 848–55.

327. Palermo GD, Schlegel PN, Hariprashad JJ et al. Fertilization and pregnancy outcome with intracytoplasmic sperm injection for azoospermic men. *Hum Reprod* 1999; 14(3): 741–8.

328. Palermo GD, Schlegel PN, Sills ES et al. Births after intracytoplasmic injection of sperm obtained by testicular extraction from men with nonmosaic Klinefelter's syndrome. *N Engl J Med* 1998; 338(9): 588–90.

329. Crosignani PG, Rubin BL. Optimal use of infertility diagnostic tests and treatments. The ESHRE Capri Workshop Group. *Hum Reprod* 2000; 15(3): 723–32.
330. Ismail MT, Sedor J, Hirsch IH. Are sperm motion parameters influenced by varicocele ligation? *Fertil Steril* 1999; 71(5): 886–90.
331. Nieschlag E, Hertle L, Fischedick A, Abshagen K, Behre HM. Update on treatment of varicocele: counselling as effective as occlusion of the vena spermatica. *Hum Reprod* 1998; 13(8): 2147–50.
332. Culha M, Mutlu N, Acar O, Baykal M. Comparison of testicular volumes before and after varicocelectomy. *Urol Int* 1998; 60(4): 220–3.
333. Asci R, Sarikaya S, Buyukalpelli R, Yilmaz AF, Yildiz S. The outcome of varicocelectomy in subfertile men with an absent or atrophic right testis. *Br J Urol* 1998; 81(5): 750–2.
334. Segenreich E, Israilov S, Shmuele J, Niv E, Baniel J, Livne P. Evaluation of the relationship between semen parameters, pregnancy rate of wives of infertile men with varicocele, and gonadotropin-releasing hormone test before and after varicocelectomy. *Urology* 1998; 52(5): 853–7.
335. Tarlatzis BC, Bili H. Intracytoplasmic sperm injection. Survey of world results. *Ann NY Acad Sci* 2000; 900: 336–44.
336. Bonduelle M, Camus M, De Vos A et al. Seven years of intracytoplasmic sperm injection and follow-up of 1987 subsequent children. *Hum Reprod* 1999; 14(suppl 1): 243–64.
337. Wennerholm UB, Bergh C, Hamberger L et al. Incidence of congenital malformations in children born after ICSI. *Hum Reprod* 2000; 15(4): 944–8.
338. Devroey P, Vandervorst M, Nagy P et al. Do we treat the male or his gamete? *Hum Reprod* 1998; 13(suppl 1): 178–85.

9

Hirsutism and virilization
Frances J Hayes, Janet E Hall

Definition

Hirsutism is the occurrence in a woman of terminal hair in a distribution characteristic of an adult male. Such androgen-dependent hair is typically coarse, dark and curly. This type of hair pattern contrasts with hypertrichosis, which is characterized by a uniform increase in soft, downy hair which is not androgen-mediated and may be familial or drug-induced. It is important for clinicians to make the distinction between androgen-dependent and androgen-independent abnormal hair growth, as the latter can only be treated by cosmetic measures and does not respond to anti-androgen therapy.

Isolated hirsutism is a common presenting complaint which, although often very distressing for the patient, rarely signifies an underlying malignancy. While initially thought to represent a purely cosmetic defect, it is now recognized that hirsutism may in fact be associated with increased morbidity due to its frequent association with characteristic metabolic abnormalities, including hyperinsulinemia, insulin resistance, and hyperlipidemia.[1] These features are linked to an increased risk of type 2 diabetes in later life and, potentially, a higher prevalence of premature cardiovascular disease.[2,3] Virilization is the combination of hirsutism with other signs of masculinization, e.g. temporal recession, increased muscle mass, clitoromegaly, deepening of the voice, or decrease in breast size. Virilization is much less common than hirsutism, but its presence always mandates a thorough evaluation, as it may reflect an underlying malignancy.

Prevalence

It has been difficult to ascertain the exact prevalence of hirsutism in the general population, owing both to ethnic variation and a lack of consistency in the definition of hirsutism. Genetic factors play an important role in determining both the number of hair follicles per unit area of skin and their sensitivity to androgens. Thus, any estimate of the prevalence of hirsutism will depend on the ethnic background of the population being studied; for example, two women of different races may have similar degrees of androgen excess yet have a markedly different phenotype in terms of hair growth.[4] In general, women of Mediterranean descent tend to have more body hair than Asian or Native American women. The second difficulty relates to the individual assessment of what constitutes hirsutism. As there is a wide spectrum in tolerance of facial and body hair, due to social and cultural factors, only a portion of hirsute women will present for medical evaluation. In those patients who come to medical attention, there is frequently a poor correlation between the perception of the patient and the physician as to what constitutes abnormal hair growth.

Location	Percentage
Arms and legs	84
Upper lip	26
Chin	10
Periareolar	17
Sternum	3
Upper abdomen	0
Upper back	0

Data derived from a cross-sectional study of 430 normal women.[5]

Table 9.1
Terminal hair distribution in normal women.

Site	Grade	Definition
1. Upper Lip	1	A few hairs at the outer margin
	2	A small moustache at the outer margin
	3	A moustache extending halfway from the outer margin
	4	A moustache extending to the midline
2. Chin	1	A few scattered hairs
	2	Scattered hairs with small concentrations
	3 and 4	Complete cover, light and heavy
3. Chest	1	Circumareolar hairs
	2	With midline in addition
	3	Fusion of these areas, with three-quarters cover
	4	Complete cover
4. Upper back	1	A few scattered hairs
	2	Rather more, still scattered
	3 and 4	Complete cover, light and heavy
5. Lower back	1	A sacral tuft of hair
	2	With some lateral extension
	3	Three-quarters cover
	4	Complete cover
6. Upper abdomen	1	A few midline hairs
	2	Rather more, still midline
	3 and 4	Half and full cover
7. Lower abdomen	1	A few midline hairs
	2	A midline streak of hair
	3	A midline band of hair
	4	An inverted V-shaped growth
8. Arm	1	Sparse growth affecting not more than a quarter of the limb surface
	2	More than this; cover still incomplete
	3 and 4	Complete cover, light and heavy
9. Forearm	1, 2, 3, 4	Complete cover of dorsal surface; 2 grades and 2 of heavy growth
10. Thigh	1, 2, 3, 4	As for arm
11. Leg	1, 2, 3, 4	As for arm

Table 9.2
Semiquantitative assessment of hirsutism using the Ferriman–Gallwey score.

An understanding of normal terminal hair distribution is essential in assessing the hirsute patient. In a cross-sectional study of 430 women presenting to hospital for non-endocrine problems in the UK,[5] Ferriman and Gallwey demonstrated that most women have terminal hair on the forearm and legs, and approximately 25% have hair on the upper lip (Table 9.1). In contrast, normal women almost never have terminal hair on the upper back or upper abdomen, and only 3% and 10% respectively have terminal hair on the sternum and chin.[5] The pattern of hair growth changes with age. Stratification of women by decades from 15 to 74 years indicates that the natural history of hirsutism is to gradually worsen until menopause, after which time body hair decreases, although facial hair continues to increase.[5]

In 1961, Ferriman and Gallwey devised what has become the most widely used scoring system for hirsutism.[5] This semiquantitative method of assessment assigns a score of 1–4 for 11 different body sites (Table 9.2). Given the frequency with which terminal hair is present on the forearm and lower leg, these two sites are often excluded, and a modified 'hormonal score' is calculated using the remaining nine body sites. Using this modified Ferriman and Gallwey method of assessment, 4.3% of the 430 women studied were hirsute if a cutoff score >7 was used.[5] In another study of 400 European college students, 9% considered themselves to have excess hair, although only 4% had sought medical evaluation and treatment for their hirsutism.[6] In a recent study of an unbiased population of women of reproductive age in the USA, 8% of white women and 7% of black women had a modified Ferriman–Gallwey score >6.[7]

Differential diagnosis

The vast majority of women presenting with hirsutism have either idiopathic hirsutism or polycystic ovary syndrome (PCOS). Features that suggest a more sinister cause of hirsutism include onset outside the decade between 15 and 25 years, rapid progression, the presence of virilizing signs, or symptoms or evidence of glucocorticoid excess.[8] In these circumstances, it is important to screen specifically for non-classic congenital adrenal hyperplasia, androgen-secreting ovarian or adrenal tumors, or Cushing's syndrome (Table 9.3).

Combined adrenal and ovarian
   Idiopathic hirsutism
   Polycystic ovary syndrome
Adrenal
   Congenital adrenal hyperplasia
   Cushing's syndrome
   Androgen-secreting adrenal tumors
Ovarian
   Androgen-secreting ovarian tumors
     Sertoli–Leydig cell
     Granulosa-theca cell
     Hyperthecosis ovarii
   Insulin resistance syndromes
Exogenous androgens
   Anabolic steroids
   Norgestrel-containing oral contraceptives
   Danazol

Table 9.3:
Differential diagnosis of hirsutism in women.

Idiopathic hirsutism and polycystic ovary syndrome

Idiopathic hirsutism and PCOS are closely related conditions, and may well form a continuum, with idiopathic hirsutism representing the milder end of the spectrum. Idiopathic hirsutism is the occurrence of hirsutism in women who continue to ovulate regularly. In contrast, the hallmark of PCOS is oligo- or anovulation associated with either clinical or biochemical evidence of androgen excess in the absence of specific underlying diseases (NIH Consensus Criteria).[9] Thus, it is the presence of menstrual abnormalities that distinguishes women with PCOS from those with idiopathic hirsutism. However, isolated hyperandrogenism with regular menstrual cycles occurs frequently in the sisters of women with PCOS.[10]

Typically, patients with idiopathic hirsutism or PCOS present between 15 and 25 years with hirsutism that is slowly progressive. Often there is a history of symptoms beginning or worsening after weight gain or discontinuation of the birth control pill. Hirsutism is accompanied by acne in approximately 25% of patients,[11] but virilization is very rare. Up to 22% of sisters of PCOS patients fulfill the diagnostic criteria for PCOS, underscoring the importance of genetic factors in the etiology of this disorder.[10] Many women with PCOS are obese and have acanthosis nigricans. Acanthosis nigricans is a cutaneous manifestation of insulin resistance, characterized by thickening and hyperpigmentation of the skin, most commonly at the nape of the neck and in the axillae, and often associated with skin tags.[12] In recent years, increasing evidence has accumulated to support an important etiologic role for insulin in the hyperandrogenism of PCOS.[1] Both insulin resistance and hyperinsulinemia have been demonstrated in women with PCOS, independent of obesity.[13–15] As a consequence of insulin resistance, glucose intolerance is common in PCOS, with 20–40% of obese PCOS women having either impaired glucose tolerance or frank diabetes,[1,16] compared with the rate of 5–10% reported in population-based studies in women of this age.[17] Unlike PCOS subjects, women with idiopathic hirsutism, even those with polycystic ovary morphology on ultrasound, tend not to be insulin resistant.[18,19] In addition to hirsutism, many women with PCOS seek medical attention because of the clinical consequences of anovulation, including oligomenorrhea, amenorrhea, dysfunctional uterine bleeding and infertility.

Congenital adrenal hyperplasia

Congenital adrenal hyperplasia (CAH) is an autosomal recessive disorder characterized by inadequate glucocorticoid production due to mutations in the enzymes involved in steroidogenesis.[20] More than 90% of cases are due to deficiency of 21-hydroxylase, the enzyme necessary to convert 17-hydroxyprogesterone to 11-deoxycortisol. The molecular basis of this disease involves a mutation in the *CYP21* gene located on chromosome 6p21.3 (for review see Speiser and White[21]). While the classic 'salt-wasting' and 'simple virilizing' forms of CAH present in the neonatal period, the phenotypic expression of CAH is now known to include a non-classic adult-onset form which may present for the first time at puberty with signs of androgen excess. The typical clinical features of late-onset CAH are hirsutism (77%) and oligomenorrhea (68%), making it indistinguishable from PCOS.[22] Approximately one-third of these patients have polycystic ovary morphology on ultrasound examination.[22] The frequency of non-classic CAH in unselected hirsute women is generally <1%.[23] However, in certain high-risk groups such as Ashkenazi Jews, the likelihood of a hirsute woman having non-classic CAH may vary from 4% to 15%.[24,25] Less commonly, non-classic CAH may be due to deficiencies in the 11-hydroxylase or 3-β-hydroxysteroid dehydrogenase enzymes.[26]

Cushing's syndrome

Hirsutism and menstrual irregularity are present in 55–80% of women with Cushing's syndrome.[27] These symptoms may be observed in Cushing's syndrome caused by pituitary adrenocorticotropic hormone (ACTH) excess (Cushing's disease), ectopic ACTH-secreting tumors or adrenal adenomas, and carcinomas. In women with hirsutism secondary to Cushing's disease, the clinical presentation is usually dominated by features of glucocorticoid excess, including facial plethora, truncal obesity, easy bruising, abdominal striae and proximal myopathy. While the development of hirsutism in patients with Cushing's disease reflects mild androgen excess, the disturbance in menstrual function correlates better with the degree of hypercortisolemia than with circulating androgen levels.[28] Thus, the mechanism underlying the menstrual abnormalities in women with Cushing's disease appears to be impaired hypothalamic secretion of gonadotropin-releasing hormone as a consequence of chronic hypercortisolemia rather than an effect of high androgen levels.[28] In ectopic ACTH-secreting tumors, hirsutism is seen in up to 70% of women.[29] In those cases due to oat cell carcinoma of the lung, the clinical course is often too rapidly progressive for the typical signs of hypercortisolemia to emerge, and the major clinical manifestations are hypertension, weakness and hyperpigmentation.[29]

Benign and malignant adrenal tumors may also hypersecrete cortisol and androgens, giving rise to Cushing's syndrome accompanied by hirsutism and virilization. Adrenal carcinomas tend to present acutely with virilization that is rapidly progressive.[30] In some of these adrenal tumors, secretion of cortisol is entirely normal.[31] In others, the anabolic effect of androgens may protect against the development of the usual catabolic features of glucocorticoid excess, e.g. easy bruising, myopathy and osteoporosis. Levels of androstenedione, dehydroepiandrosterone sulfate (DHEAS), cortisol, testosterone and urinary 17-ketosteroids tend to be markedly elevated. However, it is important to bear in mind that urinary 17-ketosteroids will be normal in the setting of the occasional adrenal tumor which secretes primarily testosterone, as the latter is responsible for less than 1% of total urinary 17-ketosteroids.[32] In addition, the absence of an elevated

DHEAS level does not exclude an adrenal tumor, as some tumors lack the sulfatase necessary to convert dehydroepiandrosterone (DHEA) to DHEAS.[31,33] Given that steroid production is often inefficient in adrenal carcinomas, there is often disproportionate elevation of steroid precursors, e.g. 11-deoxycortisol. The presence of an adrenal mass can usually be confirmed by computerized tomography. However, given the high prevalence of adrenal incidentalomas,[34] the presence of a small adrenal mass in a virilized woman does not warrant adrenalectomy unless the ovaries have been visualized and found to be free of masses.

Androgen-secreting ovarian tumors

Androgen-secreting ovarian tumors are uncommon, accounting for less than 5% of ovarian tumors.[35] The most common ovarian tumors to cause virilization are Sertoli–Leydig cell tumors, hilus cell tumors and granulosa-theca cell tumors.[35] Virilization may also result from benign tumors or cysts stimulating androgen secretion from the adjacent normal ovarian stroma or from hilus cell hyperplasia.[35,36] The typical clinical presentation is that of an abrupt onset of hirsutism and virilization, which may occur at any age. A unilateral adnexal mass may be palpable. However, many tumors, particularly hilus cell tumors, which tend to occur in postmenopausal women, are too small to allow clinical detection.

Hyperthecosis ovarii

Hyperthecosis ovarii is a benign disorder of the ovaries characterized histologically by the presence of nests of luteinized theca cells in a hyperplastic ovarian stroma. Opinion is divided as to whether hyperthecosis constitutes a distinct syndrome or whether it represents the most severe end of the spectrum of PCOS. It is manifest clinically as virilization and menstrual disturbance. While hyperthecosis may occur at any age, it is most commonly seen in postmenopausal women.[37] Insulin resistance is a prominent feature.[38,39] While there is considerable clinical overlap with PCOS, patients with hyperthecosis differ in that they are usually severely hirsute and may be virilized. In addition, while the ovaries in hyperthecosis are enlarged, they are not typically polycystic. Serum levels of testosterone and androstenedione tend to be markedly elevated. However, the slow progression of symptoms distinguishes hyperthecosis from a malignant androgen-secreting tumor. In the past, many patients with hyperthecosis required bilateral oophorectomy to halt the progressive virilization. However, there have been a number of case reports documenting improvement in hirsutism and suppression of androgen levels in women with hyperthecosis using gonadotropin-releasing hormone (GnRH) agonists.[39,40]

Insulin resistance syndromes

Several syndromes have been described that are characterized by profound insulin resistance, diabetes mellitus, acanthosis nigricans, and hyperandrogenism.[41] The type A syndrome occurs in adolescent girls and is characterized by marked virilization and very high insulin levels, due in some cases to mutations in the insulin receptor.[42] The type B syndrome is due to endogenous anti-insulin receptor antibodies and has been described in postmenopausal women who present with acanthosis nigricans and features of autoimmune disease.[43]

Normal androgen production

In women, the most potent androgens are testosterone and its metabolite, dihydrotestosterone (DHT). DHT is derived from testosterone by the action of the enzyme 5α-reductase in the skin. The greater potency of DHT results from its greater affinity for the androgen receptor. Additional circulating androgens include androstenedione, DHEA and DHEAS, which are derived primarily from the adrenal gland. These weaker androgens are more properly considered androgen precursors that require conversion to testosterone in peripheral tissues for biological activity. Approximately 50% of testosterone is derived from peripheral conversion of androstenedione, with the remainder arising in approximately equal amounts from the adrenals and ovaries. Testosterone circulates bound to sex hormone-binding globulin (SHBG) and, to a lesser extent, albumin, so that normally only 1% is free. Therefore, changes in SHBG (increased by estrogens and thyroid hormone; decreased by androgens and insulin) may alter the free or biologically active hormone. Thus, measurement of free testosterone is often a better marker of androgenic activity in obese women, who tend to have low SHBG levels due to the combination of high androgen and insulin levels.[44]

Pathophysiology

Hirsutism reflects increased androgen exposure due to an increase in serum androgen levels and/or increased sensitivity to androgens at the level of the hair follicle. An increase in serum androgen levels may result from increased ovarian or adrenal androgen secretion or both. In women with hirsutism and normal serum androgen levels, with or without menstrual irregularity, an increase in the sensitivity of the pilosebaceous unit to androgens has been invoked to explain their excess body hair. Some investigators have reported an increase in 5α-reductase activity, increased levels of the DHT metabolite 5α-androstane-3α, 17β-diol glucuronide and an increase in the number of androgen receptors in this subset of hirsute women.[45,46]

The precise glandular source of the excess androgen production in women with hirsutism is somewhat controversial, due to the difficulty in completely compartmentalizing ovarian from adrenal function. Catheterization studies have yielded conflicting results. Some studies have suggested that the ovary is the predominant source of androgen excess in women with both idiopathic hirsutism[47] and PCOS.[48] A key role for the ovary was subsequently confirmed by the demonstration that selective ovarian androgen suppression using GnRH agonists reduces serum androgens in women with PCOS to the levels seen in oophorectomized women.[49–51] However, several lines of evidence suggest that hypersecretion of adrenal androgens also contributes to hyperandrogenism in PCOS.[52] Some investigators have demonstrated a significant adrenal venous gradient for both testosterone and androstenedione.[53,54] In certain populations, approximately 50% of PCOS patients have elevated adrenal androgens, particularly DHEAS.[4,55,56] In addition, a number of studies have shown excessive androstenedione, DHEA and testosterone responses to stimulation by exogenous ACTH or metyrapone.[52,57] Recent data confirm that the elevated DHEAS levels in women with PCOS are due to intrinsic hyperresponsiveness of the adrenal cortex, rather than to abnormalities of its hypothalamic–pituitary control.[58] Whether the increased responsiveness of adrenal androgens to ACTH is secondary to an increase in the zona reticularis mass or to abnormalities in P450c17 activity has yet to be elucidated. Recent data indicate that the exaggerated adrenal response to physiological ACTH stimulation is abolished by GnRH agonist administration, suggesting that ovarian estrogen secretion may be responsible for inducing increased P450c17 activity in PCOS.[59]

The underlying mechanism for androgen excess in PCOS is still unclear. Various investigators have suggested: (1) a neuroendocrine defect characterized by increased GnRH pulse frequency and enhanced pituitary responsiveness to GnRH; (2) a primary abnormality in ovarian and/or adrenal steroidogenesis; or (3) a defect in insulin action.

The luteinizing hormone hypothesis

While the pathophysiology of PCOS awaits definitive elucidation, considerable evidence supports the importance of abnormal gonadotropin secretory dynamics in this disorder.[60] In a large unbiased sample of PCOS patients, selected independently of gonadotropin levels or ovarian morphology, all of the non-obese and 91% of the obese anovulatory subjects were found to have an elevated luteinizing hormone (LH) to follicle-stimulating hormone (FSH) ratio compared to early-follicular-phase controls.[61] It is likely that the site of the defect in gonadotropin secretion resides at the levels of both the hypothalamus (increased GnRH secretion) and the pituitary (increased gonadotropin sensitivity to GnRH).

The demonstration of an increased LH pulse frequency in most frequent sampling studies of women with PCOS,[61–64] suggests that at least a portion of the gonadotropin defect occurs at the level of the hypothalamus. One school of thought proposes that the elevated LH/FSH ratio in PCOS might result from an increased GnRH pulse frequency, based on studies of GnRH-deficient men.[65] In this model, an increase in the frequency of a fixed and physiological dose of exogenous GnRH sustained over time resulted in a similar increase in mean LH levels with little change in FSH.[66] The applicability of this 'frequency hypothesis' to PCOS is supported by the correlation between GnRH-induced LH pulse frequency and both pool LH and the LH to FSH ratio.[61] However, it is likely that additional factors such as the abnormal sex steroid milieu also contribute to the disparity in gonadotropin levels in PCOS, as estrone administration has been shown to suppress FSH levels, while having no effect on LH.[67]

In addition to a fast LH pulse frequency, PCOS is characterized by an increase in LH pulse amplitude.[61–63,68] The increased LH pulse amplitude could reflect either increased stimulation by GnRH or enhanced pituitary sensitivity. However, recent data from our group suggest that the overall quantity of GnRH is not increased in women with PCOS.[69] We used the Nal-Glu GnRH antagonist to provide a semiquantitative estimate of endogenous GnRH secretion in PCOS by determining the effect of competition between GnRH and the antagonist at the GnRH receptor. Using this approach and taking LH as a marker of GnRH action, the amount of GnRH secreted is inversely proportional to the degree of LH inhibition. The GnRH antagonist study demonstrated that the susceptibility of LH to GnRH receptor blockade is in fact similar in normal and PCOS women.[69] Therefore, it appears that it is enhanced sensitivity to endogenous GnRH rather than an increase in the overall amount of GnRH secreted that is responsible for the increase in LH pulse amplitude in PCOS. This interpretation is supported by the exaggerated response of women with PCOS both to exogenous GnRH[68] and to GnRH agonists.[70]

An understanding of the normal mechanism of ovarian androgen synthesis provides an explanation for how the increased LH levels and elevated LH to FSH ratio contribute to excess ovarian androgen production. Ovarian androgens, mainly androstenedione and, to a lesser extent, testosterone, are produced in the theca cells in response to LH stimulation. These androgens then diffuse into the granulosa cells, where they are converted to estrone and estradiol by aromatase in the presence of FSH. Therefore, in PCOS, the high LH to FSH ratio stimulates excessive production of androgenic substrates, which, in the presence of low to normal levels of FSH, are not adequately aromatized to estrogen.

The ovarian hypothesis

The ovarian hypothesis proposes that a primary defect in sex steroid synthesis or metabolism results in exaggerated ovarian androgen secretion, which in turn gives rise to anovulation. In PCOS, the ovaries have a classic morphological appearance characterized by a ring of small (≤8 mm) peripheral follicles with an increased amount of central stroma.[71] However, the demonstration of polycystic ovary morphology is not helpful in excluding other causes of hyperandrogenism, as the same ovarian morphology is seen in women with hyperandrogenism associated with other disorders, including congenital adrenal hyperplasia, adrenal tumors and exogenous androgen administration. The lack of specificity of polycystic ovary morphology for PCOS is further supported by the demonstration that 83% of women with idiopathic hirsutism, i.e. hirsutism and regular ovulatory cycles,[71] and 23% of regularly menstruating women[72] have this morphology. Interestingly, the presence of polycystic ovaries in regularly cycling women is associated with a mild elevation in both ovarian and adrenal androgens compared with women with regular cycles and normal morphology.[73]

Women with PCOS are known to have increased levels of the androgenic precursor 17-hydroxy progesterone, both basally and after stimulation with GnRH, GnRH agonists,[74] and human chorionic gonadotropin (hCG).[75] Rosenfield et al have proposed that the elevated 17-hydroxy progesterone levels seen in PCOS reflect increased activity of cytochrome P450c17, the enzyme which catalyzes the rate-limiting step in androgen biosynthesis.[76]

The insulin hypothesis

In recent years, increasing evidence has accumulated to support an important etiological role for insulin in the hyperandrogenism of PCOS.[1] A number of groups have demonstrated the presence of insulin resistance and hyperinsulinemia in PCOS women, independent of obesity.[13–15] It may seem paradoxical to invoke insulin-stimulated androgen production as a mechanism for hyperandrogenism in an insulin-resistant state like PCOS. However, it appears that while the signaling pathways that regulate carbohydrate metabolism are impaired, those involved in steroidogenesis are preserved.[1] Insulin has been shown to augment the androgen response to LH in human ovarian interstitial tissue in vitro.[77] In addition, positive correlations have been observed between circulating concentrations of androgens and insulin in many studies.[78–80] However, the most compelling evidence for the role of insulin in stimulating androgen secretion comes from studies using agents that either lower insulin levels, e.g. diazoxide,[81] or improve insulin sensitivity, e.g. metformin[82–85] and troglitazone.[86,87] All but two of these studies[84,85] documented a fall in serum androgen levels in response to a lowering of insulin, although it is possible that the decrease in androgens may be secondary to recent ovulation rather than a primary effect. The molecular basis for the insulin defect in PCOS has not yet been fully elucidated. Insulin receptor number and affinity have been shown to be normal, suggesting a post-binding defect in insulin receptor signaling.[88] In approximately 50% of women with PCOS, decreased insulin receptor autophosphorylation has been observed.[88] This is due to markedly increased basal autophosphorylation with minimal further insulin-stimulated autophosphorylation. Serine phosphorylation of the receptor impairs insulin action by inhibiting the receptor's tyrosine kinase activity. Increased insulin-independent serine phosphorylation of the insulin receptor appears to be a unique disorder of insulin action in PCOS and has not been described in other insulin-resistant states such as obesity or type 2 diabetes mellitus.[1]

Evaluation

History

A careful history is key to the evaluation of the hirsute patient by helping to exclude serious underlying disorders and by directing appropriate laboratory testing. The time course of hirsutism is one of the most critical elements of the history. Onset of symptoms outside the peripubertal period is highly suggestive of a pathological cause of hirsutism. Independent of age of onset, hirsutism that is rapidly progressive or accompanied by features of virilization is worrisome and mandates thorough evaluation. A medication history should specifically exclude use of anabolic steroids or drugs known to have androgenic side-effects (Table 9.3). Family history may suggest an increased likelihood of CAH or may be consistent with PCOS.

Physical examination

A scoring system such as that proposed by Ferriman and Gallwey is useful in documenting both the degree and distribution of androgen-dependent hair growth.[5] Skin examination should also document the presence of acne as well as clinical evidence of metabolic abnormalities, including acanthosis nigricans and xanthomata. It is important to look specifically for features of virilization, including frontal balding, increased muscle mass, and clitoromegaly. A clitoral index (length × width) >35 mm^2 is considered abnormal.[89] Blood pressure should be checked, given the increased prevalence of hypertension in Cushing's syndrome, and careful attention paid to other signs of glucocorticoid excess, including facial plethora, centripetal obesity, dorsal fat pad, supraclavicular filling, purple striae and proximal myopathy. Adrenal and ovarian masses should be sought by careful abdominal and pelvic examination.

Hormonal evaluation

Given the prevalence of hirsutism in the general population and the fact that it is rarely associated with sinister causes, there is a high potential for unnecessary investigation. It is important, therefore, to strike a balance between initiating a major diagnostic work-up in all hirsute women, and doing so little that serious underlying conditions, which require specific intervention, go unrecognized.

Diagnostic tests

Testosterone

In women presenting with the classical features of idiopathic hirsutism or PCOS as previously outlined, hormonal evaluation is usually unnecessary, because few such women have a serious underlying disorder. However, a modest evaluation may be undertaken in these circumstances to provide a baseline against which the impact of intervention can be assessed. In this clinical setting, measurement of total testosterone or an index of free testosterone such as the testosterone/SHBG ratio is the most appropriate test.

Total testosterone is the best-validated screening test for excluding an androgen-secreting ovarian tumor. It is generally accepted that a total testosterone level above 200 ng/dl (7 nmol/l) has a high sensitivity but low specificity for identifying androgen-secreting tumors.[90] Using this testosterone cutoff value alone, the yield of finding a tumor is estimated to be only about 10%.[91] This may be partly explained by the fact that over an 8-h period of frequent sampling, testosterone values may vary by up to 40%.[91] Therefore, sole reliance on the testosterone level without taking into account the clinical context may be misleading. By the same token, if testosterone levels are not markedly elevated but there is clinical evidence of virilization, further evaluation is warranted. The ovarian status of the patient is also very important, as postmenopausal women secrete lower levels of androgens. Therefore, in postmenopausal women, testosterone levels greater than 100 ng/dl and androstenedione levels of over 2 ng/ml should be investigated further.[92]

Hirsute women tend to have higher levels of free testosterone for any given level of total testosterone than do normal women, as a consequence of suppressed SHBG levels.[93] However, the assays for free testosterone are not well validated, and the results obtained may vary significantly with the method employed. As an alternative to a free testosterone measurement, an indirect index of the biologically active testosterone fraction can be reliably obtained by measuring both total testosterone and SHBG levels.

Adrenal androgens

Mild to moderate elevations in DHEAS levels are seen in many women with PCOS. However, routine measurement of DHEAS is not indicated in the evaluation of hirsute women in the absence of features suggestive of an adrenal tumor, i.e. hirsutism that is rapidly progressive or associated with virilizing features. Serum DHEAS levels greater than 700 μg/dl (19 μmol/l) are suggestive of an adrenal tumor. However, a normal DHEAS value does not exclude this diagnosis, as occasional tumors lack the sulfatase enzyme necessary to convert DHEA to DHEAS.[31,33] In addition, it is critical that DHEAS levels be interpreted in the light of the patient's age. Secretion of DHEAS begins to decline after approximately 30 years of age.[94] Therefore, age-specific reference ranges are required to interpret any DHEAS value. Urinary 17-ketosteroids are a better marker of integrated adrenal androgen secretion than DHEAS, particularly when attempting to exclude an adrenal tumor.

17-Hydroxyprogesterone (17-OHP)

If there is a suspicion of congenital adrenal hyperplasia, either because of a positive family history or because the patient is from a high-risk ethnic group, 21-hydroxylase deficiency may be excluded by measuring a basal serum level between 0700 and 0900 hours in the follicular phase of the menstrual cycle. A basal 17-OHP value less than 200 ng/dl (6 nmol/l) excludes non-classic CAH.[22] It is important to measure 17-OHP in the early morning to avoid false negative results due to the circadian decrease in 17-OHP that parallels that of cortisol and ACTH. In addition, in cycling women, the sample should be drawn in the follicular phase to avoid false positives due to increased 17-OHP production by the corpus luteum. If these conditions cannot be met or if the basal 17-OHP level obtained under these conditions exceeds 200 ng/dl, an ACTH stimulation test should be performed. A positive test consists of a 60-min value greater than 1000 ng/dl (30 nmol/l) following intravenous administration of 250 μg of ACTH.[22,95]

Ovarian ultrasound

If an ovarian tumor is suspected, the preferred method of localization is high-resolution transvaginal ultrasound, which is capable of detecting lesions as small as 2–3 mm. Suspicious findings include large or complex cysts that do not regress on repeat scanning. Ultrasound may also be used to identify the classic ovarian morphology of PCOS.[71] However, it is important to bear in mind that this morphology is not specific for PCOS.

Screening for glucocorticoid excess

Testing for Cushing's syndrome should be performed in women with clinical evidence of glucocorticoid excess and can take the form of either an overnight 1-mg dexamethasone suppression test or measurement of 24-hr urinary free cortisol. If either of these tests is positive, further evaluation should be carried out to distinguish between pituitary and adrenal causes of ACTH excess.

Assessment of metabolic abnormalities

Given the prevalence of insulin resistance in PCOS[1] and the role of hyperinsulinemia in the pathogenesis of this disorder,[13–15] it is important that patients with PCOS be screened for defects in insulin action. A single determination of either glucose or insulin levels has been shown to have a low sensitivity in detecting abnormalities in insulin action.[96,97] However, a recent study indicates that a fasting glucose/insulin ratio may be useful as a screening test for insulin resistance in obese PCOS subjects.[16] A standard 75-g oral glucose tolerance test is recommended for all obese PCOS subjects, given the high prevalence of impaired glucose tolerance in this subset of patients. A baseline lipid profile is also worth considering in these subjects, given the potential risk for premature cardiovascular disease.[2,3]

Management

The goals of treatment of the hirsute woman should be tailored to the individual patient's needs. In some women, particularly those with regular menstrual cycles and mild hirsutism, local cosmetic measures alone may be sufficient. However, in women with symptoms of significant androgen excess, i.e. severe hirsutism and menstrual irregularity, medical therapy is frequently necessary.

Cosmetic measures

Cosmetic measures are an important adjunct in the treatment of hirsutism, given that it can take up to 6 months to see a response to medical therapy. Available options include simple methods that can be performed by the woman herself, e.g. tweezing, bleaching, depilatory creams, or shaving. More sophisticated cosmetic measures such as electrolysis and laser therapy are quite expensive, but give the best long-term cosmetic results.

Weight loss

In obese PCOS women, weight loss has been shown to result in a fall in serum insulin and free testosterone levels, with a resultant improvement in both hirsutism and menstrual irregularity.[98,99] Aside from its reproductive benefits, weight loss is also helpful in the management of the impaired glucose tolerance commonly seen in PCOS and is often best accomplished in these patients in association with an exercise program.

Medical therapy

The medical treatment of hirsutism is directed at suppressing ovarian androgen secretion (oral contraceptives, GnRH analogs), blocking the actions of androgens on target organs (anti-androgens), or suppressing adrenal androgen secretion (glucocorticoids).

Oral contraceptives

Combination oral contraceptives (OCs), used alone or with other agents, form the mainstay of treatment for hirsute women not currently desirous of pregnancy. Treatment with OCs improves hirsutism and acne in 60–100% of hyperandrogenic women and also combats the effects of unopposed estrogen on the endometrium, thus preventing endometrial hyperplasia.[100] The mechanisms by which OCs correct androgen excess include stimulation of SHBG production by the liver, resulting in a decrease in serum free testosterone concentrations,[101] suppression of LH and consequently LH-dependent ovarian androgen production,[102] and inhibition of adrenal androgen secretion.[103]

To date, no birth control pill has ever been shown to be superior to another in the treatment of hirsutism. However, theoretically it makes sense to choose a formulation that contains a low dose of estrogen and a non-androgenic progestin. Third-generation progestins, e.g. desogestrel and norgestimate, offer an additional clinical advantage in that they have neutral or even beneficial effects on metabolic abnormalities with less impact on carbohydrate and lipoprotein metabolism and no significant effects on coagulation profiles.[104] OC formulations containing the anti-androgenic progestin, cyproterone acetate, are widely prescribed for the treatment of hirsutism in Europe, but are not available in the USA or Canada.

GnRH analogs

Several studies have demonstrated the efficacy of long-acting GnRH analogs in suppressing gonadotropin and consequently ovarian androgen secretion in women with androgen excess.[49–51,105] Depending on the preparation used, they are given by subcutaneous injection daily (buserelin and leuprolide), by nasal spray two or three times daily (buserelin and nafarelin), by intramuscular depot injection monthly (leuprolide) or by subcutaneous implant monthly (goserelin). Depending on the degree of gonadotropin suppression achieved with a GnRH agonist, addition of estrogen may[106,107] or may not[108,109] result in a greater improvement in hirsutism. However, independent of its effect on hirsutism scores, estrogen replacement is essential in women treated with GnRH analogs to prevent vasomotor symptoms[107,110] and to preserve bone mass.[107,111] Therefore, it is now recommended that GnRH agonists are administered in conjunction with estrogen add-back in the form of either an OC or HRT. Given the high cost of these agents and the fact that the combination of an oral contraceptive with an anti-androgen appears to be just as effective in the majority of cases, their use should be reserved for women with severe hirsutism who fail to respond to standard therapy.

Anti-androgens

Anti-androgens are an effective treatment for hirsutism when used either alone or in combination with an OC. However, in women of reproductive age, anti-androgens should be prescribed with estrogen to ensure effective contraception, given the theoretical risk that exposure of a male fetus to an anti-androgen would result in feminization.

Cyproterone acetate (CPA)

CPA is a synthetic progestin with both antigonadotropic and peripheral anti-androgenic activity. It competitively inhibits DHT binding to its receptor, decreases 5α-reductase activity in the skin, and decreases ovarian androgen secretion by inhibiting gonadotropin release.[112] While it is the most widely used anti-androgen in Europe and Canada, CPA is not available for the treatment of hirsutism in the USA. CPA may be prescribed either in conjunction with an OC or administered with ethinyl estradiol in an OC formulation called Dianette (35 μg ethinyl estradiol and 2 mg CPA). Given its long half-life and potent progestational activity, amenorrhea is common when CPA is given for more than 10 days of a birth control pill cycle. Therefore, CPA is frequently prescribed in a reverse sequential regimen at a dose of 50 mg/day for the first 10 days of a 21-day course of estrogen. Data from one study suggest that when it is used with a constant estrogen dose, there is no significant difference in the beneficial effects on hirsutism of 2, 25 or 100 mg of CPA.[113] CPA is generally well tolerated, although weight gain and edema may occur at higher doses, due to its glucocorticoid activity. Drug-induced hepatitis has been rarely reported.

Spironolactone

In addition to being an aldosterone antagonist, spironolactone acts as an anti-androgen by competitively inhibiting the binding of testosterone to the androgen receptor.[114] It also decreases testosterone biosynthesis by inhibiting ovarian and adrenal cytochrome P450c17.[115] At a dose of 50–100 mg twice daily, spironolactone is an effective treatment for hirsutism in approximately 75% of women. The commonest side-effect of therapy is menstrual irregularity, which is overcome by the addition of a birth control pill. In higher doses, spironolactone may be associated with nausea, fatigue, and hyperkalemia.

Flutamide

Flutamide is a potent non-steroidal anti-androgen. While its mechanism of action was initially thought to be selective blockade of the androgen receptor, both in vitro[116] and in vivo[117,118] studies have now shown that it also reduces androgen biosynthesis. At doses of 375–500 mg daily, flutamide causes a marked improvement in hirsutism.[119,120] Some,[117,121] but not all,[122] studies have suggested that it is more efficacious than other anti-androgens. However, a major drawback of its use in the treatment of hirsutism is its hepatotoxicity. While liver function typically returns to normal when flutamide is discontinued,[120] deaths from progressive liver failure have also been reported.[123] Therefore, flutamide is not recommended for the routine treatment of women with hirsutism.

Finasteride

Finasteride is a competitive inhibitor of the 5α-reductase type 2 isoenzyme responsible for converting testosterone to DHT. Several studies have demonstrated that finasteride at a dose of 5 mg daily is a safe and effective treatment for hirsutism.[124,125] In one randomized study comparing the efficacy of finasteride, flutamide, and CPA combined with ethinyl estradiol, finasteride was shown to be the best-tolerated agent, although slightly less effective in terms of the reductions in hirsutism score and hair diameter.[125]

Adrenal suppression

While glucocorticoids suppress adrenal androgen secretion, their efficacy in the treatment of hirsutism is a matter of debate. Some studies have demonstrated an improvement in hirsutism scores using dexamethasone 0.5 mg at night.[126] However, this beneficial effect is frequently seen at the expense of glucocorticoid side-effects, particularly weight gain. Even in women with well-defined adrenal hyperandrogenism, such as late-onset CAH, the response to anti-androgens tends to be better than to glucocorticoids.[127]

Insulin-sensitizing agents

While there are data demonstrating that improving insulin sensitivity with agents such as metformin[83] or troglitazone[86,87] lowers serum androgen levels and improves ovulatory rates, to date no published study has been of sufficient duration to evaluate the clinical effects of these agents on hair growth.

References

1. Dunaif A. Insulin resistance and the polycystic ovary syndrome: mechanism and implications for pathogenesis. *Endocrine Rev* 1997; 18: 774–800.
2. Conway GS, Agrawal R, Betteridge DJ, Jacobs HS. Risk factors for coronary artery disease in lean and obese women with the polycystic ovary syndrome. *Clin Endocrinol (Oxf)* 1992; 37: 119–25.
3. Dahlgren E, Johansson S, Lindstedt G et al. Women with polycystic ovary syndrome wedge resected in 1956 to 1965: a long-term follow-up focusing on natural history and circulating hormones. *Fertil Steril* 1992; 57: 505–13.
4. Carmina E, Koyama T, Chang L, Stanczyk FZ, Lobo RA. Does ethnicity influence the prevalence of adrenal

hyperandrogenism and insulin resistance in polycystic ovary syndrome? *Am J Obstet Gynecol* 1992; **167**: 1807–12.
5. Ferriman D, Gallwey JD. Clinical assessment of body hair growth in women. *J Clin Endocrinol Metab* 1961; **21**: 1440–7.
6. McKnight E. The prevalence of 'hirsutism' in young women. *Lancet* 1964; **i**: 410–13.
7. Knochenhauer ES, Key TJ, Kahsar-Miller M, Waggoner W, Boots LR, Azziz R. Prevalence of the polycystic ovary syndrome in unselected black and white women of the Southeastern United States: a prospective study. *J Clin Endocrinol Metab* 1998; **83**: 3078–82.
8. McKenna TJ. Screening for sinister causes of hirsutism. *N Engl J Med* 1994; **331**: 1015–16.
9. Zawadzki JK, Dunaif A. Diagnostic criteria for polycystic ovary syndrome: towards a rational approach. In: Dunaif A, Givens JR, Haseltine FP, Merriam GR, eds. *Polycystic Ovary Syndrome*. Boston: Blackwell Scientific Publications, 377–84.
10. Legro RS, Driscoll D, Strauss JF III, Fox J, Dunaif A. Evidence for a genetic basis for hyperandrogenemia in polycystic ovary syndrome. *Proc Natl Acad Sci USA* 1998; **95**: 14956–60.
11. Franks S. Polycystic Ovary Syndrome: a changing perspective. *Clin Endocrinol* 1989; **31**: 87–120.
12. Dunaif A, Hoffman AR, Scully RE et al. The clinical, biochemical and ovarian morphologic features in women with acanthosis nigricans and masculinization. *Obstet Gynecol* 1985; **66**: 545–52.
13. Burghen GA, Givens JR, Kibatchi AE. Correlation of hyperandrogenism with hyperinsulinism in polycystic ovarian disease. *J Clin Endocrinol Metab* 1980; **50**: 113–16.
14. Pasquali R, Venturoli S, Paradisi R, Capelli M, Parenti N, Melchionda N. Insulin and C-peptide levels in obese patients with polycystic ovaries. *Horm Metab Res* 1982; **14**: 284–7.
15. Chang RJ, Nakamura RM, Judd HL, Kaplan SA. Insulin resistance in nonobese patients with polycystic ovarian disease. *J Clin Endocrinol Metab* 1983; **57**: 356–9.
16. Legro RS, Finegood D, Dunaif A. A fasting glucose to insulin ratio is a useful measure of insulin sensitivity in women with polycystic ovary syndrome. *J Clin Endocrinol Metab* 1998; **83**: 2694–8.
17. Harris MI, Hadden WC, Knowler WC, Bennett PH. Prevalence of diabetes and impaired glucose tolerance and plasma glucose levels in US population aged 20–74 yr. *Diabetes* 1987; **36**: 523–34.
18. Dunaif A, Graf M, Mandeli J, Laumas V, Dobrjansky A. Characterization of groups of hyperandrogenic women with acanthosis nigricans, impaired glucose tolerance and/or hyperinsulinemia. *J Clin Endocrinol Metab* 1987; **65**: 499–507.
19. Robinson S, Kiddy D, Gelding SV et al. The relationship of insulin insensitivity to menstrual pattern in women with hyperandrogenism and insulin resistance in polycystic ovary syndrome. *Clin Endocrinol* 1993; **39**: 351–5.
20. New M, White PC, Pang S, Dupont S, Speiser PW. The adrenal hyperplasias. In: Scriver CL, Beaudet AL, Sly WS, Valle D, eds. *The Metabolic Basis of Inherited Disease*, 6th edn. New York: McGraw-Hill, 1989: 1881–918.
21. Speiser PW, White PC. Congenital adrenal hyperplasia due to steroid 21-hydroxylase deficiency. *Clin Endocrinol* 1998; **49**: 411–17.
22. Azziz R, Zacur HA. Nonclassic adrenal hyperplasia: current concepts. *J Clin Endocrinol Metab* 1994; **78**: 810–15.
23. Chetkowski RJ, DeFazio J, Shamonki I, Judd HL, Chang RJ. The incidence of late-onset congenital adrenal hyperplasia due to 21-hydroxylase deficiency among hirsute women. *J Clin Endocrinol Metab* 1984; **58**: 595–8.
24. Speiser PW, Dupont B, Rubenstein P, Piazza A, Kastelan A, New MI. High frequency of nonclassical steroid 21-hydroxylase deficiency. *Am J Hum Gen* 1985; **37**: 650–67.
25. Hawkins LA, Chasalow FI, Blethen SL. The role of adrenocorticotropin testing in evaluating girls with premature adrenarche and hirsutism/oligomenorrhea. *J Clin Endocrinol Metab* 1992; **74**: 248–53.
26. Pang S, Lerner AJ, Stoner E et al. Late-onset adrenal steroid 3β-hydroxysteroid dehydrogenase deficiency. I. A cause of hirsutism in pubertal and postpubertal women. *J Clin Endocrinol Metab* 1985; **60**: 428–39.
27. Orth DN, Kovacs WJ, DeBold CR. The adrenal cortex. In: Wilson JE, Foster DW, eds. *Williams Textbook of Endocrinology*, Philadelphia: WB Saunders Company, 1992: 489–619.
28. Lado-Abeal J, Rodriguez-Arnao J, Newell-Price JDC et al. Menstrual abnormalities in women with Cushing's disease are correlated with hypercortisolemia rather than raised circulating androgen levels. *J Clin Endocrinol Metab* 1998; **83**: 3083–8.
29. Wajchenberg BL, Mendonca BB, Liberman B et al. Ectopic adrenocorticotropic hormone syndrome. *Endocrine Rev* 1994; **15**: 752–87.
30. Luton JP, Cerdas S, Billaud L et al. Clinical features of adrenocortical carcinomas, prognostic features, and the effect of mitotane therapy. *N Engl J Med* 1990; **322**: 1195–201.
31. Derksen J, Nagesser SK, Meinders AE, Haak HR, Harm R, van de Velde CJH. Identification of virilizing adrenal tumors in hirsute women. *N Engl J Med* 1994; **331**: 968–73.
32. Maroulis GB, Manlimos FS, Abraham GE. Comparison between urinary 17-ketosteroids and serum androgens in hirsute patients. *Obstet Gynecol* 1977; **49**: 454–8.

33. Del Gaudio AD, Del Gaudio GA. Virilizing adrenocortical tumours in adult women; report of 10 patients, 2 of whom each had a tumour secreting only testosterone. *Cancer* 1993; **72**: 1997–2003.

34. Kloos RT, Gross MD, Francis IR, Korobkin M, Shapiro B. Incidentally discovered adrenal masses. *Endocrine Rev* 1995; **16**: 460–84.

35. Scully RE. Ovarian tumors with endocrine manifestations. In: DeGroot LJ, Besser GM, Cahill GF Jr et al, eds. *Endocrinology*, 2nd edn. Philadelphia: WB Saunders, 1989: 1994–2008.

36. Hayes FJ, Sheahan K, Rajendiran S, McKenna TJ. Virilization in a postmenopausal woman as a result of hilus cell hyperplasia associated with a simple ovarian cyst. *Am J Obstet Gynecol* 1997; **176**: 719–20.

37. Nagamani M, Lingold JC, Gomez LG, Garza JR. Clinical and hormonal studies in hyperthecosis of the ovaries. *Fertil Steril* 1981; **36**: 326–32.

38. Nagamani M, Van Dinh T, Kelver ME. Hyperinsulinemia in hyperthecosis of the ovaries. *Am J Obstet Gynecol* 1986; **154**: 384–9.

39. Barth JH, Jenkins M, Belchetz PE. Ovarian hyperthecosis, diabetes and hirsuties in post-menopausal women. *Clin Endocrinol* 1997; **46**: 123–8.

40. Pascale M, Pugeat M, Roberts M et al. Androgen suppressive effect of GnRH agonist in ovarian hyperthecosis and virilizing tumours. *Clin Endocrinol* 1994; **41**: 571–6.

41. Kahn CR, Flier JS, Bar RS et al. The syndromes of insulin resistance and acanthosis nigricans. *N Engl J Med* 1976; **294**: 739–45.

42. Taylor SI, Cama A, Accili D et al. Mutations in the insulin receptor gene. *Endocrine Rev* 1992; **13**: 566–95.

43. Flier JS, Kahn R, Roth J, Bar RS. Antibodies that impair insulin receptor binding in an unusual diabetic syndrome with severe insulin resistance. *Science* 1975; **190**: 63–5.

44. Nestler JE, Powers LP, Matt DW et al. A direct effect of hyperinsulinemia on serum sex hormone-binding globulin levels in obese women with polycystic ovary syndrome. *J Clin Endocrinol Metab* 1991; **72**: 83–9.

45. Horton R, Hawks D, Lobo RA. 3α, 17β-Androstanediol glucuronide in plasma. A marker of androgen action in idiopathic hirsutism. *J Clin Invest* 1982; **82**: 1203–7.

46. Serafini P, Ablan R, Lobo RA. 5α-Reductase activity in the genital skin of hirsute women. *J Clin Endocrinol Metab* 1985; **60**: 349–55.

47. Kirschner MA, Zucker IR, Jespersen D. Idiopathic hirsutism—an ovarian abnormality. *N Engl J Med* 1976; **294**: 637–40.

48. Wajchenberg BL, Achando SS, Okada H et al. Determination of the source(s) of androgen overproduction in hirsutism associated with polycystic ovary syndrome by simultaneous adrenal and ovarian venous catheterization. Comparison with the dexamethasone suppression test. *J Clin Endocrinol Metab* 1986; **636**: 1204–10.

49. Chang RJ, Laufer RM, Meldrum DR et al. Steroid secretion in polycystic ovarian disease after ovarian suppression by a long-acting gonadotropin-releasing hormone agonist. *J Clin Endocrinol Metab* 1983; **56**: 897–903.

50. Couzinet B, Le Strat N, Brailly S, Schaison G. Comparative effects of cyproterone acetate or a long-acting gonadotropin-releasing hormone agonist in polycystic ovarian disease. *J Clin Endocrinol Metab* 1986; **63**: 1031–5.

51. Steingold K, De Ziegler D, Cedars M et al. Clinical and hormonal effects of chronic gonadotropin-releasing hormone agonist treatment in polycystic ovarian disease. *J Clin Endocrinol Metab* 1987; **65**: 773–8.

52. McKenna TJ, Cunningham SK. Adrenal androgen production in polycystic ovary syndrome. *Eur J Endocrinol* 1995; **133**: 383–9.

53. Stahl NL, Teeslink CR, Greenblatt RB. Ovarian, adrenal and peripheral testosterone levels in the polycystic ovary syndrome. *Am J Obstet Gynecol* 1973; **117**: 194–200.

54. Farber M, Millan VG, Turksoy RN, Mitchell GW Jr. Diagnostic evaluation of hirsutism in women by selective bilateral adrenal and ovarian venous catheterization. *Fertil Steril* 1978; **38**: 283–8.

55. Wild RA, Umstot ED, Anderson RN, Ranney GB, Givens GR. Androgen parameters and their correlation with body weight in one-hundred thirty-eight women thought to have hyperandrogenism. *Am J Obstet Gynecol* 1983; **146**: 602–5.

56. Hoffman DI, Clove K, Lobo RA. Prevalence and significance of elevated dehydroepiandrosterone sulphate levels in anovulatory women. *Fertil Steril* 1984; **42**: 76–81.

57. Lucky AW, Rosenfield RL, McGuire J, Rudy S, Helke J. Adrenal androgen hyperresponsiveness to adrenocorticotropin in women with acne and/or hirsutism: adrenal enzyme defects and exaggerated adrenarche. *J Clin Endocrinol Metab* 1986; **62**: 840–8.

58. Azziz R, Black V, Hines GA, Fox LM, Boots LR. Adrenal androgen excess in the polycystic ovary syndrome: sensitivity and responsivity of the hypothalamic–pituitary axis. *J Clin Endocrinol Metab* 1998; **83**: 2317–28.

59. Gonzalez F, Chang L, Horab T, Stanczyk FZ, Crickard K, Lobo RA. Adrenal dynamic responses to physiologic and pharmacologic adrenocorticotropic hormone stimulation before and after steroid modulation in women with polycystic ovary syndrome. *Fertil Steril* 1999; **71**: 439–44.

60. Hall JE. Polycystic ovarian disease as a neuroendocrine disorder of the female reproductive axis. *Endocrinol Metab Clin North Am* 1993; **22**: 75–92.

61. Taylor AE, McCourt B, Martin KA et al. Determinants of abnormal gonadotropin secretion in clinically

defined women with polycystic ovary syndrome. *J Clin Endocrinol Metab* 1997; **82**: 2248–56.
62. Burger CW, Korsen T, van Kessel H, van Dop PA, Caron FJM, Schoemaker J. Pulsatile luteinizing hormone patterns in the follicular phase of the menstrual cycle, polycystic ovarian disease (PCOD) and non-PCOD secondary amenorrhea. *J Clin Endocrinol Metab* 1985; **61**: 1126–32.
63. Waldstreicher J, Santoro NF, Hall JE, Filicori M, Crowley WF Jr. Hyperfunction of the hypothalamic–pituitary axis in women with polycystic ovarian disease: indirect evidence for partial gonadotrope desensitization. *J Clin Endocrinol Metab* 1988; **66**: 165–72.
64. Imse V, Holzapfel G, Hinney B, Kuhn W, Wuttke W. Comparison of luteinizing hormone pulsatility in the serum of women suffering from polycystic ovarian disease using a bioassay and five different immunoassays. *J Clin Endocrinol Metab* 1992; **74**: 1053–61.
65. Hall JE, Taylor AE, Hayes FJ, Crowley WF Jr. Insights into hypothalamic–pituitary dysfunction in polycystic ovarian syndrome. *J Endocrinol Invest* 1998; **21**: 602–11.
66. Spratt DI, Finkelstein JS, Butler JP, Badger TM, Crowley WF Jr. Effects of increasing the frequency of low doses of gonadotropin-releasing hormone (GnRH) on gonadotropin secretion in GnRH-deficient men. *J Clin Endocrinol Metab* 1987; **64**: 1179–86.
67. Chang RJ, Mandel FP, Lu JKH, Judd HL. Enhanced disparity of gonadotropin secretion by estrone in women with polycystic ovarian disease. *J Clin Endocrinol Metab* 1982; **54**: 490–4.
68. Rebar R, Judd HL, Yen SSC, Rakoff J, Vandenberg G, Naftolin F. Characterization of the inappropriate gonadotropin secretion in polycystic ovary syndrome. *J Clin Invest* 1976; **57**: 1320–9.
69. Hayes FJ, Taylor AE, Martin KM, Hall JE. Use of a GnRH antagonist as a physiologic probe in polycystic ovary syndrome: assessment of neuroendocrine and androgen dynamics. *J Clin Endocrinol Metab* 1998; **83**: 2343–9.
70. Barnes RB, Rosenfield RL, Burstein S, Ehrmann DA. Pituitary–ovarian responses to nafarelin in the polycystic ovary syndrome. *N Engl J Med* 1989; **320**: 559–65.
71. Adams J, Polson DW, Franks S. Prevalence of polycystic ovaries in women with anovulation and idiopathic hirsutism. *BMJ* 1986; **293**: 355–9.
72. Polson DW, Adams J, Wadsworth J, Franks S. Polycystic ovaries—a common finding in normal women. *Lancet* 1988; **i**: 870–2.
73. Adams JM, Taylor AE, Crowley WF Jr, Hall JE. Polycystic ovarian morphology: significance in women with regular ovulatory cycles. In: Program of the 10th International Congress of Endocrinology, San Francisco, 1996: OR26-2.
74. Ehrmann DA, Rosenfield RL, Barnes R, Brigell DF, Sheikh Z. Detection of functional ovarian hyperandrogenism in women with androgen excess. *N Engl J Med* 1992; **327**: 157–62.
75. Ibanez L, Hall JE, Potau N, Carrascosa A, Prat N, Taylor AE. Ovarian 17-hydroxyprogesterone responsiveness to GnRH agonist challenge in women with polycystic ovary syndrome is not mediated by LH hypersecretion: evidence from GnRH agonist and human chorionic gonadotropin stimulation testing. *J Clin Endocrinol Metab* 1996; **81**: 4103–7.
76. Rosenfield RL, Barnes RB, Cara JF, Lucky AW. Dysregulation of cytochrome P450c17α as the cause of polycystic ovarian syndrome. *Fertil Steril* 1990; **53**: 785–91.
77. Barbieri RL, Makris A, Ryan KJ. Insulin stimulates androgen accumulation in incubations of human ovarian stroma and theca. *Obstet Gynecol* 1984; **64**(suppl): 73S–80S.
78. Nestler JE, Strauss J III. Insulin as an effector of human ovarian and adrenal steroid metabolism. *Endocrinol Metab Clin North Am* 1991; **20**: 807–23.
79. Poretsky L, Kalin MF. The gonadotropic function of insulin. *Endocrine Rev* 1987; **8**: 132–41.
80. Dunaif A, Mandeli J, Fluhr H, Dobrjansky A. The impact of obesity and chronic hyperinsulinemia on gonadotropin release and gonadal steroid secretion in the polycystic ovary syndrome. *J Clin Endocrinol Metab* 1988; **66**: 131–9.
81. Nestler JE, Barlascini CO, Matt DW et al. Suppression of serum insulin by diazoxide reduced serum testosterone levels in obese women with polycystic ovary syndrome. *J Clin Endocrinol Metab* 1989; **68**: 1027–32.
82. Velazquez EM, Mendoza SG, Hamer T, Sosa F, Glueck CJ. Metformin therapy in polycystic ovary syndrome reduces hyperinsulinaemia, insulin resistance, hyperandrogenemia and systolic blood pressure, while facilitating normal menses and pregnancy. *Metabolism* 1994; **43**: 647–54.
83. Nestler JE, Jakubowicz D. Decrease in ovarian cytochrome P450c17alpha activity and serum free testosterone after reduction of insulin secretion in polycystic ovary syndrome. *N Engl J Med* 1996; **335**: 617–23.
84. Acbay O, Gundogdu S. Can metformin reduce insulin resistance in polycystic ovary syndrome? *Fertil Steril* 1996; **65**: 946–9.
85. Ehrmann DA, Cavaghan M, Imperial J, Sturis J, Rosenfield R, Polonsky KS. Effects of metformin on insulin secretion, insulin action and ovarian steroidogenesis in women with polycystic ovary syndrome. *J Clin Endocrinol Metab* 1997; **82**: 524–30.
86. Dunaif A, Scott D, Finegood D, Quintana B, Whitcomb R. The insulin sensitising agent troglitazone improves metabolic and reproductive abnormalities in the polycystic ovarian syndrome. *J Clin Endocrinol Metab* 1996; **81**: 3299–306.

87. Ehrmann D, Schneider DJ, Sobel BE et al. Troglitazone improves defects in insulin action, insulin secretion, ovarian steroidogenesis, and fibrinolysis in women with polycystic ovary syndrome. *J Clin Endocrinol Metab* 1997; **82**: 2108–16.
88. Dunaif A, Xia J, Book C, Schenker E, Tang Z. Excessive insulin receptor serine phosphorylation in cultured fibroblasts and in skeletal muscle: a potential mechanism for insulin resistance in the polycystic ovary syndrome. *J Clin Invest* 1995; **96**: 801–10.
89. Tagatz GE, Kopher RA, Nagel TC, Okagaki T. The clitoral index: a bioassay of androgenic stimulation. *Obstet Gynecol* 1979; **54**: 562–4.
90. Meldrum DR, Abraham GE. Peripheral and ovarian venous concentrations of various steroid hormones in virilizing ovarian tumors. *Obstet Gynecol* 1979; **54**: 36–43.
91. Friedman CI, Schmidt GE, Kim MH, Powell J. Serum testosterone concentrations in the evaluation of androgen-producing tumors. *Am J Obstet Gynecol* 1985; **153**: 44–9.
92. Surrey ES, de Ziegler D, Gambone JC, Judd HL. Preoperative localization of androgen-secreting tumors: clinical, endocrinologic, and radiologic evaluation of ten patients. *Am J Obstet Gynecol* 1988; **158**: 1313–22.
93. Rosenfield RL. Plasma testosterone binding globulin and indexes of the concentration of unbound plasma androgens in normal and hirsute subjects. *J Clin Endocrinol Metab* 1971; **32**: 717–28.
94. Zumoff B, Rosenfeld RS, Strain GW, Levin J, Fukushima DK. Sex differences in the twenty-four hour mean plasma concentrations of dehydroepiandrosterone (DHA) and dehydroepiandrosterone sulfate (DHAS) and the DHA to DHAS ratio in normal adults. *J Clin Endocrinol Metab* 1980; **51**: 330–3.
95. New MI, Lorenzen F, Lerner AJ et al. Genotyping steroid 21-hydroxylase deficiency: hormonal reference data. *J Clin Endocrinol Metab* 1983; **57**: 320–6.
96. Laakso M. How good a marker is insulin level for insulin resistance? *Am J Epidemiol* 1993; **137**: 959–65.
97. American Diabetes Association. Consensus Development Conference on Insulin Resistance. *Diabetes Care* 1998; **21**: 310–14.
98. Kiddy DS, Hamilton-Fairley D, Bush A et al. Improvement in endocrine and ovarian function during dietary treatment of obese women with polycystic ovary syndrome. *Clin Endocrinol* 1992; **36**: 105–11.
99. Pasquali R, Casimirri F, Vicennati V. Weight control and its beneficial effect on fertility in women with obesity and polycystic ovary syndrome. *Hum Reprod* 1997; **12**(suppl): 82–7.
100. Burkman RT Jr. The role of oral contraceptives in the treatment of hyperandrogenic disorders. *Am J Med* 1995; **98**(suppl 1A): 130S–6S.
101. Wieland RG, Zorn EM, Hallberg MC. Differential studies on the mechanism of serum androgen and androgen-binding abnormalities in hirsutism. *Am J Obstet Gynecol* 1973; **117**: 983–6.
102. Givens JR, Andersen RN, Wiser WL, Fish SA. Dynamics of suppression and recovery of plasma FSH, LH androstenedione and testosterone in polycystic ovarian disease. *J Clin Endocrinol Metab* 1974; **38**: 727–35.
103. Wild RA, Umstot ES, Andersen RN, Givens JR. Adrenal function in hirsutism. II. Effect of an oral contraceptive. *J Clin Endocrinol Metab* 1982; **54**: 676–81.
104. Speroff L, DeCherney A. Evaluation of a new generation of oral contraceptives. The Advisory Board of the New Progestins. *Obstet Gynecol* 1993; **81**: 1034–47.
105. Andreyko JL, Monroe SE, Jaffe RB. The treatment of hirsutism with a gonadotropin-releasing hormone agonist (Nafarelin). *J Clin Endocrinol Metab* 1986; **63**: 854–9.
106. Heiner JS, Greendale GA, Kawakami AK et al. Comparison of a GnRH agonist and a low dose oral contraceptive given alone or together in the treatment of hirsutism. *J Clin Endocrinol Metab* 1995; **80**: 3412–18.
107. Carmina E, Janni A, Lobo RA. Physiological estrogen replacement may enhance the effectiveness of the gonadotropin releasing hormone agonist in the treatment of hirsutism. *J Clin Endocrinol Metab* 1994; **78**: 126–30.
108. Tiitinen A, Simberg N, Stenman UH, Ylikorkala O. Estrogen replacement does not potentiate gonadotropin-releasing hormone agonist-induced androgen suppression in treatment of hirsutism. *J Clin Endocrinol Metab* 1994; **79**: 447–51.
109. Elkind-Hirsch KE, Anania C, Mack M, Malinak R. Combination gonadotropin-releasing hormone agonist and oral contraceptive therapy improves treatment of hirsute women with ovarian hyperandrogenism. *Fertil Steril* 1995; **63**: 970–8.
110. Morcos RN, Abdul-Malak ME, Shikora E. Treatment of hirsutism with a gonadotropin-releasing hormone agonist and estrogen replacement therapy. *Fertil Steril* 1994; **61**: 427–31.
111. Falsetti L, Pasinetti E. Treatment of moderate and severe hirsutism by gonadotropin-releasing hormone agonists in women with polycystic ovary syndrome and idiopathic hirsutism. *Fertil Steril* 1994; **61**: 817–22.
112. Neumann F, Von Berswordt-Wallrabe R, Eiger W, Steinbeck H, Hahn JD, Kramer M. Aspects of androgen-dependent events as studied by antiandrogens. *Recent Prog Horm Res* 1970; **26**: 337–410.
113. Barth JH, Cherry CA, Wojnarowska F, Dawber RPR. Cyproterone acetate for severe hirsutism: results of a double-blind dose-ranging study. *Clin Endocrinol (Oxf)* 1991; **35**: 5–10.

114. Corvol P, Michaud A, Menard J, Freifeld M, Mahoudeau J. Antiandrogenic effects of spironolactone: mechanism of action. *Endocrinology* 1975; **97**: 52–8.
115. Menard RH, Guenther TM, Kon H, Gillette JR. Studies on the destruction of adrenal and testicular cytochrome P-450 by spironolactone. Requirement for the 7alpha-thio group and evidence for the loss of the heme and apoproteins of cytochrome P-450. *J Biol Chem* 1979; **254**: 1726–33.
116. Ayub M, Levell MJ. Inhibition of rat testicular 17α-hydroxylase and 17,20 lyase activities by antiandrogens (flutamide, hydroxyflutamide, Ru23908, cyproterone acetate) in vitro. *J Steroid Biochem* 1987; **28**: 43–7.
117. Cusan L, Dupont A, Gomez J-L, Tremblay RR, Labrie F. Comparison of flutamide and spironolactone in the treatment of hirsutism: a randomized controlled trial. *Fertil Steril* 1994; **61**: 281–7.
118. De Leo V, Lanzetta D, D'Antona D, La Marca A, Morgante G. Hormonal effects of flutamide in young women with Polycystic ovary syndrome. *J Clin Endocrinol Metab* 1998; **83**: 99–102.
119. Couzinet B, Pholsena M, Young J, Schaison G. The impact of a pure anti-androgen (flutamide) on LH, FSH, androgens and clinical status in idiopathic hirsutism. *Clin Endocrinol (Oxf)* 1993; **39**: 157–62.
120. Moghetti P, Castello R, Negri C et al. Flutamide in the treatment of hirsutism: long-term clinical effects, endocrine changes, and androgen receptor behavior. *Fertil Steril* 1995; **64**: 511–17.
121. Pazos F, Escobar-Morreale HF, Balsa J, Sancho JM, Varela C. Prospective randomized study comparing the long-acting gonadotropin-releasing hormone agonist triptorelin, flutamide, and cyproterone acetate, used in combination with an oral contraceptive, in the treatment of hirsutism. *Fertil Steril* 1999; **71**: 122–8.
122. Fruzetti F, Bersi C, Parrini D, Ricci C, Genazzani AR. Treatment of hirsutism: comparisons between different antiandrogens with central and peripheral effects. *Fertil Steril* 1999; **71**: 445–51.
123. Wysowski DK, Freiman JP, Tourtelot JB, Horton, ML III. Fatal and nonfatal hepatotoxicity associated with flutamide. *Ann Intern Med* 1993; **118**: 860–4.
124. Moghetti P, Castello R, Magnani CM, Tosi F, Negri C. Clinical and hormonal effects of the 5 alpha-reductase inhibitor finasteride in idiopathic hirsutism. *J Clin Endocrinol Metab* 1994; **79**: 1115–21.
125. Venturoli S, Marescalchi O, Colombo FM et al. A prospective randomized trial comparing low dose flutamide, finasteride, ketoconazole, and cyproterone acetate–estrogen regimens in the treatment of hirsutism. *J Clin Endocrinol Metab* 1999; **84**: 1304–10.
126. Loughlin T, Cunningham S, Moore A, Culliton M, Smyth PPA, McKenna TJ. Adrenal abnormalities in polycystic ovary syndrome. *J Clin Endocrinol Metab* 1986; **62**: 142–7.
127. Spritzer P, Billaud L, Thalabard JC et al. Cyproterone acetate versus hydrocortisone treatment in late-onset adrenal hyperplasia. *J Clin Endocrinol Metab* 1990; **70**: 642–5.

10

Autoimmune disease
Anthony P Weetman

Introduction

Autoimmunity is a common cause of endocrine disease; Table 10.1 lists the approximate frequency of the most important disorders in the UK population. In most cases, there is a lymphocytic infiltration of the target organ and T-cell-mediated destruction of the target endocrine cells, with autoantibodies probably playing only a secondary role in tissue injury.[1,2] A notable exception is the production of antibodies to the thyroid-stimulating hormone (TSH) receptor (TSH-R), causing Graves' disease if they bind to stimulatory regions on the receptor and exacerbating hypothyroidism if they bind instead to regions which are involved in mediating the effects of TSH. The clear, primary pathogenic role of these antibodies is demonstrated by their effects following transplacental passage, in particular neonatal thyrotoxicosis.[3]

Autoimmune endocrinopathies in general are multifactorial, and a shared genetic predisposition accounts for the frequent coexistence of these disorders, and other autoimmune diseases, in families as autoimmune polyglandular syndrome (APS) type 2,[4] dealt with later. In particular, HLA-DR3 is frequently found in such patients of Caucasian origin, and polymorphisms in the *CTLA-4* gene, believed to be important in regulating T-cell function, may also be shared.[5] Different HLA alleles are associated with autoimmune endocrinopathies in non-Caucasians. Genome screening and linkage analysis are now beginning to reveal other genetic loci which may be involved, especially in Graves' disease, but these remain to be confirmed and their contribution is likely to be small. Only 20–30% of monozygotic twins are concordant for Graves' disease. Endogenous factors, notably sex steroids, play an important role, as these disorders are 4–10 times commoner in women. Finally, stress, diet, infections and toxins have all been implicated as environmental factors, especially in animal models, which have contributed profoundly to our understanding of pathogenesis.[6] Although less well characterized, similar mechanisms underlie autoimmune disease in other endocrine glands.

	Approximate prevalence
Graves' disease	1:50
Autoimmune hypothyroidism	1:100
Postpartum thyroiditis	1:20
Addison's disease	1:10 000
Premature ovarian failure	1:100

Table 10.1
The frequency of major autoimmune endocrinopathies in Caucasian women.

Graves' disease

This section concentrates on uncomplicated Graves' disease; subsequent sections deal with the disease in children and in pregnancy and with thyroid-associated ophthalmopathy (TAO) and dermopathy.

Clinical assessment

The signs and symptoms produced by excess thyroid hormones in Graves' disease are the same as those in any cause of hyperthyroidism (Figure 10.1; Table 10.2).

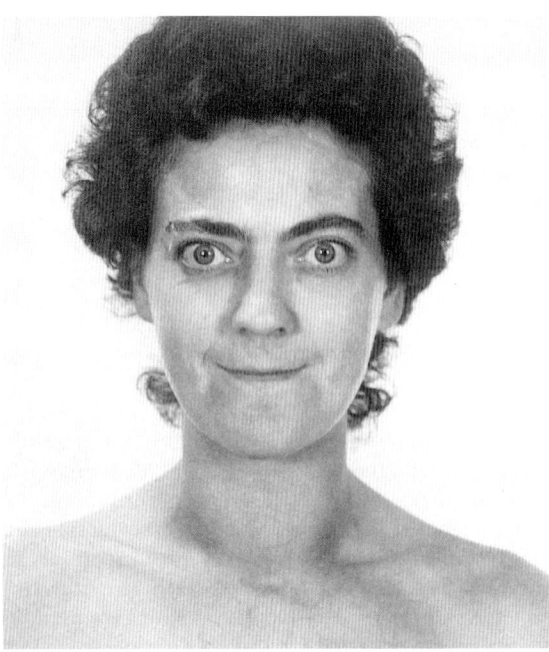

Figure 10.1
Typical appearance of Graves' disease. There is a diffuse goiter and moderate ophthalmopathy.

	Approximate prevalence (%)
Palpitations; tachycardia (atrial fibrillation in the elderly)	100
Fine tremor	95
Heat intolerance; sweating	90
Irritability and nervousness; hyperkinesia	90
Loss of weight; increased appetite (rarely weight gain)	85
Muscle weakness and wasting; fatigue	75
Dyspnea	70
Diarrhea	20
Anorexia	10
Pruritus	10
Gynecomastia	10

Table 10.2
Main symptoms and signs of thyrotoxicosis in Graves' disease in descending order of frequency.

However, the presence of these is variable, depending particularly on age and duration of disease, as well as the severity of the hyperthyroidism. Although weight loss is usual, in 5–10% of patients there may be weight gain due to the increased appetite. β-blockers given for thyrotoxic symptoms or for a coincidental condition can mask features. Atrial fibrillation typically occurs in the elderly; sinus tachycardia is usually present in younger patients. Pre-existing angina may be made worse by hyperthyroidism, and migraine can also be exacerbated.

The patient often notices heat intolerance and excessive sweating; the palms are warm and moist, whereas in anxiety, an important differential diagnosis, they are cool and moist. Pruritus, onycholysis and hair loss may also be reported. The hair loss is diffuse, although alopecia areata and totalis may occur, as these are associated autoimmune disorders. Thyrotoxic hair loss is reversible, but improvement lags far behind successful treatment, which can distress the patient.

The main neurological features are irritability, hyperactivity and a fine tremor, best detected by feeling the outstretched fingers. In contrast, apathetic thyrotoxicosis with depression and inanimation is sometimes found in the elderly. There is usually hyperreflexia, and muscle wasting with proximal myopathy can be marked, particularly in Asians, in whom TAO is uncommon.[7] Another important ethnic feature is periodic paralysis, which is a common presentation in Chinese, especially young males.[8] Chorea and bulbar palsy are rare manifestations of Graves' disease.

Oligomenorrhea or amenorrhea in women, and impotence and gynecomastia in men, are reflections of the effect of excessive thyroid hormones on the pituitary–gonadal axis, particularly through the increased level of sex hormone-binding globulin. Thirst, polyuria and diarrhea are variable. Osteoporosis, due to the direct effect of thyroid hormone on bones, has been demonstrated by body composition analyses, and bone mineral content reverses much more slowly than the loss of lean body mass after treatment.[9] The risk of fracture is increased and is sustained after treatment, and increased mortality from cardiovascular and cerebrovascular disease have also been shown, despite treatment with radioiodine.[10,11]

Graves' disease specifically causes a diffuse painless thyroid enlargement, the resulting goiter usually being palpable and distinguishable from toxic nodular thyroid disease. However, diffuse goiter also occurs in the less common causes of thyrotoxicosis, such as destructive thyroiditis and TSH-secreting tumors. Moreover, nodular thyroid disease can coexist with

Features associated with Graves' disease
  Diffuse goiter
  Thyroid-associated ophthalmopathy
  Thyroid-associated dermopathy (pretibial myxedema)
  Thyroid acropachy
Presence of other autoimmune disease (e.g. vitiligo, alopecia areata, type 1 diabetes mellitus)
Family history of thyroid or other autoimmune disease (especially autoimmune polyglandular syndrome type 2)
Persistent thyrotoxicosis (>4 weeks)

Table 10.3
Clinical features useful in the diagnosis of Graves' disease.

Graves' disease, and when they are autonomous this is called the Marine–Lenhart syndrome.[12] Thyroid cancer is more aggressive when it arises in the context of Graves' disease, due to the stimulatory action of TSH-R antibodies.[13] The overall frequency of thyroid cancer is possibly also increased slightly.[12]

A number of other clinical features help to distinguish Graves' disease from other types of thyrotoxicosis (Table 10.3). Rarely, lymphoid hyperplasia (thymus, spleen, lymph nodes) occurs and is reversible with treatment; I am aware of one patient having an unnecessary thymectomy from ignorance of this.

Investigation

Once the diagnosis is suspected, it is necessary to demonstrate the presence of thyrotoxicosis and to establish that Graves' disease is the cause, which in

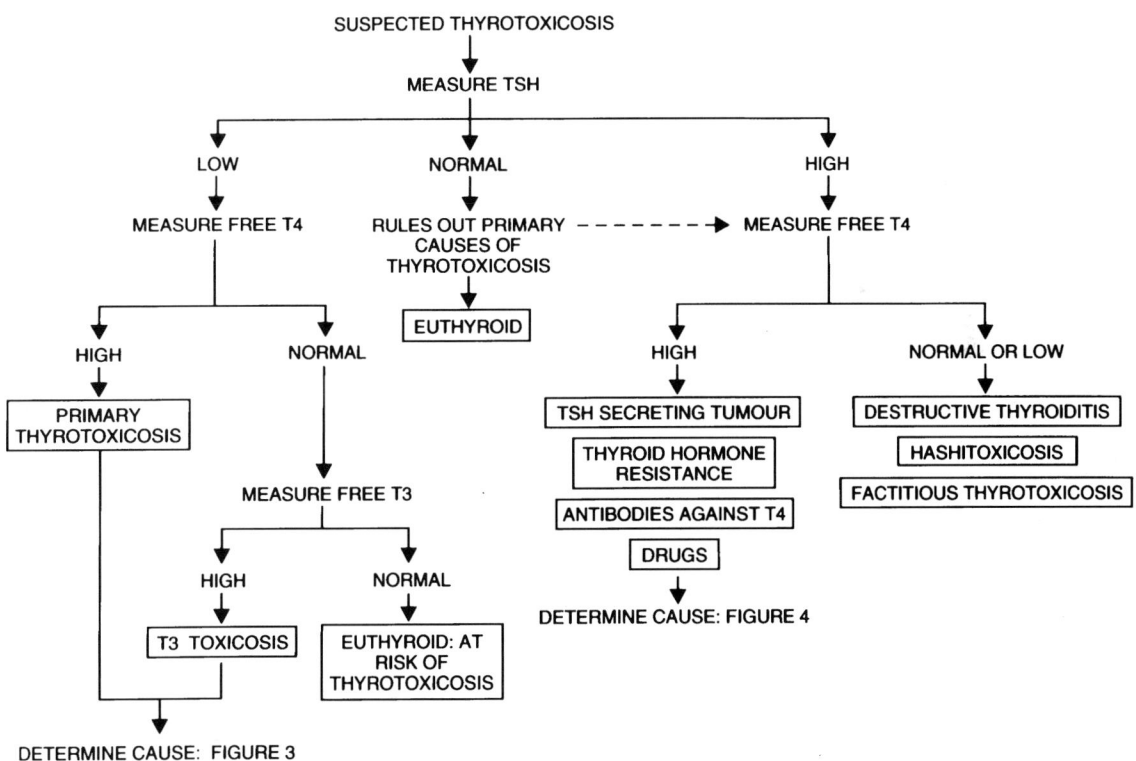

Figure 10.2
Sequence of tests to determine whether a patient has thyrotoxicosis. The dotted line indicates that this step is not always indicated, although some laboratories measure TSH and free thyroxine (T4) simultaneously.

AUTOIMMUNE DISEASE

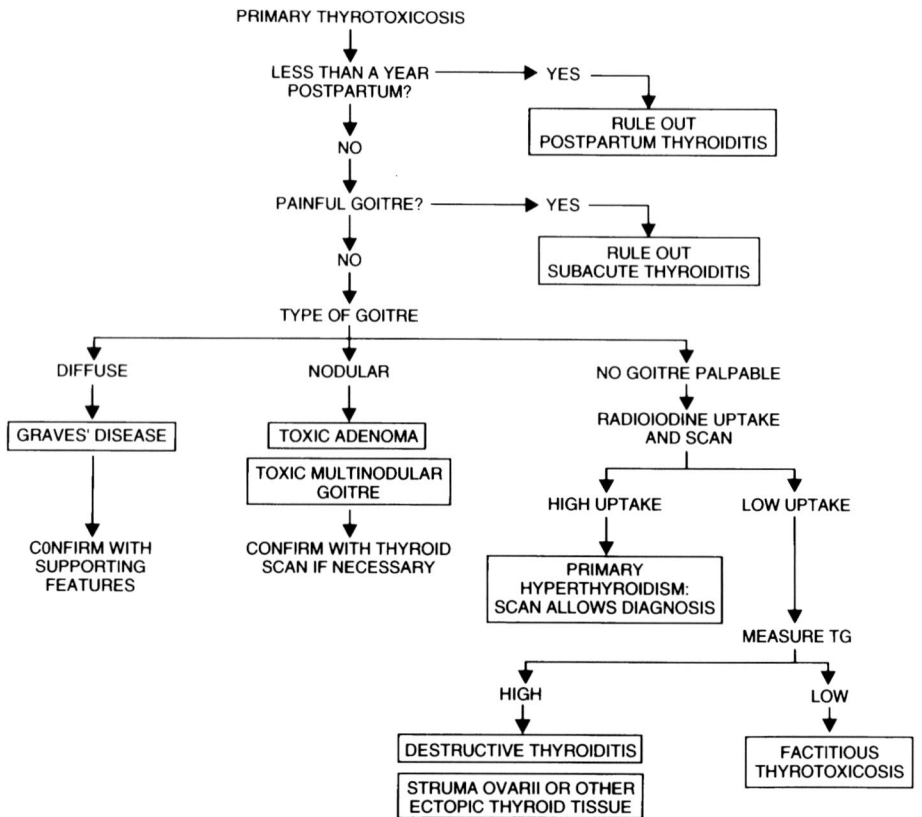

Figure 10.3
Sequence of investigations determining the cause of primary thyrotoxicosis. TG, thyroglobulin.

Recent treatment of thyrotoxicosis (any modality);[a] TSH can remain low for months after treatment of Graves' disease

Thyroid-associated ophthalmopathy;[a] may precede biochemical and clinical thyrotoxicosis by months or years

Multinodular goiter;[a] such patients are at risk of future thyrotoxicosis

Non-thyroidal illness; any severe illness, including psychiatric disorders

Pregnancy; hCG has mild thyroid stimulatory activity in the first trimester, rarely sufficient to cause transient 'gestational' thyrotoxicosis

Pituitary disease; free T4 levels are the only accurate guide to thyroid status in pituitary disease

Relatives of patients with Graves' disease;[a] at risk of developing Graves' disease

[a]Often termed subclinical hyperthyroidism.
T4, thyroxine.

Table 10.4
Situations in which the TSH may be low but the patient is not thyrotoxic.

80% of thyrotoxic patients is the case. A summary of the investigations used to confirm thyrotoxicosis and to determine the etiology is given in Figures 10.2 and 10.3. In all patients, TSH levels will be undetectable using so-called second-generation assays capable of detecting values as low as 0.04 mU/l, although up to 10% of patients will have values above 0.01 mU/l by third-generation assays.[14] The availability of sensitive TSH assays has replaced the thyrotropin-releasing hormone (TRH) test, sometimes used when there was a diagnostic problem, but it is important to be aware that a low TSH alone is inadequate to confirm the diagnosis (Table 10.4).

The development of robust analog immunoradiometric and chemiluminescent assays has allowed the measurement of free triiodothyroxine (T3) and free thyroxine (T4) levels to become readily available, and these assays have all but replaced assays for total T3 and T4, which are subject to major problems if there are abnormalities in thyroid hormone-binding proteins.[15] The exact sequence of thyroid testing usually depends on local laboratory practice. Our strategy in screening for thyroid dysfunction is to perform free T4 estimation only on samples with abnormal TSH values (unless pituitary disease is suspected) and, if the TSH is suppressed but free T4 normal, to go on to free T3 testing, to pick up the 5% or so of patients with T3 toxicosis. However, other laboratories offer different protocols, such as initial free T3 testing instead of free T4, and the local strategy should therefore be discussed and agreed between biochemist and endocrinologist. Anomalies can arise when using free T4 as an initial screening strategy, and when TSH is detectable in patients with a high free T4, the diagnosis is clearly not Graves' disease (Figure 10.4).

The diagnosis, once thyrotoxicosis is confirmed, is usually based on clinical features (Table 10.3), although the presence of antibodies to thyroglobulin (TG) and/or thyroid peroxidase (TPO; previously called the microsomal antigen) provides useful supplementary evidence, being found in around 80% of patients. At least 90% of Graves' patients have readily detectable TSH-R stimulatory antibodies, depending on the sensitivity of the assay used[16] (Table 10.5), but these assays are expensive, not widely available and tend to

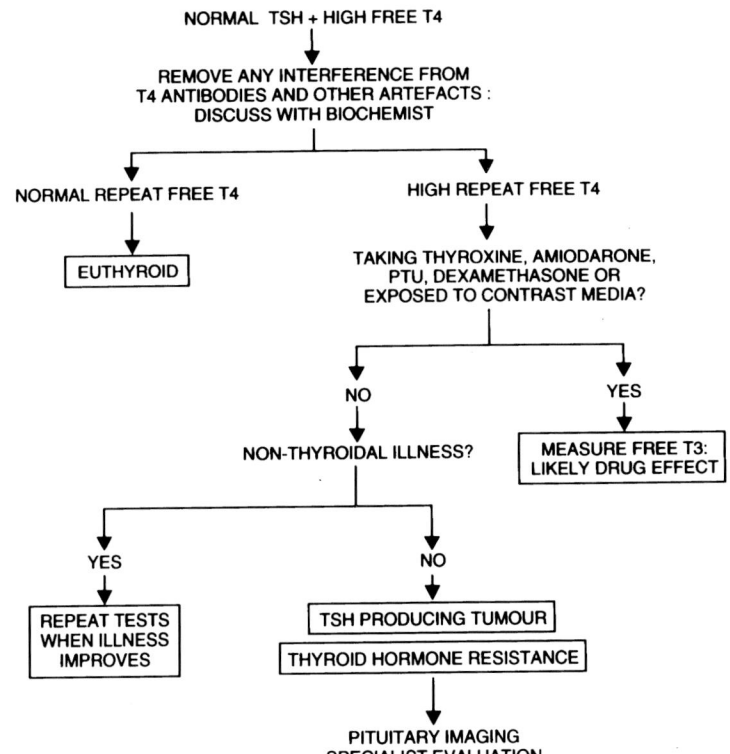

Figure 10.4
Sequence of tests to determine the cause of an elevated free T4 level with a normal (or high) TSH level. If total T4 is measured, thyroid hormone-binding protein anomalies must be ruled out by measuring free T4 first. PTU, propylthiouracil.

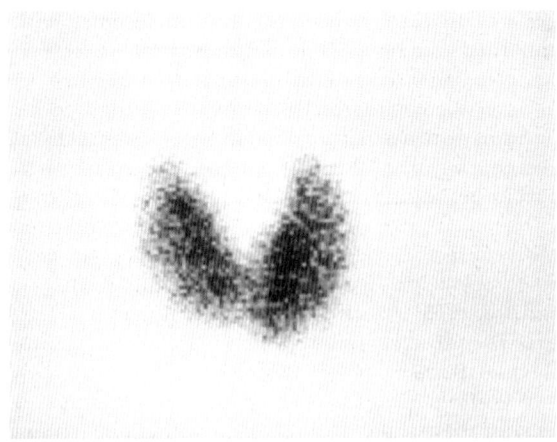

Figure 10.5
Diffuse goiter with increased radioiodine uptake demonstrated by thyroid scintiscanning.

be used for research purposes rather than confirming the diagnosis of Graves' disease in routine clinical practice. However, they may be useful in some patients with TAO, and in pregnant Graves' patients, as discussed later. If it is essential to confirm the diagnosis, e.g. because a diffuse goiter cannot be felt confidently, the best test is a ^{99m}Tc (or radioiodine) scan,[17] which will show a diffuse goiter with increased isotope uptake (Figure 10.5). This investigation will rule out unsuspected nodular thyroid disease and will also demonstrate the low and often patchy isotope uptake typical of subacute and postpartum thyroiditis, and factitious thyrotoxicosis. However, a similar scan appearance to Graves' disease occurs rarely with TSH- and human chorionic gonadotropin (hCG)-secreting tumors.

Management

A number of different management strategies are used, with marked geographical variation, particularly in the initial use of anti-thyroid drugs in Europe and radioiodine in the USA.[18,19] Obviously, the final decision rests with the patient, after a careful explanation of the risks and benefits of each treatment, but in general anti-thyroid drugs are used initially to improve thyroid status (over 4–8 weeks) and in an extended course thereafter to achieve remission in 40–50% of patients, with radioiodine being used instead of an extended course of drugs in patients who have relapsed (second courses of drugs achieve remission in less than 10% of cases), who are elderly or who have cardiac complications.[20] Other details are considered under the appropriate headings below.

Antibody	Acronym	Comment
TSH-R-stimulating antibodies	TSAb	Cause Graves' disease. Require bioassay to determine functional activity; usually involves measuring antibody-mediated cyclic AMP production by thyroid cells or cells transfected with TSH-R
Thyroid-blocking antibodies	TBAb	Cause hypothyroidism. Require bioassay to determine functional activity, measuring any antibody-mediated reduction in cyclic AMP production by thyroid cells (or TSH-R-transfected cells) stimulated with TSH
TSH-binding inhibiting immunoglobulins	TBII	Commercially available assay of antibody-mediated inhibition of binding of radiolabeled TSH to TSH-R. Measures both TSAb and TBAb and therefore gives no information on function

Table 10.5
Main types of assay for TSH-R antibodies.

Anti-thyroid drugs

Thiourylene drugs are derivatives of thionamides which inhibit iodine organification and hence interupt thyroid hormone synthesis. Carbimazole (CBZ) is rapidly converted to methimazole, and these are both popular first choices in Europe, whereas propylthiouracil (PTU) is preferred in North America, but there is little to choose beween these agents in most cases. PTU has the additional action of inhibiting the type 1 deiodinase enzyme which converts T4 to T3, and therefore T3 falls more rapidly with PTU than CBZ, but this is only of importance in severe thyrotoxicosis (Chapter 16), and the benefit is offset by the large number of 50-mg tablets that need to be taken initially (starting dose 150 mg tds or qds). CBZ is made as both 5-mg and 20-mg tablets (starting dose 20 mg bd or tds), so compliance is likely to be better. The serum half-life of methimazole is 6–9 h, whereas that of PTU is 75 min: once euthyroidism is restored, CBZ can be taken in a single daily dose, whereas PTU must be taken in divided doses. Finally, it is important to be aware that PTU doses must be reduced with renal failure.

The principal action of anti-thyroid drugs is to inhibit the action of TPO in iodine organification and iodotyrosyl coupling. However, on its own this would be insufficient to induce remission in what is an immunological disease, and there is evidence that these drugs also inhibit the intrathyroidal immune responses necessary to sustain the autoimmune process, as a result of which TSH-R antibodies decrease, sufficiently so in some patients for remission to be achieved.[21] For this reason, it is essential that the diagnosis of Graves' disease is confirmed before prolonged drug treatment is given, as remission will not be achieved in nodular thyroid disease or other causes of thyrotoxicosis. The place of anti-thyroid drugs in these disorders is generally to produce biochemical control until definitive treatment with radioiodine is given.

Considerable effort has been made to identify factors which would predict outcome after anti-thyroid drugs, with a view to reserving this treatment for those patients most likely to enter remission. Not unexpectedly, those with the highest TSH-R antibody levels do worst, but the sensitivity and specificity of this are too poor to have clinical value,[22] and no other useful markers have emerged. The best predictor is goiter size, those with the largest goiters almost always relapsing.[23]

Anti-thyroid drugs can be given in two distinct ways, each designed to avoid hypothyroidism. First, the high initial starting dose is gradually reduced as the patient becomes euthyroid, so that after 2–3 months the patient is maintained on 5–20 mg CBZ/day (or 50–200 mg PTU/day). This is called the titration regimen. The second method, the block-replace regimen, continues the high dose of anti-thyroid drugs used initially and adds in T4 to achieve euthyroidism. In practice, the patient takes 20 mg CBZ tds (or 150 mg PTU 100 mg qds) for 3–4 weeks (in some centers, and especially with mild disease, the initial CBZ dose is 20 mg bd, and the initial PTU dose 100 mg qds). At review, the CBZ dose is lowered to 40 mg once a day (PTU 100 mg qds) and a free T4 measurement is made; if it is normal, T4 100 µg/day is also commenced, and if it is still abnormal, the introduction of T4 is delayed by 1–2 weeks, depending on the severity of the thyrotoxicosis. Four weeks after starting T4, the serum free T4 level is measured and the T4 dosage is adjusted if necessary to achieve normal levels, but the anti-thyroid drug dose remains static. Once free T4 levels are normal, a check need only be made every 2 months or so, provided that both CBZ and T4 are being taken.

Which regimen is chosen depends on personal experience, and remission rates appear to be similar, with the proviso that maximum remission is achieved with only 6 months' treatment with the block-replace regimen, while the titration regimen must be continued for 18–24 months to achieve the same remission rate.[24,25] Euthyroidism is also more certainly achieved with the block-replace regimen, both because there is no need to adjust drug levels continuously, with the potential for underdosage or overdosage, and because compliance is likely to be better, with a fixed regimen generally of three tablets daily (2×20 mg CBZ plus 100 µg T4) compared to varying numbers of CBZ tablets (multiples of 5 mg) over time. For these reasons, I prefer the block-replace regimen.

Once treatment stops, patients should be followed up to detect early evidence of relapse. Around two-thirds of relapses occur within a year of stopping treatment. My policy is to review patients at 6 weeks, 3 months, 6 months, 9 months and a year after stopping treatment (or ask the general practitioner (GP) to arrange thyroid function tests at these times) and thereafter to enrol the patient in a computerized follow-up scheme for annual thyroid function tests in general practice. This will not only detect late relapse, which can occur up to 15 years after stopping treatment,[26] but also late hypothyroidism due to supervening, coincident autoimmune thyroiditis, which occurs in 5–20% of patients.[27] It is also worth pointing out that TSH levels may give misleading information in the early stages after treatment (Table 10.4), and free T3 and/or T4 measurements provide the best guide to thyroid status. Recent interest has focused on attempts to minimize relapse by continuing T4 treatment alone to lower TSH levels, after a period of administering the block-replace regimen, the idea being to suppress intrathyroidal autoimmune events which might depend on TSH, such as expression of autoantigen.[28] The initial encouraging results have proved impossible to reproduce, and this cannot therefore be recommended.[29]

The side-effects of anti-thyroid drugs are given in Table 10.6. They are partly dose and time related, with most complications occurring within the first 3 months of treatment. The commonest problem is a rash, and the usual advice is to switch drugs, generally using PTU instead of CBZ. The most serious side-effect is agranulocytosis, with anti-thyroid drugs being the commonest group of drugs responsible for this. The frequency is around 1 in 3000 users per year. All patients must be given written instructions about the need to stop treatment, recording that this has been done in the notes, and have a full blood count if suggestive symptoms (sore throat, fever, mouth ulcers) appear. Granulocyte counts usually recover spontaneously, but affected patients should be admitted for monitoring and broad-spectrum antibiotic treatment; colony-stimulating factor treatment has inconsistent benefit.[30] Agranulocytosis can occur after administering a second or subsequent course of anti-thyroid drugs in patients who have had no problems with their initial course. The place of routine monitoring of white cell counts in patients receiving anti-thyroid drugs is uncertain, but this is not normal UK practice.[31]

Other drugs

Propranolol and other β-blocker drugs are useful to ameliorate symptoms while awaiting the results of other anti-thyroid treatments. The usual dose is 20–40 mg of propranolol qds, dosage being adjusted to maintain a normal heart rate. The dose is gradually reduced as euthyroidism is achieved. Lithium carbonate controls thyrotoxicosis through its inhibitory action on adenylate cyclase; paradoxically, the drug can also stimulate autoimmune responses, including the precipitation of Graves' disease.[32] It is very much a second-line drug, useful only in controlling disease temporarily if CBZ or PTU cannot be given. The usual dose is 300–450 mg tds, with close monitoring of serum levels. Potassium perchlorate is another rarely used agent which reduces intrathyroidal iodine. It has a much greater risk of inducing agranulocytosis and aplastic anemia than CBZ. Its main use is to control amiodarone-induced thyrotoxicosis, at doses of 200 mg qds and usually in combination with CBZ and steroids, but used alone it can also produce remission in Graves' disease.[33]

Finally, large doses of stable iodine temporarily block thyroid hormone synthesis, and this action is useful in preparing patients for surgery or in thyroid storm. Traditionally, Lugol's iodine (5% iodine, 10% potassium iodide) is used, 0.1–0.3 ml tds, but 60-mg KI tablets or a saturated solution of KI can also be used. After 1–3 weeks of iodide treatment, the thyroid escapes from control and thyrotoxicosis can then be exacerbated.

Common
　Rash
　Arthralgia
　Fever
　Pruritus
　Nausea
　Headache
Uncommon or rare
　Agranulocytosis; thrombocytopenia; aplastic anemia
　Vasculitis; SLE-like syndrome; lymphadenopathy
　Rhinitis; conjunctivitis
　Diarrhea
　Jaundice; hepatic failure
　Enlargement or inflammation of salivary glands
　Induction of insulin autoimmune syndrome (insulin antibodies producing hypoglycemia)
　Loss of taste
　Alopecia
　Edema (rarely due to nephrotic syndrome)

SLE, systemic lupus erythematosus.

Table 10.6
Main side-effects of anti-thyroid drugs.

Radioiodine

There is general agreement that radioiodine is the best primary treatment for older patients (greater than 40 or 50 years old, depending on center) with Graves' disease and for adult patients who have relapsed after anti-thyroid drugs.[18–20] In many centers radioiodine is used infrequently, if at all, in children and adolescents (see below), and of course it is contraindicated in pregnancy and during breastfeeding. Pregnancy should be avoided for 4 months after treatment.[34] Radioiodine, like all radiation, carries a risk of genetic damage to germ cells, but this is negligible (an estimated increase of 0.005% in malformations after a typical dose, which delivers approximately the same amount of radiation as a barium enema), and therefore patients can be reassured about subsequent fertility. Nonetheless, some patients wish to avoid any exposure to medical radiation, and their wishes must obviously be respected. There is no overall increased risk of cancer.[11,34] Perhaps the most difficult problem is the requirement for a treated patient to minimize close contact with children and pregnant women, due to their radiosensitivity[34] (Table 10.7). This proves impossible to arrange for many mothers, and it can be difficult to reassure a woman that radioiodine is very safe while at the same time she cannot be within a meter of her child for 3 weeks! The Royal College of Physicians of London has published valuable guidelines on the advice which needs to be given to patients (in written form) and also practical details on treatment and follow-up, and these are essential reading for anyone involved with administering radioiodine.[34]

Precaution	Administered activity of ^{131}I (MBq)			
	200	400	600	800
Avoid journeys on public transport	0	0	3	6
Stay off work when travel to/from work is by public transport, even though work does not involve close contact with other people	0	0	3	6
Stay off work when travel is by private transport and work does not involve close contact with other people	0	0	0	0
Avoid places of entertainment or close contact with other people	1	5	9	12
Stay off work (when it involves close contact with other people)	1	5	9	12
Avoid non-essential close personal contact with children and pregnant women. Avoid work that involves close contact with children and pregnant women or work of a radiosensitive nature	14	21	24	27

Reproduced from the Radioiodine Audit Subcommittee of the Royal College of Physicians Committee on Diabetes and Endocrinology and the Research Unit of the Royal College of Physicians,[34] with permission.

Table 10.7
Number of days for which patients should take special precautions according to the activity of radioiodine administered.

There is a very small but important risk of thyroid storm after radioiodine, and radioiodine treatment is slow to work: for these two reasons, it seems best to treat patients with anti-thyroid drugs prior to giving ^{131}I. My own policy is to give 40 mg carbimazole daily for 4 weeks to all but young patients without any complications, although if relapse is detected soon after cessation of anti-thyroid drugs, there is probably no need to retreat. Others prepare the majority of patients with propranolol alone, reserving anti-thyroid drugs for those with severe thyrotoxicosis or atrial fibrillation and possibly cardiac failure.[35] Anti-thyroid drugs should be stopped at least 2 days prior to radioiodine. There is evidence that pre-, and particularly post-radioiodine treatment with anti-thyroid drugs increases the rate of unsuccessful treatment,[36,37] but this effect is readily countered by increasing the dose of radioiodine given. A recent retrospective survey of 93 patients found that pretreatment with PTU, but not methimazole, reduced the efficacy of radioiodine, even if the PTU was discontinued up to 7 weeks prior to radioiodine.[38] Patients who are ill with hyperthyroidism, or who have cardiac complications, should have CBZ beginning 3 days after ^{131}I, although, in the majority of patients, no treatment or propranolol will suffice.[34]

The method of treatment varies markedly between UK centers,[39] a finding which led to the recent development of guidelines.[34] In essence, there are three broad strategies: (1) calculation of the dose based on tracer isotope studies and other factors; (2) estimation of dose based on clinical grounds, including gland size; and (3) use of a fixed dose, often with the aim of deliberate ablation.[35,39] Prospective surveys, as well as the practical issues of cost-effectiveness and simplicity of treatment, have led to the conclusion that elaborate dosimetry is not worthwhile,[40,41] and even when deliberate fixed-dose ablation is attempted, hypothyroidism is only achieved in two-thirds of patients in the first year, at the expense of overdosing some patients.[42] The present recommendations are therefore that doses of radioiodine are given based on clinical features[34,35] (Table 10.8). Before giving radioiodine, it is important to check that the patient is continent (otherwise it is necessary to arrange inpatient disposal of urine via a catheter) and that the patient has not been exposed to excess stable iodine (amiodarone, contrast media), as this prevents radioiodine uptake. The special case of accompanying TAO is considered below.

Complications of radioiodine, apart from hypothyroidism, are rare, but include transient radiation thyroiditis and hypoparathyroidism. Salivary gland inflammation may also occur. The incidence of hypothyroidism varies depending on the dose regimen used, but, in general, the greater the success rate (cure after a single dose of ^{131}I), the higher the rate of hypothyroidism. For example, graded doses of radioiodine give a hypothyroidism rate of around 10% in the first year, with retreatment in up to 20%, whereas the deliberate ablation regimen gives a 1-year relapse rate of 4% and hypothyroidism in 64%.[42,43] Whatever the strategy, the key point is that hypothyroidism continues to occur indefinitely after ^{131}I, so that all patients need follow-up. My own policy is to review patients at 1½, 3, 6, 9 and 12 months after treatment and then arrange computerized follow-up via the GP. It is also important to note that hypothyroidism occurring up to 6 months after treatment can be temporary, and may result from radiation damage to TPO or immunological changes.[44] Finally, uncontrolled hyperthyroidism within 6 months of treatment should be controlled with anti-thyroid drugs, a second dose only being given if the patient remains hyperthyroid off drug treatment at 6 months after the first dose of ^{131}I. This is because radioiodine is slow to work in some patients. Recurrence after surgery is best dealt with using radioiodine, although it should be noted that such patients have a high sensitivity to this treatment and frequently develop hypothyroidism.[45]

Surgery

The advantages and disadvantages of surgery, most often subtotal thyroidectomy for Graves' disease, are shown in Table 10.9. There are few absolute indications for surgical treatment of Graves' disease,[46] although in centers performing frequent thyroidectomy, the efficacy

---

Graves' disease—no/small goiter, 200 MBq
Graves' disease—moderate/large goiter, 400 MBq
Toxic adenoma—400 MBq (600 MBq if severe hyperthyroidism)
Toxic multinodular goiter—uncomplicated, 600 MBq
Hyperthyroidism of any cause plus severe medical complications (including heart failure, atrial fibrillation), 800 MBq

Table 10.8
Suggested guidelines for radioiodine dosage.

> Benefits
>   Rapid cure of hyperthyroidism
>   No adverse effect on ophthalmopathy
>   Can be used in pregnancy (second trimester) if patient is intolerant of anti-thyroid drugs
>   Definitive diagnosis of any coincidental thyroid nodule
>   Resolves cosmetic problems with large goiter
> Risks
>   Anesthesia; need careful preoperative treatment
>   Postoperative complications:
>   Hemorrhage
>   Laryngeal edema
>   Recurrent laryngeal nerve damage
>   Hypoparathyroidism
>   Scar
>   Recurrence (should be less than 5%)
>   Hypothyroidism

Table 10.9
Summary of the benefits and risks of surgical treatment for Graves' disease.

of this treatment is established.[47] The only factor which determines outcome, in terms of thyroid function, is the remnant size,[48] and most surgeons would advocate removal of sufficient thyroid tissue to give recurrence rates below 5%, although this is associated with a high risk of hypothyroidism (around 20–40% at 1 year), which continues to increase with time.[47] This means that all postsurgical patients should be offered annual follow-up after close follow-up in the year after surgery.

Meticulous control of hyperthyroidism prior to surgery is essential, and many surgeons continue to use stable iodine in the preoperative period. My own policy is to favor surgery in the following circumstances: (1) patient's own preference for radioiodine, after anti-thyroid drug relapse; (2) treatment of Graves' disease in pregnancy, childhood or adolescence in patients intolerant of anti-thyroid drugs; (3) after inconclusive fine needle aspiration biopsy of a nodule in Graves' disease and (4) first-line treatment of patients with severe TAO and a large goiter, as these are very likely to relapse after CBZ.

Graves' disease in children and adolescents

This is uncommon, and clinical features may be subtle, so that the duration of symptoms and the degree of hyperthyroidism are usually greater than in older patients, in turn requiring longer to achieve remission after anti-thyroid drugs.[49] The best treatment is probably an extended course of anti-thyroid drugs, with additional courses if relapse occurs, particularly if there are educational milestones which require stable thyroid function. As already indicated, surgery is usually preferred to radioiodine when such patients are intolerant of drugs, or when this can be planned around a convenient time in those who have repeatedly relapsed after anti-thyroid drugs.

Graves' disease in pregnancy

Ideally, Graves' disease should be dealt with prior to planned pregnancy, as active Graves' disease causes infertility and a higher frequency of intrauterine growth retardation, miscarriage and stillbirth than normal. If pregnancy occurs, careful monitoring every 2–4 weeks is needed to ensure euthyroidism and monitor the fetus, which is at risk of neonatal thyrotoxicosis due to the transplacental transfer of TSH-R-stimulating antibodies (TSAb). The best treatment is a titration regimen of anti-thyroid drugs using the lowest dose of PTU possible to maintain free T4 levels in the upper half of the reference range. The block-replace regimen should not be used, as anti-thyroid drugs readily cross the placenta, but T4 much less so, thus risking fetal hypothyroidism. PTU is preferable to CBZ, as methimazole, the active metabolite of CBZ, has been associated (albeit controversially) with the fetal skin defect aplasia cutis, but no such cases have been reported with the equally efficacious PTU.[50]

The natural history of Graves' disease in pregnancy is for remission during the last trimester, associated with a fall in TSAb, and at this stage PTU can usually be stopped. It is recommended that maternal TSH-binding inhibiting immunoglobulins (TBII) or, ideally, TSAb levels are checked at the beginning of the third trimester, as high levels predict neonatal thyrotoxicosis, as does a persistent fetal heart rate of >160/min.[51] Management of fetal and neonatal thyrotoxicosis is highly specialized, but one important practical point is that all babies at risk should have urgent thyroid function tests at birth to exclude hyperthyroidism, repeated 4–7 days later if the mother has been taking anti-thyroid drugs up to delivery, as these can mask hyperthyroidism in the neonate until metabolized. Breastfeeding is possible with anti-thyroid drugs, using the lowest possible dose in a titration regimen. The baby's free T4 should be monitored if high doses of drugs are used.

Thyroid-associated ophthalmopathy (TAO)

Around 90% of patients with TAO have Graves' disease; 5% have autoimmune hypothyroidism and 5% are euthyroid at presentation, although subtle evidence of thyroid autoimmunity (thyroid antibodies, abnormal TSH levels, goiter) is found in the majority of the latter.[52] Conversely, signs of TAO are present in 50–60% of Graves' patients, but imaging techniques demonstrate disease in the majority of those without clinical evidence of TAO. This range of associations has led to the terminology being changed from Graves' ophthalmopathy to TAO. The pathogenesis is believed to be primarily a cytokine-mediated activation of extraocular muscle fibroblasts, leading to edema and fibrosis. It is presumed that autoreactive T cells are the main source of cytokines, and these accumulate in the extraocular muscles in response to an unknown autoantigen shared or cross-reactive with the thyroid. The most likely candidate shared autoantigen is the TSH-R, which is expressed by orbital preadipocyte fibroblasts. Supporting this idea is the development of orbital pathology in mice receiving TSH-R-primed T cells.[53] Further details of this complex autoimmune response can be found elsewhere.[52,54]

Smoking is associated with an increased risk of TAO; conversely, Asians with Graves' disease are less likely than Western Caucasians to develop TAO, suggesting the operation of genetic susceptibility factors.[7] The increased prevalence of smoking in men may explain the higher than expected frequency of TAO in older men with Graves' disease.[55] Management of severe TAO is best carried out in specialist centers with the close collaboration of an ophthalmologist interested in this condition, and only a brief account will be given of this aspect of management.

Class	Signs and symptoms
0	**N**o physical signs or symptoms
1	**O**nly signs (upper lid retraction and lag, stare), no symptoms
2	**S**oft tissue involvement (conjunctival or periorbital edema, enlarged lacrimal glands, excess tears, grittiness, discomfort, photophobia)
3	**P**roptosis
4	**E**xtraocular muscle involvement (diplopia, usually looking up and out)
5	**C**orneal involvement (stippling, ulceration, necrosis)
6	**S**ight loss (due to compressive optic neuropathy)

Table 10.10
Main clinical features of TAO, listed according to the NO SPECS classification scheme—although this is a useful mnemonic, it should be noted that patients do not necessarily progress from one class to the next, and that this scheme gives no information on disease activity.

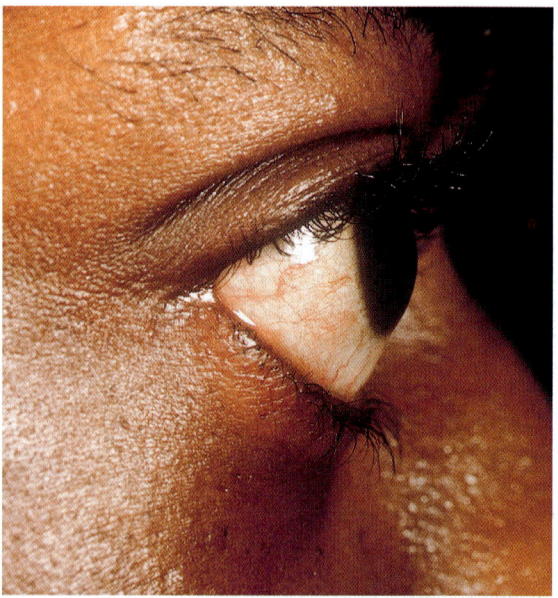

Figure 10.6
Thyroid-associated ophthalmopathy (TAO), showing lid retraction, periorbital edema, chemosis, scleral injection and proptosis. Image courtesy of Dr PMG Bouloux.

Component	Assessment technique
Eyelids	Measurement of maximum fissure width
Cornea	Rose bengal or fluorescein staining
Extraocular muscles	Hess chart, Maddox rod test or similar; muscle thickness can be measured by CT, MRI or ultrasound scans; intraocular pressure measurement (looking downward)
Proptosis	Exophthalmometry (or CT/MR measurements)
Optic nerve	Color vision, visual acuity, visual fields
Activity	Assign points for retrobulbar pain at rest, pain on eye movement, eyelid erythema, conjunctival injection, chemosis, caruncle swelling, eyelid edema
Patient self-assessment	Scales (from best to worst) for appearance, acuity, discomfort and diplopia

Table 10.11
Evaluation of the severity of TAO, based on the classification proposed by the International Thyroid Associations.

Clinical assessment and investigation

The main signs and symptoms are given in Table 10.10 and Figure 10.6. A number of classification schemes have been devised to record physical signs; present recommendations include an assessment of disease activity (Table 10.11), as this predicts outcome after immunosuppressive treatment.[56] The differential diagnosis, particularly of unilateral signs found in 5% of TAO patients, includes orbital pseudotumor (myositis), arteriovenous malformations, granulomatous disease (including Wegener's granulomatosis and sarcoidosis) and a retrobulbar tumor (including glioma, lymphoma, leukemia and metastases). If the diagnosis is in any doubt, CT or MRI will reveal the generally enlarged extraocular muscles, with sparing of the tendinous insertions, typical of TAO (Figure 10.7).[57] In all patients suspected of having TAO, it is obviously essential to measure TSH (and thyroid hormones if the TSH is abnormal) and TG plus TPO antibodies.

Management

A wide range of management approaches is evident in Europe, testifying to the rather inadequate clinical trials often conducted in TAO.[58] Further complications are the variable natural history of the disease, with an overall tendency for worsening over 6–18 months, and stabilization or, sometimes, improvement thereafter, and the effects of coincident thyroid dysfunction and treatment on TAO. What is clear is that physicians underestimate how great an impact even modest TAO has on a patient's life,[59] and the cornerstones of management are a clear explanation of likely outcome (including the caveat that resolution of concurrent thyroid disease will not necessarily be paralleled by resolution of TAO) and treatments, reassurance, sympathy and recognition of the distress the condition causes. The patient should be urged to stop smoking.

For mild to moderate disease, simple measures often relieve symptoms. These include sleeping propped up,

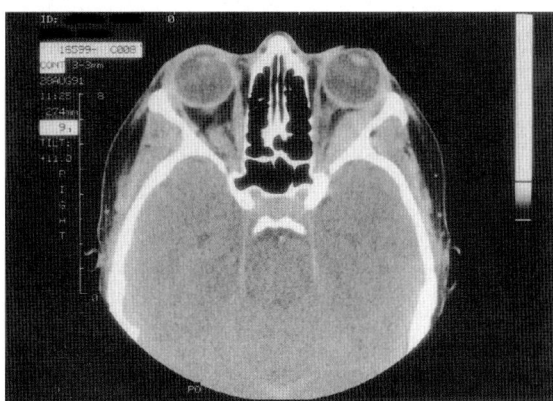

Figure 10.7
Coronal CT scan of the orbit showing TAO; note the enlarged extraocular muscles.

to relieve periorbital edema, use of dark glasses, protection of the eyes from irritants, and the use of lubricants such as hypromellose eye drops through the day and simple eye ointment last thing at night. If lid closure is incomplete, the cornea can be protected during sleep by using tape applied across the closed lids from the nose. Sometimes, periorbital edema responds to Moduretic, one or two tablets daily, or a similar diuretic. Guanethedine eye drops (preferably 1–2% solution, applied twice daily) may relieve lid lag and improve appearance, but many patients find that they cause too much stinging and conjunctival vasocongestion. Diplopia can be relieved by use of opaque spectacle lenses or prisms, pending corrective surgery once disease has stabilized, and surgery also plays a major role in correcting cosmetic problems such as lid lag and proptosis.[60] Careful ophthalmological monitoring is needed to judge the best time to operate.

Severe or congestive ophthalmopathy is an emergency requiring urgent inpatient specialist treatment to preserve vision. The usual treatment is prednisolone 60–100 mg/day, tapered over a few weeks to doses of 10–20 mg, which need to be given for around 6 months to ensure remission.[61] Some centers use intravenous methylprednisolone boluses to initiate treatment.[62] It is clear that there is no consensus over optimal steroid treatment.[58] With such treatments, the risks of peptic ulceration, diabetes and infection are high. If vision continues to deteriorate, then surgical decompression of the orbit, initially using the transethmoidal route, is needed to reverse the compressive optic neuropathy, although this is usually followed by diplopia, requiring corrective surgery when the disease is stable.[52,63] An alternative is to add cyclosporin A or other immunosuppressive agents to prednisolone; this is not as reliable as surgery, but may be considered if the main problem is with congestive changes rather than neuropathy.[64] Radiotherapy to the orbit is also used in this type of patient in certain centers, with results at least as good as those with steroids, but without such severe side-effects.[66] Similar outcomes have been reported with octreotide and intravenous immunoglobulins, but both are expensive and seem, at present, to offer little advantage.[66,67]

With regard to thyroid status, it seems that maintaining euthyroidism (including avoidance of iatrogenic hypothyroidism) has a beneficial effect on eye signs.[68] Considerable debate has focused on the possible effects of treatment for Graves' hyperthyroidism on TAO, and a detailed discussion can be found elsewhere.[52,69] In summary, anti-thyroid drugs have no adverse effects (and some even claim a benefit over radioiodine, via rapid control of thyroid status). Subtotal thyroidectomy is also without overall effect on TAO, and although there are claims that total thyroidectomy is beneficial, there are no good data to support this,[58] and of course there are more risks with a more extensive operation. Radioiodine has clearly been associated with a small risk of worsening of TAO, usually of only mild or modest degree,[70,71] and this has led many to avoid radioiodine when patients have moderately severe TAO (proptosis, diplopia) or congestive ophthalmopathy.[58] Interestingly, some authorities have taken an opposite stance, claiming that ablative doses of ^{131}I are beneficial.[70] An alternative to avoiding any possible risk by not using ^{131}I in a patient with TAO is to give prophylactic steroids.[72] My own practice is not to use radioiodine in congestive TAO, or, if possible, in patients with recent-onset, moderate TAO, instead treating such patients with the block-replace anti-thyroid drug regimen. With stable eye disease, or if a patient with moderate TAO particularly desires radioiodine, I give prednisolone 40 mg/day for 2 weeks from the day of radioiodine administration, reducing to 30 mg, 20 mg and then 10 mg every 2 weeks, and thereafter 5 mg for 2 weeks before stopping. Subtotal thyroidectomy is a reasonable alternative in this situation. As in all aspects of TAO, it is clear that there is no overall best option for dealing with hyperthyroidism, with local experience and policies dictating strategy.[58]

Thyroid dermopathy

This term is preferable to pretibial myxedema, because other sites may be involved, particularly when areas of skin away from the classical pretibial region (Figure 10.8) are traumatized. Thyroid acropachy resembles clubbing, and probably shares a similar pathogenesis with thyroid dermopathy (Figure 10.9).[73] Dermopathy is found in 1–2% of Graves' patients, almost always in association with clinically obvious TAO,[74] with acropachy being even less common but always associated with dermopathy. As with TAO, it is thought that dermopathy is caused by T cells through cytokine-mediated activation of fibroblasts.[75] The typical appearance is of painless, symmetrical plaques over the anterior and lateral aspects of the shins; the lesions are not inflamed, and the edematous skin comprising the plaque does not pit. There is sometimes associated localized hair growth, and the skin is pink to purple,

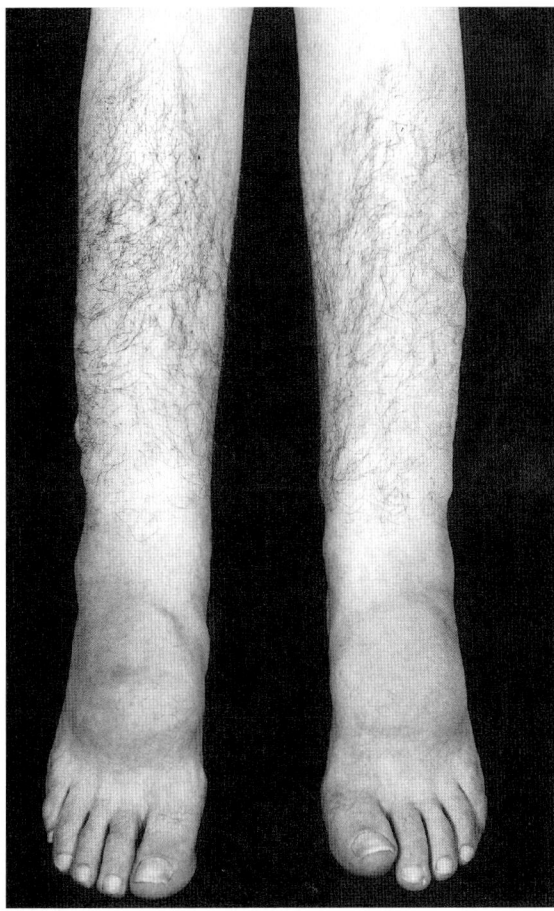

Figure 10.8
Thyroid dermopathy affecting the shins and dorsum of the feet.

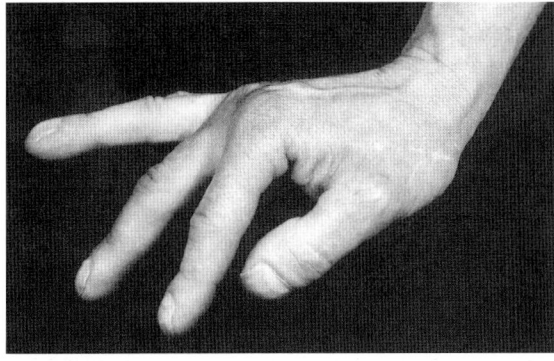

Figure 10.9
Thyroid acropachy.

turning brown in long-standing cases. Less commonly, the lesions are nodular, or the whole lower leg may become swollen, and separate lesions can appear on the dorsum of the foot, related to trauma from footwear, which make shoe wearing uncomfortable or even impossible. Diagnosis is rarely a problem but, in cases of doubt, skin biopsy is useful.[76]

Treatment is not required unless the lesions are causing a problem due to cosmetic effects, tenderness from repeated trauma, or difficulty in wearing shoes, and spontaneous resolution often occurs. Surgical excision is generally followed by recurrence, often with additional scarring, and should be avoided. Small, discrete lesions often respond to intradermal injections of corticosteroids, but more generalized disease needs topical corticosteroids (betamethasone, clobetasol), sometimes applied under occlusive dressings. Response is slow and may be incomplete. Some patients respond to octreotide, but the exact place of this remains to be established.[77]

Autoimmune hypothyroidism

By far the commonest cause of spontaneous hypothyroidism in iodine-sufficient countries, autoimmune hypothyroidism is the result of a usually prolonged, autoimmune process leading to specific destruction of thyroid follicular cells. The main components of this response are T-cell-mediated, and include the actions of specific cytotoxic T cells and T-cell-derived cytokines, which alter the metabolic function and surface molecule expression of thyroid cells.[6,78] TG and TPO antibodies may amplify damage but do not initiate it, as shown by the absence of thyroid dysfunction in neonates born to mothers with high levels of these antibodies. Around 10% of patients have blocking antibodies which interfere with TSH signaling through the TSH-R (Table 10.5), and these do play a pathogenic role, as their transplacental passage causes transient neonatal hypothyroidism.[79] It is thought that fluctuations in the level of these blocking antibodies may account for the spontaneous remission of hypothyroidism seen in some patients,[80] and in rare cases the coincident production of TSAb can lead to a confusing picture of alternating hypo- and hyperthyroidism.[81] However, the natural history in most patients is for inexorable destruction of thyroid tissue, and trials of withdrawal of T4 treatment are not worthwhile.

Table 10.12
Main clinical features of autoimmune hypothyroidism.

> Symptoms
>   Tiredness
>   Cold intolerance; hypothermia
>   Dry skin and lifeless hair (will not take a 'perm')
>   Weight gain, despite poor appetite
>   Constipation
>   Poor memory and somnolence; rarely psychosis
>   Impotence (unusual)
>   Hoarse voice
>   Menorrhagia; later oligomenorrhea or amenorrhea
>   Arthralgia, myalgia and paresthesiae
> Signs
>   Periorbital edema, puffy face and sometimes ankle edema
>   Dry, yellowish skin with cool peripheries
>   Bradycardia
>   Diffuse hair loss
>   Delayed relaxation of ankle joints; carpal tunnel syndrome
>   Cerebellar ataxia (rare)
>   Encephalopathy (rare; steroid responsive)
>   Effusions; pleural, pericardial, ascites, hydrocele (rare)
>   Galactorrhea (rare)
> In childhood
>   Delayed development
>   Delayed or, rarely, precocious puberty

Clinical assessment

The typical signs and symptoms of hypothyroidism are given in Table 10.12, although these are often not clear in the elderly, in whom depression or psychosis may sometimes be suspected instead. Other rare neurological complications include myopathy, sensory and/or motor polyneuropathy and steroid-responsive encephalopathy, the latter being associated with the presence of thyroid antibodies rather than biochemical hypothyroidism. Because of the slow progression, patients may present only with a goiter (Hashimoto's thyroiditis), which is typically firm or hard, and often irregular (bosselated) to the extent that a malignancy may be considered. The overall frequency of thyroid epithelial cell malignancy is probably not increased or decreased in Hashimoto's thyroiditis, and any suspicious nodule should be subjected to fine needle aspiration biopsy.[82] Lymphoma of the thyroid occurs almost exclusively in the setting of Hashimoto's thyroiditis, and although very uncommon, this is another reason to take nodular lesions in this context seriously.[83] Diagnosis of lymphoma can sometimes be made on aspiration biopsy, but confirmation usually requires large needle or open biopsy, and management requires specialist referral to achieve staging and determine which combination of chemotherapy, radiation and, less often, surgery should be used.[84] Pain in a Hashimoto goiter suggests lymphoma, but rarely thyroid tenderness can be due to uncomplicated thyroiditis.[84] This is difficult to manage; it usually settles with T4 treatment and aspirin, but corticosteroids are sometimes effective in severe forms, and, in extreme circumstances, thyroidectomy may be needed.

Patients without a goiter (atrophic thyroiditis; primary myxedema) tend only to present late in disease when hypothyroidism is causing symptoms. It is still unclear whether Hashimoto's and atrophic thyroiditis are simply different stages in the same disease process or have distinct etiologies. Certainly, Hashimoto goiters tend to reduce and may disappear with T4 treatment, but this can take months.[85] Amiodarone, lithium, excess iodine and certain therapeutic cytokines (α-interferon, interleukin-2 and granulocyte/macrophage colony-stimulating factor) can all precipitate autoimmune hypothyroidism. Treatment is unaltered in the presence of these drugs, but, if they are stopped, remission may occur.

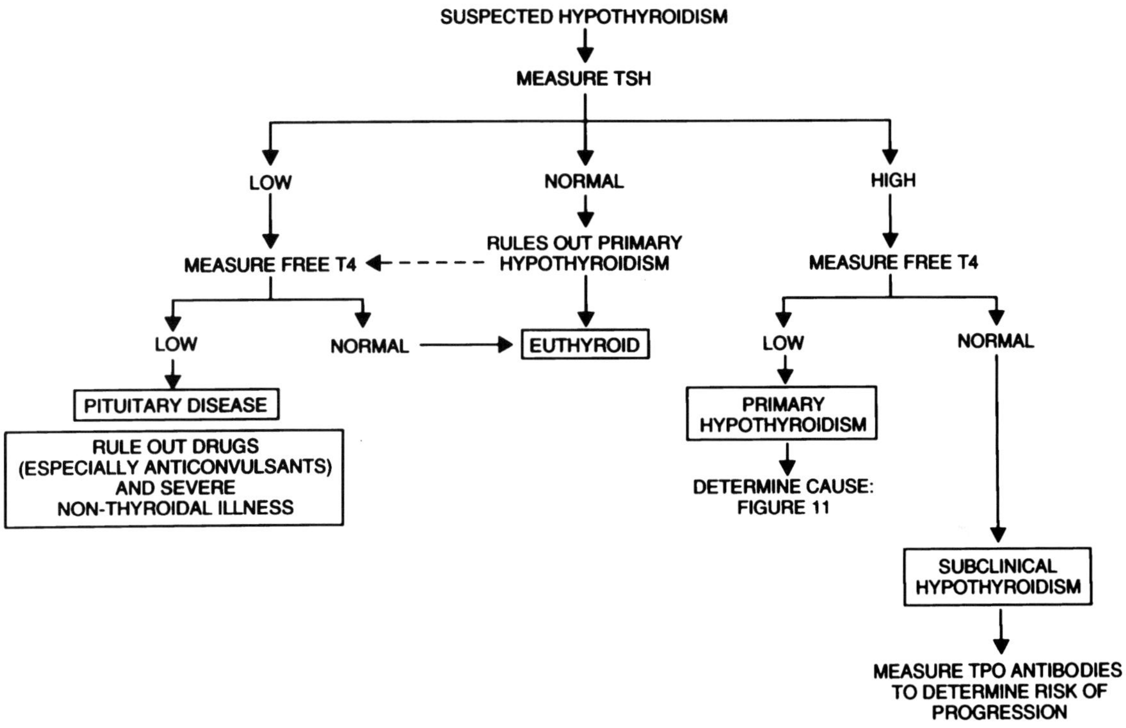

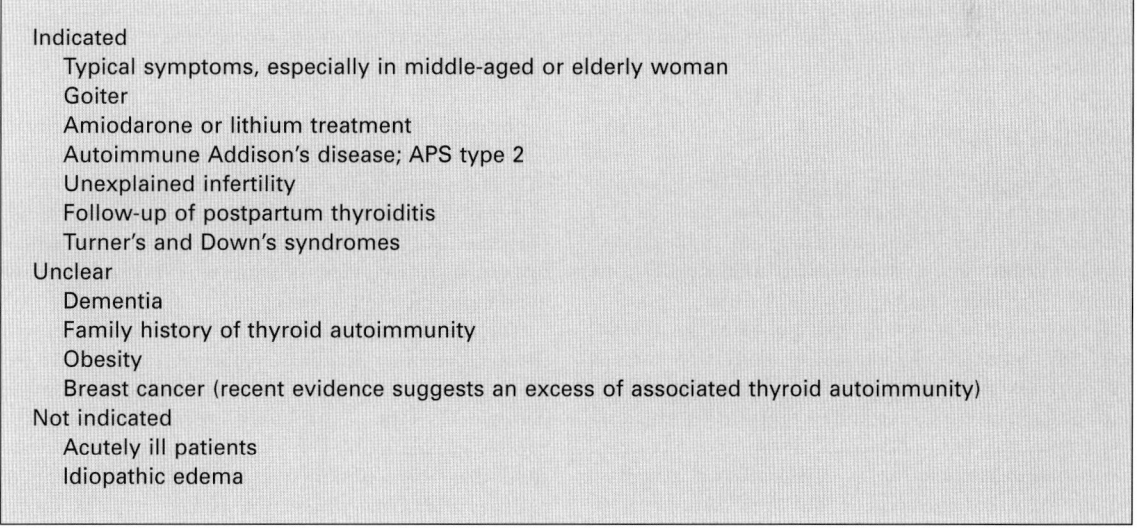

Figure 10.10
Testing strategy for primary hypothyroidism. The dotted line indicates that this step is not always indicated.

Indicated
    Typical symptoms, especially in middle-aged or elderly woman
    Goiter
    Amiodarone or lithium treatment
    Autoimmune Addison's disease; APS type 2
    Unexplained infertility
    Follow-up of postpartum thyroiditis
    Turner's and Down's syndromes
Unclear
    Dementia
    Family history of thyroid autoimmunity
    Obesity
    Breast cancer (recent evidence suggests an excess of associated thyroid autoimmunity)
Not indicated
    Acutely ill patients
    Idiopathic edema

Table 10.13
Indications for screening for autoimmune hypothyroidism.

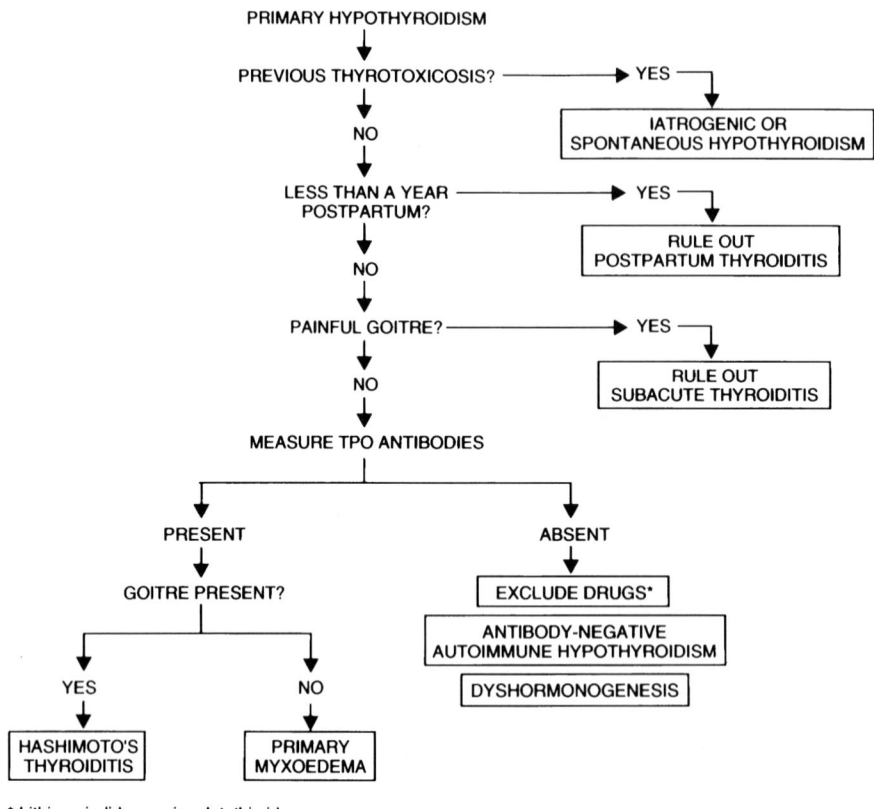

Figure 10.11
Sequence of investigations for determining the cause of primary hypothyroidism in developed, iodine-sufficient countries. Iodine deficiency is the commonest cause of hypothyroidism worldwide.

Investigations

The diagnosis of primary hypothyroidism is readily confirmed by measuring the TSH (usually >20 mU/l) and free T4; free T3 is unreliable as a marker of hypothyroidism and is not measured routinely (Figure 10.10). The other major causes of primary hypothyroidism are usually readily distinguished by clinical features (Figure 10.11), and the etiology is confirmed by demonstrating high levels of TG and/or TPO antibodies. Since TG antibodies are rarely present in the absence of TPO antibodies, some have advocated measuring only the latter.[86] Occasionally, patients have no serum thyroid antibodies,[87] but these can usually be diagnosed on clinical grounds and, if necessary, fine needle aspiration biopsy. A normochromic, normocytic or occasionally microcytic anemia often accompanies hypothyroidism and responds slowly to T4 treatment alone. The presence of a macrocytosis may also be due to hypothyroidism alone, but the coincident occurrence of pernicious anemia should also be borne in mind. Untreated Addison's disease is sometimes accompanied by transient hypothyroidism, which resolves with hydrocortisone replacement.

The frequency of autoimmune hypothyroidism and the insidious way in which symptoms present have led to suggestions that routine screening should be performed. This is probably worthwhile in some patient groups (Table 10.13), but it must be emphasized that there is no place for routine screening of patients with acute illness, due to the frequent abnormalities in thyroid function tests in this setting.[88] On the other hand, the non-specific symptoms of hypothyroidism, especially lethargy, weight gain and poor

	Serum TSH	Serum T4
Subclinical hypothyroidism[a]		
Grade 1	>Upper limit of reference range but <10 mU/l	Normal
Grade 2	10.1–20 mU/l	Normal
Grade 3	>20 mU/l	Normal
Clinical or overt hypothyroidism	>Upper limit of reference range	Low

[a]Symptoms are increasingly likely the higher the TSH level; the term mild hypothyroidism is sometimes used to indicate subclinical hypothyroidism plus symptoms.

Table 10.14
Definition of hypothyroidism.

concentration, mean that many thyroid function tests are performed, and these often pick up subclinical hypothyroidism (Table 10.14). Detailed surveys have shown that around 10% of the population over 55 years have subclinical hypothyroidism, and thyroid antibodies are also frequent (5–10% of women, depending on assay) in patients with normal or only mildly raised TSH levels.[89,90] There is an annual risk of progression to overt hypothyroidism of 2–3% per year in women with subclinical hypothyroidism or detectable thyroid antibodies and of 4–5% if both abnormalities are present; risks are five times greater in men with these findings.[90] The implications for treatment are discussed later.

Management

Treatment can be initiated with 50–100 μg T4 daily, in the absence of cardiovascular problems in the young or middle-aged patient. Otherwise, the starting dose is 25 μg/day or alternate days. It is not worth measuring TSH levels or adjusting dosage before 2 months, as TSH levels may still be falling before then. Symptoms may take even longer to improve, and the patient should be advised that any weight loss will be minor unless dieting is commenced. However, if the 25 μg dose is used to initiate treatment, the patient should be reviewed at 2–3 weeks and if all is well (particularly no worsening of angina) the dose of T4 can then be increased to 50 μg.

The aim of treatment is to normalize TSH levels, and this is usually achieved with T4 doses of 100–150 μg daily. Requirements of 200 μg/day or more suggest poor compliance, and a tactful enquiry may reveal this. One important reason for poor compliance is worsening of angina, and this should be asked about specifically. Attention to antianginal treatment, especially with the appropriate dose of β-blocker, may allow improved tolerance. If the issue is remembering to take tablets, advise the patient to count out a week's supply and take whatever is left at the end of a week all at once, before repeating the tablet count for the next week. As the half-life of T4 is 7 days, this strategy is often successful and is not associated with periods of hypothyroidism; indeed, the week's supply can safely be taken all at once,[91] and, rarely, patients find this easier than taking tablets daily. Deterioration in health after starting T4 suggests concurrent Addison's disease; it is best to start hydrocortisone without T4 initially with this disease combination.[92]

Once the TSH is normal, the patient should be offered regular follow-up to check TSH levels, usually every 1–3 years, and often done by computerized register. In pregnancy, daily T4 requirements increase by 25–50 μg in the last trimester, and patients intending to become pregnant should ensure normal TSH levels prior to conception, as the miscarriage rate and other obstetric complications are higher than normal in hypothyroidism; there is also evidence that even mild thyroid failure in the first trimester of pregnancy can cause intellectual impairment in the fetus.[93] TSH should also be checked once pregnancy is confirmed and at the beginning of the second and third trimester. T4 requirements may decline by 25–50 μg/day in the elderly. There is no place for T3 treatment in hypothyroidism, as this needs to be taken three or four times daily, and even then is associated with fluctuating serum levels.[94] The only exception is myxedema coma. A recent trial has suggested that the combination of

T3 and T4 may be a more satisfactory replacement than T4 alone, but the long-term effects of this are not known and, at present, such a combination should be regarded as experimental.[94]

There are no adverse effects of T4 when the TSH is kept within the reference range. However, T4 treatment sufficient to suppress the TSH should be avoided, as the risk of atrial fibrillation is increased.[95] There is probably little risk to bone from excessive T4, for although bone mineral density declines, particularly in the postmenopausal woman, there is no increase in fracture rate.[96] It is those women who have had a period of primary hyperthyroidism and then iatrogenic hypothyroidism who lose most bone with excessive T4 treatment.[97] Nonetheless, it is best practice to ensure normal TSH levels, irrespective of osteoporosis risk. Accidental or deliberate overdosage with T4 carries surprisingly little risk, especially in the young.[94]

Whether subclinical hypothyroidism warrants treatment has been debated extensively, but surprisingly few trials have informed that debate.[88] Based on the natural history of the disease,[89] it is clear that the minimum that should be offered is regular follow-up (this also includes those individuals with detectable thyroid antibodies but normal TSH). The risks of overt hypothyroidism are so great with the combination of an elevated TSH and positive thyroid antibodies that T4 treatment should be instituted forthwith. My own policy for patients with antibody-negative, subclinical hypothyroidism is to treat with T4 if there are suggestive symptoms and provided that the elevation of TSH has been sustained over 2–3 months; treatment is continued if symptoms improve over 3 months; otherwise, annual follow-up alone is commenced. It remains to be established whether thyroxine treatment will prevent the associated development of atherosclerosis.[90]

Postpartum thyroiditis

Postpartum thyroiditis (PPT) is defined as the occurrence of transient thyroid dysfunction in the year after delivery.[98] It is the result of an unexplained enhancement of the autoimmune response after pregnancy and is associated with a rise in TPO antibody levels at this time (Figure 10.12). Women with strongly positive TPO antibodies antepartum are at increased risk of developing PPT,[99] which has led to suggestions that antibody screening should be performed on all pregnant women, as 1 in 20 will develop PPT.[100] However, this frequency is based on repeated biochemical testing rather than symptomatic disease, which is less common, and only a half to two-thirds of the women who are TPO antibody positive will develop PPT.[101] At present, therefore, routine screening is not recommended.[102]

Clinical assessment

The initial descriptions of PPT focused on clinical manifestations that mimicked subacute thyroiditis, with the key difference that the small firm, diffuse goiter of PPT is not tender. In both conditions, there is a destructive process, leading initially to thyrotoxicosis, caused by release of stored thyroid hormone and lasting up to 4 weeks, and then a phase of hypothyroidism, lasting 1–3 months (Figure 10.12). However, careful prospective studies have shown that this pattern occurs in only a third of patients: 20% have only a thyrotoxic phase, and the remainder only hypothyroidism.[101] The peak time for the development of hypothyroidism is around 18 weeks postpartum, but poor memory and other symptoms may appear in TPO antibody-positive women weeks before the onset of biochemical hypothyroidism. There is an association between postpartum depression and TPO antibody positivity in the postpartum period, raising the possibility that some interaction between the neuroendocrine and immune systems is responsible.[103] In general, the clinical features of thyrotoxicosis and hypothyroidism in PPT are mild, in comparison to those due to sustained Graves' disease or autoimmune hypothyroidism.

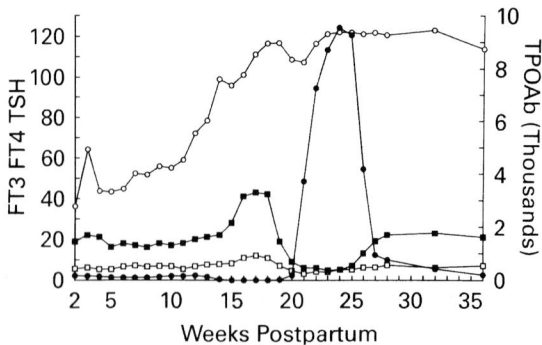

Figure 10.12
Typical changes of TPO antibodies (○) TSH (●), free T3 (□) and free T4 (■), with initial thyrotoxicosis and later hypothyroidism, in a patient with postpartum thyroiditis. From Lazarus et al,[101] with permission.

Diagnosis

Diagnosis of PPT depends largely on the clinical features, once thyroid dysfunction has been established with TSH and free T4 measurements. Strongly positive TPO antibodies clearly do not exclude Graves' disease or Hashimoto's thyroiditis arising in the postpartum period, a time of increased risk for these conditions, but are helpful in ruling out subacute thyroiditis. Moreover, the absence of TPO antibodies does not exclude PPT, particularly the isolated thyrotoxicosis form.[102]

The thyrotoxic phase of PPT is not associated with TAO or thyroid dermopathy, and Graves' disease can also sometimes be distinguished from PPT by the presence of a prior history (usually relapse after anti-thyroid drugs) and thyrotoxicosis of more than 4 weeks' duration. A definitive diagnosis can be made by performing a ^{99m}Tc thyroid uptake measurement, usually with a scan, which shows increased uptake in hyperthyroid Graves' disease, but low uptake in the destructive thyrotoxicosis of PPT. Breastfeeding need only be discontinued for a day for this test. Prolonged and severe hypothyroidism suggests Hashimoto's or atrophic thyroiditis rather than the hypothyroid phase of PPT, but an exact diagnosis is not necessary, as treatment is the same, namely T4 replacement up to a year after delivery. At this stage, T4 is withdrawn and TSH checked at 4–6 weeks to identify permanent hypothyroidism.

The place of routine antepartum screening for PPT was considered above, but patients with type 1 diabetes mellitus constitute a special case, with a frequency of PPT three times higher than normal.[104] In addition, metabolic control is poor in pregnant diabetic women who are TPO antibody-positive.[105] It is therefore worth checking TPO antibodies and TSH at the beginning of pregnancy in all women with type 1 diabetes, and following those who have abnormalities with repeat TSH testing in the second and third trimesters and at 2, 4 and 6 months postpartum.

Management

Thyrotoxic symptoms usually resolve quickly, but if these are troublesome, propranolol 20 mg tds should be started, with doubling of the dose if necessary. Very little of this β-blocker enters breast milk, and treatment is usually only for 1–3 weeks, so breastfeeding is safe, but the infant heart rate should be monitored as a precaution if the mother is taking high doses. There is no place for CBZ or other anti-thyroid drugs in the destructive thyroiditis of PPT; hence the need for distinguishing this from Graves' disease. Follow-up in the weeks after an episode of PPT thyrotoxicosis is needed in anticipation of a hypothyroid phase.

If hypothyroid symptoms are very mild, reassurance and follow-up may be all that are needed, but because of the demands of a new baby, T4 is often indicated. The aim is to restore normal TSH levels. At a year after delivery, T4 is stopped and TSH re-checked 4–6 weeks later to confirm that hypothyroidism has been transient. All women who have had PPT should be offered annual follow-up, as 20–30% develop permanent hypothyroidism in the subsequent 5 years.[106] PPT recurs in subsequent pregnancies, and therefore such women should be offered follow-up during any future postpartum period.

Addison's disease

Tuberculosis is still the commonest cause of primary adrenal failure worldwide, as it was in Thomas Addison's London over 100 years ago, but now autoimmunity accounts for 80–90% of cases in the UK.[107] Rarer causes are shown in Table 10.15. Although autoimmune Addison's disease is most likely to be T cell mediated, by analogy with other destructive autoimmune disorders, direct proof is lacking, due to the rarity of the condition and the impossibility of access to the lymphocytes infiltrating the adrenal cortex. A variety of autoantibodies have been described which fall into two classes: adrenal-specific (directed against the cytochrome P450 21-hydroxylase enzyme) and those reacting with any steroid-producing tissue (directed against the P450 17α-hydroxylase and side-chain cleaving enzymes).[107] The pathogenic role of these antibodies is uncertain, but they are valuable diagnostic tools. Using the best immunofluorescence assays, or the recently developed immunoprecipitation assays, adrenal antibodies can be found in 80–90% of patients with autoimmune Addison's disease, but are absent in non-autoimmune cases.[108]

Clinical assessment

The clinical features (Table 10.16) are highly variable, depending on whether the patient presents acutely or with chronic, slowly progressive disease.[109] The latter

AUTOIMMUNE DISEASE

Autoimmune destruction
Infection
  Tuberculosis
  Fungal infection
  AIDS
  Cytomegalovirus
Congenital
  Adrenoleukodystrophy
  Adrenal hyperplasia or hypoplasia
  Inactivating ACTH receptor mutation
Drugs (metyrapone, ketoconazole, mitotane, suramin, etomidate)
Hemorrhage
  Waterhouse–Friedrichsen syndrome after infection, especially meningococcal
  Antiphospholipid syndrome
  Warfarin
Infiltration
  Metastases
  Amyloidosis
  Sarcoidosis
  Hemochromatosis

ACTH, adrenocorticotropic hormone.

Table 10.15
Causes of primary adrenal failure (Addison's disease).

Increased pigmentation, especially skin creases, recent scars and inside cheeks
Fatigue, weakness
Depression
Nausea and weight loss
Postural hypotension
Salt craving
Abdominal pain, vomiting, diarrhea
Confusion leading to coma
Amenorrhea; decreased libido
Loss of axillary and pubic hair in postmenopausal women
Associated autoimmune disorders; vitiligo, alopecia, thyroid disease, type 1 diabetes mellitus (25–50% of patients)

Table 10.16
Clinical manifestations of Addison's disease.

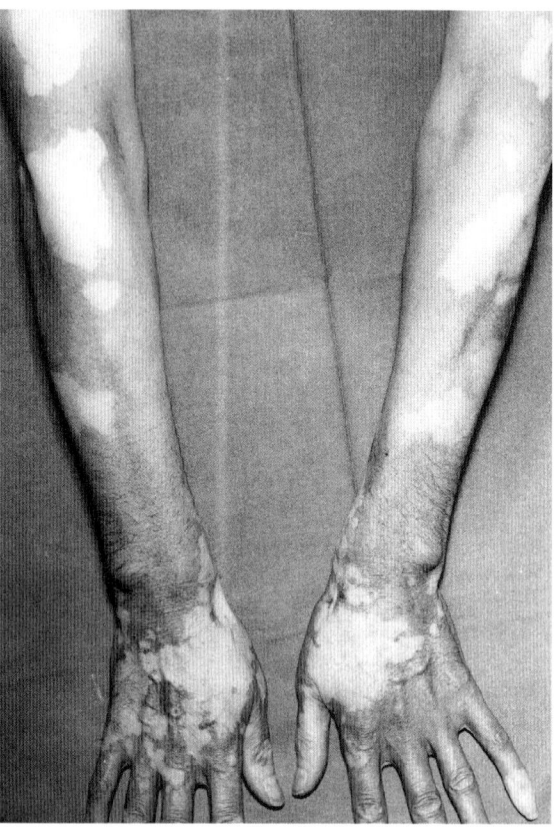

Figure 10.13
Increased pigmentation in a patient with Addison's disease and associated with vitiligo.

is insidious and the patient may be suspected of having anorexia nervosa or depression. Increased pigmentation (Figure 10.13) should always raise suspicion of Addison's disease, and of course the occurrence of Addison's disease as part of APS type 1 and 2 should prompt careful screening in patients with another autoimmune endocrinopathy who have suggestive symptoms.

The most important part of assessing the acutely ill patient is to think of the possibility of Addison's disease in the first place. Missing the diagnosis could easily result in death, and therefore empirical glucocorticoid treatment, until the diagnosis is confirmed, is essential whenever Addison's disease is suspected. Key features are hypotension resistant to dopamine, confusion, vomiting, abdominal symptoms and ultimately coma.

Diagnosis

Clues to the diagnosis are the presence of hyponatremia, hyperkalemia, raised urea and creatinine, hypoglycemia, hypercalcemia, a normochromic, normocytic anemia, eosinophilia and neutropenia. Definitive diagnosis depends on demonstrating a low cortisol, excluding secondary adrenal failure due to pituitary disease and determining the etiology. Random cortisol values are not particularly helpful, but in the setting of an acutely ill patient, a value below 200 nmol/l, together with an adrenocorticotropic hormone (ACTH) level of >80 ng/l, is diagnostic, while a cortisol level of >550 nmol/l excludes Addison's disease; blood should be stored for retrospective analysis, and treatment commenced immediately in this setting. Cortisol levels of <100 nmol/l and >525 nmol/l, at 8–9 a.m, are also sometimes used to demonstrate or exclude chronic Addison's disease.[110] If cortisol values are between these extremes, further testing is needed. The next step is the short Synacthen test, which involves giving 250 μg synthetic ACTH intravenously or intramuscularly at 8–10 a.m. and measuring cortisol at 0, 30 and 60 min; failure to produce levels of 550 nmol/l or above confirms hypoadrenalism. The further diagnosis of primary adrenal failure is usually via the long Synacthen test, in which 1 mg of depot Synacthen is given intramuscularly and cortisol measured at 0, 30, 60, 90, 120 min and 4, 6, 8, 12 and 24 h. In secondary but not primary adrenal failure, cortisol rises over this time period, a slow response (>12 h) indicating adrenocorticol atrophy secondary to chronic ACTH deficiency. Measuring ACTH levels is also very helpful in distinguishing between primary and secondary failure.[110]

Adrenocortical antibodies (to 21-hydroxylase) can be demonstrated in over three-quarters of patients with autoimmune Addison's disease, with high specificity. Antibody-positive individuals with normal cortisol levels are at risk of developing adrenal failure and must be followed up.[111] In the absence of adrenal antibodies or other evidence suggesting APS type 1 or 2, other causes of adrenal failure (Table 10.15) must be excluded. These are usually obvious from the clinical history but tuberculosis in particular must be ruled out. Chest and abdominal X-rays are useful, but CT scanning of the adrenal is the best initial investigation, as the adrenals are atrophic with autoimmune Addison's disease and usually enlarged with tuberculosis and other infiltrative conditions.[112]

Management

Emergency treatment for an Addisonian crisis consists of an intravenous or intramuscular injection of 100 mg hydrocortisone, followed by an intravenous infusion of 4 mg/h or 6-hourly intramuscular boluses of 50–100 mg. At least a liter of normal saline should be infused over 4 h, and the rate should then be adjusted according to the response, especially blood pressure. Any hypercalcemia usually corrects spontaneously, but glucose supplementation is needed if there is hypoglycemia.

Once the patient is better, or from the outset in less severely ill patients, treatment is with oral hydrocortisone. The usual dose is 20–30 mg/day in divided doses, usually taken on waking, at lunchtime and teatime, and with the highest dose in the morning (e.g. 10 mg followed by two doses of 5 mg/day). Twice-daily treatment is less satisfactory,[113] and it is also best to avoid giving the last dose too late in the day, in order to mimic the normal pattern of glucocorticoid. Urine cortisol measurements are unsatisfactory when used alone as a guide to assessing the adequacy of glucocorticoid dosage, whereas timed serum levels through the day provide useful information.[114,115] Anticonvulsant drugs and rifampicin increase hydrocortisone clearance, and estrogens raise cortisol-binding globulin levels, both of which need to be taken into account in monitoring cortisol replacement. Cortisone acetate has been replaced by hydrocortisone.

In addition, fludrocortisone is needed to replace aldosterone (in the emergency setting, the high dose of parenteral hydrocortisone obviates the need for this). The usual dose is 50–200 μg daily as a single dose; the response is tailored by ensuring a normal blood pressure and no edema, together with measurement of urea and electrolytes and plasma renin, which should be in the upper half of the reference range.[115] Recent evidence suggests that dehydroepiandrosterone replacement improves well-being and sexuality in women with adrenal insufficiency but long-term safety data are not yet available.[116]

All patients require a careful explanation of the principles of their treatment, and written instructions should be given about the need to double hydrocortisone doses during any illness and the need to seek medical attention if medication cannot be taken because of vomiting. A steroid card must be issued, with instructions about its use, and ideally a MedicAlert bracelet or necklace should be worn. Patients who are traveling should be given ampoules of hydrocortisone with syringes and needles for use in an emergency; both the patient and traveling companion must be instructed in the technique of intramuscular injection. The same advice applies to patients living in remote locations.

Pregnancy generally causes no problems in Addison's disease, and medication does not usually need adjustment, but the stress of labor requires temporary doubling of steroid doses. Patients should be reviewed annually to ensure that optimum replacement is being given and to assess the possibility that other autoimmune disorders are developing. A minimum check would be an enquiry about general health and periods, plus TSH, glucose and full blood count (or vitamin B_{12} levels and antibody testing for pernicious anemia).

Premature ovarian failure

This is considered in detail in Chapter 8. There are two autoimmune aspects to this condition, defined as menopause before the age of 40. First, there is a clear association with autoimmune Addison's disease, as around 10% of such women have premature ovarian failure due to an autoimmune response against steroid cell antigens shared between ovary and adrenal.[108,117] However, because of the rarity of Addison's disease, this accounts for only a small fraction of women with premature ovarian failure, in many of whom the diagnosis by exclusion is idiopathic ovarian failure. It has been assumed that some of these women have a different type of autoimmune response, against ovary-specific autoantigens, and this second type of etiology is not associated with Addison's disease. The evidence for this assumption is circumstantial, comprising a higher frequency of coincident autoimmune disorders than expected, the presence of ovarian antibodies in a small proportion of patients (but also in other disorders, suggesting a lack of specificity), and the infrequent finding of a lymphocytic oophoritis in ovarian biopsies.[118,119] At present, therefore, there is no consensus on how much autoimmunity contributes to premature ovarian failure unassociated with Addison's disease, and a strong case can be made against ovarian biopsy for diagnosis, particularly as the prognostic value of this is far from clear.[120] Moreover, the absence of a lymphocytic infiltrate does not exclude an autoimmune etiology, as the disease could be 'burnt-out' by the time of biopsy.[119]

Management is detailed in Chapter 6: Hormone replacement therapy is the only treatment needed unless fertility is required. Unfortunately, empirical immunosuppression with corticosteroids, with or without ovulation induction, has had only modest success,[121–123] and has not been subjected to a controlled trial. Spontaneous remission has been well documented in some patients, and may occur after giving replacement glucocorticoids for coincident Addison's disease,[124] which therefore should be excluded in all patients.

Lymphocytic hypophysitis

This is a rare disorder, reviewed in detail elsewhere.[125–127] Women are affected seven times more frequently than men, and are particularly at risk in the peripartum or postpartum period, presenting with features of either a sellar mass, anterior pituitary hormone deficiency (especially ACTH), or both. In non-peripartum women, the most frequent symptom is amenorrhea, and in men loss of libido. There may be associated autoimmune endocrinopathies which give a clue to the diagnosis. The only certain way to make the diagnosis is pituitary biopsy, but this is not indicated routinely, as spontaneous remission occurs in many patients. Pituitary antibody testing has no clinical role in diagnosis currently, as tests are neither specific nor sensitive.[128]

Treatment consists of hormone replacement as necessary and close monitoring of the size of the pituitary lesion with contrast-enhanced MRI. Transsphenoidal surgery is needed in the case of visual failure due to chiasmal compression, although some have advocated a short course of high dose prednisolone (60 mg/day) initially, to determine whether surgery is necessary.[127] Some cases of idiopathic diabetes insipidus may be due to a lymphocytic infundibuloneurohypophysitis, but the frequency of this remains to be determined, and no specific treatment directed at the autoimmune process is yet indicated.[129]

Autoimmune polyglandular syndrome (APS) type 1

This is a rare, autosomal recessive disorder, caused by mutations in the *AIRE* (autoimmune regulator) gene on chromasome 21.[130] It is believed that this gene encodes a protein expressed in the thymus which determines thymic stromal organization in a way essential for the induction of self-tolerance.[131] The diagnosis is based on

Table 10.17
Clinical features of APS type 1.

	Approximate frequency (%)
Major components	
Chronic mucocutaneous candidiasis	80–100
Hypoparathyroidism	80
Addison's disease	70
Other features	
Enamel hypoplasia	80
Gonadal failure	10 men; 60 women
Nail dystrophy	50
Keratopathy	40
Tympanic membrane calcification	30
Vitiligo	30
Alopecia	30
Malabsorption	20
Insulin-dependent diabetes mellitus	10
Hypothyroidism	10
Pernicious anemia	10
Chronic active hepatitis	10

the distinctive clinical features (Table 10.17), including the presence of at least two of the three major components, namely chronic mucocutaneous candidiasis, hypoparathyroidism and Addison's disease,[132–133] appearing in this order in childhood or, occasionally, in later life.

The presentation and management of Addison's disease in APS type 1 are as for the isolated type. Chronic mucocutaneous candidiasis affects the nails (70%), skin (10%) and oropharynx or esophagus (20%); it responds well to ketoconazole, but often this needs to be prolonged and repeated. Hypoparathyroidism presents with circumoral paresthesiae, tetany (including carpopedal spasms) or seizures; depression and other mental changes may be prominent. Cataracts, calcification of the basal ganglia and a prolonged Q–T interval on ECG may also occur. Diagnosis depends on demonstrating low serum calcium and parathyroid hormone

Table 10.18
Clinical features of APS type 2.

Major endocrinopathies
   Autoimmune thyroid disease (Graves' disease, primary myxedema, Hashimoto's thyroiditis, postpartum thyroiditis)
   Type 1 diabetes mellitus
   Addison's disease
   Premature ovarian failure
Other endocrinopathies
   Lymphocytic hypophysitis
   Lymphocytic infundibuloneurohypophysitis
Other features
   Vitiligo
   Alopecia or leukotrichia
   Pernicious anemia
   Celiac disease/dermatitis herpetiformis
   Myasthenia gravis
   Serositis

levels, and excluding other causes of hypoparathyroidism. Treatment is with vitamin D, and I prefer alfacalcidol in this situation, as doses are easily titrated against calcium levels, due to the short half-life of this preparation. The usual adult dose for hypoparathyroidism is 1–2 µg a day, and calcium levels should be checked weekly if dosage adjustments are made. Patients require close, specialist follow-up because of the wide range of complications and the need for family screening once diagnosed (Table 10.17).

Autoimmune polyglandular syndrome (APS) type 2

The key features of APS type 2 are shown in Table 10.18, but the exact definition of APS type 2 is unclear.[4,132] A reasonable compromise is to regard the presence in a patient of two or more of the endocrinopathies in Table 10.18 as definite APS type 2, while one endocrinopathy plus one or more of the associated features suggests APS type 2 and the need for follow-up. This is an autosomal dominant disorder, strongly associated with the HLA-A1, -B8, -DR3 haplotype and polymorphisms of the CTLA-4 gene.[134] The assessment, diagnosis and management of each individual component follows standard lines for the isolated disorder. The importance of the syndrome is that both the patient and family should be screened clinically and biochemically on an annual basis, to ensure that individual disease components are recognized.

References

1. Jones DEJ, Diamond AG. The basis of autoimmunity: an overview. *Baillière's Clin Endocrinol Metab* 1995; **9**: 1–24.
2. Parijs LV, Abbas AK. Homeostasis and self-tolerance in the immune system: turning lymphocytes off. *Science* 1998; **280**: 243–8.
3. Vassart G, Dumont JE. The thyrotropin receptor and the regulation of thymocyte function and growth. *Endocrine Rev* 1992; **13**: 596–611.
4. Weetman AP. Autoimmunity to steroid-producing cells and familial polyendocrine autoimmunity. *Baillière's Clin Endocrinol Metab* 1995; **9**: 157–74.
5. Tomer Y, Davies TF. The genetics of familial and non-familial hyperthyroid Graves' disease. In Rapoport B, McLachlan SM, *Graves' Disease. Pathogenesis and Treatment*. Boston: Kluwer Academic Publishers, 2000; pp18–41.
6. Weetman AP, McGregor AM. Autoimmune thyroid disease: further developments in our understanding. *Endocrine Rev* 1994; **15**: 788–829.
7. Tellez M, Cooper J, Edmonds C. Graves' ophthalmopathy in relation to cigarette smoking and ethnic origin. *Clin Endocrinol* 1992; **36**: 291–4.
8. Ko GTC, Chow CC, Yeung VTF et al. Thyrotoxic periodic paralysis in a Chinese population. *Q J Med* 1996; **89**: 463–8.
9. de la Rosa RE, Hennessey JV, Tucci JR. A longitudinal study of changes in body mass index and total body composition after radioiodine treatment for thyrotoxicosis. *Thyroid* 1997; **7**: 401–5.
10. Hall P, Lundell G, Holm L-E. Mortality in patients treated for hyperthyroidism with iodine-131. *Acta Endocrinol* 1993; **128**: 230–4.
11. Franklyn JA, Maisonneuve P, Sheppard MC et al. Mortality after the treatment of hyperthyroidism with radioactive iodine. *N Engl J Med* 1998; **338**: 712–18.
12. Carnell NE, Valente WA. Thyroid nodules in Graves' disease: classification, characterization, and response to treatment. *Thyroid* 1998; **8**: 647–652.
13. Pellegriti G, Belfiore A, Guiffrida D et al. Outcome of differentiated thyroid cancer in Graves' disease. *J Clin Endocrinol Metab* 1998; **83**: 2805–9.
14. Ito M, Takamatsu J, Yoshida S et al. Incomplete thyrotroph suppression determined by third generation thyrotropin assay in subacute thyroiditis compared to silent thyroiditis or hyperthyroid Graves' disease. *J Clin Endocrinol Metab* 1997; **82**: 616–19.
15. Surks MI, Chopra IJ, Mariash CN et al. American Thyroid Association guidelines for use of laboratory tests in thyroid disorders. *JAMA* 1990; **263**: 1529–32.
16. McKenzie JM, Zakarija M. The clinical use of thyrotropin receptor antibody measurements. *J Clin Endocrinol Metab* 1989; **69**: 1093–6.
17. Maisey MN. Thyroid imaging. In: Wheeler MH, Lazarus JH, eds. *Diseases of the Thyroid*. London: Chapman & Hall, 1994: 130–52.
18. Glinoer D, Hesch D, Lagasse R et al. The management of hyperthyroidism due to Graves' disease in Europe in 1986. Results of an international survey. *Acta Endocrinol* 1987; **115**: 1–23.
19. Solomon B, Glinoer D, Lagasse R et al. Current trends in the management of Graves' disease. *J Clin Endocrinol Metab* 1990; **70**: 1518–24.
20. Vanderpump MPJ, Ahlquist JAO, Franklyn JA et al. Consensus statement for good practice and audit measures in the management of hypothyroidism and hyperthyroidism. *BMJ* 1996; **313**: 539–44.
21. Ratanachaiyavong S, McGregor AM. Immunosuppressive effects of antithyroid drugs. *Clin Endocrinol Metab* 1985; **14**: 449–66.
22. Feldt-Rasmussen U, Schleusener H, Carayon P. Meta-analysis evaluation of the impact of thyrotropin receptor antibodies on long term remission after medical

therapy of Graves' disease. *J Clin Endocrinol Metab* 1994; **78**: 98–102.

23. Schleusener H, Schwander J, Fischer C et al. Prospective multicentre study on the prediction of relapse after antithyroid drug treatment in patients with Graves' disease. *Acta Endocrinol (Copenh)* 1989; **120**: 689–701.

24. Allannic H, Fauchet R, Orgiazzi A et al. Antithyroid drugs and Graves' disease: a prospective randomized evaluation of the efficacy of treatment duration. *J Clin Endocrinol Metab* 1990; **70**: 675–9.

25. Weetman AP, Pickerill AP, Watson PF et al. Treatment of Graves' disease with the block-replace regimen of antithyroid drugs: the effect of treatment duration and immunogenetic susceptibility on relapse. *Q J Med* 1994; **87**: 337–41.

26. Hedley AJ, Young RE, Jones SJ et al. Antithyroid drugs in the treatment of hyperthyroidism of Graves' disease: long-term follow-up of 434 patients. *Clin Endocrinol* 1989; **31**: 209–18.

27. Tamai H, Kasagi K, Takaichi Y et al. Development of spontaneous hypothyroidism in patients with Graves' disease treated with antithyroidal drugs: clinical, immunological, and histological findings in 26 patients. *J Clin Endocrinol Metab* 1989; **69**: 49–53.

28. Hashizume K, Ichikawa K, Sakurai A et al. Administration of thyroxine in treated Graves' disease: effects on the level of antibodies to thyroid-stimulating hormone receptors and on the risk of recurrence of hyperthyroidism. *N Engl J Med* 1991; **324**: 947–53.

29. McIver B, Rae P, Beckett G et al. Lack of effect of thyroxine in patients with Graves' hyperthyroidism who are treated with an antithyroid drug. *N Engl J Med* 1996; **334**: 220–4.

30. Escobar-Morreale HF, Bravo P, Garcia-Robles R et al. Methimazole-induced severe aplastic anemia: unsuccessful treatment with recombinant human granulocyte–monocyte colony-stimulating factor. *Thyroid* 1997; **7**: 67–70.

31. Toft AD, Weetman AP. Screening for agranulocytosis in patients treated with antithyroid drugs. *Clin Endocrinol* 1998; **49**: 271.

32. Barclay ML, Brownlie BEW, Turner JG et al. Lithium associated thyrotoxicosis: a report of 14 cases with statistical analysis of incidence. *Clin Endocrinol* 1994; **40**: 759–64.

33. Wenzel KW, Lente JR. Similar effects of thionamide drugs and perchlorate on thyroid-stimulating immunoglobulins in Graves' disease: evidence against an immunosuppressive action of thionamide drugs. *J Clin Endocrinol Metab* 1984; **58**: 62–9.

34. The Radioiodine Audit Subcommittee of the Royal College of Physicians Committee on Diabetes and Endocrinology and The Research Unit of the Royal College of Physicians. *The Use of Radioiodine in the Management of Hyperthyroidism*. London: Royal College of Physicians of London, 1995.

35. Farrar JJ, Toft AD. Iodine-131 treatment of hyperthyroidism: current issues. *Clin Endocrinol* 1991; **35**: 207–12.

36. Velkeniers B, Cytryn R, Vanhaelst L et al. Treatment of hyperthyroidism with radioiodine: adjunctive therapy with antithyroid drugs reconsidered. *Lancet* 1988; **i**: 1127–9.

37. Tuttle JM, Patience T, Budd S. Treatment with propylthiouracil before radioactive iodine therapy is associated with a higher treatment failure rate than therapy with radioactive iodine alone in Graves' disease. *Thyroid* 1995; **5**: 243–7.

38. Imseis RE, Vanmiddlesworth L, Massie JD et al. Pretreatment with propylthiouracil but not methimazole reduces the therapeutic efficacy of iodine-131 in hyperthyroidism. *J Clin Endocrinol Metab* 1998; **83**: 685–7.

39. Hedley AJ, Lazarus JH, McGhee SM et al. Treatment of hyperthyroidism by radioactive iodine. *J R Coll Physicians Lond* 1992; **26**: 348–51.

40. Hardisty CA, Jones SJ, Hedley AJ et al. Clinical outcome and costs of care in radioiodine treatment of hyperthyroidism. *J R Coll Physicians Lond* 1990; **24**: 36–42.

41. Jarlev AE, Hegedüs L, Kristensen LØ et al. Is calculation of the dose in radioiodine therapy of hyperthyroidism worthwhile? *Clin Endocrinol* 1995; **43**: 325–9.

42. Kendall-Taylor P, Keir MJ, Ross WM. Ablative radioiodine therapy for hyperthyroidism: long term follow up study. *BMJ* 1984; **289**: 361–3.

43. Goolden AWG, Steward JSW. Long-term results from graded low dose radioactive iodine therapy for thyrotoxicosis. *Clin Endocrinol* 1986; **24**: 217–22.

44. Aizawa Y, Yoshida K, Kaise N et al. The development of transient hypothyroidism after iodine-131 treatment in hyperthyroid patients with Graves' disease: prevalence, mechanism and prognosis. *Clin Endocrinol* 1997; **46**: 1–5.

45. Vestergaard H, Laurberg P. Radioiodine treatment of recurrent hyperthyroidism in patients previously treated for Graves' disease by subtotal thyroidectomy. *J Intern Med* 1992; **231**: 13–17.

46. Weetman AP. The role of surgery in primary hyperthyroidism. *J R Soc Med* 1998; **91**: 7–11.

47. Patwardhan NA, Moront M, Rao S et al. Surgery still has a role in Graves' hyperthyroidism. *Surgery* 1993; **114**: 1108–13.

48. Ozaki O, Ito K, Mimura T et al. Factors affecting thyroid function after subtotal thyroidectomy for Graves' disease: case control study by remnant-weight matched-pair analysis. *Thyroid* 1997; **7**: 555–9.

49. Shulman DI, Muhar I, Jorgensen V et al. Autoimmune hyperthyroidism in prepubertal children and adolescents: comparison of clinical and biochemical features at diagnosis and responses to medical therapy. *Thyroid* 1997; **7**: 755–60.

50. Mandel SJ, Brent GA, Larsen PR. Review of antithyroid drug use during pregnancy and report of a case of aplasia cutis. *Thyroid* 1994; 4: 129–33.
51. Wallace C, Couch R, Ginsberg J. Fetal thyrotoxicosis: a case report and recommendations for prediction, diagnosis and treatment. *Thyroid* 1995; 5: 125–8.
52. Burch HB, Wartofsky L. Graves' ophthalmopathy: current concepts regarding pathogenesis and management. *Endocrine Rev* 1993; 14: 747–93.
53. Many M-C, Costagliola S, Detrait M, et al. Development of an animal model of autoimmune thyroid eye disease. *J Immunol* 1999; 162: 4966–4974.
54. McGregor AM. Has the target autoantigen for Graves' ophthalmopathy been found? *Lancet* 1998; 352: 595–6.
55. Perros P, Crombie AL, Matthews JNS et al. Age and gender influence on the severity of thyroid-associated ophthalmopathy: a study of 101 patients attending a combined thyroid–eye clinic. *Clin Endocrinol* 1993; 38: 367–72.
56. Mourits MP, Prummel MF, Wiersinga WM et al. Clinical activity score as a guide in the management of patients with Graves' ophthalmopathy. *Clin Endocrinol* 1997; 47: 9–14.
57. Hosten N, Sander B, Cordes M et al. Graves' ophthalmopathy: MR imaging of the orbits. *Radiology* 1989; 172: 759–62.
58. Weetman AP, Wiersinga WM. Current management of thyroid-associated ophthalmopathy in Europe. Results of an international survey. *Clin Endocrinol* 1998; 49: 21–8.
59. Gerding MN, Terwee CB, Dekker FW et al. Quality of life in patients with Graves' ophthalmopathy is markedly decreased: measurement by the medical outcomes study instrument. *Thyroid* 1997; 7: 885–9.
60. Char DH. *Thyroid Eye Disease*. Boston: Butterworth-Heinmann.
61. Bartalena L, Pinchera A, Marcocci C. Management of Graves' ophthalmopathy: reality and perspectives. *Endocr Rev* 2000;21:168–199.
62. Kendall-Taylor P, Crombie AL, Stephenson AM et al. Intravenous methylprednisolone pulse therapy in the treatment of Graves' ophthalmopathy. *BMJ* 1988; 297: 1574–8.
63. Fatourechi V, Bergstralh EJ, Garrity JA et al. Predictors of response to transantral orbital decompression in severe Graves' ophthalmopathy. *Mayo Clin Proc* 1994; 69: 841–8.
64. Prummel MF, Mourits MP, Berghout A et al. Prednisone and cyclosporine in the treatment of severe Graves' ophthalmopathy. *N Engl J Med* 1989; 321: 1353–9.
65. Prummel MF, Mourits MP, Blank L et al. Randomised double-blind trial of prednisone versus radiotherapy in Graves' ophthalmopathy. *Lancet* 1993; 342: 949–54.
66. Kung AWC, Michon J, Tai KS et al. The effect of somatostatin versus corticosteroid in the treatment of Graves' ophthalmopathy. *Thyroid* 1996; 6: 381–4.
67. Baschieri L, Antonelli A, Nardi S et al. Intravenous immunoglobulin versus corticosteroid in treatment of Graves' ophthalmopathy. *Thyroid* 1997; 7: 579–85.
68. Prummel MF, Wiersinga WM, Mourits MP et al. Influence of abnormal thyroid function on the severity of accompanying Graves' ophthalmopathy. *Arch Intern Med* 1990; 150: 1098–101.
69. Wiersinga WM. Preventing Graves' ophthalmopathy. *N Engl J Med* 1998; 338: 121–2.
70. DeGroot LJ, Gorman CA, Pinchera A et al. Radiation and Graves' ophthalmopathy. *J Clin Endocrinol Metab* 1995; 80: 339–49.
71. Bartalena L, Marcocci C, Bogazzi F et al. Relation between therapy for hyperthyroidism and the course of Graves' ophthalmopathy. *N Engl J Med* 1998; 338: 73–8.
72. Bartalena L, Marcocci C, Bogazzi F et al. Use of corticosteroids to prevent progression of Graves' ophthalmopathy after radioiodine therapy for hyperthyroidism. *N Engl J Med* 1989; 321: 1349–52.
73. Smith TJ, Bahn RS, Gorman CA. Connective tissue, glycosaminoglycans, and diseases of the thyroid. *Endocrine Rev* 1989; 10: 336–91.
74. Fatourechi V, Pajouhi M, Fransway AF. Dermopathy of Graves' disease (pretibial myxedema). Review of 150 cases. *Medicine* 1994; 73: 1–7.
75. Heufelder AE, Bahn RS, Scriba PC. Analysis of T-cell antigen receptor variable region gene usage in patients with thyroid-related pretibial dermopathy. *J Invest Dermatol* 1995; 105: 372–8.
76. Somach SC, Helm TN, Lawlor KB et al. Pretibial mucin. Histologic patterns and clinical correlation. *Arch Dermatol* 1993; 129: 1152–6.
77. Chang TC, Kao SCS, Huang KM. Octreotide and Graves' ophthalmopathy and pretibial myxoedema. *BMJ* 1992; 304: 158.
78. Arscott PL, Baker JR Jr. Apoptosis and thyroiditis. *Clin Immunol Immunopathol* 1998; 87: 207–17.
79. Matsuura N, Yamada Y, Nohara Y et al. Familial neonatal transient hypothyroidism due to maternal TSH-binding inhibitor immunoglobulins. *N Engl J Med* 1980; 303: 738–41.
80. Takasu N, Yamada T, Takasu M et al. Disappearance of thyrotropin-blocking antibodies and spontaneous recovery from hypothyroidism in autoimmune thyroiditis. *N Engl J Med* 1992; 326: 513–18.
81. Kosugi S, Ban T, Akamizu T et al. Use of thyrotropin receptor (TSHR) mutants to detect stimulating TSHR antibodies in hypothyroid patients with idiopathic myxedema, who have blocking TSHR antibodies. *J Clin Endocrinol Metab* 1993; 77: 19–24.
82. McKee RF, Krukowski ZH, Matheson NA. Thyroid neoplasia coexistent with chronic lymphocytic thyroiditis. *Br J Surg* 1993; 80: 1303–4.

83. Matsuzuka F, Miyauchi A, Katayama S et al. Clinical aspects of primary thyroid lymphoma: diagnosis and treatment based on our experience of 119 cases. *Thyroid* 1993; **3**: 93–9.

84. Zimmerman RS, Brennan MD, McConahey WM et al. Hashimoto's thyroiditis. An uncommon cause of painful thyroid unresponsive to corticosteroid therapy. *Ann Intern Med* 1986; **104**: 355–7.

85. Hegedüs L, Hansen JM, Feldt-Rasmussen U et al. Influence of thyroxine treatment on thyroid size and anti-thyroid peroxidase antibodies in Hashimoto's thyroiditis. *Clin Endocrinol* 1991; **35**: 235–8.

86. Nordyke RA, Gilbert FI Jr, Miyamoto LA et al. The superiority of antimicrosomal over antithyroglobulin antibodies for detecting Hashimoto's thyroiditis. *Arch Intern Med* 1993; **153**: 862–5.

87. Baker JR, Lukes YG, Smallridge RC et al. Seronegative Hashimoto thyroiditis with thyroid autoantibody production localised to the thyroid. *Ann Intern Med* 1988; **108**: 26–30.

88. Weetman AP. Hypothyroidism: screening and subclinical disease. *BMJ* 1997; **314**: 1175–8.

89. Vanderpump MPJ, Tunbridge WMG, French JM, et al. The incidence of thyroid disorders in the community: a twenty-year follow-up of the Whickham survey. *Clin Endocrinol* 1995; **43**: 55–68.

90. Hak AE, Pols HAP, Visser TJ, et al. Subclinical hyperthyroidism is an independent risk factor for atherosclerosis and myocardial infarction in elderly women: the Rotterdam study. *Ann Int Med* 2000; **132**: 270–278.

91. Grebe SKG, Cooke RR, Ford HC, et al. Treatment of hypothyroidism with once weekly thyroxine. *J Clin Endocrinol Metab* 1997; **82**: 870–875.

92. Lindsay RS, Toft AD. Hypothyroidism. *Lancet* 1997; **349**: 413–417.

93. Haddow JE, Palomaki GE, Allan WC, et al. Maternal thyroid deficiency during pregnancy and subsequent neuropsychological development of the child. *New Engl J Med* 1999: **341**: 549–555.

94. Bunevicius R, Kazanavicius G, Zalinkevicius R, et al. Effects of thyroxine as compared with thyroxine plus triiodothyronine in patients with hypothyroidism. *New Engl J Med* 1999; **340**: 424–429.

95. Sawin CT, Geller A, Wolf PA et al. Low serum thyrotropin concentrations as a risk factor for atrial fibrillation in older persons. *N Engl J Med* 1994; **331**: 1249–52.

96. Faber J, Galloe AM. Changes in bone mass during prolonged subclinical hyperthyroidism due to L-thyroxine treatment: a meta-analysis. *Eur J Endocrinol* 1994; **130**: 350–6.

97. Grant DJ, McMurdo MET, Mole PA et al. Is previous hyperthyroidism still a risk factor for osteoporosis in post-menopausal women? *Clin Endocrinol* 1995; **43**: 339–45.

98. Lazarus JH, Kokandi A: Thyroid disease in relation to pregnancy. *Clin Endocrinol* 2000; **53**: 265–278..

99. Jansson R, Bernander S, Karlsson A et al. Autoimmune thyroid dysfunction in the post-partum thyroid period. *J Clin Endocrinol Metab* 1984; **58**: 681–7.

100. Gerstein HC. A methodologic overview of the literature. *Arch Intern Med* 1990; **150**: 1397–400.

101. Lazarus JH, Hall R, Othman S et al. The clinical spectrum of postpartum thyroid disease. *Q J Med* 1996; **89**: 429–35.

102. Amino N, Tada H, Hidaka Y, et al. Screening for postpartum thyroiditis. *J Clin Endocrinol Metab* 1999; **84**: 1813–1821.

103. Harris B, Othman S, Davies JA et al. Association between postpartum thyroid dysfunction and thyroid antibodies and depression. *BMJ* 1992; **305**: 152–7.

104. Alvarez-Marfany M, Roman SH, Drexler AJ et al. Long-term prospective study of postpartum thyroid dysfunction in women with insulin dependent diabetes mellitus. *J Clin Endocrinol Metab* 1994; **79**: 10–16.

105. Fernandez-Soto L, Gonzalez A, Lobon JA et al. Thyroid peroxidase autoantibodies predict poor metabolic control and need for thyroid treatment in pregnant IDDM women. *Diabetes Care* 1997; **20**: 1524–8.

106. Othman S, Phillips DIW, Parkes AB et al. A long-term follow-up of postpartum thyroiditis. *Clin Endocrinol* 1990; **32**: 559–64.

107. Weetman AP. Autoantigens in Addison's disease and associated syndromes. *Clin Exp Immunol* 1997; **107**: 227–9.

108. Betterle C, Volpato M, Pedini B, et al. Adrenal-cortex autoantibodies and steroid-producing cells autoantibodies in patients with Addison's disease: comparison of immunofluorescence and immunoprecipitation assays. *J Clin Endocrinol Metab* 1999; **84**: 618–622.

109. Oelkers W. Adrenal insufficiency. *N Engl J Med* 1996; **335**: 1206–12.

110. Grinspoon SK, Biller BMK. Laboratory assessment of adrenal insufficiency. *J Clin Endocrinol Metab* 1994; **79**: 923–31.

111. De Bellis A, Bizzarro A, Rossi R et al. Remission of subclinical adrenocortical failure in subjects with adrenal autoantibodies. *J Clin Endocrinol Metab* 1993; **76**: 1002–7.

112. Vita JA, Silverberg SJ, Goland RS et al. Clinical clues to the cause of Addison's disease. *Am J Med* 1985; **78**: 461–6.

113. Groves RW, Tomas GC, Houghton BJ et al. Corticosteroid replacement therapy: twice or thrice daily? *J R Soc Med* 1988; **81**: 514–16.

114. Peacey SR, Guo CY, Robinson AM et al. Glucocorticoid replacement therapy: are patients overtreated and does it matter? *Clin Endocrinol* 1997; **46**: 255–61.

115. Oelkers W, Diederich S, Bahr V. Diagnosis and therapy surveillance in Addison's disease: rapid adrenocorticotropin (ACTH) test and measurement of plasma ACTH, renin activity and aldosterone. *J Clin Endocrinol Metab* 1992; 72: 259–64.
116. Arlt W, Callies F, Van Vlijmen JC, et al. Dehydroepiandrosterone replacement in women with adrenal insufficiency. *New Engl J Med* 1999: 341: 1013–1020.
117. Betterle C, Volpato M. Adrenal and ovarian autoimmunity. *Eur J Endocrinol* 1998; 138: 16–25.
118. Wheatcroft N, Weetman AP. Is premature ovarian failure an autoimmune disease? *Autoimmunity* 1997; 25: 157–65.
119. Fox H. The pathology of premature ovarian failure. *J Pathol* 1992; 167: 357–63.
120. Khastgir G, Abdalla H, Studd JWW. The case against ovarian biopsy for the diagnosis of premature menopause. *Br J Obstet Gynaecol* 1994; 101: 96–8.
121. Corenblum B, Rowe T, Taylor PJ. High-dose, short-term glucocorticoids for the treatment of infertility resulting from premature ovarian failure. *Fertil Steril* 1993; 59: 988–91.
122. Blumenfeld Z, Halachmi S, Peretz BA et al. Premature ovarian failure—the prognostic application of autoimmunity on conception after ovulation induction. *Fertil Steril* 1993; 59: 750–5.
123. Barbarino-Monnier P, Gobert R, Fuillet-May F et al. Ovarian autoimmunity and corticotherapy in an in vitro fertilization attempt. *Hum Reprod* 1995; 10: 2006–7.
124. Cowchok FS, McCabe JL, Montgomery BB. Pregnancy after corticosteroid administration in premature ovarian failure (polyglandular endocrinopathy syndrome). *Am J Obstet Gynaecol* 1988; 158: 118–19.
125. Thodou E, Asa SL, Kontogeorgos G et al. Lymphocytic hypophysitis: clinicopathological findings. *J Clin Endocrinol Metab* 1995; 80: 2302–11.
126. Jenkins PJ, Chew SL, Lowe DG et al. Lymphocytic hypophysitis: unusual features of a rare disorder. *Clin Endocrinol* 1995; 42: 529–34.
127. Sawers HA, Bevan JS. Pituitary autoimmunity. In: Weetman AP, ed. *Endocrine Autoimmunity and Associated Conditions*. Dordrecht: Kluwer Academic Publishers, 1998: 223–41.
128. Crock PA. Cytosolic autoantigens in lymphocytic hypophysitis. *J Clin Endocrinol Metab* 1998; 83: 609–18.
129. Imura H, Nakao K, Shimatsu A et al. Lymphocytic infundibuloneurohypophysitis as a cause of central diabetes insipidus. *N Engl J Med* 1993; 329: 683–9.
130. Peterson P, Nagamine K, Scott H et al. APECED: a monogenic autoimmune disease providing new clues to self-tolerance. *Immunol Today* 1998; 19: 384–6.
131. Zuklys S, Balciunaite G, Agarwal A, et al. Normal thymic architecture and negative selection are associated with *Aire* expression, the gene defective in the autoimmune-polyendocrinopathy-candidiasis-ectodermal dystrophy (APECED). *J Immunol* 2000; 165: 1976–1983.
132. Neufeld M, Maclaren NK, Blizzard RM. Two types of autoimmune Addison's disease associated with different polyglandular autoimmune (PGA) syndromes. *Medicine* 1981; 60: 355–62.
133. Betterle C, Greggio NA, Volpato M. Autoimmune polyglandular syndrome type 1. *J Clin Endocrinol Metab* 1998; 83: 1049–55.
134. Vaidya B, Imrie H, Greatch DR, et al. Association analysis of the cytotoxic T lymphocyte antigen-4 (CTLA-4) and autoimmune regulator-1 (AIRE-1) genes in sporadic autoimmune Addison's disease. *J Clin Endocrinol Metab* 2000; 85: 688–691.

11

Non-autoimmune thyroid disease
Soo-Mi Park, Luca Persani, Paolo Beck-Peccoz, Krishna Chatterjee

Introduction

Thyroid hormones (thyroxine (T4), triiodothyronine (T3)) regulate many cellular processes, including growth, the basal metabolic rate, myocardial contractility and functional differentiation of the central nervous system. The synthesis of thyroid hormones is controlled by hypothalamic thyrotropin-releasing hormone (TRH) and pituitary thyroid-stimulating hormone (TSH). TSH exerts its effect on the thyroid gland via a transmembrane receptor, mediating cellular growth and hormone production. In turn, T4 and T3 regulate TRH and TSH synthesis as part of a negative feedback loop.

This chapter considers human disorders in which this feedback axis is dysregulated. First, the functional effects of TSH receptor gene mutations are considered: somatic activating TSH receptor mutations cause thyroid autonomy with toxic adenomas or multinodular goiter; germline activating TSH receptor mutations are associated with non-autoimmune hyperthyroidism. In both cases, elevated circulating thyroid hormones are associated with suppressed pituitary TSH secretion, reflecting normal feedback sensitivity of the pituitary–thyroid axis.

In contrast, hyperthyroid or euthyroid individuals may rarely present with elevated T4 and T3 levels accompanied by normal, non-suppressed circulating TSH. Two uncommon disorders are involved in the differential diagnosis of this biochemical entity: resistance to thyroid hormone (RTH) associated with loss-of-function mutations in the thyroid hormone receptor β gene; or TSH-secreting pituitary tumors (TSH-omas). This chapter describes the clinical features, differential diagnosis and management of RTH and TSH-omas.

TSH receptor mutations and thyroid disease

TSH receptor action

The TSH receptor (TSHR) plays a critical role in the development and function of the thyroid gland. It appears early in thyroid organogenesis, with expression being detected at the onset of thyroid differentiation after the gland has migrated down to its final position from its origin in the foramen cecum. It regulates the function of the thyroid by mediating the effects of pituitary TSH. Recent studies indicate that abnormalities of the TSH receptor play a role in the etiology of both overactive and underactive thyroid states.

TSHR is a transmembrane receptor on thyroid follicular cells, belonging to a subfamily of heptahelical G protein-coupled receptors. Its structure consists of seven transmembrane segments, three extracellular and three intracellular loops, an extracellular N-terminal domain, and an intracytoplasmic C-terminal tail (Figure 11.1).

The actions of TSH on the thyroid follicular cell occur principally by receptor-mediated activation of the α subunit of the stimulatory guanine nucleotide-binding protein (Gsα) to which it preferentially couples. Adenylyl cyclase is then activated, leading to subsequent generation of intracellular cyclic adenosine monophosphate (cAMP).[1] At 5–10-fold higher circulating TSH levels, the receptor also couples to the q subunit of guanine nucleotide-binding protein α (Gq), activating the phospholipase C regulatory cascade to stimulate the production of inositol phosphate.[2] The cAMP pathway regulates expression of the thyroglobulin and thyroperoxidase genes, thyrocyte growth and thyroid hormone secretion, whereas the inositol

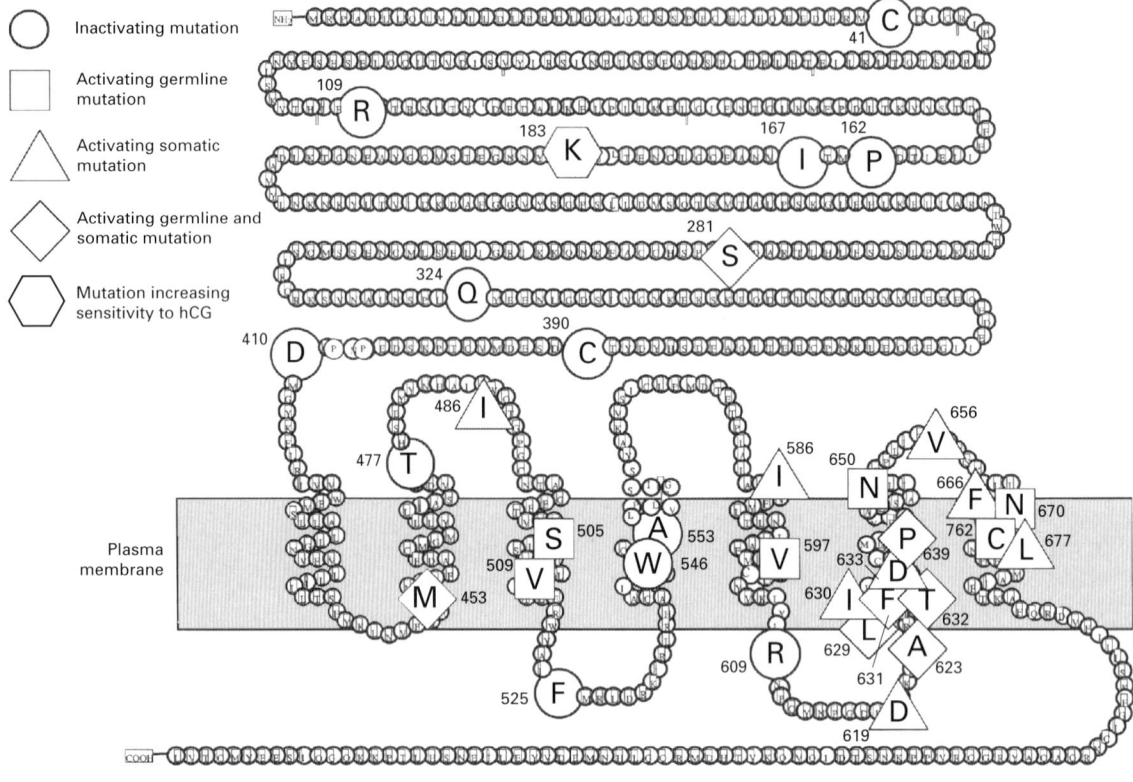

Figure 11.1
A schematic representation of the TSH receptor, showing the location of mutations associated with human disease. For clarity, deletion and frameshift mutations have not been shown. hCG, human chorionic gonadotropin.

phosphate pathway is primarily involved in control of organification of iodine and hormone synthesis.[1]

Somatic activating mutations of the TSH receptor and autonomously functioning thyroid adenomas

Autonomously functioning thyroid adenomas may occur as either solitary or multiple nodules leading to hyperthyroidism. In principle, a somatic mutation affecting the TSH signaling pathway in a single thyroid epithelial cell would lead to continuous stimulation of the cAMP pathway and a growth advantage, allowing it to expand clonally, leading to the formation of a thyroid adenoma that synthesizes and secretes thyroid hormones autonomously. Consistent with this notion, evidence indicates that the majority of thyroid adenomas are clonal in origin.[3] The autonomous function of these adenomas leads to suppression of TSH secretion with quiesence of the surrounding extranodular tissue, manifesting as 'hot' areas on a 'cold' background on radionuclide imaging.

The first somatic mutations in the TSH receptor leading to toxic adenomas were described in the third intracellular loop of the receptor (Figure 11.1) and found as a result of screening the large tenth exon of the gene encoding the transmembrane regions.[4]

Mutation	Nucleotide change	Germline or somatic	Frequency[a]
K183R[b]	AAA→AGA	G	2
S281N	AGC→AAC	G+S	1+2
S281I	AGC→ATC	S	1
S281T	AGC→ACC	S	2
M453T	ATG→ACG	G+S	1+2
I486M	ATC→ATG	S	2
I486F	ATC→TTC	S	2
S505N	ACC→AAC	G	1
S505R	AGC→AGA	G	1
V509A	GTG→GCG	G	1
I586T	ATC→ACC	S	5
V597L	GTC→CTC	G	1
D619G	GAT→GGT	S	7
Δ613–621 (YNPGDKDTK)	ΔTACAACCCAGG GGACAAAGATACCAAA	S	1
A623V	GCC→GTC	G+S	1+7
A623S	GCC→TCC	S	7
A623I	GCC→ATC	S	1
L629F	TTG→TTT	G+S	1+2
	TTG→TTC	S	1
I630L	ATC→CTC	S	5
F631I	TTC→ATC	S	1
F631L	TTC→CTC	S	1
F631Y	TTC→TAC	S	7
L631F	CTC→TTC	G	1
T632I	ACC→ATC	G+S	1+21
T632A	ACC→GCC	S	1
D633A	GAC→GCC	S	1
D633H	GAC→CAC	S	3
D633Y	GAC→TAC	S	3
D633E	GAC→GAG	S	2
	GAC→GAA	S	4
P639S	CCA→TCA	S	1
N650Y	ACC→TAC	G	1
V656F	GTT→TTT	S	1
F666S	TTC→TCC	S	1
N670S	AAC→AGC	G	1
C672Y	TGT→TAT	G	1
L677V	CTG→GTG	S	1
Δ658–661 (NSKI)	(ΔAACTCCAAAATC)	S	1

[a] Refers to number of published cases with germline mutations (first figure) or toxic adenomas with somatic mutations (second figure).
[b] A gain-of-function mutation associated with receptor responsiveness to human chorionic gonadotropin.

Table 11.1
Gain-of-function human TSH receptor mutations.

Additional mutations found subsequently were not restricted to these regions but also involved the N-terminal extracellular domain (Figure 11.1 and Table 11.1).[5–9] There are several 'hot spots' within which activating mutations in the TSHR cluster have been identified: the third intracellular loop, a cluster of residues from 629 to 633 in transmembrane segment VI, and five residues (Ser 281, Ile 486, Ile 586, Ala 623, Phe 631, and Asp 633). These regions are thought to play a critical role in maintaining the structure and conformation of the TSH receptor and are also important in receptor interaction with Gs and therefore signal transduction.[10] So far, 40 different activating mutations involving 25 amino acid residues in TSHR have been reported (Table 11.1). Functional characterization of these mutants using transfection assays has revealed that they all mediate constitutive elevation of intracellular cAMP levels, independent of circulating TSH.[4,7–9,11,12]

There is a large variation in the frequency of activating TSHR mutations in autonomously functioning adenomas, ranging from as little as 0% up to 80%,[4–8] depending upon the methodology used for mutation screening (e.g. sequencing versus single-strand conformation polymorphism analysis), the extent of the receptor gene screened (e.g. only exon 10 versus all coding exons), the tube of tissue examined (e.g. frozen versus paraffin-embedded), and quantity of tissue sampled (surgical specimen versus fine-needle aspiration biopsy). Other factors may also influence the frequency of TSHR gene mutations, including genetic background and dietary iodine. In areas with iodine-sufficient diets, hyperthyroidism due to Graves' disease is much more common than that due to autonomously functioning thyroid adenomas, whereas in iodine-deficient areas, thyroid adenomas and toxic multinodular goiters constitute a greater proportion of the underlying cause (10% and 48% respectively versus Graves' disease).[13] Thus iodine deficiency appears to favor either the development or clinical expression of autonomous thyroid adenomas and toxic multinodular goiters. Interestingly, in Japan, an iodine-sufficient area, the incidence of TSH receptor mutations in both hyperfunctioning adenomas and toxic multinodular goiters is low.[14,15] Multiple hyperfunctioning adenomas in the same thyroid gland have been demonstrated to be associated with identical or different somatic TSH receptor mutations.[7]

A significant proportion of hyperfunctioning nodules in toxic multinodular goiters, including those with histological features of true thyroid adenomas as well as hyperplastic nodules, have also been reported to contain activating mutations in the TSH receptor gene,[8,16] whereas such mutations are not present in non-functioning cold nodules within a multinodular goiter.[16] Furthermore, even microscopic areas of euthyroid goiters from patients in iodine-deficient areas have been reported to contain activating TSHR mutations, suggesting that toxic thyroid nodules may originate from such small autonomous areas.[17]

Somatic mutations in other components of the cAMP signaling pathway leading to constitutive activation of cAMP production might also be expected to induce thyroid adenoma formation, but to date only activating mutations in Gsα have been reported in up to 38% of toxic adenomas.[18] A search for mutations in protein kinase A, another key component of the cAMP pathway, in both thyroid adenomas and pituitary tumors, revealed none, suggesting that mutations in the gene encoding this protein may not play a significant oncogenic role in thyroid and pituitary neoplasms.[19]

Clinical features of hyperthyroidism may take from months to greater than a decade to develop, depending on how long it takes for an adenoma to grow large enough to cause thyroid dysfunction. This depends partly on dietary iodine intake, growth potential and the genetic makeup of the individual. An unusual case of congenital hyperthyroidism due to a solitary toxic adenoma associated with a somatic mutation in the thyrotropin receptor has been described.[9]

Somatic activating mutations of the TSH receptor and differentiated thyroid cancer

Constitutively activating mutations in the TSHR as well as mutations in Gsα have been demonstrated in a very small proportion of differentiated thyroid tumors, including follicular and Hurthle cell carcinoma.[20,21] Most of the mutations in the TSH receptor gene found in these malignant tumors have been previously described in autonomously functioning adenomas.

However, experimental models involving chronic activation of cellular cAMP, e.g. by transgenic expression of constitutively active Gsα in the thyroid, result in enhanced thyrocyte growth leading to cellular hyperplasia but not carcinogenesis.[22] This suggests that rather than being directly causal, constitutive TSHR or Gsα gene mutations may act synergistically in concert with additional oncogenic mutations in the development of thyroid carcinoma. In support of such a model, *ras* oncogene mutations have been reported to coexist with TSH receptor mutations in a thyroid carcinoma.[20]

Germline activating mutations of the TSH receptor and congenital, sporadic or autosomal dominant, non-autoimmune, hyperthyroidism

Familial cases of persistent neonatal hyperthyroidism and autosomal dominant, non-autoimmune hyperthyroidism were first characterized clinically over 20 years ago.[23] Heterozygous, germline, activating mutations in the TSH receptor gene were associated with cases of hereditary non-autoimmune hyperthyroidism more recently,[24] and numerous different TSHR mutations have been identified in many families (Table 11.1). In addition to mutations previously described in thyroid adenomas, novel codon substitutions have been found, with the majority localizing to transmembrane domains of TSHR. Activating germline mutations in the TSH receptor gene occurring de novo in sporadic cases of non-autoimmune hyperthyroidism have also now been reported.

As with somatic mutations identified in thyroid adenomas, the germline mutant TSH receptors have been shown to mediate constitutive activation of the cAMP pathway in vitro.[11,24–27] Most germline and somatic mutants activated only the cAMP pathway, but a subset (including I468M, A623I, I568T, T632I and I486F) were also capable of activating the phospholipase C-dependent signaling cascade. No obvious functional differences between somatic and germline activating mutants in vitro or in clinical phenotype between patients with hyperfunctioning nodules and families with germline mutations has been observed. A model in which the wild-type TSH receptor isomerizes between an active and inactive state, with activating somatic or germline TSHR mutations shifting the equilibrium towards the active conformation of the receptor in the absence of ligand, has been proposed.

Autosomal dominant non-autoimmune hyperthyroidism is defined clinically by the familial occurrence of thyroid autonomy in two or more generations, with a slight excess preponderance (two-fold) in women over men. The onset of thyrotoxicosis varies from as early as the fetal/neonatal period, leading to fetal tachycardia, intrauterine growth retardation and low birthweight, up to 23 years of age, depending on modifying factors, including genetic background and dietary goitrogen or iodine intake. Neonatal hyperthyroidism can result in advanced bone age, premature craniosynostosis, hepatosplenomegaly and cholestasis, lymphadenopathy and thrombocytopenia.[25,26,28] Microcephaly may be present, with later developmental delay and speech disturbance.[9] Homogeneous diffuse thyroid enlargement in childhood becomes multinodular in later life. Interestingly, exophthalmos confirmed by CT or MRI scanning has been described in some sporadic cases of congenital hyperthyroidism, possibly representing constitutive activity of TSHR, which is now known to be also expressed in retro-orbital tissue.[26,28] In many cases thyrotoxicosis is refractory to medical therapy or subtotal thyroidectomy, with patients requiring further ablative surgery or radioiodine treatment.

Graves' disease is the main differential diagnosis of familial non-autoimmune hyperthyroidism. Helpful features which suggest the latter include a history of familial thyrotoxicosis (although familial clustering of Graves' is well recognized), an earlier age of onset of hyperthyroidism, a greater proportion of affected males, moderate and diffuse goiter, and an absence of extrathyroidal disease manifestations such as pretibial myxedema. Negative thyroid microsomal and anti-TSH receptor antibody levels, refractoriness of hyperthyroidism to therapy and absence of lymphocytic infiltrate in the thyroid are added diagnostic features. The identification of a TSHR gene mutation in suspected cases is helpful because it enables a definitive diagnosis leading to appropriate treatment with total thyroid ablation to prevent recurrent thyrotoxicosis. In addition, genetic counseling of family members harboring a receptor mutation but who are not yet clinically symptomatic might be useful.

Germline inactivating mutations of the TSH receptor and congenital hypothyroidism with TSH resistance

Congenital hypothyroidism (CH) is detected in 1 in 4000 live births, making it the most common congenital endocrine anomaly. Early thyroxine therapy following neonatal screening prevents serious neurodevelopmental and intellectual sequelae. CH results primarily from defects in development of the thyroid gland leading either to agenesis (40%), or maldescent (ectopy 40%), or hypoplasia (5%). In other cases, CH is associated with either a goiter due to dyshormonogenesis (10%) or a normal thyroid gland.

During mouse embryogenesis, the TSH receptor is expressed after the migration of the thyroid gland to its final position, suggesting that it might play a developmental role. Further evidence for a role of the TSH signaling pathway is provided by the observation that pituitary glycoprotein hormone α-subunit gene null mice exhibit thyroid hypoplasia and that human TSH deficiency due to homozygous mutation in the TSHβ subunit gene is associated with thyroid dysgenesis. The TSH receptor gene is directly implicated by the discovery that a homozygous loss-of-function TSHR mutation in the *hyt/hyt* mouse causes hypothyroidism and thyroid hypoplasia.[29]

Resistance of the thyroid gland to TSH was first suspected in patients presenting with CH, normal-sized thyroid glands and high serum levels of biologically active TSH with evidence of impaired end-organ response such as decreased uptake of radioiodine and thyroglobulin synthesis.[30] The molecular basis of TSH resistance in humans was first described in 1995 in three siblings who were compound heterozygous for two different loss-of-function mutations in the extracellular domain of TSHR.[31] Their heterozygous parents were biochemically and clinically euthyroid. Since then, 13 different loss-of-function TSH receptor mutations have been identified in 10 other families with recessively inherited TSH resistance (Figure 11.1, Table 11.2).[32-38] In functional studies, most of these mutant receptors exhibited an impaired or absent intracellular cAMP response to TSH stimulation. In five families,[31,32] receptor abnormalities were associated with euthyroid hyperthyrotropinemia, with normal serum thyroid hormone but elevated TSH levels, consistent with fully compensated TSH resistance; borderline hypothyroidism was seen in two families,[33,34] with elevated serum TSH associated with slightly subnormal thyroid hormone levels suggesting partial resistance; finally, markedly elevated TSH and low thyroid hormone levels, consistent with severe resistance, have been reported in four families.[35-38]

Fully compensated TSH resistance is associated with euthyroidism, normal thyroglobulin levels and a normal or slightly enlarged eutopic thyroid gland on

Mutation[a]	Nucleotide change	Number of cases[b]
C41S	TGC→TCC	1
R109Q	CGG→CAG	2
P162A	CCT→GCT	5
I167D	ACC→CCC	3
G→C(+3)IVS6[c]		1
Q324X	CAG→TAG	2
C390W	TGT→TGG	2
Δ406fs→TGG420X	Δnucleotides 1217–1234, iCACG	1
D410N	GAC→AAC	2
T477I	ACT→ATT	1
F525L	TTC→TTA	1
W546X[b]	TGG→TAG	5
A553T[b]	GCC→ACC	4
R609X	CGA→TGA	6
Δ655	ΔAC	1

[a] fs, frameshift; i, insertion; Δ, deletion.
[b] Number of affected cases includes unpublished data from authors.
[c] Splicing mutation at position +3 of the intervening sequence in intron 6, affecting the splice donor site.

Table 11.2
Loss-of-function TSH receptor mutations

ultrasound or radioisotope scanning. Partially compensated TSH resistance is characterized by similar features but with higher TSH and lower thyroid hormone levels. Furthermore, administration of even large doses of thyroxine fails to fully suppress TSH secretion, but may result in biochemical and clinical thyrotoxicosis.[33] Severe TSH resistance may present at birth with classic features of CH, such as prolonged jaundice, hoarse cry and macroglossia. Ultrasound and radionuclide scanning usually suggests a severely hypoplastic or even apparently absent thyroid gland, with thyrogobulin levels being undetectable or measurable. This latter finding suggests that remnants of thyroid tissue which cannot be visualized by imaging may remain.

Resistance to TSH has also been described in families without mutations in the TSHR gene,[39] and abnormalities in the TSH signaling pathway downstream of the receptor might be expected to be implicated. Thus, germline loss of function mutations in the Gsα gene have been reported to produce resistance to TSH even in the heterozygous state.[40] However, as Gsα is ubiquitously expressed, the phenotype often includes defects in other pathways, including parathyroid hormone and gonadotropin resistance, together with somatic and skeletal abnormalities, constituting a syndrome called Albright's hereditary osteodystrophy. Reduced TSH receptor expression due to gene promoter abnormalities or defects in other downstream factors beyond Gs (e.g. G protein-coupled receptor kinase 5 (GRK5)) have been postulated but have yet to be described.

TSH receptor mutation in familial gestational hyperthyroidism

Human chorionic gonadotropin (hCG) is another member of the glycoprotein hormone family that includes TSH, luteinizing hormone (LH) and follicle-stimulating hormone (FSH). The CG receptor shares homology with TSHR, and there is also evidence for some specificity spillover in their ligands, with hCG exhibiting weak agonist action on the TSH receptor. Thus, stimulation of the thyroid gland by desialylated or elevated hCG is thought to mediate gestational thyrotoxicosis and hyperthyroidism associated with trophoblastic disease respectively.

Studies of a family where both mother and daughter had recurrent gestational hyperthyroidism with normal serum hCG levels have elucidated another mechanism.[41] The proband gave a history of two full-term pregnancies, both associated with hyperthyroidism and hyperemesis gravidarum. Clinical and biochemical thyrotoxicosis was present but without ophthalmopathy or circulating anti-TSH receptor antibodies to suggest Graves' disease, and the hyperthyroidism resolved postpartum. Both mother and daughter were heterozygous for a missense mutation (K183R) in the extracellular domain of TSHR, and functional studies indicated that this receptor mutant was more sensitive to CG than the wild-type receptor. Such abnormal sensitivity of this mutant receptor to circulating hCG was suggested to mediate the recurrent gestational thyrotoxicosis.

Resistance to thyroid hormone

Thyroid hormone receptor action

The regulation of physiological processes by thyroid hormones is mediated by changes in expression of specific target genes in different tissues. Thus, the feedback effects of thyroid hormones on TSH production are mediated by inhibition of hypothalamic TRH and pituitary TSHα and β subunit gene expression. Conversely, target genes which are induced by thyroid hormone include malic enzyme and sex hormone-binding globulin (SHBG) in the liver, myosin heavy chain and sodium–calcium ATPase in myocardium, myelin basic protein in brain, and sodium–potassium ATPase in skeletal muscle. The regulation of target genes by thyroid hormone is mediated by a nuclear receptor (TR), which is a member of the steroid nuclear receptor superfamily of proteins. Via a central zinc finger domain, the receptor binds to specific regulatory DNA sequences (so-called thyroid response elements—TREs), usually located in the promoter regions of target genes. Although TR can bind these sequences as a monomer or homodimer, it usually interacts preferentially as a heterodimer with another nuclear receptor partner—the retinoid X receptor (RXR). It is now recognized that, in the absence of hormone, many promoters are repressed or 'silenced' by unliganded receptor. Hormone binding to the C-terminal domain of TR results in relief of repression followed by ligand-dependent activation of gene transcription (see Figure 11.4a). Recently, specific cofactor complexes which mediate silencing and transcription activation functions have been isolated: a family of co-repressor proteins (nuclear receptor co-repressor, N-CoR; silencing mediator for RAR/TR,

SMRT) interact with unliganded TR, but dissociate following T3 binding; conversely, a number of putative coactivator proteins (steroid receptor coactivator 1 (SRC-1), CREB-binding protein (CBP), CBP-associated factor (pCAF)) that are recruited by TR and other nuclear receptors in a hormone-dependent manner have also been identified (Figure 11.4a).

In humans, two highly homologous thyroid hormone receptors, denoted TRα and TRβ, are encoded by separate genes on chromosomes 17 and 3 respectively. Alternate splicing generates three major receptor isoforms (TRα1, TRβ1, TRβ2), which are widely expressed but with differing tissue distributions: TRα1 is most abundant in the central nervous system, myocardium and skeletal muscle; TRβ1 is predominant in liver and kidney; and the TRβ2 isoform is most highly expressed in the pituitary and hypothalamus.

Definition of RTH

The syndrome of RTH is characterized by reduced responsiveness of target tissues to circulating thyroid hormones. Thus, resistance to thyroid hormone action in the hypothalamic–pituitary–thyroid axis gives rise to the biochemical hallmark of RTH, with inappropriate pituitary TSH secretion driving T4 and T3 production to establish a new equilibrium with high serum levels of thyroid hormones together with a non-suppressed TSH.

RTH was first described in 1967 in two siblings with high circulating thyroid hormone levels who were clinically euthyroid and exhibited a number of other abnormalities, including deaf-mutism, delayed bone maturation with stippled femoral epiphyses and short stature, as well as dysmorphic facies, winging of the scapulae and pectus carinatum.[42] It is now clear that some of these features are unique to this kindred, in which the disorder was recessively inherited.

The prevalence of RTH is approximately 1 in 50 000, and about 400 cases have been described to date. The disorder is usually dominantly inherited and associated with variable clinical features. Many patients with RTH are either asymptomatic or have non-specific symptoms and may be noted to have a goiter, prompting testing of thyroid function, which suggests the diagnosis. In these individuals, classified as exhibiting generalized resistance (GRTH), the high thyroid hormone levels are thought to compensate for ubiquitous tissue resistance, resulting in a euthyroid state.[43] In contrast, a subset of individuals with the same biochemical abnormalities exhibit thyrotoxic clinical features: in adults, these can include weight loss, tremor, palpitations, insomnia and heat intolerance; in children, failure to thrive, accelerated growth and hyperkinetic behavior have also been noted. When the latter clinical entity was first described, patients were thought to have 'selective' or predominant pituitary resistance to thyroid hormone action (PRTH), with preservation of normal hormonal responses in peripheral tissues.[44]

However, a careful comparison of the clinical and biochemical characteristics of individuals classified clinically as having either GRTH or PRTH indicates that there may be significant overlap between these entities. For example, there are no differences in age, sex ratio, frequency of goiter or levels of free T4, free T3 or TSH between patients with the two types of disorder. Significantly, features such as tachycardia, hyperkinetic behavior and anxiety have been documented in individuals with GRTH. Conversely, serum SHBG—a hepatic index of thyroid hormone action—is normal in patients with PRTH, suggesting that tissue resistance is not solely confined to the pituitary–thyroid axis in this group. Indeed, in some cases, hypothyroid features such as growth retardation, delayed dentition or bone age in children, or fatigue and hypercholesterolemia in adults, may coexist with thyrotoxic symptoms in the same individual. Nevertheless, the absence or presence of overt thyrotoxic symptoms, signifying either GRTH or PRTH, is a clinical distinction which will probably remain useful as a guide to the most appropriate form of treatment (see below).

Clinical features

A palpable goiter is the commonest presenting feature, being present in up to 65% of individuals, especially adult females. Although the enlargement is usually diffuse, following surgical attempts to correct the biochemical abnormality, which are often unsuccessful, recrudescence of multinodular gland enlargement and thyroid dysfunction occurs. Interestingly, fewer children with RTH born to affected mothers exhibit thyroid enlargement (35%) compared to offspring born of unaffected mothers (87%), suggesting that maternal hyperthyroxinemia may protect against goiter formation.[45] The biological activity of circulating TSH has been shown to be significantly enhanced in RTH, and it has been suggested that this may explain the occurrence of marked goiter and very elevated serum thyroid hormones with normal levels of immunoreactive TSH in some cases.[46]

The combination of palpitations and a resting tachycardia (75% of GRTH, nearly all PRTH) with goiter has often led to a misdiagnosis of Graves' disease for RTH, particularly before the availability of sensitive TSH assays. We have analyzed cardiac function in RTH, and although the heart rate is not significantly different from that of controls, some indices of myocardial contractility are in the hyperthyroid range. Atrial fibrillation is commoner in older subjects with RTH, but we have not documented more frequent mitral valve prolapse as suggested by others.[45]

Childhood short stature (height <5th centile) has been noted in 18% and delayed bone age (>2 SD) in 29% in both GRTH and PRTH, but final adult height is often not affected. In adults, we have measured bone mineral density and documented a reduction which is more marked in the femoral neck (mean Z score –0.41) than lumbar spine (mean Z score –0.24). The basal metabolic rate is variably altered in RTH, being normal in many cases but elevated particularly in childhood. This may account for the abnormally low body mass index seen in approximately one-third of children.

Recently, neuropsychological abnormalities have been documented in patients with RTH. First, a history of attention deficit hyperactivity disorder (ADHD) in childhood was elicited more frequently (75%) in patients with RTH compared to their unaffected relatives (15%).[47] Children and adults with RTH have been found to exhibit problems with language development, manifested by poor reading skills and problems with articulation. Frank mental retardation (IQ < 60) is quite uncommon, but 30% of patients show mild learning disability (IQ < 85). A direct comparison of individuals with ADHD and RTH versus ADHD alone indicates an association with lower non-verbal intelligence and academic achievement in the former group. Indeed, in detailed analyses of one family, RTH co-segregates with lower IQ rather than ADHD. However, when cohorts of unselected children with ADHD were screened biochemically using thyroid function tests, no cases of RTH were found, suggesting that the latter disorder is unlikely to be a common cause of hyperactivity. MRI shows anomalies of the Sylvian fissure or Heschl's gyri more frequently in RTH, but these features do not correlate with ADHD.

Significant hearing loss has been documented in 21% of RTH cases: in the majority, audiometry indicated a conductive defect, probably related to an increased incidence of recurrent ear infections in childhood; abnormal otoacoustic emissions, suggestive of cochlear dysfunction, were also documented in those with hearing deficit.[48]

Recurrent pulmonary and upper respiratory tract infections occur more often in RTH, and affected individuals have reduced circulating immunoglobulin levels. Intrauterine growth retardation has been observed in two neonates with RTH. Pubertal development, fertility and overall survival are not adversely affected by the disorder. The major clinical features that are recognized in association with RTH are summarized in Table 11.3.

Elevated serum free thyroid hormones
Non-suppressed TSH with enhanced bioactivity
Goiter
Growth retardation, short stature
Low body mass index in childhood
Attention deficit hyperactivity disorder, low IQ
Tachycardia, atrial fibrillation, heart failure
Ear, nose and throat infections and hearing loss
Osteopenia

Table 11.3
Features of RTH.

Differential diagnosis

The hallmark of RTH is elevated serum thyroid hormones together with non-suppressed TSH levels. However, as shown in Table 11.4, a variety of different conditions can be associated with hyperthyroxinemia and detectable TSH levels. An algorithm which enables the differential diagnosis of this diagnostic entity is shown in Figure 11.2. Initially, it is helpful to determine whether the free thyroid hormones (FT4, FT3) are also raised, excluding an elevated total T4 due to an increase in serum binding proteins. The use of an equilibrium dialysis or direct 'two-step' method to assay FT4 usually excludes artefactual elevation due to dysalbuminemia or the presence of antiiodothyronine (anti-T4, anti-T3) antibodies. If the measured TSH falls linearly with serial dilution of serum, a spurious result due to anti-TSH antibodies is unlikely. Other causes (neonatal period, systemic illness, drugs) are excluded by recognition of the abnormal clinical context or

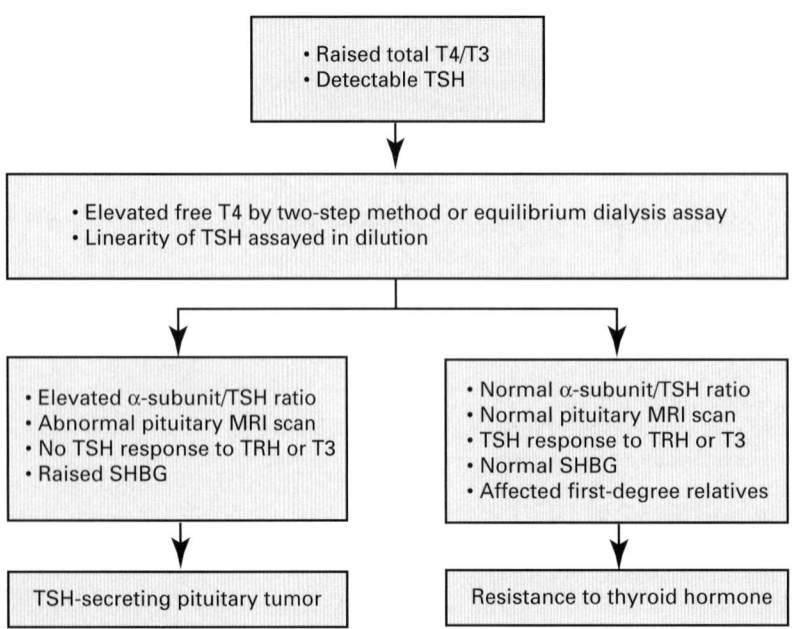

Figure 11.2
An algorithm for the investigation of elevated circulating thyroid hormones with non-suppressed pituitary TSH secretion.

Raised serum binding proteins
Familial dysalbuminemic hyperthyroxinemia
Anti-iodothyronine/anti-TSH antibodies
Non-thyroidal illness (including acute psychiatric disorders)
Neonatal period
Iatrogenic thyroxine replacement therapy, drugs (e.g. amiodarone, heparin)
TSH-secreting pituitary tumor
Resistance to thyroid hormone

Table 11.4
Causes of raised serum T4 with non-suppressed TSH.

documenting subsequent normalization of thyroid function following recovery or drug withdrawal.

The main differential diagnosis of RTH is from a TSH-secreting pituitary tumor, and this distinction can be difficult, particularly when the former is associated with hyperthyroid features. There are no significant differences in age, sex, FT4, FT3 or TSH levels between the two groups of patients (Table 11.5). Pituitary imaging may show an obvious macroadenoma, but the occurrence of pituitary 'incidentalomas' or thyrotroph hyperplasia following inappropriate thyroid ablation in RTH can lead to diagnostic difficulties. Dynamic tests of the pituitary–thyroid axis can be helpful. Circulating TSH shows a normal or exaggerated response to TRH and is suppressed following T3 administration in patients with RTH, whereas TSH secretion from autonomous tumors is unresponsive. However, the specificity of such dynamic testing is not absolute (Table 11.5). Likewise, the molar ratio of serum glycoprotein hormone α subunit to TSH is normal in RTH and elevated with most (but not all) TSH-omas. In our experience, two additional investigations are of value: (1) serum SHBG is almost invariably normal in RTH, but often elevated into the thyrotoxic range with TSH-secreting tumors; (2) similar thyroid function test abnormalities in first-degree relatives are virtually diagnostic of RTH, as the disorder is familial in 80–90% of cases (Table 11.5).

In addition to clinical signs and symptoms, the measurement of indices of thyroid hormone action are of use in evaluating the differing responses of various target organs and tissues to elevated circulating thyroid hormones in RTH (Table 11.6). Although these measurements are most useful in assessing the effects of marked thyroid hormone excess states such as overt hyperthyroidism, they may be less discriminatory in individuals with borderline thyroid dysfunction or in hypothyroidism. In order to improve the sensitivity and specificity of these parameters, it has been

Parameter[a]	TSH-omas	RTH	P
Female/male ratio	1.3	1.4	NS
Familial cases	0%	84%	<0.0001
TSH (mU/l)	3.0±0.5	2.3±0.3	NS
FT4 (pmol/l)	38.8±4.0	29.9±2.4	NS
FT3 (pmol/l)	14.0±1.2	11.3±0.9	NS
SHBG (nmol/l)	117±18	61±4	<0.0001
Lesions on CT or MRI	100%	6%	<0.0001
High α-subunit levels	69%	3%	<0.0001
High α-subunit/TSH molar ratio	81%	2%	<0.0001
Blunted TSH response to TRH stimulation	94%	2%	<0.0001
Abnormal TSH response to T3 suppression[b]	100%	100%	NS

[a] Data presented are from untreated patients with an intact pituitary–thyroid axis studied at the Institute of Endocrine Sciences.
[b] Werner's test: 80–100 μg T3 administered daily for 8–10 days followed by measurement of TSH response to TRH. Although complete suppression of basal and TRH-stimulated TSH levels has never been recorded in either group, RTH subjects exhibit greater inhibition of TSH secretion than patients with TSH-omas.

Table 11.5
Differential diagnosis of TSH-secreting adenomas (TSH-omas) versus resistance to thyroid hormones (RTH).

Central	
Pituitary	TSH
Peripheral	
General	Basal metabolic rate
Hepatic	Sex hormone-binding globulin, ferritin, cholesterol
Muscle	Creatine kinase, ankle jerk relaxation time
Cardiac	Sleeping pulse rate, systolic time interval, diastolic isovolumic relaxation time
Bone	Height, bone age, bone density, alkaline phosphatase, osteocalcin, pyridinium crosslinks
Hematological	Soluble interleukin-2 receptor
Lung	Angiotensin-converting enzyme

Table 11.6
Markers of thyroid hormone action.

suggested that RTH patients are assessed following the administration of graded supraphysiological doses of T3 (50, 100 and 200 μg/day, each given for a period of 3 days) with comparison of any change in indices to baseline values and responses in normal subjects.[43]

Molecular genetics

Following the cloning of thyroid hormone receptors, RTH was shown to be tightly linked to the TRβ gene locus in a single family.[49] This prompted analysis of the gene in other cases, and a growing number of receptor mutations have since been associated with the disorder. In keeping with the dominant inheritance of RTH, affected individuals are heterozygous for mutations in the TRβ gene which occur de novo in approximately 10% of sporadic cases. Over 80 different defects, including point mutations, in-frame deletions and frameshift insertions, have been documented to date, all of which localize to three mutation clusters within the hormone-binding domain of the receptor (Figure 11.3).

Based on the supposition that PRTH was associated with selective pituitary resistance, it had been hypothesized that this disorder might be associated with defects

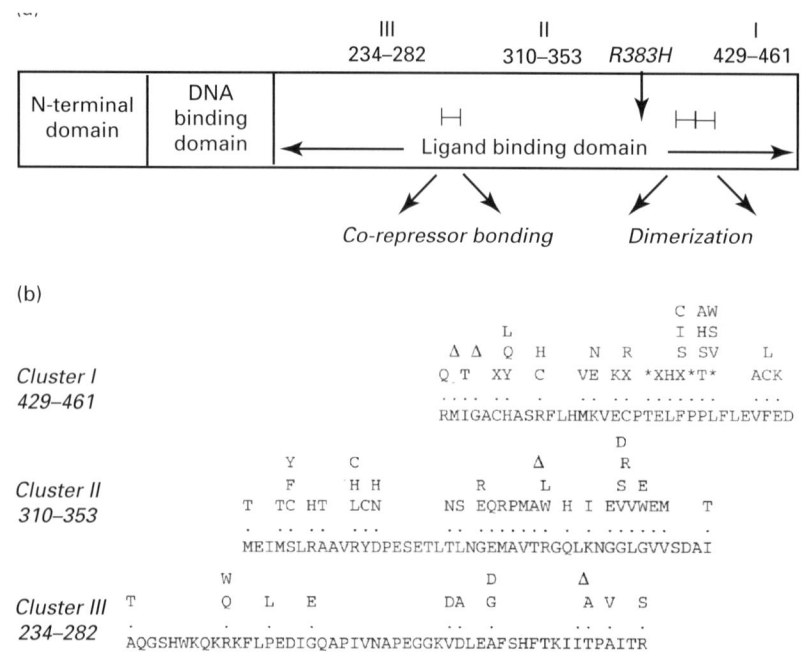

Figure 11.3
The domains of TRβ, showing that, with one exception (R383H), resistance to thyroid hormone mutations localize to three clusters within the ligand-binding domain (LBD). The receptor defects in each cluster include missense mutations in frame codon deletions (Δ), premature termination codons (X) and frameshift (*) mutations.

in the pituitary type II 5′-deiodinase enzyme or the TRβ2 receptor isoform. However, TRβ gene mutations have also been documented in PRTH.[50] Receptor mutations occurring in individuals with PRTH have also been documented in cases of GRTH in unrelated kindreds. Furthermore, even within a single family, the same receptor mutation can be associated with abnormal thyroid function and thyrotoxic features consistent with PRTH in some individuals, but similar biochemical abnormalities and a lack of symptoms indicative of GRTH in other members. Overall, these findings indicate that GRTH and PRTH represent differing phenotypic manifestations of a single genetic entity.

In a small number of cases, clearcut biochemical evidence of RTH is not associated with a mutation in the coding region of TRβ1. Several explanations have been postulated to account for such cases, including the existence of somatic TRβ1 mutations whose expression is limited so as to be undetectable in peripheral blood leukocyte DNA. In some families or sporadic cases, mutations in TRβ2 and defects at the TRα locus have also been excluded. This raises the possibility of novel, non-receptor mechanisms by which thyroid hormone action could be disrupted to produce the RTH phenotype. In one case, TRβ bound aberrantly to an 84-kDa protein from patient fibroblast nuclear extracts, raising the possibility of abnormal receptor interaction with a cofactor. Patients with Rubinstein–Taybi syndrome, a disorder associated with defects in the nuclear receptor coactivator CBP, exhibit a number of somatic abnormalities (broad thumbs, mental retardation, short stature), yet have normal thyroid function. Disruption of the steroid receptor coactivator 1 (SRC-1) gene in mice results in resistance to thyroid and steroid hormones, raising the possible existence of a homologous human defect.[51] However, recent studies in several families excluded defects in both coactivators (SRC-1, ACTR) and co-repressors (NCOR, SMRT) by linkage and sequence analysis.[52]

Properties of mutant receptors

In keeping with their location in the hormone-binding domain, the ability of mutant receptors to bind T3 is moderately or markedly reduced and their ability to activate or repress target gene expression is impaired. A subset of receptor mutations which exhibit normal hormone binding but markedly reduced transcriptional function involve residues that are critical for mediating TR interaction with coactivators.

In the first documented family with RTH, in which the disorder was recessively inherited, both affected siblings were found to be homozygous for a complete deletion of the TRβ receptor gene.[53] Significantly, their heterozygous parents, harboring a deletion of one TRβ allele, were completely normal, with no evidence of thyroid dysfunction. This suggested that a simple lack of functional β receptor, as a consequence of the single deleted TRβ allele, was insufficient to generate the resistance phenotype. This observation led to the hypothesis that the mutant receptors in dominantly inherited RTH are not simply functionally impaired, but are also capable of inhibiting wild-type receptor action. Indeed, experiments indicate that, when co-expressed, the mutant proteins are able to inhibit the function of their wild-type counterparts in a 'dominant negative' manner[54] (Figure 11.4b). Further clinical and

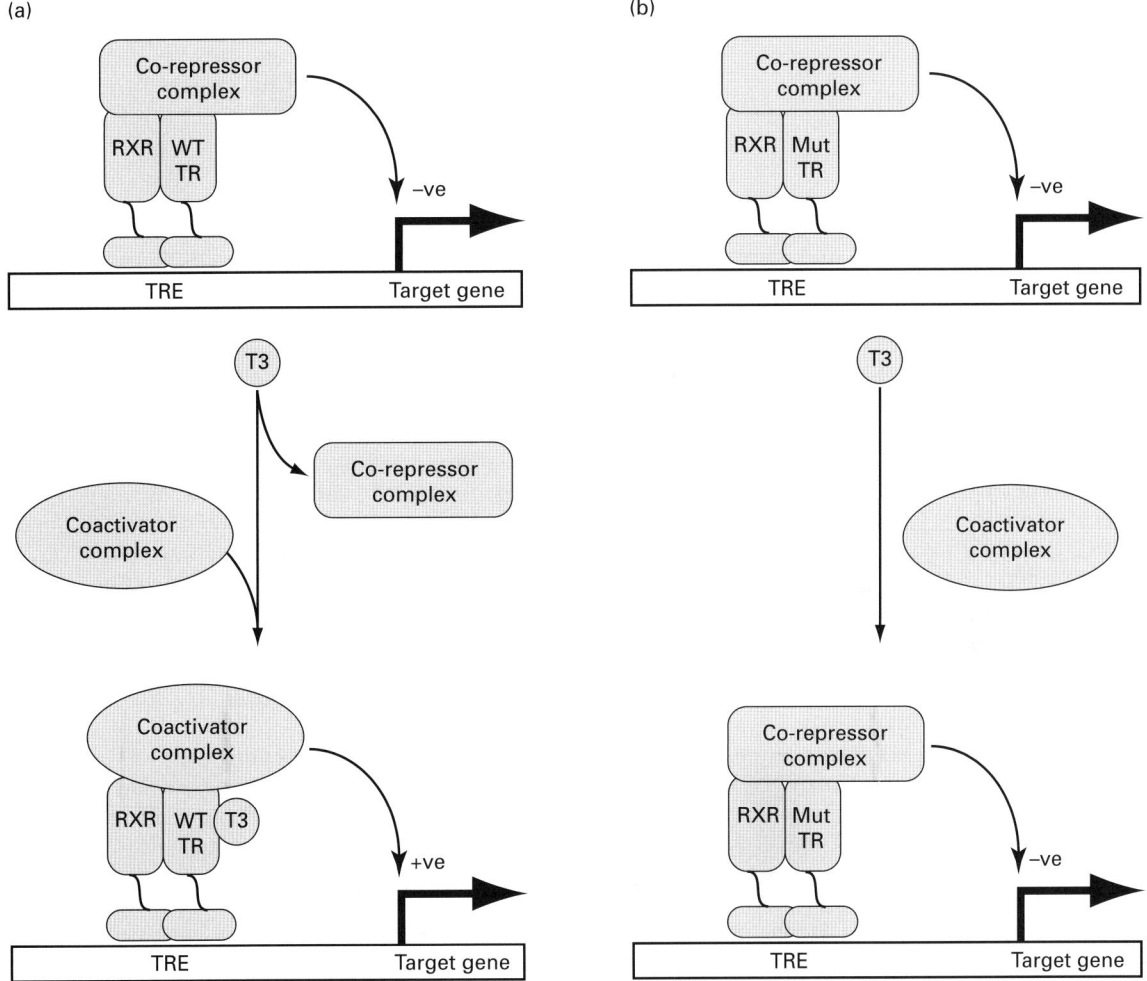

Figure 11.4
Possible mechanism for dominant negative inhibition by resistance to thyroid hormone mutants. (a) Wild-type TR action on target genes. The unliganded RXR–TR heterodimer recruits a co-repressor complex to silence basal gene transcription. Receptor occupancy by ligand (T3) promotes co-repressor dissociation followed by binding of a coactivator complex which leads to target gene activation. (b) Mutant receptor action. The primary defect in mutant receptors is failure to release co-repressor and/or recruit coactivator. Occupancy of promoter thyroid response elements (TREs) by mutant receptor–co-repressor complexes results in inhibition of target gene expression.

genetic evidence to support this hypothesis is provided by a unique childhood case in which severe biochemical resistance with marked developmental delay, growth retardation and cardiac hyperthyroidism proved fatal due to heart failure following septicemia. This individual was homozygous for a point mutation in both alleles of the TRβ gene, and the extreme phenotype presumably reflects the compound effect of two dominant negative mutant receptors.[55]

Pathogenesis of variable tissue resistance

The ability to exert a dominant negative effect within the hypothalamic–pituitary–thyroid axis is a key property of RTH mutant receptors which generates the characteristically abnormal thyroid function tests that lead to the identification of the disorder. One study has shown that, for a subset of RTH mutants, there is a correlation between their functional impairment in vitro and the degree of central pituitary resistance as quantified by the degree of elevation in serum free T4 in vivo.[56] On this biochemical background, the variable clinical phenotypes may be due to variable degrees of peripheral resistance in different individuals, as well as variable resistance in different tissues within a single subject. A number of factors might contribute to such variable tissue resistance.

One factor may be the differing tissue distributions of receptor isoforms. The hypothalamus/pituitary and liver express predominantly TRβ2 and TRβ1 receptors respectively, whereas TRα1 is the major species expressed in myocardium. Therefore, mutations in the TRβ gene are likely to be associated with pituitary and liver resistance, as exemplified by normal SHBG and non-suppressed TSH levels, while the tachycardia and cardiac hyperthyroidism often seen in RTH may represent retention of myocardial sensitivity to thyroid hormones mediated by a normal α receptor (Figure 11.5). Another factor which may regulate the degree of tissue resistance is the relative expression of mutant versus wild-type TRβ alleles. Although one study has suggested that both alleles are expressed equally, another showed marked differences, with overexpression of mutant receptor messenger RNA in skin correlating with the degree of skeletal tissue resistance. The dominant negative inhibitory potency of mutant receptors has been shown to differ with target gene promoter context and is a further variable which may influence the degree of resistance.

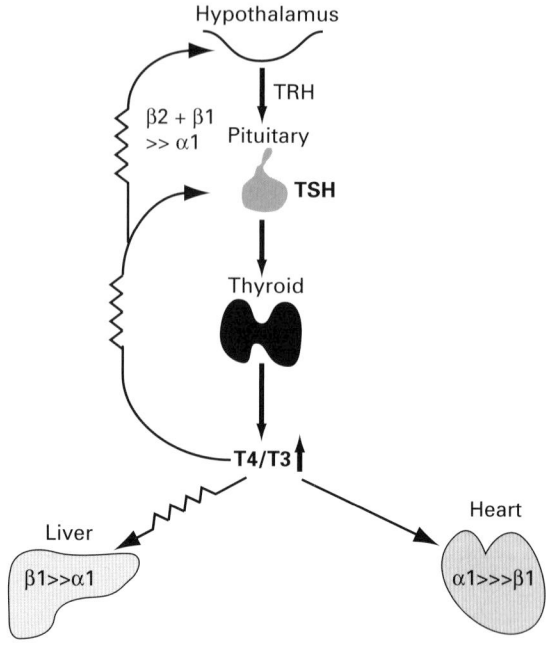

Figure 11.5
The influence of tissue distribution of thyroid hormone receptor isoforms on the phenotype of resistance to thyroid hormone. TRβ2 and TRβ1 are the predominant isoforms in pituitary and hypothalamus, generating resistance in the feedback axis and the characteristic abnormalities of thyroid function. The abundance of TRα1 in myocardium is associated with retention of cardiac sensitivity to thyroid hormones.

Attempts to correlate the clinical phenotype of RTH with the nature of the underlying receptor mutation have been confounded by three factors: first, the imprecision of clinical criteria used to define GRTH and PRTH; second, the apparently spontaneous temporal variation in thyrotoxic features in some cases of RTH; and third, the relatively small number of individuals with any given mutation that have been identified hitherto. Nevertheless, some interesting associations are emerging from the published literature. The first patient described with PRTH was found to harbor an R338W receptor mutation, and the same phenotype has been associated with the majority of cases with substitutions at this codon. When tested in vitro, this mutant exhibits dominant negative activity with the negatively regulated pituitary TSHα subunit gene promoter, but is a relatively poor inhibitor of wild-type receptor action in other TRE contexts.[54] A patient harboring the R383H receptor mutation, which is impaired mainly in the regulation of the TRH and TSH genes, exhibited predominantly central resistance following T3 administration. Some RTH receptor mutants (R338W or L, V349M, R429Q, I431T) associated with PRTH have been shown to exert a greater dominant negative effect in a TRβ2 than TRβ1 context.

Finally, non-receptor-mutation-related factors may influence the phenotype. For example, a deleterious R316H mutation was associated with normal thyroid function in some members of one kindred, but abnormal thyroid hormone levels in an unrelated family, suggesting that other genetic variables can modulate the effect of mutant receptors on the pituitary–thyroid axis.

Management

The management of RTH is complex, as variable resistance makes it difficult to maintain euthyroidism in all tissues. In general, the presence or absence of overt thyrotoxic or hypothyroid features is a useful guide to the need for therapy. In most individuals, the receptor defect is compensated by high circulating thyroid hormone levels, leading to a clinically euthyroid state not associated with abnormalities other than a goiter. Inappropriate thyroid ablation with surgery or radioiodine to correct the biochemical abnormality is often unsuccessful, with recrudescence of the goiter and disruption of the pituitary–thyroid axis which renders the RTH patient hypothyroid. This is one context in which thyroxine replacement in supraphysiological dosage is indicated. Other circumstances, such as hypercholesterolemia in adults or developmental delay and growth retardation in children, may also warrant the administration of supraphysiological doses of L-T4 to overcome a higher degree of resistance in certain tissues. While successful in some cases, such therapy needs careful monitoring of other peripheral indices of thyroid hormone action (e.g. heart rate, BMR, bone markers) to avoid the adverse cardiac effects or excess catabolism associated with overtreatment.

On the other hand, a reduction in thyroid hormone levels may be of benefit in the management of patients with thyrotoxic symptoms. However, the adminstration of conventional anti-thyroid drugs usually causes a further rise in serum TSH with consequent thyroid enlargement and may also induce pituitary thyrotroph hyperplasia, with a theoretical risk of inducing autonomous neoplasms in either organ. Accordingly, agents which inhibit pituitary TSH secretion, yet are devoid of peripheral thyromimetic effects, are used to reduce thyroid hormone levels. The most widely used agent is 3,3,5-triiodothyroacetic acid (TRIAC), a thyroid hormone analog which has been shown to be beneficial in both childhood and adult cases.[57,58] This compound has two interesting properties which make it an attractive therapeutic option in RTH: first, in vivo, it exerts predominantly pituitary and hepatic thyromimetic effects—target tissues which are relatively refractory to thyroid hormones in RTH; second, it exhibits a higher affinity for TRβ than TRα in vitro. A dose of 1.4–2.8 mg is used, and a recent study suggested that twice-daily administration might inhibit TSH secretion more effectively.[59] The use of TRIAC in one pregnancy controlled maternal thyrotoxic symptoms but may have induced fetal goiter. However, TRIAC treatment is not always successful, and dextrothyroxine (D-T4) is another agent which has been shown to be effective in some cases.[60] The dopaminergic agent bromocriptine, or the somatostatin analog octreotide, have been used but, unlike TSH-omas, pituitary TSH secretion is not subject to their inhibitory effects. In view of the spontaneous variation in thyrotoxic symptoms in RTH, periodic cessation of thyroid hormone-lowering therapy and re-evaluation of the clinical status of the patient is advisable. Thyroid ablation followed by subphysiological thyroxine replacement can be used in rare circumstances such as RTH associated with life-threatening thyrotoxic cardiac failure.

The treatment of RTH with thyrotoxic manifestations (e.g. failure to thrive) in childhood also requires careful monitoring to ensure that any reduction in thyroid hormone levels is not associated with growth retardation or adverse neurological sequelae. Indeed, control of cardiac and sympathetic overactivity with β-blockade may be the safest course in this context. A recent study showed that L-T3 therapy improved hyperactivity in nine children with ADHD and RTH, including three individuals who were unresponsive to methylphenidate.[61]

In the future, development of thyroid hormone analogs with greater thyromimetic activity on mutant versus normal TRβ receptors,[62] or receptor isoform-specific antagonists, might represent a more rational therapeutic approach.

TSH-secreting pituitary tumors

Definition

The term central hyperthyroidism refers to a form of thyrotoxicosis due to excessive stimulation of the thyroid gland by TSH. This condition represents a rare cause of hyperthyroidism, since thyroid hormone excess results most frequently from autoantibody stimulation or primary disorders of the thyroid. Typically, patients with central hyperthyroidism have normal or elevated TSH levels in the presence of high thyroid hormone concentrations. The most frequent cause of central hyperthyroidism is a TSH-secreting pituitary adenoma (TSH-oma). However, a subset of patients with predominant PRTH with retention of peripheral sensitivity may also present with signs and symptoms of hyperthyroidism together with biochemcial findings similar to those found in TSH-oma. In the past, as they are characterized by disruption of the negative feedback mechanism that usually leads to suppression of TSH secretion, the above unusual syndromes were classified as hyperthyroidism with 'inappropriate secretion of TSH'.

Epidemiology

TSH-omas are rare tumors,[63,64] accounting for about 0.5–1% of all pituitary adenomas, with an estimated prevalence of about one case per million. However, this figure is probably an underestimate, as the number of reported cases of TSH-omas has tripled in the last decade, with, for example, in increase in occurrence from less than 1% to 2.8% in the period 1989–91 in a large surgical series of pituitary tumors.[65] This increase in reported cases of TSH-omas is principally due to the introduction of ultrasensitive immunometric assays for TSH as a first-line test for the evaluation of thyroid function. Thus, many patients previously thought to have Graves' disease could now be correctly diagnosed as having either a TSH-oma or, alternatively, PRTH, based on the finding of measurable serum TSH levels in the presence of elevated thyroid hormone concentrations.[43,64,66]

Although most cases are diagnosed between the third and the sixth decade of life, TSH-omas have been observed in patients of any age, from 11 to 84 years, with equal frequency in men and women. Familial occurrence of TSH-omas has been reported only as part of the multiple endocrine neoplasia type 1 syndrome (MEN 1).

Pathology

Almost all TSH-omas originate from pituitary thyrotrophs, with only a single report of an ectopic nasopharyngeal TSH-secreting tumor.[67] TSH-omas are almost always benign, and malignant transformation to carcinoma with multiple metastases has been reported in only one patient.[68] The great majority are macroadenomas, with a diameter of more than 10 mm, with about 15% being microadenomas. Extrasellar extension in supra- and/or parasellar directions is present in more than two-thirds of cases, with frequent diffuse invasiveness into the surrounding structures. Significantly, the occurrence of invasive macroadenomas is particularly high in patients with a history of previous thyroid ablation with surgery or radioiodine (Figure 11.6). Such aggressive transformation of the tumor resembles that occurring in corticotroph adenomas after adrenalectomy for Cushing's disease, leading to Nelson's syndrome.

By light microscopy, tumoral thyrotrophs appear chromophobic, though they occasionally stain with either basic or acid dyes. They may show nuclear atypia and mitoses, thus sometimes being mistakenly diagnosed as pituitary malignancy or metastasis from distant carcinomas.[69] By electron microscopy, these tumors are mostly monomorphous, characterized by a poorly developed Golgi apparatus and a low number of small secretory granules mainly located under the plasma membrane.[69,70]

About 75% of TSH-omas secrete TSH alone, often accompanied by an unbalanced hypersecretion of pituitary glycoprotein hormone α subunit. Hypersecretion of growth hormone and/or prolactin (PRL), resulting in acromegaly and/or amenorrhea–galactorrhea syndrome, occurs in about 25% of tumors, whereas the occurrence of mixed TSH/gonadotropin-secreting adenomas is rare and ACTH co-secretion has not been documented to date.

Immunocytochemical studies show the presence of TSHβ and/or α subunit in the great majority of cases. In addition, double immunostaining has documented the existence of mixed TSH/α subunit adenomas, composed of one cell type secreting α subunit alone and another co-secreting α subunit and TSH.[70] In addition to α subunit, TSH frequently colocalizes with other pituitary hormones in the same tumoral cell, but

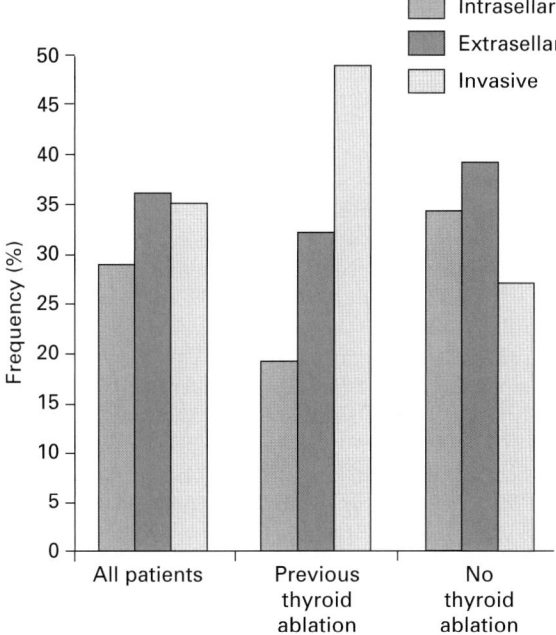

Figure 11.6
The effects of previous thyroid ablation on the size of TSH-secreting tumors. Note the significant increase of invasive tumors in patients with previous thyroid ablation. Data have been calculated from 264 reported cases (169 with intact thyroid and 95 with previous ablation). 'Intrasellar' refers to both micro- and macroadenomas confined to the fossa, 'extrasellar' to macroadenomas with suprasellar extension, and 'invasive' to invasive macroadenomas.

without the latter immunopositivity necessarily resulting in excess hormone secretion.

As with most other pituitary tumors, the pathogenesis of TSH-omas remains largely unknown. Screening studies for genetic abnormalities have yielded negative results.[71] However, the data available concern a relatively low number of tumors and are too preliminary to definitively rule out transcription factor or gene expression abnormalities in TSH-omas.[71–73]

Clinical manifestations

Patients with TSH-oma present with signs and symptoms of hyperthyroidism that are sometimes milder than expected on the basis of circulating thyroid hormone levels. In particular, cardiac thyrotoxicosis with atrial fibrillation and/or cardiac failure are rare features in these patients. Signs and symptoms of hyperthyroidism are frequently associated with those related to the mass effects of the pituitary adenoma, and the latter often predominate. Visual field defects are present in about 40%, headache in 20% and partial or total hypopituitarism in about 25% of patients. Most patients have a long history of thyroid dysfunction, often misdiagnosed as Graves' disease, and about one-third have had inappropriate thyroidectomy or radio-iodine thyroid ablation.[63,64,74,75] In some acromegalic patients, signs and symptoms of hyperthyroidism may be clinically missed, as they are overshadowed by those of acromegaly. The presence of a goiter, frequently uni- or multinodular (about 72% of reported cases), is the rule. Even following previous thyroidectomy, remnant thyroid residue may regrow as a consequence of TSH hyperstimulation. However, progression of thyroid nodules to functional autonomy or differentiated carcinoma seems to be infrequent.[76,77] Bilateral exophthalmos has been documented in rare patients who subsequently developed concomitant autoimmune thyroid disease, while unilateral exophthalmos due to orbital invasion by pituitary tumor was reported in three patients with TSH-omas.

Diagnosis

Serum thyroid hormone and TSH levels
Serum TSH levels in patients with TSH-oma may be elevated or in the normal range, whereas total and free thyroid hormone levels are definitely high (Table 11.5). The findings of normal immunoreactive TSH in the presence of high levels of FT4 and FT3 is probably due to the increased biological activity of circulating TSH molecules in TSH-oma.[78,79] The differential diagnosis of hyperthyroxinemia with non-suppressed TSH levels and its further investigation are described in the section on resistance to thyroid hormone.

Pituitary glycoprotein hormone α subunit
A helpful diagnostic tool in the diagnosis of TSH-omas is the determination of levels of α subunit common to each of the pituitary glycoprotein hormones.[63,64] Secretion of the α subunit in these tumors is not only in excess of TSHβ subunit but also in excess of the intact TSH molecule, resulting in an α subunit/TSH molar ratio generally higher than 1. An elevated ratio can also occur in normal subjects (e.g. euthyroid postmenopausal

women).[80] In some patients with TSH-omas, normal absolute α subunit levels may yet be associated with an elevated α subunit/TSH molar ratio (Table 11.5).[74,75]

Indices of thyroid hormone action on peripheral tissues

Measurements of parameters of peripheral thyroid hormone action are helpful in quantifying hyperthyroid tissue responses.[43,64,66,75] Some of these parameters (e.g. SHBG and ICTP) have been used to differentiate hyperthyroid patients with TSH-oma from those with PRTH (Table 11.5), since the former have elevated levels of these indices, whereas they are usually in the normal range in patients with PRTH.[81,82]

Dynamic testing

In the past, several stimulatory and inhibitory tests have been suggested as useful in the diagnosis of TSH-oma. Classically, the T3 suppression test has been used, with failure to completely suppress TSH secretion after T3 administration (80–100 μg/day for 8–10 days) being strongly supportive of a TSH-oma (Table 11.5). It is also worth noting that the T3 suppression test is particularly sensitive and specific in patients with previous thyroid ablation.[74,75] In 83% of TSH-oma patients, TSH levels do not increase after TRH injection. This lack of TSH response to TRH may also be useful in making the unusual diagnosis of TSH-oma coexisting with primary hypothyroidism.[83] In the majority of TSH-oma patients, TSH secretion can be inhibited by administration of native somatostatin or its analogs, and these tests may be helpful in predicting the efficacy of long-term medical treatment with these agents.[73,84]

Imaging studies

Pituitary imaging studies, particularly nuclear magnetic resonance imaging (MRI) or high-resolution computed tomography (CT), are mandatory when making a diagnosis of TSH-oma. With macroadenomas accounting for the majority of cases, plain skull radiographs may also reveal abnormalities of the sella turcica. Various degrees of suprasellar extension or sphenoid sinus invasion are present in two-thirds of cases.

Differential diagnosis

In a patient with signs and symptoms of hyperthyroidism, the presence of elevated thyroid hormone and detectable TSH levels rule out primary hyperthyroidism. When the existence of central hyperthyroidism is confirmed and artefactual biochemical measurement is excluded, several further diagnostic steps are useful in differentiating a TSH-oma from PRTH.[43,64,66] First, the presence of neurological signs and symptoms (visual defects, headache) or clinical features of concomitant hypersecretion of other pituitary hormones points to the presence of a TSH-secreting pituitary lesion, and abnormalities on MRI or CT scan would strongly support this. Nevertheless, the differential diagnosis may be difficult if the pituitary adenoma is too small to be detected by pituitary imaging, or conversely if there is the confusing occurrence of 'false-positive' abnormalities such as an empty sella or pituitary incidentalomas. In such cases, elevated α subunit levels or raised α subunit/TSH molar ratio or TSH unresponsiveness to TRH stimulation and/or to T3 suppression tests favor the presence of a TSH-oma. In contrast to RTH, familial cases of TSH-oma have never been documented. However, the apparent coexistence of TSH-oma and RTH has been recently reported in a young Japanese woman, although the latter was not confirmed genetically by identifying a TRβ gene mutation.[85] Nonetheless, the occurrence of TSH-omas in RTH patients is theoretically possible and should therefore be carefully considered.[86]

Treatment, outcome and follow-up

Surgical resection is the recommended therapy for TSH-secreting pituitary tumors. However, complete resection of large tumors, which represent the majority of TSH-omas, can be particularly difficult due to the local invasion that is frequently present. Preparation of the patient prior to surgery includes the administration of anti-thyroid drugs or octreotide together with propranolol to restore euthyroidism. If surgery is contraindicated or declined, or in cases of surgical failure, pituitary radiotherapy may be undertaken with a recommended dose of either 45 Gy fractionated at 2 Gy/day or a single 10–25-Gy dose via stereotactic radiosurgery. The criteria for cure in patients with TSH-omas treated surgically or with radiotherapy have not been clearly established, due to the rarity of the disease and the great heterogeneity of clinical parameters used. Clinical remission of hyperthyroidism, with normalization of elevated thyroid hormones, TSH, α subunit or α subunit/TSH molar ratio and disappearance of neurological symptoms represent useful criteria of a good therapeutic response. In addition, in our experience, undetectable TSH levels 1 week after surgery are likely to predict complete adenomectomy, provided that anti-thyroid therapy was stopped at least 10 days before surgery.[75] The most sensitive and specific test to document the complete removal of the adenoma remains the T3 suppression test. In fact, only patients in whom T3 administration completely inhibits basal and TRH-stimulated TSH secretion appear to be truly cured.[75] No data on the recurrence rates of TSH-oma in patients judged to be cured after surgery or radiotherapy have been reported.

Although earlier diagnosis has improved the surgical cure rate, failure or an incomplete response to surgery requires postoperative adjunctive medical therapy in order to control persistent hyperthyroidism. Dopamine agonists such as bromocriptine have been used in some TSH-omas with variable results, positive effects being observed mainly in some patients with mixed PRL/TSH-secreting tumors. Currently, the mainstay for medical management of TSH-omas comprise long-acting somatostatin analogs, such as octreotide or lanreotide.[84,87,88] Treatment with these analogs leads to a reduction of TSH and α subunit secretion in almost all cases, with restoration of the euthyroid state in the majority of them. During octreotide therapy, tumor shrinkage occurs in about one-half of patients and visual improvement in 75%.[87] Resistance to octreotide treatment has been documented in only 4% of cases. Whether somatostatin analog treatment might be an alternative to surgery and irradiation as first-line therapy in older patients with TSH-oma remains to be established.

References

1. Vassart G, Dumont JE. The thyrotropin receptor and the regulation of thyrocyte function and growth. *Endocrine Rev* 1992; 13(3): 596–611.
2. Van Sande J, Raspe E, Perret J et al. Thyrotropin activates both the cyclic AMP and the PIP2 cascades in CHO cells expressing the human cDNA of TSH receptor. *Mol Cell Endocrinol* 1990; 74(1): R1–6.
3. Krohn K, Fuhrer D, Holzapfel HP, Paschke R. Clonal origin of toxic thyroid nodules with constitutively activating thyrotropin receptor mutations. *J Clin Endocrinol Metab* 1998; 83(1): 130–4.
4. Parma J, Duprez L, Van Sande J et al. Somatic mutations in the thyrotropin receptor gene cause hyperfunctioning thyroid adenomas. *Nature* 1993; 365(6447): 649–51.
5. Duprez L, Hermans J, Van Sande J, Dumont JE, Vassart G, Parma J. Two autonomous nodules of a patient with multinodular goiter harbor different activating mutations of the thyrotropin receptor gene. *J Clin Endocrinol Metab* 1997; 82(1): 306–8.
6. Parma J, Duprez L, Van Sande J et al. Diversity and prevalence of somatic mutations in the thyrotropin receptor and Gs alpha genes as a cause of toxic thyroid adenomas. *J Clin Endocrinol Metab* 1997; 82(8): 2695–701.
7. Fuhrer D, Holzapfel HP, Wonerow P, Scherbaum WA, Paschke R. Somatic mutations in the thyrotropin receptor gene and not in the Gs alpha protein gene in 31 toxic thyroid nodules. *J Clin Endocrinol Metab* 1997; 82(11): 3885–91.
8. Holzapfel HP, Fuhrer D, Wonerow P, Weinland G, Scherbaum WA, Paschke R. Identification of constitutively activating somatic thyrotropin receptor mutations in a subset of toxic multinodular goiters. *J Clin Endocrinol Metab* 1997; 82(12): 4229–33.
9. Kopp P, Muirhead S, Jourdain N, Gu WX, Jameson JL, Rodd C. Congenital hyperthyroidism caused by a solitary toxic adenoma harboring a novel somatic mutation (serine281-->isoleucine) in the extracellular domain of the thyrotropin receptor. *J Clin Invest* 1997; 100(6): 1634–9.
10. Farid NR, Kascur V, Balazs C. The human thyrotropin receptor is highly mutable: a review of gain-of-function mutations. *Eur J Endocrinol* 2000; 143(1): 25–30.
11. Van Sande J, Parma J, Tonacchera M, Swillens S, Dumont J, Vassart G. Somatic and germline mutations of the TSH receptor gene in thyroid diseases. *J Clin Endocrinol Metab* 1995; 80(9): 2577–85.
12. Tonacchera M, Van Sande J, Cetani F et al. Functional characteristics of three new germline mutations of the thyrotropin receptor gene causing autosomal dominant toxic thyroid hyperplasia. *J Clin Endocrinol Metab* 1996; 81(2): 547–54.
13. Laurberg P, Pedersen KM, Vestergaard H, Sigurdsson G. High incidence of multinodular toxic goitre in the elderly population in a low iodine intake area vs. high incidence of Graves' disease in the young in a high iodine intake area: comparative surveys of thyrotoxicosis epidemiology in East-Jutland Denmark and Iceland. *J Intern Med* 1991; 229(5): 415–20.
14. Takeshita A, Nagayama Y, Yokoyama N et al. Rarity of oncogenic mutations in the thyrotropin receptor of autonomously functioning thyroid nodules in Japan. *J Clin Endocrinol Metab* 1995; 80(9): 2607–11.
15. Tanaka K, Nagayama Y, Takeshita A et al. Low incidence of the stimulatory G protein alpha-subunit mutations in autonomously functioning thyroid adenomas in Japan. *Thyroid* 1996; 6(3): 195–9.
16. Tonacchera M, Chiovato L, Pinchera A et al. Hyperfunctioning thyroid nodules in toxic multinodular goiter share activating thyrotropin receptor mutations

with solitary toxic adenoma. *J Clin Endocrinol Metab* 1998; **83**(2): 492–8.
17. Krohn K, Wohlgemuth S, Gerber H, Paschke R. Hot microscopic areas of iodine-deficient euthyroid goitres contain constitutively activating TSH receptor mutations. *J Pathol* 2000; **192**(1): 37–42.
18. Russo D, Arturi F, Suarez HG et al. Thyrotropin receptor gene alterations in thyroid hyperfunctioning adenomas. *J Clin Endocrinol Metab* 1996; **81**(4): 1548–51.
19. Esapa CT, Harris PE. Mutation analysis of protein kinase A catalytic subunit in thyroid adenomas and pituitary tumours. *Eur J Endocrinol* 1999; **141**(4): 409–12.
20. Russo D, Arturi F, Schlumberger M et al. Activating mutations of the TSH receptor in differentiated thyroid carcinomas. *Oncogene* 1995; **11**(9): 1907–11.
21. Spambalg D, Sharifi N, Elisei R, Gross JL, Medeiros-Neto G, Fagin JA. Structural studies of the thyrotropin receptor and Gs alpha in human thyroid cancers: low prevalence of mutations predicts infrequent involvement in malignant transformation. *J Clin Endocrinol Metab* 1996; **81**(11): 3898–901.
22. Michiels FM, Caillou B, Talbot M et al. Oncogenic potential of guanine nucleotide stimulatory factor alpha subunit in thyroid glands of transgenic mice. *Proc Natl Acad Sci USA* 1994; **91**(22): 10488–92.
23. Hollingsworth DR, Mabry CC. Congenital Graves disease. Four familial cases with long-term follow-up and perspective. *Am J Dis Child* 1976; **130**(2): 148–55.
24. Duprez L, Parma J, Van Sande J et al. Germline mutations in the thyrotropin receptor gene cause non-autoimmune autosomal dominant hyperthyroidism. *Nature Genet* 1994; **7**(3): 396–401.
25. Tonacchera M, Agretti P, Rosellini V et al. Sporadic nonautoimmune congenital hyperthyroidism due to a strong activating mutation of the thyrotropin receptor gene. *Thyroid* 2000; **10**(10): 859–63.
26. de Roux N, Polak M, Couet J et al. A neomutation of the thyroid-stimulating hormone receptor in severe neonatal hyperthyroidism. *J Clin Endocrinol Metab* 1996; **81**(6): 2023–6.
27. Kopp P, van Sande J, Parma J et al. Brief report: congenital hyperthyroidism caused by a mutation in the thyrotropin-receptor gene. *N Engl J Med* 1995; **332**(3): 150–4.
28. Schwab KO, Sohlemann P, Gerlich M et al. Mutations of the TSH receptor as cause of congenital hyperthyroidism. *Exp Clin Endocrinol Diabetes* 1996; **104**(suppl 4): 124–8.
29. Stein SA, Oates EL, Hall CR et al. Identification of a point mutation in the thyrotropin receptor of the hyt/hyt hypothyroid mouse. *Mol Endocrinol* 1994; **8**(2): 129–38.
30. Codaccioni JL, Carayon P, Michel-Bechet M, Foucault F, Lefort G, Pierron H. Congenital hypothyroidism associated with thyrotropin unresponsiveness and thyroid cell membrane alterations. *J Clin Endocrinol Metab* 1980; **50**(5): 932–7.
31. Sunthornthepvarakul T, Gootschalk ME, Hayashi Y, Refetoff S. Resistance to thyrotropin caused by mutations in the thyrotropin-receptor gene. *N Engl J Med* 1995; **332**: 155–60.
32. de Roux N, Misrahi M, Brauner R et al. Four families with loss of function mutations of the thyrotropin receptor. *J Clin Endocrinol Metab* 1996; **81**(12): 4229–35.
33. Clifton-Bligh RJ, Gregory JW, Ludgate M et al. Two novel mutations in the thyrotropin (TSH) receptor gene in a child with resistance to TSH. *J Clin Endocrinol Metab* 1997; **82**: 1094–100.
34. Biebermann H, Schoneberg T, Krude H, Schultz G, Gudermann T, Gruters A. Mutations of the human thyrotropin receptor gene causing thyroid hypoplasia and persistent congenital hypothyroidism. *J Clin Endocrinol Metab* 1997; **82**(10): 3471–80.
35. Abramowicz MJ, Duprez L, Parma J, Vassart G, Heinrichs C. Familial congenital hypothyroidism due to inactivating mutation of the thyrotropin receptor causing profound hypoplasia of the thyroid gland. *J Clin Invest* 1997; **99**(12): 3018–24.
36. Gagne N, Parma J, Deal C, Vassart G, Van Vliet G. Apparent congenital athyreosis contrasting with normal plasma thyroglobulin levels and associated with inactivating mutations in the thyrotropin receptor gene: are athyreosis and ectopic thyroid distinct entities? *J Clin Endocrinol Metab* 1998; **83**(5): 1771–5.
37. Tiosano D, Pannain S, Vassart G et al. The hypothyroidism in an inbred kindred with congenital thyroid hormone and glucocorticoid deficiency is due to a mutation producing a truncated thyrotropin receptor. *Thyroid* 1999; **9**(9): 887–94.
38. Tonacchera M, Agretti P, Pinchera A et al. Congenital hypothyroidism with impaired thyroid response to thyrotropin (TSH) and absent circulating thyroglobulin: evidence for a new inactivating mutation of the TSH receptor gene. *J Clin Endocrinol Metab* 2000; **85**(3): 1001–8.
39. Xie J, Pannain S, Pohlenz J et al. Resistance to thyrotropin (TSH) in three families is not associated with mutations in the TSH receptor or TSH. *J Clin Endocrinol Metab* 1997; **82**(12): 3933–40.
40. Levine MA, Jap TS, Mauseth RS, Downs RW, Spiegel AM. Activity of the stimulatory guanine nucleotide-binding protein is reduced in erythrocytes from patients with pseudohypoparathyroidism and pseudopseudohypoparathyroidism: biochemical, endocrine, and genetic analysis of Albright's hereditary osteodystrophy in six kindreds. *J Clin Endocrinol Metab* 1986; **62**(3): 497–502.
41. Rodien P, Bremont C, Sanson ML et al. Familial gestational hyperthyroidism caused by a mutant thyrotropin receptor hypersensitive to human chorionic gonadotropin. *N Engl J Med* 1998; **339**(25): 1823–6.

REFERENCES

42. Refetoff S, De Wind LT, De Groot LJ. Familial syndrome combining deaf-mutism, stippled epiphyses, goiter and abnormally high PBI: possible target organ refractoriness to thyroid hormone. *J Clin Endocrinol Metab* 1967; 27: 279–94.
43. Refetoff S, Weiss RE, Usala SJ. The syndromes of resistance to thyroid hormone. *Endocrine Rev* 1993; 14: 348–99.
44. Gershengorn MC, Weintraub BD. Thyrotropin-induced hyperthyroidism caused by selective pituitary resistance to thyroid hormone. A new syndrome of inappropriate secretion of TSH. *J Clin Invest* 1975; 56: 633–42.
45. Brucker-Davis F, Skarulis MC, Grace MB et al. Genetic and clinical features of 42 kindreds with resistance to thyroid hormone. *Ann Intern Med* 1995; 123: 572–83.
46. Persani L, Asteria C, Tonacchera M, Vitti P, Chatterjee VKK, Beck Peccoz P. Evidence for the secretion of thyrotropin with enhanced bioactivity in syndromes of thyroid hormone resistance. *J Clin Endocrinol Metab* 1994; 78: 1034–9.
47. Hauser P, Zametkin AJ, Martinez P et al. Attention deficit-hyperactivity disorder in people with generalized resistance to thyroid hormone. *N Engl J Med* 1993; 328: 997–1001.
48. Brucker-Davis F, Skarulis MC, Pikus A et al. Prevalence and mechanisms of hearing loss in patients with resistance to thyroid hormone. *J Clin Endocrinol Metab* 1996; 81(8): 2768–72.
49. Usala SJ, Bale AE, Gesundheit N et al. Tight linkage between the syndrome of generalized thyroid hormone resistance and the human c-erbA β gene. *Mol Endocrinol* 1988; 2: 1217–20.
50. Adams M, Matthews CH, Collingwood TN et al. Genetic analysis of twenty-nine kindreds with generalised and pituitary resistance to thyroid hormone. *J Clin Invest* 1994; 94: 506–15.
51. Weiss RE, Xu J, Ning G, Pohlenz J, O'Malley BW, Refetoff S. Mice deficient in the steroid receptor coactivator 1 (SRC-1) are resistant to thyroid hormone. *EMBO J* 1999; 18(7): 1900–4.
52. Pohlenz J, Weiss RE, Macchia PE et al. Five new families with resistance to thyroid hormone not caused by mutations in the thyroid hormone receptor β gene. *J Clin Endocrinol Metab* 1999; 84(11): 3919–28.
53. Takeda K, Sakurai A, De Groot LJ, Refetoff S. Recessive inheritance of thyroid hormone resistance caused by complete deletion of the protein-coding region of the thyroid hormone receptor-β gene. *J Clin Endocrinol Metab* 1992; 74: 49–55.
54. Collingwood TN, Adams M, Tone Y, Chatterjee VKK. Spectrum of transcriptional dimerization and dominant negative properties of twenty different mutant thyroid hormone β receptors in thyroid hormone resistance syndrome. *Mol Endocrinol* 1994; 8: 1262–77.
55. Ono S, Schwartz ID, Mueller OT, Root AW, Usala SJ, Bercu BB. Homozygosity for a dominant negative thyroid hormone receptor gene responsible for generalized resistance to thyroid hormone. *J Clin Endocrinol Metab* 1991; 73(5): 990–4.
56. Hayashi Y, Weiss RE, Sarne DH et al. Do clinical manifestations of resistance to thyroid hormone correlate with the functional alteration of the corresponding mutant thyroid hormone β receptors? *J Clin Endocrinol Metab* 1995; 80: 3246–56.
57. Beck Peccoz P, Piscitelli G, Cattaneo MG, Faglia G. Successful treatment of hyperthyroidism due to non-neoplastic pituitary TSH hypersecretion with 3,5,3′-triiodothyroacetic acid (TRIAC). *J Endocrinol Invest* 1983; 6: 217–23.
58. Radetti G, Persani L, Molinaro G et al. Clinical and hormonal outcome after two years of TRIAC treatment in a child with thyroid hormone resistance. *Thyroid* 1997; 7(5): 775–8.
59. Ueda S, Takamatsu J, Fukata S et al. Differences in response of thyrotropin to 3,5,3′-triiodothyronine and 3,5,3′-triiodothyroacetic acid in patients with resistance to thyroid hormone. *Thyroid* 1996; 6: 563–70.
60. Hamon P, Bovier-LaPierre M, Robert M, Peynaud D, Pugeat M, Orgiazzi J. Hyperthyroidism due to selective pituitary resistance to thyroid hormones in 15-month-old boy: efficacy of D-thyroxine therapy. *J Clin Endocrinol Metab* 1988; 67: 1089–93.
61. Weiss RE, Stein MA, Refetoff S. Behavioral effects of liothyronine (L-T3) in children with attention deficit hyperactivity disorder in the presence and absence of resistance to thyroid hormone. *Thyroid* 1997; 7: 389–93.
62. Ye HF, O'Reilly KE, Koh JT. A subtype-selective thyromimetic designed to bind a mutant thyroid hormone receptor implicated in resistance to thyroid hormone. *J Am Chem Soc* 2001; 123(7): 1521–2.
63. Greenman Y, Melmed S. Thyrotropin-secreting pituitary tumors. In: Melmed S, ed. *The Pituitary*. Boston: Blackwell Science, 1995: 546.
64. Beck-Peccoz P, Brucker-Davis F, Persani L, Smallridge RC, Weintraub BD. Thyrotropin-secreting pituitary tumors. *Endocrine Rev* 1996; 17: 610–38.
65. Mindermann T, Wilson CB. Thyrotropin-producing pituitary adenomas. *J Neurosurg* 1993; 79(4): 521–7.
66. Beck-Peccoz P, Asteria C, Mannavola D. Resistance to thyroid hormone. In: Braverman LE, ed. *Contemporary Endocrinology: Diseases of the Thyroid*. Totowa, NJ: Humana Press, 1997; 199.
67. Cooper DS, Wenig BM. Hyperthyroidism caused by an ectopic TSH-secreting pituitary tumor. *Thyroid* 1996; 6(4): 337–43.
68. Mixson AJ, Friedman TC, Katz DA et al. Thyrotropin-secreting pituitary carcinoma. *J Clin Endocrinol Metab* 1993; 76(2): 529–33.
69. Bertholon-Gregoire M, Trouillas J, Guigard MP, Loras B, Tourniaire J. Mono- and plurihormonal thyrotropic pituitary adenomas: pathological, hormonal and clinical studies in 12 patients. *Eur J Endocrinol* 1999; 140(6): 519–27.

70. Terzolo M, Orlandi F, Bassetti M et al. Hyperthyroidism due to a pituitary adenoma composed of two different cell types, one secreting alpha-subunit alone and another cosecreting alpha-subunit and thyrotropin. *J Clin Endocrinol Metab* 1991; 72(2): 415–21.

71. Boggild MD, Jenkinson S, Pistorello M et al. Molecular genetic studies of sporadic pituitary tumors. *J Clin Endocrinol Metab* 1994; 78(2): 387–92.

72. Dong Q, Brucker-Davis F, Weintraub BD et al. Screening of candidate oncogenes in human thyrotroph tumors: absence of activating mutations of the G alpha q, G alpha 11, G alpha s, or thyrotropin-releasing hormone receptor genes. *J Clin Endocrinol Metab* 1996; 81(3): 1134–40.

73. Takano K, Ajima M, Teramoto A, Hata K, Yamashita N. Mechanisms of action of somatostatin on human TSH-secreting adenoma cells. *Am J Physiol* 1995; 268(4 Pt 1): E558–64.

74. Brucker-Davis F, Oldfield EH, Skarulis MC, Doppman JL, Weintraub BD. Thyrotropin-secreting pituitary tumors: diagnostic criteria, thyroid hormone sensitivity, and treatment outcome in 25 patients followed at the National Institutes of Health *J Clin Endocrinol Metab* 1999; 84(2): 476–86.

75. Losa M, Giovanelli M, Persani L, Mortini P, Faglia G, Beck-Peccoz P. Criteria of cure and follow-up of central hyperthyroidism due to thyrotropin-secreting pituitary adenomas. *J Clin Endocrinol Metab* 1996; 81(8): 3084–90.

76. Gasparoni P, Rubello D, Persani L, Beck-Peccoz P. Unusual association between a thyrotropin-secreting pituitary adenoma and a papillary thyroid carcinoma. *Thyroid* 1998; 8(2): 181–3.

77. Abs R, Stevenaert A, Beckers A. Autonomously functioning thyroid nodules in a patient with a thyrotropin-secreting pituitary adenoma: possible cause–effect relationship. *Eur J Endocrinol* 1994; 131(4): 355–8.

78. Beck-Peccoz P, Persani L. Variable biological activity of thyroid-stimulating hormone. *Eur J Endocrinol* 1994; 131(4): 331–40.

79. Magner J, Klibanski A, Fein H et al. Ricin and lentil lectin-affinity chromatography reveals oligosaccharide heterogeneity of thyrotropin secreted by 12 human pituitary tumors. *Metabolism* 1992; 41(9): 1009–15.

80. Beck-Peccoz P, Persani L, Faglia G. Glycoprotein hormone α-subunit in pituitary adenomas. *Trends Endocrinol Metab* 1992; 3: 41.

81. Beck Peccoz P, Roncoroni R, Mariotti S et al. Sex hormone-binding globulin measurement in patients with inappropriate secretion of thyrotropin (IST): evidence against selective pituitary thyroid hormone resistance in nonneoplastic IST. *J Clin Endocrinol Metab* 1990; 71: 19–25.

82. Persani L, Preziati D, Matthews CH, Sartorio A, Chatterjee VKK, Beck Peccoz P. Serum levels of carboxyterminal cross-linked telopeptide of type I collagen (ICTP) in the differential diagnosis of the syndromes of inappropriate secretion of TSH. *Clin Endocrinol* 1997; 47: 207–14.

83. Langlois MF, Lamarche JB, Bellabarba D. Long-standing goiter and hypothyroidism: an unusual presentation of a TSH-secreting adenoma. *Thyroid* 1996; 6(4): 329–35.

84. Losa M, Magnani P, Mortini P et al. Indium-111 pentetreotide single-photon emission tomography in patients with TSH-secreting pituitary adenomas: correlation with the effect of a single administration of octreotide on serum TSH levels. *Eur J Nuclear Med* 1997; 24(7): 728–31.

85. Watanabe K, Kameya T, Yamauchi A et al. Thyrotropin-producing microadenoma associated with pituitary resistance to thyroid hormone. *J Clin Endocrinol Metab* 1993; 76(4): 1025–30.

86. Safer JD, Colan SD, Fraser LM, Wondisford FE. A pituitary tumor in a patient with thyroid hormone resistance: a diagnostic dilemma. *Thyroid* 2001; 11(3): 281–91.

87. Chanson P, Weintraub BD, Harris AG. Octreotide therapy for thyroid-stimulating hormone-secreting pituitary adenomas. A follow-up of 52 patients. *Ann Intern Med* 1993; 119(3): 236–40.

88. Kuhn JM, Arlot S, Lefebvre H et al. Evaluation of the treatment of thyrotropin-secreting pituitary adenomas with a slow release formulation of the somatostatin analog lanreotide. *J Clin Endocrinol Metab* 2000; 85(4): 1487–91.

12

Multinodular goiter, toxic adenoma and thyroiditis
Arie Berghout, Alex F Muller

Non-toxic goiter is a visible or palpable benign enlargement of the thyroid gland in a euthyroid subject. A non-toxic goiter can consist of a single solitary nodule or of multiple nodules, and in the latter case it is called multinodular goiter.

Prevalence

The prevalence is high, as demonstrated in the Framingham study (6.4% in females and 1.5% in males) and the Whickham survey, UK (10% in females and 2% in men).[1,2] The prevalence is higher in iodine-deficient than in iodine-sufficient areas (rising to about 30%).[3,4] Furthermore, ultrasound and autopsy studies have revealed an even greater prevalence of thyroid nodules.[5]

Pathology

Most goiters consist of nodules, cysts, and areas of hemorrhage and calcification. Single nodules and adenomas, as well as most nodules in multinodular goiters, are monoclonal in origin. The early literature suggests that diffuse goiters precede nodular goiters and that thyroid-stimulating hormone (TSH) is involved in the earlier phases of growth.[6] Evidence for this hypothesis is lacking. Current opinion favors a continuous pathophysiological process operating on the background of the natural heterogeneity and polyclonality of human thyroid cells,[4,7,8] where, in addition to TSH and iodine, growth factors and goitrogens are also involved in the evolution of thyroid nodules. Thus a widely divergent picture emerges, with both mono- and polyclonal nodules within one goiter.

With the advances in molecular biology, attention has recently focused on genetic alterations that can explain thyroid growth. In autonomously functioning thyroid adenomas, activating mutations of the TSH receptor and Gs α genes have been demonstrated. Multinodular goiters are functionally and morphologically heterogeneous, and thus appear polyclonal.[9] However, most nodules are monoclonal in origin.[10,11] As the family history in patients with multinodular goiter is often positive, genetic research could be of clinical benefit in the future. Indeed, a germline polymorphism of codon 727 of the human TSH receptor was found to be associated with toxic multinodular goiter,[12] and a familial form of goiter has been found with a link to markers on chromosome 14q.[13,14] However, these findings are not universal, and other studies have failed to confirm the presence of these non-functional mutations. Furthermore, these mutations may be secondary phenomena and thus not etiologically related to adenoma or goiter formation.

Clinical presentation

In about 50% of patients, the goiter is detected by the patient, and in the remaining cases by relatives or a physician.[15] Seventy-one per cent of the patients have symptoms largely due to neck discomfort (61%), cosmetic complaints (19%) and dyspnea (17%). Fear of malignancy is expressed by 17% of patients,[15] which is probably an underestimate, as it represents only those patients volunteering their concerns.

Diagnosis

Diagnosis is primarily by inspection and palpation. The availability of ultrasonography has led to frequent coincidental detection of thyroid nodules and cysts.[5]

Although in most cases goiters are associated with an increased thyroid volume, this is not always the case, as single thyroid nodules may be visible and palpable in thyroid glands with normal volumes.[16]

The estimation of thyroid size by inspection and palpation is too inaccurate, and for this purpose should no longer be applied; instead, ultrasonography has become an indispensable tool for precise estimation of goiters or nodules.[15,17] In a research setting, thyroid volume should be measured ultrasonographically, and in cases of substernal extension—especially in cases of trachea compression—thyroid volume should be measured by MRI.[18] An iodine uptake scan can confirm the diagnosis of multinodular goiter, but is too inaccurate for measurement of thyroid volume.[18]

Most patients—and their physicians—wish to exclude thyroid carcinoma. The frequency of thyroid cancer is higher in solitary, rapidly growing nodules, in children, probably in males, and in subjects with a history of neck irradiation, particularly in childhood.[19,20] The prevalence of cancer in 'all' thyroid nodules is reported to be 5–6.5%,[20,21] but these figures include papillary microcarcinomas, whose malignant potential is low; the prevalence of cancer, including papillary microcarcinomas, rises to 10% in autopsy series.[22,23] In goiters removed at surgery, carcinoma is found in 5–15%.[24,25] Fortunately, the number of occult carcinomas far exceeds the number of clinically overt carcinomas. In general, the risk of clinically important carcinoma is considered to be small, and more aggressive therapy for non-toxic goiter is therefore not justified. Since the introduction of fine needle aspiration biopsy (FNA), the numbers of thyroidectomies for non-toxic goiter have declined dramatically.[26] FNA is now the first diagnostic procedure in the evaluation of solitary or dominant nodules.[27] The value of ultrasonography in differentiating between benign and malignant nodules has not been convincingly demonstrated. Scintigraphy adds little diagnostic value.[28] FNA cytology is a simple outpatient procedure. Although estimates of the specificity and sensitivity of this diagnostic test have not been performed (because this would require a consecutive prospective study, with FNA and histology to be performed in all cases), some studies report 'adequate samples' in 90–97% of all aspirations.[29–31] Ultrasound-guided aspirations are only slightly better than conventional aspirations.[32,33] The test result can be benign, suspicious, malignant or non-diagnostic. Surgery is indicated in cases of malignancy or suspicion of neoplasia. FNA cannot discriminate between follicular adenoma and follicular carcinoma, so all follicular neoplasms should be excised. FNA can yield diagnostic cytology for medullary thyroid carcinoma, thyroid lymphoma, anaplastic carcinoma and other rare malignancies or non-neoplastic conditions. In cases of a non-diagnostic FNA result, surgery should be considered.

Molecular markers are being increasingly studied in cytological samples from thyroid nodules, and the data are promising.[34] Thus, staining for galectin-3, a lectin-related molecule, and TPO may improve the differentiation between follicular adenomas and carcinomas.[35,36] Hopefully, these molecular methods will further increase the diagnostic accuracy of FNA and reduce unnecessary thyroidectomies.

Thyroid function

Thyroid function should preferably be measured by a single measurement of serum TSH by immunoradiometric assay, followed by free thyroxine (T4) and also triiodothyronine (T3).[15,37] The natural history of goiter is characterized by increases of volume at a rate of about 4% per year.[15] Concomitant with the increase in size, TSH values decline, and initially serum T3 levels rise, followed by T4 levels. In a study of 102 consecutive patients with multinodular goiter performed in the Amsterdam area several years ago, serum total T3 was higher but free T4 not different compared to 50 healthy adults.[15] This phenomenon is indicative of the evolution of 'autonomy' of thyroid function and eventual development of hyperthyroidism.[15] In a follow-up study of 64 patients with subclinical multinodular goiter, overt hyperthyroidism developed in 28%.[38] However, these studies were cross-sectional, and serum TSH was measured by radioimmunoassays. Thus, prospective, longitudinal studies with assessment of thyroid function by ultrasensitive TSH-IRMA and thyroid volume by ultrasound are urgently needed. Toxic multinodular goiter is often complicated by atrial fibrillation.[39] Furthermore, a recent study found increased cardiovascular mortality in elderly people with low serum thyrotropin.[40] In the last decade, several publications have focused on the cardiac effects of low serum TSH. One study found increased heart rate and left ventricular mass, and impaired diastolic function, in patients on T4 suppressive therapy ('subclinical thyrotoxicosis').[41] These findings, however, were not confirmed by others.[42] Very recently, abnormalities in heart rate and function, similar to patients with subclinical thyrotoxicosis due to T4 treatment, were also found in patients with 'endogenous' subclinical hyperthyroidism caused by a multinodular goiter or an autonomously functioning thyroid nodule.[43] In this study, the mean serum T4 and T3 values were elevated (suggesting an advanced state of subclinical hyperthyroidism) compared to patients with subclinical hyperthyroidism in whom only mean serum T3 was increased. These patients were selected on the basis of a low or suppressed serum TSH level.[43] However, in most patients with multinodular goiter, serum TSH levels often vary between the limit of detection of the assay and the lower end of the normal range, while serum T3 and T4 levels are within the normal range. The clinical significance of this minor suppression of serum TSH level is unknown.

In a recent controlled study of 26 patients with multinodular goiter, we were unable to confirm cardiac abnormalities described by others,[37] but serum cholesterol levels were significantly lower in patients with multinodular goiter (mean serum TSH of 0.6 mU/l) compared to controls (mean serum TSH 2.4 mU/l). Other metabolic parameters such as sex hormone-binding globulin (SHBG), ferritin or creatinine, which are influenced by thyroid hormones, were not altered. Similar changes in circulating lipids have been found in another study of subjects with subclinical hyperthyroidism.[44] In that study, free T4 was higher compared to controls, but still within normal limits.[44] In another study of 44 patients with clinically euthyroid goiter, plasma levels of bone gla protein and SHBG were found to be higher compared to controls in those patients with a low TSH.[45] A study of 27 consecutive patients with multinodular goiter reported elevated levels of serum osteocalcin which correlated with free T4 levels.[46] An important question is whether endogenous subclinical hyperthyroidism in patients with a goiter and subclinical thyrotoxicosis due to exogenous T4 therapy are two different entities. In both of these clinical situations, plasma TSH levels are low or suppressed. In endogenous subclinical hyperthyroidism, first total T3 and later both total T3 and free T4 become elevated—within the normal range—while in subclinical thyrotoxicosis due to T4 suppressive treatment, only free T4 is elevated.[41] In both situations, TSH is suppressed because the pituitary responds to plasma levels of T4, which enters the thyrotrophs and is locally converted to T3, as well as to T3 derived directly from the plasma pool.[47] In contrast, many tissues, such as the liver, appear to be sensitive mainly to the plasma T3 concentration. Furthermore, the activity and type of deiodinases and the expression of nuclear T3 receptor isoforms differ between pituitary and other organs such as liver and kidney.[48,49] The situation in the human heart is largely unknown. In neonatal rats, cardiac muscle takes up mostly T3 but not T4.[50] The conversion of T4 to T3 in human cardiac myocytes has thus far been demonstrated only indirectly by the presence of type II deiodinase mRNA.[51] In summary, the manifestation of cardiac and metabolic effects seems to depend upon the degree of increased thyroid function, which is a feature of the natural course of 'non-toxic' goiter. However, it is not known at present whether preventive or early treatment—by means of radioactive iodine—is effective.

Treatment

The following management options are available: no treatment, thyroid hormones, surgery and radioactive iodine. The aim of treatment is reduction of goiter size and prevention of toxic multinodular goiter. Given that the goiter is an incidental finding in the majority of cases, most experts would advise no treatment and some form of follow-up and monitoring. Thyroid hormone suppressive therapy has been advocated in the past and has been widely applied, based on the theoretical consideration that TSH is involved in the pathogenesis of goiter formation. Although this assumption may be partially true, the pathogenesis is far more complicated (as outlined above), and TSH suppression does not necessarily lead to goiter reduction. In a double-blind randomized trial comparing L-thyroxine and placebo in patients with non-toxic multinodular goiter, a mean reduction of goiter size (measured by ultrasonography)

Causes of hyperthyroidism
    Graves' disease
    Toxic multinodular goiter
    Toxic adenoma
    Gestational hyperthyroidism
    Trophoblastic disorders
    TSH-producing pituitary adenoma
    Iodine- or drug-induced hyperthyroidism

Causes of thyrotoxicosis
    L-thyroxine therapy
    Subacute thyroiditis
    Postpartum thyroiditis

Table 12.1
Causes of hyperthyroidism and thyrotoxicosis.

of 25% was observed in about 60% of the patients. However, thyroid volume rose to baseline after discontinuation of thyroxine therapy.[52] From the patients' perspective, this result is disappointing; the reduction in goiter size is not clinically significant, and necessitates lifelong medical treatment with a dubious and potentially harmful outcome, as adverse effects on the heart have been reported in patients on long-term T4 suppressive therapy.[39,41] Interestingly, similar results have been reported from non-randomized trials.[53] The data from randomized trials on the effects of suppressive thyroid hormone therapy of solitary benign nodules are contradictory.[54–56] The same concerns about medical therapy as discussed for multinodular goiters apply for solitary nodules, and this practice is not recommended.

Surgery is appropriate when patients express a preference and in cases of suspicious or non-diagnostic findings at FNA.

Radioiodine therapy has emerged in recent years as the most attractive treatment modality for non-toxic multinodular goiter. It has been applied mostly in elderly patients with large, obstructive goiters and in whom surgery was considered a less desirable option. The efficacy of this treatment as evaluated by MRI is excellent.[57,58] Both obstructive symptoms and thyroid volume decrease significantly in nearly all patients. Most patients are treated with doses of 3–15 MBq/g thyroid tissue.[59] Possibly, the efficacy of such treatment is enhanced by the use of recombinant hTSH, although clinicians must be aware of the risk of inducing transient hyperthyroidism following injection of this drug.[60] However, a caveat of radioactive iodine therapy is the rare occurrence of a Graves'-like hyperthyroidism, a severe form of thyrotoxicosis induced by TSH receptor autoantibodies.[61] The onset of this form of hyperthyroidism is insidious and can occur even months after therapy. As radioactive iodine is given notably to elderly patients who are susceptible to cardiac rhythm disturbances, physicians should be well aware of this dangerous complication and adopt an appropriate follow-up strategy.

Toxic adenoma and toxic multinodular goiter

Toxic adenomas are single hyperfunctioning thyroid nodules in patients with hyperthyroidism; the function of the remainder of the thyroid gland is suppressed. Toxic adenomas are pathogenetically different from multinodular goiters, with a dominant, i.e. hyperfunctioning, single nodule. Unlike toxic adenomas, toxic multinodular goiters represent the end stage of longstanding multinodular goiters. The diagnosis of toxic adenoma is made in a patient with a single palpable nodule and characteristic scintigraphic features. Scintigraphy reveals uptake of iodine in the nodule, with no, or reduced, uptake in the remaining thyroid. Patients are usually older and female, and the nodule is often more than 3 cm in diameter. About 10–20% of all patients with solitary nodules present with hyperthyroidism. As with toxic multinodular goiter, the hyperthyroidism associated with toxic adenomas is preceded by a phase of subclinical hyperthyroidism (see above).

Pathogenesis

In selected cases of toxic adenoma and in some families with toxic multinodular goiter, gain-of-function somatic mutations of the TSH receptor, and mutations in the genes coding for G proteins, have been demonstrated.[62–64]

Treatment

The preferred treatment of toxic adenoma is radioactive iodine: there is virtually no long-lasting remission of hyperthyroidism after treatment with thionamides. The same holds true for toxic multinodular goiter. In addition to treating the hyperthyroid state, radioiodine also reduces the size of adenoma or goiter: this can take some time, however, and repeated doses are often necessary.[65] Treatment with radioactive iodine can be given de novo with beta-blocker cover if necessary, or after pretreatment with thionamides. The relative merits of these approaches have not been evaluated. In patients with Graves' disease, recent studies have indicated that pretreatment with thionamides or the prescription of thionamides after treatment with radioactive iodine is not better or even worse in terms of outcome of treatment.[66] Moreover, elevation of TSH levels due to pretreatment with thionamides could induce hypothyroidism via enhanced uptake of radioiodine in the surrounding tissue. Generally, the risk of hypothyroidism seems to be low, although long-term follow-up is warranted.[67] Interestingly, the old belief that radioactive iodine could aggravate the symptoms of hyperthyroidism in unprepared patients (with Graves' disease) has turned out not to be true.[66,68] However, this has not been studied in patients with toxic adenoma or toxic multinodular goiter.

Other disorders that cause thyrotoxicosis

The first trimester of a normal pregnancy is associated with a decline in serum TSH levels, while serum free T4 levels remain unchanged.[69] This phenomenon is explained by the thyroid-stimulating effect of human chorionic gonadotropin (hCG), which peaks in the first weeks of pregnancy.[70,71] If hCG rises above physiological levels, clinical hyperthyroidism can ensue.[70] Interestingly, this is observed in hyperemesis gravidarum and molar pregnancy.[72,73] The severity of vomiting correlates with serum free T4 and hCG concentrations.[74] hCG stimulates the thyroid via binding of beta-hCG to the TSH receptor. The affinity of binding is influenced by the degree of sialylation of hCG.[75] In cases of molar pregnancy, hCG levels are particularly high (often 10 000–30 000 IU/l), and therefore hyperthyroidism is frequent.[76] Although very rare, hyperthyroidism has been observed in patients with testicular carcinoma.[77,78]

Hyperthyroidism due to metastatic differentiated thyroid carcinoma is extremely rare.[79] Hyperthyroidism due to TSH-producing adenomas is discussed elsewhere in this book.

Thyroiditis

The hallmark of thyroiditis is thyroid inflammation. Thyroid inflammation can be due to different causes: physical factors (palpation, radiation), microorganisms and autoimmunity. In this section, we will focus on subacute granulomatous thyroiditis, subacute lymphocytic thyroiditis and postpartum thyroiditis. Riedel's thyroiditis and infectious thyroiditis will be discussed only briefly.

Hashimoto's disease and Graves' disease are discussed extensively elsewhere in this book, and will thus not be covered here.

Subacute granulomatous thyroiditis

This form of thyroiditis is known by several names: subacute (Quervain's) thyroiditis,[80] subacute non-suppurative thyroiditis, pseudotuberculous thyroiditis, giant cell thyroiditis, pseudo-giant cell thyroiditis, or struma granulomatosa.

Epidemiology

The incidence of subacute granulomatous thyroiditis is reported to be one-fifth to one-eighth of the incidence of Graves' disease.[81,82] Assuming that the incidence of Graves' disease for women in iodine-replete areas is 0.8/1000 per year, we estimate the incidence of subacute granulomatous thyroiditis in women to be approximately 0.1/1000 per year.[2,83] Of 151 094 patients who were treated for thyroid disease between 1970 and 1993 at a large Japanese thyroid referral center (Ito Hospital, Saitama, Japan), 2.2% had subacute granulomatous thyroiditis. Unfortunately, the incidence of Graves' disease was not quoted in this population.[84]

Subacute granulomatous thyroiditis develops most frequently between the third and sixth decades, with a mean age of 44 years.[84–86] The male/female ratio is reported to be in the range of 1 to 3–9.7;[87,88] this large variation is thus far unexplained.

Given the presumed viral etiology (see below), it is not surprising that in the majority of patients the disease is diagnosed in the summer season.[84,86] Also, some disease clusters have been reported and are described below.[89–92]

Etiology

Several studies have investigated the etiology of subacute granulomatous thyroiditis. These studies support the notion that subacute granulomatous thyroiditis is caused by a viral infection or a postviral inflammatory process. Many authors maintain—albeit without citing supportive data—that subacute granulomatous thyroiditis is frequently preceded by an upper respiratory infection, and often has a viral prodromal phase characterized by fatigue, malaise, muscle pains and fever without leukocytosis. A self-limiting course within weeks or months is the rule.[85,87,93]

Indirect evidence from case series for a viral origin has also emerged from studies in which viral antibodies were measured in cases of subacute granulomatous thyroiditis. Eylan et al reported 11 cases of subacute granulomatous thyroiditis occurring during a mumps epidemic. Circulating antibodies to mumps virus were found in each case; moreover, mumps virus was grown from thyroid specimens obtained in two cases.[91] Subsequently, others have also reported an association between mumps virus infections and subacute granulomatous thyroiditis.[87,93] In several other studies, subacute granulomatous thyroiditis was associated with the presence of antibodies to several other viral pathogens (for review see Volpe et al[93]). An epidemic of subacute granulomatous thyroiditis involving 23 persons was described in The Netherlands, but no etiological pathogen could be identified.[89]

In the course of subacute granulomatous thyroiditis, autoimmune phenomena have also been described. Approximately 50% of patients with subacute granulomatous thyroiditis have thyroid autoantibodies; however, they are generally transient and their titer is low.[85] Moreover, circulating and intrathyroidal antigen-binding T cells are also observed in subacute granulomatous thyroiditis.[87,94–97] As these phenomena are transient, they are unlikely to be the primary disruptive events in the pathogenesis of subacute granulomatous thyroiditis.

Genetic associations have also been described in subacute granulomatous thyroiditis. Most important are the genes of the major histocompatibility complex (MHC) region located on the short arm of chromosome 6. MHC comprises the antigen-presenting molecules located on the cell membranes of antigen-presenting cells. HLA-B35 and HLA-B67 have been reported to be strongly associated with subacute granulomatous thyroiditis.[98–102] Interestingly, Oshako et al found that patients with the HLA-B67 phenotype more often became euthyroid after transient thyrotoxicosis followed by hypothyroidism than patients with the HLA-B35 phenotype.[101] Moreover, in patients with the HLA-B35 phenotype, the onset of thyroiditis was distributed evenly throughout the year, whereas in the patients with the HLA-B67 haplotype, there was a seasonal variation, with onset mainly during the summer and autumn.[101]

Collectively, the above evidence supports a viral etiology—either direct or indirect—for subacute granulomatous thyroiditis, and is consistent with subacute granulomatous thyroiditis being the result of a 'final common pathway' occurring after a viral infection in genetically susceptible individuals.

Clinical course

Biochemically, subacute granulomatous thyroiditis is characterized by a transient thyrotoxic phase occurring in about 75% of cases,[84,85,103] during which symptoms are usually mild compared with Graves' disease.[104] Nevertheless, thyrotoxic symptoms such as heat intolerance, palpitations, nervousness and increased sweating can occur.[89] The thyrotoxic phase of subacute granulomatous thyroiditis is due to leakage of thyroid hormones from destroyed thyrocytes, and is therefore self-limiting, usually lasting 2–10 weeks.[85,89] In a minority of cases, the thyrotoxic phase is followed by a transient hypothyroid phase.[85,93]

Subsequent permanent hypothyroidism seems to be a rare event. Nikolai et al could find no cases of hypothyroidism in their 1–15 years of follow-up of 124 patients who had suffered an episode of subacute granulomatous thyroiditis. Thyrotropin-releasing hormone (TRH) testing was done in a subgroup of 20 patients, 6 of whom had exaggerated peak TSH values, implying impaired thyroid reserve.[103] Although considered to be a rare event, permanent hypothyroidism has been described after an episode of subacute granulomatous thyroiditis.[85,93,105]

Is recovery possible? The question of recurrence of subacute granulomatous thyroiditis after complete recovery has been specifically addressed by Iitaka et al. These authors surveyed their database of 3344 patients who experienced an episode of subacute granulomatous thyroiditis between 1970 and 1993. They concluded that late recurrences arise in at least 2% of cases. The mean latency period ($\pm$SD) between the first and second episodes of subacute granulomatous thyroiditis was 14.5 ± 4.5 years.[84]

Diagnosis, treatment and follow-up

The diagnosis of subacute granulomatous thyroiditis is fairly straightforward and is primarily clinical. The most prominent symptom of subacute granulomatous thyroiditis is pain in the region of the thyroid,[85,87] frequently described as a sore throat.[104] Indeed, most authors consider it a condition sine qua non for the diagnosis to be made.[84,101] Frequently, the pain radiates to the jaw and ear.[85] Other reported symptoms are: malaise, fatigue, myalgia and arthralgia.[85,93] Physical signs include fever and a small to medium-sized diffuse goiter that is nearly always painful on palpation.[85,93] Further diagnostic confirmation can be obtained by finding a raised erythrocyte sedimentation rate, above 40 mm/h in 97% of patients,[84] and a reduced or absent iodine uptake (usually <2%).[84,85] Other reported findings are mild anemia and a leukocytosis.[85]

With respect to late recurrences, it should be noted that although the biochemical severity of thyrotoxicosis is similar to that of the previous event(s), the erythrocyte sedimentation rate (ESR) is lower and RAIU higher, indicating a less severe inflammatory response.[84]

The differential diagnosis of pain in the thyroid region comprises primarily acute pharyngitis and, within the spectrum of thyroid disorders, acute infectious thyroiditis and hemorrhage into a pre-existing thyroid nodule or cyst. As the treatments for these disorders differ considerably, it is of paramount importance to establish a precise diagnosis. Symptoms can be localized to the thyroid by finding a painful goiter. Thyroid function testing should be performed, as thyrotoxicosis is the rule in subacute granulomatous thyroiditis, whereas acute infectious thyroiditis and hemorrhage into a pre-existent thyroid nodule do not present with thyroid dysfunction. Moreover, acute infectious thyroiditis—but not hemorrhage into a pre-existent thyroid nodule—is generally accompanied by more prominent systemic manifestations, including a markedly elevated ESR, than subacute granulomatous thyroiditis. In cases of doubt, a needle aspiration of the thyroid—with or without ultrasound guidance—can be of diagnostic value.

Measurement of radioactive iodine uptake will confirm the destructive nature of the thyrotoxicosis, but is usually not indicated. In exceptional cases where the cervical pain is not a prominent feature and Graves' disease is being considered as a plausible diagnosis, thyroid scintigraphy is valuable in distinguishing between these conditions.

The treatment of subacute granulomatous thyroiditis consists of relief of pain and thyrotoxic symptoms. Treatment is not indicated in asymptomatic cases of subacute granulomatous thyroiditis. Moreover, we are unaware of studies showing that permanent hypothyroidism after subacute granulomatous thyroiditis can be prevented by treatment of subacute granulomatous thyroiditis. If treatment is considered, non-steroidal anti-inflammatory drugs or corticosteroids are the drugs of choice.[84,85,106] Our strategy is to start with a non-steroidal anti-inflammatory drug (e.g. aspirin 600 mg 3–6 times daily), and if it yields insufficient pain relief within 3 days, to switch to corticosteroids.[84,107] A typical dose regimen consists of a starting dose of prednisone 40 mg/day (as a single dose), which should lead to a significant reduction in pain within 48 h. We advocate a dose reduction to 30 mg after 4 days, followed by a dose reduction of 5 mg each week, and a total course of treatment of about 7 weeks. With respect to thyrotoxicosis, 4–6 weeks of treatment with a beta-blocker (e.g. 40–120 mg propranolol or 25–50 mg atenolol daily) is usually beneficial in symptomatic cases. Antithyroid drug therapy is ineffective and should not be given, because there is no increased thyroid hormone synthesis. After weeks to months, the thyroid dysfunction resolves.

It is our opinion that symptomatic hypothyroidism should always be treated with L-thyroxine replacement therapy. We give full replacement, and stop thyroxine after 2 months to see whether remission has occurred.

Regarding follow-up, permanent hypothyroidism is the most important sequel of subacute granulomatous thyroiditis. Permanent hypothyroidism develops in less than 10% of patients immediately after an episode of subacute granulomatous thyroiditis. We are unaware of the development of hypothyroidism after a previous recovery from an episode of subacute granulomatous thyroiditis, and therefore long-term follow-up of patients whose biochemical status has been restored seems unnecessary.

Lymphocytic thyroiditis: subacute lymphocytic thyroiditis and postpartum thyroiditis

We suggest that subacute lymphocytic thyroiditis and postpartum thyroiditis should be considered as the same disease, and variants of chronic autoimmune (Hashimoto's) thyroiditis. If subacute lymphocytic thyroiditis manifests itself in the first year after delivery, the term postpartum thyroiditis is more appropriate. To complicate matters, subacute lymphocytic thyroiditis has several synonyms: 'silent thyroiditis', 'hyperthyroiditis', 'atypical thyroiditis' and 'lymphocytic thyroiditis with spontaneously resolving hyperthyroidism'.

Epidemiology

The prevalence of subacute lymphocytic thyroiditis varies widely. In various studies, subacute lymphocytic thyroiditis accounts for 0–23% of all cases of thyrotoxicosis.[108–113] Because of the close temporal association with parturition—which facilitates prospective studies—more data are available on the epidemiology of postpartum thyroiditis than for other variants. The reported prevalence of postpartum thyroiditis varies widely, from 1.1% to 21.1% (Table 12.2).[114] A critical appraisal of the available literature concluded that the prevalence of postpartum thyroiditis in iodine-sufficient areas ranges between 5% and 7%.[114]

Subacute lymphocytic thyroiditis can occur at virtually any age. It has been described in 5–93-year-olds.[85,108] There is a slight female predominance, with a female/male ratio of 3:2 to 2:1.[85]

Post-partum thyroid dysfunction (PPTD) occurs more frequently in patients with type I diabetes mellitus. The incidence of PPTD in patients with type I diabetes mellitus is at least 15%.[114–116]

Table 12.2
Epidemiological data on postpartum thyroiditis. Reproduced with permission. © The Endocrine Society. Muller AF, Drexhage HA, Berghout A. Endocrine Rev 2001; 22: 605–30.

Reference	Year	Country	No. in source population	Inclusion criteria	No. included	Time of inclusion and last fu	No. of source population included (%)/last fu (%)	Prevalence of TD (n)
Amino[12]	1982	Japan	507 consecutive F who delivered	TD, Tab+ or G	63	3 month pp/6 month pp	63 (12)/63 (12)	5.5% (28/507)
Jansson[24]	1984	Sweden	644 consecutive F who delivered	Informed consent	460	2 month pp/5 month pp	460 (71)/460 (71)	6.5% (30/460)
Freeman[20]	1986	USA	216 F at routine pp visits	Informed consent	212	4–8 weeks pp/8–12 weeks pp	212 (98)/44 (21)	1.9% (4/212)
Lervang[27]	1987	Denmark	694 F who delivered	Informed consent	591	3 month pp/12 month pp	591 (85)/23 (4)	3.9% (23/591)
Nicolai[29]	1987	USA	238 F who delivered	Informed consent	238	Delivery/3 month pp	238 (100)/154 (65)	6.7% (16/238)
Hayslip[23]	1988	USA	1034 F who delivered	Tab+	63	2nd day pp/6 month pp	63 (6)/51 (5)	3.3% (34/1034)
Vargas[35]	1988	USA	261 F completing 1 year fu	Informed consent	261	Delivery/12 month pp	261 (100)/261 (100)	21.1% (55/261)
Fung[21]	1988	UK	901 F attending an antenatal clinic	Tab+ (Tab-co's)	100 (132)	1st trimester/pp	220 (24)/82 (9)	16.7% (49/220)[a]
Rajatanavin[31]	1990	Thailand	812 F who delivered	Tab+	812	6 weeks pp/12 month pp	812 (100)/67 (8)	1.1% (9/812)
Rasmussen[32]	1990	Denmark	1163 F in the 1st trimester	Tab+ (Tab-co's)	36 (20)	1st trimester/12 month pp	56 (5)/56 (5)	3.3%,9 (33% of 10% Tab)
Roti[33]	1991	Italy	372 F who delivered	Informed consent	219	1 month pp/12 month pp	219 (59)/42 (11)	8.7% (19/219)
Walfish[36]	1992	Canada	1376 F who delivered	Informed consent	1376	Delivery/12 month pp	1376 (100)/300 (22)	5.9% (81/1376)
Stagnaro-Green[34]	1992	USA	552 F in the 1st trimester	Tab+ (Tab-co's)	38 (32)	1st trimester/6 month pp	60 (11)/60 (11)	8.8%[a,b]
Harris[22]	1992	UK	1248 F attending an antenatal clinic	Tab+ (Tab-co's)	145 (229)	2nd trimester/8 month pp	374 (30)/374 (30)	5.0% (62/1248)[a,c]
Pop[30]	1993	Netherlands	382 pregnant F	Informed consent	303	3rd trimester/8 month pp	303 (79)/293 (77)	7.2% (21/293)
Kuijpens[26]	1998	Netherlands	448 pregnant F	Informed consent	310	1st trimester/9 month pp	310 (69)/291 (65)	5.2% (15/291)
Kent[25]	1999	Australia	1816 F who delivered	Informed consent	748	6 month pp/6 month pp	748 (41)/748 (41)	10.3% (76/739)
Lucas[28]	2000	Spain	757 pregnant F	Informed consent	605	Delivery/12 month pp	605 (80)/444 (59)	7.4% (45/605)
Barca[37]	2000	Brazil	830 pregnant F with no TD, no G/C/N, Tab–	Informed consent	800	1st trimester/12 month pp	800 (96)/335 (40)	14.6% (49/335)
Sakaihara[38]	2000	Japan	4072 pregnant F in a screening program	–	4072	1st trimester/3 month pp	1161/4072	6.5% (76/1161)

fu, follow up; Tab, thyroid antibodies; TD, thyroid dysfunction; TF, thyroid function; F, females; pp, postpartum; G/C/N, goiter, cysts or nodules.
[a]Estimated prevalence.
[b]33% of 18% Tab+ and 3% of 82% Tab–.
[c]43% of 12% Tab+ and 0% of 78% Tab–.

Etiology

Subacute lymphocytic thyroiditis and postpartum thyroiditis should—in our view—be conceptualized as acute phases of autoimmune thyroid destruction in the context of an existing and ongoing process of thyroid autosensitization (Figure 12.1). The following arguments support this view: (1) a strong relationship between the presence of thyroid autoantibodies and subacute lymphocytic thyroiditis and postpartum thyroiditis;[108,114,117] (2) the histology of subacute lymphocytic thyroiditis and postpartum thyroiditis (both focal organized and diffuse destructive lymphocytic thyroiditis with folliculolysis and disruption);[114,118,119] (3) the presence of circulating activated T cells in patients with subacute lymphocytic thyroiditis and postpartum thyroiditis;[114,119] (4) the association between specific MHC haplotypes and risk of subacute lymphocytic thyroiditis and postpartum thyroiditis;[85,114] and (5) the fact that subacute lymphocytic thyroiditis and postpartum thyroiditis frequently lead to permanent autoimmune thyroid failure.[103,114]

At present, the initiating event in silent thyroiditis and postpartum thyroiditis remains unknown. Immunotherapy with interferon-α and interleukin-2 can induce thyroid autoantibodies and a clinical picture similar to that of lymphocytic thyroiditis.[120–123] In postpartum thyroiditis, it is clear that, following the profound pregnancy-associated immunomodulation, there is a rebound effect leading to aggravation of thyroid autoimmunity during the puerperal period, which plays an important role in the pathogenesis of this condition.[114] These observations indicate that a sudden change in 'immunohomeostasis' plays an important role in the initiation of the disorder.

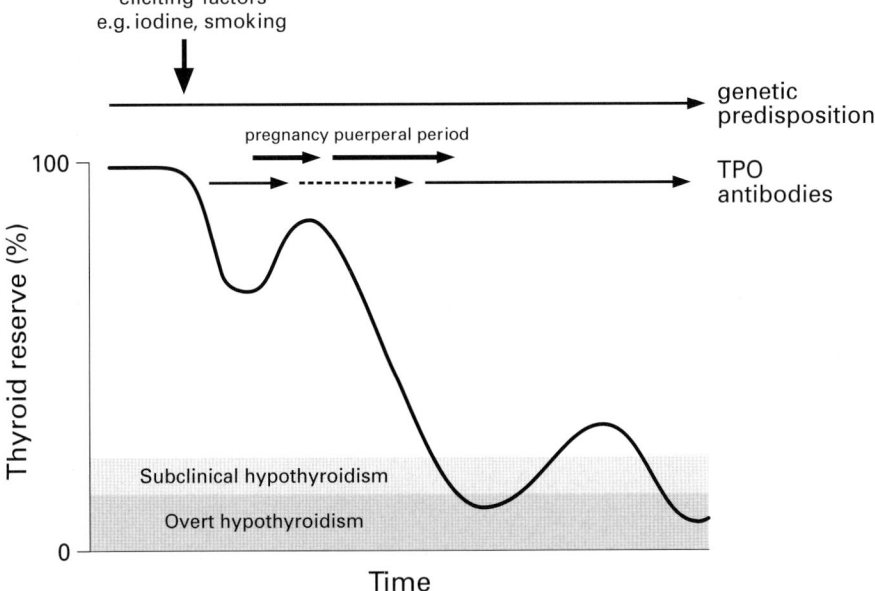

Figure 12.1
*A scheme depicting the gradual loss of thyroid reserve over time (often years) due to thyroid autoimmune mechanisms. On the basis of a genetic predisposition for endocrine and thyroid autoreactivity, an insult on the level of the thyroid (leading to the attraction of antigen-presenting cells (APCs)), and various other eliciting factors (e.g. smoking), a thyroid autoimmune reaction is initiated. Thyroid antibodies (e.g. TPO antibodies) are markers of the ongoing thyroid autosensitization process. Pregnancy—in the case of postpartum thyroiditis—ameliorates the process, while the puerperal period aggravates thyroid autoimmunity. If thyroid reserve was already considerably compromised before pregnancy, or if the transient autoimmune attack in the puerperal period is severe enough, subclinical hypothyroidism and even overt hypothyroidism will develop.
Reproduced with permission. © The Endocrine Society. Muller AF, Drexhage HA, Berghout A. Endocrine Rev 2001; 22: 605–30.*

Iodine has been implicated in several ways. Most important is iodine excess in autoimmune-prone individuals.[124–126] Following the introduction of iodine supplementation to a population, a rise in thyroid autoantibodies and a higher incidence of lymphocytic thyroiditis has been observed.[127–131] In goitrous NOD mice, OS chickens and BB-DP rats, a high iodine intake induces a rise in the titer of thyroid autoantibodies and an outburst or acceleration of lymphocytic thyroiditis.[132–134] Several potential pathogenic mechanisms have been proposed to explain iodine-induced thyroid autoimmunity.

Besides iodine, other environmental factors such as toxins and cigarette smoking have also been implicated as pathogenic factors in the development of thyroid autoimmunity.[114]

In subacute lymphocytic thyroiditis and postpartum thyroiditis, the rapid destruction of thyroid follicles is most frequently followed by a recovery of thyroid function. It is at present largely unclear how the immune system generally regains equilibrium after activation. The same applies to the recovery phase after subacute lymphocytic thyroiditis and postpartum thyroiditis. The observation that apoptosis of T cells can be induced by exposure to large amounts of antigen is very interesting in this respect. The transient nature of subacute lymphocytic thyroiditis and postpartum thyroiditis might thus be due to the induction of clonal apoptosis of thyroid-specific T cells that may follow the release of thyroid antigens into the circulation when many thyrocytes lose their integrity.[114,135] In postpartum thyroiditis, the development of immunotolerance to microchimeric cells (which enter the maternal circulation during pregnancy and delivery)[136,137] and a possible immunomodulatory role of prolactin are alternative ways in which the immune system might regain equilibrium.[135,138–142]

Clinical course

Subacute lymphocytic thyroiditis and postpartum thyroiditis classically run a biphasic course: a thyrotoxic phase is followed by a hypothyroid phase. The disease can also present as either transient thyrotoxicosis or hypothyroidism. The duration of thyrotoxicosis is variable, and can be 1–2 months. The onset of thyrotoxicosis in postpartum thyroiditis is variable, ranging from the first to the sixth month postpartum. During the thyrotoxic phase, the physical symptoms are usually mild compared to Graves' thyrotoxicosis and toxic multinodular goiter. The thyrotoxic phase is due to leakage of thyroid hormones from destroyed thyrocytes and is therefore self-limiting.[85,114,117]

In order to delineate the prevalence of permanent hypothyroidism after an episode of subacute lymphocytic thyroiditis, Nikolai et al assessed thyroid function 1–15 years after an initial disease period in 54 patients. Three patients (6%) became hypothyroid.[103] In a recent review, we reported that permanent hypothyroidism ensues in 12–61% of patients after an initial episode of postpartum thyroiditis.[114] The wide variation in the prevalence of hypothyroidism—both between subacute lymphocytic thyroiditis and postpartum thyroiditis as well as 'within' postpartum thyroiditis—is currently unexplained. We have already pointed out the scarcity of long-term data with regard to subacute lymphocytic thyroiditis. Moreover, genetic and environmental factors also play a role (see above).

Diagnosis, treatment and follow-up

It is our experience that the thyrotoxic phase of subacute lymphocytic thyroiditis and postpartum thyroiditis are frequently misdiagnosed as Graves' disease. Because management and follow-up of subacute lymphocytic thyroiditis and postpartum destructive thyrotoxicosis and Graves' disease differ, it is important to establish an accurate diagnosis. Clinical features have been discussed in the previous section, but it is important to note that symptoms and the presence of a goiter are not helpful in differentiating subacute lymphocytic thyroiditis and postpartum destructive thyrotoxicosis from Graves' disease. The presence of ophthalmopathy, however, points to a diagnosis of Graves' disease.[143] Diagnosis is further based on the presence of TSH-R antibodies—denoting Graves' disease—and thyroid scintigraphy, with an elevated uptake in Graves' disease and a suppressed uptake in cases of lymphocytic thyroiditis.[143]

It is important to be aware that thyrotoxicosis in patients with a previous history of Graves' disease does not necessarily represent relapse: postpartum thyroiditis can be superimposed on Graves' disease. Momotani et al systematically followed 96 episodes of postpartum thyrotoxicosis in the first year after delivery in women with a history of Graves' disease: in 26 cases, radioiodine uptake was low (<10%) during the thyrotoxic phase, indicating destructive postpartum thyroiditis.[144] Indeed, the diagnosis of postpartum destructive thyrotoxicosis (i.e. postpartum thyroiditis) is best established by the presence of a low radioiodine uptake. Thyroid scintigraphy should therefore be part of the diagnostic work-up. During breastfeeding, however, the administration of iodine-131 is contraindicated. When iodine-123 is used, breastfeeding should be stopped for 3 days.[145,146] By using technetium (^{99m}Tc) pertechnetate, interruption of breastfeeding for only 24 h is required.[145,147]

Serum thyroglobulin (Tg) has been proposed as useful in the differential diagnosis of postpartum thyroiditis.[148] However, as serum Tg concentrations are also elevated in nearly all patients with Graves' disease, it follows that the determination of the serum Tg concentration is not helpful in differentiating lymphocytic destructive thyrotoxicosis from Graves' disease.[149] With respect to treatment, it is important to keep in mind that the thyrotoxicosis is destruction-induced and therefore self-limiting. Thus, antithyroid drug therapy should not be given. In symptomatic cases, a short course of beta-blockade may be beneficial, e.g. 40–120 mg propranolol or 25–50 mg atenolol daily, until serum free T4 concentrations are normal. In cases of hypothyroidism, we strongly advise treatment with L-thyroxine replacement therapy. Spontaneous recovery of thyroid function should not be awaited. Instead, it is reasonable to stop thyroxine after 2–6 months to see whether remission has occurred. If so, we advise discontinuation of treatment followed by yearly assessment of thyroid function.

The prevalence of permanent—clinically overt—hypothyroidism after an episode of lymphocytic thyroiditis (i.e. after a transient exacerbation of a pre-existing and ongoing process of autoimmune thyroiditis) is sufficiently high (see above) to warrant yearly determination of TSH levels. Moreover, mild thyroid failure—e.g. due to lymphocytic thyroiditis—is increasingly recognized as a serious health problem, particularly in women of childbearing age.[114] Existing thyroid autoimmunity increases the probability of spontaneous fetal loss.[114] In addition, there are indications that maternal thyroid failure due to autoimmune thyroiditis during pregnancy—often mild and subclinical—leads to permanent and significant impairment in neuropsychological performance of the offspring.[114] Finally, there is now emerging evidence that, as women age, subclinical hypothyroidism—e.g. as a sequel of lymphocytic thyroiditis—predisposes them to cardiovascular disease.[114]

Riedel's thyroiditis

Riedel's thyroiditis is also known as Riedel's struma, fibrous thyroiditis or invasive thyroiditis.[150]

It is a rare disorder affecting predominantly middle-aged women.[151] Less than 200 cases have been reported.[151–153]

What causes the disease is unknown. As it is sometimes associated with fibrosis in other areas (retroperitoneum, mediastinum, orbitae) and organs (lung, heart, bile ducts, parotid and lacrimal glands) it is considered a rare manifestation of systemic collagenosis.[154] Indeed, on histology, the thyroid gland is densely infiltrated with connective tissue, with inflammatory cells, especially lymphocytes, eosinophils and plasma cells, present.[154,155]

The clinical hallmark is an unusually hard thyroid gland that is often diffusely enlarged and attached to adjacent skeletal muscles, nerves, blood vessels and trachea.[151] Other symptoms include anterior neck pain, dysphagia, tracheal compression with dyspnea and hoarseness.[152] As thyroid infiltration progresses, hypothyroidism is reported to occur in 30–40% of cases.[156] In exceptional cases, even hypoparathyroidism can ensue.[152,157–159] Carcinomas with extensive fibrosis and sclerosing lymphomas should be ruled out; this is best achieved by surgical biopsy. However, in patients unfit for surgery, cytology and MRI may be helpful in the differential diagnosis.[154,160] Systemic steroids can stabilize the fibrosis and alleviate symptoms.[161–163] Hypothyroidism should be treated with L-thyroxine replacement therapy. Considering the progressive nature of the fibrotic process, long-term follow-up with yearly determination of thyroid function seems logical.

Infectious thyroiditis

Infection of the thyroid gland is a rare event. Most thyroid infections involve pyogenic bacteria, although all sorts of infectious agents have been described.[164–166]

Infectious thyroiditis is often observed in two age groups: in children under age 10, when the infection frequently reaches the thyroid via a fistula from the left pyriform sinus, and in young and middle-aged adults, in whom underlying thyroid disease—goiter, thyroiditis, adenoma or carcinoma—seems to be a predisposing factor.[164,165]

Infectious thyroiditis should be considered whenever there are systemic signs of infection accompanied by neck pain. Signs often include a uni- or bilateral tenderness to palpation, local erythema and warmth, dysphagia and dysphonia.[166] Thyroid function is usually normal. The differential diagnosis comprises:

infection of neck cysts (thyroglossal duct cyst, cystic hygroma, branchial cleft cyst), subacute thyroiditis, hemorrhages in a nodule, and, in cases of slowly growing infectious agents, diffuse goiter or carcinoma. If infectious thyroiditis is suspected, a causal diagnosis is best established by needle aspiration or surgical excision of the involved thyroid. This will enable drainage as well as initiation of antibiotic therapy based on direct staining and culture results. In children—and in adults with recurrent episodes of suppurative thyroiditis—antibiotic cover should be directed against oropharyngeal flora, as in these groups infection is most likely caused by a fistula from the pyriform sinus. In these cases, barium swallow or CT scanning should be performed after recovery. In cases of pyriform fistulae, fistulectomy should be performed.[166] There is no reason to advocate long-term follow-up after appropriate treatment for infectious thyroiditis.

References

1. Vander JB, Gaston EA, Dawber TR. The significance of non-toxic thyroid nodules. Final report of a 15-year study of the incidence of thyroid malignancy. *Ann Intern Med* 1968; 69(3): 537–40.
2. Vanderpump MP, Tunbridge WM, French JM et al. The incidence of thyroid disorders in the community: a twenty-year follow-up of the Whickham Survey. *Clin Endocrinol (Oxf)* 1995; 43(1): 55–68.
3. Berghout A, Wiersinga WM, Smits NJ, Touber JL. Determinants of thyroid volume as measured by ultrasonography in healthy adults in a non-iodine deficient area. *Clin Endocrinol (Oxf)* 1987; 26(3): 273–80.
4. Gutekunst R, Smolarek H, Wachter W, Scriba PC. Goiter epidemiology. IV. Thyroid volumes in German and Swedish school children. *Dtsch Med Wochenschr* 1985; 110(2): 50–4.
5. Woestyn J, Afschrift M, Schelstraete K, Vermeulen A. Demonstration of nodules in the normal thyroid by echography. *Br J Radiol* 1985; 58(696): 1179–82.
6. Studer H, Ramelli F. Simple goiter and its variants: euthyroid and hyperthyroid multinodular goiters. *Endocrine Rev* 1982; 3(1): 40–61.
7. Derwahl M, Studer H. Nodular goiter and goiter nodules: where iodine deficiency falls short of explaining the facts. *Exp Clin Endocrinol Diabetes* 2001; 109(5): 250–60.
8. Studer H, Peter HJ, Gerber H. Toxic nodular goiter. *Clin Endocrinol Metab* 1985; 14(2): 351–72.
9. Ramelli F, Studer H, Bruggisser D. Pathogenesis of thyroid nodules in multinodular goiter. *Am J Pathol* 1982; 109(2): 215–23.
10. Aeschimann S, Kopp PA, Kimura ET et al. Morphological and functional polymorphism within clonal thyroid nodules. *J Clin Endocrinol Metab* 1993; 77(3): 846–51.
11. Apel RL, Ezzat S, Bapat BV, Pan N, LiVolsi VA, Asa SL. Clonality of thyroid nodules in sporadic goiter. *Diagn Mol Pathol* 1995; 4(2): 113–21.
12. Gabriel EM, Bergert ER, Grant CS, van Heerden JA, Thompson GB, Morris JC. Germline polymorphism of codon 727 of human thyroid-stimulating hormone receptor is associated with toxic multinodular goiter. *J Clin Endocrinol Metab* 1999; 84(9): 3328–35.
13. Bignell GR, Canzian F, Shayeghi M, Stark M et al. Familial non-toxic multinodular thyroid goiter locus maps to chromosome 14q but does not account for familial nonmedullary thyroid cancer. *Am J Hum Genet* 1997; 61(5): 1123–30.
14. Neumann S, Willgerodt H, Ackermann F et al. Linkage of familial euthyroid goiter to the multinodular goiter-1 locus and exclusion of the candidate genes thyroglobulin, thyroperoxidase, and Na+/I− symporter. *J Clin Endocrinol Metab* 1999; 84(10): 3750–6.
15. Berghout A, Wiersinga WM, Smits NJ, Touber JL. Interrelationships between age, thyroid volume, thyroid nodularity and thyroid function in patients with sporadic non-toxic goiter. *Au J Med* 1990; 89(5): 602–8.
16. Berghout A, Wiersinga W, Smits NJ, Touber JL. The value of thyroid volume measured by ultrasonography in the diagnosis of goitre. *Clin Endocrinol* 1988; 28: 409–14.
17. Hegedus L, Perrild H, Poulsen LR et al. The determination of thyroid volume by ultrasound and its relationship to body weight, age, and sex in normal subjects. *J Clin Endocrinol Metab* 1983; 56(2): 260–3.
18. Huysmans DA, de Haas MM, van den Broek WJ et al. Magnetic resonance imaging for volume estimation of large multinodular goiters: a comparison with scintigraphy. *Br J Radiol* 1994; 67(798): 519–23.
19. Belfiore A, La Rosa GL, Padova G, Sava L, Ippolito O, Vigneri R. The frequency of cold thyroid nodules and thyroid malignancies in patients from an iodine–deficient area. *Cancer* 1987; 60(12): 3096–102.
20. Belfiore A, Giuffrida D, La Rosa GL et al. High frequency of cancer in cold thyroid nodules occurring at young age. *Acta Endocrinol (Copenh)* 1989; 121(2): 197–202.
21. Werk EE Jr, Vernon BM, Gonzalez JJ, Ungaro PC, McCoy RC. Cancer in thyroid nodules. A community hospital survey. *Arch Intern Med* 1984; 144(3): 474–6.
22. Harach HR, Franssila KO, Wasenius VM. Occult papillary carcinoma of the thyroid. A 'normal' finding in Finland. A systematic autopsy study. *Cancer* 1985; 56(3): 531–8.
23. Sampson RJ, Woolner LB, Bahn RC, Kurland LT. Occult thyroid carcinoma in Olmsted County, Minnesota: prevalence at autopsy compared with that in Hiroshima and Nagasaki, Japan. *Cancer* 1974; 34(6): 2072–6.
24. Koh KB, Chang KW. Carcinoma in multinodular goiter. *Br J Surg* 1992; 79(3): 266–7.

25. McCall A, Jarosz H, Lawrence AM, Paloyan E. The incidence of thyroid carcinoma in solitary cold nodules and in multinodular goiters. *Surgery* 1986; 100(6): 1128–32.
26. Berghout A, Hoogendoorn D, Wiersinga WM. A diminishing number of thyroid operations in The Netherlands in 1972–1986. *Ned Tijdschr Geneeskd* 1989; 133(26): 1313–17.
27. Belfiore A, La Rosa GL. Fine-needle aspiration biopsy of the thyroid. *Endocrinol Metab Clin North Am* 2001; 30(2): 361–400.
28. Gharib H, Goellner JR. Fine-needle aspiration biopsy of the thyroid: an appraisal. *Ann Intern Med* 1993; 118(4): 282–9.
29. Gharib H. Fine-needle aspiration biopsy of thyroid nodules: advantages, limitations, and effect. *Mayo Clin Proc* 1994; 69(1): 44–9.
30. Jayaram G. Fine needle aspiration cytologic study of the solitary thyroid nodule. Profile of 308 cases with histologic correlation. *Acta Cytol* 1985; 29(6): 967–73.
31. La Rosa GL, Belfiore A, Giuffrida D et al. Evaluation of the fine needle aspiration biopsy in the preoperative selection of cold thyroid nodules. *Cancer* 1991; 67(8): 2137–41.
32. Carmeci C, Jeffrey RB, McDougall IR, Nowels KW, Weigel RJ. Ultrasound-guided fine-needle aspiration biopsy of thyroid masses. *Thyroid* 1998; 8(4): 283–9.
33. Danese D, Sciacchitano S, Farsetti A, Andreoli M, Pontecorvi A. Diagnostic accuracy of conventional versus sonography-guided fine-needle aspiration biopsy of thyroid nodules. *Thyroid* 1998; 8(1): 15–21.
34. Ippolito A, Vella V, La Rosa GL, Pellegriti G, Vigneri R, Belfiore A. Immunostaining for Met/HGF receptor may be useful to identify malignancies in thyroid lesions classified suspicious at fine-needle aspiration biopsy. *Thyroid* 2001; 11(8): 783–7.
35. Gasbarri A, Martegani MP, Del Prete F, Lucante T, Natali PG, Bartolazzi A. Galectin-3 and CD44v6 isoforms in the preoperative evaluation of thyroid nodules. *J Clin Oncol* 1999; 17(11): 3494–502.
36. Lange M, Feldt-Rasmussen U, Christensen L, Blichert-Toft M. Thyroperoxidase immunostaining in evaluation of thyroid nodules. *Clin Endocrinol (Oxf)* 2000; 52(6): 797.
37. Berghout A, Van de Wetering J, Klootwijk P, Hennemann G. Cardiac and metabolic effects in patients with clinically euthyroid goiter. Submitted, 2002.
38. Elte JW, Bussemaker JK, Haak A. The natural history of euthyroid multinodular goiter. *Postgrad Med J* 1990; 66(773): 186–90.
39. Sawin CT, Geller A, Wolf PA et al. Low serum thyrotropin concentrations as a risk factor for atrial fibrillation in older persons. *N Engl J Med* 1994; 331(19): 1249–52.
40. Parle JV, Maisonneuve P, Sheppard MC, Boyle P, Franklyn JA. Prediction of all-cause and cardiovascular mortality in elderly people from one low serum thyrotropin result: a 10-year cohort study. *Lancet* 2001; 358(9285): 861–5.
41. Biondi B, Fazio S, Carella C et al. Cardiac effects of long term thyrotropin-suppressive therapy with levothyroxine. *J Clin Endocrinol Metab* 1993; 77(2): 334–8.
42. Shapiro LE, Sievert R, Ong L et al. Minimal cardiac effects in asymptomatic athyreotic patients chronically treated with thyrotropin-suppressive doses of L-thyroxine. *J Clin Endocrinol Metab* 1997; 82(8): 2592–5.
43. Biondi B, Palmieri EA, Fazio S et al. Endogenous subclinical hyperthyroidism affects quality of life and cardiac morphology and function in young and middle-aged patients. *J Clin Endocrinol Metab* 2000; 85(12): 4701–5.
44. Parle JV, Franklyn JA, Cross KW, Jones SR, Sheppard MC. Circulating lipids and minor abnormalities of thyroid function. *Clin Endocrinol (Oxf)* 1992; 37(5): 411–14.
45. Faber J, Perrild H, Johansen JS. Bone Gla protein and sex hormone-binding globulin in non-toxic goiter: parameters for metabolic status at the tissue level. *J Clin Endocrinol Metab* 1990; 70(1): 49–55.
46. Mudde AH, Bastiaanse AJ, Jonkers H. Is there a relationship between thyroid function and serum osteocalcin in women with multinodular goiter? A preliminary report. *Neth J Med* 1990; 37(1–2): 17–20.
47. Larsen PR. Thyroid–pituitary interaction: feedback regulation of thyrotropin secretion by thyroid hormones. *N Engl J Med* 1982; 306(1): 23–32.
48. Hodin RA, Lazar MA, Chin WW. Differential and tissue-specific regulation of the multiple rat c-erbA messenger RNA species by thyroid hormone. *J Clin Invest* 1990; 85(1): 101–5.
49. Silva JE, Dick TE, Larsen PR. The contribution of local tissue thyroxine monodeiodination to the nuclear 3,5,3′-triiodothyronine in pituitary, liver, and kidney of euthyroid rats. *Endocrinology* 1978; 103(4): 1196–207.
50. Everts ME, Verhoeven FA, Bezstarosti K et al. Uptake of thyroid hormones in neonatal rat cardiac myocytes. *Endocrinology* 1996; 137(10): 4235–42.
51. Croteau W, Davey JC, Galton VA, St Germain DL. Cloning of the mammalian type II iodothyronine deiodinase. A selenoprotein differentially expressed and regulated in human and rat brain and other tissues. *J Clin Invest* 1996; 98(2): 405–17.
52. Berghout A, Wiersinga WM, Drexhage HA, Smits NJ, Touber JL. Comparison of placebo with L-thyroxine alone or with carbimazole for treatment of sporadic non-toxic goiter. *Lancet* 1990; 336(8709): 193–7.
53. Ross DS. Thyroid hormone suppressive therapy of sporadic non-toxic goiter. *Thyroid* 1992; 2(3): 263–9.
54. Gharib H, James EM, Charboneau JW, Naessens JM, Offord KP, Gorman CA. Suppressive therapy with levothyroxine for solitary thyroid nodules. A double-blind controlled clinical study. *N Engl J Med* 1987; 317(2): 70–5.

55. Papini E, Petrucci L, Guglielmi R et al. Long-term changes in nodular goiter: a 5-year prospective randomized trial of levothyroxine suppressive therapy for benign cold thyroid nodules. *J Clin Endocrinol Metab* 1998; 83(3): 780–3.
56. Zelmanovitz F, Genro S, Gross JL. Suppressive therapy with levothyroxine for solitary thyroid nodules: a double-blind controlled clinical study and cumulative meta-analyses. *J Clin Endocrinol Metab* 1998; 83(11): 3881–5.
57. Hegedus L, Hansen BM, Knudsen N, Hansen JM. Reduction of size of thyroid with radioactive iodine in multinodular non-toxic goiter. *BMJ* 1988; 297(6649): 661–2.
58. Huysmans DA, Hermus AR, Corstens FH, Barentsz JO, Kloppenborg PW. Large, compressive goiters treated with radioiodine. *Ann Intern Med* 1994; 121(10): 757–62.
59. Huysmans DA, Buijs WC, van de Ven MT et al. Dosimetry and risk estimates of radioiodine therapy for large, multinodular goiters. *J Nucl Med* 1996; 37(12): 2072–9.
60. Lawrence JE, Emerson CH, Sullaway SL, Braverman LE. The effect of recombinant human tsh on the thyroid (123)i uptake in iodide treated normal subjects. *J Clin Endocrinol Metab* 2001; 86(1): 437–40.
61. Nygaard B, Faber J, Veje A, Hegedus L, Hansen JM. Appearance of Graves'-like disease after radioiodine therapy for toxic as well as non-toxic multinodular goiter. *Clin Endocrinol (Oxf)* 1995; 43(1): 129–30.
62. Tonacchera M, Vitti P, Agretti P et al. Activating thyrotropin receptor mutations in histologically heterogeneous hyperfunctioning nodules of multinodular goiter. *Thyroid* 1998; 8(7): 559–64.
63. Tonacchera M, van Sande J, Parma J et al. TSH receptor and disease. *Clin Endocrinol (Oxf)* 1996; 44(6): 621–33.
64. Parma J, Duprez L, van Sande J et al. Diversity and prevalence of somatic mutations in the thyrotropin receptor and Gs alpha genes as a cause of toxic thyroid adenomas. *J Clin Endocrinol Metab* 1997; 82(8): 2695–701.
65. Nygaard B, Hegedus L, Nielsen KG, Ulriksen P, Hansen JM. Long-term effect of radioactive iodine on thyroid function and size in patients with solitary autonomously functioning toxic thyroid nodules. *Clin Endocrinol (Oxf)* 1999; 50(2): 197–202.
66. Burch HB, Solomon BL, Cooper DS, Ferguson P, Walpert N, Howard R. The effect of antithyroid drug pretreatment on acute changes in thyroid hormone levels after (131)I ablation for Graves' disease. *J Clin Endocrinol Metab* 2001; 86(7): 3016–21.
67. Ross DS, Ridgway EC, Daniels GH. Successful treatment of solitary toxic thyroid nodules with relatively low-dose iodine-131, with low prevalence of hypothyroidism. *Ann Intern Med* 1984; 101(4): 488–90.
68. Burch HB, Solomon BL, Wartofsky L, Burman KD. Discontinuing antithyroid drug therapy before ablation with radioiodine in Graves disease. *Ann Intern Med* 1994; 121(8): 553–9.
69. Berghout A, Endert E, Ross A, Hogerzeil HV, Smits NJ, Wiersinga WM. Thyroid function and thyroid size in normal pregnant women living in an iodine replete area. *Clin Endocrinol (Oxf)* 1994; 41(3): 375–9.
70. Nisula BC, Taliadouros GS. Thyroid function in gestational trophoblastic neoplasia: evidence that the thyrotropic activity of chorionic gonadotropin mediates the thyrotoxicosis of choriocarcinoma. *Am J Obstet Gynecol* 1980; 138(1): 77–85.
71. Nisula BC, Morgan FJ, Canfield RE. Evidence that chorionic gonadotropin has intrinsic thyrotropic activity. *Biochem Biophys Res Commun* 1974; 59(1): 86–91.
72. Goodwin TM, Montoro M, Mestman JH, Pekary AE, Hershman JM. The role of chorionic gonadotropin in transient hyperthyroidism of hyperemesis gravidarum. *J Clin Endocrinol Metab* 1992; 75(5): 1333–7.
73. Goodwin TM, Montoro M, Mestman JH, Perkary AE, Hershman JM. The role of chorionic gonadotropin in transient hyperthyroidism of hyperemesis gravidarum. *Trans Assoc Am Physicians* 1991; 104: 233–7.
74. Goodwin TM, Montoro M, Mestman JH. Transient hyperthyroidism and hyperemesis gravidarum: clinical aspects. *Am J Obstet Gynecol* 1992; 167(3): 648–52.
75. Hoermann R, Amir SM, Ingbar SH. Evidence that partially desialylated variants of human chorionic gonadotropin (hCG) are the factors in crude hCG that inhibit the response to thyrotropin in human thyroid membranes. *Endocrinology* 1988; 123(3): 1535–43.
76. Berghout A, Endert E, Wiersinga WM, Touber JL. The application of an immunoradiometric assay of plasma thyrotropin (TSH–IRMA) in molar pregnancy. *J Endocrinol Invest* 1988; 11(1): 15–19.
77. Chowdhury TA, Tanchel BM, Jaganathan RS, Dodson PM. A toxic testicle. *Lancet* 2000; 355(9220): 2046.
78. Orgiazzi J, Rousset B, Cosentino C, Tourniaire J, Dutrieux N. Plasma thyrotropic activity in a man with choriocarcinoma. *J Clin Endocrinol Metab* 1974; 39(4): 653–7.
79. Paul SJ, Sisson JC. Thyrotoxicosis caused by thyroid cancer. *Endocrinol Metab Clin North Am* 1990; 19(3): 593–612.
80. De Quervain F. Die akute nicht eiterige thyreoiditis und die beteiligungder schilddruse an akute intoxikationen und infektionen überhaupt. *Mitteilungen grenzgebieten med chirurg* 1904; 2: 1–165.
81. Nikolai TF. Lymphocytic thyroiditis with spontaneously resolving hyperthyroidism. *Thyroid Today* 1989; 2: 1.
82. Woolner LB, McConahey WM, Bears OH. Granulomatous thyroiditis (De Quervain thyroiditis). *J Clin Endocrinol Metab* 1957; 17: 202.
83. Tunbridge WM, Evered DC, Hall R et al. The spectrum of thyroid disease in a community: the Whickham survey. *Clin Endocrinol (Oxf)* 1977; 7(6): 481–93.

84. Iitaka M, Momotani N, Ishii J, Ito K. Incidence of subacute thyroiditis recurrences after a prolonged latency: 24-year survey. *J Clin Endocrinol Metab* 1996; 81(2): 466–9.
85. Lazarus JH. Silent thyroiditis and subacute thyroiditis. In: Braverman LE, Utiger RD, eds. *Werner and Ingbar's The Thyroid: a Fundamental and Clinical Text*. Philadelphia: Lippincott-Raven, 1996: 577–91.
86. Martino E, Buratti L, Bartalena L et al. High prevalence of subacute thyroiditis during summer season in Italy. *J Endocrinol Invest* 1987; 10(3): 321–3.
87. Tomer Y, Davies TF. Infection, thyroid disease, and autoimmunity. *Endocrine Rev* 1993; 14(1): 107–20.
88. Volpe R. Subacute thyroiditis. In: Burrow GN, Oppenheimer JH, Volpe R, eds. *Thyroid Function and Disease*. Philadelphia: WB Saunders, 1989: 179.
89. de Bruin TW, Riekhoff FP, de Boer JJ. An outbreak of thyrotoxicosis due to atypical subacute thyroiditis. *J Clin Endocrinol Metab* 1990; 70(2): 396–402.
90. Sheba C, Bank H. Prevention of mumps thyroiditis. *N Engl J Med* 1968; 279(2): 108–9.
91. Eylan E, Zmucky R, Sheba C. Mumps virus and subacute thyroiditis. Evidence for a causal association. *Lancet* 1957; 1: 1062–3.
92. Hung W. Mumps thyroiditis and hypothyroidism. *J Pediatr* 1969; 74(4): 611–13.
93. Volpe R, Row VV, Ezrin C. Circulating viral and thyroid antibodies in subacute thyroiditis. *J Clin Endocrinol Metab* 1967; 27(9): 1275–84.
94. Chartier B, Bandy P, Wall JR. Fc receptor-bearing blood mononuclear cells in thyroid disorders: increased levels in patients with subacute thyroiditis. *J Clin Endocrinol Metab* 1980; 51(5): 1014–18.
95. Galluzzo A, Giordano C, Andronico F, Filardo C, Andronico G, Bompiani G. Leukocyte migration test in subacute thyroiditis: hypothetical role of cell-mediated immunity. *J Clin Endocrinol Metab* 1980; 50(6): 1038–41.
96. Wall JR, Gray B, Greenwood DM. Total and 'activated' peripheral blood T lymphocytes in patients with thyroid disorders. *Acta Endocrinol (Copenh)* 1977; 85(4): 753–9.
97. Totterman TH. Distribution of T-, B-, and thyroglobulin-binding lymphocytes infiltrating the gland in Graves' disease, Hashimoto's thyroiditis, and de Quervain's thyroiditis. *Clin Immunol Immunopathol* 1978; 10(3): 270–7.
98. Buc M, Nyulassy S, Hnilica P, Busova B, Stefanovic J. The frequency of HLA-Dw1 determinant in subacute (de Quervain's) thyroiditis. *Tissue Antigens* 1979; 14(1): 63–7.
99. Farid NR, Bear JC. The human major histocompatibility complex and endocrine disease. *Endocrine Rev* 1981; 2(1): 50–86.
100. Nyulassy S, Hnilica P, Buc M, Guman M, Hirschova V, Stefanovic J. Subacute (de Quervain's) thyroiditis: association with HLA-Bw35 antigen and abnormalities of the complement system, immunoglobulins and other serum proteins. *J Clin Endocrinol Metab* 1977; 45(2): 270–4.
101. Ohsako N, Tamai H, Sudo T et al. Clinical characteristics of subacute thyroiditis classified according to human leukocyte antigen typing. *J Clin Endocrinol Metab* 1995; 80(12): 3653–6.
102. Yeo PP, Chan SH, Aw TC et al. HLA and Chinese patients with subacute (De Quervain's) thyroiditis. *Tissue Antigens* 1981; 17(2): 249–50.
103. Nikolai TF, Coombs GJ, McKenzie AK. Lymphocytic thyroiditis with spontaneously resolving hyperthyroidism and subacute thyroiditis. Long-term follow-up. *Arch Intern Med* 1981; 141(11): 1455–8.
104. Weihl AC, Daniels GH, Ridgway EC, Maloof F. Thyroid function tests during the early phase of subacute thyroiditis. *J Clin Endocrinol Metab* 1977; 44(6): 1107–14.
105. Greene JN. Subacute thyroiditis. *Am J Med* 1971; 51(1): 97–108.
106. Volpe R. The management of subacute (DeQuervain's) thyroiditis. *Thyroid* 1993; 3(3): 253–5.
107. Yamamoto M, Saito S, Sakurada T et al. Effect of prednisolone and salicylate on serum thyroglobulin level in patients with subacute thyroiditis. *Clin Endocrinol (Oxf)* 1987; 27(3): 339–44.
108. Nikolai TF, Brosseau J, Kettrick MA, Roberts R, Beltaos E. Lymphocytic thyroiditis with spontaneously resolving hyperthyroidism (silent thyroiditis). *Arch Intern Med* 1980; 140(4): 478–82.
109. Williams I, Ankrett VO, Lazarus JH, Volpe R. Aetiology of hyperthyroidism in Canada and Wales. *J Epidemiol Community Health* 1983; 37(3): 245–8.
110. Schorr AB, Miller JL, Shtasel P, Rose LI. Low incidence of painless thyroiditis in the Philadelphia area. *Clin Nucl Med* 1986; 11(6): 379–80.
111. Vitug AC, Goldman JM. Silent (painless) thyroiditis. Evidence of a geographic variation in frequency. *Arch Intern Med* 1985; 145(3): 473–5.
112. Woolf PD, Daly R. Thyrotoxicosis with painless thyroiditis. *Am J Med* 1976; 60(1): 73–9.
113. Dorfman SG, Cooperman MT, Nelson RL, Depuy H, Peake RL, Young RL. Painless thyroiditis and transient hyperthyroidism without goiter. *Ann Intern Med* 1977; 86(1): 24–8.
114. Muller AF, Drexhage HA, Berghout A. Postpartum thyroiditis and autoimmune thyroiditis in women of childbearing age: recent insights and consequences for antenatal and postnatal care. *Endocrine Rev* 2001; 22(5): 605–30.
115. Alvarez-Marfany M, Roman SH, Drexler AJ, Robertson C, Stagnaro-Green A. Long-term prospective study of postpartum thyroid dysfunction in women with insulin dependent diabetes mellitus. *J Clin Endocrinol Metab* 1994; 79(1): 10–16.
116. Gerstein HC. Incidence of postpartum thyroid dysfunction in patients with type I diabetes mellitus. *Ann Intern Med* 1993; 118(6): 419–23.

117. Woolf PD. Transient painless thyroiditis with hyperthyroidism: a variant of lymphocytic thyroiditis? *Endocrine Rev* 1980; 1(4): 411–20.
118. Mizukami Y, Michigishi T, Nonomura A et al. Postpartum thyroiditis. A clinical, histologic, and immunopathologic study of 15 cases. *Am J Clin Pathol* 1993; 100(3): 200–5.
119. Mizukami Y, Michigishi T, Hashimoto T et al. Silent thyroiditis: a histologic and immunohistochemical study. *Hum Pathol* 1988; 19(4): 423–31.
120. Ronnblom LE, Alm GV, Oberg KE. Autoimmunity after alpha-interferon therapy for malignant carcinoid tumors. *Ann Intern Med* 1991; 115(3): 178–83.
121. Vialettes B, Guillerand MA, Viens P et al. Incidence rate and risk factors for thyroid dysfunction during recombinant interleukin-2 therapy in advanced malignancies. *Acta Endocrinol (Copenh)* 1993; 129(1): 31–8.
122. Schwartzentruber DJ, White DE, Zweig MH, Weintraub BD, Rosenberg SA. Thyroid dysfunction associated with immunotherapy for patients with cancer. *Cancer* 1991; 68(11): 2384–90.
123. Preziati D, La Rosa L, Covini G et al. Autoimmunity and thyroid function in patients with chronic active hepatitis treated with recombinant interferon alpha-2a. *Eur J Endocrinol* 1995; 132(5): 587–93.
124. Drexhage HA. Autoimmunity and thyroid diseases. In: Monaco F, Satta MA, Shapiro B, Troncone L, eds. *Thyroid Diseases: Clinical Fundamentals and Therapy*. Boca Raton, Fla: CRC Press, 1993: 491–505.
125. Kahaly GJ, Dienes HP, Beyer J, Hommel G. Iodide induces thyroid autoimmunity in patients with endemic goiter: a randomised, double-blind, placebo-controlled trial. *Eur J Endocrinol* 1998; 139(3): 290–7.
126. Tajiri J, Higashi K, Morita M, Umeda T, Sato T. Studies of hypothyroidism in patients with high iodine intake. *J Clin Endocrinol Metab* 1986; 63(2): 412–17.
127. Boukis MA, Koutras DA, Souvatzoglou A, Evangelopoulou A, Vrontakis M, Moulopoulos SD. Thyroid hormone and immunological studies in endemic goiter. *J Clin Endocrinol Metab* 1983; 57(4): 859–62.
128. Boukis MA, Koutras DA, Souvatzoglou A et al. Iodine-induced autoimmunity. In: Hall R, Kobberling J, eds. *Thyroid Disorders Associated with Iodine Deficiency and Excess*. New York: Raven Press, 1985: 217–21.
129. Doufas AG, Mastorakos G, Chatziioannou S et al. The predominant form of non-toxic goiter in Greece is now autoimmune thyroiditis. *Eur J Endocrinol* 1999; 140(6): 505–11.
130. Laurberg P, Nohr SB, Pedersen KM et al. Thyroid disorders in mild iodine deficiency. *Thyroid* 2000; 10(11): 951–63.
131. Tsatsoulis A, Johnson EO, Andricula M et al. Thyroid autoimmunity is associated with higher urinary iodine concentrations in an iodine-deficient area of Northwestern Greece. *Thyroid* 1999; 9(3): 279–83.
132. Allen EM, Appel MC, Braverman LE. The effect of iodide ingestion on the development of spontaneous lymphocytic thyroiditis in the diabetes-prone BB/W rat. *Endocrinology* 1986; 118(5): 1977–81.
133. Bagchi N, Brown TR, Urdanivia E, Sundick RS. Induction of autoimmune thyroiditis in chickens by dietary iodine. *Science* 1985; 230(4723): 325–7.
134. Many MC, Maniratunga S, Denef JF. The non-obese diabetic (NOD) mouse: an animal model for autoimmune thyroiditis. *Exp Clin Endocrinol Diabetes* 1996; 104(suppl 3): 17–20.
135. Davies TF. The thyroid immunology of the postpartum period. *Thyroid* 1999; 9(7): 675–84.
136. Weetman AP. The immunology of pregnancy. *Thyroid* 1999; 9(7): 643–6.
137. Nelson JL. Microchimerism and scleroderma. *Curr Rheumatol Rep* 1999; 1(1): 15–21.
138. Abramson J, Stagnaro-Green A. Thyroid antibodies and fetal loss: an evolving story. *Thyroid* 2001; 11(1): 57–63.
139. Imaizumi M, Pritsker A, Unger P, Davies TF. Identification of fetal cells within the thyroid—potential influence of microchimerism on autoimmune thyroiditis. *Endocrine J* 2000; 47(8): 256.
140. Klintschar M, Schwaiger P, Mannweiler S, Regauer S, Kleiber M. Evidence of fetal microchimerism in Hashimoto's thyroiditis. *J Clin Endocrinol Metab* 2001; 86(6): 2494–8.
141. Reber PM. Prolactin and immunomodulation. *Am J Med* 1993; 95(6): 637–44.
142. Reichlin S. Neuroendocrinology. In: Wilson JD, Foster DW, Kronenberg HM, Larsen PR, eds. *Williams Textbook of Endocrinology*. Philadelphia: WB Saunders, 1998: 165–248.
143. Kendall-Taylor P. Investigation of thyrotoxicosis. *Clin Endocrinol (Oxf)* 1995; 42(3): 309–13.
144. Momotani N, Noh J, Ishikawa N, Ito K. Relationship between silent thyroiditis and recurrent Graves' disease in the postpartum period. *J Clin Endocrinol Metab* 1994; 79(1): 285–9.
145. Cavalieri RR, McDougall IR. In vivo isotopic tests and imaging. In: Braverman LE, Utiger R, eds. *Werner and Ingbar's The Thyroid: a Fundamental and Clinical Text*. Philadelphia: Lippincott-Raven, 1996: 352–76.
146. Romney BM, Nickoloff EL, Esser PD, Alderson PO. Radionuclide administration to nursing mothers: mathematically derived guidelines. *Radiology* 1986; 160(2): 549–54.
147. Lervang HH, Askaa S, Ostergaard Kristensen HP. Technetium Tc 99m uptake in postpartum thyrotoxicosis. *Arch Intern Med* 1987; 147(5): 994–7.
148. Parkes AB, Black EG, Adams H et al. Serum thyroglobulin: an early indicator of autoimmune postpartum thyroiditis. *Clin Endocrinol (Oxf)* 1994; 41(1): 9–14.
149. Filetti S, Belfiore A, Amir SM et al. The role of thyroid-stimulating antibodies of Graves' disease in differenti-

ated thyroid cancer. *N Engl J Med* 1988; 318(12): 753–9.
150. Riedel BMCL. Die chronische, zur bildung eisenharter tumoren fuhrende entzundung der schilddruse. 1896; *Verh Dtsch Ges Chir* 25: 101.
151. Schwaegerle SM, Bauer TW, Esselstyn CB Jr. Riedel's thyroiditis. *Am J Clin Pathol* 1988; 90(6): 715–22.
152. de Lange WE, Freling NJ, Molenaar WM, Doorenbos H. Invasive fibrous thyroiditis (Riedel's struma): a manifestation of multifocal fibrosclerosis? A case report with review of the literature. *Q J Med* 1989; 72(268): 709–17.
153. Girod DA, Bigler SA, Coltrera MD. Riedel's thyroiditis: report of a lethal case and review of the literature. *Otolaryngol Head Neck Surg* 1992; 107(4): 591–5.
154. LiVolsi VA. Pathology. In: Braverman LE, Utiger R, eds. *Werner and Ingbar's The Thyroid: a Fundamental and Clinical Text*. Philadelphia: Lippincott-Raven, 1996: 497–520.
155. Heufelder AE, Goellner JR, Bahn RS, Gleich GJ, Hay ID. Tissue eosinophilia and eosinophil degranulation in Riedel's invasive fibrous thyroiditis. *J Clin Endocrinol Metab* 1996; 81(3): 977–84.
156. Barsano CP. Other forms of primary hypothyroidism. In: Braverman LE, Utiger R, eds. *Werner and Ingbar's The Thyroid, a Fundamental and Clinical Text*. Philadelphia: Lippincott-Raven Publishers, 1996: 768–78.
157. Best TB, Munro RE, Burwell S, Volpe R. Riedel's thyroiditis associated with Hashimoto's thyroiditis, hypoparathyroidism, and retroperitoneal fibrosis. *J Endocrinol Invest* 1991; 14(9): 767–72.
158. Chopra D, Wool MS, Crosson A, Sawin CT. Riedel's struma associated with subacute thyroiditis, hypothyroidism, and hypoparathyroidism. *J Clin Endocrinol Metab* 1978; 46(6): 869–71.
159. McRorie ER, Chalmers J, Campbell IW. Riedel's thyroiditis complicated by hypoparathyroidism and hypothyroidism. *Scott Med J* 1993; 38(1): 27–8.
160. Perez Fontan FJ, Cordido CF, Pombo FF, Mosquera OJ, Villalba MC. Riedel thyroiditis: US, CT, and MR evaluation. *J Comput Assist Tomogr* 1993; 17(2): 324–5.
161. Lo JC, Loh KC, Rubin AL, Cha I, Greenspan FS. Riedel's thyroiditis presenting with hypothyroidism and hypoparathyroidism: dramatic response to glucocorticoid and thyroxine therapy. *Clin Endocrinol (Oxf)* 1998; 48(6): 815–18.
162. Tutuncu NB, Erbas T, Bayraktar M, Gedik O. Multifocal idiopathic fibrosclerosis manifesting with Riedel's thyroiditis. *Endocrine Pract* 2000; 6(6): 447–9.
163. Vaidya B, Harris PE, Barrett P, Kendall-Taylor P. Corticosteroid therapy in Riedel's thyroiditis. *Postgrad Med J* 1997; 73(866): 817–19.
164. Berger SA, Zonszein J, Villamena P, Mittman N. Infectious diseases of the thyroid gland. *Rev Infect Dis* 1983; 5(1): 108–22.
165. Brook I. The swollen neck. Cervical lymphadenitis, parotitis, thyroiditis, and infected cysts. *Infect Dis Clin North Am* 1988; 2(1): 221–36.
166. Basgoz N, Swartz MN. Infections of the thyroid gland. In: Braverman LE, Utiger R, eds. *Werner and Ingbar's The Thyroid: a Fundamental and Clinical Text*. Philadelphia: Lippincott-Raven, 1996: 1049–56.

13

Calcium disorders and bone diseases
Laura Masi, Alberto Falchetti, Luigi Gennari, Maria Luisa Brandi

Primary hypoparathyroidism

Introduction

Hypocalcemia is a disorder that can be asymptomatic or may present as an emergency case. The concentration of calcium (Ca) in the extracellular fluid is crucial for many physiological functions. In normal conditions, the range is maintained constant between 8.5 and 10.5 mg/dl (2.25–2.6 mmol/l). The total content of Ca in plasma consists of about 35% protein-bound Ca (mostly albumin-bound Ca: 70–90%), 15% phosphate- and citrate-complexed Ca, and 50% ionized Ca.[1] It is only the ionized portion of calcium that is physiologically important, regulating neuromuscular contractility, the activity of several enzymes, coagulation and a variety of other cellular reactions. The regulation of plasma Ca concentration is so precise that it normally fluctuates by <0.025 mmol/l in either direction from its 'set' value. The parathyroid glands are extremely sensitive to small changes in the serum ionized Ca level. Parathyroid hormone (PTH), through its acute effects on bone and on kidney, is responsible for the regulation of the serum Ca levels. The most common causes of hypocalcemia include hypoparathyroidism (HP), deficiency or abnormal metabolism of vitamin D, and acute or chronic renal failure.

Idiopathic HP is manifested by hypocalcemia with low or absent PTH levels. It is often a part of autoimmune disease associated with deficient function of an endocrine gland (adrenal, thyroid and ovaries). Sometimes, isolated HP may occur, the mode of inheritance varying in each kindred. Finally, congenital aplasia of the parathyroid glands may occur.

Clinical features of hypocalcemia

The signs and symptoms of acute hypocalcemia result from enhanced neuromuscular irritability. Muscle cramps are often experienced by hypocalcemic patients, especially in the lower back, legs and feet. In severe hypocalcemia, carpopedal spasm, laryngospasm and bronchospasm may also develop. Severe hypocalcemia may be accompanied by prolongation of the QT interval on the electrocardiogram. Patients with chronic hypocalcemia due to idiopathic HP or pseudohypoparathyroidism (PHP) also have calcification of the basal ganglia and extrapyramidal neurological symptoms.

Hypoparathyroidism

HP is a clinical disorder that manifests when PTH is insufficient to maintain extracellular fluid calcium in the normal range.

The clinical manifestations of HP include latent or evident neuromuscular irritability due to hypocalcemia (tetany). Manifestations are more likely to appear when the plasma Ca level is falling rapidly than during steady hypocalcemia. Low concentrations of magnesium (Mg) and hydrogen (alkalosis) and high concentrations of potassium (K) predispose to tetany. Chronically, patients may manifest muscle cramps, pseudopapilledema, extrapyramidal signs, mental retardation and personality disturbances, as well as cataracts, dry skin, alopecia and abnormal dentition.

Tetany
Tetany refers to the entire complex of manifestations of increased neural excitability. A typical attack of tetany begins with increased tingling, which starts in the

fingertips, around the mouth and sometimes in the feet. The muscles then feel tense and go into spasm in the same pattern as the sensory symptoms. The hand and forearms are the parts of the body most commonly involved. Sometimes, atypical tetany may occur in patients with mild hypocalcemia. They may have frequent mild tingling and cramps instead of clearly defined attacks of tetany, and may have carpal spasm during prolonged use of the hand and forearm. Seizures resembling epilepsy may occur, but in these cases hypocalcemia is frequently associated with characteristic changes in the electroencephalogram.[2] Signs of latent tetany remain useful in diagnosis and in adjusting therapy. Chvostek's sign is elicited by tapping the facial nerve with a fingertip as a hammer, 1–2 cm anterior to the earlobe just below the zygomatic process. A grade 1 sign (twitching of the upper lip) can be found in >25% of normal children. Trousseau's sign is evoked by sphygmomanometer cuff on the upper arm when inflated to above the systolic pressure for up 3 min. A positive response is seen, with the development of carpal spasm, typically within 2 min. The severity of spasm is such that even the examiner is unable to overcome it. Only the severe grade of the sign is abnormal with certainty, because the milder grade occurs in a small percentage of normal subjects. The sign depends on induction of ischemia of the ulnar nerve.

Basal ganglia calcification

In patients with HP and with PHP, small irregular areas of calcification may be observed in the basal ganglia in skull radiographs (Figure 13.1) and CT scans.[3]

Papilledema

In patients with untreated HP, there may be swelling of the optic disks. The papilledema is usually benign and subsides within a few days of normocalcemia.

Cataracts

These are common in chronic hypocalcemia. They appear as punctate opacities in the lens and they may develop more in the posterior pole than in the anterior pole. Within 5–10 years, they become confluent. Control of hypocalcemia arrests their progression.

Dental and dermal manifestations

The skin may be dry, and the hair coarse, dry and easily shed. Eruption of teeth may be delayed, and their roots may be blunted (Figure 13.2).

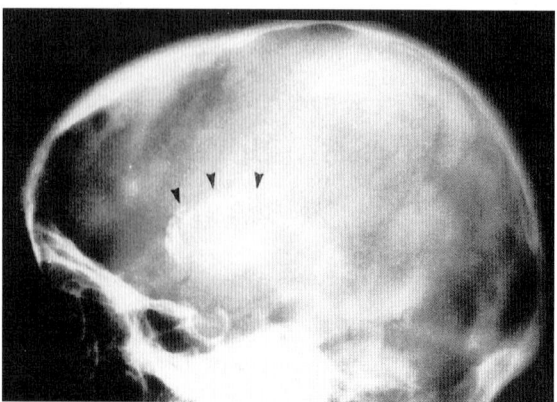

Figure 13.1
Skull radiograph: calcifications (black arrows) of the basal ganglia in a patient affected by pseudohypoparathyroidism. (From Gennari C, Avioli LV (eds) Atlante delle Malattie Dell'osso, Vol. II. Parma: Chiesi Farmaceutici S.p.A., 1992.)

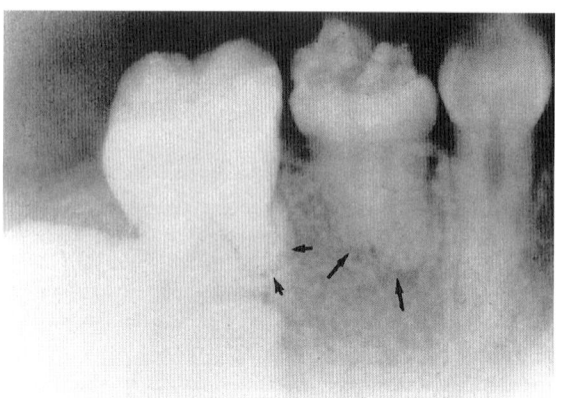

Figure 13.2
Abnormal eruption of teeth in a patient affected by hypoparathyroidism. (From Gennari C, Avioli LV (eds) Atlante delle Malattie Dell'osso, Vol. II. Parma: Chiesi Farmaceutici S.p.A., 1992.)

Cardiovascular disorders

A prolongation of the QT interval on the electrocardiogram may be observed in patients with hypocalcemia. Congestive heart failure may occur in patients with HP.[4]

Biochemically, the HP is characterized by hypocalcemia and hyperphosphatemia in the presence of

> **Table 13.1**
> Causes of hypoparathyroidism.
>
> Failure of parathyroid gland development
>   Isolated hypoparathyroidism (X-linked, autosomal recessive)
>   DiGeorge syndrome
>   Kenny–Caffey syndrome
>   Mitochondrial neuromyopathies (Kearns–Sayre syndrome)
>   GCMB gene mutation GATA3 gene mutation
> Destruction of the parathyroid glands
>   Surgical
>   Polyglandular autoimmune disease (APACED)
>   Radiation
>   Metal overload (iron, copper)
>   Granulomatous infiltration
>   Neoplastic invasion
> Reduced parathyroid gland function due to altered regulation
>   Primary (autosomal dominant—calcium-sensing receptor mutation, PTH gene mutation; autosomal recessive—PTH gene mutation)
>   Secondary (maternal hyperparathyroidism, hypomagnesemia)
> Impaired PTH action
>   Hypomagnesemia
>   Pseudohypoparathyroidism

normal renal function. The amount of urinary Ca is reduced, although Ca excretion is high relative to the plasma Ca level. Serum PTH is low or undetectable, except in cases of PTH resistance (PHP) in which case it is elevated or high normal. The serum level of 1,25-dihydroxyvitamin D is usually low or normal. Finally, nephrogenous cyclic adenosine monophosphate (cAMP) excretion is low. Urinary cAMP and phosphorus excretion both increase markedly after administration of exogenous bioactive PTH, except in PHP.

The causes of HP can be classified as: (1) failure of parathyroid gland development; (2) destruction of the parathyroid glands; (3) reduced parathyroid gland function due to altered regulation; and (4) impaired PTH action (Table 13.1).

Failure of the parathyroid glands

Congenital agenesis or hypoplasia of the parathyroid glands can produce HP that manifests in the newborn period. This may occur as isolated HP or be associated with thymic aplasia and immunodeficiency and congenital conotruncal cardiac anomalies. Several genetic and environmental factors are responsible for this syndrome, which is characterized by a developmental field defect of the third and fourth pharyngeal pouches.[5] This condition is known as DiGeorge syndrome. Detection of the microdeletion of chromosomal band 22q11.21–q11.23 by using fluorescence in situ hybridization is diagnostic, but a negative result does not completely exclude the possibility of a 22q abnormality.[6] A small group of patients have been shown to carry deletions on the short arm of chromosome 10.[7] Finally, karyotypic abnormalities on other chromosomes have also been reported. It is probable that other genetic loci will be identified as being important for parathyroid development. The term CATCH indicates a complex disorder characterized by cardiac anomalies, abnormal facies, thymic aplasia, cleft palate and hypocalcemia with 22q deletion. All patients with unexplained HP in infancy should be karyotyped for 22q11 or 10p microdeletions and evaluated for other occult anomalies.

The clinical manifestations occur in the neonatal period, mostly because of cardiac problems (90% of recorded patients have had a cardiac defect), and in some cases as convulsions. In addition, infections are rare causes of early death in these patients, but a high susceptibility to infections becomes more important with increasing age. Most of the patients have low T-cell counts or evidence of thymus aplasia. In 50% of the patients, B-lymphocyte counts are supernormal. In

71%, total blood lymphocyte counts are normal. Many patients have hypergammaglobulinemia.[8]

Sometimes, HP is associated with rare syndromes such as Barakat syndrome (HP, nerve deafness and renal dysplasia), the Kenney–Caffey syndrome (HP, growth retardation, slender long bones, macrocephaly, delayed closure of the anterior fontanelle, eye abnormality)[9] and Kearns–Sayre syndrome (ophthalmoplegia, retinal degeneration, cardiac conduction defects).

Destruction of the parathyroid glands

The surgical ablation of the parathyroid gland is the most frequent cause of HP. The resulting HP can be transient or permanent and sometimes may not develop for many years. Transient and reversible postoperative hypocalcemia following parathyroid surgery can be due to (1) edema or hemorrhage into the parathyroid, (2) hungry bone syndrome, or (3) hypomagnesemia.[10]

HP may also occur as an autoimmune disorder called type I polyglandular syndrome (APS-1). It can be sporadic or familial, transmitted by an autosomal recessive mutant gene located in chromosome 21q22.3.[11] The triad characteristic of this syndrome is represented by HP, adrenal insufficiency and mucocutaneous candidiasis. The clinical onset of the three principal components of the syndrome typically follows a predictable pattern, in which mucocutaneous candidiasis first appears, followed by HP and adrenal insufficiency. Antibodies against parathyroid and adrenal tissue have been demonstrated in many patients.[12] HP appears at ages 2–4 years, and Addison's disease appears at ages 10–14 years. Other manifestations can occur in these patients, such as intestinal fat malabsorption, gastric parietal cell failure with vitamin B_{12} malabsorption, chronic hepatitis, dermal vasculitis, insulin-dependent diabetes mellitus, primary hypogonadism, autoimmune thyroiditis, alopecia (totalis or areata), and ocular disease (keratopathy, iritis, retinitis pigmentosa).

Reduced parathyroid gland function due to altered regulation

Primary alterations of parathyroid function may be due to genetic defects. Activating mutations of the Ca-sensing receptor (CaSR) (i.e. a receptor with a decreased set-point for extracellular Ca concentrations) cause a functional HP with hypocalcemia and hypercalciuria. In cases in which the mutations are transmitted through several generations, the picture is one of familial autosomal dominant HP.

Isolated HP has also been described with a single base substitution in exon 2 of the PTH gene.[13] The autosomal recessive isolated HP has usually arisen in families with consanguineous marriages. Abnormalities of the PTH gene have been described, and in one family a donor splice site mutation at exon 2 of the PTH gene has been identified.[14]

Secondary causes of HP include maternal HP and/or hypomagnesemia. The infant generally develops hypocalcemia within the first 3 weeks of life.

Pseudohypoparathyroidism
Impaired PTH action

PHP describes a heterogeneous syndrome characterized by biochemical HP, increased plasma levels of PTH, and unresponsiveness of target tissues to the biological actions of PTH. In the initial classical description of PHP, Albright et al focused on the failure of patients with this syndrome to show either a calcemic or a phosphaturic response to administered parathyroid extract.[15]

Types of PHP

Several kinds of basic defects have indeed been identified in PHP. The PTH receptor is coupled by heterotrimeric guanine nucleotide-binding regulatory proteins (G proteins) to signal effector molecules localized to the inner surface of the plasma membrane.[16] Characterization of the molecular basis for PHP commenced with the observation that cAMP mediates many of the actions of PTH on kidney and bone and that administration of biologically active PTH to normal subjects leads to a significant increase in the urinary excretion of nephrogenous cAMP.[17] Table 13.2 shows the various causes of PHP.

PHP type Ia
Albright's original description of PHP emphasized PTH resistance, the biochemical hallmark of this disorder. Resistance to PTH alone would be consis-

	PHP Ia	PPHP	PHP Ib	PHP Ic	PHP II
Phenotype	AHO	AHO	Normal	AHO	Normal
Response to PTH:					
Urinary cAMP	Low	Normal	Low	Low	Normal
Urinary phosphate	Low	Normal	Low	Low	Low
Serum Ca	Low	Normal	Low	Low	Low
Hormone resistance	Multiple	No	Only to PTH	Multiple	Only to PTH
Gsα activity	Reduced	Reduced	Normal	Normal	Normal
Molecular defect	Mutation Gsα gene	Mutation Gsα gene	PTH receptor (?)	Unknown	Unknown

Table 13.2
Various forms of pseudohypoparathyroidism.

tent with a defect in the cell-surface receptor specific for PTH. Sometimes, patients with PHP type I display resistance to multiple hormones whose effects are mediated by cAMP. In addition, cell membranes from most of these patients have an approximately 50% reduction in expression or activity of Gsα protein. The constellation of developmental and somatic defects are collectively termed Albright's hereditary osteodystrophy (AHO).[15] Patients with AHO who lack apparent hormone resistance have been classified as having pseudopseudohypoparathyroidism (PPHP). Gsα deficiency in patients with AHO results from heterozygous inactivating mutations in the *GNAS1* gene, a complex gene that maps to 20q13.2.[18] Most AHO patients with decreased G_s bioactivity have an approximately 50% decrease in expression of Gsα mRNA and protein.[19] Similar decreases in G_s bioactivity and Gsα expression are present in both PHP Ia and PPHP. However, the mechanism by which some patients with heterozygous *GNAS1* mutations develop multihormone resistance (PHPIa) while others do not (PPHP) has remained ill-defined. A possible role for imprinting in the pathogenesis of AHO has been suggested.[20] Genomic imprinting is an epigenetic phenomenon affecting some genes, whereby one allele has partial or total loss of expression. If the paternal allele *GNAS1* is imprinted (poorly expressed), then maternal transmission of a null mutation would result in little or no Gsα expression and would be associated with hormone resistance (PHP Ia). In contrast, paternal transmission should result in a similar level of Gsα expression to that found in normals and should not be associated with a defect in hormone action (PPHP).[21]

PHP type Ia is characterized by the following clinical picture.

AHO is characterized by short stature, round face, depressed nasal bridge, stocky or obese body and bone anomalies. The latter consist of brachymetacarpia of, in decreasing order of prevalence, metacarpals IV (Figure 13.3), V, I, III and rarely, and never alone, II, and brachymetatarsia of IV, V, III and I. Hand and foot abnormalities are not generally apparent before 4 years of age, and the typical phenotype may not present until school age. Ossified plaques and nodules, called

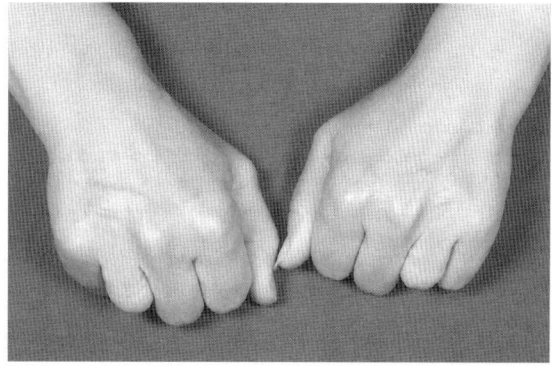

Figure 13.3
Brachymetacarpia of the IVth finger (black arrows) in a patient with PHP Ia.

osteomas, occur frequently in subcutaneous tissues, brain and heart. Calcification of the basal ganglia has been observed in up to 10% of adult patients. Finally, dental abnormalities are common. A mild to moderate mental retardation occurs in about 50–70% of patients. Spinal cord compression has developed as a result of abnormal vertebral fusion. Some patients have completely normal habitus.

Biochemical signs are characterized by hypocalcemia, which develops only after the first years of life and may alternate with normocalcemia. PTH levels show an inverse correlation with plasma Ca levels. In some patients, the secretion of PTH may be suppressed secondary to calcitriol deficiency. Resistance to other hormones is frequent. Clinically, HP as a result of thyroidal resistance is the most common. The thyroid-stimulating hormone (TSH) response to thyrotropin-releasing hormone (TRH) is exaggerated in nearly all patients. Clinical hypogonadism may be present, particularly in females, due to ovarian gonadotropin resistance. Growth hormone (GH) secretion is usually normal. Most patients with PHP have the AHO habitus but no endocrine abnormality.

PHP type Ib

People with PHP type Ib have normal habitus and intelligence. There is normal G_s activity and hormone resistance is limited to PTH. Short stature is common, and prolactin deficiency may occur. These patients have a severe osteitis fibrous cystica with bone pain which resolves only after parathyroidectomy.

PHP type II

These individuals have biochemical features of HP, with a normal cAMP response, but an abnormal phosphaturic response to PTH. Type II PHP may develop with vitamin D deficiency. Sjögren's syndrome may include type II PHP, presumably by an autoimmune mechanism.

The diagnosis of PHP requires the PTH test to be performed with biosynthetic fragments of human PTH, with determination of plasma and/or urinary cAMP responses (Table 13.3).

Subject should be in a fasting state, and active urine output should be initiated and maintained by the ingestion of 200 ml water/h, beginning 2 h before the PTH infusion.

Baseline: Urine collection (60 min before PTH infusion)

Infusion of PTH fragment (200 units in an adult and 3 units/kg body weight in children over the age of 3 years) intravenously over 10 min.

Time 0: Urine collection, blood collection
Time +30 min: Urine collection
Time +60 min: Urine collection
Time +120 min Urine collection, blood collection

Urine samples should be analyzed for cAMP, phosphorus and creatinine concentration.
Blood samples should be analyzed for serum creatinine and phosphorus concentrations.

Response
The response (cAMP : nmol/l glomerular filtrate (GF)) during the first 30 min from the start of PTH infusion differentiates patients with PHP type I from patients with hypoparathyroidism and from normal subjects.

Normal subjects: 10- to 20-fold increase in urinary cAMP
Patients with hypoparathyroidism: 10- to 20-fold increase in urinary cAMP
Patients with PHP type Ia: low increase in urinary cAMP
Patients with PPHP: normal response

Table 13.3
Synthetic PTH infusion test.

Therapy

Acute therapy

The correction of the hypocalcemic state depends on the clinical severity of the condition. A patient who is convulsing or has laryngeal stridor or severe tetany should be given a prompt intravenous injection of 10% calcium gluconate solution (0.25 ml/kg over >2 min). A continuous infusion should then follow (1.7 ml/kg) of the 10% solution over 6–12 h.[22] Oral administration of Ca salts is quite efficient for the control of hypocalcemia and is preferable to prolonged infusion.

Long-term therapy

The principal goal of therapy in HP and PHP is to restore the serum Ca and phosphate. If therapy is successful, HP does not disturb the patient's life, and long-term complications are avoided. One of the most important problems with the restoration of normocalcemia is the development of hypercalciuria, with a resulting predilection for renal stone formation. In addition to medication, therapy must include the regular intake of relatively large amounts of fluid. In patients with PHP, in contrast to those with HP, therapy should maintain plasma Ca at the high normal level. The basic differences between these two conditions dictating this difference in therapy are as follows: (1) normocalcemia causes hypercalciuria in HP but not in PHP; and (2) in PHP, even low normal calcemia is associated with secondary hyperparathyroidism, which may harm the skeleton.

If serum is normalized but phosphate remains greater than 1.9 mmol/l, a non-absorbable antacid may be added to reduce the hyperphosphatemia and prevent ectopic calcification.

Calcium and calciferol sterol are the main agents available. The dose of sterol must be carefully adjusted and frequently monitored, because the serum Ca may change, even after long periods of steady normocalcemia.

Vitamin D (D_2 and D_3 are identical in effect) has a slow, prolonged and cumulative action. The use of these sterols involves a risk of severe prolonged hypercalcemia because they are stored in adipose tissue. Calcitriol and $1\alpha(OH)D$ are the fastest and shortest-acting vitamin D derivatives. In a comparative study of therapy in adults with HP or PHP, the mean daily dosages were similar for calcitriol (1.5 μg) and dihydrotachysterol (DHT) (450 μg).[23] In contrast, more $1\alpha(OH)D$ was required in HP (4 μg) than in PHP (2 μg). The full effect of DHT is reached in 10–20 days, and in moderate hypercalcemia the DHT intake is discontinued for a few days and restarted only when a repeat serum Ca is normal (Table 13.4).

Close monitoring of urine Ca, serum Ca and serum phosphate are required in the first month.

Patients with PHP type Ia will frequently manifest resistance to other hormones in addition to PTH, and may display clinical evidence of hypothyroidism or gonadal dysfunction.

Sterol	Average dosage (μ/kg/day)	Average $t_{\frac{1}{2}}$ (days)
$1,25(OH)_2D_3$	0.03	1
$1\alpha(OH)D$	0.06	2
DHT	20	7
$25(OH)D$	4	15
D_2 and D_3	50	30

Table 13.4 Calciferol sterols.

Primary hyperparathyroidism

Introduction

Primary hyperparathyroidism (PHPT) represents the major cause of hypercalcemia in outpatient subjects. Before the 1970s, PHPT was suspected and diagnosed in patients presenting with traditionally associated features such as hypercalcemia, renal stones, and bone fractures. Recently, due to the worldwide introduction of multichannel analyzers in clinical biochemistry laboratories, serum Ca levels are routinely evaluated.[24,25] Thus, PHPT has become a relatively 'common' disease. It rarely presents as the 'bones, stones, groans' picture accounting for bone alterations, renal stones and psychic disorders as described by Albright. More frequently, the patient with PHPT is asymptomatic. Its incidence is between 1:500 and 1:1000.[26] It can occur at all ages, but most frequently presents during the sixth decade of life, with the ratio of affected women/men = 3:1.[27] When PHPT presents at young age (children, adolescents, young adults), physicians are strongly recommended to investigate for a familial form of PHPT, such as MEN 1 and/or MEN 2A.

PHPT produces hypercalcemia due to the hypersecretion of PTH by one or more parathyroid glands. About 80% of cases of PHPT are due to a solitary, benign adenoma. Less frequently, multiple adenomas, hyperplasia of all parathyroid glands and carcinoma occur. The latter represents no more than 0.5% of PHPT cases,[28] while hyperplasia can be seen in 15–20% of PHPT patients. Parathyroid hyperplasia is commonly associated with multiple endocrine neoplasia type 1 and 2 syndromes.

Pathophysiological aspects

PHPT pathophysiology can be briefly summarized as follows:

1. Proliferative disorder caused by alterations of several genetic mechanisms with clonal loss or gain of cell function, as clearly demonstrated by molecular genetic studies.[29–35]
2. Extracellular Ca set-point disorder causing the loss of normal feedback control of PTH production and secretion by extracellular Ca concentrations.[34]

Finally, in a few patients, a past history of external neck irradiation in childhood should also be taken into consideration.

Clinical classification

In the context of a Consensus Conference held at the National Institutes of Health (NIH),[36–37] a clinical classification of PHPT has been proposed:

1. Severe PHPT.
2. Symptomatic and complicated PHPT.
3. Asymptomatic, but complicated PHPT.
4. Asymptomatic and uncomplicated PHPT.

The term asymptomatic indicates PHPT forms without clinical evidence or symptoms or biochemical anomalies previously referred to. The frequency of asymptomatic PHPT ranges from 20% to 50% of total cases. The complicated form encompasses cases in which a potentially dangerous functional defect due to PTH hypersecretion is evident, such as occult calculosis, hypercalciuria, osteopenia, and hypertension both in the presence and absence of symptoms. The severe form represents a life-risk situation and comprises <1% of total cases.[38]

Complicated asymptomatic PHPT represents the most difficult form to be defined, due to the several possibilities of differential diagnoses of causes accounting for both osteopenia and peptic ulcer. In such a situation, physicians have to face some problems: (1) evaluation of the most accurate method, demonstrating the best cost–benefit ratio, to diagnose PHPT; (2) evaluation of the real need for neck surgery compared to long-term accurate clinical follow-up of asymptomatic patients; and (3) identification of the best and safest follow-up procedure for these patients. For patients over 50 years of age exhibiting mild hypercalcemia, with bone and renal function substantially conserved, an accurate clinical survey can be proposed, until the indications for surgery appear (Table 13.5).

According to these guidelines, approximately 50% of typical PHPT patients will meet the criteria to undergo surgery.[39]

Clinical presentation of asymptomatic PHPT

These patients are most frequently detected using routine biochemical screening. Specific symptoms are generally lacking. Patients often report a sense of weakness without signs of neuromuscular disorders.[40] Other 'aspecificities', such as depression, difficulty in concentrating and several other deficits, might very often be described.[41] Such symptomatology is extremely difficult to quantify. About 30% of asymptomatic patients have a slight reduction of

---

Calcemia >3 mmol/l or >0.25 mmol/l above the upper limits of normal
Marked hypercalciuria >400 mg/day
Bone density >−2 SD when compared to age- and sex-matched controls
An episode of acute PHPT with life-threatening hypercalcemia
Clear clinical evidence of PHPT: calculosis, fibrous cystic osteitis, neuromuscular disorders (rare)
Age <50 years

Table 13.5.
Guidelines for neck surgery.

bone mass. Table 13.6 summarizes indications for investigations of phosphorus–calcium metabolism.

Diagnostic set of PHPT patients

According to the Consensus Conference, PHPT diagnosis can be established on the presence of both a persistent hypercalcemia (after eliminating possible artefacts) and inappropriately high circulating levels of PTH, measured as intact molecule. The following steps are advised:

1. Laboratory investigations to confirm the diagnosis: Ca, phosphate, PTH (at least two independent determinations on different days), gastrin, urinary Ca and phosphate excretion.
2. When anamnesis is indicative, laboratory tests to exclude/include endocrinopathies (i.e. MEN 1, MEN 2, familial isolated hyperparathyroidism (FIHP)).
3. Evaluation of organ damage (kidneys, bone, heart, vessels) secondary to PHPT.
4. Evaluation of other possible associated disorders (i.e. chronic atrophic gastritis, neoplasms, thyroid disorders).
5. Imaging for localization (e.g. ultrasound (US), scintigraphy). This may be used for the evaluation of specific cases prior to surgery.

Useful notes for clinical practice

In several clinical circumstances, patients with PHPT present a real normocalcemic state or only a mild and intermittent hypercalcemia, the so-called 'normocalcemic PHPT'. In other circumstances, we can find patients with normal values of PTH also compatible with a diagnosis of PHPT. Patients exhibiting concomitant malabsorption and/or vitamin D deficiency might present with bone disease but with normal blood Ca values, 'PHPT masked by vitamin D deficiency'. Bone disease may be present as fibrous cystic osteitis (Figure 13.4), variably accompanied by

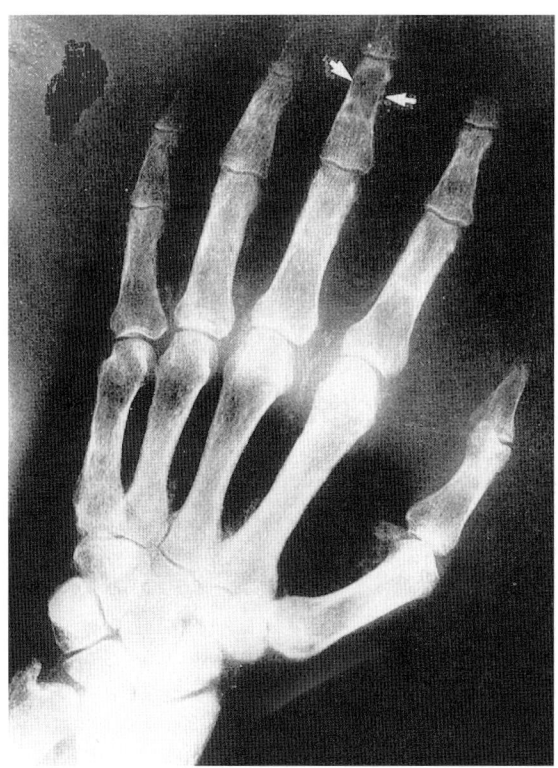

Figure 13.4
Osteolytic area of the phalanx (white arrows) in a patient affected by PHPT. (From Gennari C, Avioli LV (eds) Atlante delle Malattie Dell'osso, Vol. II. Parma: Chiesi Farmaceutici S.p.A., 1992.)

Familial anamnesis
  Renal stones
  Recurrent peptic ulcers
  Pancreatitis
  Osteoporosis with bone fractures
  Other endocrinopathies (pituitary, thyroid, adrenal)
Physiological anamnesis
  Asthenia, weakness
  Thirst increasing
  Appetite decreasing
  Weight loss in last year
  Polyuria
  Stypsis
Remote and near-pathological anamnesis
  Duodenal or gastric peptic ulcer
  Renal stones
  Pancreatitis
  Depression, intellectual weariness
  Fractures
  Hypertension

Table 13.6
Suspect elements for PHPT in outpatient visit.

osteomalacia. Other bone manifestations of PHPT include subperiosteal resorption of the distal phalanges (Figure 13.5), tapering of the distal clavicles, a 'salt and pepper' appearance of the skull, bone cysts (Figure 13.4), brown tumors, pathological fractures of the long bones and loss of lamina dura of the teeth.[42] PHPT-related bone disease is, however, quite unusual, occurring in less than 5% of patients.[38] Bone mineral density (BMD) measurements by dual emission X-ray absorptiometry (DEXA) has become a gold standard technique to assess the bone involvement in PHPT and to monitor the efficacy of the treatment. The anatomical sites exhibiting the most striking losses of BMD are mainly represented by the femoral neck and mid-radius.

Patients affected by mild PHPT and renal disease constitute the more frequent and difficult problem. Typically, these patients exhibit a mild and intermittent hypercalcemic state with oscillation of calcemia of 0.125–1.25 mmol/l, average 2.52–2.55 mmol/l. Such a situation can be identified only after repeating serum Ca evaluations. The diagnosis of PHPT has to be considered in any patient exhibiting renal stones and with an average value of calcemia greater than 2.5 mmol/l in three determinations in fasting patients.

Asymptomatic PHPT follow-up

Patients with asymptomatic PHPT exhibit serum Ca levels not usually higher than 0.25 mmol/l above the upper limits of normal. They should be regularly followed by evaluating calcemia and urinary Ca excretion. There should also be an assessment of possible organ damage, including kidney (renal functionality), bone (BMD evaluation, bone turnover markers), and cardiovascular (blood pressure measurement).

It is now possible to confidently assess whether a patient will develop progressively severe disease or remain in a stable state.[43]

Imaging in PHPT

Imaging investigations may help surgeons in gland/s localization. Imaging techniques do not accurately identify parathyroid glands of normal size, but they do identify the glands in cases of hyperplasia and adenoma.[44]

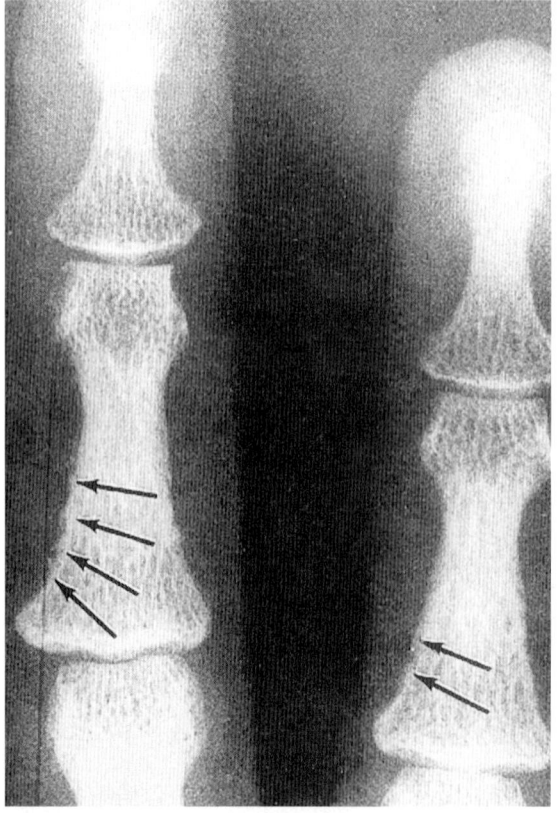

Figure 13.5
Subperiosteal resorption of the distal phalanges (black arrows) in a patient affected by PHPT. (From Gennari C, Avioli LV (eds) Atlante delle Malattie Dell'osso, Vol. II. Parma: Chiesi Farmaceutici S.p.A., 1992.)

Lack of a clear distinction between thyroid and parathyroid nodules
Small size and the generally ellipsoidal shape of pathological parathyroids (with at least two of the three axes exhibiting dimensions <1 cm)
Frequent coexistence of goiter and thyroiditis interfering with diagnostic procedures
Possibility of ectopic localization of parathyroid glands

Table 13.7
Difficulties in parathyroid imaging evaluation.

In persistent or recurrent postsurgery PHPT, preoperative localization of hyperplastic/adenomatous glands is required. Reoperation is complicated by the alteration of anatomy and presence of fibrous tissue that follows previous surgery.[45]

Several parathyroid imaging techniques are used, including US, scintigraphy, CT and MR, but no single technique is fully reliable. For first operations, many surgeons prefer direct surgical exploration, which, in expert hands, is successful in 90–95% of cases. The main difficulties of parathyroid imaging evaluation are briefly summarized in Table 13.7.

US doppler

US permits the direct visualization of enlarged pathological glands. As for other anatomical regions, parathyroid US always remains an operator-dependent technique. Owing to the superficial disposition of parathyroid glands, the use of a high-frequency probe (7.5–10 MHz) is required.[46–48]

US can be used for fine needle aspiration (FNA) biopsy for cytological examination.[49]

Doppler examination enables parathyroid gland vascularization to be viewed. The power color doppler can be helpful in differential diagnosis, with vascular structures and/or thyroid nodular lesions both exhibiting peripheral capsular flows.[50]

Parathyroid scintigraphy

The most frequent nuclear medicine techniques for the detection of parathyroid enlargement consist of double-tracer and double-phase scintigraphy. The former takes advantage of the different kinetics of the two radiotracers, while the latter utilizes a unique radiotracer which exhibits a different releasing time from healthy to hyperplastic/adenomatous tissue.

The most common tracer is represented by technetium-99m-2-methoxy-isobutyl-isonitrile (^{99m}Tc-MIBI), whose intracellular accumulation depends on both the number and activity of mitochondria.[51–55] Moreover, MIBI accumulation is proportional to blood-flow and capillary permeability. Reported data demonstrate a high diagnostic accuracy for the double-tracer technique, 67–100% in cases of adenoma and 56–100% for hyperplasia. The advantages offered by the double-phase method are mainly represented by the minor dose of radiation for the patient, the less time required, and the lack of image subtraction artefacts.

To date, parathyroid scintigraphy represents one of the most accurate techniques in the detection of parathyroid hyperplasia–adenoma. It has the advantage of enabling ectopic parathyroids to be identified.

In a general context, parathyroid scintigraphy exhibits two major limitations, which depend upon the glands' size and the possibility of false-positive results. For glands weighing less than 300 mg the method's sensitivity greatly decreases. This is clearly demonstrated by the lower sensitivity of this technique in localized parathyroid glands. False positivity is a problem in the presence of nodular thyroid disease, which has a similar uptake of radiotracer to the parathyroid glands.

In the last 2 years, another cationic complex, tetrofosmin, labeled with ^{99m}Tc, has been used for imaging. Both the sensitivity and specificity data reported in the literature overlap with those of ^{99m}Tc-MIBI scintigraphy.[54,55] A more recent experimental method consists of tomography with ^{99m}Tc-MIBI or tetrofosmin (SPECT). This technique provides improved spatial resolution, enabling the identification of smaller glands and their differentiation from thyroid nodules.[56,57]

Computerized tomography (CT)

Classical CT is rarely used in preoperative localization of parathyroid glands, because of the presence of artefacts. It is, however, useful for the localization of ectopic mediastinal glands. Spiral CT has generated new interest in this form of imaging for parathyroid disease. The possibility of evaluating arterial perfusion offers the opportunity of looking for parathyroid contrastographic features, providing differential diagnosis with thyroid and lymph node diseases.[45,58]

Magnetic resonance (MR)

Parathyroid tissue does not exhibit a pattern signal significantly different from that of the thyroid tissue. Thus, structural and morphological alterations of hyperplastic/neoplastic parathyroid tissue are not easily identified with this technique.[59–64]

Therapeutic approaches to PHPT

Neck surgery

Neck surgery still remains the primary and definitive therapy of PHPT. The goal of surgery is represented by both parathyroid hyperfunction resolution and stable euparathyroid condition restoration. Thus, it is mandatory to perform in all patients an accurate bilateral cervical exploration, looking for at least four parathyroid glands.

Surgical strategy differs for adenomas and hyperplasias. Removal of a parathyroid adenoma cures the disease.[65–67] More difficulties occur with parathyroid hyperplasia. This is often associated with inherited diseases such as MEN 1, MEN 2A and FIHP syndromes. For parathyroid hyperplasia, three different possible approaches have been described:

1. Total parathyroidectomy (TPTX) with autotransplantation of a parathyroid remnant in the nondominant forearm. This is associated with a risk of permanent/temporary HP (0–30%). The risk of permanent hypofunction can be minimized if the surgery is performed by a skilled neck surgeon. Conversely, there is a minor risk of recurrence of parathyroid hyperfunction (0–20%). In this situation, the autotransplanted tissue fragment can be removed.
2. TPTX with the deliberate aim of producing permanent HP which is then treated medically.
3. Subtotal parathyroidectomy (SPTX) with a $3-3\frac{1}{2}$ removal of parathyroid hyperplastic tissue, leaving on site no more than 50 mg of tissue, with a higher risk of local persistent or recurrent PHPT (up to 50% of cases), but with a very low risk of postsurgery HP (0–10%).

When the surgeon faces a MEN-associated PHPT or an FIHP, in both TPTX and SPTX techniques, a transcervical thymectomy must be performed.[68–74]

Until a few years ago, after the surgical localization of whole parathyroid tissue, its intrasurgical macroscopic evaluation took a long time. Actually, the opportunity of performing intraoperative PTH measurement makes it possible to avoid the neck bilateral exploration, especially in cases of adenoma, and to decrease the duration of surgery.[75–81] A decrease of 70% of basal PTH levels after 15 minutes from gland removal can exclude the presence of a second adenoma or hyperplasia. Adenomatous PHPT surgery can achieve normalization of calcemia in 95–98% of cases.

Unsuccessful surgery is most frequently the result of an inexperienced surgeon. Other causes include ectopic adenoma, multiple adenomas or supranumerary glands.[82] Reoperation of a persistent or recurrent case of PHTP may present serious difficulties.

Medical management

The recommended approach to PHPT is surgical. Some patients can, however, for several reasons be managed conservatively. It is mandatory to give them some precise instructions, such as an appropriate water balance, active life, and careful use of diuretics (avoid thiazides). Dietary Ca intake should be moderate (it is not necessary to avoid dairy products). Dietary Ca restriction is not advised, because of parathyroid gland stimulation. Difficulty in clinical management occurs for patients with PHPT masked by vitamin D deficiency.[83] They can be recognized by mild hypercalcemia and low 25(OH)D and 1-25(OH)2D$_3$ levels. As such, vitamin D deficiency can exacerbate the associated bone disease. Vitamin D deficiency does, however, moderate the hypercalcemia limiting the Ca intestinal absorption and its removal from bone. The correction of vitamin D deficiency can aggravate hypercalcemia, although it may be beneficial for bone disease. Controlled studies in this field have not yet been performed.

Theoretically, estrogens might have a potential beneficial role in asymptomatic PHPT treatment, through both their anti-PTH effect and prevention of bone loss.[84–86]

Bisphosphonates, such as alendronate and risedronate, might be helpful in inhibiting bone reabsorption, and reducing serum Ca levels. Available data to date indicate that neither ethidronate nor clodronate are efficacious in chronic treatment.[87]

New medical therapeutic approaches

Availability of an effective pharmacological therapy could benefit not only the asymptomatic patients, but also those patients in whom surgery is not suitable due to intercurrent diseases and recurrent or persistent PHPT. The discovery of a Ca-sensing receptor in parathyroid cells, whose activation decreases PTH secretion, has opened up an exciting area of research for medical therapy of PHPT. Molecules able to mimic the Ca effect could activate the receptor and then inhibit parathyroid function. In 1993, a role for PTH secretion inhibition by 'calcium mimetics' was described. In fact, a compound named NPS R568 can be given orally. Recent studies have demonstrated encouraging results for this molecule in reduction of both calcemic and PTH levels, without any important adverse events. Such molecules have a great potential for medical treatment of primary or secondary hyperparathyroidism.[88–92]

Other causes of hypercalcemia

Pathogenesis

Hypercalcemia develops when the amount of Ca in the blood exceeds the amount eliminated by urine. This

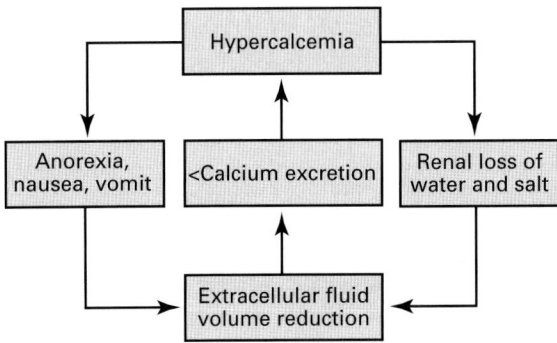

Figure 13.6
Scheme of pathogenic mechanisms of hypercalcemia.

can happen in: (1) accelerated bone resorption (more frequent);[93] (2) excessive gastrointestinal reabsorption exceeding both the urinary excretion and the capacity of the skeleton to accept Ca; and (3) less frequently, when a normal aliquot of Ca enters the extracellular fluid but there is a concomitant impairment of both renal Ca excretion and bone mineralization (Figure 13.6).

Accelerated bone turnover

This frequently represents the first event in hypercalcemia, the osteoclast cells (OCs) being the target for PTH, PTHrP and $1,25(OH)_2D_3$.[94–95] Several human cytokines may exhibit a similar effect on OCs in different diseases (IL-1α, IL-1β, TNF-α, TGF-α), but their capacity to cause hypercalcemia in human diseases has not yet been elucidated.[96]

Excessive gastrointestinal reabsorption

This represents a rarer situation and may play a role in hypercalcemic states characterized by vitamin D excess (i.e. lymphoma, vitamin D intoxication).

In both the above situations, the kidney always constitutes the most important defense against hypercalcemia, and generally, hypercalciuria precedes hypercalcemia. The latter occurs when the renal threshold for Ca is overcome.[97]

PTH and PTHrP both cause an increase of both bone resorption and Ca absorption by the renal distal tubule. In addition, hypercalcemia impairs antidiuretic hormone (ADH) action at the distal tubule level, producing nephrogenic diabetes insipidus. The first mechanism may also be impaired, due to nausea and vomiting worsening the state of dehydration (Figure 13.6). In consequence, the decrease of extracellular fluid (ECF) volume concomitant with the reduction of glomerular filtration rate exacerbates the hypercalcemic state.

Clinical features

Clinical presentation may involve different organs, and both signs and symptoms are quite similar irrespective of etiology.[98] A great variability of presentation exists, depending on the Ca plasma level and the rate of rise. Mild symptomatology is frequent in the context of chronic hypercalcemia. Symptoms generally do not appear with plasma Ca levels >75 mmol/l. Symptoms will be always present when the serum Ca is >3.5 mmol/l.

Neurological symptoms

These are often predominant in hypercalcemic states and, depending on plasma Ca levels, they may vary from weakness (very common), sleepiness, difficulty in concentration, depression, confusion, to coma.

Gastrointestinal symptoms

The most common symptoms are constipation, anorexia, nausea and vomiting. Less frequently, patients may have symptoms of peptic ulcer or pancreatitis.

Renal symptoms

Polyuria, often associated with polydipsia, renal stones and nephrocalcinosis, represents the classical clinical features of renal involvement. Renal stones are present in 15–20% of HPT cases and nephrocalcinosis is prevalently present in chronic hypercalcemia.

Cardiac symptoms

Hypercalcemia increases the myocardium's repolarization rate, narrows the QT interval, and may produce bradycardia and first-degree AV block. There is increased sensitivity to digoxin.

Differential diagnosis

Table 13.8 details the most frequent clinical conditions associated with hypercalcemia.

- More common
    - PHPT malignancies
        - PTHrP production
            - Lung
            - Esophagus
            - Head–neck
            - Kidney
            - Ovary
            - Bladder
        - Ectopic calcitriol
            - Lymphoma
        - Metastatic osteolysis
            - Myeloma
            - Breast
        - Local or ectopic factors
- Less common
    - Endocrine diseases (thyrotoxicosis)
    - Granulomatous diseases (sarcoidosis)
    - Drugs
        - Vitamin D
        - Thiazides
        - Lithium
        - Estrogens and anti-estrogens
        - Androgens (therapy breast cancer)
        - Aminophylline
        - Vitamin A
        - Aluminum intoxication (CRF)
    - Miscellaneous
        - Immobilization
        - ARF and CRF
        - Parenteral nutrition
- Rare
    - Endocrine diseases (pheochromocytoma, VIPoma, FHH, Addison's disease)
    - Granulomatous diseases (calcitriol excess)
        - Tuberculosis
        - Histoplasmosis
        - Coccidiomycosis
        - Leprosy
- Miscellaneous
    - Milk-alkali syndrome
    - Hypophosphatasia

ARF, acute renal failure; CRF, chronic renal failure; FHH, familial hypocalciuric hypercalcemia

Table 13.8
Most frequent clinical conditions associated with hypercalcemia.

Particular forms of hypercalcemia

Humoral hypercalcemia of malignancy (HHM)

This is a distinct clinical syndrome where hypercalcemia is secondary to tumoral factors, particularly PTHrP. HMM is the most frequent cause of malignancy-associated hypercalcemia (Figure 13.7). Usually, the tumor exhibits scarce or absent skeletal involvement, and hypercalcemia disappears when the tumor is treated or removed. Unfortunately, such tumors usually have an unfavorable prognosis (exceptions are represented by pheochromocytoma and some malignancies of the insular pancreas). The most frequent HHM causes are squamous carcinomas (head, neck, lung, esophagus, skin, etc.). Biochemically and histologically, HHM syndromes exhibit features common to PHPT (hypercalcemia, hypophosphatemia, increase of nephrogenic cAMP and high bone turnover). They differ, however, in that circulating levels of $1,25(OH)_2D_3$ are increased in PHPT, with a consequent increase in the intestinal absorption of Ca. Moreover, in contrast to HMM, patients with PHPT exhibit a moderate rate of hypercalciuria. Hypercalcemia in HHM patients depends on both the skeletal and renal components, as detailed above. Breast cancer may also be responsible for HMM. Hypercalcemia may also occur as a result of skeletal metastasis.[99] Generally, hypercalcemia is present in all cases of solid tumors associated with extensive bone destruction.

Hypercalcemia in the context of hematological malignancies

Myeloma

All patients affected by myeloma exhibit bone destruction, but hypercalcemia is present in only 20–40% of cases. Impaired renal function is quite common in myeloma (Bence-Jones' nephropathy, recurrent infec-

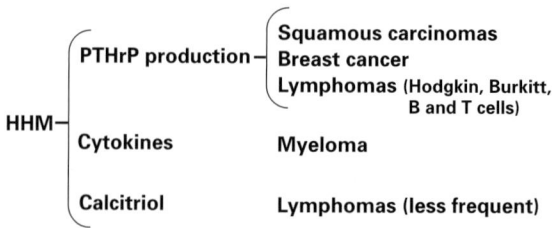

Figure 13.7
Particular conditions determining hypercalcemia.

tions, amyloidosis). Hypercalcemia develops from bone destruction by increased osteoclast activity due to tumoral cytokines (lymphotoxin, IL-6 and IL-1).[100–102] Bone alkaline phosphatase does not increase, because of scarce or absent bone formation. The recommended therapy is represented by pamidronate, careful monitoring of renal function, or alkylating drugs (treatment of primary disease) and corticosteroids.[103]

Lymphomas

Hypercalcemia occasionally occurs in Hodgkin's disease, and B-cell, T-cell and Burkitt's lymphomas.[104] It is probably due to the production of PTHrP by tumour cells,[105] although in a few cases it can be secondary to $1,25(OH)_2D_3$ production by neoplasm.[95,106]

Drug-sustained hypercalcemia
Vitamin D and correlated compounds

The daily recommended dose of vitamin D consists of 400–800 UI/day. The amount of vitamin D required to produce hypercalcemia is >50 000 UI/week. Hypercalcemia is usually well controlled after discontinuation of vitamin D, dietary Ca restriction and adequate hydration. If hypercalcemia persists, corticosteroids should be administered. It is important to bear in mind that the biological half-life of vitamin D is extremely long (weeks to months), whereas that of its metabolites is quite short (hours to days).

Alkali excess

Although less frequent than in the past, such a condition results from renal damage secondary to excessive ingestion of Ca and antacids (milk or calcium carbonate). Patients at risk are those affected by senile osteoporosis or subjects who have undergone long periods of parenteral nutrition. The pathogenic mechanism could be briefly summarized as: hypercalcemia → bicarbonate retention → alkalosis → renal calcium retention → severe hypercalcemia.[107]

The most important biochemical defects are represented by hypercalcemia, hyperphosphatemia, metabolic acidosis, and signs of renal impairment. The renal damage can be reversible, if readily recognized, after alkali suspension.

Hypercalcemia in granulomatous disorders

Hypercalcemia occurs in about 10% of patients suffering from sarcoidosis. Fifty per cent of patients will develop hypercalciuria in the course of the disease.[108] It is well known that the hypercalcemia is a result of increased production of $1,25(OH)_2D_3$. Recently, in other granuloma-forming diseases and lymphoproliferative disorders, high serum $1,25(OH)_2D_3$ concentrations have also been demonstrated. In both granulomatous and lymphoproliferative diseases, the source of $1,25(OH)_2D_3$ synthesis is extrarenal, generally lacking any physiological regulation.[109–111] The extrarenal sources of $1,25$-$(OH)_2D$ have been described as being the macrophage cells in sarcoidosis[112] and tumour cells in lymphoproliferative disorders.

Hypercalcemia in infants and children

Five particular hypercalcemic conditions are mentioned in Table 13.9. For their specific treatment, refer to specialized textbooks and international literature. Ionized Ca values in healthy infants and young children are similar to those of adults, with an average of ±2 SD, corresponding to 1.21 ± 0.13 mM. In newborns, the normal ionized Ca level depends on postnatal age. Generally, in the first 72 h after delivery, ionized Ca increases from 1.4 mM to 1.2 mM. Such a decrement is higher in premature infants.

Therapeutic approaches

The treatment will depend on the hypercalcemic values reached and on the presence/absence of related clinical manifestations. Generally, patients exhibiting plasma Ca levels of <3 mmol/l are asymptomatic and do not need medical intervention. Conversely, when Ca levels are ≥3.5 mmol/l, treatment should be given, regardless of symptoms. For intermediate Ca values of 3–3.5 mmol/l, physicians should be aggressive in the presence of hypercalcemic-related signs and symptoms.

It is extremely important to take into account the cause of hypercalcemia in order to decide the treatment strategy.

General principles

These are represented by the decrease of plasma Ca levels and the increase of its urinary excretion.[113,114] Patients must be hydrated with physiological saline solution to correct the deficit of the ECF volume (a 24–48 h continuous infusion of 3–4 l of 0.9% NaCl generally decreases the calcemia by approximately 0.25–0.75 mmol/l. Rehydration enhances the Ca urinary excretion by increasing the glomerular filtration and decreasing the reabsorption of Ca and sodium in both proximal and distal tubules.

Special points: (1) it can correct hypercalcemia only if Ca levels are moderately elevated; (2) attention to elder patients and to patients with cardiovascular and renal

> Williams' syndrome[231]
>   Hypercalcemia during the first year of age associated with cardiovascular malformations and elfic facies
>   Deletions of elastin gene on chromosome 7q
>   Pathogenic hypothesis: impaired control of vitamin D metabolism
> Idiopathic infantile hypercalcemia (IIH)[231]
>   Most children are born of mothers who have received very high vitamin D supplementation. However, cases in the absence of such supplementation have been described.
>   Incidence is increased
>   Children severely affected exhibit common features with Williams' syndrome, including cardiovascular alterations and dysmorphisms. Differential diagnosis is difficult. Hyperacusia may be present in IIH, but it is absent in Williams' syndrome
>   Pathogenic hypotheses: increased sensitivity to vitamin D. Recently, PTHrP levels have been reported in the context of hypercalcemia
> Subcutaneous liponecrosis[231]
>   Association between liponecrosis and significant birth trauma has been reported
>   Histological examination shows the presence of inflammatory infiltrate enriched in mononucleated cells and calcium crystals
>   Hypercalcemia has also been reported in children with subcutaneous liponecrosis and important traumas or disseminated varicella
>   Pathogenic hypothesis: increase of calcitriol and/or PGE
> Jensen's syndrome[231]
>   Hypercalcemia in newborns with rickets-like skeleton is a form of metaphyseal dysplasia caused by mutation of the PTH/PTHrP receptor gene on chromosome 3p22–21.1
>   Skeletal X-rays show patches of calcified cartilage in the distal part of long bones and more rarely at the skull and spinal levels
>   Hypercalcemia is a life-long disorder
> Hypophosphatasia[231]
>   It is a very rare form of inherited rickets or osteomalacia
>   Missense mutations of non-tissue-specific alkaline phosphatase (ALP) gene on chromosome 1p36.1–p34 or regulatory defects
>   Four different types have been described: perinatal, infantile, adolescent and adult
>   Reduction of ALP activity
>   Alterations of phospho-compound metabolism with their increase
>   Therapy recommended: calcium dietary restriction and/or glucocorticoids

Table 13.9
Causes of hypercalcemia in infants and children.

functional impairment; (3) in some circumstances, a loop diuretic (10–20 mg frusemide/l) can be added—it acts on the thick ascending part of Henle's loop, inhibiting Ca and sodium reabsorption, and moreover, it attenuates the risks of hypernatremia and volume overloading that can accompany saline infusion; (4) thiazides must be avoided because they decrease Ca urinary excretion.

Patients with renal failure or severe hypercalcemia may benefit from dialysis (peritoneal or hemodialysis).

Specific therapy
Bisphosphonates

Bisphosphonates have to be administered intravenously in at least 500 ml of volume for >4 h in order to prevent nephrotoxicity due to Ca-bisphosphonate precipitation. Pamidronate (60–90 mg in a single infusion) represents the powerful bisphosphonate for this specific treatment.

The most common side-effects are fever (about 20% of cases) and muscle pain the day after the treatment.

Normally, such effects can be prevented by pretreatment with aminoacetophene.

Occasional side-effects consist of transient leukopenia, light asymptomatic hypocalcemia (10%) and hypophosphatemia (10–30%), especially in patients treated with higher doses.

Both pamidronate and clodronate can reduce the progression of skeletal metastasis. Bisphosphonates can prevent the development of hypercalcemia in patients affected by breast cancer. Monthly infusion of pamidronate reduces the skeletal complications of multiple myeloma.

Calcitonin
Calcitonin reduces osteoclastic bone resorption with a rapid effect and increases Ca urinary excretion. Calcemia decreases by 0.5 mmol/l in 2–6 h when administered at a dosage of 4–8 UI/kg intramuscularly or subcutaneously every 8 h. Unfortunately, the hypocalcemic effect is transient and the calcemia is only rarely normalized. Calcitonin seems to be more efficient when combined with bisphosphonates or plycamicin.[113]

Plycamicin (mithramicin)
This is a cytotoxic antibiotic blocking RNA synthesis in the osteoclasts, and consequently inhibiting bone resorption. When administered at doses of 15–25 µg/kg in 4 h, it reduces calcemia within 12 h, achieving the nadir value in 48–72 h. Normally, a single dose is sufficient, but it can be repeated at 24–48-h intervals.

Nausea is quite common, but bone marrow, liver and renal toxicity (especially when repeated) represent the most important side-effects. Thus, it is not a suitable therapy for correcting chronic hypercalcemia.

Gallium nitrate
Originally used as an anticancer drug, this has also been approved by the FDA for the treatment of hypercalcemia. Its mechanism of action is still unclear, but it is thought to adsorb hydroxyapatite crystals[93] reducing their solubility, thus inhibiting bone resorption. Moreover, it also has a direct inhibitory action on osteoclasts.[115] When administered as a continuous intravenous infusion for 5 days at doses of 200 mg/m²/day, it is able to normalize the calcemia in most patients. However, calcemia decreases very slowly, reaching the nadir 3 days after infusion. Its use is contraindicated in renal failure or in combination with nephrotoxic drugs. Reductions of both plasma phosphate and hemoglobin concentrations have been described.

Glucocorticoids
These have been used for several years for the treatment of hypercalcemic conditions, especially if secondary to hematological tumors (lymphomas, myeloma). They are also effective in vitamin D toxicity or in granulomatous diseases, in which hypercalcemia is mediated by the actions of $1,25(OH)_2D_3$. The usual dose is 200–300 mg/day of intravenous hydrocortisone, or its equivalent, for 3–5 days.

Osteoporosis

Introduction
Osteoporosis is the most prevalent metabolic bone disease in developed countries and is defined as a systemic skeletal disease characterized by low bone mass and microarchitectural deterioration of bone tissue with a consequent increase in bone fragility and susceptibility to non-traumatic fracture.[116] A non-traumatic fracture is arbitrarily defined as one resulting from trauma equal to or less than a fall from a standing height. In the preclinical state, the disease is characterized simply by a low bone mass without fractures. An important characteristic of osteoporosis is a normal mineral/collagen ratio, which distinguishes it from osteomalacia, a disease characterized by a relative deficiency of mineral in

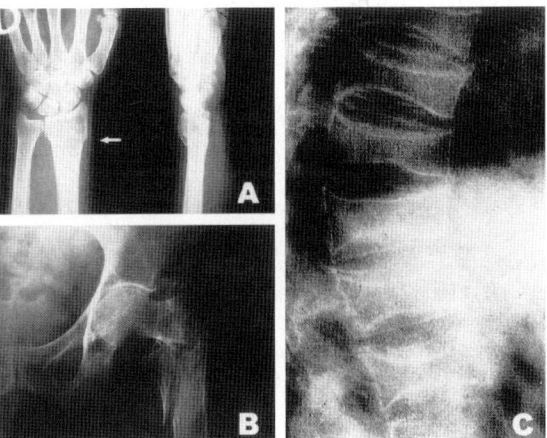

Figure 13.8
Typical osteoporotic fractures at the wrist (A), hip (B), and vertebral bodies (C). (From Gennari C, Avioli LV (eds) Atlante delle Malattie Dell'osso, Vol. I. Parma: Chiesi Farmaceutici S.p.A., 1992.)

relation to collagen. Osteoporotic fractures may affect any part of the skeleton except the skull. Most commonly, fractures occur in the distal forearm (Colle's fracture), thoracic and lumbar vertebrae, and proximal femur (Figure 13.8). The incidence of osteoporotic fractures increases with age, is higher in whites than in blacks, and is higher in women than in men. The female/male ratio is about 1.5:1 for Colle's fractures, 7:1 for vertebral fractures, and 2:1 for hip fractures. Because most osteoporotic fractures, except hip fractures, do not require admission to the hospital, it is difficult to obtain precise knowledge on the true prevalence of this disease.

Osteoporosis in the elderly has become a major public health problem for most industrialized societies as the average age of the population increases. Its significance will dramatically increase during the years to come. It has been calculated that the lifetime risk in women of 50 years is about 16% for hip fractures, 15% for wrist fractures, and 32% for vertebral fractures,[117] and that the costs related to hip fractures may double during the next 25 years.[118] Because bone loss accelerates after menopause, osteoporosis and osteoporotic fractures are much commoner among elderly women than among men. The prevalence of osteoporosis is reported to be lower in blacks than in Caucasian populations of European or Asiatic ancestry.[119] However, significant risk has been reported in people of all ethnic backgrounds. The prevention and treatment of osteoporosis is therefore of major importance for health organizations in all countries.

Bone metabolism and pathogenesis of osteoporosis

Bone is a vascularized skeletal tissue made up of an organic matrix, a mineral phase (calcium hydroxyapatite) and bone cells (osteoclasts, osteoblasts and osteocytes). The organic matrix is composed of fibers of collagen (chiefly type 1 collagen), elastin and other proteins. Apart from its ability to provide structural integrity, bone has several biochemical functions, bone itself serving as a Ca reservoir and its marrow as a hemopoietic organ. The constant renewal of bone tissue is the source of a number of biochemicals excreted into body fluids and the circulation. Bone formation by osteoblasts has two phases: synthesis of bone matrix, including the formation of a network of collagenous fibers, and mineralization of the matrix. Osteoclasts, in contrast, bring about bone resorption, which also consists of two simultaneous processes: dissolution of hydroxyapatite crystals and proteolysis of the matrix. Anatomically, bone can be divided into cortical (compact) and spongy (cancellous) parts. In spongy bone, the interconnecting trabecular structures increase resistance to mechanical load. Bone is constantly being remodeled, and the processes of formation and resorption of bone tissue are coupled. The cycle is initiated by resorption of old bone, recruitment of osteoblasts, deposition of new matrix and mineralization of that newly deposited matrix. Thus, remodeling provides a mechanism for bone self-repair and adaptation to stress, by a process of renewal of old bone and replacement with new bone. The annual bone turnover rates in adult women are about 2–5% in cortical bone and 15–25% in trabecular bone and cortical surfaces, the latter two types being metabolically most active. Spongy and cortical bones also differ in their hormonal sensitivity: the vertebral spine, which is rich in spongy bone, responds to hormonal treatments more strongly than appendicular bones with cortical bone dominance.[120]

The two most significant determinants of bone mass are the peak bone mass attained at about 30 years of age and the rate of bone loss after this.[121] These in turn are controlled by genetic, hormonal, nutritional and environmental factors, which are thus centrally involved in the pathogenesis of osteoporosis. Thus, a bone mass below average for age can be considered a consequence of inadequate accumulation of bone in young adult life (low peak bone mass) or of excessive rates of bone loss or, in some circumstances, of both conditions. In the lifelong process of bone turnover, formation is dominant in the growth period. Bone mass peaks at or before 30 years of age, sometimes even in the late teenage years.[122] At peak, the activity of bone-forming cells equals that of the resorbing cells, and skeletal size remains unchanged. Soon afterwards, bone mass begins to decrease, the average annual loss becoming about 0.3–0.5% by the fifth decade of life. In women after menopause, bone loss accelerates to about 2% (range 1–5%) for 5–10 years, stabilizing thereafter to about 1% per year, so that by age 65–70, bone loss is still above the premenopausal level.[123] During her lifetime, a normal woman will lose approximately half of her spinal bone and about a third of her cortical bone tissue. The postmenopausal decrease of estrogen is responsible for the increased bone-remodeling rate by enhancing the activity of both osteoblasts and, particularly, osteoclasts.[121] This remodeling unbalance results in irreversible bone loss. The increase in bone loss with age in women is made up of two components: an exponential, postmenopausal, estrogen-related component that lasts for 5–10 years, and a linear, age-related component[120] (Figure 13.9). This latter, slower phase of bone loss affects men, starting at about age 55 years, and has been attributed to age-related factors such as a reduction in renal Ca absorption as well as in intestinal Ca absorption and to a vitamin D deficiency status, mainly due to a decreased renal 1α-hydroxylase, all resulting in an increase in circulating PTH levels. Estrogen-related bone loss causes type I osteoporosis, characterized by loss of spongy bone tissue and fractures in spongy bones, such as crush fractures of the vertebral spine. Age-related bone loss due to declining activity of osteoblasts causes type II osteoporosis (senile osteoporosis), resulting in thinning of trabeculae and loss of cortical bone tissue, which also becomes porous. This predisposes to fractures of both spongy and cortical bones, and particularly of the femoral neck. In line with this classification, cross-sectional[124] and longitudinal[125] studies have shown that bone loss from the spine exceeds that from appendicular bones, at least during the early postmenopausal years. In elderly women, however, the age-related factor dominates. On average, a 70-year-old woman has lost 11% of her bone mass through lack of estrogen and 18% as a function of age. It has been calculated[126] that the opposite contributions of peak bone mass and postmenopausal bone loss to the risk of osteoporotic fracture are approximately equal at 75 years, the age when women enter the period of substantially increased risk for hip fracture. A number of diseases and drugs have been clearly related to accelerated bone loss, causing secondary osteoporosis. Their effects are superimposed on those described earlier. For example, a woman starting on corticosteroid therapy is more likely to have an osteoporotic fracture if she has low BMD resulting from low peak bone mass and the accelerated bone loss of the menopause. However, bone strength depends not only on bone mass: its quality, which seems to deteriorate with aging, is another important component. Changes in the microarchitectural quality of bone have not yet been well characterized, but are recognized as being due to inefficiency in the remodeling process.[127]

Classification of osteoporosis

Osteoporosis is commonly classified into 'primary' or 'idiopathic', and 'secondary', the latter being osteoporosis for which a clearly identifiable etiologic mechanism is recognized. Primary osteoporosis is further characterized into 'idiopathic juvenile osteoporosis', 'idiopathic osteoporosis of the young adult' and 'involutive osteoporosis', which comprises 'postmenopausal' or 'type I osteoporosis' and 'senile' or 'type II osteoporosis'. A clinical classification of osteoporosis is given in Table 13.10.

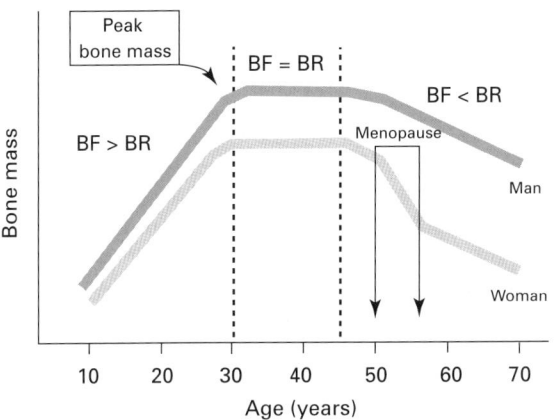

Figure 13.9
Bone mass and age in males and females. BF, bone formation; BR, bone resorption.

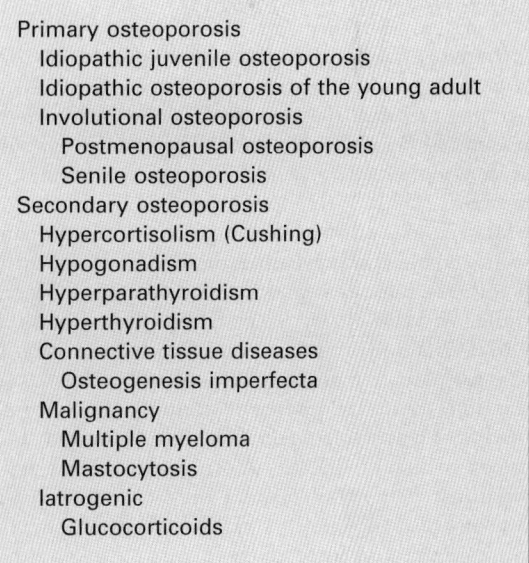

Table 13.10.
Clinical classification of osteoporosis.

Depending on bone remodeling, the disease is also classified into 'high-turnover' or 'low-turnover' osteoporosis. It is known that the excessive bone loss that characterizes the pathogenesis of osteoporosis results from abnormalities in the bone-remodeling cycle. It appears that with each cycle there is a slight, imperceptible deficit in bone formation. The total bone loss is therefore a function of the number of cycles active at any one time. Conditions that increase the rate of activation of the bone-remodeling process increase the proportion of the skeleton undergoing remodeling at any one time, thus increasing the rate of bone loss. These circumstances characterize high-turnover osteoporosis. Most of the secondary causes of osteoporosis are associated with this increased rate of activation of the bone-remodeling cycle. In other circumstances, excessive bone loss can occur when activation of the skeleton is not increased and even when activation of the skeleton might be decreased. This gives rise to the concept of low-turnover osteoporosis and is typical of the normal aging process. In this case, there appears to be a progressive impairment of signaling between bone resorption and bone formation, such that with every cycle of remodeling there is an increase in the deficit between resorption and formation, because osteoblast recruitment is inefficient.

Genetic factors
   Race (Caucasian/Asian)
   Sex (female)
   Familial prevalence (father > mother > brother with osteoporosis)
   Constitutional habitus (low BMI, thin skin)
Nutritional factors
   Low calcium intake
   High caffeine
   High sodium
   High animal protein
   High alcohol
Lifestyle factors
   Cigarette use
   Low physical activity
Endocrine factors
   Sex hormone status (amenorrhea/hypogonadism)
   Menopausal age (early menopause, ovariectomy)

Table 13.11
Proposed risk factors for osteoporosis.

Diagnosis of osteoporosis

Clinical evaluation of the risk of osteoporosis

Bone loss is asymptomatic, and symptoms related to fractures are often the first sign of osteoporosis. Some anamnestic data, clinical signs and lifestyle factors such as smoking, excessive alcohol consumption or physical inactivity (Table 13.11) have been associated with low BMD and may assist in assessing the risk of osteoporosis[121] and thus in preventing the occurrence of osteoporotic fractures. It is possible that the risk of fracture could be reduced by identifying these factors in individuals and recommending appropriate lifestyle changes. Hyperthyroidism, hyperparathyroidism and the long-term use of corticosteroids or thyroidal hormones may also enhance bone loss. A simple clinical estimation of the risk of osteoporosis, however, is often inaccurate. Only about a third of the women at real risk for osteoporosis can be identified by the clinical indicators listed above.

Genetic factors certainly play a major role in the pathogenesis of osteoporosis. There is clear evidence of genetic modulation of bone parameters, including bone density, bone size and bone turnover. It has been postulated that, at any particular age and phase of life, genetic factors explain about 70% of the variance in bone phenotype. Hormonal factors, diet and lifestyle interact with the genetic regulators of bone, over time, to determine net bone mass. Common allelic variations at several candidate genes, such as vitamin D receptor and collagen type I α1 genes, have been recently reported to be implicated in the genetic determination of bone phenotype.[128]

Clinical manifestations of osteoporosis

Osteoporosis is often called the 'silent disease', because bone loss generally occurs without symptoms. If not prevented, or if left untreated, the disease can progress painlessly until a bone breaks. Thus, in many cases the first symptom is a broken bone. Any bone can be affected, but of special concern are fractures of the wrist (Figure 13.8A), hip (Figure 13.8B), spine (Figure 13.8C) and, sometimes, ribs, even though the latter are more common in cases of osteomalacia or osteoporomalacia. Collapsed vertebrae may initially be felt or seen in the form of severe back pain, loss of height, or spinal deformities such as kyphosis (Figure 13.10) or stooped

OSTEOPOROSIS

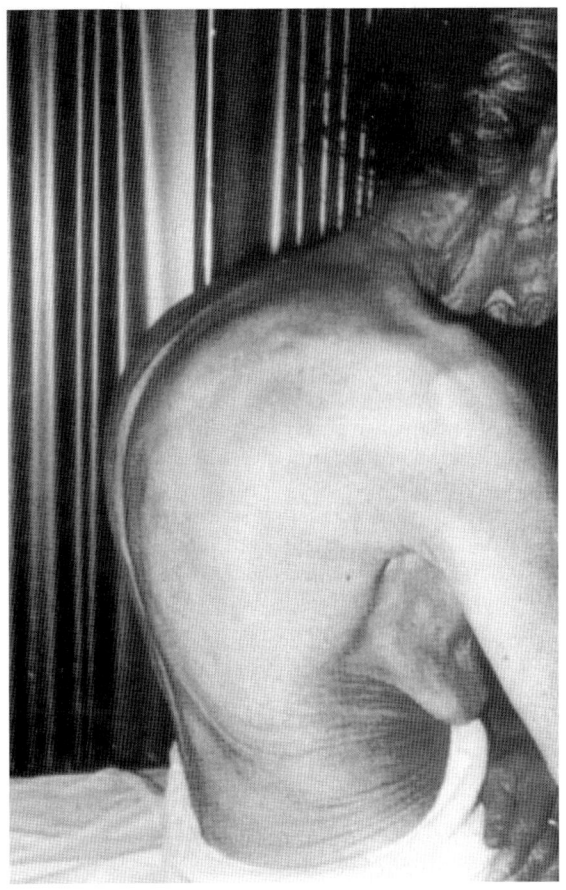

Figure 13.10
Severe kyphosis due to vertebral collapse in an elderly woman affected by osteoporosis. (From Gennari C, Avioli LV (eds) Atlante delle Malattie Dell'osso*, Vol. I. Parma: Chiesi Farmaceutici S.p.A., 1992.)*

posture. Surveys of spinal radiographs in older subjects suggest that many vertebral fractures have occurred in the absence of acute symptoms. Generally, the acute skeletal pain after an osteoporotic vertebral fracture should dissipate within 4–6 weeks. If skeletal pain persists much beyond this, other causes for the fracture (i.e. metastatic diseases, multiple myeloma) should be considered. As the number of vertebrae involved increases and the severity of individual vertebral deformities progresses, anatomical changes become more pronounced, giving rise to chronic pain. The progressive loss of stature results in progressive shortening of the paraspinal musculature; that is, the paraspinal muscles are actively contracted, resulting in the pain of muscle fatigue. This is the major determinant of the chronic back pain in spinal osteoporosis. Careful clinical examination reveals that the spine itself is not tender, and most patients indicate that the pain is paraspinal. The pain worsens with prolonged standing and is often relieved by walking. Fractures of the proximal femur are devastating both to the health of the affected individual and to society. In elderly women, there is a 12–30% reduction in expected survival after this fracture,[129] and the mortality is even greater in men.[130] Age and pre-fracture conditions are important indicators of outcome, as the increased mortality after a hip fracture is probably the result of an interaction between pre-existing conditions and the fracture itself.[131] Hip fracture almost always requires hospitalization and major surgery. It can impair a person's ability to walk unassisted and may cause prolonged or permanent disability. Essentially, permanent nursing home care is needed in an important fraction of patients.[132]

Measurement of bone mineral density, bone resorption and bone formation

The measurement of BMD, an index of bone mass, gives information on the biophysical, static condition of bone, whereas biochemical markers are indicators of the rate of bone turnover and thus reflect functional activity of the bone tissue. Biophysical and biochemical bone measurements can be used separately or together for evaluating bone tissue in different physiological and pathological conditions and during therapies affecting bone. In clinical practice, the current approach to evaluation of osteoporotic patients involves documentation of bone mass (commonly by DEXA), documentation of fractures if present, a diligent search for secondary causes, and then an evaluation of the biochemistry of bone remodeling.

Bone mineral density

The strength of bone is closely correlated with its mineral density. In general, the lower the BMD, the higher the risk for fracture. Overall, 75–85% of the variance in the ultimate strength of bone tissue is accounted for by changes in BMD. Other risk factors are predictive of fracture, but the risk is either not so objectively quantifiable as bone mass or is not modifiable.[133] Reliable measurement of the bone mineral content is therefore essential in the diagnosis of osteoporosis. All patients suspected of having osteoporosis, with or without fractures, should have measurement of bone mass. The only possible exception is the patient with far advanced disease both clinically and radiographically. BMD can be evaluated by several biophysical methods. All are painless, non-invasive and safe and are becoming more readily available. Although bone mass can be measured at multiple anatomical sites, BMD measurements are best made at the main fracture sites in osteoporotic patients—lumbar spine, femoral neck and distal forearm. BMD value is compared to two standards known as 'age-matched' and 'young normal'. The age-matched reading (expressed as Z score) compares the observed BMD value with what is expected in individuals of the same sex, age and size. The young normal reading (expressed as T score) compares the observed BMD value with the optimal peak bone density of a healthy young adult of the same sex. At any site, the result may also be given as a percentage of the reference mean. The T score, the number of standard deviations above or below the mean of healthy subjects aged 20–40, has been recently recommended by the World Health Organization (WHO) as the main parameter for diagnosis of osteoporosis.[134] According to the WHO criteria, four main categories have been established:[134]

1. *Normality*: T-score up to 1 SD lower than the mean reference BMD.
2. *Osteopenia*: T score >1 SD but <2.5 SD lower than the reference mean.
3. *Osteoporosis*: T score ≤2.5 SD than the reference mean.
4. *Severe osteoporosis*: T score as in osteoporosis, plus one or more fractures.

The diagnosis of osteopenia is clinically important, independent of any fracture risk implications. This diagnostic category represents the range of bone density for which prevention strategies have to be initiated, particularly in postmenopausal women or when secondary conditions associated with bone loss are present.

In the last decade, several studies and clinical trials have confirmed that BMD measurements are highly effective in assessing the fracture risk, confirming a diagnosis of osteoporosis and monitoring the effect of treatment.

Ultrasound

The use of US for the assessment of skeletal status has been of continued interest in recent years, because it has been demonstrated that US parameters may give information not only on bone mass, but also on bone structure. Ultrasonographic parameters, velocity (speed of sound or SOS) and attenuation (broadband ultrasound attenuation or BUA) are currently measured at the patella, the fingers, the tibia and the heel, with different instruments. Standardized coefficients of variation have shown good precision for both SOS and BUA. US parameters are positively correlated with BMD in vivo, although the correlations, even if statistically significant, are moderate. In this respect, there is now general agreement that US and DEXA measure different aspects of bone and, consequently, a high correlation between them should not be expected. In recent years, it has been demonstrated that US can be used to discriminate normal from osteoporotic patients and can independently predict vertebral and femoral fractures. Moreover, US recently appeared to be useful in monitoring the response to different treatments in osteoporotic patients as well as in the diagnosis of metabolic diseases different from osteoporosis, such as PHPT. Indeed, the absence of ionizing radiation, the portability of the equipment and its cost-effectiveness make US assessment an attractive option for future screening and managing of osteoporotic patients

Quantitative computed tomography

Quantitative computed tomography (QCT) has become an established technique for measuring BMD in the axial spine and appendicular skeleton. Because it provides cross-sectional images, QCT provides separate measurements of trabecular and cortical bone BMD, as well as true volumetric mineral density in grams per cubic centimeter. In recent years, QCT has been used for assessment of vertebral fracture risk, measurement of age-related bone loss and follow-up of osteoporosis. Recent technical developments, such as fast three-dimensional data acquisition, high-resolution image acquisition and processing techniques seem to provide additional information about bone strength and trabecular microarchitecture.

Radiographic assessment of osteoporosis

If an osteoporotic fracture is suspected, it is imperative that a radiograph is taken of the appropriate part of the skeleton. Conversely, there is no clear indication for a radiograph of the skeleton if fracture is not suspected. In clinical practice, the diagnosis of osteoporosis is often made by X-rays, albeit with low sensitivity, since bone loss is only apparent when bone mass has decreased by about 40%. The sites most commonly used in the assessment of patients are the spine, hip and hands.

Scintigraphy

The most commonly used tracer for bone imaging is methylene diphosphonate (MDP) labeled with ^{99m}Tc, a radionuclide available in all nuclear medicine departments. The exact mechanism of localization of this compound in bone is not fully understood, but it is probable that it is chemiadsorbed to hydroxyapatite crystals of bone. Under normal conditions, approximately 30% of an injected dose of ^{99m}Tc-MDP remains in the skeleton, with the majority of uptake being within the first hour. The remaining tracer is cleared by renal excretion. Imaging is usually performed at 3 or 4 h, when the ratio between bone activity and background activity is maximal. The degree of accumulation in bone is dependent on local bloodflow and, to a greater extent, on the degree of osteoblastic activity and hence bone formation. A bone scan is therefore a functional map of bone turnover which may be either focal or generalized throughout the skeleton. In clinical practice, bone scintigraphy is most widely used in malignancy to assess skeletal metastases, while it has no role in the diagnosis of uncomplicated osteoporosis. In some circumstances, bone scan has been used in established osteoporosis to diagnose vertebral, pelvic and rib fractures. The characteristic scintigraphic appearance of a fracture is of intense, linearly increased tracer uptake at the affected site.

Biochemical assessment of bone turnover

The bone-remodeling cycle is characterized by two opposite but finely coupled processes, bone formation and bone resorption. Most metabolic bone diseases, including osteoporosis, are the consequence of an unbalancing of these two processes. Although the status of bone turnover is not pathognomonic of any particular disorder, biochemical evaluation of bone formation and resorption may provide useful information in clinical practice. The biochemical markers of bone turnover are based on the measurement of either enzymatic activities characteristic of the bone-forming or -resorbing cells, such as alkaline or acid phosphatase, or bone matrix components released into the circulation during bone apposition or resorption. Markers of bone formation are serum total or bone-specific alkaline phosphatase, serum osteocalcin, and serum type I collagen C-terminal (PICP) and N-terminal (PINP) propeptides. Markers of bone resorption are urinary hydroxyproline, serum tartrate-resistant acid phosphatase, urinary hydroxylysine glycosides, and pyridinoline crosslinks (urinary N-terminal and C-terminal-to-helix crosslinks, termed respectively NTX and CTX, and serum C-terminal-to-helix crosslinks or ICTP). Table 13.12 lists currently available biochemical markers of bone resorption and formation. Although this classification of markers implies that each parameter is an indicator of either formation or resorption, this phase specificity should not be assumed to be very strict. Because of the coupling between bone formation and resorption, whenever bone turnover is increased both processes are accelerated and thus markers of both phases are increased. Some general limitations to the clinical application of these biochemical parameters must be kept in mind, as they cannot discriminate whether changes in remodeling rates are the result of remodeling activity in the whole skeleton, reflecting systemic conditions, or represent a dilution of the marker produced at extremely high rates by focal disorders (e.g. Paget's disease of bone). Moreover, in some circumstances, circulating levels of these markers can be influenced by factors other than bone turnover. Depending on the parameter considered, liver uptake and metabolism, renal excretion,

---

Bone formation
  Serum
    Alkaline phosphatase
    Bone-specific alkaline phosphatase
    Osteocalcin or bone Gla-protein
    C-terminal propeptide of type I collagen (PICP)
    N-terminal propeptide of type I collagen (PINP)

Bone resorption
  Urine
    Hydroxyproline
    Free and total pyridinolines
    Free and total deoxypyridinolines
    N-telopeptide of collagen crosslinks (NTX)
    C-telopeptide of collagen crosslinks (CTX)

  Serum
    Tartrate-resistant acid phosphatase (TRAP)
    Crosslinked C-telopeptide of type I collagen (ICTP)

Table 13.12
Currently available bone biochemical markers.

trapping in the bone tissue or uptake by osteoblasts may significantly affect the results. To date, there is increasing evidence that biochemical markers of bone turnover form a useful adjunct in predicting the rate of bone loss and the response to therapy, while they are not the standard diagnostic tool for the diagnosis of osteoporosis. It has been demonstrated that changes in these markers after only 3 months of therapy are significantly related to changes in bone mass after 24 months of therapy.[135] The markers may also provide confidence for defining the most appropriate therapeutic intervention and for dose adjustments. Theoretically, patients with high-turnover osteoporosis, with increased levels of resorption and formation markers, should be experiencing bone loss at an accelerated rate and should respond best to therapy with drugs that inhibit bone resorption. By contrast, those with low- or normal-turnover osteoporosis should have bone markers in the physiological range, should not be losing bone at an accelerated rate, should respond less to antiresorptive therapy, and should be treated preferentially with drugs that primarily enhance bone formation. Because osteoporosis may be the only manifestation of many of the secondary causes listed in Table 12.1, it is also appropriate to perform simple screening analyses, looking for these causes in each patient. A biochemical profile should include information about renal and hepatic function, PHPT, and possible malnutrition. A hematological profile might also provide clues to the presence of myeloma and malnutrition. The precise role of hyperthyroidism in the pathogenesis of accelerated bone loss and osteoporosis remains unresolved; however, it seems prudent to also obtain a sensitive TSH assay in all patients with documented bone loss. A 24-h urinary collection for measurement of Ca (which should always be accompanied by assessment of creatinine and sodium) is useful in detecting patients with hypercalciuria, which may be the end result of excess skeletal loss. Conversely, a very low level of urinary Ca (below 50 mg for 24 h) may be indicative of the presence of vitamin D malnutrition or malabsorption. In this respect, biochemical evaluation of serum 25(OH)D or 1,25(OH)$_2$D levels may also be recommended.

Bone biopsy and histomorphometry

In recent years, the study of bone biopsies has provided important information on the pathogenesis and treatment of osteoporosis. A needle bone biopsy is currently carried out in the iliac crest about 2 cm behind the anterior superior spine. The indications for bone biopsy are relatively limited in routine clinical practice. For obvious reasons, non-invasive methods are preferred. However, bone biopsy may be the only way of excluding osteomalacia, and this is actually the main indication for biopsy outside the area of clinical research. In fact, neither X-ray examination nor bone densitometry are able to differentiate osteoporosis from osteomalacia or osteoporomalacia. In some selected circumstances and doubtful cases, the histomorphometric measurement of trabecular bone volume, which provides the degree of osteopenia and the evaluation of connectivity, can be very useful in obtaining further morphological information and in assessing precise criteria of therapy and prognosis. The histological study of the biopsy can be completed by histochemical, ultrastructural and electron-microscopic examination. Moreover, dynamic histomorphometry enables the changes in bone to be quantified, differentiating high-turnover from low-turnover osteoporosis. The calcification process of the bone matrix can be evaluated on the basis of tetracycline uptake. It is known that the deposition of tetracyclines only occurs in areas of bone mineralization,[136] where they remain until they are removed by osteoclastic resorption. Because tetracyclines are fluorescent under ultraviolet light, their presence in bone is easy to demonstrate. A time-spaced, double administration of tetracyclines induces two linear fluorescent markers in the ossification areas. The two markers define the area of bone that has been deposited and calcified during the time that has elapsed between the first and the second tetracycline administrations, and the measurement of the interval between the markers indicates the amount of bone synthesized by osteoblasts in that period. The finding can be used to calculate bone formation rate. Occasionally, unsuspected disease, including mastocytosis, myelomatosis, hyperparathyroidism, sarcoidosis, hemochromatosis and apudomas, is first diagnosed at bone biopsy.

Prevention and treatment of osteoporosis

Osteoporosis is a preventable and, in its early phases, treatable disease. Maximizing peak bone mass during childhood and early adulthood is the most cost-effective way of reducing the risk of an osteoporotic fracture. An adequate intake of Ca (approximately 1000–1200 mg/day), moderate weight-bearing exercise and the maintenance of normal body weight are important elements in building up strong bones and preserving skeletal strength life-long.[137,138] Avoidance of smoking and alcohol are also beneficial; indeed, smoking may totally negate the normal protection from hip fractures induced by female sex hormones.[139] Another practical method is to use antiresorptive drugs or agents which stimulate bone formation, such as bisphosphonates (Table 13.13). Estrogen replacement therapy (ERT) is the treatment of choice for prevention of bone loss in early postmenopausal or younger women lacking ovarian estradiol secretion. Transdermal estradiol is as effective as oral estrogen in preventing bone loss, and ERT has also been shown to reduce the risk of coronary heart disease[140] as well as the risk of neurodegenerative disorders (i.e. Alzheimer's disease) in women after menopause. However, before embarking on treatment of patients with a low BMD, other differential diagnoses (mainly hyperparathyroidism or osteomalacia) should be considered.

Estrogen

Estrogen alone or in combination with progestogen has a central position in all strategies aimed at preventing and treating postmenopausal osteoporosis.[141] The epidemiological data indicating that estrogens may reduce the risk of ischemic heart disease as well as the risk of Alzheimer's disease are additional preventive benefits for estrogen replacement therapy. Estrogen acts directly on estrogen receptors α and β in bone cells, suppressing bone remodeling, especially bone resorption, by decreasing the frequency of activation of the bone-remodeling cycle. Estrogen also modulates Ca homeostasis by decreasing the sensitivity of bone to PTH and by activating Ca absorption by the intestine in concert with the action of $1,25(OH)_2D$.[123] Indirect mechanisms of estrogen action on bone, such as changes in 1-α-hydroxylase and calcitonin secretory reserve, as well as on local factors, are still under investigation. Estrogen significantly reduces bone loss in all postmenopausal women,[137,138,141] especially in the 5–10 years after menopause. The rate of bone loss decreases to premenopausal levels, being maximally 0.3–0.5% a year. This treatment is beneficial not only immediately after menopause but also in established osteoporosis,[137] where it may increase bone mass, i.e. in the vertebral spine, by more than 5%.[123] ERT is effective in preventing osteoporotic fractures.[137,138,141] In several case–control studies[142–148] it decreased the risk of hip fracture by 21–66%, with, in one study, significant reduction in the number of hip fractures after 6–9 years of therapy.[144] Transdermal administration of estrogen is as effective as oral treatment, for example, in reducing the frequency of crush fractures of the vertebral spine by 61%.[149] Short-term complications of ERT include breast tenderness and vaginal bleeding. Long-term complications include occasional weight gain, venous thrombosis, and, rarely, an idiosyncratic increase in blood pressure. Moreover, estrogen given unopposed by progestogens increase the risk of endometrial hyperplasia and carcinoma. There is more doubt about the effect of estrogen on breast cancer, but long-term therapy (>10–15 years) may increase the risk slightly (from 10% to 30%).[150] To diminish the possible negative effect of long-term estrogen treatment, minimal effective doses are used: 0.625 mg/day of conjugated estrogen, 2 mg of 17β-estradiol orally or 0.05 mg transdermally, and 1 mg of estradiol valerate, have been shown to have a bone-sparing effect. If the patient has gone through a natural menopause and still has uterus, combination or sequential therapy with progestin is used to protect the endometrium. There is no rationale at present for progestins in patients who have undergone hysterectomy. All patients should have mammography and endometrial evaluation (by US) before therapy is initiated and every 1–2 years during treatment. There is no evidence that progestogens oppose estrogen in its action on bone. A meta-analysis of the relevant published data revealed that the risk of hip fracture and its related mortality relative to non-users of hormone replacement therapy (HRT) was

Inhibitors of bone resorption
  Estrogens
  Calcitonins
  Bisphosphonates
  Selective estrogen receptor modulators (SERMs)
  Calcium
  Vitamin D and its metabolites
  Tibolone
  Ipriflavone
  Thiazide diuretics
  Phytoestrogens
Stimulators of bone formation
  Fluorides
  Anabolic steroids
  Parathyroid hormone fragments

Table 13.13
Current available medications used in the prevention and/or treatment of osteoporosis

similar for estrogen-alone or estrogen-plus-progestogen users, namely 0.75.[151] In addition, it has also been speculated that progestogens, at least 19-nortestosterone derivatives, may positively affect bone independently of estrogen.[152] The main contraindication to ERT is the presence or history of an estrogen-dependent tumor, especially breast malignancy. Other relative contraindications include undiagnosed vaginal bleeding, a prior history of endometrial malignancy, active thromboembolic disease, and grossly abnormal liver or renal function. Hypertension and diabetes are not contraindications but must be controlled before therapy is started. How long should ERT be given in order to give adequate protection from osteoporotic fracture during the last third of a woman's life? The Framingham study[153,154] revealed that, by 80 years of age, women who had taken estrogen for 10 years or less after menopause had lost 27% of their bone mass, and those never treated 30%, whereas in those who had used ERT throughout the postmenopausal period the loss was about 10%. Hence, the benefit of adopting ERT during the immediate postmenopausal period appears to be lost in a few years after the suspension of treatment. Consequently, estrogen therapy should continue for longer than 10 years and, if possible, lifelong if it is to counteract osteoporosis effectively. A recent study of 9704 women[149] also showed that, for long-term protection against fractures, estrogen should be initiated soon after menopause and continued indefinitely. In cases with a fracture as a first sign of osteoporosis, ERT should be started immediately and sustained lifelong.[154] The bone-sparing efficacy of ERT in the elderly might be expected to be marginal, since the bone loss at that age may be predominantly due to a deficit of vitamin D, with consequent impaired bone formation. Evidence from longitudinal studies has, however, shown that long-term estrogen continues to slow bone loss even in elderly women[155] and also protects women over 75 from hip fractures.[156]

Calcium and vitamin D

All treatment or prevention strategies for osteoporosis should include Ca intake. Although an adequate intake of Ca should be obtained from nutritional sources, in practice it is difficult for many people to achieve the recommended dietary intake. Self-imposed calorie restriction and the avoidance of cholesterol commonly results in limited consumption of milk and other dairy products. Other sources of Ca include green vegetables, nuts, and certain fish. Recommendations for Ca intake include an intake of 800 mg until age 10, 1200 mg during adolescence, and 1000 mg thereafter, increasing to 1200 mg during pregnancy and lactation, and to 1500 mg if at increased risk for osteoporosis or if over age 65. Commonly, most individuals require from 500 to 1000 mg/day as a supplement to dietary sources to achieve these intakes. Ca cannot increase bone mass, but it can slow down bone loss in postmenopausal women. Ca is especially necessary as a supplement to ERT and other antiresorptive treatments if the dietary intake of Ca is insufficient.

Vitamin D exerts a key role in Ca homeostasis, mainly because of its role in facilitating intestinal Ca absorption. Most patients with established osteoporosis show lower Ca absorption than their age-matched controls, either because of a deficit in $1,25(OH)_2D$ or a relative (and perhaps genetically determined) resistance to active metabolites of vitamin D. The malabsorption of Ca in osteoporotic patients may be corrected by pharmacological doses of vitamin D or physiological doses of vitamin D metabolites. Most clinical studies have used calcitriol 0.5 μg/day or 1-α-hydroxyvitamin D_3 (alphacalcidol) 1.0 μg/day. Alphacalcidol is a prodrug which has to be metabolized in the liver before the active compound, $1,25(OH)_2D$ is formed. Calcitriol in established vertebral osteoporosis is able to normalize Ca absorption and to inhibit bone loss, with about 65% reduction in the rate of new vertebral fractures.[137,157] A recent study[158] showed suppression of bone loss and significant reduction of fracture incidence in elderly women given 1200 mg Ca plus 20 μg (800 IU) vitamin D per day. In elderly women, high Ca intake plus vitamin D treatment can also decrease serum PTH and consequently reduce bone turnover.[159] These results stress the importance of vitamin D metabolites in the prevention and treatment of osteoporosis in elderly women. Over-treatment, however, may induce hypercalciuria and hypercalcemia.

Calcitonin

In the past, calcitonin has been used to treat women who have declined ERT or who have been unable to take it due to contraindications. Bisphosphonates and raloxifene represent valid alternatives. All these drugs are also effective in older women with established osteoporosis. However, they are relatively expensive. Calcitonin, a peptide hormone produced by the parafollicular cells of the thyroid, regulates Ca homeostasis by inhibiting bone resorption through specific and direct suppressive effects on osteoclastic receptors.[160] This action appears to be related to alteration of the internal structure of osteoclasts, and probably to a decrease in the rate of osteoclast formation by blocking of the fusion of mononuclear marrow cells.[161] Calcitonin can be used intranasally, subcutaneously or, less often, by intravenous injection, without significant side-effects. Transient facial flushing and nausea, occasional vomiting, diarrhea and mild inflammation at the injection site represent the main adverse effects; very rarely, they necessitate drug discontinuation.[162] Four species of calcitonin—salmon, human, eel and an analog of eel calcitonin—are available for therapeutic administration. Salmon calcitonin is the most potent: 50–100 UI given intramuscularly has been found to prevent postmenopausal bone loss and even to increase vertebral bone mass.[163] Conflicting results have been published regarding the optimal nasal dosage for preventing postmenopausal bone loss.[164] In established involutional osteoporosis, the recommended dose of nasal salmon calcitonin may be 200 UI/day. The treatment should be administered discontinuously.[165] Calcitonin treatment has been demonstrated to be specifically effective in osteoporotic patients with high bone turnover.[166] However, a potential decrease in therapeutic effectiveness with prolonged treatment has been reported and is presumably due to the development of neutralizing antibodies, downregulation at receptor sites or a counterregulatory mechanism.[167,168] Calcitonin often has potent analgesic activity,[169] which may be particularly beneficial in patients suffering from metabolic bone diseases characterized by excessive bone turnover, such as Paget's disease of bone and postmenopausal osteoporosis. Pain relief precedes any change in biochemical indices of bone turnover. Calcitonin is thus recommended, especially for women suffering pain due to osteoporotic fractures.

Bisphosphonates

Bisphosphonates are potent inhibitors of bone resorption. They are all derivatives of pyrophosphate, are specific for the skeleton and are not metabolized by the body.[170] The biological effects of bisphosphonates on Ca metabolism were originally ascribed to their physicochemical effects on hydroxyapatite crystals. Although such effects contribute to the overall action of bisphosphonates on bone, their effects on bone cells are probably of greater importance, particularly for the more potent compounds.[171] They have been shown to increase bone mass in postmenopausal osteoporosis, and to reduce the incidence of fractures.

Etidronate was the first clinically available bisphosphonate. It has been used in several clinical trials to stabilize and increase bone mass and also to possibly reduce fracture rate.[172] The treatment regimen for etidronate is 400 mg/day orally for 2 weeks, followed by a 10–12 week etidronate-free period, during which supplementation with Ca is recommended. There is evidence from long-term treatment of Paget's disease that large doses of or longer duration of therapy with etidronate may result in a mineralization defect, and a consequent increased risk of developing osteomalacia. This drawback is not apparent with newer compounds such as alendronate, which inhibits bone resorption 1000 times more potently than etidronate. It could become a low-cost alternative to estrogen, particularly in older women with established osteoporosis and osteoporotic fracture.

Alendronate is an aminobisphosphonate for which extensive clinical trials have been completed worldwide. It is approved for the treatment of osteoporosis in most countries. Treatment with alendronate in postmenopausal women has been demonstrated to be effective in reducing bone loss and the incidence of hip, vertebral and wrist fractures to about 30–50%.[173–175] The recommended dosage of alendronate is 10 mg/day. In common with other bisphosphonates, oral absorption of alendronate is very poor (<1%). Absorption is further impaired if alendronate is taken with food, any liquid except water, or Ca supplements. These problems can be avoided if patients take the medication first thing in the morning, with water, and delay breakfast for at least 30 min. The major side-effects of alendronate are upper gastrointestinal disturbances and esophagitis in a small proportion of patients.

Selective estrogen receptor modulators (SERMs)

Raloxifene is a novel agent approved for the prevention and treatment of postmenopausal osteoporosis. This drug is a non-steroidal benzothiophene compound which appears to act through the estrogen receptor pathway, producing estrogen-agonist effects on bone and low-density lipoprotein cholesterol but estrogen-antagonist effects on breast, endometrium and hypothalamus. Preliminary evidence indicates that raloxifene reduces the incidence of breast cancer, but more time is needed to establish and confirm this important observation. The clinical effects of this drug have been assessed in a large randomized trial in European women.[176] The recommended dose for prevention of bone loss is 60 mg daily.[177] Concomitant food intake does not appreciably affect bioavailability. Adverse events of raloxifene include the persistence of hot flushes, which in clinical trials occurred more frequently with raloxifene than with placebo, and leg cramps. Similar to estrogen, raloxifene is associated with a low but statistically significant increased risk of venous thrombosis. For this reason, it is contraindicated in women with an active or past history of venous thrombosis or embolism and should not be used during periods of immobilization. Moreover, raloxifene may cause fetal harm and is contraindicated in women who are or may become pregnant.

Tamoxifen, the most commonly prescribed synthetic anti-estrogen for the treatment of breast cancer, has been shown to produce estrogen agonist effects on the skeleton. In postmenopausal women with breast cancer, it has been reported that tamoxifen preserved spinal bone mass;[178] however, this effect was not universally confirmed.[179]

Other treatments

Other anti-osteoporotic agents include steroidal (progestogens, androgens, anabolic steroids, tibolone) and non-steroidal (sodium fluoride, PTH fragments, GH and thiazide diuretics) compounds.

Anabolic steroids have been developed from androgens to decrease the virilizing effect and retain the anabolic action. In the past few years, they have received attention as therapeutic agents for osteoporosis. Effects of anabolic steroids on bone result from a combined direct action on osteoblast bone formation and indirect effects mediated by mechanical forces caused by muscle strength improvement.[180]

Nandrolone (19-nortestosterone) is an anabolic steroid given by injection at a dosage of 50 mg every 2–3 weeks, and may sometimes be used to treat involutional osteoporosis. Virilization effects, hoarsening and sodium retention represent the main adverse effects of nandrolone; they are in any case dose related and reversible.

Sodium fluoride has been used in several countries to treat osteoporosis. It is mitogenic for osteoblasts and works by directly increasing bone formation. In contrast to antiresorptive agents, which produce early gains in BMD followed by a plateau phase and in some circumstances by a slow decrease, fluoride produces dramatic, sustained, linear increases in spinal BMD, averaging 9% per year for 4 years.[181]

Fluoride can be given as the sodium salt, as a slow-release preparation, and as a monofluorophosphate. Two hundred milligrams of disodium monofluorophosphate is equivalent to 36 mg sodium fluoride or 16.4 mg of fluoride ion. Although there is debate about the optimal dose, most studies show increases of bone mass with doses of 20–30 mg fluoride ion daily.[182] The main problem with fluoride is the narrow therapeutic window, with toxic doses leading to production of bone that is histologically abnormal, undermineralized, and more dense but less strong than normal.[183]

Several studies over the past decades have established that intermittent injections of PTH can increase trabecular bone mass in rats and other animals.[184] Preliminary data in humans, showing considerable increases in cancellous bone, make PTH a promising alternative for the treatment of osteoporosis in the future.

The presence of reduced BMD in patients with adult-onset GH deficiency and the evidence for skeletal growth factor deficiency in elderly people,[185] raised the possibility that human recombinant GH may have a role in the treatment of involutional osteoporosis. However, at present, the role of GH therapy in osteoporosis remains to be established.

Thiazide diuretic agents may be useful in some circumstances to lower the urinary excretion of Ca and to improve Ca balance. The use of these agents has been associated with a reduction in the risk of hip fracture.[186]

Treatment of osteoporosis in men

Ensuring adequate Ca and vitamin D intake is an essential foundation for preserving and enhancing bone mass in men who have osteoporosis. Although several pharmacological approaches are being evaluated, to date there are no controlled trials of osteoporosis therapies in men. However, small studies with calcitonin, bisphosphonates and PTH suggest that they may be useful in men as well. Testosterone replacement increases bone mass in hypogonadal men, and if there are no contraindications, it should be considered as a useful means of preventing the increased fracture risk associated with testicular dysfunction.

Paget's disease of bone

Introduction

Paget's disease of bone (PDB) is a chronic disorder which typically results in enlarged and deformed bones in one or more regions of the skeleton. Excessive bone breakdown and formation can cause the bone to weaken. As a result, bone pain, arthritis, noticeable deformities and fractures can occur. Paget's disease is most common in Caucasian people of European descent, but it also occurs in African-Americans. It is rare in people of Asian descent. Both men and women are affected, in a sex ratio of about three men to one woman. Paget's disease is rarely diagnosed in people under age 40. Because there are no large population studies, the actual prevalence of Paget's disease is not specifically known. Until now, it has been suggested that Paget's disease may occur in up to 3% of the US population over age 60 and in up to 10% of elderly people from European countries.[187] Recent research suggests, however, that Paget's disease may occur in a smaller percentage of people, perhaps 1.3% of the US population over age 60. It is important to emphasize the localized nature of Paget's disease. It may be monostotic, affecting only a single bone or a proportion of a bone, or may be polyostotic, involving two or more bones. Sites of disease are often asymmetric. In most instances, sites affected with Paget's disease at the time of diagnosis are the only ones that will show pagetic change over time. Although progression of disease within a given bone may occur, the sudden appearance of new sites of involvement some years after the initial diagnosis is uncommon.

Etiopathogenesis

The cause of Paget's disease is still unknown. Research findings suggest that Paget's disease may be caused by a slow-acting viral infection of bone, a condition which is present for many years before symptoms appear. There are also data supporting a hereditary hypothesis, since the disease may appear in more than one member of a family. Current evidence suggests that both environmental and genetic factors are involved in Paget's disease. How the virus and the genetic factors are intertwined in Paget's disease is not yet clear. Genetic factors may increase an individual's chance of getting the disease. The individuals with a genetic predisposition to Paget's disease may be more susceptible to viral infection. Another explanation is that the genetic version of the disease represents only one group of Paget's disease patients and that the other patients have a type of Paget's disease that requires viral exposure.

Viral hypothesis

For many years, it has been thought that a group of viruses in the Paramyxovirus family may cause Paget's disease. Pagetic changes in bone remodeling may occur as a result of a viral infection of osteoclasts. Viral inclusions have been described in the nuclei and cytoplasm of osteoclasts at pagetic sites.[188,189] The virus particles resemble members of the Paramyxovirus family, including respiratory syncytial, measles or canine distemper viruses. A recent report that erythroid cells from patients affected with Paget's disease express viral mRNA suggests the existence of some generally quiescent hematopoietic stem cells as the primary host for viral infection.[190] However, conflicting results have emerged from investigations using RNA extraction and polymerase chain reaction techniques, with some reporting the presence of viral RNA in pagetic bone, and others failed to detect this.[191,192] Results from a recent study demonstrated that expression of measles virus nucleocapsid transcript in normal osteoclast precursors enhanced formation of mature osteoclasts that showed many of the characteristics of pagetic osteoclasts, further supporting the role of a viral infection in the pathogenesis of Paget's disease.[193] Compared with osteoclasts from non-transfected cells, osteoclasts formed from normal precursors transfected with measles virus nucleocapsid gene have increased numbers of nuclei per multinucleated cell, increased sensitivity to $1,25(OH)_2D$, increased bone-resorbing capacity, enhanced IL-6 production, increased RANK expression and increased NF-κB signaling in the absence of RANK ligand.

Hereditary factors

It has been observed for many years that people with Paget's disease often have a relative who also has the disease. According to several clinical series, 15% to 40% of pagetic patients have a positive family history of the disorder.[194,195] Although conceivably compatible with some environmental factors being active when relatives are growing up together, such familial clusters strongly suggest the presence of a genetic predisposition. Genetic analyses of multiple affected kindreds support an autosomal dominant pattern of inheritance.[196] The existence of families with few affected members could be due to incomplete penetrance and variable expressivity of the PDB gene. Furthermore, interaction with other factors, either genetic or exogenous, appears to be necessary for disease expression. Sex-specific distribution in familial groups reveals that occurrence of the disease is clearly more frequent in males than in females, with a male/female ratio of about 4:1.[195] Moreover, the proportion of both early-onset and polyostotic cases is significantly higher among familial than sporadic PDB patients.[195] Higher frequencies of both Mokenberg-type vascular calcification and green and blue eye color in familial Paget's disease has also been reported.[195] Linkage analysis in some PDB families has shown evidence of linkage to a region on chromosome 18q (18q21–22), co-segregating with the rare Paget's disease-like bone dysplasia named familial expansile osteolysis (FEO).[197,199] Subsequent analyses in other kindreds, however, have not shown any evidence of linkage to the 18q21–22 locus, providing evidence for genetic heterogeneity.[199] Two different tandem duplications in exon I of the gene encoding the receptor for osteoclast differentiation factor (ODFR or RANK), in chromosome 18q22.1, have been recently discovered in FEO families and in one PDB family.[200] These duplications (respectively of bases 84–101 in FEO, and of bases 75–101 in PDB) are activating mutations, resulting in increased constitutive RANK signaling. Both duplications shared an identical 3-endpoint at base 101 and were thought to have arisen by reverse slippage during DNA replication.

Pathophysiology

The characteristic feature of the disease is increased resorption followed by an increase in bone formation. It is generally believed that the primary cellular abnormality in Paget's disease is in the osteoclasts, while the osteoblasts are intrinsically normal,[201] even though this has not been proven conclusively.[202] Pagetic osteoclasts are markedly increased in number as well as in size and contain up to 100 nuclei per cell.[203] Moreover, pagetic osteoclast precursors are hyper-responsive to $1,25(OH)_2D$ and produce increased amounts of IL-6.[204] The marrow microenvironment also appears to be abnormal and has an enhanced capacity to induce osteoclast formation compared with the normal marrow microenvironment.[204,205] It has been recently discovered that levels of RANK ligand mRNA, which may be the common mediator for the effects of other osteoclastogenic factors on osteoclast formation,[206] are significantly elevated in the stromal cell line derived from patients with Paget's disease compared to that from normal individuals.[204]

Generally, the evolution of the disease follows three major phases. In the early phase, termed the 'osteolytic phase', bone resorption predominates and there is a concomitant increased vascularity of involved bones. In this phase, body Ca balance may be negative, and the typical radiological picture is represented by an advancing lytic wedge or 'blade of grass' lesion (Figure 13.11) in a long bone (i.e. femur or tibia) or by osteoporosis circumscripta, as seen in the skull ('salt and pepper') (Figure 13.12). Commonly, the excessive resorption of pagetic bone is followed closely by formation of new bone. During this second phase of the disease, the new bone that is made is structurally abnormal, presumably because of the accelerated nature of the remodeling process. Newly deposed collagen fibers are laid down in a disorganized rather than a linear fashion, creating the so-called 'woven bone'. Such a woven pattern is not specific for Paget's disease, but it reflects a high rate of bone turnover. With time, the hypercellularity at the affected bone may diminish, leading to development of a sclerotic, less vascular pagetic mosaic without evidence of active bone turnover. This is the so-called 'sclerotic' or 'burned-out' phase of Paget's disease. Typically, all these three phases of the disease can be seen at the same time at different sites in a single pagetic patient.

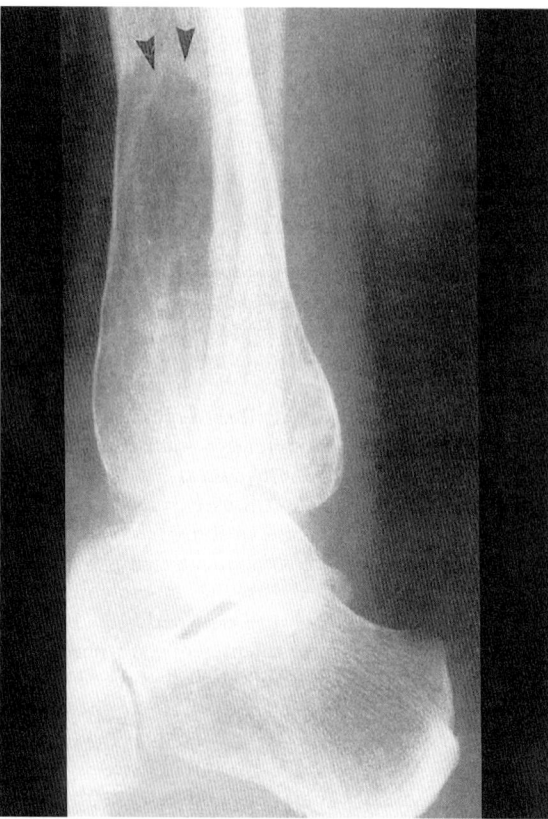

Figure 13.11
Typical radiological picture of the advancing lytic wedge (blade of grass) of the osteolytic phase of Paget's disease. (From Gennari C, Avioli LV (eds) Atlante delle Malattie Dell'osso, Vol. II. Parma: Chiesi Farmaceutici S.p.A., 1992.)

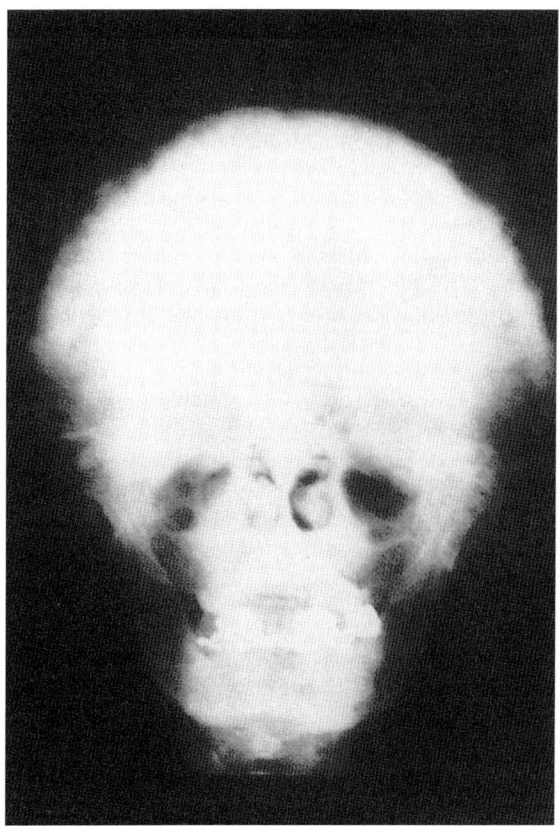

Figure 13.12
Radiological picture of pagetic lesion of the skull. (From Gennari C, Avioli LV (eds) Atlante delle Malattie Dell'osso, *Vol. II. Parma: Chiesi Farmaceutici S.p.A., 1992.)*

Diagnosis

Many patients who have Paget's disease do not know they have it, since the disease may be so mild that is not detected. Sometimes, the patient's doctor is alerted to the possibility of Paget's disease when physical deformities appear (e.g. enlargement of the skull or bowing of the tibia) or when a blood test reveals an elevated level of alkaline phosphatase. Occasionally, the patient's symptoms are confused with arthritis or other disorders. In other cases, the diagnosis is made only after complications have developed.

Clinical presentation

Localized bone pain is the most common symptom that brings a patient with Paget's disease to a physician. Pain varies greatly from patient to patient, depending on the location and extent of the disease. Also, the pain associated with Paget's disease can take many forms. It may arise from increased vascularity, from distortion of the periosteum due to disorganized remodeling, or from a focus of mechanical stress. The first phase of Paget's disease involves thinning of the bone, which is being aggressively resorbed; this is called 'lytic disease'. This process can cause small breaks (microfractures) in the bone that are painful, especially when they involve weight-bearing bone. Alternatively, another source of pain can arise from involvement of nerves covering affected bones. Patients usually describe this pain as a deep pain which is most symptomatic at night and may lessen during the day. When Paget's disease reaches the end of a long bone, the cartilage may degenerate. Deformed pagetic bones also damage the adjacent joints. Both of these situations result in osteoarthritis. Osteoarthritis is common among patients with Paget's disease and can be quite painful. Periarticular pain may be the presenting feature in 50% of cases.[207] It commonly affects bone around major joints such as the hip and knee, as well as those of the spine, with narrowing of the joint spaces and the formation of osteophytes. When bones are deformed, the muscles contract at abnormal angles, causing muscle pain. A variety of abnormalities and neurological complications can be associated with Paget's disease of the skull and spinal column. Skull deformity may result in enlargement of the vault, with a characteristic appearance particularly of the forehead (frontal bossing) or of the maxilla (leontiasis osseum). Basilar invagination is also common. It does not result in outwardly visible changes but is apparent radiologically and may cause symptoms due to internal hydrocephalus or long tract signs from brainstem compression. Cranial nerves may become compressed as they emerge from their foramina adjacent to pagetic bone. The auditory and ocular nerves seem to be particularly at risk. These changes usually occur in association with obvious radiological features of skull involvement. Pain radiating from the lower back into the legs (sciatica) can also occur because of the overgrowth of bone or the compression of disks.

Bowing of weight-bearing bones is a common feature of Paget's disease. It occurs most frequently in the femur, tibia, and forearm. Since bone deformity is usually acquired later in life and is often asymmetrical, it has relatively good diagnostic specificity. This type of deformity in the femur or tibia is often associated with stress fractures on the convex surface of the bowed bone. These may present as localized areas of bone pain or tenderness and may also extend to produce a complete transverse fracture. The radiographic appearances are diagnostic and are easily distinguished from other types of stress fracture such as those typical of osteomalacia. Symmetrical bowing deformity of the lower limbs may be confused with other metabolic bone diseases, such as the consequences of childhood rickets, but radiographs and biochemistry can confirm the cause.

Biochemistry

Paget's disease is characteristically associated with an increase in bone turnover but normal concentrations of serum Ca, phosphate, PTH and vitamin D metabolites. Over recent years, various markers of bone turnover have been indicated for the diagnosis of Paget's disease. Among these, bone-specific alkaline phosphatase (BAP) seems to have the best diagnostic accuracy as a measure of increased bone turnover of pagetic bone. Considering its simplicity and low cost, total serum alkaline phosphatase (SAP) concentration is still a credible alternative. The range of SAP that is considered normal varies considerably, depending on the laboratory used for the test. A typical normal range for a person over the age of 60 may range from 20 to 120 units. Provided that there is no evidence of liver disease, a mild increase in SAP level (up to twice the normal level) might indicate Paget's disease as well as another problem, such as a healing fracture. An SAP level two or more times higher than normal strongly suggests Paget's disease, especially if serum Ca and phosphate, as well as renal function, are normal. In addition to their use in diagnosis, both BAP and SAP measurements are important tools for monitoring a patient's response to treatment for Paget's disease. The main advantage for BAP over total SAP is in the assessment of localized or monostotic disease: BAP but not SAP concentration will often be raised and can be used to monitor the response to treatment. BAP is also particularly useful when liver function tests are abnormal and the hepatic contribution to total SAP concentration is uncertain. Although osteocalcin is a specific gene product of the osteoblast and is generally considered a specific marker of bone formation, it lacks sensitivity in Paget's disease. Other markers of bone formation, such as PINP and PICP, which are released into circulation during the conversion of type I procollagen into collagen, have proved to have different sensitivities in Paget's disease. Only about 45% of patients with active disease have raised PICP values.[208]

Conversely, recent data with serum PINP suggest that this marker of collagen synthesis has good sensitivity in pagetic patients, but the amount of data available is still limited.[209,210] Among the various biochemical markers of bone resorption, the most sensitive ones in Paget's disease are collagen type I-related peptides. These include the urinary N-telopeptide (NTX) and the C-telopeptide (CTX), which can be assayed in both serum and urine. Measurements of plasma tartrate-resistant acid phosphatase and of urinary excretion of free pyridinoline and deoxypyridinoline or of hydroxyproline seem to be less sensitive.[209–210] The low cost and general availability of urinary hydroxyproline testing, however, makes it an acceptable alternative for monitoring of active polyostotic Paget's disease. It has, however, poor sensitivity in limited disease. In extensive and active disease, most markers of bone turnover will be abnormal, and the choice of resorption marker can then be based on cost and availability. It has recently been demonstrated that the CTX of the α1 chain of collagen type I contains a sequence site susceptible to β-isomerization, a non-enzymatic post-transcriptional modification believed to be associated with aging of proteins.[211] Non-isomerized (α-CTX) and β-isomerized (β-CTX) forms arising from degradation of type I collagen CTX can now be measured in urine independently by specific immunoassays.[212,213] Measurement of the α-CTX/β-CTX ratio provides an index of the degree of β-isomerization of bone matrix and has recently been shown to be abnormally high in untreated pagetic patients, returning to normal values under bisphosphonate treatment.[214,215] This novel marker of bone quality could prove to be very useful in the monitoring of pagetic patients.

Radiography and scintigraphy

Radiographs of painful or deformed bones are usually diagnostic, showing the characteristic mixed appearance of areas of lysis due to increased osteoclastic resorption with sclerosis (Figure 13.13) from excessive osteoblastic bone formation. In the early stages of the disease, the changes may be predominantly lytic, with flame-shaped resorption fronts in the long bones or osteoporosis circumscripta in the skull. A characteristic appearance that distinguishes Paget's disease from other conditions is the increased diameter of affected bones, particularly those of the spine or the shafts of long bones.

Scintigraphy (Figure 13.14) is a sensitive but non-specific method of detecting areas of skeletal abnormality and is the best way of assessing the skeletal

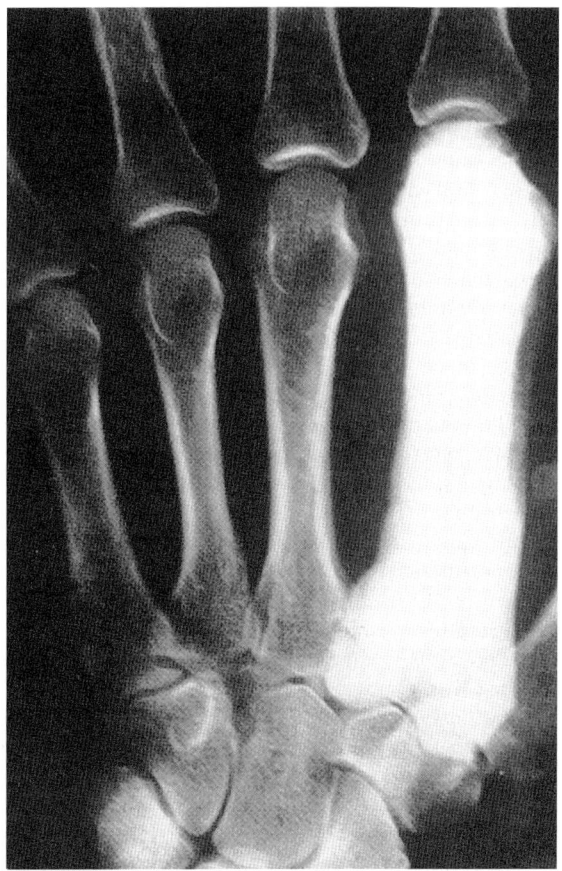

Figure 13.13
Increased diameter and density at the metacarpal level in monostotic Paget's disease. (From Gennari C, Avioli LV (eds) Atlante delle Malattie Dell'osso, Vol. II. Parma: Chiesi Farmaceutici S.p.A., 1992.)

distribution of Paget's disease. Although some sites may be asymptomatic, it is important that they are identified, because they may be susceptible to complications, such as fracture.

Differential diagnosis

In most cases, the diagnosis of Paget's disease can be made from the combination of symptoms, characteristic radiographic appearances, and raised concentrations of bone alkaline phosphatase or of other bone turnover markers. In some circumstances, the diagnosis may be difficult. A single sclerotic vertebra may cause uncertainty, and the differential diagnosis includes vertebral hemangioma, malignancy, and other infiltrations such

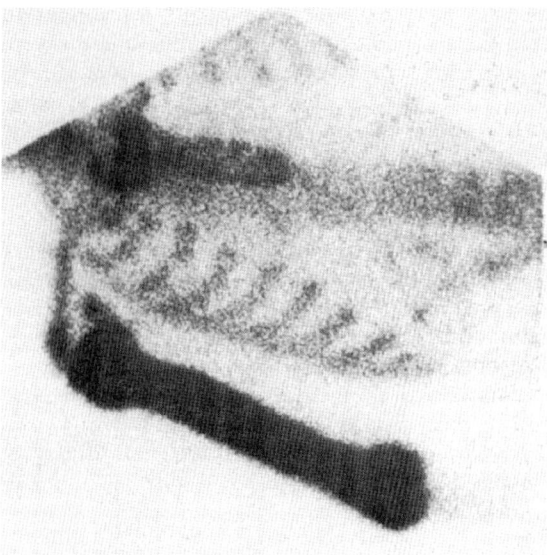

Figure 13.14
Typical ^{99m}Tc-MDP scan of a patient affected with polyostotic Paget's disease. (From Gennari C, Avioli LV (eds) Atlante delle Malattie Dell'osso, Vol. II. Parma: Chiesi Farmaceutici S.p.A., 1992.)

as sarcoidosis, osteomyelitis, or vertebral compression fractures. Vertebral hemangioma may show an increase in vertical trabeculation, but the end plates and neural arches are rarely affected, whereas they often are in Paget's disease. Vertebral size is usually normal, but collapse may occur. Hemangiomas are usually solitary, and other areas of abnormality, e.g. on a bone scan, would make this diagnosis unlikely. Bone biochemistry may sometimes be unhelpful, because it could be normal in both hemangioma and monostotic Paget's disease. Collapsed osteoporotic vertebrae may appear mildly sclerotic and cause confusion with Paget's disease, although the vertebrae commonly expand in the anteroposterior or lateral directions. Moreover, osteoporosis is a generalized condition, while Paget's disease is focal, and this is usually helpful in diagnosis. Bone scintigraphy may be unhelpful, since a recently collapsed vertebra and Paget's disease both show increased uptake. Malignancy, either primary or secondary, as well as infiltrations due to sarcoidosis or infection, may cause diagnostic difficulties, particularly if systemic features of the primary condition are absent or inconspicuous. In all these conditions, bone scintigraphy is of limited value, since increased uptake will generally be shown. Biochemical or hematological abnormalities, and particularly hypercalcemia, anemia, raised sedimentation rate, or hypoalbuminemia, may point to a systemic illness. Concentrations of bone markers may also be raised in both conditions. Where doubt remains, bone biopsy is indicated. Fibrous dysplasia may cause diagnostic problems, although the polyostotic form is usually easy to distinguish from Paget's disease, because it generally presents in childhood with fractures and long bone deformity. Small solitary lesions of fibrous dysplasia may go unrecognized until early adult life, when they may cause diagnostic confusion with monostotic Paget's disease. The condition is usually asymptomatic unless a fracture occurs but, like Paget's disease, may be associated with increased uptake on isotope scans. Biopsy of the affected lesion may be needed when the clinical features are equivocal.

Complications of Paget's disease

Bloodflow may be markedly increased in extremities involved with Paget's disease. When the disease is widespread and involves several bones, the increased bloodflow may be associated with high cardiac output and rarely with high-output heart failure. There are also reports suggesting an increased incidence of calcific aortic disease.[216] Pathologic fractures may occur at any stage, even though they are more common in the lytic phase of the disease. They particularly involve long bones with active areas of advancing lytic disease (i.e. the femoral shaft or the subtrocanteric area), and may occur spontaneously or following slight trauma. In some circumstances, Paget's disease of bone may be associated with involvement of the central and peripheral nervous system.[217] Neurological complications of the spine are relatively common, occurring in 4–10% of patients,[218,219] while the neurological complications of cranial disease, excluding auditory involvement, are rare. Irreversible hearing loss occurs in 13% of patients.[220] Interestingly, recent studies strongly support the hypothesis of cochlear pathology due to structural and/or density changes in cochlear capsule bone as the cause of hearing loss.[221] Newer imaging modalities such as CT and MRI have improved our ability to evaluate neurological symptoms in the context of Paget's disease. Hyperuricemia, gout, and osteoarthritis are all possible complications of Paget's disease. Subchondral bone enlargement, bowing of the long bones and softening of the subchondral bone may all alter the involved articular cartilage, leading to or precipitating osteoarthritis in pagetic patients.[222] One of the most serious complications of Paget's disease is neoplastic degeneration of pagetic bone with an increased incidence of sarcomas, especially in polyostotic cases of the disease. The majority of these tumors are classified as osteosarcomas, although fibrosarcomas and chondrosarcomas may also be seen. Approximately 1% of pagetic patients develop osteosarcoma, the risk being several thousand-fold higher than in the general population. It has been estimated that 20% of patients with osteosarcoma over the age of 60 have Paget's disease as a predisposing condition.[223] This significantly contributes to the mortality and morbidity of Paget's disease patients. The sarcomas most frequently arise in the femur, tibia, humerus, skull, mandibula and pelvis, and rarely occur in vertebrae. Typically, pagetic osteosarcomas are osteolytic, in contrast to the sclerotic appearance of radiation-induced osteosarcomas. Current treatment regimens emphasize maximal resection of tumor mass and chemotherapy. However, the prognosis, is generally poor and ablative surgery is rarely successful. Death from massive local extension or from pulmonary metastases occurs in the majority of cases in 1–3 years. Benign giant-cell tumor may also occur in pagetic bone. Radiographic evaluation of lesion, as well as bone biopsy, may be useful in the diagnosis. These tumors may show great sensitivity to glucocorticoids, and, in many instances, the mass may shrink or even disappear after treatment with dexamethasone or prednisone.[224]

Medical therapy for Paget's disease of bone

Most pagetic patients do not have symptoms, since the disease is localized. However, appropriate treatment should be given not only to symptomatic patients but also to any patient with a pagetic lesion in a high-risk location, even if the patient is asymptomatic. High-risk locations include the skull, spine, weight-bearing bones, pelvis and areas near major joints. The treatment objective is to control symptoms and reduce the risk of long-term complications. A reduction in bone turnover will reduce disease progression and, therefore, the risk of complications. Absolute indications for therapy are listed in Table 13.14 and include persistent bone pain, neural compression, rapidly progressive deformity resulting in disabling disturbance of

> Any symptomatic pagetic lesion (pain)
> Asymptomatic lesions in high-risk locations
>   Weight-bearing bone lesions
>   Lesions affecting the skull and/or the spine
>   Periarticular bone lesions
> Prior to surgical intervention in pagetic bone
> Immobilization

Table 13.14
Indications for treatment of Paget's disease of bone.

posture, hypercalcemia, severe hypercalciuria with or without renal stones, high-output congestive heart failure and repeated fractures. The use of antipagetic therapy before elective orthopedic surgery on pagetic bone also is recommended. Preoperative reduction in the flow of blood to bone has been advanced as an indication for antiresorptive therapy to reduce the risk of bleeding and improve the mechanical properties of bone.

Two major classes of drugs, calcitonin and bisphosponates, are approved by the Food and Drug Administration (FDA) in the USA as well as in several countries for the treatment of Paget's disease. Both classes of drugs suppress the abnormal bone cell activity that is associated with Paget's disease. Paget's disease is generally considered to be in remission until bone turnover has increased by more than 25% above the minimum achieved after treatment. Although bone turnover measurements after treatment may lie within the normal range for the population, they may nevertheless be greater than the value before the patient developed Paget's disease. The duration of remission achieved with bisphosphonates is considerably longer than that achieved by calcitonin.

Calcitonin

Calcitonin has been now largely superseded by the advent of bisphosphonates. It may still be useful in patients who cannot tolerate oral bisphosphonates because of gastrointestinal side-effects or who prefer to avoid intravenous therapy with pamidronate. Moreover, it may occasionally be needed to reduce bone bloodflow before surgery. The recommended dose of salmon calcitonin is 50–100 units daily or three times per week for 6–18 months, given subcutaneously. Repeat courses can be given after brief rest periods. The administration of porcine, salmon and human calcitonins for prolonged periods to pagetic patients induces a decrease in alkaline phosphatase and causes variable decrease in bone pain due to suppression of the pagetic lesion and the replacement of pagetic bone with normal lamellar bone. There is also an independent, centrally mediated analgesic effect. Calcitonin induces improvement in neurological symptoms and a decrease in elevated cardiac output. Patients with moderate to severe disease may require indefinite treatment courses to maintain a 50% reduction in the biochemical indices and symptomatic relief, while milder or monostotic disease may allow discontinuation of treatment for prolonged periods. Escape from the efficacy of treatment may sometimes occur, due to either a downregulation of calcitonin receptors or as a consequence of the development of neutralizing antibodies. The main side-effects are nausea or flushing of the skin.

Bisphosponates

The introduction of these potent antiresorptive drugs has led to a drastic improvement in the treatment of Paget's disease. The potency of the bisphosphonates and the sustained control of disease activity which they produce has resulted in them replacing calcitonin as the drug of first choice. Etidronate, pamidronate, tiludronate, alendronate and risedronate are currently licensed for this indication in the USA and in several European countries. None of the bisphosphonates should be used in the presence of severe kidney failure. As a rule, oral bisphosphonates should be taken on an empty stomach, with no food, beverages (except water) or other medications (including dietary supplements) for up to 2 h beforehand. An adequate dietary Ca intake (1000–1500 mg daily) and vitamin D intake (400 units) are recommended during bisphosphonate use, unless there is a history of hemolithiasis. It is important to know that the drugs discussed above differ in potency. Some drugs are more appropriate for people with mild Paget's disease, while others are better suited for people with severe disease.

Etidronate was the first bisphosphonate to have been used clinically for Paget's disease. It is given by mouth in a daily dose of 400 mg (approximately 5 mg/kg body weight) for a 6-month period, followed by at least 6 months of no treatment. Etidronate is moderately effective in reducing bone turnover by about 40–60% and producing clinical improvement, but in many patients responses are incomplete. Larger doses over shorter periods (10 mg/kg body weight for 3 months or 20 mg/kg body weight for 1 month) have also been shown to be effective, and bone turnover will be reduced in a dose-dependent fashion. Occasionally, some patients may experience diarrhea. Moreover, higher doses (>10 mg/kg body weight) may be associated with defective mineralization leading to osteomalacia and fractures. For this reason, etidronate treatment is not recommended for treating severe Paget's disease and is contraindicated in the presence of advancing lytic changes in a weight-bearing bone.

Tiludronate is about 10 times more potent than etidronate. It is given orally as a 40-mg daily dose for 3 months. This dose usually leads to normal levels of SAP after 3 months in 30–40% of moderately affected subjects.[225] It is generally well tolerated, with a minority of patients experiencing mild upper gastrointestinal disturbances. In clinical trials with tiludronate, bone biopsy showed no evidence of defective mineralization. This drug may represent an attractive choice in patients with mild disease.

Pamidronate is administered intravenously, since it is poorly absorbed and may have a local irritant effect on the upper gastrointestinal tract. Pamidronate is approximately 100 times more potent than etidronate. Current recommendations are to give three daily infusions of 30 mg weekly or a 60-mg single infusion, both doses being diluted in 500 ml normal saline or 5% dextrose in water, at an infusion rate of not more than 20 mg/h. The greater potency of this drug allows a majority of patients to experience normalization of pagetic indices rather than only partial suppression.[226] Two to four 60–90-mg doses may suffice in moderate disease, while total doses in the range of 300–500 mg, given over a number of weeks, may be required for severe cases. Side-effects include a low grade of fever the day after the first infusion, and the possibility of mild hypocalcemia, hypophosphatemia and lymphopenia. The rapid onset of symptomatic improvement as well as the overall potency of pamidronate make it the drug of choice for cases with neurological compression syndromes, for severe and painful lytic disease, and for pretreatment of active Paget's disease before elective surgery.

Alendronate is an orally administered bisphosphonate that is 700 times more potent than etidronate. The recommended dose is 40 mg daily for 6 months, i.e. four times the recommended dosage for treating osteoporosis. The patient should be instructed to take the drug in the morning, on an empty stomach, with about 8 oz of water, and not to lie down for at least 30 min after the dose. Alendronate is not associated with mineralization problems at therapeutically effective doses. In clinical trials, alendronate led to a normalized SAP in over 63% of patients, compared with 17% for etidronate.[227] Some patients taking alendronate may experience upper or lower gastrointestinal or esophageal symptoms, or less commonly oesophageal ulceration. For these reasons, the drug should be used with caution by patients who have disorders affecting the esophagus.

Risedronate is more than 1000 times more potent than etidronate. It is given orally, in a single 30-mg dose for 2–3 months, with a follow-up measurement of SAP 1 month later. If the value fails to normalize, an additional 2 months of therapy are suggested. Two to three month courses of risedronate therapy led to a nearly 80% reduction in bone turnover markers in about 50–70% of patients.[228] Like alendronate, risedronate is taken with 8 oz of water, in the morning, with no food intake and no lying down for 30 min after the dose. Mild upper gastrointestinal upset may occur in 15% of patients. A few cases of iritis have also been reported.

Other therapies

Pain associated with Paget's disease is often alleviated by treating the Paget's disease itself. However, nonsteroidal anti-inflammatory drugs such as ibuprofen and naproxen, as well as newer drugs of the same class, can be used to treat pain related to Paget's disease. Aspirin and acetaminophen can also be used. Surgery may be necessary when severe pain is not controlled by medication. Elective joint replacement, although more complex in Paget's disease than in typical osteoarthritis, may be successful in relieving refractory pain. Occasionally, osteotomy is performed to correct bowing deformity. All cases of serious neurological disturbances require immediate neurological and neurosurgical consultation.

Osteomalacia

Osteomalacia represents defective bone matrix mineralization occurring after the cessation of growth and involving only the bone and the growth plate.

Vitamin D and calcium deficiency

Deficiencies of vitamin D, Ca, or phosphate due to inadequate nutritional intake or malabsorption may result in defective bone mineralization. The main natural sources of vitamin D in foods are fish and liver, while the main natural sources of Ca and phosphate are represented by milk and dairy products. The most biologically active vitamin D metabolite, $1,25(OH)_2D_3$ (calcitriol), is synthesized in the kidney by hydroxylation of 25(OH)D produced by the liver. Calcitriol enhances Ca and phosphate absorption from the small intestine. In the presence of vitamin D deficiency, intestinal Ca and phosphate absorption are reduced, causing hypocalcemia followed by a consequent hyperparathyroid state. Consumption of cereals and other grain products, high in phytate, can result in intraluminal calcium phytate formation and consequent Ca malabsorption.[229]

Clinical manifestation

Diffuse bone pain is the most common manifestation of osteomalacia, especially in the hip area. Other clinical manifestations of osteomalacia are mainly represented by hypotonia, muscle weakness and, in severe cases, tetany. Deformity of the back, including kyphosis and lordosis, may be present, as may an increased risk of bone fractures (Figure 13.15). Radiologically, the long bones exhibit thin cortical radiolucent lines (stress fractures). The pelvis and ribs are the most frequently affected areas.[230] A decreased BMD is also observed. Biochemical findings include low or normal serum Ca and phosphate and elevated SAP. Serum levels of 25(OH)D are low and PTH levels are elevated in presence of hypocalcemia. Chronic hypophosphatemia exhibits similar radiological manifestations to those seen in both Ca and vitamin D deficiency. Since the serum Ca levels are in the normal range, secondary hyperparathyroidism is not an accompanying clinical feature. Consequently, bone mass is not decreased.

Oncogenic osteomalacia

In most cases, a tumour has been documented as causing the osteomalacia, because the metabolic distur-

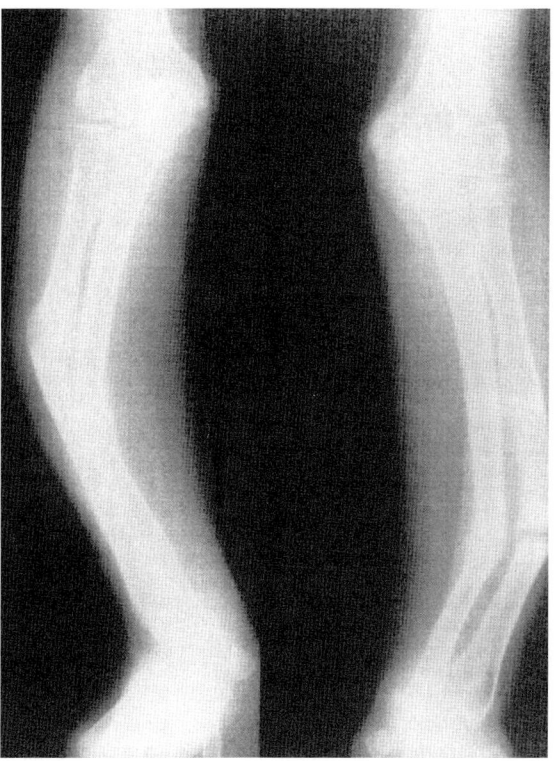

Figure 13.15
Pathological fractures of radius and ulna in a patient affected by intestinal malabsorption. (From Gennari C, Avioli LV (eds) Atlante delle Malattie Dell'osso, Vol. II. Parma: Chiesi Farmaceutici S.p.A., 1992.)

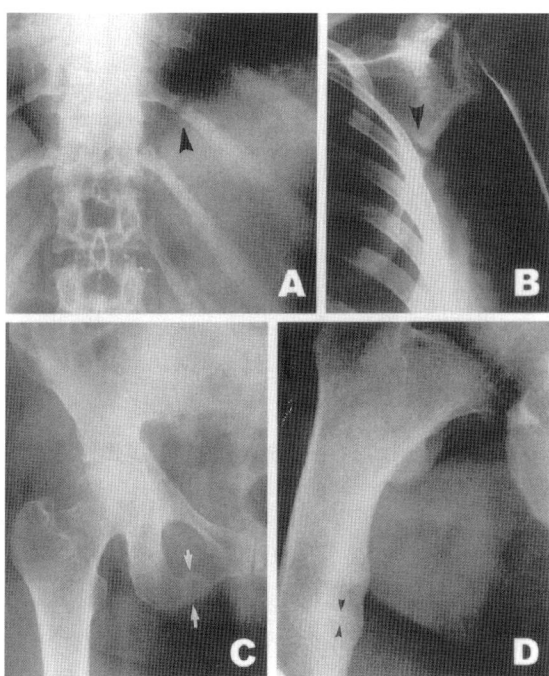

Figure 13.16
Pseudofractures (arrows) of ribs (A), scapula (B), pelvis (C) and femoral diaphysis (D). (From Gennari C, Avioli LV (eds) Atlante delle Malattie Dell'osso, Vol. II. Parma: Chiesi Farmaceutici S.p.A., 1992.)

bances improve or completely disappear on removal of the tumor. Patients usually present with vague symptoms, including bone and muscle pain and muscle weakness. Fractures of long bone are occasionally reported. In younger patients, fatigue, gait disturbances, slow growth and skeletal abnormalities occur. The biochemical findings characterizing this disorder include hypophosphatemia and an abnormally low renal tubular maximum for the reabsorption of phosphate per liter of glomerular filtrate resulting in phosphate wasting. The serum levels of $25(OH)D_3$ are normal and $1,25(OH)_2D_3$ are generally inappropriately normal relative to the hypophosphatemia. Alkaline phosphatase is high. X-ray abnormalies include osteopenia, pseudofractures (Figure 13.16) and coarsened trabeculae.

The responsible tumors are mainly represented by neoplasms of mesenchymal origin.

Drugs disrupting the vitamin D endocrine system
  Cholestyramine (inhibition of vitamin D absorption)
  Phenytoin (alteration of vitamin D metabolism)
  Phenobarbital (alteration of vitamin D metabolism)
  Rifampicin (alteration of vitamin D metabolism)
  Cadmium (alteration of vitamin D metabolism)
  Glucocorticoids (alteration of vitamin D metabolism)
Drugs disrupting phosphate homeostasis
  Aluminum-containing antacid (inhibition of phosphate absorption)
  Cadmium (induction of renal phosphate wasting)
  Lead (induction of renal phosphate wasting)
Drugs disrupting bone mineralization
  Aluminum
  Fluoride
  Bisphosphonates

Table 13.15
Drugs inducing osteomalacia

Drug-induced osteomalacia

Numerous drugs can cause osteomalacia by several mechanisms, as summarized in Table 13.15.

References

1. Moore EW. Ionized calcium in normal serum, ultrafiltrates, and whole blood determined by ion-exchange electrodes. *J Clin Invest* 1970; 49: 318.
2. Swash M, Rowan AJ. Electroencephalographic criteria for hypocalcemia and hypercalcemia. *Arch Neurol* 1972; 26: 218–28.
3. Illum F, Duppont E. Prevalence of CT-detected calcification in the basal ganglia in idiopathic hypoparathyroidism and pseudohypoparathyroidism. *Neuroradiology* 1985; 27: 32–7.
4. Aryanpur I, Farhoudi A, Zangeneh F. Congestive heart failure secondary to idiopathic hypoparathyroidism. *Am J Dis Child* 1974; 127: 738–9.
5. Lammer EJ, Optiz JM. The DiGeorge anomaly as a developmental field defect. *Am J Med Genet Suppl* 1986; 2: 113–27.
6. Lindsay EA, Halford S, Wadey R, Scambler PJ, Baldini A. Molecular cytogenetic characterization of the DiGeorge syndrome region using fluorescence in situ hybridization. *Genomics* 1993; 17: 403–7.
7. Gottilieb S, Driscoll DA, Punnett HH, Sellinger B, Emanuel BS, Budarf ML. Characterization of 10p deletions suggests two non overlapping regions contribute to the DiGeorge syndrome phenotype. *Am J Hum Genet* 1998; 62: 495–8.
8. Haire RN, Buell RD, Litman RT et al. Diversification, not use, of the immunoglobulin VH gene repertoire is restricted in DiGeorge syndrome. *J Exp Med* 1993; 178: 825–34.
9. Fanconi S, Fischer JA Weiland P et al. Kenney syndrome: evidence for idiopathic hypoparathyroidism in two patients and for abnormal parathyroid hormone in one. *J Pediatrics* 1986; 109: 489–92.
10. Goltzman D, Cole DEC. Hypoparathyroidism. In: Favus MJ, ed. *Primer on the Metabolic Bone Diseases and Disorders of Mineral Metabolism*, 4th edn. Philadelphia: Lippincott Wiliams & Wilkins, 1999; 226–30.
11. Aaltonen J, Bjorses P, Sandkuijl L, Perheentupa J, Peltonen L. An autosomal locus causing autoimmune polyglandular disease type I assigned to chromosome 21. *Nature Genet* 1994; 8: 23–87.
12. Blizzard RM, Chee D, Davis W. The incidence of parathyroid and other antibodies in the sera of patients with idiopathic hypoparathyroidism. *Clin Exp Immunol* 1966; 1: 119.
13. Arnold A, Horst SA, Gardella TJ, Baba H, Levine MA, Kronenberg HM. Mutations of the signal peptide

14. Parkinson DB, Takker RV. A donor splice site mutation in the parathyroid hormone gene is associated with autosomal recessive hypoparathyroidism. *Nature Genet* 1992; 1: 149–52.
15. Albright F, Burnett CH, Smith PH. Pseudohypoparathyroidism: an example of 'Seabright–Bantam syndrome.' *Endocrinology* 1942; 30: 922–32.
16. Levine MA. Parathyroid hormone resistance syndrome. In: Favus MJ, ed. *Primer on the Metabolic Bone Diseases and Disorders of Mineral Metabolism*, 4th edn. Philadelphia: Lippincott Williams & Wilkins, 1999; 230–5.
17. Chase LR, Melson GL, Aurbach GD. Pseudohypoparathyroidism: defective excretion of 3′,5′-AMP in response to parathyroid hormone. *J Clin Invest* 1969; 48: 1832–44.
18. Levine MA, Modi WS, Obren SL. Mapping of the gene encoding the alpha subunit of the stimulatory protein of adenyl cyclase (GNAS1) to 20q13.2–q13.3 in human in situ hybridization. *Genomics* 1991; 11: 478–9.
19. Carter A, Bardin C, Collins R, Simons C, Bray P, Spiegel A. Reduced expression of multiple forms of the α subunit of the stimulatory GTP-binding protein in pseudohypoparathyroidism type Ia. *Proc Natl Acad Sci USA* 1987; 84: 7266–9.
20. Davies SJ, Hughes HE. Imprinting in Albright's hereditary osteodystrophy. *J Med Genet* 1993; 30: 101–3.
21. Weinstein LS, Yu S. The role of genomic imprinting of Gsα in the pathogenesis of Albright's hereditary osteodystrophy. *Trends Endocrinol Metab* 1999; 10: 81–5.
22. Marx SJ. Hypoparathyroidism. In: Krieger DT, Bardin CW, eds. *Current Therapy in Endocrinology and Metabolism*. Toronto: BC Decker, 1985; 329–33.
23. Okano K, Furukawa Y, Morii H, Fujita T. Comparative efficacy of various vitamin D metabolites in the treatment of various types of hypoparathyroidism. *J Clin Endocrinol Metab* 1982; 55: 238–43.
24. Heath H. Clinical spectrum of primary hyperparathyroidism: evolution with changes in medical practice and technology. *J Bone Mineral Res* 1991, 6(2): S63–70.
25. Leifsson BG, Ahren BO. Serum calcium and survival in a large health screening program. *J Clin Endocrinol Metab* 1996; 81(6): 2149–53.
26. Silverberg SJ. Diagnosis, natural history, and treatment of primary hyperparathyroidism. *Cancer Treat Res* 1997; 89: 163–81.
27. Wermers RA, Khosla S, Atkinson EJ, Hodgson SF, O'Fallon WM, Melton LJ 3rd. The rise and fall of primary hyperparathyroidism: a population-based study in Rochester, Minnesota, 1965–1992. *Ann Intern Med* 1997; 15: 126(6): 433–40.
28. Wynne AG, Van Heerden J, Carney JA, Fitzpatrick LA. Parathyroid carcinoma: clinical and pathologic features in 43 patients. *Medicine (Baltimore)* 1992; 71(4): 197–205.
29. Arnold A. Molecular mechanisms of parathyroid neoplasia. *Endocrinol Metab Clin North Am* 1994; 23(1): 93–107.
30. Hsi ED, Zukerberg LR, Yang WI, Arnold A. Cyclin D1/PRAD1 expression in parathyroid adenomas: an immunohistochemical study. *J Clin Endocrinol Metab* 1996; 81(5): 1736–9.
31. Chandrasekharappa SC, Guru SC, Manickam P et al. Positional cloning of the gene for multiple endocrine neoplasia-type 1. *Science* 1997; 18: 276(5311): 404–7.
32. Heppner C, Kester MB, Agarwal SK et al. Somatic mutation of the MEN1 gene in parathyroid tumours. *Nature Genet* 1997; 16(4): 375–8.
33. Cryns VL, Yi SM, Tahara H, Gaz RD, Arnold A. Frequent loss of chromosome arm 1p DNA in parathyroid adenomas. *Genes Chromosomes Cancer* 1995; 13(1): 9–17.
34. Hosokawa Y, Pollak MR, Brown EM, Arnold A. Mutational analysis of the extracellular Ca(2+)-sensing receptor gene in human parathyroid tumors. *J Clin Endocrinol Metab* 1995; 80(11): 3107–10.
35. Falchetti A, Becherini L, Martineti V et al. Telomerase repeat amplification protocol (TRAP): A new molecular marker for parathyroid carcinoma. *Biochem Biophys Res Commun* 1999; 265(1): 252–5.
36. Consensus Development Statement. *J Bone Mineral Res* 1991; 6(2): S9–13.
37. Consensus Development Conference Panel. Diagnosis and management of asymptomatic primary hyperparathyroidism. *Ann Intern Med* 1991; 114: 593–7.
38. Bilezikian JP, Silverberg SJ. Primary hyperparathyroidism: still evolving? *J Bone Miner Res* 1997; 12(9): 1538.
39. Sosa J, Powe NR, Levine MA, Udelsman R, Zeiger MA. Thresholds for surgery and surgical outcomes for patients with primary hyperparathyroidism: a national survey of endocrine surgeons. *J Clin Endocrinol Metab* 1998; 83(8): 2658–65.
40. Turken SA, Cafferty M, Silverberg SJ et al. Neuromuscular involvement in mild, asymptomatic primary hyperparathyroidism. *Am J Med* 1989; 87(5): 553–7.
41. Solomon BL, Schaaf M, Smallridge RC. Psychologic symptoms before and after parathyroid surgery. *Am J Med* 1994; 96(2): 101–6.
42. Silverberg SJ, Shane E, Jacobs TP, Siris E, Bilezikian JP. A 10-year prospective study of primary hyperparathyroidism with or without parathyroid surgery. *N Engl J Med* 1999; 341(17): 1249–55.
43. Clark OH. Asymptomatic primary hyperparathyroidism: is parathyroidectomy indicated? *Surgery* 1994; 116(6): 947–53.

44. Haines GA, Miller DL, Turton DB, Ghosh BC. Preoperative localization in patients with difficult re-explorations for hyperparathyroidism. *J Surg Oncol* 1996; 61(1): 66–7.
45. Doppman JL, Skarulis MC, Chen CC et al. Parathyroid adenomas in the aortopulmonary window. *Radiology* 1996; 201: 456–62.
46. Arkles BL, Jones T, Hicks RJ, De Luise MA, Chou ST. Impact of complementary parathyroid scintigraphy and ultrasonography on the surgical management of hyperparathyroidism. *Surgery* 1996; 120: 845–51.
47. Solbiati L, Rizzatto G. In: *Ultrasound of Superficial Structures*. Churchill Livingstone, 1995.
48. Tziakoury C, Eracleous E, Skannavis S, Pierides A, Symeonides P, Gourtsoyannis N. Value of ultrasonography, CT and MR imaging in the diagnosis of primary hyperparathyroidism. *Acta Radiol* 1996; 37: 720–6.
49. Bergenfelz A, Forsberg L, Hederstrom E, Ahren B. Preoperative localization of enlarged parathyroid glands with ultrasonically guided fine needle aspiration for parathyroid hormone assay. *Acta Radiol* 1991; 32(5): 403–5.
50. Gooding GAW, Clark OH. Use of color doppler imaging in the distinction between thyroid and parathyroid lesions. *Am J Surgery* 1992; 164: 51–6.
51. Coakley AJ. Parathyroid imaging. *Nuclear Med Commun* 1995; 16: 522–33.
52. McBiles M, Lambert AT, Cote MG, Kim SY. Sestamibi parathyroid imaging. *Semin Nuclear Med* 1995; XXV(3): 221–34.
53. Taillefer R. 99mTc Sestamibi parathyroid scintigraphy. *Nuclear Med Ann* 1995; 55–79.
54. Aigner RM, Fueger GF, Nicoletti R. Parathyroid scintigraphy: comparison of technetium 99m methoxy-isobutyl isonitrile and technetium 99m tetrofosmin studies. *Eur J Med* 1996; 23(6): 693–6.
55. Gallowitsch HJ, Mikosch P, Kresnik E, Gomez I, Lind P. Technetium 99m tetrofosmin parathyroid imaging. Results with double-phase study and SPECT in primary and secondary hyperparathyroidism. *Invest Radiol* 1997; 32(8): 459–65.
56. Moka D, Voth E, Larena-Avellaneda A et al. SPECT parathyroid gland scintigraphy for the preoperative localization of small parathyroid gland adenoma. *Nuklearmedizin* 1998; 37(1): 61.
57. Billotey C, Sarfati E, Aurengo A et al. Advantages of SPECT in 99mTc-MIBI parathyroid scintigraphy. *J Nuclear Med* 1996; 37(11): 1773–8.
58. Wegener OH. In: *Whole Body Computed Tomography*, Vol. 6. Blackwell Scientific Publications, 158–9.
59. Auffermann WA, Gooding GAW, Okerlund MD et al. Diagnosis of recurrent hyperparathyroidism: comparison of MR imaging and other imaging techniques. *Am J Radiol* 1987; 150: 1027–33.
60. Kneeland JB, Krubsach AJ, Lawson TL et al. Enlarged parathyroid glands: high-resolution local coil MR imaging. *Radiology* 1987; 162: 143–6.
61. McDermott VG, Mendez Fernandez RJ, Meakem III TJ, Stolpen AH, Spritzer CE, Gefter WB. Preoperative imaging in hyperparathyroidism: results and factors affecting parathyroid detection. *Am J Radiol* 1996; 166: 705–10.
62. Nakahara H, Noguchi S, Marakami N et al. Gadolinium-enhanced MR imaging of thyroid and parathyroid masses. *Radiology* 1997; 202: 765–72.
63. Seelos KC, De Narco WB, Clark OH, Higgings CB. Persistent and recurrent hyperparathyroidism: assessment with gadopentate dimeglumine-enhanced MR imaging. *Radiology* 1990; 177: 373–8.
64. Spritzer CE, Gefter WB, Hamilton R, Greenberg BM, Axel L, Kressel HY. Abnormal parathyroid glands: high-resolution MR imaging. *Radiology* 1987; 487–91.
65. Ljunghall S, Hellman P, Rastad J, Akerrstrom G. Primary hyperparathyroidism: epidemiology, diagnosis and clinical picture. *World J Surg* 1991; 15: 681–7.
66. Thompson NW. Surgical anatomy of hyperparathyroidism. *Prog Surg* 1986; 18: 59–79.
67. Hooghe L, Kinnaert P, van Geertruyden J. Surgical anatomy of hyperparathyroidism. *Acta Chir Belg* 1992; 92: 1–9.
68. Esselstyn CB, Levin HS. A technique for parathyroid surgery. *Surg Clin North Am* 1975; 55: 1047.
69. Irvin III GL, Dembrow VD, Prudhomme DL. Operative monitoring of parathyroid glands hyperfunction. *Am J Surg* 1991; 162: 299.
70. Herrera M, Grant C, van Heerden JA, Fitzpatrick LA. Parathyroid autotransplantation. *Arch Surg* 1992; 127: 825.
71. Sepanati A, Young AE. Parathyroid autotransplantation. *Br J Surg* 1990; 77: 1171.
72. O'Riordain DS, O'Brian T, Grant CS, Weaner A, Gharib H, van Heerden JA. Surgical management of primary hyperparathyroidism in multiple endocrine neoplasia type 1 and 2. *Surgery* 1993; 114(6): 1031.
73. Janson S, Tisell LE. Total parathyroidectomy and parathyroid transplantation into subcutaneous fat tissue in the treatment of hyperparathyroidism in multiple endocrine neoplasia type 1. *Acta Chir Aust* 1994; 26(suppl 112): 23.
74. Mallette LE, Eisenberg KL, Schwaitzberg SD, Noon GP. Factors that influence the assessment of parathyroid graft function. *Ann Surg* 1984; 199(2): 192.
75. Nussbaum SR, Thompson AR, Hutcheson K, Gaz RD, Wang CA. Intraoperative measurement of parathyroid hormone in the surgical management of hyperparathyroidism. *Surgery* 1988; 104: 1121–6.
76. Davies CH, Demeure MJ, Ast J, Edis AJ. Study of intact (1–84) parathyroid hormone secretion in patients undergoing parathyroidectomy. *World J Surg* 1990; 14: 355–60.

77. Bergenfelz A, Norden NE, Ahren B. Intraoperative fall in plasma levels of intact parathyroid hormone after removal of one enlarged parathyroid gland in hyperparathyroid patients. *Eur J Surg* 1991; **157**: 109–12.
78. Ryan MF, Jones SR, Barnes AD. Clinical evaluation of a rapid parathyroid hormone assay. *Ann Clin Biochem* 1992; **29**(Pt 1): 48–51.
79. Duquenne M, Weryha G, Kaminsky P, De Talance N, Mathieu P, Leclere J. Serum parathormone profile during surgical treatment of hyperfunctioning parathyroid adenoma: a multicompartmental model. *J Bone Mineral Res* 1994; **9**: 1371–5.
80. Manin M, de la Cruz VC, Martinez JP, Barrodera ML, Ortega G. Intraoperative serum parathyroid hormone measurement in the surgical treatment of hyperparathyroidism. *Med Clin (Barc)* 1997; **109**(6): 201–6.
81. Locchi F, Tommasi M, Brandi ML, Tonelli F, Meldolesi U. Model of iPTH clearance after parathyroid adenomectomy. *Eur J Nucl Med* 1998; **25**(8): PS-726, 1165.
82. Levin KE, Clark OH. The reason for failure in parathyroid operations. *Arch Surg* 1989; **124**: 911–5.
83. Lumb GA, Stanbury SW. Parathyroid function in vitamin D deficiency and vitamin D deficiency in primary hyperparathyroidism. *Am J Med* 1974; **56**: 833–9.
84. Selby PL, Peacock M. Ethinyl estradiol and norethindrone in the treatment of primary hyperparathyroidism in postmenopausal women. *N Engl J Med* 1986; **314**: 1481–5.
85. Coe FL, Favus MJ, Parks JH. Is estrogen preferable to surgery for menopausal women with primary hyperparathyroidism? *N Engl J Med* 1986; **314**: 1508–9.
86. Marcus R. Estrogens and progestins in the management of primary hyperparathyroidism. *J Bone Mineral Res* 1991; **6**(suppl 2): S125–9.
87. Reasner CA, Stone MD, Hosking DJ, Ballah A, Mundy GR. Acute changes in calcium homeostasis during treatment of primary hyperparathyroidism with risedronate. *J Clin Endocrinol Metab* 1993; **77**: 1067–71.
88. Steffey ME, Fox J, van Wagenen BC, Del Mar EG, Balandrin MF, Nemeth EF. Calcimimetics: structurally and mechanistically novel compounds that inhibit hormone secretion from parathyroid cells. *J Bone Mineral Res* 1993; **8**(suppl 1): S175a.
89. Ott SM. Calcimimetics—new drugs with the potential to control hyperparathyroidism. *J Clin Endocrinol Metab* 1998; **83**(4): 1080–2.
90. Collins MT, Skarulis MC, Bilezikian JP, Silverberg SJ, Spiegel AM, Marx SJ. Treatment of hypercalcemia secondary to parathyroid carcinoma with a novel calcimimetic agent. *J Clin Endocrinol Metab* 1998; **83**(4): 1083–8.
91. Silverberg SJ, Bone HG, Marriott TB et al. Short-term inhibition of parathyroid hormone secretion by a calcium-receptor agonist in patients with primary hyperparathyroidism. *N Engl J Med* 1997; **337**(21): 1506–10.
92. Antonsen JE, Sherrard DJ, Andress DL. A calcimimetic agent acutely suppresses parathyroid hormone levels in patients with chronic renal failure. *Kidney Int* 1998; **53**: 223–7.
93. Attie MF. Treatment of hypercalcemia. *Endocrinol Metab Clin North Am* 1989; **18**: 807–28.
94. Halloran BP, Nissenson BA, eds. *Parathyroid Hormone-Related Protein: Normal Physiology and its Role in Cancer*. Boca Raton, Florida: CRC Press, 1992.
95. Adams JS, Fernandez M, Gacad MA et al. Vitamin D metabolite-mediated hypercalcemia and hypercalciuria in patients with AIDS and non-AIDS associated lymphoma. *Blood* 1989; **73**: 235–9.
96. Mundy GR. Hypercalcemic factors other than parathyroid hormone-related protein. *Endocrinol Metab Clin North Am* 1989; **18**: 795–805.
97. Harinck HI, Bijvoet OL, Plantingh AS et al. Role of bone and kidney in tumor-induced hypercalcemia and its treatment with bisphosphonate and sodium chloride. *Am J Med* 1987; **82**: 1133–42.
98. Stewart AF, Broadus AE. Mineral metabolism. In: Felig P, Baxter JP, Broadus AE, Frohman LA, eds. *Endocrinology and Metabolism*. New York: McGraw-Hill, 1987; 1376–421.
99. Roberts MM, Stewart AF. Humoral hypercalcemia of malignancy. In: Favus MJ, ed. *Primer on the Metabolic Bone Diseases and Disorders of Mineral Metabolism*, 4th edn. Philadelphia: Lippincott Williams & Wilkins, 1999: 203–7.
100. Garrett IR, Durie BG, Nedwin GE et al. Production of the bone resorbing cytokine lymphotoxin by cultured human myeloma cells. *N Engl J Med* 1987; **317**: 526–32.
101. Bataille R, Jourdan M, Zhang XG, Klein B. Serum levels of interleukin-6, a potent, myeloma cell growth factor as a reflection of disease severity in plasma cell dyscrasias. *J Clin Invest* 1989; **84**: 2008–11.
102. Cozzolino F, Torcia M, Aldinucci D et al. Production of interleukin-1 by bone marrow myeloma cells. *Blood* 1989; **74**(1): 387–90.
103. Binstock ML, Mundy GR. Effects of calcitonin and glucocorticoids in combination with hypercalcemia of malignancy. *Ann Intern Med* 1980; **93**: 269–72.
104. Canellos GP. Hypercalcemia in malignant lymphoma and leukemia. *Ann NY Acad Sci* 1974; **230**: 240–6.
105. Motokura T, Fukumoto S, Matsumoto T et al. Parathyroid hormone related protein in adult T-cell leukemia–lymphoma. *Ann Intern Med* 1989; **111**: 484–8.
106. Breslau NA, McGuire JL, Zerwekh JE, Frenkel EP, Pak CYC. Hypercalcemia associated with increased serum calcitriol levels in three patients with lymphoma. *Ann Intern Med* 1984; **100**: 107.

107. Orwoll ES. The milk-alkali syndrome: current concepts. *Ann Intern Med* 1982; **97**: 242–8.
108. Studdy PR, Bind R, Neville E, James DG. Biochemical findings in sarcoidosis. *J Clin Pathol* 1980; **33**: 528–33.
109. Sandler LM, Wineals CG, Fraher LJ, Clemens TL, Smith R, O'Riordan JLH. Studies of the hypercalcemia of sarcoidosis: effects of steroids and exogenous vitamin D3 on the circulating concentrations of 1,25-dihydroxyvitamin D3. *Q J Med* 1984; **53**: 165–80.
110. Meyrier A, Valeyre D, Bouillon R, Paillard F, Battesti JP, Georges R. Resorptive versus absorptive hypercalciuria in sarcoidosis: correlations with 25-hydroxyvitamin D3 and 1,25-dihydroxyvitamin D3 and parameters of disease activity. *Q J Med* 1985; **54**: 269–81.
111. Insogna KL, Dreyer BE, Mitnick M, Ellison AF, Broadus AE. Enhanced production rate of 1,25-dihydroxyvitamin D in sarcoidosis. *J Clin Endocrinol Metab* 1988; **66**: 72–5.
112. Adams JS, Singer FR, Gacad MA et al. Isolation and structural identification of 1,25-dihydroxyvitamin D3 produced by cultured alveolar macrophages in sarcoidosis. *J Clin Endocrinol Metab* 1985; **60**: 960–6.
113. Bilezikian JP. Management of acute hypercalcemia. *N Engl J Med* 1992; **326**: 1196–203.
114. Grill V, Murray RM, Ho PW et al. Circulating PTH and PTHrP levels before and after treatment of tumor induced hypercalcemia with pamidronate disodium. *J Clin Endocrinol Metab* 1990; **74**: 1468–70.
115. Hall TJ, Chambers TJ. Gallium inhibits bone resorption by a direct action on osteoclasts. *Bone Miner* 1990; **8**: 211–6.
116. Consensus Development Conference. Diagnosis, prophylaxis, and treatment of osteoporosis. *Ann Intern Med* 1993; **94**: 646–50.
117. Cummings SR, Black DM, Newitt MC et al. Bone density at various sites for prediction of hip fractures. *Lancet* 1993; **341**: 72–5.
118. Sambrook PN. The treatment of postmenopausal osteoporosis. *N Engl J Med* 1995; **333**: 1495–6.
119. Avioli LV, Lindsay R. The female osteoporotic syndromes. In: Avioli LV, Krane SM, eds. *Metabolic Bone Disease*, 2nd edn. Philadelphia: WB Saunders Company, 397–451.
120. Nordin BEC, Need AG, Chatterton BE, Horowitz M, Morris HA. The relative contributions of age and years since menopause to postmenopausal bone loss. *J Clin Endocrinol Metab* 1990; **70**: 83–8.
121. Dempster DW, Lindsay R. Pathogenesis of osteoporosis. *Lancet* 1993; **i**: 797–801.
122. Theintz G, Busch B, Rizzoli R et al. Longitudinal monitoring of bone mass accumulation in healthy adolescents; evidence for a marked reduction after 16 years of age at the level of lumbar spine and femoral neck in female subjects. *J Clin Endocrinol Metab* 1992; **75**: 1060–5.
123. Heaney RP. Estrogen–calcium interactions in the postmenopause: a quantitative description. *Bone Mineral* 1990; **11**: 67–84.
124. Riggs BL, Wahner HW, Dunn WL. Mazess RB, Offord KP, Melton LJ III. Differential changes in bone mineral density of the appendicular and axial skeleton with aging. Relationship to osteoporosis. *J Clin Invest* 1931; **67**: 328–35.
125. Genant HK, Cann CE, Ettinger S, Gordan GS. Quantitative computed tomography of vertebral spongiosa: a sensitive method for detecting early bone loss after oophorectomy. *Ann Intern Med* 1982; **97**: 699–705.
126. Hui SI, Slemenda CW, Johnston CC Jr. The contribution of bone loss to postmenopausal osteoporosis. *Osteoporosis Int* 1990; **1**: 30–4.
127. Marcus R. The nature of osteoporosis. *J Clin Endocrinol Metab* 1996; **81**: 1–5.
128. Eisman JA. Genetics of osteoporosis. *Endocrine Rev* 1999; **20**: 788–804.
129. Cummings SP, Kelsey JL, Nevitt MC, O'Dowd KJ. Epidemiology of osteoporosis and osteoporotic fractures. *Epidemiol Rev* 1985; **7**: 178–208.
130. Jacobsen SJ, Goldberg J, Miles TP, Brody JA, Streis W, Rimm AA. Race and sex differences in mortality following fracture of the hip. *Am J Public Health* 1992; **82**: 1147–50.
131. Nevitt MC. Epidemiology of osteoporosis. *Rheum Dis Clin North Am* 1994; **20**: 535–59.
132. Chrischilles EA, Butler CD, Davis CS, Wallace RB. A model of lifetime osteoporosis impact. *Arch Intern Med* 1991; **151**: 2026–32.
133. Cummings SR, Nevitt MC, Browner WS et al. Risk factors for hip fracture in white women. *N Engl J Med* 1995; **332**: 767–73.
134. World Health Organization. Assessment of fracture risk and its application to screening for postmenopausal osteoporosis. Report of a WHO study group. *WHO Tech Rep Ser* 1994; **843**: 1–129.
135. Garnero P, Shih WJ, Gineyts E, Karpf DB, Delmas PD. Comparison of new biochemical markers of bone turnover in late postmenopausal women in response to alendronate treatment. *J Clin Endocrinol Metab* 1994; **79**: 1693–700.
136. Teitelbaum SL, Nichols SH. Tetracycline-based morphometric analysis of trabecular bone kinetics. In: Meunier PJ, ed. *Bone Histomorphometry* Paris: Armour Montagu, 1977; 311–19.
137. Riggs BL, Melton LJ. The prevention and treatment of osteoporosis. *N Engl J Med* 1992; **327**: 620–7.
138. Lindsay R. Prevention and treatment of osteoporosis. *Lancet* 1993; **i**: 801–5.
139. Kiel DP, Baron JA, Anderson JJ et al. Smoking eliminates the protective effect of oral estrogens on the risk

140. Barrett-Connor E, Bush TL. Estrogen and coronary heart disease in women. *JAMA* 1991; **265**: 1861–967.
141. Barzel US. Estrogens in the prevention and treatment of postmenopausal osteoporosis. *Am J Med* 1988; **85**: 847–50.
142. Paganini-Hill A, Ross RK, Gerkins VR et al. Menopausal estrogen therapy and hip fractures. *Ann Intern Med* 1981; **95**: 28–31.
143. Hutchinson TA, Polansky SM, Feinstein AR. Postmenopausal oestrogens protect against fractures of hip and distal radius. *Lancet* 1979; **ii**: 705–9.
144. Weiss NS, Ure CL, Ballard JH et al. Decreased risk of fractures of the hip and lower forearm with postmenopausal use of estrogen. *N Engl J Med* 1930; **303**: 1195–203.
145. Kreiger N, Kelsey JI, Holford TR. An epidemiologic study of hip fracture in postmenopausal women. *Am J Epidemiol* 1982; **116**: 141–8.
146. Kiel DP, Feison DT, Anderson JJ et al. Hip fracture and the use of estrogens in postmenopausal women: the Framingham study. *N Engl J Med* 1987; **317**: 1169–74.
147. Naessen T, Persson I, Adami HO et al. Hormone replacement therapy and the risk for first hip fracture. *Ann Intern Med* 1990; **113**: 95–103.
148. Kanis JA, Johnell O, Gullberg B et al. Evidence for efficacy of drugs affecting bone metabolism in preventing hip fracture. *BMJ* 1992; **305**: 1124–8.
149. Lufkin EG, Wahner HW, O'Fallon WM et al. Treatment of postmenopausal osteoporosis with transdermal estrogen. *Ann Intern Med* 1992; **117**: 1–9.
150. Hulka BS. Hormone replacement therapy and the risk of breast cancer. *Cancer* 1990; **40**: 289–96.
151. Grady D, Rubin SM, Petitti DB et al. Hormone therapy to prevent disease and prolong life in postmenopausal women. *Ann Intern Med* 1992; **117**: 1016–37.
152. Horowitz M, Wishart IM, Need AG, Morris HA, Nordin BEC. Effects of norethisterone on bone related biochemical variables and forearm bone mineral in postmenopausal osteoporosis. *Clin Endocrinol (Oxf)* 1993; **39**: 649–55.
153. Felson DT, Zhang Y, Hannan MT, Kiel DP, Wilson PWF. The effect of postmenopausal estrogen therapy on bone density in elderly women. *N Engl J Med* 1993; **329**: 1141–6.
154. Ettinger B, Grady D. The waning effect of postmenopausal estrogen therapy on osteoporosis. *N Engl J Med* 1993; **329**: 1192–3.
155. Ensrud KE, Palermo L, Black DM et al. Hip and calcaneal bone loss increase with advancing age: longitudinal results from the study of osteoporotic fractures. *J Bone Mineral Res* 1995; **10**: 1778–87.
156. Cauley JA, Seeley DG, Ensrud K, Ettinger B, Black D, Cummings SR. Estrogen replacement therapy and fractures in older women. *Ann Intern Med* 1995; **122**: 9–16.
157. Tilyard MW, Spears GFS, Com B, Thomson J, Dovey S. Treatment of postmenopausal osteoporosis with calcitriol or calcium. *N Engl J Med* 1992; **326**: 357–68.
158. Chapuy MC, Arlot ME, Duboeuf F et al. Vitamin D3 and calcium to prevent hip fractures in the elderly woman. *N Engl J Med* 1992; **327**: 1637–42.
159. McKane WR, Khosla S, Egan KS, Robins SP, Burritt MF, Riggs BL. Role of calcium intake in modulating age-related increases in parathyroid function and bone resorption. *J Clin Endocrinol Metab* 1996; **81**: 1699–703.
160. Singer FR, Melvin KEW, Mills BG. Acute effects of calcitonin on osteoclasts in man. *Clin Endocrinol (Oxf)* 1976; **5**: 333–40.
161. Nicholson GC, Mosley JM, Sexton PM et al. Abundant calcitonin receptors in isolated rate osteoclasts. Biochemical and autoradiographic characterization. *J Clin Invest* 1986; **78**: 355–70.
162. Wimalawansa SJ. Long and short term side effects and safety of calcitonin in man: a prospective study. *Calcif Tissue Int* 1993; **52**: 90–3.
163. Ostergaard K, Riis BJ, Christiansen C. Effect of salcatonin given intranasally on early postmenopausal bone loss. *BMJ* 1989; **299**: 477–9.
164. Stevenson JC, Lees B, Ellerington MC et al. Postmenopausal osteoporosis: a double blind placebo controlled study. *J Bone Miner Res* 1992; **7(S1)**: 325.
165. Overgard K. Effect of intranasal salmon calcitonin therapy on bone mass and bone turnover in early postmenopausal women: a dose–response study. *Calcif Tissue Int* 1994; **55**: 82–6.
166. Civitelli R, Gonnelli S, Zacchei S et al. Bone turnover in postmenopausal osteoporosis: effects of calcitonin treatment. *J Clin Invest* 1988; **82**: 1268–74.
167. Gruber HE, Ivey JL, Baylink DJ et al. Long-term calcitonin therapy in postmenopausal osteoporosis. *Metabolism* 1984; **33**: 295–303.
168. Muff R, Dambacher MA, Fisher JA. Formation of neutralizing antibodies during intranasal synthetic salmon calcitonin treatment of postmenopausal osteoporosis. *Osteoporosis Int* 1991; **1**: 72–5.
169. Lyritis GP, Tsakalakos N, Magiasis B et al. Analgesic effect of salmon calcitonin in osteoporotic vertebral fractures. *Calcif Tissue Int* 1991; **49**: 369–72.
170. Fleish H. The possible use of bisphosphonates in osteoporosis. In: De Luca HF, Mazess R, eds. *Osteoporosis: Physiological Basis, Assessment and Treatment*. New York: Elsevier, 1990: 323–30.
171. Russell RG, Rogers MJ, Frith JC et al. The pharmacology of bisphosphonates and new insights into their mechanisms of action. *J Bone Miner Res* 1999; **14**(suppl 2:) 53–65.
172. Storm T, Thamsborg G, Steiniche T, Genant HK, Sorensen OH. Effect of intermittent cyclical etidronate

therapy on bone mass and fracture rate in women with postmenopausal osteoporosis. *N Engl J Med* 1990; **322**: 1265–71.
173. Leiberman UA, Weiss SR, Broll J et al. Effect of alendronate on bone mineral density and the incidence of fracture in postmenopausal osteoporotic women. *N Engl J Med* 1995; **333**: 1437–43.
174. Black DM, Cummings SR, Karpf DB et al. Randomized trial of effect of alendronate on risk of fractures in women with existing vertebral fractures. *Lancet* 1996; 1535–41.
175. Karpf DB, Shapiro DR, Seeman E et al. Prevention of non-vertebral fractures by alendronate: a meta-analysis. *JAMA* 1997; **277**: 1159–64.
176. Delmas PD, Bjarnason NH, Mitlak BH et al. Effects of raloxifene on bone mineral density, serum cholesterol concentrations, and utrine endometrium in postmenopausal women. *N Engl J Med* 1997; **337**: 1641–7.
177. Anonymous. Raloxifene for postmenopausal osteoporosis. *Med Lett Drugs Ther* 1998; **40**: 29–30.
178. Ryan WG, Wolter J, Bagdade JD. Apparent beneficial effect of tamoxifen on bone mineral content in patients with breast cancer: a preliminary study. *Osteoporosis Int* 1991; **2**: 39–41.
179. Neal AJ, Evans K, Hoskin PJ. Does long-term administration of tamoxifen affect bone mineral density? *Eur J Cancer* 1993; **29A**: 1971–3.
180. Dequeker J, Geusens P. Anabolic steroids, muscle function and bone. In: Duursma SA, Raymarkers JA, Scheven BAA, eds. *Update on Osteoporosis*. Utrecht: Stichting Education Permanente, 1990: 69–76.
181. Riggs BL, Hodgson SF, O'Fallon WM et al. Effect of fluoride treatment on the fracture rate in postmenopausal women with osteoporosis. *N Engl J Med* 1990; **322**: 802–9.
182. Dure-Smith BA, Kraenzkin ME, Farley SM, Libanti CR, Schultz EE, Baylink DJ. Fluoride therapy for osteoporosis: a review of dose response, duration of treatment, and skeletal sites of action. *Calcif Tissue Int* 1991; **49(S)**: S64–7.
183. Sogaard CH, Mosekilde L, Richards A, Mosekilde LE. Marked decrease in trabecular bone quality after five years of sodium fluoride therapy, assessed by biochemical testing of iliac crest biopsies in osteoporotic patients. *Bone* 1994; **15**: 393–9.
184. Dempster DW, Cosman F, Parisien M et al. Anabolic actions of parathyroid hormone on bone. *Endocrine Rev* 1993; **14**: 690–709.
185. Boonen S, Aerssens J, Broos P et al. Age-related bone loss and senile osteoporosis: evidence for both secondary hyperparathyroidism and skeletal growth factor deficiency in the elderly. *Aging Clin Exp Res* 1996; **7**: 414–22.
186. Thiazide effect on the mineral content of bone. *N Engl J Med* 1990; **322**: 286–90.

187. Barker DJP, Chamberlain AT, Guyer PB, Gardner MJ. Paget's disease of bone: the Lancashire focus. *BMJ* 1980; **280**: 1105–7.
188. Rebel A, Bregeon C, Basle M, Malkani K, Patezour A, Filmon R. Osteoclastic inclusions in Paget's disease of bone. *Rev Rhum Mal Osteoartic* 1942; **42(637)**: 641.
189. Mills BG, Singer FR. Nuclear inclusions in Paget's disease of bone. *Science* 1976; **194**: 201–2.
190. Reddy SV et al. Measles virus nucleocapsid transcript expression is not restricted to the osteoclast lineage in patients with Paget's disease of bone. *Exp Hematol* 1999; **27**: 1528–32.
191. Ralston SH, Digiovine FS, Gallacher SJ, Boyle IT, Duff GW. Failure to detect paramyxovirus sequences in Paget's disease of bone using polymerase chain reaction. *J Bone Miner Res* 1991; **6**: 1243–8.
192. Birch MA, Taylor W, Fraser WD, Ralston SH, Hart CA, Gallagher JA. Absence of paramyxovirus RNA in cultures of pagetic bone cells and in pagetic bone. *J Bone Miner Res* 1994; **9**: 11–16.
193. Kurihara N, Reddy SV, Menaa C, Anderson D, Roodman GD. Osteoclasts expressing the measles virus nucleocapsid gene display pagetic phenotype. *J Clin Invest* 2000; **105**: 607–614.
194. Siris ES, Canfield RE, Jacobs TP. Paget's disease of bone. *Bull NY Acad Med* 1980; **56**: 285–304.
195. Morales-Piga AA, Rey-Rey JS, Corres-Gonzalez J, Garcia-Sagredo JM, Lopez-Abente G. Frequency and characteristics of familial aggregation of Paget's disease of bone. *J Bone Miner Res* 1995; **10**: 663–70.
196. McKusick VA. Paget's disease of bone. In: *Heritable Disorders of Connective Tissue*. St Louis, MO: CV Mosby, 1972; 718–23.
197. Hughes AE, Shearman AM, Weber JL et al. Genetic linkage of familial expansile osteolysis to chromosome 18q. *Human Mol Genet* 1994; **3**: 359–61.
198. Cody JD, Singer FR, Roodman GD et al. Genetic linkage of Paget disease of bone to chromosome 18q. *Am J Human Genet* 1997; **61**: 1117–22.
199. Haslam SI, Van Hul W, Morales-Piga A et al. Paget's disease of bone: evidence for a susceptibility locus on chromosome 18q and for genetic heterogeneity. *J Bone Miner Res* 1998; **13**: 911–17.
200. Mutations in TNFRSF11A, affecting the signal peptide of RANK, cause familial expansile osteolysis. *Nature Genet* 2000; **24**: 45–8.
201. Rebel A, Basle M, Pouplard A, Malkani K, Filmon R, Lepetezour A. Bone tissue in Paget's disease of bone: ultrastructure and immunocytology. *Arthritis Rheum* 1980; **23**: 1104–14.
202. Robey PG, Bianco P. The role of osteogenic cells in the pathophysiology of Paget's disease. *J Bone Miner Res* 1999; **14(suppl 2)**: 9–16.
203. Krane S. Paget's disease of bone. *Calcif Tissue Int* 1986; **38**: 309–17.

204. Reddy SV, Menaa C, Singer FR, Demulder A, Roodman GD. Cell biology of Paget's disease. *J Bone Miner Res* 1999; 14(suppl 2): 3–8.
205. Demulder A, Takahashi S, Singer FR, Hosking DJ, Roodman GD. Evidence for abnormalities in osteoclast precursors and the marrow microenvironment in Paget's disease. *Endocrinology* 1993; 133: 1978–82.
206. Yasuda H, Shima N, Nakagawa N et al. Osteoclast differentiation factor is a ligand for osteoprotegerin/osteoclastogenesis-inhibitory factor and is identical to TRANCE/RANKL. *Proc Natl Acad Sci USA* 95: 3597–602.
207. Meunier PJ, Salson C, Mathieu L et al. Skeletal distribution and biochemical parameters of Paget's disease. *Clin Orthop* 1987; 217: 37–44.
208. Alvarez L, Guanebens N, Peris P et al. Discriminative value of biochemical markers of bone turnover in assessing the activity of Paget's disease. *J Bone Miner Res* 1995; 10: 458–65.
209. Alvarez L, Peris P, Pons N et al. Relationship between biochemical markers of bone turnover and bone scintigraphy indices in assessment of Paget's disease activity. *Arthritis Rheum* 1997; 40: 461–8.
210. Delmas PD. Biochemical markers of bone turnover in Paget's disease of bone. *J Bone Miner Res* 1999; 14(suppl 2): 66–9.
211. Fledelius C, Johnsen AH, Cloos P, Bonde M, Qvist P. Characterization of urinary degradation products derived from type I collagen: identification of a β-isomerised aspartyl residue within the C-telopeptide (α1) region. *J Biol Chem* 1997; 272: 9755–63.
212. Bonde M, Qvist P, Fledelius C, Riis BJ, Christiansen C. Immunoassay for quantifying type I collagen degradation products in urine evaluated. *Clin Chem* 1994; 40: 2022–5.
213. Bonde M, Fledelius C, Qvist P, Christiansen C. Coated tube radioimmunoassay for C-telopeptides of type I collagen to assess bone resorption. *Clin Chem* 1996; 42: 1639–44.
214. Garnero P, Fledelius C, Gineyts E, Serre CM, Vignot E, Delmas PD. Decreased β-isomerization of C-telopeptides of α1 chain of type I collagen in Paget's disease of bone. *J Bone Miner Res* 1997; 12: 1407–15.
215. Garnero P, Gineyts E, Schaffer AV, Seaman J, Delmas PD. Measurement of urinary excretion of non-isomerised and β-isomerised forms of type I collagen breakdown products to monitor the effects of the bisphosphonate zolendronate in Paget's disease. *Arthritis Rheum* 1998; 41: 354–60.
216. Strickenberger SA, Schulman SP, Hutchins GM. Association of Paget's disease of bone with calcific aortic valve disease. *Am J Med* 1987; 82: 953–6.
217. Poncelet A. The neurologic complications of Paget's disease. *J Bone Miner Res* 1999; 14(suppl 2): 88–91.
218. Hadjipavlou A, Lander P. Paget disease of the spine. *J Bone Joint Surg Am* 1991; 73: 1376–81.
219. Hartman JT, Dohn DF. Paget's disease of the spine and cord or nerve-root compression. *J Bone Joint Surg Am* 1966; 48: 1079–84.
220. Ooi CG, Fraser WD. Paget's disease of bone. *Postgrad Med* 1997; 73: 69–74.
221. Monsell EM, Cody DD, Bone HG, Divine GW. Hearing loss as a complication of Paget's disease of bone. *J Bone Miner Res* 1999; 14(suppl 2): 92–5.
222. Altman RD. Arthritis in Paget's disease of bone. *J Bone Miner Res* 1999; 14(suppl 2): 85–7.
223. Huvos AG. Osteogenic sarcoma of bones and soft tissues in older persons. A clinicopathologic analysis of 117 patients older than 60 years. *Cancer* 1986; 57: 1442–9.
224. Jacobs TP, Michelsen J, Polay J, D'Adamo AC, Canfield RE. Giant cell tumor in Paget's disease of bone: familial and geographic clustering. *Cancer* 1979; 44: 742–7.
225. McClung MR, Tou CPK, Goldstein NH, Picot C. Tiludronate therapy for Paget's disease of bone. *Bone* 1995; 17: 493S–6S.
226. Siris ES. Perspectives: a practical guide to the use of pamidronate in the treatment of Paget's disease. *J Bone Miner Res* 1994; 9: 303–4.
227. Siris E, Weinstein RS, Altman R et al. Comparative study of alendronate vs. etidronate for the treatment of Paget's disease of bone. *J Clin Endocrinol Metab* 1996; 81: 961–7.
228. Siris E, Chines AA, Altman RD et al. Risedronate in the treatment of Paget's disease: an open-label, multicenter study. *J Bone Miner Res* 1998; 13: 1032–8.
229. Stamp TCB. Factors in human vitamin D nutrition and in the production and cure of classical rickets. *Proc Nutr Soc* 1975; 34: 119–30.
230. Sandstead HH. Clinical manifestations of certain classical deficiency disease. In: Goodhart RS, Shils ME, eds. *Modern Nutrition in Health and Disease*, 6th edn. Philadelphia: Lea & Febiger, 1980: 693–6.
231. Langman CB. Hypercalcemic syndrome in infants and children. In: Favus MS, ed. *Primer on the Metabolic Bone Diseases and Disorders of Mineral Metabolism*, 4th edn. Philadelphia: Lippincott Williams & Wilkins, 1999: 219–23.

14

Endocrinology and systemic disease
R Andrew James, Richard Quinton, Steven G Ball

Introduction

The endocrine system interacts intimately with all other bodily functions under normal physiological conditions. It provides a biological rheostat to maintain homeostasis at the cellular, tissue and organ level. Similarly, in pathological states, the endocrine system can be both the disrupter and the disrupted. Hormonal responses to a wide variety of environmental stimuli are crucial to survival. In this chapter we analyze how the endocrine system reacts and interacts with a variety of disease states which are recognized for their endocrine manifestations.

HIV disease and endocrine dysfunction

Infection with the human immunodeficiency virus (HIV) has only been recognized as a biological entity since 1981. Since that time, protean manifestations of the disease, its complications and the consequences of its treatment have become realized. We still have much to learn about interactions between physiology and pathophysiology and how these translate to disease progression. HIV disease illustrates how the endocrine and immune systems are intimately linked.[1,2] HIV disease and its complications and treatments can affect every function of the endocrine system. Potential effects include: the risk of direct damage to endocrine tissue by the HIV virus, opportunistic infection, malignant infiltration of endocrine organs, the metabolic response to severe illness with activation of cytokine cascades, and the endocrine side-effects of an increasing array of antiviral drug therapies (Table 14.1).

Cachexia/malnutrition
Weight loss/redistribution
Psychological stress
Drug and alcohol abuse
Chronic/acute infection
Associated malignancy
Secondary hemorrhage/infarction
Treatment medications
Coincident conditions
Genetic predisposition, e.g. autoimmune disease, diabetes mellitus

Table 14.1
Factors influencing endocrine status in the HIV-infected individual.

Two viral subtypes, HIV-1 and HIV-2, have been recognized, each having the potential of progressing to acquired immunodeficiency syndrome (AIDS), characterized by weight loss, multiple opportunistic infections and the occurrence of unusual neoplasms such as high-grade lymphomas and Kaposi's sarcoma. The primary target for the HIV is the $CD4^+$ T cells, where it has a cytopathic effect. HIV particles have been found in other cell types, including neuronal, epithelial and human carcinoma cell lines, but there is no evidence as yet for a direct destructive effect on endocrine tissue.

Although the course followed by an infected individual is difficult to predict, and response to antiretroviral therapy varies, the ultimate outcome is invariably death from sepsis or neoplasia. One of the most potent clinical manifestations of HIV is a profound wasting syndrome that is characteristic of the later stages of the disease. Through studying individuals with progressive disease, disturbances of adrenal, gonadal and thyroid function have been recognized, along with disruption of lipid and energy metabolism. Hypercortisolemia, hypogonadism and apparent thyroid dysfunction are commonly found, along with hypertriglyceridemia and increased resting energy expenditure.[3] Relative adrenal insufficiency is also being increasingly recognized. Whether endocrine disturbances are primary manifestations of HIV infection or secondary to the severity of immune deficiency, acquired sepsis or drug therapy is not always easy to distinguish, though certain characteristic features emerge. At every stage of HIV progression clear abnormalities of immune status are seen. These are mainly related to the depletion of $CD4^+$ T lymphocytes and are accompanied by characteristic changes in cytokine levels. Cytokine expression is intimately involved with the endocrine system, in particular, elements of the stress response.

Relative hypercortisolemia with suppression of the pituitary–gonadal axis are common early adaptations to any severe illness. However, in HIV infection this response can readily become maladaptive, contributing further to adverse weight loss, changes in body composition and anorexia. Even in asymptomatic seropositive patients, there is a degree of hypercortisolemia and catabolism with weight loss that exceeds the clinical severity of the stage of their disease.[4] These effects are likely to be the result of cytokine overproduction; for example, the systemic levels of interferon-alpha (IFN-α) correlate with both disease progression and hypertriglyceridemia.[5,6]

The hypothalamic–pituitary–adrenal (HPA) axis in HIV disease

There have been variable reports of both subclinical and overt under- and over-function of the HPA axis in HIV disease. Early stages of the disease appear to correspond with overactivation of this axis, whereas in more advanced disease with AIDS or AIDS-related complex (ARC), patients can have relative or absolute adrenal insufficiency. There is some research to suggest that HIV infection confers a degree of cortisol resistance even in the presence of an apparently hyperfunctioning pituitary–adrenal axis.[7] Presentation with postural hypotension and hyponatremia is a relatively rare occurrence (4%),[8] though a diminution of adrenal reserve can be found in 2–10% of patients when evaluated using a standard synthetic adrenocorticotropic hormone (ACTH) (250 μg) stimulation test.[9,10]

Although it is difficult to generalize, it appears that baseline adrenal function is increased, whereas the adrenocortical reserve to stress is impaired or blunted in HIV disease. Clearly, the response seen in a given individual may depend on the stage of disease, the coincident infection or neoplasm, and the balance of elaborated cytokines, which are known to both initiate and modify the stress response.

Demonstrable adrenal insufficiency in HIV-infected subjects, if not related to drug therapy, is most commonly due to destruction of adrenal tissue by sepsis or neoplasia. Cytomegalovirus (CMV) displays adrenal tropism, is found in 33–88% of AIDS patients at autopsy, and can account for up to 50% of the microscopic glandular destruction.[11,12] However, to correlate these changes with functional integrity is more difficult. One of the most comprehensive studies undertaken in HIV-related adrenal disease involving 41 subjects dying of AIDS, showed CMV adrenalitis to be present in 50% of subjects, with the medulla more severely involved than the cortex. However, prior functional adrenal insufficiency was more difficult to ascribe to the degree of pathological damage.[13] Secondary hypoadrenalism due to hypothalamic–pituitary damage has been described in HIV-infected individuals due to disseminated infection with *Toxoplasma gondii*, CMV and *Cryptococcus neoformans*, either alone or in combination.[14,15] In addition, in an autopsy series on patients succumbing to AIDS/ARC, 11% had adenohypophyseal necrosis of undetermined origin.[16]

The progression of HIV disease is characterized by severe immunodepression and worsening cachexia. The immunodepression is largely attributed to a dramatic drop in the number of circulating $CD4^+$ cells. The weight loss is mainly due to a reduced fat-free mass with a redistribution of adipose tissue in a viscero-truncal pattern. In the absence of direct pituitary–adrenal insufficiency, serum cortisol levels are elevated at all stages of HIV infection; conversely, dihydroepiandrostenedione (DHEA) levels decline with advancing disease and become lower than in HIV-negative controls when the $CD4^+$ count reaches <500.[17] Although these findings are consistently reported in the current literature, cause and effect is more difficult to discern. In addition, even patients with biochemical hypercortisolemia can present with Addisonian features (hypotension, hyponatremia, mucocutaneous melanosis), reaffirming a degree of cortisol resistance. This has been partially borne out at the tissue level, with monocytes from these individuals showing lower receptor affinity for glucocorticoid (high

K_d for tritiated dexamethasone in vitro), but higher receptor density than control patients or normal individuals.[18] These patients may also appear to be increasingly pigmented, due to increased ACTH secretion and higher levels of IFN-α, both of which have melanocyte-stimulating properties.

Within the physiological range, cortisol is both a modulator and an enhancer of the immune response. Pathological excess or deficiency is detrimental to the functional integrity of the immune system. How these factors interact with cytokine modulation and disease progression has yet to be fully elucidated. Similarly, when an extreme physiological response becomes a maladaptive mechanism is a difficult question to answer. One autopsy series reported an increased number of and enhanced staining for ACTH-producing cells in the anterior pituitary of HIV-infected individuals,[19] indicating chronic overactivation of the stress axis.

Pharmacological doses of steroids may be used as adjuvant treatment for certain HIV-associated diseases such as pneumocystis pneumonia. Their use may predispose to secondary adrenal insufficiency after withdrawal, or reveal underlying primary adrenal insufficiency. As a group, HIV-infected individuals are more likely to be illicit drug users. Methadone in high doses is known to depress the pituitary–adrenal axis, and this should be taken into account as a secondary cause of hypoadrenalism in HIV-infected drug users.[20] Replacement or therapeutic doses of steroids should be used rationally and with caution in HIV-infected patients, as excess steroid exposure can have an immunodepressive effect. There is some evidence to suggest an increased incidence of CMV infection in AIDS patients receiving corticosteroids.[21]

The hypothalamic–pituitary–gonadal (HPG) axis in HIV disease

The ability to retain normal reproductive function in males and females relies on relative health. Hence, during ill-health such as sepsis, altered nutritional status or rapid changes in body weight, the reproductive axis is one of the first endocrine systems to shut down. It appears that the degree of gonadal dysfunction for both sexes is related to the stage of HIV infection, with 76% of men experiencing reduced libido and 26% of women with amenorrhea.[9,22] Decreased spermatogenesis is a universal finding among male AIDS patients, due to non-specific local inflammatory changes in the testis.[23] Later, there is an increasing proportion with hypogonadotrophic hypogonadism as their disease progresses.[24] Primary testicular involvement with CMV is most commonly seen, but associated infection with *Toxoplasma* and malignant involvement with Kaposi's sarcoma are also described. The incidence of lymphoma and germ cell neoplasms may also be increased.[25] Similar infectious and neoplastic agents can give rise to hypothalamic–pituitary dysfunction, causing or compounding the gonadal deficiency. It appears that increased cytokine levels, in particular tumor necrosis factor alpha (TNF-α), have a generally suppressive effect on the HPG axis, and also contribute to gonadal dysfunction.

Effects of HIV on thyroid status

While baseline thyroid function tests are normal in the majority of patients with asymptomatic HIV infection, as the disease progresses to AIDS, defects in thyroid status become apparent. With progressive illness, a 'sick euthyroid syndrome' develop, with a decline in triiodothyroxine (T3) level, the severity of which appears to correlate with the metabolic status of patients presenting with different stages of HIV infection.[26] The combination of severe infection, low body mass and a depressed T3 level is predictive of the worst outcome. The effects of cytokines on thyroid hormone status and peripheral conversion of thyroxine (T4) to T3 is likely to be complex, invoking the same arguments proposed to explain 'non-thyroidal illness'. Involvement of the thyroid gland in HIV infected individuals with opportunistic infections such as *Mycobacterium avium*, *Pneumocystis carinii*, *Cryptococcus neoformans*, *Aspergillus fumigatus* and CMV has been reported without obvious endocrine dysfunction.[27] Similarly, malignant infiltration of the thyroid gland with Kaposi's sarcoma has been recorded. The incidence of primary autoimmune thyroid disease appears to be no greater in HIV-infected individuals than in the background population. Treatment of Kaposi's sarcoma with IFN-α can induce or exacerbate autoimmune thyroid dysfunction, with the occurrence of both hypo- and hyperthyroidism.

HIV and the pancreas

Asymptomatic lesions of the pancreas are frequently discovered at autopsy and are characteristically due to disseminated infection from CMV, tuberculosis (TB) and cryptococcus, or neoplasms such as Kaposi's sarcoma and lymphoma. These may cause varying degrees of pancreatic exocrine and endocrine dysfunction. Toxic drug effects include hypoglycemia with pentamidine, and elevated amylase levels with the nucleoside reverse transcriptase inhibitors, didanosine, lamivudine, stavudine and zalcitabine. The protease inhibitors indinavir, nelfinavir, ritonavir and saquinavir are associated with hyperglycemia, hyperlipidemia and lipodystrophy.

Water and electrolyte disturbance and HIV disease

A variety of electrolyte disturbances can occur with HIV infection. These can include sodium, potassium, magnesium and calcium imbalance.

Sodium imbalance

Hyponatremia is a common finding in sick hospitalized patients, particularly those with HIV disease, its complicating infections and neoplasms. Up to 30% of HIV patients will be hypovolemic and have an inadequate short ACTH stimulation test, indicating relative adrenal insufficiency as a contributing factor to their hyponatremia.[2] This situation, once recognized, is readily corrected with appropriate steroid replacement therapy. The syndrome of inappropriate antidiuretic hormone (SIADH) secretion is also common and results in a hypervolemic hyponatremia due to excessive water retention, i.e. non-osmotic antidiuretic hormone (ADH) secretion. The prevalence of SIADH-associated hyponatremia increases with increasing degree of sickness in patients with progressive HIV disease.[28] SIADH can occur with any atypical pulmonary or intracranial infection or neoplasm and is a good example of a maladaptive neuroendocrine reponse to systemic disease. ADH is elaborated inappropriately and not adequately cleared from the circulation, resulting in a more prolonged antidiuretic action and a dilutional hyponatremia. Treatment is directed at the underlying cause, with gentle fluid restriction in the interim depending on the clinical situation. Hyponatremia of any cause can be complicated by electrolyte loss through diarrhea and vomiting, altered renal function and inappropriate intravenous fluid regimens.

Pseudohyponatremia can occur with certain methods of sodium estimation due to lipid-laden serum, severe hypergammaglobulinemia or nephrotic syndrome, all of which have been described in HIV-infected individuals.

Hypernatremia can occur due to dehydration, poor oral intake and high-output diarrheal states. Nephrogenic diabetes insipidus has been described associated with foscarnet therapy resulting in hypernatremia.[29] In situations of both hypo- and hypernatremia, accurate attention to fluid balance and appropriate intravenous fluid replacement, when indicated, are key to resolving the metabolic disturbance.

Potassium imbalance

Despite the propensity for nausea, vomiting and diarrheal states associated with HIV disease, hypokalemia appears to be an infrequent occurrence. Hyperkalemia is more often reported, the cause of which can be multifactorial. Mild hyperkalemia can occur in association with relative adrenal insufficiency, often associated with a mild hyponatremia and acidosis. Alternatively, renal lesions frequently seen in HIV disease, such as nephritis, glomerular sclerosis and drug-induced tubular dysfunction, can all lead to high serum potassium levels. One of the most common causes is long-term treatment with antibiotic regimens containing trimethoprim, which is structurally related to the potassium-sparing diuretic amiloride.[30] Similarly, pentamidine can cause adverse potassium retention through a renal tubular mechanism.

Calcium and magnesium imbalance

Disorders of calcium and magnesium status are occasionally seen in HIV patients. Hypocalcemia has been recorded in 18% of AIDS patients,[31] and causes can be multiple, including calcium malabsorption and vitamin D deficiency. Pentamidine can cause hypomagnesemia due to renal tubular Mg^{2+} wasting resulting in a resistant hypocalcemia due to insufficient parathyroid hormone (PTH) release. Ketoconazole can impair the synthesis of 1,25-dihydroxyvitamin D and contribute to hypocalcemia. Hypercalcemia is rarely reported in the absence of lymphoma or granulomatous disease in HIV-infected subjects.

Lipid disturbance in HIV infection

Differences in free (non-esterified) fatty acid concentrations, triglyceride and cholesterol levels in HIV-infected individuals vary greatly, due to individual genetic background, disease stage, nutritional status and antiretroviral treatment strategies. However, more consistent patterns of lipid abnormalities are seen in the later stages (IV) of the disease, with a considerable increase in circulating triglycerides, and a fall in cholesterol and free fatty acid (FFA) levels. These changes correlate to a certain degree with the production of lipogenic cytokines (interleukin-1 (IL-1), TNF and INF-α). Concurrent azidothymidine (AZT) treatment appears to exaggerate these changes.[32]

Endocrine effects of drug therapies in HIV

Current therapies used in HIV patients are known to have endocrine and metabolic effects. Pentamidine used to counteract *Pneumocystis cariniae* infection has a cytolytic effect on the endocrine pancreas, causing inappropriate insulin release and hypoglycemia. Chronic β-cell destruction can go on to overt insulin deficiency and hyperglycemia with all the well-known metabolic consequences of diabetes mellitus.[33]

The imidazole antifungal agent ketoconazole, if given long term, is known to inhibit early P450-dependent enzymatic steps in both adrenal and gonadal steroidogenesis.[34] In addition, it impairs 1,25-dihydroxyvitamin D synthesis in the kidney, thereby having a potential adverse effect on calcium status.[35] The triazole derivatives such as itraconazole, the allylamine agent terbinafine and amphotericin do not have such an adverse effect on steroidogenesis. Trimethoprim, often used as antibiotic prophylaxis as part of a sulfonamide combination (Septrin) in HIV-infected individuals, can result in hyperkalemia, especially with impaired renal function.[30] This is due to its structural similarity to amiloride, the potassium-conserving diuretic. Rifampicin is an inducer of hepatic enzymes which accelerates the metabolism of corticosteroids and may contribute to a relative adrenal insufficiency.

Highly active antiretroviral therapy which includes protease inhibitors may exacerbate weight redistribution, which is characteristically truncal/visceral,[3] reminiscent of the body habitus seen in Cushing's syndrome.

Megesterol acetate, a synthetic progestational steroid, has been studied as an appetite-stimulating and anabolic agent for use in AIDS wasting in males. An 800 mg/day dose gave a significant increase in caloric intake and subsequent weight gain with increased wellbeing over a control group treated with placebo. Weight gain was mainly attributable to increased fat mass. These trials have so far been short term, and whether the effects are sustainable has yet to be determined.[3] In addition, megesterol acetate has several adverse side-effects that may limit its use. It has significant glucocorticoid activity, potentially causing a cushingoid appearance with impaired glucose tolerance or even diabetes mellitus. Owing to its suppressive effect on the HPA axis, rapid cessation after long-term use could precipitate adrenal insufficiency. Megesterol can also suppress the HPG axis, resulting in a worsening of hypogonadism. Testosterone supplementation is indicated in males with AIDS wasting and documented hypogonadism. In this group, it appears to have a sustained beneficial effect on wellbeing and lean body mass without deleterious side-effects. No additional benefit was derived in trials looking at testosterone analogs such as oxandrolone or nandrolone, and with the knowledge that these synthetic agents can cause liver dysfunction, their use cannot be recommended.[3]

Growth hormone (GH) has anabolic effects which could be of potential use in HIV-infected individuals with wasting or during a septic episode. AIDS patients tend to have high serum GH concentrations with relatively low levels of insulin-like growth factor-1 (IGF-1), suggesting an intrinsic resistance to GH, possibly related to chronic disease and malnutrition. Early trials suggest that the dose required for an anabolic effect are higher than those used for standard GH replacement therapy. Side-effects such as edema, arthralgia, myalgia and worsening glucose tolerance were frequent dose-limiting factors. Although GH is approved for short-term use at a dose of 0.1 mg/kg in the USA for patients with AIDS wasting, its use will need to be carefully monitored and should perhaps be reserved for patients whose wasting process is resistant to other forms of intervention. In male patients with associated hypogonadism, testosterone administration appears to improve GH sensitivity, with a significant benefit on lean body mass.[36]

Drugs such as thalidomide and pentoxifylline are thought to have a modulatory effect on inflammatory cytokines and have been studied in AIDS subjects, where they appear to have an anabolic effect. However, the exact mechanism behind this effect and the potential for long-term efficacy of such treatment remains to be validated.

Practical evaluation of the pituitary–adrenal axis in HIV disease

If adrenocortical insufficiency is suspected in a patient with HIV due to presenting features such as confusion, hypotension, hyponatremia, hyperkalemia and acidosis, then prompt diagnosis and management is critical. In the acute situation, a random cortisol with ACTH can be diagnostic, prior to the administration of parenteral intramuscular or intravenous hydrocortisone 100 mg. The serum cortisol should be appropriately elevated for the degree of stress (i.e. >650 nmol/l) and, if not, the ACTH will help indicate whether the insufficiency is of pituitary or adrenal origin. Appropriate steroid cover can then be administered for the duration of the acute illness with consideration of a continuous steroid infusion in an ITU setting.[37] If time allows, a more formal short ACTH stimulation test should be performed for diagnostic accuracy and to better predict the need for long-term steroid management.[38] However, in the context of acute hypothalamic–pituitary insufficiency, the short ACTH test can be falsely reassuring,[39] and should be interpreted in the clinical context if intracranial disease is suspected.

Dysfunctional thyroid status in a HIV-infected individual would seem to be no different from that in other, non-HIV-infected, sick patients, as in the 'sick-euthyroid syndrome'. However, caution should be used in interpreting thyroid-stimulating hormone (TSH) values in isolation in patients receiving the following drugs: high-dose glucocorticoids, intravenous dopamine in an intensive care facility, somatostatin analogs for HIV-related diarrhea, or methadone. Each of these agents can suppress TSH secretion and mask true underlying primary thyroid failure.[20]

Summary of the clinical evaluation of the HIV patient

A basic nutritional evaluation with optimization of protein, fat and carbohydrate intake with attention to vitamin and mineral supplements is essential in the care of the HIV patient. A thorough screen for opportunist and parasitic infections, especially those affecting the gastrointestinal tract, is mandatory. Screening of males for hypogonadism is a worthwhile evaluation, with early testosterone supplementation by injection or transdermal routes. Synthetic testosterone analogs are of no additional benefit and may be detrimental to hepatic function. Similarly, oral testosterone supplements may cause unwanted hepatotoxicity in this group of patients. Patients over the age of 50 who are receiving testosterone supplementation should have monitoring of prostate-specific antigen (PSA) levels. Anabolic and appetite-stimulating steroids such as megestrol acetate may be beneficial if other therapies have failed, but side-effects with long-term use need to be monitored. Although high-dose GH as licensed in the USA may have its indications in patients with severe weight loss where other therapies have proved ineffective, its use cannot be widely recommended based on currently available data. Use of cytokine modulators and androgenic steroids in female AIDS subjects similarly remains experimental. Aggressive treatment of patients with multiple antiviral regimens which include protease inhibitors appears to be associated with a peculiar redistribution of fat mass in the visceral/truncal regions and a metabolic syndrome of insulin resistance and hypertriglyceridemia.[40]

Adrenoleukodystrophy

Adrenoleukodystrophy (ALD) is a rare metabolic disorder with neurological and endocrine manifestations. Though it has historically been classified into four subtypes (neonatal, childhood-cerebral, adult-onset adrenomyeloneuropathy, and adrenal/endocrine-only phenotypes), ALD is a spectrum disorder. Up to six overlapping phenotypes have been recognized. Nevertheless, the historic classification can be useful in a clinical context. Neonatal ALD differs from the other forms in that it is not inherited as an X-linked recessive trait.

Clinical features

The neurological features of the disease dominate the clinical picture of ALD.

Neonatal ALD affects both male and female newborns. Symptoms include mental retardation, seizures, retinal degeneration, hypotonia, hepatomegaly and adrenal insufficiency. It is rapidly progressive, and leads to early death.

Onset of the childhood-cerebral form is generally between 4 and 10 years of age. It affects only boys. Common symptoms heralding presentation include behavioral changes such as withdrawal, aggression, poor memory and deterioration in school performance. These are followed by subsequent neurological features that include seizures, learning difficulties and progressive dementia, visual and hearing loss, dysphagia and disturbance of gait and coordination. The neurological course is progressive, with death usually occurring within 1–10 years after onset of symptoms.

The adult-onset adrenomyeloneuropathy variant typically has an onset between the ages of 21 and 35 years. Common neurological symptoms at presentation include stiffness and weakness of the lower limbs. Subsequent progression may lead to the development of a spastic paraparesis and ataxia. A myeloneuropathy or peripheral neuropathy may dominate. Higher function can also be affected. Progression of the disease is less rapid than that found in the childhood form.

Female heterozygote carriers of X-linked ALD occasionally present with mild neurological disease. This may be manifest as a spastic paraparesis, ataxia, myeloneuropathy or peripheral neuropathy. The prevalence of occult neurological disease in carriers of X-linked ALD is high on formal testing.[41]

Endocrinopathy in ALD

Adrenal insufficiency is the most important endocrine manifestation of ALD. It is the only apparent manifestation in 8% of patients with X-linked disease. Recent data suggest that as many as 35% of males with presumed idiopathic primary adrenal failure and who are negative for adrenal autoantibodies have ALD.[42] The majority of such patients have magnetic resonance imaging or electrophysiological evidence of occult neurological disease, suggesting that the adrenal-only phenotype may be erroneous. Adrenal insufficiency rarely develops in female heterozygote carriers of X-linked ALD, though subtle subclinical reductions in adrenal reserve have been reported.[43] However, the high prevalence of occult neurological disease in carriers suggests that expression of adrenal disease may be dependent on the sensitivity of the method used to determine adrenal reserve.

Testicular function is commonly impaired in ALD. Leydig and/or Sertoli cell dysfunction is demonstrable in up to 82% of patients with the adult adrenomyeloneuropathy variant.[44] However, such defects may be subtle or partially compensated, as indicated by normal levels of total testosterone but elevated gonadotropins, and may not require replacement therapy. As with other aspects of the disease, gonadal dysfunction may not be apparent at presentation but may develop and progress over time.

Pathophysiology

Patients with ALD have high levels of saturated very long chain fatty acids (VLCFAs), particularly hexacosanoic acid (C26:0), both in body fluids and in tissues in which there is normally a high lipid turnover (such as those synthesizing steroid hormones). This accumulation is due to a block in VLCFA metabolism: a consequence of a defect in either peroxisomal β-oxidation, or peroxisome biogenesis. Inability to metabolize VLCFAs leads to the formation of characteristic dense, leaflet or needle-like lipid inclusions within macrophages and Schwann cells of the nervous system, and similar inclusions within adrenocortical and Leydig cells. Within the nervous system, there is also multi-focal inflammatory demyelination. The relationship of the defect in VLCFA metabolism to the inflammatory demyelination remains to be clarified.

The gene responsible for X-linked ALD (X-ALD) maps to Xq28 and is composed of 10 exons. It encodes a 745 amino acid peroxisomal membrane transport protein (ALDP), a member of a superfamily of membrane transporters (ABC transporters) which have in common an ATP-binding cassette. ALDP is closely related to several other peroxisome membrane proteins: ALD-related protein (ALDRP), PMP70 and PMP70-related protein, which may share overlapping functions, leading to a limited functional redundancy in ALDP-dependent processes.[45,46] There is a functional interaction between ALDP and these related peroxisome membrane proteins. ABC transporters commonly have two functional components subserved within the same protein. ALDP and its relatives are half-transporters, functional through the formation of homo- or heterodimers with each other.[47] This intimate functional relationship of ALDP with other peroxisome proteins has key implications, both as a potential mechanism for variable disease expression and as a potential target for therapy.

Over 110 different mutations in the X-ALD gene have been identified, 50% being missense mutations.[48,49] Though they are distributed across the full length of the gene, there is some clustering of mutations in the region coding for the ALDP nucleotide-binding domain. The most common mutation in many populations is an AG dinucleotide deletion at position 1081–1082.[50] There is no clear genotype–phenotype correlation. Moreover, the various phenotypes of X-linked ALD commonly occur within the same kindred, despite transmission of identical mutations in the X-ALD gene.[51] This would suggest additional genetic and/or environmental influences capable of modifying disease expression.

Though apparently a key factor in peroxisomal VLCFA β-oxidation, the function of ALDP and its precise role in this process remains to be determined.[52] Moreover, there remains some doubt as to the role of

VLCFA accumulation in the pathogenesis of ALD. Mice with targeted deletion of the X-ALD gene show reduced VLCFA β-oxidation, high circulating VLCFA levels, and typical lipid inclusions. However, they do not express a neurological phenotype.[53,54] This suggests that other modifying factors, genetic and/or environmental, must be involved in the expression of ALD. It may be that the defect in VLCFA metabolism is an epiphenomenon. Alternatively, it has been proposed that VLCFA deposition may trigger an inflammatory response that is a major determinant of neurological disease expression.[55] Genetic and environmental disease modifiers may impact through modification of this response. The importance of disease modifiers in expression of ALD is emphasized by the variation in disease expression within a single kindred.

In contrast to the other ALD variants, neonatal ALD is caused by a defect in peroxisome biogenesis rather than peroxisome membrane transport. This is brought about by a failure of peroxisomal matrix protein import, a process mediated by the products of the genes *PEX1* and *PEX6*, commonly mutated in this form of the disease.[56]

Diagnosis

From an endocrine perspective, the diagnosis of ALD must be considered in anyone presenting with adrenal insufficiency, either concurrent with or on a background of progressive neurological symptoms and signs, or with a family history of neurological disease or adrenal failure. Similarly, ALD should be considered in those individuals initially presenting with adrenal failure who subsequently develop a progressive neurological syndrome.

Should ALD be considered in all individuals presenting with adrenal failure in the absence of suggestive neurological symptoms, signs and family history? Recent data suggest that the prevalence of ALD is likely to be higher than previous estimates. Given the implications for both the patient and their family, there is a strong case for considering the diagnosis of ALD in any patient with adrenal failure who is adrenal antibody negative and has no other features of autoimmune disease. This is particularly so in those patients below 15 years of age. It is increasingly likely that combinations of genetic and endocrine screening will detect presymptomatic endocrinopathy.

The hallmark confirmation of ALD is through the measurement of circulating VLCFAs. However, exclusion by biochemical testing alone can be unreliable. The development of robust molecular screening tools to identify mutations in the X-ALD gene can aid in both the diagnosis and the determination of carrier status in X-linked ALD.[57]

Patients diagnosed with ALD from their neurological disease must be screened at presentation, and regularly thereafter for adrenal and gonadal dysfunction. Similar endocrine screening is required for as yet asymptomatic male X-ALD mutation carriers identified through genetic screening programs.

Management

Supportive therapy

There is currently no cure for ALD. The majority of current management is supportive. Adrenal and testicular failure requires standard replacement therapy. Patients should be offered appropriate genetic counselling. As patients with ALD may require the expertise of several healthcare professionals, such care may best be delivered through a coordinated multidisciplinary team approach.

Dietary treatment

Dietary treatment with a 4:1 mixture of glyceroltrioleate and glyceroltrierucate ('Lorenzo's oil') normalizes plasma VLCFA concentrations in patients with ALD. However, it neither ameliorates nor arrests the rapid progression of neurological symptoms in cerebral variants. Recent data indicate that it has no impact on the development or progression of endocrine manifestations of the disease.[58]

Bone marrow transplantation

The aim of bone marrow transplantation (BMT) in ALD is reconstitution of ALDP expression in bone marrow-derived cells, normalization of plasma VLCFAs, and facilitation of myelin remodeling. The role of BMT in the management of ALD remains to be clarified.

Future therapy

Identification of the X-ALD gene as the genetic basis of X-linked ALD has driven the development of gene therapy paradigms with potential applications in the treatment of ALD. Retroviral-mediated transfer of the X-ALD gene can normalize VLCFA metabolism in ALD cells in vitro.[59] Considerable improvements in current vector efficiency and targeting are required to transfer this approach to a clinical setting.

The close functional relationship between ALDP and ALDRP, and the possible overlap in function of these proteins, has focused attention on the possibility of restoring peroxisomal function in X-linked ALD not by restoring ALDP, but by stimulating overexpression of ALDRP, so-called complementation. Retroviral transfer of the ALDRP gene can rescue VLCFA metabolism in ALD cells in vitro in a similar manner to that observed with the ALD gene.[60] In addition, pharmacological stimulation of ALDRP expression and peroxisome proliferation with 4-phenylbutyrate or fenofibrate can rescue VLCFA metabolism in X-ALD null-mice.[61] Such pharmacological complementation approaches provide viable alternatives to gene transfer strategies for the development of novel treatments.

Inflammatory, granulomatous and infectious disease affecting the endocrine system

Sarcoidosis

Sarcoidosis is a multisystem disease characterized by epithelioid cell granulomas in many tissues. The spectrum of presentation can be broad, from a transient affliction in certain individuals to chronic and debilitating disease in others. It most commonly affects young adults presenting with an acute illness manifest by erythema nodosum, uveitis and/or bilateral hilar lymphadenopathy. A more indolent presentation involves pulmonary infiltrates, and parotid, cardiac and neurological involvement.[62] The specific etiology is uncertain, though PCR analysis of cutaneous sarcoid lesions has demonstrated mycobacterial DNA to be present in 80% of lesions in one series.[63] The diagnosis is often made on clinical grounds initially, supported by histological evidence of widespread non-caseating epithelioid cell granulomas in more than one organ. The Kveim test, although diagnostically helpful, is no longer used. Non-specific inflammatory markers such as the erythrocyte sedimentation rate (ESR) are elevated, and serial measurement of angiotensin-converting enzyme activity (ACE) are helpful as part of diagnosis and monitoring of disease activity, though elevated levels are not entirely specific for the disease. A negative tuberculin test at 1:100 is a feature in up to two-thirds of patients with sarcoidosis. The course and prognosis of the disease correlate with the presenting features, suggesting that the outcome is related to the host immune response to the condition.

The main endocrine manifestations are: (1) hypercalcemia with hypercalciuria (covered elsewhere in this book); and (2) hormone deficiency due to direct endocrine gland involvement. Sarcoidosis involving every organ in the body with the possible exception of the adrenal gland has been described with variable functional consequences. Apart from hypercalcemia, a primary endocrine presentation with sarcoidosis is rare. However, as the most common endocrine manifestation is with pituitary and/or hypothalamic involvement and hypopituitarism, an awareness of this mode of presentation is crucial to the correct diagnosis and management of the patient. This is especially important when other more obvious clinical indicators of sarcoidosis are not evident if the diagnosis is not to be missed. A patient may present with the symptoms of endocrine deficiency yet have only lupus pernio as the cutaneous manifestation of indolent sarcoidosis of the hypothalamic–pituitary axis. Sarcoid granulomas in the brain and pituitary account for less than 7% of all cases. Patients may present with headache due to meningeal involvement, raised intracranial pressure and papilledema due to obstructive hydrocephalus, in addition to variable anterior and posterior pituitary deficiency syndromes. Hyperprolactinemia may be the only indication of pituitary involvement. Macroscopic appearances of infiltration as delineated by CT or MRI do not always correlate with functional deficit. Diabetes insipidus (DI) as a presenting feature with or without associated anterior pituitary dysfunction is quite characteristic of sarcoid granuloma of the pituitary. Therefore, any patient presenting with polyuria and polydipsia with other clinical or biochemical features of sarcoidosis should have a full pituitary evaluation. Similarly, in patients diagnosed as having DI, sarcoidosis should be considered in the differential diagnosis as a cause. Hypothalamic infiltration can lead to more widespread endocrine deficit in addition to causing somnolence, megaphagia with weight gain, altered thirst perception, fluctuations in body temperature and personality change, all of which can prove very difficult to manage.

Experience indicates that patients with hypothalamic– pituitary sarcoidosis most commonly have indolent cutaneous involvement (lupus pernio) as an associated clinical sign. Having performed a full anterior and posterior pituitary evaluation, treatment of hypothalamic–pituitary sarcoidosis is directed at the cause, using high doses of steroids to counteract the granulomatous process and replacement of deficient hormones, e.g. hydrocortisone, thyroxine, testosterone/estrogen and desmopressin (1-desamino-8-D-arginine vasopressin). Hypothalamic–pituitary function requires periodic re-evaluation, especially after a period of steroid therapy at treatment doses, as granuloma involution may result in a functional recovery. High-dose steroid regimens are used to treat manifestations of sarcoidosis in other organs such as lung, parotid and eye. It is important to be aware of possible underlying pituitary–adrenal insufficiency, as abrupt cessation of high-dose steroids could precipitate an Addisonian crisis. Although sarcoid granulomata can be found in other endocrine organs such as the pancreas and thyroid, they are not known to cause any functional impairment of hormone production. The adrenal glands seem to be peculiarly spared by sarcoid infiltration, perhaps as a result of their intrinsic steroid-producing capacity. In the absence of hypothalamic–pituitary involvement, sarcoidosis does not usually affect fertility or the outcome of pregnancy. As with many other immune-mediated diseases, sarcoidosis characteristically improves during pregnancy but may relapse in the post-partum period.

Langerhan's cell histiocytosis (LCH) and variants

Langerhan's cell histiocytosis is the collective term now used for several disease complexes previously recognized in the literature, which include histiocytosis X, Letterer–Siwe disease, Hand–Schueller–Christian disease and eosinophilic granuloma. The common pathological finding is the presence of the Langerhan's cells in affected tissues which are characteristically S100 protein positive and contain intracytoplasmic inclusion bodies called Birbeck granules. It is a rare condition and can present in several different clinical ways. More than half of the cases present in children between the ages of 1 and 15, the rest occurring in adults even into the 6th decade.[64] The most frequent endocrine dysfunction is DI, followed by growth retardation as a result of hypothalamic–pituitary infiltration.[65] It occurs equally in males and females. Locally occurring disease has a better prognosis than disseminated lesions, which may display overtly malignant behavior. The prevalence of DI in the pediatric age group with histiocytosis varies between 5% and 50% in different series. In adults, the diagnosis of DI may precede detectable bone and soft tissue involvement by several months.[66] Short stature in children with LCH is due to GH insufficiency associated with DI and primarily resulting from hypothalamic–pituitary infiltration or involvement from adjacent meninges.

Other endocrine deficiencies as a result of the disease rather than the treatment are relatively rare but include hyperprolactinemia, hypogonadism and panhypopituitarism.[65] In one series of 47 patients with DI, eight had associated GH deficiency, and six had panhypopituitarism.[67] The diagnosis of DI is no different from that of any cause of this endocrine dysfunction, with a carefully conducted water deprivation test in borderline clinical cases. The important thing is to recognize histiocytosis within the differential diagnosis of adults and especially children presenting with symptoms of polyuria and polydipsia. In patients presenting with panhypopituitarism, it is important to remember that institution of appropriate steroid replacement therapy may reveal an underlying tendency to DI. MRI is the imaging modality of choice to define the extent of hypothalamic, pituitary and central nervous system (CNS) involvement. There are few reports of LCH involving other endocrine organs, apart from thyroid infiltration, which was initially diagnosed as thyroid carcinoma until the disease presented in the gingiva and the histology was critically reviewed.[68]

Optimal treatment of this rare condition is not universally agreed. The morbidity and mortality may largely depend on individual organ dysfunction or degree of systemic spread. Spontaneous remission has been reported, and surgical excision has been successful for solitary bone lesions and one case of an isolated hypothalamic granuloma.[69] In patients presenting with DI and hypothalamic involvement, early fractionated radiotherapy has been advocated, with a resultant improvement in posterior pituitary function. Late-presenting lesions with established DI appear not to respond so effectively.[70] High-dose steroids can transiently improve DI as well as bone and visceral lesions. Chemotherapy in more advanced disease has little to offer. As the endocrine dysfunction associated with hypothalamic–pituitary LCH is not often reversible, prompt recognition of functional deficits and institution of appropriate replacement therapy is crucial.[71]

Erdheim–Chester disease (ECD) and Rosai–Dorfman disease (RDD) are two atypical forms of histiocytosis that are worthy of mention, as they have been reported to present with manifestations within the endocrine system. ECD is characterized by exuberant histiocyte proliferation, which can occur in the hypothalamic–pituitary region, resulting in hyperprolactinemia, anterior pituitary dysfunction and DI. Bilateral adrenal infiltration has also been reported. One of the characteristic features of ECD is histiocytic infiltration without Langerhan's cells, no staining for S100, and an absence of Birbeck inclusion granules. The common presenting clinical features are symmetrical long bone osteosclerosis, unilateral exophthalmos and DI. Patients tend to be older at presentation and have a worse prognosis than that of LCH.[72] RDD is a benign systemic proliferative disorder of histiocytes that resemble the sinus histiocytes of lymph nodes with lymphophagocytosis (emperiopolesis). It presents as massive lymphadenopathy, typically bilateral and painless with fever and a polyclonal hyperglobulinemia. Cutaneous lesions are present in 43% of cases.[73] RDD has been reported to present as a pituitary mass with DI and anterior pituitary failure.[74]

Wegener's granulomatosis

Wegener's granulomatosis (WG) is a rare midline granulomatous disorder of uncertain etiology which can involve the pituitary gland. It can present as a pituitary mass with visual failure, disrupted anterior pituitary function and DI.[75] The lesion is best demonstrated by MRI, where loss of the normal posterior pituitary T1 hyperintensity appears to correlate with the incidence of DI.[76] A positive antineutrophil cytoplasmic antibody (cANCA) is diagnostic but can be negative in the early stages of the disease. Treatment is based on replacement of hormone deficiencies, high-dose steroids and cyclophosphamide.

Sheehan's syndrome and head trauma (Simmond's disease)

Sheehan's syndrome is the occurrence of spontaneous infarction of the normal pituitary gland after obstetric hemorrhage. The mechanism is thought to be occlusive arteriospasm with vascular congestion and thrombosis. Clinically, it is recognized as a failure of lactation following a birth complicated by a severe postpartum hemorrhage often requiring transfusional resuscitation. With improvements in obstetric practice, Sheehan's syndrome is becoming a rare condition. Pituitary infarction produces variable dysfunction that may be temporary or permanent; DI is rarely seen in this context.

Head trauma resulting in selective or total pituitary dysfunction, as recognized by Simmond,[77] has recently been highlighted as an under-represented cause of hormone deficit.[78] In a recent review of the world literature, 367 cases have been described. The male to female ratio is 5:1, with approximately 60% occurring in the 11–29-year age group, reflecting the population most at risk of trauma to the head. Seventy-one per cent of cases present clinically with a hormone deficiency within 1 year of the traumatic event, though late recognition after 20 years or more is described. Road traffic and sporting accidents feature highly as a cause and should be asked for in the history of any patient presenting with unexplained anterior or posterior pituitary dysfunction. Hormone deficiencies can be isolated, though multiple and reversible defects have been described. The gonadotroph appears to be most vulnerable, with transient or sustained amenorrhea being a common presentation among females. Both hypo- and hyperprolactinemia can occur, the latter due to stalk disruption as a result of the trauma. Radiological evaluation can be normal in 6.6–7.7%, or can show features suggestive of previous traumatic events such as a small atrophic pituitary, hypodense areas or an empty sella. The occurrence and duration of coma but not skull fracture seem to be important predictive factors. Subarachnoid hemorrhage or aneurysm clipping, particularly of the anterior communicating artery, can result in damage to perforating vessels that supply the hypothalamus. This can give rise to isolated DI, which can be further complicated by infarction of the thirst center. The clinical picture is one of adipsic DI, where the patient is at constant risk of hypernatremic dehydration. Management of this condition is difficult and involves a predetermined dose of DDAVP with an obligatory daily fluid intake estimated from an accurate, fasting early-morning body weight. Serum sodium needs to be measured every 2–3 weeks, or more frequently during a destabilizing event.[79] Vascular or structural damage to the hypothalamus can also result in a hypothalamic syndrome of somnolence, hyperphagia and temperature dysregulation. These features are often irreversible and are particularly difficult to treat.

Lymphocytic hypophysitis

Lymphocytic hypophysitis is a rare disorder, predominantly, though not exclusively, affecting females during the postpartum period. It is characterized by a lymphocytic infiltration, probably of autoimmune origin, with varying degrees of functional destruction. Lymphocytic hypophysitis can also present with mass effect, acute visual field defect[80] and, occasionally, cranial nerve palsies. MRI appearances are of an enhancing expanded lesion occupying the whole of the pituitary fossa, often extending up into the stalk and having a suprasella extension. Histological features can vary from a predominantly lymphocytic infiltration to a more granulomatous appearance. Treatment is with high-dose steroids and anterior pituitary support, though surgical decompression may be indicated if this does not result in a rapid improvement in mass effect.[81] Granulomatous disease of the pituitary appears to be associated with an older age at presentation and a more insidious onset. Anterior pituitary dysfunction, including DI, is a characteristic feature. Presentation with painful ophthalmoplegia and visual impairment (Tolosa–Hunt syndrome) and Takayasu's arterial occlusive disease have both been reported.[82,83]

Systemic lupus erythematosis

Systemic lupus erythematosis (SLE) is a multisystem autoimmune-mediated disease that is more prevalent in females. SLE appears to be hormone responsive, with a 'flare' of disease activity associated with estrogen therapy and pregnancy in about 50% of patients.[84] Lupus nephritis, presence of antiphospholipid antibodies and a previous history of pregnancy loss appear to increase the risk of complications during pregnancy and worsen fetal loss. A possible factor stimulating immune responses is prolactin, which has been found to be elevated in SLE patients of both sexes and has been linked to disease activity in several studies. The physiological hyperprolactinemia of lactation also seems to influence the postpartum behavior of SLE. Most autoimmune diseases benefit from the immune tolerance of pregnancy, but SLE is unusual in having a contrary effect. Prolactin is closely related to the cytokine family and appears to undergo an important interaction with the immune system. A link has been proposed between autoimmune disease activity and elevated prolactin levels, with isolated reports of bromocriptine treatment resulting in remission of SLE.[85] Elevated basal prolactin levels in male patients with SLE have been proposed to cause the observed decrease in testosterone levels in this disease.[86]

In the absence of direct hypothalamic–pituitary involvement with SLE, there does not appear to be any major functional deficit of the endocrine system. However, detailed dynamic endocrine testing has revealed the cortisol response after hypoglycemia to be significantly lower in SLE patients compared to controls in regular menstruating female subjects who had not previously had any steroid exposure.[87]

A recognized feature of SLE is the antiphospholipid syndrome (Hughes syndrome). Individuals with this antibody have an increased tendency for hemorrhagic infarction and necrosis of the adrenal glands. Females have an increased incidence of fetal loss in early pregnancy. Patients have a prolonged partial thromboplastin with IgM and IgG anticardiolipin antibodies.[88] Adrenal infarction can be unilateral or bilateral and present at the time of surgery, pregnancy or intercurrent disease. Clinical features are flank pain and hypotensive circulatory collapse consistent with acute adrenal insufficiency. Early recognition of this situation is crucial to the successful management of the crisis with prompt steroid replacement.

Fibrosing conditions and the endocrine system

Riedel's thyroiditis, fibrosing pituitary pseudotumor, retroperitoneal fibrosis, Peyronie's disease of the penis and sclerosing cholangitis are all conditions sharing similar pathological features. They can occur in isolation or in combination and have been described as a familial multifocal fibrosclerosis syndrome.[89] Pathological examination characteristically reveals a low-grade inflammatory infiltrate with poorly formed granulomas and an intense fibrotic component. Presenting features and complications depend on the affected organ and the intensity of fibrosis. Riedel's thyroiditis presents as a stony hard goiter, often with local compressive symptoms as the dense fibrous tissue involves the mediastinal structures. The local inflammation can be severe enough to cause thrombosis of the internal jugular veins, and in one case progression to a superior sagittal sinus thrombosis.[90] Treatment is with high-dose steroids, heparin for thrombotic complications and, in certain cases, decompressive surgery. Fibrosing lesions involving the orbit and progressing to involve the anterior pituitary have been described which have been accompanied by anterior pituitary failure.[91] This rare condition may be part of a spectrum of inflammatory, autoimmune or low-grade neoplastic processes allied to lymphocytic hypophysitis or histiocytosis. Transsphenoidal biopsy is often necessary to make this important diagnosis. Treatment is directed at replacing hormone deficits with high-dose steroids, surgery and radiotherapy, all having been used with varying degrees of success.[91]

Infectious conditions and the endocrine system

Specific infiltration of endocrine organs with infectious agents is actually rare. Involvement of the pituitary gland is most commonly quoted in the literature. Infectious agents that have presented as a pituitary mass and anterior pituitary dysfunction include tuberculosis, systemic mycoses (histoplasmosis, blastomycosis, coccidioidomycosis), opportunistic pathogens in immunocompromised people such as *Aspergillus* and mucormycosis, and abscess-forming bacteria. HIV-infected patients have presented with disseminated infection due to *Toxoplasma*, *Cryptococcus* and CMV involving the pituitary gland. Management is aimed at diagnosis, surgical evacuation where indicated, replacement of deficient hormones, and aggressive treatment of the underlying cause.

Metabolic disorders affecting the endocrine system

Hemochromatosis

Hemochromatosis is a genetic or acquired disorder of iron overload with selective deposition of iron in certain endocrine organs, leading to a toxic effect which results in hormone deficiency. Patients with the genetic disorder may have an endocrinopathy as their prime presenting feature. The most common endocrine deficits are diabetes mellitus (bronze diabetes), hypogonadism, hypothyroidism and hypoparathyroidism, occurring alone or in combination. In secondary disorders of iron overload such as transfusion-dependent disease (marrow aplasias, thalassemias), patients should be monitored on a regular basis to look for an evolving endocrinopathy. With untreated iron overload, liver cirrhosis can develop, with further detrimental effects on the function of the endocrine system. Treatment is based on recognition of an endocrine deficiency and appropriate replacement therapy. While venesection to deplete iron stores may halt the progression of an endocrinopathy, there is no evidence that endocrine function can be restored by this treatment.[92]

Significant clinical involvement in the pituitary–adrenal axis is rarely seen in conditions of iron overload,[93] although, on detailed dynamic testing, subtle defects in ACTH reserve have been reported in certain patient groups.[94] Although histologically iron is selectively deposited in the zona glomerulosa, a functional mineralocorticoid deficiency rarely occurs.[95] The pituitary–gonadal axis appears to be particularly sensitive to the toxic effects of iron overload, with selective deposition in both the end organ (testis) and the pituitary gonadotroph. This dysfunction is more clearly recognized in men, as females of reproductive age have menstruation as a physiological form of iron depletion. The predilection of iron for the gonadotroph is thought to relate to selective expression of the transferrin receptor in this pituitary cell population.[96] In children with thalassemia major requiring multiple blood transfusions there is clinical evidence of short stature and pubertal delay despite desferoxamine therapy. On endocrine evaluation, hormone deficits were multiple, but defects in gonadal, GH secretion and thyroid function were most common.[97]

Cirrhosis

Hepatic dysfunction with cirrhosis can be the end result of many diseases and toxins which affect the liver. There are several endocrine disturbances characteristically associated with chronic liver dysfunction. Testicular atrophy, impotence and gynecomastia are found in more than 50% of males with cirrhosis, due to altered androgen synthesis and availability, increased sex hormone-binding globulin (SHBG), and increased estrogen levels. These changes may be compounded when the cause of the cirrhosis is alcohol, as this has a direct toxic effect on the Leydig cell and further impairs testosterone synthesis. With progressive liver failure, hepatic clearance of steroid hormones is impaired, resulting in hyperaldosteronism and fluid retention, which give rise to a dilutional hyponatremia. Alcohol in particular can enhance activation of the stress axis, which, along with impaired hepatic clearance of cortisol, results in a pseudo-Cushingoid appearance.

Neoplastic and paraneoplastic conditions

Metastatic spread of cancer to endocrine organs is often found at postmortem, although in life a functional deficit is rarely seen. As endocrine tissue is rich in hormones and growth factors, it provides a favorable environment to support growth of the malignant cell. Many non-endocrine tumors are hormone dependent. The adrenal glands are most commonly involved in metastatic disease, particularly from disseminated breast cancer.[98,99] Small and large cell lung cancers are the most common secondary lesions of the adrenal glands, followed by metastatic deposits of renal carcinoma. Metastatic disease to the adrenal is frequently bilateral, and there is hence an increased risk of functional hypoadrenalism. Occasionally, infarction of metastatic tissue within the adrenal can precipitate an acute adrenal insufficiency. The pituitary[100] and thyroid glands are next most frequently involved, with the pancreas, parathyroid and pineal glands being least affected. Metastases to the pituitary gland are rarely found in isolation without other more commonly found sites such as lung, liver, brain or bone marrow being evident on post-mortem examination. Tumor-to-tumor metastases have been described, such as breast carcinoma to pheochromocytoma and prolactinoma, renal carcinoma to adrenal adenoma, gastric carcinoma to prolactinoma, and prostatic carcinoma to a non-functioning pituitary adenoma.[101]

Endocrine effects from pituitary metastases are very variable, though the occurrence of DI in a patient with a pituitary mass that does not have features of a granuloma or a craniopharyngioma should raise a suspicion of a metastasis from a non-endocrine primary. Similarly, patients presenting with III, IV, V or VI nerve palsies and a pituitary mass should be regarded as possibly having secondary malignant disease. A presentation with both nerve involvement and DI is almost pathognomonic of a pituitary metastasis. Although anterior pituitary dysfunction is not a constant feature, hyperprolactinemia due to stalk compression is a common finding on endocrine evaluation. The most common tumors to metastasize to the pituitary are breast followed by bronchus, colon, kidney and prostate. Infiltration, as opposed to metastatic spread, into endocrine organs is also a well-recognized phenomenon, especially by lymphomas, leukemias and sarcomas. Non-Hodgkin's lymphoma is the most common of these malignancies to involve the pituitary, often with a functional consequence, most commonly DI.

Parasellar lesions can often present with an endocrine deficit due to extension into the pituitary substance, e.g. optic nerve gliomas, neurofibromas, schwannomas, parasellar meningiomas, and nasopharyngeal carcinomas. Rare tumors arising within the pituitary gland which characteristically present with an endocrine deficit are hemangiopericytomas and hemangioendotheliomas. These are difficult to resect but are fortunately radiosensitive, though the functional endocrine deficit is invariably permanent. Treatment of any head or neck tumor with radiotherapy can have a long-term functional consequence for the function of the pituitary gland. This is becoming an increasingly important area of endocrinology as more childhood malignancies are treated and cured by craniospinal irradiation requiring long-term adolescent and adult endocrine surveillance. Similarly, chemotherapy regimens can cause lasting damage to reproductive end organs. The thyroid gland is commonly involved by metastatic disease on postmortem examination, but this is rarely associated with a premorbid defect in thyroid function. At postmortem examination of patients with malignant disease, thyroid involvement was reported in up to 26.4% of cases.[102] The most commonly found lesion was metastatic renal cell carcinoma, with lesions from breast, bronchus and colon also occurring. Squamous cell carcinomas from primaries in the lungs, esophagus and larynx have also been reported. Non-Hodgkin's lymphoma also has a predilection for thyroid tissue, where it can cause diagnostic difficulty with primary thyroid neoplasms. Metastatic deposits in the parathyroid glands have been described at postmortem but are rare and do not characteristically cause a functional deficit. The pineal gland is often neglected as an endocrine organ, but primary tumors of germinomatous origin most frequently occur within the gland. Metastatic deposits from testis, ovary or thymus have been rarely described, in addition to isolated case reports of small cell and adenocarcinoma occurring within the pineal from other primary sites.[101]

Neoplastic tissue from a variety of sources can have the ability to produce 'ectopic' or 'embryological hormones' in addition to elaborating cytokines which can have a distant endocrine effect. These are grouped together under the heading of paraneoplastic disease. Although the primary tumors may not belong to the classical endocrine system, histological analysis often reveals a neuroendocrine origin. Neuroendocrine cells are dispersed throughout the tissues of the body and, under normal physiological conditions, probably subserve a local paracrine effect. There are several well-recognized paraneoplastic conditions involving the endocrine system. Humoral hypercalcemia results from the elaboration of a PTH-like peptide (PTHrp). Hypocalcemia due to the release of osteoblastic factors from certain tumors, notably breast cancer, has been described. Cushing's syndrome from ectopic production of proopiomelanocortin (POMC)/ACTH-like peptides is described with small cell lung cancers, and bronchial and gut carcinoids. Ectopic vasopressin production causing SIADH is also common in small cell lung cancer. Hypoglycemia from tumoral overproduction of insulin-like growth factors has been described in several neoplastic conditions.

Tumors derived from several organs often display a de-differentiated or fetal phenotype and elaborate several useful tumor markers, e.g. carcinoma embryonic antigen (CEA), α-fetoprotein (AFP), human chorionic gonadotropin (HCG), CA-125 and CA19-9. Tumors secreting excess amounts of HCG, such as choriocarcinoma and teratomas, can have an interesting endocrine effect, due to the molecular similarity between HCG and TSH. Patients harboring these tumors can present with thyrotoxicosis due to cross-reactivity of high circulating levels of HCG competing for the TSH receptor. This situation is analogous to hyperemesis gravidarum/gestational thyrotoxicosis occurring in the early stages of pregnancy in certain predisposed individuals.

Cachexia is a common occurrence with many underlying neoplasms and probably relates to the elaboration of excess cytokines such as TNF-α. Cytokine elaboration by a variety of malignancies can have several diverse effects on the endocrine system. Perhaps the best recognized syndrome is POEMS (polyneuropathy, organomegaly, endocrinopathy, monoclonal gammopathy and skin changes). POEMS seems to be related to Castleman's disease, a rare syndrome of lymph node hyperplasia often localized to the mediastinum. Other vascular and cutaneous lesions such as Kaposi's sarcoma have been co-related. The POEMS syndrome is also known in the literature as Crow–Fucase syndrome, Takatsukis syndrome and PEP (polyneuropathy, endocrinopathy and plasma cell dyscrasia). The syndrome seems to occur most commonly in the Japanese, with gonadal dysfunction as the most common endocrinopathy. Amenorrhea is the most common feature in females of reproductive age, while 70% of men present with gynecomastia and impotence. Thyroid dysfunction, glucose intolerance, adrenocortical insufficiency, hypercalcemia and hyperprolactinemia have been less consistently described in this syndrome. The predominant cytokine is IL-6, which may account in part for some of the observed endocrine disturbances.

Hypoglycemia in adult life
Glucose homeostasis

The human body's supply of nutrients fluctuates widely, depending on food intake and metabolic demand, e.g. exercise, fever or trauma. Glucose homeostasis is, however, tightly regulated. In euglycemic adults, the mean arterial glucose concentration is largely maintained between 4.0 and 8.0 mmol/l, with a mean of around 5.0 mmol/l. Even during vigorous exercise[103] or after up to 60 h of fasting,[104] glucose levels do not usually fall to 3.0 mmol/l, and they rarely rise above 9.0 mmol/l after meals.[105] Adult males are particularly resistant to hypoglycemia, even with prolonged starvation.[106]

Insulin is the principal modulator of glucose homeostasis, stimulating peripheral glucose uptake and suppressing hepatic glucose output. A falling arterial glucose level initially suppresses pancreatic insulin secretion. Secretion of insulin-counterregulatory hormones is then stimulated if plasma glucose continues to fall to the lower limit of the normal range. Glucagon stimulates both glycogenolysis[107] and gluconeogenesis,[108] and inhibits glycolysis.[109] Catecholamines, particularly adrenaline, also stimulate glycogenolysis[108] and gluconeogenesis,[110] as well as promoting glucagon secretion.[111] GH and cortisol have a permissive effect on glucose metabolism, promoting the effects of glucagon and inhibiting those of insulin.[112]

The consequences of any perturbation of glucose homeostasis are severe. Even borderline hyperglycemia, as experienced by patients with impaired glucose tolerance, is associated with an elevated cardiovascular morbidity and mortality.[113] In diabetes mellitus, the cardiovascular risk is greater still, and more extreme long-term hyperglycemia is associated with a greater prevalence of neuropathic and microvascular complications.[114] By contrast, the effects of hypoglycemia are rather immediate, principally with the onset of potentially devastating cerebral dysfunction.

Physiological effects of hypoglycemia

Glucose is essentially the exclusive fuel used by the CNS, because the alternative substrates are either poorly transported across the blood–brain barrier or circulate at low plasma concentrations. The CNS is virtually dependent upon circulating glucose levels, because its cells do not synthesize glucose and can store only a few minutes' supply. Glucose uptake by the CNS is independent of insulin and depends upon the concentration gradient across the blood–brain barrier; at arterial plasma concentrations below 3.0 mmol/l, uptake becomes rate limiting for utilization.[115] Electrophysiological and psychometric studies suggest that cerebral function becomes impaired at an arterial plasma glucose level of around 2.6 mmol/l,[116,117] with neuroglycopenic and autonomic symptoms usually occurring at about the same time.[118] Severe or prolonged hypoglycemia may cause convulsions, permanent damage to the CNS and, eventually, death.

Detection of hypoglycemia was historically considered to be an exclusive function of the brain, particularly the hypothalamus.[119–121] However, recent data have shown that glucose sensors in the hepatic portal vein play an equally important role in initiating the counterregulatory response to hypoglycemia, particularly at lower glucose concentrations and with hypoglycemia of gradual onset.[122–124]

Although the venous plasma glucose concentration is usually measured in clinical settings, the cognitive and neurohumoral response to hypoglycemia has been studied in relation to arterial or arterialized venous samples. Readings of plasma glucose concentration are around 10% lower with venous rather than arterial or capillary sampling. Furthermore, readings from whole blood are about 15% below plasma samples, due to the lower glucose content of red blood cells relative to plasma.[125] Pocket glucometers, measuring glucose concentration in capillary whole blood, will thus tend to read approximately 5% below the actual venous plasma glucose level.

Schwartz et al[126] and Mitrakou et al[118] demonstrated a hierarchy of responses to decreasing plasma glucose concentrations. The threshold arterial glucose concentration for suppression of endogenous insulin secretion with the onset of counterregulatory hormone secretion is around 3.8 mmol/l. The onset of autonomic warning symptoms occurs at about 3.2 mmol/l, with acute neuroglycopenic symptoms and cognitive dysfunction occurring at glucose levels of around 2.8 mmol/l and 2.7 mmol/l, respectively. The counterregulatory humoral response to hypoglycemia is itself graded, with increased secretion initially of adrenaline, glucagon and GH, then cortisol and, finally, as overt hypoglycemic symptoms develop, noradrenaline.

Diagnosis of hypoglycemia

Autonomic symptoms and altered behavior, the classic symptoms of hypoglycemia, are non-specific and also occur in a number of other disorders, including thyrotoxicosis and primary psychiatric disease. Nevertheless, the diagnosis must always be considered in any patient with a history of episodic behavioral disturbance, particularly when punctuated by clouding of consciousness.

The biochemical definition of hypoglycemia is ultimately based on function, being the venous plasma glucose level at which the counterregulatory neurohumoral response is well underway, there is subtle cerebral dysfunction secondary to neuroglycopenia, and most individuals have begun to experience symptoms of autonomic activation (Table 14.2). In an adult, that point will usually be around 2.5 mmol/l,[127] although, in the UK, the cutoff point is traditionally taken to be 2.2 mmol/l during the endocrine investigation of hypoglycemia. Indeed, venous glucose concentrations can fall to 2.2 mmol/l during fasting in some women without symptoms of hypoglycemia.[128] Moreover, the sensitivity of the insulin hypoglycemia test in the assessment of anterior pituitary ACTH–cortisol and GH counterregulatory reserve has itself been validated on the basis of a fall in plasma glucose to 2.2 mmol/l.

It must be reiterated that the venous plasma glucose concentration is only a surrogate marker for cerebral arterial and hepatic portal venous glucose levels. Autonomic symptoms may be attenuated in individuals who have previously been exposed to hypoglycemia,[129–131] but the complete absence of neuroglycopenic symptoms excludes real cerebral or portal venous hypoglycemia. Although the precise symptoms of hypoglycemia vary from person to person, they are nevertheless consistent between episodes for any individual.[132]

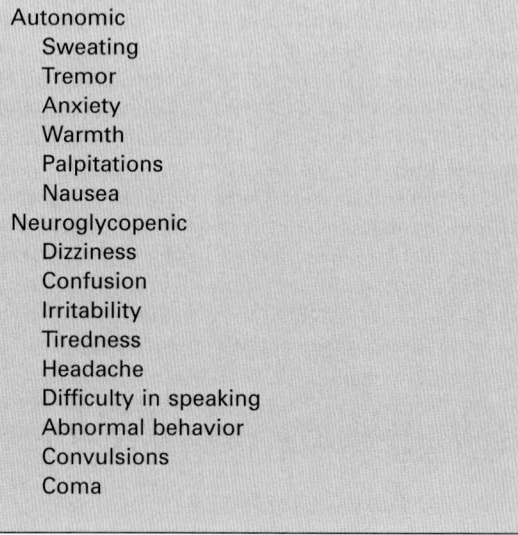

Autonomic
   Sweating
   Tremor
   Anxiety
   Warmth
   Palpitations
   Nausea
Neuroglycopenic
   Dizziness
   Confusion
   Irritability
   Tiredness
   Headache
   Difficulty in speaking
   Abnormal behavior
   Convulsions
   Coma

Table 14.2
Symptoms of hypoglycemia.[132]

Investigation of hypoglycemia

The clinical presentation of hypoglycemia determines the necessary direction and extent of evaluation. The diagnostic approach to a healthy-looking patient, with a history of episodic symptoms suggestive of hypoglycemia, is summarized in Table 14.3, and that for a sick, hospitalized patient in Table 14.4.

- Observe during fasting or, if reactive hypoglycemia suspected, during/after test meal
- If venous plasma glucose drops to less than 2.2 mmol/l, associated with neuroglycopenic ± autonomic clinical features, proceed as per Table 14.4.

Table 14.3
Elective evaluation of possible hypoglycemic episodes in an otherwise well patient.

- Identify venous plasma glucose of less than 2.2 mmol/l, associated with symptoms
- Take contemporaneous samples for further analysis (and resuscitate patient):
    Sulfonylurea screen (blood or urine)
    Cortisol (should be >550 nmol/l with hypoglycemia)
    fT4 and TSH
    Prothrombin time/INR, liver function tests and blood alcohol level
    Insulin, C-peptide and proinsulin
    Keep spare serum frozen
- Physical examination, chest radiograph, abdominal and pelvic ultrasonography
- When the presumptive diagnosis is non-islet cell tumor hypoglycemia, send plasma and, if possible, tumor specimen to specialist center for analysis (liaise with local biochemistry department regarding sample storage and transportation)

Table 14.4
Urgent evaluation of possible spontaneous hypoglycemia in a sick patient.

The finding of an abnormally low capillary blood glucose reading in a drowsy, unconscious or psychiatrically disturbed patient by nursing staff, using a glucometer and test strip, represents the typical in-hospital scenario. Interrogation of witnesses, physical examination or careful reading of past medical records may immediately reveal an obvious cause of hypoglycemia, e.g. intentional, inadvertent or iatrogenic insulin or sulfonlyurea overdose, alcohol intoxication, paracetamol poisoning or other cause of liver failure, renal failure, cardiogenic shock or cerebral malaria. In this situation, it is quite appropriate to proceed directly to treatment with intravenous glucose, a sugary drink, or a meal or snack, or a combination of these, depending on the patient's conscious level and capacity to cooperate. However, the opportunity to accurately document and biochemically define a spontaneous hypoglycemic episode can all too easily be missed when glucose is administered too precipitously in the emergency situation.

In the absence of any obvious precipitant, treatment should be deferred just long enough to enable venous blood to be drawn, a citrated sample for laboratory measurement of plasma glucose to be obtained, and a 10-ml clotted sample to be spun down and frozen for subsequent analysis. Spontaneous hypoglycemia can be eliminated from the differential diagnosis if the venous plasma glucose concentration is found to be normal, at a time when the patient is symptomatic. On the other hand, should the venous plasma glucose concentration be less than 2.2 mmol/l, with symptoms alleviated by the administration of glucose, the 'spare' plasma sample can be analyzed further, as per Table 14.4, for cortisol and alcohol levels, thyroid and liver function tests, and insulin, proinsulin and C-peptide levels. Sulfonylurea screening should also be performed on a urine specimen.

Elective admissions for evaluation of possible hypoglycemia in apparently well individuals, as described in Table 14.3, typically occur in two different contexts: first, where there is a high index of suspicion on the basis of the history, ideally with objective corroboration of at least one episode, witnessed by a friend, relative or physician; and second, where the index of suspicion is low, but the patient requires reassurance, having perhaps been uncritically labeled with hypoglycemia by a referring physician. Arranging for a patient to undergo a prolonged observed in-hospital fast involves fairly complex logistics, requiring the understanding and collaboration of on-call medical, nursing and laboratory staff. A pragmatic approach might be to reserve 72-h fasts for patients in whom there is a high index of suspicion and perform 24-h fasts in other cases, but this is perhaps controversial.

Non-islet cell tumor hypoglycemia

Hypoglycemia produced by tumors other than insulinomas is referred to as non-islet cell tumor hypoglycemia (NICTH). This can essentially be subdivided into tumors secreting forms of IGF-II, which represent the majority of cases, malignancies producing TNF or other hypoglycemic cytokines, and, arguably, where there is overwhelming metastatic destruction of the liver parenchyma. To date, there has been a single convincing reported case of NICTH secondary to ectopic secretion of insulin.[133]

NICTH may be the presenting feature of a previously undiagnosed malignancy, or it may only become evident during the terminal stages of disease. The incidence of NICTH in the developed world has been estimated to be around one case per 10^6 patient years,[134] though it is likely that many cases go undiagnosed. The symptoms of neuroglycopenia may be erroneously ascribed to etiologies such as cerebral metastases, opiate analgesia or terminal illness. Furthermore, the incidence of hepatoma and nasopharyngeal carcinoma, tumors specifically associated with NICTH, is considerably higher in the developing world.[135]

Once NICTH has revealed itself, its progress is usually both rapid and relentless, sometimes requiring enormous amounts of intravenous glucose (up to 2000 g/24 h) for its alleviation.[134] Isotopic studies of glucose utilization in NICTH have demonstrated a 50% reduction in hepatic glucose output coupled with a 4-6-fold increase in peripheral glucose uptake, largely by skeletal muscle rather than the tumor itself.[136] The underlying tumor is almost invariably identifiable at presentation, either on physical examination or with simple imaging (chest radiograph or abdominal ultrasonography). However, indium-111 labeled octreotide scintigraphy may be useful in locating tumors containing somatostatin receptors and which are either relatively small or obscured by the pelvis.[137]

Most cases of NICTH result from overproduction of a high molecular weight form of IGF-II ('big' IGF-II) by the tumor. Big IGF-II results from incomplete processing of proIGF-II, with a truncated form of the proIGF-II E domain retained instead of being completely cleaved.[138–143] IGFs-I and -II are peptides structurally similar to proinsulin, with insulin-like actions on glucose metabolism in liver and skeletal muscle. These actions are mediated by the type 1 IGF receptor, a heterodimer structurally related to the insulin receptor. Both IGFs-I and -II can produce hypoglycemia in human volunteers when administered in sufficiently large doses, yet only big IGF-II has been definitely linked to NICTH. It has recently been suggested that, in NICTH, the biological effects of big IGF-II are not in fact mediated by the type 1 IGF receptor itself, but largely by the insulin receptor and possibly also by heterodimers of the insulin/type 1 IGF receptor.[135]

In normal human serum, 70–80% of IGF-II circulates as a 150-kDa ternary complex with a specific binding protein (IGFBP-3) and an acid-labile-subunit (ALS). In this form, IGF-II is largely confined to the intravascular space and is thus excluded from target cell receptors. Of circulating IGF-II, 20–30% is bound as a 60-kDa binary complex with IGFBP-3 and less than 2% is present in the free form.[144] Under normal circumstances, the IGFs are thus prevented from exerting a significant physiological hypoglycemic or antilipolytic action, even though they circulate at concentrations many hundreds of times that of insulin.

Where no specific assay for big IGF-II is available, total plasma levels of IGF-II often appear normal in NICTH. However, concentrations of the 150-kDa complex will be markedly reduced as a result of several factors. First, production of IGF-I, IGFBP-3 and ALS is reduced, probably as a result of inhibition of GH secretion by tumor-derived big IGF-II. Second, as a consequence of its relatively poor binding affinity for the ALS, big IGF-II circulates predominantly as 50–60-kDa binary complexes with IGFBP-2, -3 and -6.[145–147] These are able to traverse the capillary endothelium more readily, allowing greater binding of big IGF-II to receptors.[148] Finally, inhibition of GH and glucagon secretion by IGF-II will tend to blunt the counterregulatory response to hypoglycemia.

A molar ratio of IGF-II/IGF-I greater than 10:1 (ratio is normally around 3:1), with undetectable levels of insulin, C-peptide and proinsulin and reduced levels of IGFBP-3, is virtually pathognomonic of NICTH.[142]

Although no tumor class appears to be exempt, NICTH has classically been associated with large retroperitoneal or thoracic fibrosarcomas. Even in these tumors, hypoglycemia is relatively rare, being present in 3% of benign and 11% of malignant tumors at any time in their evolution.[149] Among the series of 68 consecutive cases of IGF-II-mediated NICTH reported by Marks and Teale,[134] the majority (45.6%) were carcinomas, most frequently of the lung, pancreas and stomach, 33.8% were sarcomas or fibromas, and 5.9% were hepatomas (Table 14.5). Unlike insulinomas, where hypoglycemia is invariably the presenting feature, the diagnosis of neoplasia will often already have been made by the time hypoglycemia appears. The occurrence of hypoglycemia in terminally ill patients with disseminated carcinomatosis has traditionally been attributed to liver failure secondary to overwhelming metastatic destruction.[150] More recently, it has been suggested that, in many of these cases, hypoglycemia might be mediated by inflammatory cytokines, such as TNF and IL-1 and IL-6, secreted by the tumor.[151] Hypersecretion of these cytokines probably also underlies the hypoglycemia that may occur with end-stage heart failure, overwhelming sepsis and *Falciparum* malaria parasitemia,[152–154] although quinine-stimulation insulin secretion might also play a role.[155] Hematological malignancies are very rarely associated with NICTH,[156] with overproduction of IGF-II in some cases[157] and of cytokines in others.[158]

Treatment of non-islet cell tumor hypoglycemia

Solid tumors rarely weigh less than 1 kg, and progression of hypoglycemia is continuous and relentless rather than episodic. First-line treatment involves restoring euglycemia by frequent feeding and intra-

Islet cells
    Insulinoma
    Islet cell hyperplasia
Drugs and toxins
    Insulin, sulfonylureas
    Quinine, pentamidine
    Quinidine, disopyramide
Endocrine disease
    ACTH, GH or TSH deficiency
    Adrenocortical insufficiency
    Severe hypothyroidism
Reactive
    Post-gastric surgery
    Alcohol
    Idiopathic postprandial
Autoimmune
    Insulin receptor autoantibodies
    Autoimmune insulin syndrome
Metabolic stress
    Sepsis, e.g. *Falciparum* malaria
    Pregnancy
    Starvation
IGF-II-secreting tumors
    Mesenchymal
        Fibroma
        Mesothelioma
        Fibrosarcoma
        Hemangiopericytoma
        Leiomyosarcoma
    Mesenchymal (continued)
        Neurofibroma
        Rhabdomyosarcoma
        Hemangioendothelioma
        Histiocytoma
    Carcinomas
        Lung (small and squamous cell)
        Pancreatic
        Gastric
        Hepatoma
        Adrenal
        Esophagus
        Renal
Laboratory artefact
    Hemolytic crisis
    Polycythemia
    Leukemia
Hematological malignancy
    Lymphoma
    Leukemia
    Myeloma
Organ failure
    Severe chronic liver disease
    Acute liver failure
    Denervated transplant liver
    Acute pancreatitis
    End-stage renal failure
    Renal dialysis
    End-stage cardiac failure

Table 14.5
Causes of hypoglyglycemia in adults.

venous infusion of glucose, sometimes coupled with overnight nasogastric feeding. However, the large amounts required usually make this impractical for more than a few days. Complete removal of a benign or locally invasive tumor is curative, eliciting a rise in IGF-1 and IGFBP-3 levels and restoring physiological secretion of insulin and GH. IGF-II levels also fall, resulting in normalization of the IGF-II/IGF-I molar ratio.[134] However, most tumors causing NICTH are metastatic or infiltrative and typically involve elderly patients, for whom the survival period will be relatively brief. Surgical debulking often reduces or even eliminates hypoglycemia, but is only indicated where medical therapy has failed in a patient who, if only euglycemia could be restored, would have a good chance of spending several months outside hospital.

Large doses of glucocorticoids, such as prednisolone 30 mg daily or more, may produce remarkable improvements in glucose homeostasis, with restoration of endogenous GH responsiveness, a rise in ALS and IGFBP-3 levels, and a fall in both total and free big IGF-II. Incremental doses of recombinant human GH (r-hGH) (up to 36 units daily given subcutaneously) initially have a similar clinical effect on NICTH, but this is not always sustained, and improvements in biochemical markers are less profound. Nevertheless, r-hGH is still useful in combination with glucocorticoids or chemotherapy, or as a second-line treatment when glucocorticoid monotherapy has failed.[137,159–161] Use of glucagon has been limited by its short duration of action and the prominence of nausea as a side-effect.[162]

Other causes of hypoglycemia

The possibility of sample misidentification or laboratory error should always be considered where biochemical hypoglycemia has apparently occurred in the absence of symptoms. Where multichannel analyzers are used to process non-citrated blood samples, delayed analysis can result in spuriously low plasma glucose concentrations due to glycolysis, particularly in patients with leukemia[163] or hemolytic crisis.[164] This occurs as a result of excessive glycolysis by leukocytes and nucleated erythrocytes, respectively. Whole blood glucose values may be artefactually low in polycythemic patients, due to the lower glucose content of erythrocytes compared to plasma.[165]

Factitial hypoglycemia encompasses surreptitious self-administration of insulin or sulfonylurea, typically by a healthcare professional,[166] malicious administration to an unsuspecting victim, or the unwitting ingestion of a sulfonylurea due to a dispensing error. Sulfonylureas can be detected by screening blood or urine, and abuse of insulin by a non-diabetic can be differentiated from insulinoma by demonstrating suppressed levels of proinsulin and C-peptide. The presence of insulin antibodies is strong evidence for repeated injection of insulin.[167] However, antibodies to insulin also occur in the rare autoimmune insulin syndrome.[168,169] Affected patients typically have a history of Graves' disease, rheumatoid arthritis or SLE, and develop polyclonal antibodies to insulin, which bind to and activate the insulin receptor, causing hypoglycemia.[170] Monoclonal antibodies to insulin have been observed to cause hypoglycemia in a patient with multiple myeloma.[171] Hypoglycemia due to antibodies to the insulin receptor is described as a rare phenomenon in patients with a previous history of insulin-resistant diabetes mellitus.[170]

Food-stimulated or reactive or postprandial hypoglycemia occurs in 5–37% of patients who have undergone surgery to the stomach and/or the vagus nerve.[172,173] There does appear to be a small number of patients with idiopathic reactive hypoglycemia.[174] Such patients are usually advised to eat 'little and often', avoiding foods rich in fat or refined sugar. However, the diagnosis can almost invariably be excluded once autonomic symptoms, postulated to have been hypoglycemic in origin, are found to bear no relationship to any significant plasma glucose nadir. If necessary for reassurance, glucose levels can be measured in relation to a test meal, but most patients with autonomic symptoms following meals ('postprandial syndrome') are said to exhibit psychological problems.[175–177]

Severe reactive hyperinsulinemic hypoglycemia occurs within 3–4 h in up to 30% of healthy volunteers following ingestion of a mixture of alcohol (50 g), sucrose (60 g) and quinine, taken as gin and tonic.[178] This effect is exacerbated rather than relieved by simultaneous consumption of carbohydrate-rich snacks. Alcohol can also induce fasting hypoglycemia. Even moderate amounts (>30 g) taken by fasting or malnourished subjects are capable of inducing hypoglycemia 6–36 h later as a result of suppression of gluconeogenesis. Signs of hypoglycemia, such as stupor, unconsciousness, disorientation and aggression, can easily be mistaken for simple alcohol intoxication, even though the blood alcohol level is usually under 20 mmol/l.[179]

The oral glucose tolerance test has no place in the evaluation of patients with suspected reactive hypoglycemia. Over 10% of healthy individuals record venous plasma glucose nadirs less than 2.7 nmol/l, temporally unrelated to any autonomic symptoms[180]—a phenomenon which is especially evident in patients on carbohydrate-restricted diets.[181]

During pregnancy, mean fasting venous plasma glucose levels fall by approximately 10–15%, particularly at night, and pregnant women are more sensitive to food restriction.[182,183] Hypoglycemia may also be a presenting feature of previously unrecognized primary adrenocortical insufficiency, ACTH deficiency (either selective or in association with GH deficiency) and, more rarely, hypothyroidism.[184]

Conclusion

The causes of hypoglycemia of adult onset are well defined and the diagnostic process involves three stages: first, acting on clinical suspicion and confirming hypoglycemia by measuring plasma glucose concentration during a spontaneous neuroglycopenic episode; second, determining the etiology of hypoglycemia through a careful history, examination and biochemical investigation; and finally, anatomical localization of a responsible lesion or identification of a systemic metabolic etiology. Provided that appropriate biochemical investigations are performed at the time of autonomic or neuroglycopenic symptoms, it rarely becomes necessary to admit patients for prolonged observed inpatient food deprivation.

Hypercalcemia of malignancy

Introduction

The relative frequency of cancer as a cause of hypercalcemia will vary according to local circumstances, e.g. primary care versus hospitalized patients, or district hospital versus tertiary referral center. However, population-based studies indicate that malignancy is responsible for around 35% of cases of hypercalcemia, compared with 55% caused by primary hyperparathyroidism.[185] Table 14.6 illustrates the underlying tumor in 72 consecutive cases of hypercalcemia of malignancy (HM). It also demonstrates that, although the three commonest human cancers—lung, breast and prostate—frequently cause hypercalcemia,

	Frequency (%)
Lung	35
Breast	25
Myeloma	7
Lymphoma	6
Head and neck	6
Gastrointestinal	6
Renal	3
Prostate	3
Unknown primary	7
Others	2

Table 14.6
Etiology of hypercalcemia of malignancy in 72 consecutive patients.[236]

certain cancers cause hypercalcemia with a frequency disproportionate to their population prevalence. Thus, squamous cell carcinomas of the lung or head and neck commonly cause hypercalcemia, whereas small cell lung carcinomas and carcinomas of the gastrointestinal and female genital tracts rarely do so, despite commonly metastasizing to bone.

Because it undergoes a continuous process of remodeling under the influence of systemic hormones and local growth factors, bone is particularly vulnerable to disruption by cancer. There are two principal mechanisms by which this can occur: first, the direct local effect of tumor deposits, and second, the indirect effect of tumor-derived humoral factors acting systemically on bone and kidney to disturb calcium homeostasis. Squamous cell carcinomas classically cause hypercalcemia even in the absence of bone metastases, whereas myelomatosis is invariably associated with skeletal disease deposits. However, there is a continuum between these two mechanisms, typified by breast cancer. Bone secondaries exert at least part of their action through locally secreted factors and, where there is a high tumor load, locally secreted factors may spill over into the circulation to exert a systemic effect. Thus, the hypercalcemia which occurs in about 10% of women with breast cancer is usually in the context of late-stage metastatic bone disease, but is also associated with elevated levels of PTH-related protein (PTHrP).[186] In myeloma, discrete osteolytic lesions occur in 80% of cases, with most of the remainder exhibiting diffuse osteopenia, and hypercalcemia is present in around 30%.[187]

Parathyroid hormone-related protein and humoral hypercalcemia

PTHrP is the major mediator of humoral HM. It shares 70% sequence homology with PTH over the first 13 amino acids at the N-terminus,[188] and binds to the common PTH/PTHrP G-protein-coupled receptor,[189] although there is evidence for a separate PTHrP receptor.[190] PTH and PTHrP both stimulate adenylate cyclase in kidney and bone-derived systems,[189,191–194] and thus share similar biological properties. PTHrP not only mediates most cases of HM, through stimulation of osteoclastic bone resorption, increased renal tubular calcium reabsorption, decreased phosphate reabsorption and stimulation of 1α-hydroxylase,[195] but probably also plays a role in cancer cell survival and progression of osteolytic bone metastases.[196]

PTHrP has diverse and important functions in normal physiology and development, and these are extensively reviewed in Strewler.[197] Unlike PTH, which is a classical systemically acting hormone, PTHrP is a paracrine agent and is usually only detectable in the circulation during lactation (when it is able to maintain normocalcemia even in the context of hypoparathyroidism). PTHrP is crucial to the development of cartilage, mammary glands and teeth and also plays a physiological role in lactation, placental calcium transport, turnover of skin and hair follicles, and neuron survival within the CNS. Null mutations of the PTHrP gene in mice result in a severe and lethal form of chrondrodysplasia. Moreover, humans with the rare Blomstrand's and Janssen's chrondrodysplasias have been found to harbor inactivating and activating mutations, respectively, of the common PTH/PTHrP receptor.

PTHrP has been demonstrated in most of the tumor types associated with HM, including breast, renal and all types of squamous carcinoma.[198–200] Although detectable or elevated PTHrP levels are found in around 80% of hypercalcemic patients with solid tumors,[201] they only occur in 50% of cases associated with hematological malignancy.[202,203] Other humoral factors must therefore be involved, and extrarenal production of 1,25-dihydroxyvitamin D_3 $(1,25(OH)_2D_3)$ does appear to be a mediator in some cases of hypercalcemia.[204] More importantly, myeloma cells, which are found in close association with osteoclasts, osteoblasts and their precursor cells, have been shown to release osteoclast activating factors (OAFs) which promote active bone resorption and hence may result in hypercalcemia.[205] A number of different cytokines can potentially act as OAFs, including IL-1, IL-6, lymphotoxin, TNF-α and TGF-β. These cytokines are probably also secreted by the osteoclasts themselves, under paracrine stimulation from myeloma calls, and IL-6, in particular, seems to be a potent growth factor for myeloma.[196,206–210] Indeed, IL-6 and TNF-α have been shown to act synergistically with PTHrP to induce hypercalcemia.[211,212] More recently, a novel cDNA encoding an osteoclast differentiation factor/TNF-related activation-induced cytokine has been sequenced from squamous cell carcinoma cell lines associated with severe humoral hypercalcemia.[213]

Evaluation of presumed malignancy-related hypercalcemia

The physical examination and baseline investigations will almost always identify those patients in whom hypercalcemia is related to underlying malignant disease, although the possibility of a clinically occult squamous carcinoma of the sinuses or nasopharynx needs to be borne in mind (Table 14.7). Even with proven malignancy, it is always necessary to confirm that PTH levels are suppressed, because undiagnosed 10 hyperparathyroidism may coexist, particularly in an elderly patient. Pending the PTH assay result, a therapeutic trial of bisphosphonate therapy following intra-

---

Baseline tests
  FBC, ESR, U & Es, immunoglobulins
  Serum and urine protein electrophoresis
  fT4, TSH, PTH, PSA
  CXR
Further assessment
  Sputum cytology
  Fine needle aspiration/biopsy of any suspicious lymph node
  Bone marrow immunocytology
  ENT assessment
  Exclude adrenal insufficiency
  Abdominal and pelvic ultrasonography
  Gynecological assessment

Table 14.6

Investigation of presumed hypercalcemia of malignancy.

venous rehydration (see below) will usually distinguish HM from 1° hyperparathyroidism (where it will almost invariably have no effect on serum calcium levels). Hypercalcemia may be a feature of adrenal insufficiency, and the clinical picture of anorexia, myopathy and weight loss may mimic cachexia of malignancy. Indeed, hypoadrenalism resulting from tumor metastasis to the adrenals is probably as common as tuberculous adrenal insufficiency in developed countries. An inappropriately low-normal cortisol level in the face of systemic illness will usually suggest the diagnosis, and a synacthen test will confirm the diagnosis.

Treatment

The long-term therapy of malignancy-associated hypercalcemia should ideally include treating the underlying tumor. However, hypercalcemia may of itself be life-threatening and, in most cases, remains relatively refractory to anti-tumor therapy, even where a reduction in tumor load can be achieved. Therefore, specific treatment directed at lowering serum calcium levels is almost always indicated. Whether or not the malignancy is associated with PTHrP production, increased osteoclastic bone resorption occurs in virtually all patients with malignancy-associated hypercalcemia, and a significant number also exhibit increased renal tubular calcium absorption.[214,215]

The clinical features of hypercalcemia include neuropsychiatric disorders (confusion and drowsiness), gastrointestinal disorders (anorexia, nausea, dyspepsia, constipation, pancreatitis), cardiac arrythmias and renal disease (polyuria, polydipsia, nephrocalcinosis). An elevated serum calcium concentration induces renal tubular resistance to ADH, resulting in a degree of nephrogenic DI. Dehydration caused by increased renal water loss further exacerbates systemic hypercalcemia and, if associated with pre-existing renal disease, hyperuricemia and/or Bence Jones proteinuria, can precipitate acute renal failure. Volume expansion with intravenous saline is therefore essential first-line therapy. Hemodilution reduces serum calcium concentrations, and volume expansion increases glomerular filtration rate, with a consequent reduction in fractional tubular calcium reabsorption. However, the effect of hydration alone in normalizing serum calcium is only transient.[216]

Bisphosphonates are the current first-line agents in the treatment of hypercalcemia. They have a high affinity for hydroxyapatite, such that around half of an intravenous dose is concentrated in bone, preferentially in areas of high bone turnover. They are, however, so poorly absorbed (less than 1%) that the oral route is ineffective at treating hypercalcemia.[217] The mechanisms by which bisphosphonates inhibit bone resorption probably include induction of osteoclast apoptosis[218] and inhibition of osteoclast development, partly through recruitment of osteoblasts to produce osteoclast-inhibitory factors,[219] and partly through inhibition of tyrosine phosphatase activity.[220] Bisphosphonates are most effective in lowering serum calcium when bone metastases are present. Their effectiveness declines with higher levels of PTHrP, presumably because of the increased renal tubular reabsorption of calcium promoted by PTHrP.[221,222] Successful therapy is associated with increased levels of PTH and $1,25(OH)_2D_3$ and decreased biochemical markers of bone resorption.[223,224] A subset of lymphoma patients with hypercalcemia related to elevated levels of $1,25(OH)_2D_3$ do respond to steroid therapy, but in any case usually also respond to bisphosphonates.

The bisphosphonates disodium pamidronate and sodium clodronate, given as intravenous infusions over 2–4 h, are both licensed for the treatment of HM. A single infusion of pamidronate normalized serum calcium concentrations in 30% of patients receiving 30 mg, 61% of patients receiving 60 mg, and 100% of those receiving 90 mg.[223] At the 90 mg dose, pamidronate normalized the serum calcium level over about 4 days, with normocalcemia subsequently being maintained for about a month.[225] Prolonged therapy with fortnightly infusions of pamidronate 60 mg maintained long-term normocalcemia in the majority of patients with HM.[226] Rapid lowering of serum calcium has been achieved using combination therapy with pamidronate and subcutaneous salmon calcitonin, 200–400 MRC units twice-daily,[227,228] though this is rarely necessary in practice. Calcitonin has a transient hypocalcemic action, mediated through inhibition of osteoclastic bone resorption and of renal calcium reabsorption. The effect begins to wane after about 48 h, probably due to calcitonin receptor downregulation, by which time pamidronate has begun to take effect.

More recently, there has been a report of a patient with a metastatic malignant carcinoid tumor, presenting with severe, intractable hypercalcemia associated with elevated plasma concentrations of PTHrP and IL-6.[229] Conventional therapy with intravenous fluids and pamidronate was ineffective, but thrice-daily subcutaneous injections of octreotide 50–200 mg restored and maintained normocalcemia over a period of months, with an accompanying fall in PTHrP and IL-6 levels.

Conclusions

The process by which cancer metastasizes to bone is likely to depend on the same humoral factors responsible for HM. In order for tumor cells to grow in such a hard, mineralized tissue, they require the capacity to cause bone demineralization and destruction, and PTHrP is a major candidate factor responsible for this osteoclastic bone resorption. Indeed, Bouizar et al[230] found PTHrP expression in 37 of 38 primary breast cancers by RT-PCR, with levels of expression being correlated with subsequent development of bone metastases and hypercalcemia. It is likely that further studies of the interactions between PTHrP and OAFs will elucidate why only some PTHrP-secreting cancers result in clinical hypercalcemia.

In addition to their effect on hypercalcemia, bisphosphonates may also play a role in retarding progression of multiple myeloma and are increasingly given as standard anti-tumor therapy.[231] A 4-week course of intravenous pamidronate 60 mg daily has also been shown to reduce skeletal events and improve the quality of life in women with bone metastases from breast cancer.[232] Third-generation bisphosphonates, e.g. zolendronate or ibandronate, currently being evaluated in clinical trials appear to be over 100 times as potent as pamidronate.[233] It is hoped that these will be even more effective in treating HM and palliating painful bone metastases, and might also have a significant therapeutic action on both solid tumor metastases and myeloma.

A limitation of bisphosphonates is that they have no effect on PTHrP-induced tubular reabsorption of calcium. HM relapses more quickly following bisphosphonate therapy in patients with higher levels of renal calcium reabsorption.[215] New therapeutic modalities are therefore being explored. Osteoprotegerin (OPG) is a secreted protein from the TNF receptor family that inhibits osteoclast formation and activity and appears to be a critical regulator of bone mass and metabolism. Morony et al[234] challenged mice with various cytokines and hormones (IL-1, TNF-α, PTH, PTHrP and calcitriol), and this resulted in hypercalcemia with increased osteoclast numbers and bone resorption in the control group. However, mice treated concurrently with a recombinant form of human OPG remained normocalcemic and maintained osteoclast numbers in the normal range. A similar effect of OPG was demonstrated by Capparelli et al[235] in another murine model of HM, the PTHrP-secreting Colon-26 tumor. These potent effects of OPG in mice suggest a potential therapeutic role in the prevention and treatment of HM in humans.

Sick euthyroid syndrome

Introduction

The term 'sick euthyroid syndrome', or, in North American usage, 'euthyroid sick syndrome', refers to the anomalously low plasma concentrations of thyroid hormones commonly observed in relation to systemic disease. Although the phenomenon has been recognized for over 30 years, there is still no firm consensus on two important issues: first, whether affected patients are truly euthyroid, or whether there may instead be a degree of global or tissue-specific hypothyroidism (the neutral term, 'non-thyroidal illness syndrome' (NTIS) is therefore more apposite); and second, whether the physiological decrease in thyroid hormone levels during systemic illness is adaptive or maladaptive in nature.[237] NTIS might reflect a process of energy conservation contributing to the patient's recovery. Alternatively, the functional hypothyroid state may impair tissue function and threaten recovery. Anomalies of thyroid biochemistry form only part of the endocrine response to systemic illness, which also encompasses activation of the hypothalamic–pituitary–adrenal axis and inhibition of the hypothalamic–pituitary–gonadal axis. The adaptiveness or otherwise of the functional hypogonadotropic hypogonadism of systemic disease is likewise obscure. By contrast, hypercortisolism is clearly an adaptive response, given that patients with partial glucocorticoid deficiency, who may not be symptomatic in everyday life, can nevertheless develop hypoadrenal shock with intercurrent stress/illness unless high-dose glucocorticoid therapy is administered.

Pathophysiology of NTIS

NTIS occurs in 25–50% of hospitalized patients[238] and is most commonly characterized by an isolated reduction in total and free T3 levels.[239] These fall rapidly within 0.5–24 h of the onset of systemic illness to around 40% of normal levels.[240,241] This is accompanied by a reciprocal rise in levels of reverse T3 (rT3) as a result of reduced metabolic clearance.[242] Several animal studies point to reduced functional activity of tissue deiodinases (especially hepatic type I iodothyronine 5′-monodeiodinase, which deiodinates T4 to T3 and rT3 to T2). Impaired uptake of T4 by tissues may also play a role. Conversion of T3 to T4, by rat liver homogenates and cultured rat hepatocytes, and first-pass extraction of labeled T3 and T4 by isolated rat liver are inhibited in a dose-dependent manner by serum from patients with NTIS.[243–245]

More severe degrees of NTIS occur in relation to starvation,[246–248] sepsis,[249] trauma,[250] major surgery,[251,252] myocardial infarction,[241,253,254] bone marrow transplantation,[255] malignancy,[256] burns[257] and inflammatory disorders.[258,259] The degree of disturbance of thyroid function correlates with disease severity, and studies of patients in high-dependency and intensive care settings have found it to predict mortality.[241,249,254,258,260,261] In these patients, levels of total and, sometimes, also free T4 are reduced in association with inappropriately low (but almost invariably detectable) levels of TSH.

Two necropsy studies of NTIS patients have examined tissue levels of T3[262] and hypothalamic levels of TRH mRNA,[263] finding both to be extremely low. In rats, starvation similarly reduces hypothalamic TRH mRNA, portal TRH levels and pituitary TSH content.[264] Van den Berghe et al[265] normalized plasma levels of TSH, T4 and T3 in NTIS patients by infusing TRH 1 μg/kg per hour. The data are therefore consistent with impaired hypothalamic TRH secretion as a major component of severe NTIS. This may in part be secondary to stress/illness-induced hypercortisolemia, as glucocorticoids are recognized to suppress the hypothalamic–pituitary–thyroid axis.[266–268] Cytokines, plasma and tissue levels of which are elevated in acute and chronic disease, are also likely to play a role in NTIS, as they do in stress/illness-related hypercortisolemia. TNF-α and IL-1 both reduce basal and TSH-stimulated uptake of iodide by rat thyroid-derived cells.[269] Serum IL-6 levels are inversely associated with free T3 and T4 levels and positively associated with rT3 levels in postoperative and high-dependency medical patients.[270,271] However, the precise pathways by which the various cytokines act and interact are incompletely understood, and the results of in vitro and in vivo animal and human (normal volunteers and NTIS patients) studies are consequently often discrepant.

Practical considerations

The most frequent scenario in which endocrinologists encounter severe NTIS is in the context of a request for advice from an intensive care or high-dependency unit. The key question will usually be whether there is an organic endocrinopathy requiring thyroid hormone replacement therapy. Severely ill patients classically have levels of total or free T3 close to or below the detection limit of current assays, total T4 (where measured) significantly below the normal range, and free T4 and TSH around the lower limit of their respective normal ranges. It should first be ascertained whether or not the history, examination and/or available investigations are consistent with a possible lesion of the hypothalamus or pituitary, e.g. head trauma, intracranial hemorrhage, pituitary tumor or infarction, recent neurosurgery or relative bradycardia. An inappropriately low random plasma cortisol level or the presence of DI would be highly suggestive of a dysfunctional hypothalamo–pituitary axis. Where the clinical context is suggestive of organic secondary hypothyroidism, e.g. significantly low free T4, TSH and cortisol levels and/or putative lesion on neuroimaging, a trial of thyroxine replacement should be undertaken, with hydrocortisone cover if indicated. Inevitably, some patients with very severe NTIS and functional secondary hypothyroidism will end up being treated 'in error'. However, the mortality of such patients approaches 80% in any case, and the limited available evidence suggests no active harm, albeit no benefit, accruing to NTIS patients receiving thyroxine treatment.[272,273]

Conclusions

Neuroendocrine activation of the catecholaminergic system was long believed to be an adaptive mechanism which helped to maintain cardiac output when cardiac function was impaired. This dogma was only recently overturned with the recognition that β-adrenergic receptor antagonists significantly reduced mortality in this context. Until large randomized placebo-controlled studies of leiothyronine replacement therapy are performed, it will remain impossible to determine whether NTIS is an adaptive response, or maladaptive and therefore requiring treatment. It is fairly clear that treating NTIS patients with thyroxine imparts no benefit. That consensus also largely holds for not treating NTIS with leiothyronine, despite De Groot's well argued proposition[237] that the most logical way to uphold the principle of *primum non nocere* is precisely to restore physiological levels of T3 with replacement therapy.

References

1. Merenich JA, McDermott MT, Asp AA et al. Evidence of endocrine involvement early in the course of human immunodeficiency virus infection. *J Clin Endocrinol Metab* 1990; **70**: 566–71.
2. Grinspoon S, Bilezikian J. HIV disease and the endocrine system. *N Engl J Med* 1992; **327**: 1360–5.
3. Corcoran C, Grinspoon S. Drug therapy: treatment for wasting in patients with the acquired immunodeficiency syndrome. *N Engl J Med* 1999; **340**(22): 1740–50.
4. Christeff N, Gharakhanian S, Thobie N et al. Evidence for changes in adrenal and testicular steroids during HIV infection. *AIDS* 1992; **5**: 841–6.
5. Grunfeld C, Kotler DP, Shigenaga JK et al. Circulating interferon-alpha levels and hypertriglyceridaemia in the acquired immunodeficiency syndrome. *Am J Med* 1991; **90**: 154–62.
6. Grunfeld C, Pang M, Doerrler W et al. Lipids, lipoproteins, triglyceride clearance and cytokines in human immunodeficiency virus infection and the acquired immunodeficiency syndrome. *J Clin Endocrinol Metab* 1992; **74**: 1045–52.
7. Norbiato G, Bevilacqua M, Vago T et al. Cortisol resistance in acquired immunodeficiency syndrome. *J Clin Endocrinol Metab* 1992; **74**: 608–13.
8. Membrano L, Irony I, Dere W et al. Adrenocortical function in acquired immunodeficiency syndrome. *J Clin Endocrinol Metab* 1987; **65**: 482–7.
9. Dobs AS, Dempsey MA, Ladenson PW et al. Endocrine disorders in men infected with human immunodeficiency virus. *Am J Med* 1988; **84**: 611–16.
10. Verges B, Chavanet P, Desgres J et al. Adrenal function in HIV infected patients. *Acta Endocrinol* 1989; **121**: 633–7.
11. Donovan DS, Dluhy RG. AIDS and its effect on the adrenal gland. *Endocrinologist* 1991; **1**: 227–32.
12. Orpocher G, Mantero F. *Baillière's Clin Endocrinol Metab* 1994; **8**(4): 769–76.
13. Glasgow BJ, Steinsapir KD, Anders K, Layfield LJ. Adrenal insufficiency pathology in the acquired immune deficiency syndrome. *Am J Clin Pathol* 1984; **84**: 594–7.
14. Milligan SA, Katz MS, Craven PC et al. Toxoplasmosis presenting as panhypopituitarism in a patient with acquired immunodeficiency syndrome. *Am J Med* 1984; **77**: 760–4.
15. Sullivan WM, Kelly GG, O'Conner PG et al. Hypopituitarism associated with a hypothalamic CMV infection in a patient with AIDS. *Am J Med* 1992; **92**: 221–3.
16. Ferreira J, Vinters HV. Pathology of the pituitary gland in patients with the acquired immunodeficiency syndrome (AIDS). *Pathology* 1988; **20**: 211–15.
17. Christeff N, Gherbi N, Mammes O et al. Serum cortisol and DHEA concentrations during HIV infection. *Psychoneuroendocrinology* 1997; **22**(1): 11.8.
18. Norbiato G, Bevilacqua M, Vago T. Glucocorticoids and the immune system. *Psychoneuroendocrinology* 1997; **22**(1): 19.25.
19. Mosca L, Costanzi G, Antonacci C et al. Hypophyseal pathology in AIDS. *Histol Histopathol* 1992; **7**: 291–300.
20. Brown LS, Singer F, Killian P. Endocrine complications of AIDS and drug addiction. *Endocrinol Metab Clin North Am* 1991; **20**: 655–73.
21. Nelson MR, Erskin D, Hawkins DA, Gazzard BG. Treatment with corticosteroids—a risk factor for the development of clinical cytomegalovirus disease in AIDS. *AIDS* 1993; **7**: 375–8.
22. Widy-Wirski R, Berkley S, Downing R et al. Evaluation of the WHO Clinical Case Definition for AIDS in Uganda. *JAMA* 1988; **260**: 3286–9.
23. Chabon AB, Stenger RJ, Grabstald H. The histopathology of the testis in acquired immunodeficiency syndrome. *Urology* 1987; **29**: 658–63.
24. Croxen TS, Chapman WE, Miller LK et al. Changes in the hypothalamic–pituitary–gonadal axis in human immunodeficiency virus infected homosexual men. *J Clin Endocrinol Metab* 1989; **68**: 317–21.
25. Wilson WT, Frenkel E, Vuitch F et al. Testicular tumours in men with human immunodeficiency virus. *J Urol* 1992; **147**: 1038–40.
26. Grunfeld C, Pang M, Doerrler W et al. Indices of thyroid function and weight loss in human immunodeficiency virus infection and the acquired immunodeficiency syndrome. *Metab Clin Exp* 1993; **42**: 1270–6.
27. Lamberts M. Thyroid dysfunction in HIV infection. *Baillière's Clin Endocrinol Metab* 1994; **8**:(4) 825–35.
28. Tang WW, Kaptein EM, Feinstein EI, Massry SG. Hyponatraemia in hospitalized patients with the acquired immunodeficiency syndrome (AIDS) and the AIDS-related complex. *Am J Med* 1993; **94**: 169–74.
29. Farese RV, Schambelan M, Hollander H et al. Nephrogenic diabetes insipidus associated with foscarnet treatment of cytomegalovirus retinitis. *Ann Intern Med* 1990; **112**: 955–6.
30. Choi MJ, Fernandez PC, Patnaik A et al. Trimethoprim-induced hyperkalaemia in a patient with AIDS. *N Engl J Med* 1993; **328**: 703–6.
31. Peter SA. Disorders of serum calcium in acquired immunodeficiency syndrome. *J Natl Med Assoc* 1992; **84**: 626–8.
32. Nunez EA, Christeff N. Steroid hormone, cytokine, lipid and metabolic disturbances in HIV infection. *Baillière's Clin Endocrinol Metab* 1994; **8**(4): 803–24.
33. Perrone C, Bricaire F, Leport C et al. Hypoglycaemia and diabetes mellitus following intravenous pentamidine mesylate treatment in AIDS patients. *Diabetic Med* 1990; **7**: 585–9.

34. Loose DS, Kan PB, Hirst MA et al. Ketoconazole blocks adrenal steroidogenesis by inhibiting cytochrome P450-dependent enzymes. *J Clinl Invest* 1983; **71**: 1495–9.
35. Glass AR, Eil C. Ketoconazole-induced reduction in 1,25-dihydroxyvitamin D and total serum calcium in hypercalcaemic patients. *J Clin Endocrinol Metab* 1988; **66**: 934–8.
36. Grinspoon S, Corcoran C, Stanley T, Katznelson L. Effects of androgen administration on the growth hormone-insulin-like growth factor 1 axis in men with the acquired immunodeficiency syndrome. *J Clin Endocrinol Metab* 1998; **83**: 4251–6.
37. Lamberts SWJ, Bruining HA, de Jong FH. Drug therapy: corticosteroid therapy in severe illness. *N Engl J Med* 1997; **337(18)**: 1285.
38. Stewart PM, Corrie J, Seckl JR et al. A rational approach for assessing the pituitary–adrenal axis. *Lancet* 1988; **i**: 1208–10.
39. Hjortrup A, Kehlet H, Lindholm J, Stentoft RT. Value of the 30 minute adrenocorticotrophic (ACTH) test in demonstrating hypothalamic–pituitary–adrenocortical insufficiency after acute ACTH deprivation. *J Endocrinol Metab* 1983; **57**: 668–70.
40. Grinspoon S, Corcoran C, Miller K et al. Determinants of increased energy expenditure in HIV-infected women. *Am J Human Nutr* 1998; **70**: 299–300.
41. Restuccia D, Di Lazzaro V, Valeriani M et al. Neurophysiological abnormalities in adrenoleukodystrophy carriers. Evidence of different degrees of central nervous system involvement. *Brain* 1997; **120**: 1139–48.
42. Laureti S, Casucci G, Santeusanio F, Angeletti G, Aubourg P, Brunetti P. X-linked adrenoleukodystrophy is a frequent cause of idiopathic Addison's disease in young adult male patients. *J Clin Endocrinol Metab* 1996; **81**: 470–4.
43. El-Deiry SS, Naidu S, Blevins LS, Ladenson PW. Assessment of adrenal function in women heterozygous for adrenoleukodystrophy. *J Clin Endocrinol Metab* 1997; **82**: 856–60.
44. Brennemann W, Kohler W, Zierz S, Klingmuller D. Testicular dysfunction in adrenomyeloneuropathy. *Eur J Endocrinol* 1997; **137**: 34–9.
45. Holzinger A, Kammerer S, Berger J, Roscher AA. cDNA cloning and mRNA expression of the human adrenoleukodystrophy related protein (ALDRP), a peroxisomal ABC transporter. *Biochem Biophy Res Commun* 1997; **239**: 261–4.
46. Smith KD, Kemp S, Braiterman LT et al. X-linked adrenoleukodystrophy: genes, mutations, and phenotypes. *Neurochem Res* 1999; **24**: 521–35.
47. Liu L, Janvier K, Berteaux-Lecellier V, Cartier N, Benarous R, Aubourg P. Homo- and heterodimerisation of peroxisomal ATP-binding cassette half-transporters. *J Biol Chem* 1999; **274**: 32738–43.
48. Krasemann EW, Meier V, Korenke GC, Hunneman DH, Hanefeld F. Identification of mutations in the ALD-gene of 20 families with adrenoleukodystrophy/adrenomyeloneuropathy. *Human Genet* 1996; **97**: 194–7.
49. Dodd A, Rowland SA, Hawkes SL, Kennedy MA, Love DR. Mutations in the adrenoleukodystrophy gene. *Human Mutation* 1997; **9**: 500–11.
50. Takano H, Koike R, Onodera O, Sasaki R, Tsuji S. Mutational analysis and genotype–phenotype correlation of 29 unrelated Japanese patients with X-linked adrenoleukodystrophy. *Arch Neurol* 1999; **56**: 295–300.
51. Gartner J, Braun A, Holzinger A, Roerig P, Lenard HG, Roscher AA. Clinical and genetic aspects of X-linked adrenoleukodystrophy. *Neuropediatrics* 1998; **29**: 3–13.
52. Braiterman LT, Watkins PA, Moser AB, Smith KD. Peroxisomal very long chain fatty acid beta-oxidation activity is determined by the level of adrenoleukodystrophy protein (ALDP) expression. *Mol Genet Metab* 1999; **66**: 91–9.
53. Forss-Petter S, Werner H, Berger J et al. Targeted inactivation of the X-linked adrenoleukodystrophy gene in mice. *J Neurosci Res* 1997; **50**: 829–43.
54. Lu JF, Lawler AM, Watkins PA et al. A mouse model for X-linked adrenoleukodystrophy. *Proc Natl Acad Sci USA* 1997; **94**: 9366–71.
55. Dubois-Dalcq M, Feigenbaum V, Aubourg P. The neurobiology of X-linked adrenoleukodystrophy, a demyelinating peroxisomal disorder. *Trends Neurosci* 1999; **22**: 4–12.
56. Geisbrecht BV, Collins CS, Reuber BE, Gould SJ. Disruption of a PEX1–PEX6 interaction is the most common cause of the neurologic disorders Zellweger syndrome, neonatal adrenoleukodystrophy, and infantile Refsum disease. *Proc Natl Acad Sci USA* 1998; **95**: 8630–5.
57. Boehm CD, Cutting GR, Lachtermacher MB, Moser HW, Chong SS. Accurate DNA-based diagnostic and carrier testing for X-linked adrenoleukodystrophy. *Mol Genet Metab* 1999; **66**: 128–36.
58. van Geel B, Assies J, Haverkort E et al. Progression of abnormalities in adrenomyeloneuropathy and asymptomatic X-linked adrenoleukodystrophy despite treatment with 'Lorenzo's oil'. *J Neurol Neurosurg Psychiatry* 1999; **67**: 290–9.
59. Doerflinger N, Miclea JM, Lopez J et al. Retroviral transfer and long-term expression of the adrenoleukodystrophy gene in human CD34+ cells. *Human Gene Ther* 1998; **9**: 1025–36.
60. Flavigny E, Sanhaj A, Aubourg P, Cartier N. Retroviral-mediated adrenoleukodystrophy-related gene transfer corrects very long chain fatty acid metabolism in adrenoleukodystrophy fibroblasts: implications for therapy. *FEBS Lett* 1999; **448**: 261–4.

61. Kemp S, Wei HM, Lu JF et al. Gene redundancy and pharmacological gene therapy: implications for X-linked adrenoleukodystrophy. *Nature Med* 1998; 4: 1261–8.
62. Johns CJ, Michele TM. The clinical management of sarcoidosis. A 50-year experience at the Johns Hopkins Hospital. *Medicine* 1999; 78(2): 65–111.
63. Li N, Bajoghli A, Kubba A, Bhawan J. Identification of mycobacterial DNA in cutaneous lesions of sarcoidosis. *J Cutan Pathol* 1999; 26(6): 271–8.
64. Berry BH, Becton DL. Natural history of histiocytosis-X. *Hematol Oncol Clin North Am* 1997; 1: 23–34.
65. Braunstein GD, Kohler PO. Endocrine manifestations of histiocytosis-X. *Am J Pediatr Hematol Oncol* 1981; 3: 67–75.
66. Berry BH, Gresik MV, Humphrey GB et al. Natural history of histiocytosis-X: a Pediatric Oncology Group Study. *Med Pediatr Oncol* 1986; 14: 1–5.
67. Minehan KJ, Chen MG, Zimmerman D et al. Radiation therapy for diabetes insipidus caused by Langerhan's cell histiocytosis. *Radiat Oncol Biol Physics* 1992; 23: 519–24.
68. Wang WS, Liu JH, Chiou TJ et al. Langerhans' cell histiocytosis with thyroid involvement masquerading as thyroid carcinoma. *Jap J Clin Oncol* 1997; 27(3): 180–4.
69. d'Avella D, Giusa M, Blandino A et al. Microsurgical excision of a primary isolated hypothalamic eosinophilic granuloma. *J Neurosurg* 1997; 87(5): 768–72.
70. Rosenzweig KE, Arceci RJ, Tarbell NJ et al. Diabetes insipidus secondary to Langerhans' cell histiocytosis: is radiation therapy indicated? *Med Pediatr Oncol* 1997; 29(1): 36–40.
71. Kaltsas GA, Powles TB, Evanson J et al. *J Clin Endocrinol Metab* 2000; 85: 1370–6.
72. Veyssier-Berlot C, Cacoub P, Caparros-Lefebvre D et al. Erdheim–Chester disease. Clinical and radiological characteristics of 59 cases. *Medicine* 1996; 75(3): 157–69.
73. Huang HY, Yang CL, Chen WJ. Rosai–Dorfman disease with primary cutaneous manifestations—a case report. *Ann Acad Med Singapore* 1998; 27(4): 589–93.
74. Kelly WF, Bradey N, Scoones D. Rosai–Dorfman disease presenting as a pituitary tumour. *Clin Endocrinol* 1999; 50(1): 133–7.
75. Roberts GA, Eren E, Sinclair H et al. Two cases of Wegener's granulomatosis involving the pituitary gland. *Clin Endocrinol* 1995; 42(3): 323–8.
76. Katzman GL, Langford CA, Sneller MC et al. Pituitary involvement by Wegener's granulomatosis: a report of two cases. *Am J Radiol* 1999; 20(3): 519–23.
77. Escamilla RF, Lisser H. Simmonds disease. *J Clin Endocrinol* 1942; 2: 65–96.
78. Benvenga S, Campenni A, Ruggeri RM, Trimarchi F. Hypopituitarism second to head trauma. *J Endocrinol Metab* 2000; 85(4): 1353–61.
79. Ball SG, Vaidja B, Baylis PH. Hypothalamic adipsic syndrome: diagnosis and management. *Clin Endocrinol* 1997; 47(4): 405–9.
80. Kerrison JB, Lee AG, Weinstein JM et al. Acute loss of vision due to a suprasella mass. *Surv Ophthalmol* 1997; 41(5): 402–8.
81. Honegger J, Fahlbusch R, Bornemann A et al. Lymphocytic and granulomatous hypophysitis: experience with nine cases. *Neurosurgery* 1997; 40(4): 713–22.
82. Hama S, Arita K, Kurisu K et al. Parasellar chronic inflammatory disease presenting Tolosa–Hunt syndrome, hypopituitarism and diabetes insipidus: a case report. *Endocrine J* 1996; 43(5): 503–10.
83. Toth M, Szabo P, Racz K et al. Granulomatous hypophysitis associated with Takayasu's disease. *Clin Endocrinol* 1996; 45(4): 499–503.
84. Ostensen M. Sex hormones and pregnancy in rheumatoid arthritis and systemic lupus erythematosus. *Ann NY Acad Sci* 1999; 876: 131–43.
85. McMurray RW, Allen SH, Braun AL, Rodriguez F, Walker SE. Longstanding hyperprolactinemia associated with systemic lupus erythematosus: possible hormonal stimulation of an autoimmune disease. *J Rheumatol* 1994; 21(5): 843–50.
86. Lavalle C, Loyo E, Paniagua R et al. Correlation study between prolactin and androgens in male patients with systemic lupus erythematosus. *J Rheumatol* 1987; 14(2):268–72.
87. Gutierrez MA, Garcia ME, Rodriguez JA, Rivero S, Jacobelli S. Hypothalamic–pituitary–adrenal axis function and prolactin secretion in systemic lupus erythematosus. *Lupus* 1998; 7(6): 404–8.
88. Arnason JA, Graziano FM. Adrenal insufficiency in the antiphospholipid antibody syndrome. *Semin Arthritis Rheum* 1995; 25(2): 109–16.
89. Comings DE, Skubi KB, VanEyes J, Motulsky AG. Familial multifocal fibrosclerosis. *Ann Intern Med* 1967; 66: 884–92.
90. Vaidya B, Coulthard A, Goonetilleke A, Burn DJ, James RA, Kendall-Taylor P. Cerebral venous sinus thrombosis: a late sequel of invasive fibrous thyroiditis. *Thyroid* 1998; 8(9): 787–90.
91. Olmos PR, Falko JM, Rea GL, Boesel CP, Chakeres DW, McGhee DB. Fibrosing pseudotumor of the sella and parasellar area producing hypopituitarism and multiple cranial nerve palsies. *Neurosurgery* 1993; 32(6): 1015–21.
92. Lufkin et al. Influence of phlebotomy treatment on abnormal hypothalamic–pituitary function in genetic hemochromatosis. *Mayo Clin Proc* 1987; 62(6): 473–9.
93. Walsh CH, Murphy AL, Cunningham S, McKenna TJ. Mineralocorticoid and glucocorticoid status in idiopathic haemochromatosis. *Clin Endocrinol* 1994; 41(4): 439–43.
94. Schafer AI, Cheron RG, Dluhy R et al. Clinical consequences of acquired transfusional overload in adults. *N Engl J Med* 1981; 304(6): 319–24.

95. Hempenius LM, Van Dam PS, Marx JJ, Koppeschaar HP. Mineralocorticoid status and endocrine dysfunction in severe hemochromatosis. *J Endocrinol Invest* 1999; 22(5): 369–76.
96. Atkin SL, Burnett HE, Green VL, White MC, Lombard M. Expression of the transferrin receptor in human pituitary adenomas is confined to gonadotrophinomas. *Clin Endocrinol* 1996; 44(4): 467–71.
97. Oerter KE, Kamp GA, Munson PJ, Nienhuis AW, Cassorla FG, Manasco PK. Multiple hormone deficiencies in children with hemochromatosis. *J Clin Endocrinol Metab* 1993; 76(2): 357–61.
98. Del La Monte SM, Hutchins GM, Moore GW. Endocrine organ metastases from breast carcinoma. *Am J Pathol* 1984; 114: 131–6.
99. Seidenwurm DJ, Elmer EB, Kaplan LM et al. Metastases to the adrenal glands and the development of Addison's disease. *Cancer* 1984; 54: 552–7.
100. Teears RJ, Silverman EM. Clinicopathological review of 88 cases of carcinoma metastatic to the pituitary gland. *Cancer* 1975; 36: 216–20.
101. Lowe D. Metastatic and other extraneous neoplasms in endocrine organs. In: Sheaves R, Jenkins PJ, Wass JAH, eds. *Clinical Endocrine Oncology*. Blackwell Science, 1997: 470–4.
102. McCabe DP, Farrar WB, Petkov TM et al. Clinical and pathological correlations in disease metastatic to the thyroid gland. *Am J Surg* 1985; 52: 797–808.
103. Wahren J, Felig P, Hagenfeldt L. Physical exercise and fuel homeostasis in diabetes mellitus. *Diabetologia* 1978; 14: 213–22.
104. Consoli A, Kennedy F, Miles J, Gerich JE. Determination of Krebs cycle metabolic carbon exchange *in vivo* and its use to estimate gluconeogenesis in man. *J Clin Invest* 1987; 80: 1303–10.
105. Rizza RA, Gerich JE, Haymond MW et al. Control of blood sugar in insulin-dependent diabetes: comparison of an artificial endocrine pancreas, subcutaneous insulin infusion and intensified conventional insulin therapy. *N Engl J Med* 1980; 303: 1313–18.
106. Owen O, Reichard G. Human forearm metabolism during progressive starvation. *J Clin Invest* 1971; 50: 1536–45.
107. Cherrington A, Chiasson JL, Liljenquist JE, Jennings AS, Keller U, Lacy WW. The role of insulin and glucagon in the regulation of basal glucose production in the postabsorptive dog. *J Clin Invest* 1976; 58: 1407–18.
108. Exton JH, Park CR. The role of cyclic AMP in plasma glucose, insulin and glucagon levels. *Am J Physiol* 1968; 221: 1596–603.
109. Larner J, Lawrence JC, Walkenbach RJ, Roach PJ, Hazen RJ, Huang LC. Insulin control of glycogen synthesis. *Adv Cyclic Nucleotide Res* 1978; 9: 425–39.
110. Cahill GF. Action of adrenal cortical steroids on carbohydrate metabolism. In: Smith R, Gaebler O, Long C, eds. *The Human Adrenal Cortex*. New York: McGraw-Hill, 1955: 270–5.
111. Gerich JE, Langlois M, Noacco C, Schneider V, Forsham PH. Adrenergic modulation of pancreatic glucagon secretion in man. *J Clin Invest* 1974; 53: 1441–6.
112. Gerich JE, Davis J, Lorenzi M et al. Hormone mechanisms of recovery from hypoglycaemia in man. *Am J Physiol* 1979; 236: 380–5.
113. Jarrett RJ, Keen H. Hyperglycaemia and diabetes mellitus. *Lancet* 1976; 2(7993): 1009–12.
114. The DCCT Research Group. The effect of intensive treatment of diabetes on the development and progression of long-term complications in insulin dependent diabetes mellitus. *N Engl J Med* 1993; 329: 977–86.
115. Siesjö BK. Hypoglycaemia, brain metabolism and brain damage. *Diabetes Metabol Rev* 1988; 4: 113–14.
116. Koh THHG, Aynesley-Green A, Tarbit M, Eyre JA. Neural dysfunction during hypoglycaemia. *Arch Dis Child* 1988; 63: 1353–8.
117. Blackman JD, Towle VL, Lewis GF, Spire JP, Polonsky KS. Hypoglycaemic thresholds for cognitive dysfunction in humans. *Diabetes* 1990; 260: 828–35.
118. Mitrakou A, Ryan C, Veneman T et al. Hierarchy of glycaemic thresholds for counterregulatory hormone secretion, symptoms, and cerebral dysfunction. *Am J Physiol* 1991; 260: E67–74.
119. Frohman LA, Bernardis LL. Effect of hypothalamic stimulation on plasma glucose, insulin, and glucagon levels. *Am J Physiol* 1971; 221: 1596–603.
120. Benzo C. The hypothalamus and blood glucose regulation. *Life Sci* 1983; 32: 2509–15.
121. Frizzell RT, Jones EM, Davis SN et al. Counterregulation during hypoglycaemia is directed by widespread brain regions. *Diabetes* 1993; 42: 1253–61.
122. Donovan C, Halter J, Bergman R. Importance of hepatic glucoreceptors in sympathoadrenal response to hypoglycaemia. *Diabetes* 1991; 40: 155–8.
123. Perseghin G, Regalia E, Battezzati A et al. Regulation of glucose homeostasis in humans with denervated liver. *J Clin Invest* 1997; 100: 931–41.
124. Henever A, Bergman R, Donovan C. Novel glucosensor for hypoglycaemic detection localized to the hepatic portal vein. *Diabetes* 1997; 46: 1521–5.
125. Liu D, Moberg E, Kollkind M, Lin PE, Adamson U, Macdonald IA. Arterial, arterialized venous, venous and capillary blood glucose measurements in normal man during hyperinsulinaemic euglycaemia and hypoglycaemia. *Diabetologia* 1992; 35: 287–90.
126. Schwartz NS, Clutter WE, Shah SD, Cryer PE. Glycaemic thresholds for activation of glucose counterregulatory systems are higher than the threshold for symptoms. *J Clin Invest* 1987; 79: 777–81.
127. Marks V. Spontaneous hypoglycaemia. *BMJ* 1972; 1(797): 430–2.
128. Fajans SS, Floyd JC Jr. Fasting hypoglycemia in adults. *N Engl J Med* 1976; 294: 766–72.

129. Heller SR, Cryer PE. Reduced neuroendocrine and symptomatic responses to subsequent hypoglycaemia after 1 episode of hypoglycaemia in nondiabetic humans. *Diabetes* 1991; 40: 223–6.
130. Veneman T, Mitrakou A, Mokan M, Cryer P, Gerich J. Induction of hypoglycemia unawareness by asymptomatic nocturnal hypoglycemia. *Diabetes* 1993; 42: 1233–7.
131. Mitrakou A, Fanelli C, Veneman T et al. Reversibility of unawareness of hypoglycaemia in patients with insulinomas. *N Engl J Med* 1993; 329: 834–9.
132. Hepburn DA, Deary IJ, Frier BM, Patrick AW, Quinn JD, Fisher BM. Symptoms of acute insulin-induced hypoglycaemia in humans with and without IDDM: factor-analysis approach. *Diabetes Care* 1991; 14: 949–57.
133. Seckl MJ, Mulholland PJ, Bishop AE et al. Hypoglycaemia due to a small-cell carcinoma of the cervix. *N Engl J Med* 1999; 10: 733–6.
134. Marks V, Teale JD. Tumours producing hypoglycaemia. *Endocrine-Related Cancer* 1998; 5: 111–29.
135. Koch CA, Rother KI, Roth J. Tumor hypoglycemia linked to IGF-II. In: *Contemporary Endocrinology*, Vol. 20: *The IGF System: Molecular Biology, Physiology & Clinical Applications*. New Jersey: Totowa Press, 1999; 28: 675–98.
136. Phillips LS, Robertson DG. Insulin-like growth factors and non-islet cell tumour hypoglycaemia. *Metabolism* 1993; 42: 1093–101.
137. Perros P, Simpson J, Innes JA, Teale JD, McKnight JA. Non-islet cell tumour-associated hypoglycaemia: [111]In octreotide imaging and efficacy of octreotide, growth hormone and glucocorticosteroids. *Clin Endocrinol Oxf* 1996; 44: 727–31.
138. Megyesi K, Kahn CR, Roth J, Gorden P. Hypoglycaemia in association with extrapancreatic tumors: demonstration of elevated plasma NSILA-s by a new receptor assay. *J Clin Endocrinol Metab* 1974; 38: 931–4.
139. Gorden P, Hendricks CM, Kahn CR, Megyesi K, Roth J. Hypoglycaemia associated with non-islet cell tumor and insulin-like growth factors. A study of the tumor types. *N Engl J Med* 1981; 305: 1452–5.
140. Axelrod L, Ron D. Insulin-like growth factor II and the riddle of tumor-induced hypoglycaemia. *N Engl J Med* 1988; 319: 1477–9.
141. Lowe WL, Roberts CT, LeRoith D et al. Insulin-like growth factor-II in non-islet cell tumors associated with hypoglycaemia: increased levels of messenger ribonucleic acid. *J Clin Endocrinol Metab* 1989; 69: 1153–9.
142. Teale JD, Marks V. Inappropriately elevated plasma insulin-like growth factor-II in relation to suppressed insulin-like growth factor-I in the diagnosis of non-islet cell tumour hypoglycaemia. *Clin Endocrinol Oxf* 1990; 33: 89–97.
143. Daughaday WH, Trivedi B. Heterogeneity of serum peptides with immunoassay detected by RIA for proIGF-II E domain. *J Clin Endocrinol Metab* 1992; 75: 641–5.
144. Rajaram S, Baylink DJ, Mohan S. Insulin-like growth factor binding-proteins in serum and other biological fluids: regulation and function. *Endocrine Rev* 1997; 18: 801–31.
145. Baxter RC, Daughaday WH. Impaired formation of the ternary insulin-like growth factor-binding protein complex in patients with hypoglycaemia due to non-islet cell tumors. *J Clin Endocrinol Metab* 1991; 73: 696–702.
146. Zapf J, Futo E, Peter M, Froesch ER. Can 'big' insulin-like growth factor II in serum of tumour patients account for the development of extrapancreatic tumor hypoglycaemia? *J Clin Invest* 1992; 90: 2574–84.
147. Hoekman K, van Doorn J, Gloudemans T, Maassen JA, Schuller AG, Pinedo HM. Hypoglycaemia associated with the production of insulin-like growth factor II and insulin-like growth factor binding protein 6 by a haemangiopericytoma. *Clin Endocrinol (Oxf)* 1999; 51: 247–53.
148. Moller N, Frystyk J, Skaerbaek C et al. Systemic and regional tumour metabolism in a patient with non-islet cell tumour hypoglycaemia: role of increased levels of free insulin-like growth factors. *Diabetologia* 1996; 39: 1534–5.
149. England DM, Hocholzer L, McCarthy MJ. Localized benign and malignant fibrous tumors of the pleura. A clinicopathologic review of 223 cases. *Am J Surg Pathol* 1989; 13: 640–58.
150. Younus S, Soterakis J, Sossi AJ, Chawla SK, LoPresti PA. Hypoglycaemia secondary to metastases to the liver: a case report and review of the literature. *Gastroenterology* 1977, 72: 334–7.
151. Fitzpatrick DR, Peroni DJ, Bielefeldt-Ohmann H. The role of growth factors and cytokines in the tumorigenesis and immunobiology of malignant mesothelioma. *Am J Respir Cell Mol Biol* 1995; 12: 455–60.
152. Levine B, Kalmas J, Mayer L, Fillit HM, Packer M. Elevated circulating levels of tumor necrosis factor in severe chronic heart failure. *N Engl J Med* 1990; 323: 236–41.
153. Rockett KA, Awburn MM, Rockett EJ, Clark IA. Tumor necrosis factor and interleukin-1 synergy in the context of malaria pathology. *Am J Trop Med Hyg* 1994; 50: 735–42.
154. Elased KM, Taverne J, Playfair JH. Malaria, blood glucose, and the role of tumour necrosis factor (TNF) in mice. *Clin Exp Immunol* 1996; 105: 443–4.
155. White NJ, Warrell DA, Chanthanavich P et al. Severe hypoglycaemia and hyperinsulinaemia in falciparum malaria. *N Engl J Med* 1983; 309: 61–6.
156. Al-Hilali MM, Majer RV, Penney O. Hypoglycaemia in acute myelomonoblastic leukaemia: report of two

cases and review of published work. *BMJ* 1984; **289**: 1443–4.
157. Snowden JA, Greaves M, Page K. Reversal of diabetes associated with escape of myeloma: evidence of inappropriate IGF-II secretion. *Br J Haematol* 1994; **87**: 202–4.
158. Durig J, Fiedler W, de Wit M, Steffen M, Hossfeld DK. Lactic acidosis and hypoglycaemia in a patient with high grade non-Hodgkin's lymphoma and elevated circulating TNF-alpha. *Ann Haematol* 1996; **72**: 93–9.
159. Hunter SJ, Daughaday WH, Callender ME et al. A case of hepatoma associated with hypoglycaemia and overproduction of IGF-II (E21): beneficial effects of treatment with growth hormone and intrahepatic adriamycin. *Clin Endocrinol Oxf* 1994; **41**: 397–401.
160. Baxter RC, Holman SR, Corbould A, Stranks S, Ho PJ, Braund W. Regulation of the insulin-like growth factors and their binding proteins by glucocorticoid and growth hormone in non-islet cell tumor hypoglycaemia. *J Clin Endocrinol Metab* 1995; **80**: 2700–8.
161. Teale JD, Marks V. Glucocorticoid therapy suppresses abnormal secretion of big IGF-II by non-islet cell tumours inducing hypoglycaemia (NICTH). *Clin Endocrinol Oxf* 1998; **49**: 491–8.
162. Samaan NA, Pham FK, Sellin RV, Fernandez JF, Benjamin RS. Successful treatment of hypoglycaemia using glucagon in a patient with an extrapancreatic tumor. *Ann Intern Med* 1990; **113**: 404–6.
163. Goodenow TJ, Malarkey WB. Leukocytosis and artifactual hypoglycaemia. *JAMA* 1977; **237**: 1961–2.
164. Macaron CI, Kadri A, Macaron Z. Nucleated red blood cells and artifactual hypoglycaemia. *Diabetes Care* 1981; **4**: 113–15.
165. Arem R, Jeang MK, Blevens TC, Waddell CC, Field JB. Polycythemia rubra vera and artifactual hypoglycaemia. *Arch Intern Med* 1982; **142**: 2199–201.
166. Service FJ, Moore GL. Factitial and autoimmune hypoglycaemias. In: Service FJ, ed. *Hypoglycaemic Disorders: Pathogenesis, Diagnosis and Treatment*. Boston: GK Hall, 1983: 129.
167. Scarlett JA, Blix PM, Goldman J et al. Factitious hypoglycaemia: diagnosis by measurement of serum C-peptide immunoreactivity and insulin-binding antibodies. *N Engl J Med* 1977; **297**: 1029–32.
168. Hirata Y. Methimazole and insulin autoimmune syndrome with hypoglycemia [letter]. *Lancet* 1983; **2**(8357): 1037–8.
169. Dozio N, Sodoyez-Goffaux F, Koch M, Ziegler B, Sodoyez JC. Polymorphism of insulin antibodies in six patients with insulin-immune hypoglycaemic syndrome. *Clin Exp Immunol* 1991; **85**: 282–7.
170. Taylor SI, Barbetti F, Accili D, Roth J, Gorden P. Syndromes of autoimmunity and hypoglycaemia. *Endocrinol Metab Clin North Am* 1989; **18**: 123–43.
171. Redmon P, Pydrowski KL, Elson MK, Kay NE, Dalmasso AP, Nuttall FQ. Hypoglycaemia due to an insulin-binding monoclonal antibody in multiple myeloma. *N Engl J Med* 1992, **326**: 994–8.
172. Leichter SB, Permutt MA. Effect of adrenergic agents on postgastrectomy hypoglycaemia. *Diabetes* 1974; **24**: 1005–10.
173. Wiznitzer T, Shapira N, Stadler J, Ayalon D, Harell A. Late hypoglycaemia in patients following vagotomy and pyloroplasty. *Int Surg* 1974; **59**: 229–32.
174. Permutt MA, Kelly J, Berstein R, Alpers DH, Siegel BA, Kipnis DM. Alimentary hypoglycaemia in the absence of gastrointestinal surgery. *N Engl J Med* 1973; **288**: 1206–10.
175. Johnson DD, Dorr KE, Swenson WM, Service FJ. Reactive hypoglycaemia. *JAMA* 1980; **243**: 1151–5.
176. Anthony D, Dippe S, Hofeldt FD. Personality disorder and reactive hypoglycaemia: a quantitative study. *Diabetes* 1973; **22**: 664–75.
177. Ford CV, Bray CA, Swerdloff RS. A psychiatric study of patients referred with a diagnosis of hypoglycaemia. *Am J Psychiatry* 1976; **133**: 290–4.
178. O'Keefe SJ, Marks V. Lunchtime gin and tonic: a cause of reactive hypoglycaemia. *Lancet* 1977; **1**(8025): 1286.
179. Fishbain DA, Rotundo D. Frequency of hypoglycaemic delirium in a psychiatric emergency service. *Psychosomatics* 1988; **29**: 346–8.
180. Lev-Ran A, Anderson RW. The diagnosis of postprandial hypoglycaemia. *Diabetes* 1981; **30**: 996–9.
181. Permutt MA, Delmuz J, Stenson W. Effects of carbohydrate restriction on the hypoglycaemic phase of the glucose tolerance test. *J Clin Endocrinol Metab* 1976; **43**: 1088–93.
182. Felig P, Lynch V. Starvation in human pregnancy: hypoglycemia, hypoinsulinemia, and hyperketonemia. *Science* 1970; **170**: 990–2.
183. Victor A. Normal blood sugar variation during pregnancy. *Acta Obstet Gynecol Scand* 1974; **53**: 37–40.
184. Samaan NA. Hypoglycaemia secondary to endocrine deficiencies. *Endocrinol Metab Clin North Am* 1989; **18**: 163–83.
185. Mundy GR, Cove DH, Fisken R. Primary hyperparathyroidism: changes in the pattern of clinical presentation. *Lancet* 1980; **1**: 1317–20.
186. Percival RC, Yates AJP, Gray RE et al. Mechanisms of malignant hypercalcaemia in carcinoma of the breast. *BMJ* 1985; **291**: 776–9.
187. Kyle RA. Multiple myeloma: a review of 869 cases. *Mayo Clin Proc* 1975; **50**: 29–40. *J Clin Endocrinol Metab* 1999; **84**: 3545–50.
188. Suva LJ, Winslow GA, Wettenhall REH et al. A parathyroid hormone-related protein implicated in malignant hypercalcaemia: cloning and expression. *Science* 1987; **237**: 893–6.
189. Abou-Samra AB, Jüppter H, Force T et al. Expression cloning of a common receptor for parathyroid hormone and parathyroid hormone-related

189. peptide from rat osteoblast-like cells: a single receptor stimulates intracellular accumulation of both cAMP and inositol triphosphates and increases intracellular free calcium. *Proc Natl Acad Sci USA* 1992; **89**: 2732–6.
190. Orloff JJ, Kats Y, Urena P et al. Further evidence for a novel receptor for amino-terminal parathyroid hormone-related protein on keratinocytes and squamous carcinoma cell lines. *Endocrinology* 1995; **136**: 3016–23.
191. Moseley JM, Dieffenbach-Jagger H, Wettenhall REH et al. Parathyroid hormone-related protein of malignancy: active synthetic fragments. *Science* 1987; **238**: 1568–70.
192. Burtis WJ, Wu T, Bunch C et al. Identification of a novel 17,000-dalton parathyroid hormone-like adenylate cyclase-stimulating protein from a tumor associated with humoral hypercalcaemia of malignancy. *J Biol Chem* 1987; **262**: 7151–6.
193. Kemp BE, Moseley JM, Rodda CP et al. Parathyroid hormone-related protein of malignancy: active synthetic fragments. *Science* 1987; **238**: 1568–70.
194. Yates AJP, Gutierrez GE, Smolens P et al. Effects of a synthetic peptide of a parathyroid hormone-related protein on calcium homeostasis, renal tubular calcium reabsorption, and bone metabolism in vivo and in vitro in rodents. *J Clin Invest* 1988; **81**: 932–8.
195. Horiuchi N, Caulfield MP, Fisher JE et al. Similarity of synthetic peptide from human tumor to parathyroid hormone *in vivo* and *in vitro*. *Science* 1987; **238**: 1566–8.
196. Yin JJ, Selander K, Chirgwin JM et al. TGF-beta signaling blockade inhibits PTHrP secretion by breast cancer cells and bone metastases development. *J Clin Invest* 1999; **103**: 197–206.
197. Strewler GJ. The physiology of parathyroid hormone-related protein. *N Engl J Med* 2000; **342**: 177–85.
198. Danks JA, Ebeling PR, Hayman J et al. Parathyroid hormone-related protein: immunohistochemical localisation in cancers and in normal skin. *J Bone Miner Res* 1989; **4**: 273–8.
199. Asa SL, Henderson J, Goltzman D, Drucker DJ. Parathyroid hormone-like peptide in normal and neoplastic human endocrine tissues. *J Clin Endocrinol Metab* 1990; **71**: 1112–18.
200. Dunne FP, Lee S, Ratcliffe WA, Hutchesson AC, Bundred AJ, Heath DA. Parathyroid hormone-related protein (PTHrP) gene expression in solid tumours associated with normocalcaemia and hypercalcaemia. *J Pathol* 1993; **171**: 215–21.
201. Burtis WJ, Brady TG, Orloff JJ et al. Immunochemical characterisation of circulating parathyroid hormone-like protein in patients with humoral hypercalcaemia of malignancy. *N Engl J Med* 1990; **322**: 1106–12.
202. Firkin F, Seymour JF, Watson AM, Grill V, Martin TJ. Parathyroid hormone-related protein in hypercalcaemia associated with haematological malignancy. *Br J Haematol* 1996; **94**: 486–92.
203. Kremer R, Shustik C, Tabak T, Papavasiliou V, Goltzman D. Parathyroid-hormone-related peptide in hematologic malignancies. *Am J Med* 1996; **100**: 406–11.
204. Seymour JF, Gagel RF, Hagemeister FB, Dimopoulos MA, Cabanillas F. Calcitriol production in hypercalcaemic and normocalcaemic patients with non-Hodgkin's lymphoma. *Ann Intern Med* 1994; **21**: 633–40.
205. Mundy GR, Raisz LG, Cooper RA, Schechter GP, Salmon S. Evidence for the secretion of an osteoclast stimulating factor in myeloma. *N Engl J Med* 1974; **291**: 1041–6.
206. Garrett IR, Durie BGM, Newin GE et al. Production of lymphotoxin, a bone-resorbing cytokine, by cultured human myeloma cells. *N Engl J Med* 1987; **317**: 526–32.
207. Kawano M, Hirano T, Matsuda T et al. Autocrine generation and requirement of BSF-2/IL-6 for human multiple myelomas. *Nature* 1988; **32**: 83–5.
208. Cozzolini F, Torcia M, Aldinucci D et al. Production of interleukin-1 by bone marrow myeloma cells. *Blood* 1989; **74**: 380–7.
209. Sabatini M, Boyce BF, Aufdemorte T, Bonewald L, Mundy GR. Infusions of recombinant human interleukins 1α and 1β cause hypercalcemia in normal mice. *Proc Natl Acad Sci USA* 1988; **85**: 5235–9.
210. Sati HI, Greaves M, Apperley JF, Russell RG, Croucher PI. Expression of interleukin-1beta and tumour necrosis factor-alpha in plasma cells from patients with multiple myeloma. *Br J Haematol* 1999; **104**: 350–7.
211. De la Mata J, Uy HL, Guise TA et al. Interleukin-6 enhances hypercalcemia and bone resorption mediated by parathyroid hormone-related protein in vivo. *J Clin Invest* 1995; **95**: 2846–52.
212. Uy HL, Mundy GR, Boyce BF et al. Tumor necrosis factor enhances parathyroid hormone-related protein-induced hypercalcemia and bone resorption without inhibiting bone formation in vivo. *Cancer Res* 1997; **57**: 3194–9.
213. Nagai M, Kyakumoto S, Sato N. Cancer cells responsible for humoral hypercalcemia express mRNA encoding a secreted form of ODF/TRANCE that induces osteoclast formation. *Biochem Biophys Res Commun* 2000; **269**: 532–6.
214. Tuttle KR, Kunau RT, Loveridge N, Mundy GR. Altered renal calcium handling in hypercalcemia of malignancy. *J Am Soc Nephrol* 1991; **2**: 191–9.
215. Rizzoli R, Thiebaud D, Bundred N et al. Serum parathyroid hormone-related protein levels and response to bisphosphonate treatment in hypercalcemia of malignancy.
216. Hosking DJ, Cowley A, Bucknall CA. Rehydration in the treatment of severe hypercalcaemia. *Q J Med* 1981; **51**: 473–81.

217. Mundy GR, Wilkinson RB, Heath DA. Comparative study of available medical therapy for hypercalcemia of malignancy. *Am J Med* 1983; 74: 421–32.
218. Hughes DE, Wright KR, Uy HL et al. Bisphosphonates promote apoptosis in murine osteoclasts, *in vitro* and *in vivo*. *J Bone Mineral Res* 1995; 10: 1478–87.
219. Rodan GA, Fleisch HA. Bisphosphonates: mechanisms of action. *J Clin Invest* 1996; 97: 2692–6.
220. Schmidt A, Rutledge SJ, Endo N et al. Protein-tyrosine phosphatase activity regulates osteoclast formation and function: inhibition by alendronate. *Proc Natl Acad Sci USA* 1996, 93: 3068–73.
221. Dodwell DJ, Abbas SK, Morton AR, Howell A. Parathyroid hormone-related protein (50–69) and response to pamidronate therapy for tumour-induced hypercalcaemia. *Eur J Cancer* 1991; 27: 1629–33.
222. Walls J, Ratcliffe WA, Howell A, Bundred NJ. Response to intravenous bisphosphonate therapy in hypercalcaemic patients with and without bone metastases: the role of parathyroid hormone-related protein. *Br J Cancer* 1994; 70: 169–72.
223. Nussbaum SR, Younger J, Vandepol CJ et al. Single-dose intravenous therapy with pamidronate for the treatment of hypercalcemia of malignancy: comparison of 30-, 60-, and 90-mg dosages. *Am J Med* 1993; 95: 297–304.
224. Budayr AA, Zysset E, Jenzer A et al. Effects of treatment of malignancy-associated hypercalcemia on serum parathyroid hormone-related protein. *J Bone Mineral Res* 1994; 9: 521–6.
225. Purohit OP, Radstone CR, Anthony C, Kanis JA, Coleman RE. A randomised double blind comparison of intravenous pamidronate and clodronate in the hypercalcaemia of malignancy. *Br J Cancer* 1995; 72: 1289–93.
226. Wimalawansa SJ. Optimal frequency of administration of pamidronate in patients with hypercalcaemia of malignancy. *Clin Endocrinol Oxf* 1994; 41: 591–5.
227. Ralston SH, Alzaid AA, Gardner MD, Boyle IT. Treatment of cancer associated hypercalcaemia with combined aminohydroxypropylidene diphosphonate and calcitonin. *BMJ* 1986; 292: 1549–50.
228. Thiebaud D, Jacquet AF, Burckhardt P. Fast and effective treatment of malignant hypercalcemia. *Arch Intern Med* 1990; 151: 2125–8.
229. Barhoum M, Hutchins L, Fonseca VA. Intractable hypercalcemia due to a metastatic carcinoid secreting parathyroid hormone-related peptide and interleukin-6: response to octreotide. *Am J Med Sci* 1999; 318: 203–5.
230. Bouizar Z, Spyratos F, Deytieux S, de Vernejoul CM, Julienne A. Polymerase chain reaction analysis of parathyroid hormone-related protein gene expression in breast cancer patients and occurrence of bone metastases. *Cancer Res* 1993; 55: 3551–7.
231. Shipman CM, Rogers MJ, Apperley JF, Russell RGG, Croucher PI. Anti-tumour activity of bisphosphonates in human myeloma cells. *Leuk Lymphoma* 1999; 32: 129–38.
232. Hultborn R, Gundersen S, Ryden S et al. Efficacy of pamidronate in breast cancer with bone metastases: a randomized, double-blind placebo-controlled multi-center study. *Anticancer Res* 1999; 19: 3383–92.
233. Berenson JR, Lipton A. Bisphosphonates in the treatment of malignant bone disease. *Annu Rev Med* 1999; 50: 237–48.
234. Morony S, Capparelli C, Lee R et al. A chimeric form of osteoprotegerin inhibits hypercalcemia and bone resorption induced by IL-1beta, TNF-alpha, PTH, PTHrP, and 1,25(OH)2D3. *J Bone Mineral Res* 1999; 14: 1478–85.
235. Capparelli C, Kostenuik PJ, Morony S et al. Osteoprotegerin prevents and reverses hypercalcemia in a murine model of humoral hypercalcemia of malignancy. *Cancer Res* 2000; 60: 783–7.
236. Mundy GR, Martin TJ. The hypercalcaemia of malignancy: pathogenesis and management. *Metabolism* 1982; 31: 1247–77.
237. De Groot LJ. Dangerous dogmas in medicine: the nonthyroidal illness syndrome. *J Clin Endocrinol Metab* 1999; 84: 151–64.
238. Bermudez F, Surks MI, Oppenheimer JH. High incidence of decreased serum triiodothyronine concentration in patients with nonthyroidal disease. *J Clin Endocrinol Metab* 1975; 41: 27–40.
239. Kaptein EM, Robinson WJ, Grieb DA, Nicoloff JT. Peripheral serum thyroxine and reverse triiodotyrosine kinetics in the low thyroxine state of acute nonthyroidal illnesses. *J Clin Invest* 1982; 69: 526–35.
240. Wellby ML, Kennedy JA, Barreau PB, Roediger WE. Endocrine and cytokine changes during elective surgery. *J Clin Pathol* 1995; 47: 1049–51.
241. Vardarli I, Schmidt R, Wdowinski JM, Teuber J, Schwedes U, Usadel KH. The hypothalamo–hypophyseal thyroid axis, plasma protein concentrations and the hypophyseogonadal axis in low T_3 syndrome following myocardial infarct. *Klin Wochenschr* 1987; 65: 129–33.
242. Chopra JJ, Chopra U, Smith SR, Reza M, Solomon DH. Reciprocal changes in serum concentrations of 3,3,5′-triiodothyronine (reverse T_3) and 3,5,3′-triiodothyronine (T_3) in systemic illnesses. *J Clin Endocrinol Metab* 1975; 41: 1043–9.
243. Partridge WM, Slag MF, Morley JE, Elson MK, Shafer RB, Mietus LJ. Hepatic bioavailability of serum thyroid hormones in nonthyroidal illness. *J Clin Endocrinol Metab* 1981; 53: 913–16.
244. Chopra JJ, Huang TS, Beredo A, Solomon DH, Chua-Teco GN, Mead JF. Evidence for an inhibitor of extrathyroidal conversion of thyroxine to 3,5,3′-triiodothyronine in sera of patients with nonthyroidal illnesses. *J Clin Endocrinol Metab* 1985; 60: 666–72.

245. Vos RA, De Jong M, Bernard BF, Docter R, Krenning EP, Hennemann G. Impaired thyroxine and 3,5,3'-triiodothyronine handling by rat hepatocytes in the presence of serum from patients with nonthyroidal illness. *J Clin Endocrinol Metab* 1995; 80: 2364–70.

246. Harris AR, Fang SL, Azizi F, Lipworth L, Vagenakis AG, Braverman LE. Effect of starvation on hypothalamic–pituitary–thyroid function in the rat. *Metabolism* 1978; 27: 1074–83.

247. Hennemann G, Docter R, Krenning EP. Causes and effects of the low T_3 syndrome during caloric deprivation and non-thyroidal illness: an overview. *Acta Medic Austria Suppl* 1988; 15(1): 42–5.

248. Spalter AR, Gwirtsman HE, Demitrack MA, Gold PW. Thyroid function in bulaemia nervosa. *Biol Psychiatry* 1993; 33: 408–14.

249. Chow CC, Mak TW, Chan CH, Cockram CS. Euthyroid sick syndrome in tuberculosis before and after treatment. *Ann Clin Biochem* 1995; 32: 385–91.

250. Phillips RH, Valente WA, Caplan ES, Connor TB, Wiswell JG. Circulating thyroid hormone changes in acute trauma: prognostic implications for clinical outcome. *J Trauma* 1984; 24: 116–19.

251. Halabe CJ, Nellen HH, Barabejski GF, Chong MBA, Lifshitz GA. Thyroid function and abdominal surgery. A longitudinal study. *Arch Med Res* 1992; 23: 143–7.

252. Holland FW 2nd, Brown PS Jr, Weintraub BD, Clark RE. Cardiopulmonary bypass and thyroid function: a 'euthyroid sick syndrome'. *Ann Thorac Surg* 1991; 52: 46–50.

253. Eber B, Schumacher M, Langsteger W et al. Changes in thyroid hormone parameters after acute myocardial infarction. *Cardiology* 1995; 86: 152–6.

254. De Marinis L, Mancini A, Masala R, Torlontano M, Sandric S, Barbarino A. Evaluation of pituitary–thyroid axis response to acute myocardial infarction. *J Endocrinol Invest* 1985; 8: 507–11.

255. Vexiau P, Perez-Castiglioni P, Socie G et al. The 'euthyroid sick syndrome': incidence, risk factors and prognostic value soon after allogeneic bone marrow transplantation. *Br J Haematol* 1993; 85: 778–782.

256. Wehmann RE, Gregerman RI, Burns WH, Saral R, Santos GW. Suppression of thyrotropin in the low-thyroxine state of severe nonthyroidal illness. *N Engl J Med* 1985; 312: 546–52.

257. Herrmann F, Hambsch K, Sorger D, Hantschel H, Muller P, Nagel I. Low T_3 syndrome and chronic inflammatory rheumatism. *Z Gesamte Innere Med Grenzgebiete* 1989; 44: 513–18.

258. Vaughan GM, Mason AD, McManus WF, Pruitt BA. Alterations of mental status and thyroid hormones after thermal injury. *J Clin Endocrinol Metab* 1985; 60: 1221–5.

259. Park DJ, Cho CS, Lee SH, Park SH, Kim HY. Thyroid disorders in Korean patients with systemic lupus erythematosis. *Scand J Rheumatol* 1995; 24: 13–17.

260. Maldonaldo LS, Murata GH, Hershman JM, Braunstein GD. Do thyroid function tests independently predict survival in the critically ill? *Thyroid* 1992; 2: 119–23.

261. Slag MF, Morley JE, Elson MK, Crowson TW, Nettle FQ, Schafer RB. Hypothyroxinaemia in critically ill patients as a predictor of high mortality. *JAMA* 1981; 245: 43–5.

262. Arem R, Wiener GJ, Kaplan SG, Kim H-S, Reichlin S, Kaplan MM. Reduced tissue thyroid hormone levels in fatal illness. *Metabolism* 1993; 42: 1102–8.

263. Fliers E, Guldenaar SEF, Wiersinga WM, Swaab DF. Decreased hypothalamic thyrotropin-releasing hormone gene expression in patients with non-thyroidal illness. *J Clin Endocrinol Metab* 1997; 82: 4032–6.

264. Blake NG, Eckland JA, Foster OJF, Lightman SL. Inhibition of hypothalamic thyrotropin-releasing hormone messenger ribonucleic acid during food deprivation. *Endocrinology* 1991; 129: 2714–18.

265. Van den Berghe G, De Zegher F, Baxter RC et al. Neuroendocrinology of prolonged critical illness: effects of exogenous thyrotropin-releasing hormone and its combination with growth hormone secretagogues. *J Clin Endocrinol Metab* 1998; 53: 309–19.

266. Nicoloff JT, Fisher DA, Appleman MD Jr. The role of glucocorticoids in the regulation of thyroid function in man. *J Clin Invest* 1970; 49: 1922–9.

267. Bianco AC, Nunes MT, Hell NS, Maciel RMB. The role of glucocorticoids in the stress-induced reduction of extrathyroidal 3,5,3'triiodothyronine generation in rats. *Endocrinology* 1987; 120: 1033–8.

268. Benker G, Raida M, Olbricht T, Wagner R, Reinhardt W, Reinwein D. TSH secretion in Cushing's syndrome: relation to glucocorticoid excess, diabetes, goitre and the 'sick euthyroid' syndrome. *Clin Endocrinol Oxf* 1990; 33: 777–86.

269. Pang XP, Hershman JM, Smith V, Pekary AE, Sukowara M. The mechanism of action of tumour necrosis factor-alpha and interleukin 1 on FRTL-5 rat thyroid cells. *Acta Endocrinol Copenh* 1990; 123: 203–10.

270. Murai H, Murakami S, Ishida K, Sugawara M. Elevated serum interleukin-6 and decreased thyroid hormone levels in post-operative patients and effects of IL-6 on thyroid cell function *in vitro*. *Thyroid* 1996; 6: 601–6.

271. Boelen A, ter Platvoet SM, Wiersinga WM. Relationship between serum 3,5,3'-triiodothyronine in nonthyroidal illness. *J Clin Endocrinol Metab* 1993; 77: 1695–9.

272. Becker RA, Vaughan GM, Ziegler MG et al. Hypermetabolic low triiodothyronine syndrome of burn injury. *Crit Care Med* 1982; 10: 870–5.

273. Brent GA, Hershman JM. Thyroxine therapy in patients with severe nonthyroidal illness and lower serum thyroxine concentration. *J Clin Endocrinol Metab* 1986; 63: 1–8.

15

Disorders of fluid and electrolytes
Pierre-Marc G Bouloux

Introduction to body fluid and electrolyte composition

In lean, healthy adults 55–65% of body weight is composed of water, and 55–75% of this is intracellular, the extracellular portion comprising the intravascular (plasma) and extracellular (interstitial) compartments. The solute compositions of intracellular fluid (ICF) and extracellular fluid (ECF) are markedly different: cell membranes possess a number of transport systems which actively accumulate or expel specific solutes. Na^+ and Cl^- are predominantly extracellular, whereas intracellular fluid contains K^+, Mg^{2+} and several organic acids and phosphates. Glucose is present in significant amounts only in the ECF, being converted rapidly to glycogen or other metabolites upon insulin-induced entry into cells. HCO_3^-, though present in both compartments, is three times more concentrated in ECF. With the exception of the renal medulla, urea, being freely diffusible across cell membranes, is present in identical concentrations in ECF and ICF.

Despite marked differences in solute concentrations in ECF and ICF, total solute concentration is almost everywhere the same: this equilibrium results from the fact that most membranes separating various compartments are freely permeable to water. The exceptions to this are transcellular fluids such as intestinal secretions, sweat, tears and saliva, which are hypotonic, and urine and the renal medulla, which are hypertonic. Solute concentration is expressed in osmolality (milliosmoles of solute per kilogram of water) or osmolarity (milliosmoles of solute per liter of water).[1] Total solute concentration can be estimated by adding up the concentrations of all individual ions and solutes, but this generates higher values than those generated by depression of freezing point, since osmotic activity coefficients of electrolytes are significantly less than 1. In the case of plasma, the concentrations of K^+ and other minor solutes are usually ignored. The formula used is:

Plasma osmolality = $2(Na^+)$ + (urea) + (glucose), all expressed in mmol/l

This gives a value within 1–2% of that obtained by depression of freezing point.

Fluid balance in health

The average adult consumes 2.5–3 l of water each day, about 30% of which is derived from food or from metabolism of fat, the remainder being consumed not so much as a consequence of thirst, but through such influences as taste and other psychological factors. About 1000 mmol of solute is ingested or generated by metabolism of nutrients each day. Urinary excretion of water and solute is closely geared to control of fluid and electrolyte balance, such that almost all ingested Na^+, K^+ and Cl^- is excreted in urine. Divalent ingested solutes are excreted primarily by the gastrointestinal tract. Water excretion, regulated by antidiuretic hormone (ADH, vasopressin), is similarly closely influenced by rate of solute excretion, and cannot be reduced below a certain obligatory level required to carry the solute load. Thus, the volume of urine required depends not only on the size of the solute load, but also on the level of antidiuresis. The average 70 kg man excretes a daily solute load of 800–1200 mOsm in 1.5–2 l of urine. With maximal antidiuresis, the same solute load would require an obligatory minimum urine output of 750–1000 ml. On the other hand, with a low urine concentration (e.g. 50 mOsm/kg), up to 20 l of urine would be required to eliminate the same solute load. It is evident that restriction of Na⁺ and protein load reduces polyuria in cases of diabetes insipidus. Basal insensible water losses amount to approximately 10 ml/kg, but may double in subjects participating in outdoor activities in temperate climates, depending on such factors as dress, humidity, temperature and exercise.

Antidiuretic hormone (ADH; vasopressin)

ADH is a nonapeptide (molecular weight 1099) containing an intrachain disulfide bridge with a tripeptide tail on which the terminal carboxyl group is amidated. It has both vasopressor and antidiuretic properties, the former being mediated by V_1 receptors, and the latter by V_2 receptors. Both receptors belong to the seven transmembrane domain guanine nucleotide-binding (G) protein-coupled family of receptors. V_2 receptors are located in the distal and collecting tubules of the nephron.[2] Upon receptor occupancy with ADH, adenyl cyclase is activated with cAMP generation, and this results in preformed aquaporin-2 water channels being translocated to the luminal plasma membrane, enabling tubular water to back-diffuse down the osmotic gradient created by the hypertonic medulla (Figure 15.1). ADH has a short biological half-life, whereas dDAVP (1-desamino-8-D-arginine vasopressin), a synthetic analog, has enhanced antidiuretic potency with a prolonged duration of action and reduced pressor effects.[3]

Both vasopressin and the closely related oxytocin are synthesized and stored with their corresponding neurophysins, which dissociate upon release into plasma. Each neurophysin has a binding site, which may play a key role in the intracellular processing of the prohormone as well as storage of the hormone in intracellular granules.[4] Both vasopressin and oxytocin are released by the neurohypophysis, comprising a densely interwoven network of capillaries, pituicytes and non-myelinated fibers containing many electron-dense secretory granules. The cells of origin of these neuropeptides are the magnocellular neurons of the supraoptic and paraventricular nuclei of the hypothalamus, from which most of the axons project ventrally and caudally, terminating in the bulbous enlargements of the capillary networks scattered throughout the neurohypophysis. Both ADH and oxytocin are synthesized in the cell bodies as their precursors (pre-provasopressin and pre-prooxytocin),[5] and translocated from the cytosol into the endoplasmic reticulum, where signal peptide cleavage occurs and the prohormone folds and oligomerizes into a specific conformation that allows it to be transported to the Golgi and neurosecretory granules, which are then transported down the axons. Neuropeptides are subsequently stored in the terminals of the pars nervosa and infundibulum. Structurally, the precursor molecules contain the biologically active peptides at the N-terminus after the signal peptide, and is followed by a Gly–Lys–Arg sequence linking it to the neurophysin moiety. The neurophysin moiety of vasopressin is connected to a 39 amino acid peptide called copeptin by a single basic amino acid. This peptide is subsequently glycosylated with a mannose-rich side-chain.

Regulation of vasopressin secretion

Although vasopressin secretion is influenced by a large number of stimuli (Table 15.1), the most important stimuli are an increase in plasma osmolality, and changes in blood volume and pressure.

Osmotic stimuli
Plasma osmolality—changes in water balance, hypertonic and hypotonic states
Hyperglycemia
Hemodynamic
Changes in blood volume
Posture
Hemorrhage
Mineralocorticoid deficiency or excess
Gastrointestinal fluid losses
Cirrhosis
Nephrotic syndrome
Positive-pressure breathing
Diuretics
Changes in blood pressure
Orthostatic hypotension
Vasovagal attacks
Others
Nausea, vomiting
Ketoacidosis
Addison's disease

Table 15.1
Variable influencing vasopressin secretion

Osmoreceptor regulation of vasopressin secretion

Osmoreceptors are located in the anterolateral hypothalamus, and receive their blood supply from small perforating branches of the anterior cerebral and/or communicating arteries. With a fall in plasma osmolality below a threshold level, ADH secretion is switched off, and above this threshold ADH secretion climbs steeply in direct proportion to plasma osmolality. Thus a change of plasma osmolality of 1% increases ADH concentration by 1 pg/ml, an amount sufficient to activate V_2 receptors. Osmoregulatory sensitivity shows considerable inter-individual variation, with up to 10-fold differences in slope between adults, and these appear to be genetically determined. Other influences on this slope include blood pressure, volume, serum calcium and several drugs. Age appears to increase sensitivity. Osmoregulatory threshold also varies from person to person, from 275 to 290 mOsm/kg, and appear to be constant over time. The threshold set-point is reduced in pregnancy, as well as during the luteal phase of the menstrual cycle.[6]

Osmoregulatory mechanisms are solute-dependent. Na^+ and its anions, which contribute >95% of plasma osmotic pressure, are potent stimulators of vasopressin release. Mannitol and sucrose are also potent when infused intravenously, in contrast to urea and glucose, which are relatively neutral.

Hemodynamic influences on vasopressin secretion

Both blood pressure and volume profoundly affect vasopressin secretion. Thus, lowering of blood pressure, whatever the mechanism, will stimulate ADH release, a stimulus–secretion relationship which has an exponential characteristic. Blood pressure falls of 20–30% elicit a rise in ADH levels several times that required to maximally stimulate maximal antidiuresis.[4] Similarly, a fall in blood volume of 1–15% will roughly double the vasopressin concentration; true hypovolemia, on the other hand (e.g. in severe hemorrhage), is an extremely potent stimulus to ADH release. In contrast, a sharp rise in blood volume or pressure acutely switches off vasopressin release. The afferent limb to such reflexes originates in the pressure-sensitive receptors in the atria and in the aortic and carotid sinuses. These ascend in the vagus and glossopharyngeal nerves to the nucleus tractus solitarius, from where postsynaptic fibers carrying noradrenergic, opiodergic, GABAergic and dopaminergic terminals ascend to the lateral parabrachial, paraventricular and supraoptic nuclei.[6]

The inputs from these pathways are largely inhibitory. Changes in blood pressure or volume do not interfere with the osmoregulation of ADH release; rather, they act by shifting the set-point of ADH release in response to a given osmotic stimulus. Thus, in the presence of a hemodynamic stimulus, plasma ADH continues to respond appropriately to small changes in plasma osmolality and can still be fully suppressed if plasma osmolality falls below the lower set-point. Such an interaction ensures that the capacity to osmoregulate is not lost even in the presence of increases or decreases in blood volume or pressure.

Nausea and vomiting

Both nausea and vomiting are extremely potent stimulators of vasopressin release, probably acting through the chemoreceptor trigger zone in the area postrema of the 4th ventricle, and can be activated by ipecahuana, apomorphine, alcohol and nicotine, effecting several orders of magnitude rises in ADH. Water loading blunts the rise in ADH resulting from these stimuli.

Hypoglycemia

Acute hypoglycemia is a potent stimulus to ADH release, and seems to act through different pathways to the above. The stimulus–response relationship appears to be exponential, a decrease in glucose of 50% leading to a three-fold increase in ADH; the rate of fall of glucose is the critical element, since the rise in ADH is not sustained when hypoglycemia is persistent.

Renin–angiotensin system

Pressor doses of angiotensin II roughly double the concentration of ADH, but the magnitude of the response depends in part on the concurrent osmotic stimulus.

Miscellaneous stimuli

Pain, emotion and severe physical exercise stimulate ADH release, as do hypoxia and hypercapnia. It is unclear whether in the latter case the modest ADH release only occurs with the concomitant changes in blood pressure or nausea. There is a slight though inconstant rise in ADH at night; the main cause of reduction in urine flow during sleep, however, is the associated nocturnal reduction in solute and water intake. Except for transient increases in ADH after meals, ADH levels are remarkably constant throughout the day and night, and the lack of change despite the fall in blood pressure at night simply reflects the lack of sensitivity of ADH secretion to mild hemodynamic changes.[4]

Drugs altering vasopressin secretion

A large number of drugs influence ADH secretion, and these are listed in Table 15.2. Lithium, which antagonizes the renal effects of ADH, leads to a rise in ADH secretion, an effect independent of water balance, representing an increase in sensitivity of the osmoregulatory system. Carbamazepine inhibits ADH secretion by diminishing osmoreceptor sensitivity, an effect occurring independently of changes in blood volume or pressure; thus, its antidiuretic properties are presumably mediated directly at the level of the renal collecting tubule.

Stimulatory
  Nicotine
  Apomorphine
  Histamine
  Prostaglandin
  Cyclophosphamide (IV)
  Vincristine
  Chlorpropamide
  Clofibrate
  Carbamazepine
Inhibitory
  Flufenazine
  Haloperidol
  Kappa opioid agonists
  Alcohol
  Glucocorticoids
  Clonidine
  Phencyclidine

Table 15.2
Drugs affecting the secretion or action of ADH.

Thirst

A rise in effective osmolality of 2–3% induces thirst in most healthy adults, and is not dependent on changes in blood volume. The threshold to stimulate the urge to drink is variable in health but is around 295 mOsm/kg H_2O, a level above the threshold for vasopressin secretion, and close to the plasma ADH concentration at which maximal antidiuresis occurs.[4] Urea and glucose are ineffective at stimulating thirst. The dipsogenic center appears to be in the anterolateral hypothalamus and involve osmoreceptors. A modest decline in plasma osmolality induces a sensation of satiation and reduces the basal rate of fluid intake.

The threshold or set-points of the hypothalamic systems that osmoregulate thirst and vasopressin secretion provide a mechanism that adjusts total body water to keep plasma Na^+ remarkably constant, and their ability to effect changes in water intake or excretion prevent states of over- or underhydration.[7] Because of the reverse exponential relationship between urine osmolality and flow, the suppression of plasma ADH to levels permitting maximal antidiuresis increases the rate of water excretion up to 18 l/day.

Pharmacokinetics of vasopressin

ADH, when secreted, distributes rapidly into the extracellular compartment, the initial or mixing phase of exogenously administered ADH having a half-life of 4–8 min, and being virtually complete by 20 min. It is not bound to plasma proteins. In pregnant women, the metabolic clearance rate increases some four-fold, due to the added effect of placental vasopressinase, and this mechanism may account for rare cases of pregnancy-induced cranial diabetes insipidus in patients in whom there may exist a subclinical vasopressin deficiency. Inactivation is in the liver and kidney, and is initiated by rupture of the disulfide linkage followed by aminopeptidase cleavage of the bond between amino acid residues 1 and 2.

Vasopressin and the aquaporins

Vasopressin acts on the distal nephron V_2 receptor, with generation of cAMP, activation of protein kinase A

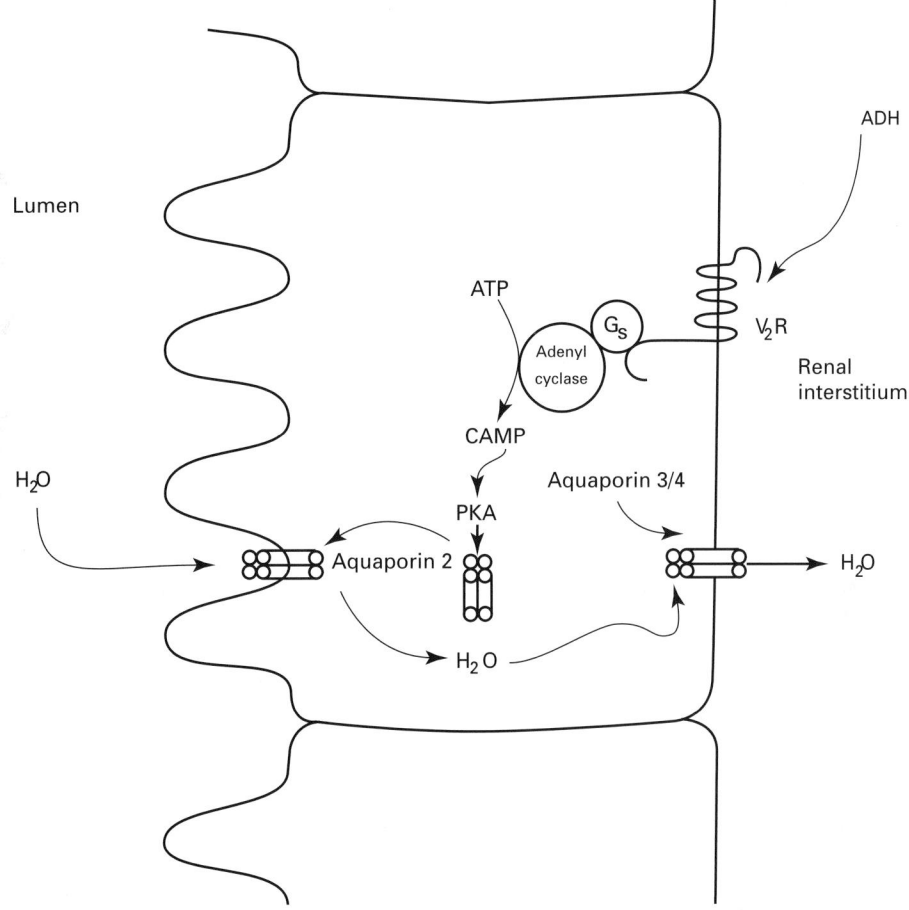

Figure 15.1
Representation of an ADH-sensitive collecting tubular cell, showing the site of action of ADH on the V_2 receptor; this is coupled to a G_s protein, and activation of adenyl cyclase leads to cAMP generation, and activation of PKA, which stimulates insertion of the tetrameric aquaporin 2 into the luminal membrane. Water is shuttled across the cell and delivered to the ADH-insensitive but constitutively active aquaporins 3 and 4, into the renal interstitial space.

(PKA), and the subsequent mobilization of aquaporin channels from intracellular vesicles to the apical plasma membrane[8,9] (Figure 15.1). Aquaporins (AQPs), of which nine have been described, constitute a family of transmembrane water channels. AQP-1, AQP-2 and AQP-4 have high permeabilities, whereas AQP-3 has much lower permeability. AQP-3 and AQP-9 also allow the passage of other solutes, including urea, glycerol and other small solutes. AQP-4 is present in osmoreceptor regions of the brain and in astrocytes.[10] AQP-2 is the ADH-responsive water channel protein specific to renal collecting ducts. Tetramers of AQP-2 are inserted into the luminal membrane, whereas the non-vasopressin-sensitive AQP-3 and AQP-4 are constitutively expressed on the adluminal membrane to allow water to follow across the tubular cell.

Diabetes insipidus

This is a syndrome characterized by the excretion of abnormally large volumes of dilute urine (polyuria) and increased fluid intake (polydipsia), usually triggered by increased thirst. Polyuria leads to urinary frequency, enuresis, nocturia and incontinence. Although osmoregulated thirst remains intact, there is a consequent increase in plasma osmolality and serum Na$^+$ which stimulates thirst, thereby stimulating drinking and the replenishment of body water. There are four main types of diabetes insipidus (DI):

1. Cranial DI (also known as central, neurogenic or vasopressin-responsive DI) is due to inadequate secretion of vasopressin.
2. Nephrogenic (or renal insensitivity to vasopressin DI.
3. Primary polydipsia—this is caused by excessive ingestion of fluids, either due to an abnormality in the thirst mechanism (dipsogenic polydipsia) or following severe emotional or cognitive dysfunction (psychogenic polydipsia).
4. Gestational DI following increased metabolism of vasopressin during pregnancy.

Cranial diabetes insipidus (CDI)

The neurohypophysis can be damaged by a large number of pathologies, including infiltrative processes, tumors, granulomatous conditions and inflammatory/infective conditions.[11,12] Familial and sporadic cases of cranial DI can occur, and both dominant and X-linked recessive inheritance have been described.[13,14]

Most cases of CDI result from destruction of the magnocellular neuronal system in the neurohypophysis. A list of pathologic processes associated with CDI is shown in Table 15.3. Most pathologic processes lead to atrophy of the pars nervosa and loss of magnocellular neurons, predominantly in the supraoptic nucleus. In the case of CDI following surgical section of the pituitary stalk, the process of retrograde degeneration of neurons whose axons have been surgically sectioned may take up to 6 weeks to become complete.[15] Axon terminals end at diverse levels along the hypothalamo-neurohypophyseal tract, and to produce symptomatic DI, around 90% of fibers must be sectioned, usually above the infundibulum. It is rare for pituitary adenomas to present with CDI when confined to the sella turcica.

Clinical features of CDI

Childhood
Nocturia and enuresis are common in children, as is slow weight gain and slow growth rate, secondary to poor calorie intake. Excessive crying and constipation may occur.

Decreased secretion of ADH due to destructive process
 Trauma (surgical, road traffic accident)
 Tumor: craniopharyngioma, germinoma, meningioma, glioma, astrocytoma affecting hypothalamus
 Metastatic deposits (lung, breast, lymphoma, leukemia, squamous carcinoma of head and neck)
 Granulomatous disorders (sarcoidosis, histiocytosis)
 Infectious processes (viral, bacterial meningitis, tuberculoma)
 Vascular—ischemic brain death, Wegener's granulomatosis
 Autoimmune hypophysitis
 Genetic—autosomal dominant disorder affecting ADH gene
 Idiopathic

Inhibition by excessive consumption of water
 Psychogenic
 Dipsogenic (reset thirst threshold)

Increased ADH metabolism
 Gestational diabetes insipidus

Table 15.3
Causes of cranial diabetes insipidus.

Adulthood
Polyuria, polydipsia, excessive thirst and increased fluid ingestion are characteristic, and may occur even in mild forms of the disease. In severe cases, polyuria of 15–20 l/day is not uncommon. Provided that the thirst mechanism is intact, patients may be able to maintain the plasma osmolality in the upper normal range. Glucocorticoid deficiency caused by either pituitary or adrenal disease impairs water excretion, due partly to persistent non-osmotic ADH secretion and partly to reduced water permeability of the distal nephron. Thus, when there is coexisting hypopituitarism, the glucocorticoid deficiency may mask underlying DI, which may manifest clinically only when glucocorticoid replacement is administered. A similar impairment of water excretion may also occur in hypothyroidism as a consequence of enhanced non-osmotic vasopressin release.

CDI may follow head injury, with some patients showing a classical triple-phase response characterized by an initial period of intensive polyuria stretching over hours or days, followed by a second phase of intensive antidiuresis (vasopressin release from degenerating axon terminals), and a third phase when polyuria and polydipsia return. Continued treatment of the first phase by dDAVP or large quantities of fluid at a time when the patient has progressed to the second phase may lead to acute profound hyponatremia.[15]

Partial cranial diabetes insipidus

Because of the large hypothalamic ADH reserve, a significant loss of magnocellular neurons is necessary before clinical manifestations of CDI occur. Such individuals can frequently be shown to be able to maximally concentrate urine following a prolonged period of water restriction, but only at the expense of a significantly raised plasma osmolality, in excess of that required to stimulate the thirst center; that is, provided the osmotic stimulus is sufficiently intense, ADH secretion sufficient to maximally concentrate urine can occur. Such patients are polydipsic and polyuric also, as a small fall in plasma osmolality sufficient to quench their thirst will switch off ADH secretion, significantly increasing free water clearance.[16]

Nephrogenic diabetes insipidus (NDI)

In NDI, the renal tubules are totally or partially resistant to vasopressin. The hereditary X-linked congenital form is uncommon; patients present shortly after birth with profound polyuria, hypernatremia and dehydration and failure to thrive, and are at risk of central nervous system (CNS) damage. At a cellular level, V_2 receptor occupancy by ADH is unable to generate cAMP.[17] The result is that the transepithelial water permeability of the collecting duct remains in its low basal state, and a large volume of hypotonic urine is formed. There have been over 70 mutations of the V_2 receptor described,[14,18] associated with NDI. Mutations of the AQP-2 gene are responsible for autosomal recessive forms of congenital NDI.[19,20] Metabolic causes of NDI include hypercalcemia (which impairs vasopressin action on the distal tubule as well as stimulating vasopressin secretion), and hypokalemia. Hypokalemia and hypercalcemia are associated with reduced expression of AQP-2, the polyuria produced being less severe than that induced by lithium. Targeting of AQP-2 to the cell membrane is also disturbed in hypercalcemia.

Intrinsic renal causes include tubulointerstitial nephropathies (drug-induced, sarcoidosis, etc.). In the case of hypokalemic and hypercalcemic NDI, renal responsivity to vasopressin may take several weeks to recover after correction of the biochemical defect.[18] One-third of patients taking lithium develop NDI, sometimes severely despite therapeutic blood lithium levels. Lithium inhibits cAMP generation in the distal nephron, augments its metabolism by stimulating phosphodiesterase activity, and impairs its intracellular action. One per thousand of the population is on lithium, and 20–30% suffer from NDI while on this treatment.[21] Studies in rats have shown that lithium induces a dramatic decrease in AQP-2 expression, probably induced by impairment in the production of cAMP. This is consistent with the presence of a cAMP-responsive element in the 5′-untranslated region of the AQP-2 gene. AQP-2 recovers only slowly following withdrawal of lithium therapy, consistent with clinical findings.

Ureteral obstruction, when relieved, may be associated with NDI. In experimental models, this appears to be due to downregulation of AQP-2 expression. The hyponatremia of cirrhosis and congestive cardiac failure are in part due to upregulation of AQP-2 expression.

Diabetes insipidus of pregnancy

Polyuria and polydipsia develop at mid-pregnancy and continue shortly after delivery. They are thought to be due to increased clearance of vasopressin by placental vasopressinase, a cysteine aminopeptidase enzyme.[22]. Characteristically, the patients fail to respond to therapeutic arginine vasopressin, the natural hormone, but do respond to dDAVP (desmopressin), which is resistant to degradation.

Primary polydipsia

Affected patients consume water in large quantities in excess of body requirements. It is important to exclude drugs which reduce salivary secretion, thereby causing a dry mouth. In some individuals, a lowered osmotic threshold for thirst sensation is demonstrable in the presence of normal osmoregulated vasopressin secretion (dipsogenic polydipsia). It is rarely associated with an underlying structural abnormality.[7] Individuals with primary polydipsia increase their fluid intake, thereby lowering plasma osmolality and switching off vasopressin secretion. Urine osmolality falls, urine output increases, and plasma osmolality stabilizes at a low value.

Diagnostic approaches to evaluation of the polyuric patient

Several investigations have been devised to distinguish between the various causes of polyuric states (both types of DI and primary polydipsia). In general, other forms of polyuria (e.g. diabetes mellitus) involve osmotic or solute diuresis, where the osmolality of the urine tends towards that of plasma, since excretion of increased volumes of water is required. Therefore, a urine specific gravity of 1.005 (osmolality of <200 mOsm/kg of water) generally rules out polyuria due to osmotic diuresis. Initially, it is important to document 24 urine volumes and basal plasma osmolality or Na^+ concentrations. Thus, if the 24-h urine volume is <2.5 l in 24 h and the plasma osmolality is in the normal reference range, a diagnosis of DI is most unlikely. The osmolality of urine in DI and primary polydipsia is low compared with that of plasma. Hypercalcemia and hypokalemia suggest NDI.

Prolonged polyuria irrespective of the cause leads to a reduction in maximum urinary renal concentrating ability, due to loss of renal interstitial solute ('medullary washout'), the reduction of renal concentrating ability being directly related to the severity of the polyuria.

Plasma and urine osmolality

Simultaneous plasma and urine osmolalities should be estimated first, since in both forms of DI, the primary problem is inappropriate water diuresis, and the urine will be less concentrated than the plasma, whereas the plasma osmolality may be higher than normal, depending on the state of hydration. In primary polydipsia, dilute plasma is associated with production of dilute urine.

Dehydration tests

These are useful in the diagnosis of CDI and NDI, and consist of a period of dehydration with measurement of plasma and urine osmolalities as well as regular weighing of the patient. This is followed by an injection of intramuscular dDAVP (1–2 μg) to observe the renal concentrating response.

In the Dashe test,[23] the patient is adequately hydrated overnight, and plasma and urine osmolalities measured basally. The patient is weighed and then water-deprived for an 8-h period. Every 2 h, urine is collected to assess volume and osmolality, blood is drawn for plasma osmolality, and the patient is weighed. The test is terminated if weight loss during the test exceeds 5% of the initial weight. At the end of the dehydration period, urine and plasma osmolality are measured, the patient is given a 2-μg dose of dDAVP, and urine is collected over the ensuing 6 h for osmolality estimation. Following the injection, patients may eat and drink ad libitum. Surreptitious drinking must be looked for during the period of dehydration. A guide to interpretation of results is given in Table 15.4.[16]

ADH vasopressin estimation

Sensitive radioimmunoassays are available, enabling estimation of plasma vasopressin levels. Levels are ideally measured during dynamic testing, either during water deprivation or with infusions of hypertonic saline (see above). Plasma levels are interpreted based on nomograms of the relationship with plasma osmolality.[24] Patients with NDI have normal or increased levels of vasopressin following water deprivation, allowing a clear distinction to be made with CDI, whereas patients with partial CDI show a smaller than normal increase in plasma ADH concentrations with dehydration or hypertonic saline infusion.

Urine osmolality (mOsm/kg)		
After dehydration	After IM dDAVP	Interpretation
<300	>750	Cranial DI
<300	<300	Nephrogenic DI
300–800	<750	Partial cranial DI Primary polydipsia

Table 15.4
Interpretation of Dashe test.

Investigation of cause of cranial diabetes insipidus

Patients with CDI require imaging to exclude a space-occupying lesion affecting the hypothalamus/ infundibular region. MRI studies usually demonstrate a bright spot in the normal posterior pituitary (high-intensity signal) on TI-weighted images, and several studies have shown that the intensity of this is related to content of the stored hormone.[25] This high-intensity spot is present in most normal subjects and absent in most patients with CDI. Occasionally, the bright spot is present early in the disease and is then lost as the disease progresses. In reported cases of primary polydipsia, the posterior pituitary bright spot is preserved, indicating persistent posterior pituitary storage of vasopressin. Widening of the stalk has been reported in several diseases associated with CDI and may also be an early sign of inflammation of the neurohypophysis.[12] A thickened stalk with absence of a posterior pituitary bright spot should prompt a thorough search for systemic diseases known to cause DI (e.g. sarcoidosis, histiocytosis).

The most common cause of CDI is idiopathic CDI, in which there is no anatomic abnormality. Tumors (e.g. craniopharyngioma, secondary deposits) are readily identifiable, as is trauma to the area due to head injury or pituitary surgery, or infiltrative diseases such as granulomatous disorders. If no suprasellar mass or systemic disease is found after 4 years of follow-up, the patient probably has idiopathic DI.

Treatment of diabetes insipidus

Central DI

The drug of choice is desmopressin acetate (1-desamino-8-arginine vasopressin) (dDAVP), a vasopressin analog which acts predominantly on the antidiuretic V_2 receptors of the kidney, with little action on the V_1 vascular receptors.[3] It is administered intranasally as a metered-dose nasal spray that delivers 10 μg per spray or via a calibrated plastic catheter in doses of 5–20 μg. Administration frequency varies between patients. In mild to moderate disease, one or two 10-μg doses may be required, usually at night. In more severe disease, 2–3 puffs may be required per 24 h. Polyuria and polydipsia are usually well controlled, but plasma osmolality should

	Cranial DI	Nephrogenic DI	Primary Polydipsia
Random PO	⇑	⇑	⇓
Random UO	⇓	⇓	⇓
UP with WD	⇔	⇔	⇓
UO after dDAVP	⇑	⇔	⇑
Plasma ADH	⇓	⇑	⇓

Table 15.5
Interpretation of diagnostic studies in polyuric states.

be monitored at regular intervals (initially 2–3-weekly) to check the appropriateness of the dose. The equivalent intramuscular dose is 1–2 μg per 24 h. An orally available form of dDAVP is now available (Desmotabs 200), and is usually given at an initial dose of 300 μg/day in three divided doses, although doses as high as 1.2 mg daily may be required. Side-effects of dDAVP include fluid retention and hyponatremia (in more severe cases with convulsions) on administration without restricting fluid intake. Abdominal pain, headache, nausea and vomiting have also been reported. More rarely, patients have suffered from epistaxis and nasal congestion when using the intranasal form. In order to avoid hyponatremia, patients are advised to withhold one dose every week or so to eliminate excess retained body water.

Nephrogenic DI

The underlying disorder must be identified and treated appropriately. In particular, familial forms must be identified early to prevent neurologic damage to the neonate by dehydration. Diuretics such as thiazides have been used with some success,[26] along with dietary salt restriction—both reduce solute loads to the kidney. Prostaglandin synthetic inhibitors may also be useful.[27] Maintaining the patient in a mild state of Na^+ depletion reduces the renal solute load, thereby enhancing proximal tubular fluid reabsorption. The fall in distal tubular flow allows some Na^+ concentration to take place with a reduction in water clearance. In partial NDI, larger doses of desmopressin may afford symptomatic relief.

Essential hypernatremia represents a form of DI due to absence of osmoreceptor input, but with intact volume receptor input. Patients excrete excess hypotonic urine, and do not sense thirst as a consequence. Serum Na^+ rises, and when the patient becomes sufficiently dehydrated, volume receptors will respond to release vasopressin and will maintain a clinical condition of hypernatremia and concentrated urine. When sufficient water to correct the volume deficit is administered, the inability to respond to elevated osmolality is demonstrated by excessive urine output.

Hyponatremic states

These are characterized by serum Na^+ levels less than 130 mmol/l and affect 3–5% of hospital patients.[28] It is important to rule out pseudohyponatremia, which occurs in patients with very high concentrations of lipids or protein, situations where these substances contribute substantially to serum volume, and where the Na^+ concentration in the water phase of the serum is in fact normal. In pseudohyponatremia, the plasma osmolality is normal.[29] By contrast, in severe hyperglycemia, plasma osmolality is raised, but Na^+ may be reduced, due to movement of water from the intracellular to the extracellular compartment.

True hyponatremia is present when there is an excess of extracellular water relative to the total Na^+ in the extracellular compartment. Total extracellular Na^+ can be:

1. reduced, resulting in extracellular hypovolemia
2. normal, with effectively normal or slightly expanded extracellular volume
3. higher than normal, associated with hypervolemia.

Examination of the patient will reveal which of these is present. In (1), hypovolemia leads to thirst, tachycardia, reduced skin turgor and orthostatic hypotension, whereas in (3), edema, raised jugular pressures and ascites may be present.

Urinary Na^+ measurement will easily distinguish between the three situations.[30] In extracellular hypovolemic hyponatremic states (e.g. resulting from persistent vomiting, diarrhea, extensive skin burns and excessive prolonged sweating and diuretic overuse), the kidney, by activating the renin–angiotensin system, will conserve Na^+ maximally (in extreme cases, urine Na^+ can fall to <1 mmol/l), whereas inappropriate Na^+ loss may be present in various renal diseases (e.g. analgesic nephropathy, chronic pyelonephritis, polycystic disease, recovery from urinary tract obstruction or acute tubular necrosis), and other disorders such as mineralocorticoid deficiency (Addison's disease, hyporeninemic hypoaldosteronism) and diuretic overuse.

Normovolemic hyponatremia is generally caused by SIAD (see below), and, more rarely, is found in beer drinker's potomania, where excessive fluid intake exceeds the kidney's capacity to excrete water.

Hypervolemic hyponatremia is most frequently seen in severe congestive cardiac failure, decompensated cirrhosis, and the nephrotic syndrome, where glomerular filtration is reduced and proximal tubular Na^+ reabsorption is stimulated.[31] With reduced afferent arteriolar perfusion, the renin-angiotensin system is stimulated, and the raised angiotensin II levels stimulate thirst. Non-osmotic-induced vasopressin secretion also contributes to water retention.

Syndromes of inappropriate antidiuresis (SIAD)

Several disorders are associated with plasma ADH concentrations which are inappropriately raised for the plasma osmolality[32] (Table 15.6). This leads to water retention in the presence of a normal fluid intake, and this leads to dilutional hyponatremia and hypoosmolality and an inappropriately raised urinary osmolality.[28,33] Overall, Na^+ balance tends to remain normal. Renal and endocrine disorders that diminish the kidney's capacity to dilute the urine must be excluded, e.g. renal failure, hypothyroidism and hypoadrenalism. The clinical picture of SIAD can be reproduced by giving high doses of vasopressin to healthy subjects receiving normal to high fluid intake. The corollary is that patients with SIAD can be treated by water restriction, which will normalize plasma osmolality and Na^+ concentration.

Lung neoplasms—bronchial carcinoma
Non-malignant lung disease—tuberculosis
Other neoplasms—lymphoma, sarcoma (e.g. duodenal, pancreatic, prostate or thymic tumors)
CNS trauma and infections (e.g. brain abscess), subarachnoid hemorrhage
Drugs stimulating vasopressin release: clofibrate, chlorpropamide, thiazides, carbamazepine, vincristine, cyclophosphamide
Endocrine diseases—adrenal insufficiency, myxedema, anterior hypopituitarism

---

Table 15.6
Conditions associated with SIAD.

Clinical manifestations of hyponatremia

Hypo-osmolality is associated with a broad spectrum of neurologic sequelae ('hyponatremic encephalopathy'), ranging from mild non-specific symptoms (headache and nausea) to more severe symptoms such as disorientation, confusion, stupor and seizures (Table 15.7). When it is severe, death can result from respiratory arrest secondary to tentorial cerebral herniation and brainstem compression.[34-37] The primary pathology is brain edema, resulting from osmotic water shifts into the brain because of decreased effective plasma osmolality. Symptoms supervene in general when serum Na^+ falls to less than 125 mmol/l, the severity of the symptoms correlating with the degree of hyponatremia, although for any one individual the degree of hyponatremia precipitating symptoms is not easily predicted.[38] The rate of onset of hyponatremia plays a key role in symptom generation; the more rapid the development, the more severe the symptoms. Non-neurologic metabolic disorders such as hypoxia, hypercapnia, acidosis and hypercalcemia can also affect the level of plasma osmolality at which CNS symptoms supervene. Conversely, slow evolution of hyponatremia is associated with fewer symptoms.[39] This is because, under such circumstances, the brain can counteract the osmotic swelling by excreting intracellular solutes, including K^+ and organic osmolytes, a process termed osmotic regulation. Most reports of death with hyponatremia have concerned postoperative patients in whom it developed rapidly as a result of postoperative fluid retention of hypotonic fluid infusions. Menstruating women and young children are particularly at risk.

Mild	Moderate	Severe
Anorexia	Change of personality	Drowsiness
Headache	Cramps	Reduced reflexes
Nausea	Muscle weakness	Convulsions
Vomiting	Ataxia	Coma
Lethargy		Death

Table 15.7
Clinical features of hyponatremia

Diagnosis of SIAD

The criteria of diagnosis include:

1. Hyponatremia, with hypo-osmolality of plasma (<280 mOsm/kg).
2. Failure to maximally dilute the urine (urine osmolality >60 mOsm/kg).
3. Euvolemia—no evidence of fluid depletion, postural hypotension, or dry mucous membranes (including absence of congestive cardiac failure, cirrhosis, and nephrotic syndrome).
4. Absence of renal, adrenal and thyroid underactivity.

Urine Na^+ usually exceeds 20 mmol/day, probably as a consequence of atrial natriuretic factor secretion. Plasma ADH levels are detectable when they should be suppressed.

Causes of SIAD

Causes of SIAD are listed in Table 15.6. Malignant neoplasms associated with ectopic ADH secretion include bronchial carcinoma, and pancreatic and duodenal tumors. Non-malignant conditions include pulmonary diseases such as tuberculosis and pneumonia; in the case of the former, bioassayable ADH has been identified from tuberculous lung lesions. In other disorders involving the chest, vasopressin release appears to be pituitary in origin. CNS lesions are associated with SIAD, and include surgical trauma, anesthesia, pain, opiates and anxiety. Endocrine disorders include hypopituitarism, especially isolated adrenocorticotropic hormone (ACTH) deficiency and hypothyroidism.[40] All of these conditions can lead to dilutional hyponatremia, particularly with fluid loading.

The majority of patients with euvolemic hyponatremia are suffering from SIAD. Surgery and anesthesia are potent causes of SIADH.[41]

Treatment of hyponatremia

This depends upon the underlying cause, which must be identified by careful history, examination and investigation. Adrenal insufficiency, hypothyroidism and renal disease should be sought, the hypovolemia corrected, and appropriate fluid and hormone replacement administered. When associated with a drug, the latter should be withheld. In the context of a bronchial neoplasm, where the prognosis is poor, treatment may be more complicated. The general principles of treatment include the following:[41,42]

1. Fluid restriction: usually 500 ml/day will lead to normalization of plasma Na⁺ within a few days. Chronically, however, this may be difficult to enforce.
2. Demeclocycline antagonizes the effects of vasopressin at the renal level and can be given at a dose of 600–1200 mg/day. Alternatively, the more toxic lithium carbonate (600–1800 mg/day) may be used. The NDI effects of these drugs may take up to 6 weeks to develop.[43]
3. Frusemide in a dose of 40–80 mg orally together with salt supplementation (3 g/day).[44]
4. Hypertonic saline infusion is reserved for severe symptomatic hyponatremia in the emergency situation.

Rate of correction of hyponatremia

Too rapid a correction of hyponatremia can cause brain demyelination associated with severe morbidity and mortality.[45-47] The decision to correct hyponatremia depends upon the balance of risk versus benefit. The factors that determine the decision to treat actively include:

1. severity of hyponatremia
2. duration of hyponatremia
3. patients' symptomatology.

Neither encephalopathy nor myelinolysis are likely in patients whose serum Na⁺ remains >120 mmol/l, although in rare cases severe symptoms have developed at higher serum Na⁺ levels, especially if the fall of Na⁺ has been rapid. When acute (<48 h), symptoms usually supervene if hyponatremia is severe (<120 mmol/l). In such patients, the risk of neurologic complications from the hyponatremia far exceeds the small risk of complications from correction of the hyponatremia, and correction should be relatively rapid. With more chronic hyponatremia, where symptoms are relatively mild, demyelination can occur with rapid correction. It is not necessary to correct these patients rapidly, and fluid restriction is the preferred treatment in these cases.

Problems arise in patients in whom the duration of the hyponatremia is indeterminate. In such patients, the hyponatremia may have been present for a sufficiently long time to allow brain volume regulation, but not enough to prevent some residual brain edema and neurologic symptomatology.[48] Consequently, complications from both the hyponatremia and its correction may be present. A controlled and limited correction of hyponatremia is indicated in such cases, with a maximum rate of correction of 0.5–2 mmol/l per hour as long as the total magnitude of correction does not exceed 18–25 mmol/l in the first 48 h.[41] In moderately symptomatic patients, the lower rates of correction are preferable[37,41] (0.5 mmol/l/h), while those with more severe symptoms will benefit from more rapid (1–2 mmol/l/h) correction. In cases of clinical volume depletion, including known diuretic use and/or a spot urine of 30 mmol/l, it is preferable to infuse isotonic saline at 50–100 ml/h, depending on the degree of hypovolemia. Where SIAD is the likely diagnosis (i.e. no volume depletion or diuretic use) and the spot urine >30 mmol/l, 3% NaCl should be used instead, the rate of infusion being calculated from the following equation:

Body weight (kg) × desired correction rate (mmol/l/h) = ml/h of 3% NaCl to infuse

Serum Na⁺ should be monitored at frequent intervals (at least 3–4-hourly) during the active phase of treatment to adjust therapy, and acute treatment should be interrupted once the following endpoints are reached:

1. The patient's symptoms are abolished.
2. A safe serum Na⁺ (>120 mmol/l) level has been reached.
3. A total magnitude of correction of 15–20 mmol/l has been achieved.

Disorders of potassium balance

Potassium is the most abundant intracellular cation, and is necessary for a large number of cellular functions, including cell volume regulation, cell polarity, receptor-mediated endocytosis and electrical excitability, RNA synthesis, protein synthesis, hormone secretion, vascular reactivity, acid–base balance, and apoptosis. Severe derangement of K⁺

balance can lead to life-threatening cardiac dysrhythmias and muscular paralysis. Dietary K$^+$ intake in Western societies ranges between 50 and 150 mmol/24 h, although homeostasis can be maintained with intakes as high as 500 mmol/day. The kidney is the most important organ for K$^+$ excretion, although in renal failure gastrointestinal losses may increase.[49,50]

Regulation of potassium homeostasis

Potassium homeostasis is regulated by a combination of K$^+$ intake, excretion and cellular transport. K$^+$ is present in most foods, and in health, K$^+$ excretion reflects intake, with around 90% eliminated by the kidneys and 8–10% in stool. Cellular K$^+$ transport involves both uptake and efflux, cellular uptake being essential for homeostasis and thereby preventing large changes in serum K$^+$ (internal balance).[51] Thus, an infusion of 50 mmol of K$^+$ to a healthy individual will only increase serum K$^+$ by about 1 mmol, even though less than 50% is excreted in the urine within the first 6 h; this is mediated by cellular uptake, a process termed 'extrarenal potassium homeostasis'.[52]

Cellular potassium transporters and ion channels

Internal K$^+$ homeostasis depends upon active cellular uptake and passive cellular efflux. Active uptake depends upon the activity of the ouabain/digoxin-sensitive Na$^+$/K$^+$-ATPase, which maintains the intracellular Na$^+$ concentration at 10–20 mmol/l, and the intracellular K$^+$ concentration at 80–120 mmol/l, through active extrusion of Na$^+$ in exchange for K$^+$, a process dependent on ATP hydrolysis. During this process, three Na$^+$ are extruded in exchange for two K$^+$. In gastric mucosa and colonic epithelial cells and intercalated collecting duct cells in the kidney, K$^+$ absorption depends on ion motive pumps that exchange extracellular K$^+$ for intracellular protons or hydronium ions by the use of H$^+$/K$^+$-ATPases, resulting in alkalinization of the cytosol.

In the thick ascending loop of Henle, K$^+$ uptake is via the Na$^+$/K$^+$/2Cl$^-$ cotransporter family of proteins, which are inhibited by frusemide and bumetanide. As they are electroneutral transporters, K$^+$ entry against its concentration gradient is achieved using the energy derived from the chemical gradient for Na$^+$ and Cl$^-$ and does not require ATP hydrolysis.

Potassium efflux is largely passive but regulated by cell membrane K$^+$ channels, and this is crucial to establishing the resting membrane potential. An increase in extracellular K$^+$, which retards K$^+$ efflux, will reduce (make the interior less electronegative) the membrane potential.

Internal potassium balance

The proportion of intra- to extracellular K$^+$ is influenced by pH and plasma bicarbonate separately, with a rise in either (i.e. alkalosis) increasing intracellular at the expense of extracellular K$^+$. Conversely, in acidosis, hyperkalemia occurs because of an exchange of H$^+$ for K$^+$ in cells, although inhibition of Na$^+$/K$^+$-ATPase may also play a role. The magnitude of the change in extracellular K$^+$ depends on the cause of the pH change, with metabolic acidosis (e.g. hyperchloremic acidosis) causing an increase of K$^+$ of 0.6–0.8 mmol per 0.1 unit fall in pH, whereas respiratory acidosis is only associated with a 0.1 mmol/l change for a 0.1 fall in pH.

Hormones regulating potassium

Aldosterone is released with a rise in K$^+$, and this increases renal and, to a lesser extent, colonic K$^+$ excretion.[53] Insulin increases cellular K$^+$ uptake in vivo, in a dose-dependent manner, into skeletal muscle.[54] An increase in K$^+$ increases insulin release per se, an important mechanism for extrarenal homeostasis, with K$^+$ being driven into liver and muscle cells. Adrenergic stimuli such as an increase in circulating adrenal drives K$^+$ into cells, particularly muscle, through stimulation of β_2 receptors and subsequent stimulation of Na$^+$/K$^+$-ATPase.[55] Heavy exercise releases K$^+$ from muscle into extracellular fluid, and this can cause a rise of K$^+$ of as much as 50% after 10–15 min, falling rapidly in the post-exercise period. The exercise-induced rise in K$^+$ is exaggerated by β-blockade. Finally, hyperosmolar states caused, for instance, by hyperglycemia or mannitol infusion, tend to increase K$^+$ by some 0.6 mmol/l per 10 mOsm/kg increase in osmolality.

External potassium balance

This is mainly regulated by the kidney, with a small contribution from the gastrointestinal tract; the latter route of elimination assumes greater importance in renal failure.

Renal potassium handling

Filtered K^+ reabsorption is effectively complete by the end of the proximal tubule, but K^+ re-enters the tubule in the pars recta and the thin descending limb of the loop of Henle (emanating from reabsorption in the collecting ducts via medullary tissue). It is reabsorbed in the thick ascending loop via the frusemide/bumetanide-blockable $Na^+/K^+/2Cl^-$ cotransporter. A high medullary concentration of K^+ tends to decrease Na^+ reabsorption in the thick ascending limb. The greater delivery of Na^+ to the distal tubule also favors kaliuresis, in part due to Na^+ concentration and tubular flow rates.[56]

Aldosterone enhances Na^+ reabsorption and K^+/H^+ secretion in the cortical collecting ducts by increasing Na^+/K^+-ATPase activity in the basolateral membranes and by increasing the conductance of K^+ of the principal collecting tubular cells. Alkalosis increases the uptake of K^+ in the basolateral membranes, and the conductance of the luminal membranes of the distal nephron promotes kaliuresis, such that alkalotic states are associated with enhanced K^+ excretion.

Potassium adaptation

The kidney can excrete as much as 10–20 times the normal amount of K^+ that it normally does. With chronic high-K^+ intake, distal tubular secretion is enhanced and Na^+/K^+-ATPase activity is increased, this being only partly dependent on aldosterone action.

Hypokalemia

There are many causes of hypokalemia, as listed in Table 15.8. It is commonly caused by gastrointestinal disorders, vomiting, diarrhea or renal K^+ wasting, usually induced by diuretics, aldosterone excess (hyperaldosteronism) or, more rarely, Liddle's syndrome (pseudohyperaldosteronism). Endocrine causes include hyperaldosteronism, phaeochromocytoma, ectopic ACTH secretion associated with Cushing's syndrome, and 11β-hydroxysteroid dehydrogenase deficiency—these are all associated with secondary hypertension, mild alkalosis and a kaliuresis. A subgroup of patients have inherited hypokalemia with metabolic alkalosis, inherited as an autosomal recessive trait. In Bartter's syndrome, described over 35 years ago, there is renal salt wasting, an elevated plasma renin activity and hyperplasia of the juxtaglomerular apparatus, and hypercalciuria. In Gitelman's syndrome, patients have a similar abnormality but in association with hypocalciuria and hypomagnesemia.

Clinical features of hypokalemia

A fall in extracellular K^+ causes an increase in the intraextracellular K^+ ratio, which causes hyperpolarization across excitable membranes, such as in heart muscle. There is an increased risk of dysrhythmia, ranging from unifocal extrasystoles to ventricular tachycardia and ventricular fibrillation. When K^+ falls below 3.0 mmol/l, ST depression occurs, as does flattening of T waves, and U waves become prominent. Marked hypokalemia causes skeletal muscle weakness with depressed reflexes. Respiratory muscles can be affected, and frank rhabdomyolysis may occur after exercise in K^+-depleted patients, although more often there is an increase in CPK levels without obvious myalgia. Smooth muscle in the intestine is also affected, causing constipation and, less frequently, ileus. Hypokalemia may cause NDI, a fall in glomerular filtration rate, a tendency to Na^+ retention, and a urinary phosphate leak with hypophosphatemia. Metabolic alkalosis may be accentuated by increased renal acid secretion, and patients occasionally complain of paresthesiae. When chronic, vacuolation of tubular cells occurs in both proximal and distal tubular cells, which may lead to a chronic tubulointerstitial nephropathy.[51]

Diuretic overuse

Loop diuretics block K^+ reabsorption in the ascending loop of Henle by inhibiting the $Na^+/K^+/2Cl^-$ cotransporter and are thus also chloruretic, and lead to hypokalemia as well as calcium wastage. Thiazide diuretics block the Na^+/Cl^- cotransporter in the distal convoluted tubule. Both will lead to secondary hyperaldosteronism with consequent K^+ wastage and alkalosis.

Investigation of hypokalemia

This depends on the suspected underlying cause, but it is useful to identify those causes associated with renal K$^+$ loss—such as renal tubulopathies, hyperaldosteronism, syndromes of apparent mineralocorticoid excess, Cushing's syndrome, glucocorticoid resistance, 17α-hydroxylase deficiency, and Liddle's syndrome—from those causes where there is increased intracellular uptake of K$^+$.

Treatment

Treatment of hypokalemia depends on the underlying cause, and the treatment of the endocrine causes associated with hypertension have been discussed elsewhere.

Gitelman's syndrome

The electrolyte changes characteristic of this autosomal recessive condition resemble those of patients taking thiazide diuretics: patients suffer from hypokalemic alkalosis, absence of hypertension, hypocalciuria, hypomagnesemia, and presentation after 8 years of age and mutations of the distal tubular Na$^+$/Cl$^-$ cotransporter have been described in this condition.[59]

Bartter's syndrome

These patients differ from those with Gitelman's syndrome in having a hypercalciuric form of hypokalemic alkalosis. Patients have nephrocalcinosis and usually present shortly after birth with severe dehydration. The biochemical findings in Bartter's syndrome resemble those of patients on loop diuretics (frusemide and bumetanide), which act on the Na$^+$/K$^+$/2Cl$^-$ cotransporter in the thick ascending loop of Henle (TAL), and mutations of this transporter have been reported.[57,58] The result is that Na$^+$ reabsorption is severely impaired (30% of filtered Na$^+$ is reabsorbed in the TAL) in the TAL, causing hypovolemia, activation of the renin–angiotensin system, and consequent hypokalemic alkalosis.

The reabsorption of approximately 25% of filtered calcium in the TAL is coupled to Na$^+$/K$^+$/2Cl$^-$ activity, whose loss of activity therefore results in calcium wastage and nephrocalcinosis. An apical ATP-sensitive K$^+$

Intracellular potassium shifts
  Alkalosis
  Intravenous insulin
  β$_2$-adrenergic stimulation
  Theophylline intoxication
  Periodic paralysis
  Barium salt poisoning
  Glue sniffing
  Chloroquine intoxification
Renal wasting
  Metabolic and respiratory alkalosis
  Diuretic use
Solute diuresis
  Glucose
  Urea
  Mannitol
  Saline
  Carbenecillin
  Penicillin
Hyperaldosteronism
  Primary (Conn's syndrome, nodular hyperplasia)
  Secondary
  Hemangiopericytoma (renin-secreting tumor)
  Renal tubulopathy
  Mineralocorticoid excess
  11β-Hydroxylase deficiency
  Bartter's syndrome
  Gitelman's syndrome
  Magnesium depletion
  11β-Hydroxysteroid dehydrogenase deficiency
  Liquorice abuse
  Carbenoxolone
  Renal tubular acidosis
  Ureterosigmoidostomy
  Gentamicin
  Amikacin
  Tobramycin
  Cisplatinum
  Amphotericin
  Ectopic ACTH syndrome
Gastrointestinal loss
  Vomiting from pyloric stenosis
  Bulimia nervosa
  Ileostomy
  VIPoma
  Chloride diarrhea
  Villous adenoma of the rectum
  Purgative abuse

Table 15.8
Causes of hypokalemia

channel recycles K^+ back into the lumen (and is critical to the function of the $Na^+/K^+/2Cl^-$ cotransporter).

Primary tubular disorders such as cystinosis closely mimic Bartter's syndrome, as do laxative abuse and vomiting, all of which can cause urinary K^+ wasting, particularly when alkalosis and hypokalemia are severe. With severe vomiting, there is a rebound Cl^--retaining state, whereas in Bartter's syndrome, there is excessive urinary Cl^- loss. Diuretic abuse, notably with loop diuretics, precisely mimics Bartter's syndrome.

Treatment

In asymptomatic patients with mild chemical disturbance, simply increasing the intake of K^+ may suffice. Spironolactone, amiloride and triamperene may also be used. Indomethacin, in doses of up to 2 mg/kg per day, has the greatest effect in reducing the hyperaldosteronism, although K^+ levels are rarely normalized.[51]

Hypokalemic periodic paralysis (HPP)

In this condition, hypokalemia is associated with profound weakness. In Western countries, most cases are due to familial periodic paralysis, whereas in Asian populations, thyrotoxic periodic paralysis is most commonly associated with this illness. In HPP, hypokalemia and paralysis are due to an acute shift of K^+ into cells, whereas in cases where HPP is not present, an excessive excretion of K^+ is usually an important etiologic factor.[51] In cases of HPP, the transtubular K^+ gradient (TTKG: (urine/plasma K^+)/(urine/plasma osmolality) is low (<2). The normal renal response when hypokalemia is due to non-renal causes is a TTKG <2, whereas a TTKG >5 reflects a net secretion of K^+ in the cortical collecting ducts.[58]

Treatment of HPP

Thyrotoxicosis must be excluded as an underlying cause, and in the acute emergency situation a potassium chloride infusion may be required, but caution is required to avoid rebound hyperkalemia upon recovery. The administration of a β-blocker has been shown to prevent future attacks of HPP.[60]

Hyperkalemia

This is potentially lethal, primarily because of its effect on cardiac conduction. Management requires exclusion of pseudohyperkalemia, assessment of the urgency of treatment, the identification of the cause, and institution of the appropriate therapy. Hyperkalemia occurs when K^+ intake exceeds excretion or when the distribution between intracellular and extracellular K^+ is perturbed. Chronic hyperkalemia only occurs when there is impairment of renal excretion.

Pseudohyperkalemia

This usually occurs where blood has been allowed to clot and centrifuged to obtain the K^+ level, K^+ release occurring from several of the formed elements of the blood. The commonest cause is, however, hemolysis, and is detected in the laboratory by a pink tinge to the serum. K^+ release other than from red cells may occur in situations where there is an excessive number of white cells ($>70 \times 10^3$) or platelet counts $>10^6$. Pseudohyperkalemia can be excluded by the simultaneous measurement of plasma and serum K^+ concentrations, and diagnosed when the latter exceeds plasma levels by >0.3 mmol/l.

Excess potassium intake or potassium release

The healthy kidney can eliminate several hundred millimoles of K^+ daily, and increased intake per se is unlikely to cause hyperkalemia. However, in the presence of impairment of renal K^+ excretion due to intrinsic kidney disease or drugs (Table 15.9), excess intake may precipitate hyperkalemia.

Tissue necrosis

Hyperkalemia depends upon the mass and rate of tissue lysis, occurring most frequently with rhabdomyolysis and ischemia of the extremities or bowel. Rhabdomyolysis occurs most frequently in association with crush injuries, seizures, electrical shock, cocaine ingestion, sepsis, ischemia, and excessive exertion. It may also occur in association with severe hypokalemia. Acute renal failure is a known complication of rhabdomyolysis.

> **Causes of hyperkalemia**
> **Excessive intake of potassium** (e.g. in oranges)
> **Reduced/impaired renal excretion**
>   Acute renal failure
>   Chronic renal failure
>   Pseudohypoaldoateronism
> **Endocrine causes**
>   Addison's Disease
>   Hyporeninaemic hypoaldosteronism
>   21-hydroxylase deficiency
>   3-hydroxysteroid dehydrogenase deficiency
> **Drugs**
>   Amiloride
>   Triamterene
>   Spironolactone
>   ACE inhibitors
>   Angiotensin II receptor inhibitors
> **Tissue release of potassium**
>   Acidosis
>   Rhabdomyolysis
>   Massive tumour necrosis
>   Hyperkalaemic periodic paralysis
>   Malignant hyperthermia syndrome
>   Familial hyperkalaemic acidosis
> **Pseudohyperkalaemia**
>   Haemolysed blood sample
>   Leukaemia with high white cell count

Table 15.9
Causes of hyperkalemia

Acid–base disturbances

Several forms of metabolic acidoses caused by organic acids can be associated with hyperkalemia: these acids include β-hydroxybutyric acid and lactic acid. However, the degree of hyperkalemia is less severe than hyperkalemia associated with HCl or NH_4Cl administration. In type IV renal tubular acidosis, hyperkalemia may be present, and is frequently secondary to the use of nonsteroidal anti-inflammatory agents. Hyporeninemic hypoaldosteronism is also a cause of hyperkalemia.

Mineralocorticoid deficiency

This is most frequently seen in association with primary adrenal failure (Addison's disease), particularly during an Addisonian crisis. The coexistence of hyponatremia, hyperkalemia, low bicarbonate and raised urea and creatinine should suggest the presence of Addison's disease. Other causes of endocrine hyperkalemia include diabetic ketoacidosis, 21-hydroxylase deficiency, hyporeninemic hypoaldosteronism, 18-oxidase deficiency, and pseudoaldosteronism.

Hyperosmolality

Hypertonicity causes redistribution of K^+ into the extracellular space, and this is part of the explanation for the hyperkalemia associated with diabetic ketoacidosis.

Drugs

Inhibitors of aldosterone production, as well as the competitive aldosterone antagonist spironolactone, and ACE inhibitors may be associated with hyperkalemia. Amiloride and triampterene inhibit the distal tubular Na^+/Cl^--transporter and cause hyperkalemia. After renal transplantation, cyclosporin A may cause hyperkalemia (K^+ 6.0–7.1 mmol/l) and acidosis out of proportion to glomerular filtration rate and dietary intake. The condition is probably a variant of hyporeninemic hypoaldosteronism.

Treatment of hyperkalemia

This again depends on the cause: whether it is acute or chronic, whether it is stable or increasing, and, most importantly, whether there are any pathognomonic changes on the ECG.[61] Stable concentrations of 6.0 may not require treatment, whereas levels >6.5 with associated ECG changes constitute a medical emergency. If ECG changes are absent or involve only the P waves, intravenous glucose (50 g) and insulin (10–20 units) (Actrapid) will lower plasma K^+ by about 1 mmol/l within 20–30 min, the effect persisting for 1–2 h. With more ominous ECG changes, 10–30 ml intravenous calcium gluconate (10%) will correct the ECG, but the effect is short-lived.[62] A cation exchange resin in the calcium or sodium phase given in a dose of 15–20 g three or four times daily can also be given by mouth or by retention enema; these bring down K^+ within 1–2 h. Hemodialysis or peritoneal dialysis may be required in severe cases. Mineralocorticoid deficiency responds well to 0.1–0.2 mg fludrocortisone daily, the failure of such doses to correct the hyperkalemia suggesting an underlying renal tubular defect.

References

1. Gennari FJ. Serum osmolality: uses and limitations. *N Engl J Med* 1984; 310: 102–5.
2. Jard S. Vasopressin receptors. In: Czernichow P, Robinson AG, eds. *Frontiers of Hormone Research*, Vol. 13, *Diabetes Insipidus in Man*. Basel: Karger, 1985: 89–104.
3. Richardson DW, Robinson AG. Desmopressin. *Ann Intern Med* 1985; 103: 228.
4. Vokes T, Robinson GL. Physiology of secretion of vasopressin. In: Czernikow P, Robertson AG, eds. *Frontiers of Hormone Research*, Vol. 13, *Diabetes Insipidus in Man*. Basel: Karger, 1985.
5. Richter D. Molecular events in the expression of vasopressin and oxytocin and their cognate receptors. *Am J Physiol* 1988; 255: F207–19.
6. Zerbe RL, Robinson GL. Osmotic and non-osmotic regulation of thirst and vasopressin secretion. In: Maxwell MH, Kleeman CR, Narin RG, eds. *Clinical Disorders of Fluid and Electrolyte Metabolism*, 4th edn. New York: McGraw-Hill, 1987.
7. Robertson GL. Disorders of thirst in man. In: Ramsay D, ed. *Thirst: Physiological and Psychological Aspects*. London: Springer-Verlag, 1991: 453.
8. Deen PMT, Verdijk MAJ, Knoers NVAM et al. Requirement of human renal water channel aquaporin-2 for vasopressin-dependent concentration of urine. *Science* 1994; 264: 92.
9. Hayashi M, Sasaki S, Tsuganezawa H et al. Role of vasopressin V2 receptor in acute regulation of aquaporin-2. *Kidney Blood Press Res* 1996; 19: 32–7.
10. Agre P, Bonhivers M, Borgnia MJ. The aquaporins, blueprints for cellular plumbing systems. *J Biol Chem* 1998; 273: 14659–62.
11. Greger NG, Kirkland RT, Clayton GW, Kirkland JL. Central diabetes insipidus: 22 years' experience. *Am J Dis Child* 1986; 140: 551–4.
12. Imura H, Kazuwa N, Shimatsu A et al. Lymphocytic infundibuloneurohypophysitis as a cause of central diabetes insipidus. *N Engl J Med* 1993; 329: 683.
13. Bahnsen U, Oosting P, Swaab DF et al. A missense mutation in the vasopressin–neurophysin precursor gene cosegretates with human autosomal dominant neurohypophyseal diabetes insipidus. *EMBO J* 1992; 11: 19.
14. Bichet DG, Birnbaumer M, Lonergan M et al. Nature and recurrence of AVPR2 mutations in X-linked nephrogenic diabetes insipidus. *Am J Hum Genet* 1994; 55: 278.
15. Verbalis JG, Robinson AG, Moses AM. Postoperative and post-traumatic diabetes insipidus. In: Czernikow P, Robinson AG, eds. *Frontiers in Hormone Research*, Vol. 13, *Diabetes Insipidus in Man*. Basel: Karger, 1986.
16. Miller et al. Recognition of partial defects in antidiuretic hormone secretion. *Ann Intern Med* 1970; 73: 721–9.
17. Knoers N, van den Ouweland A, Dreesen J et al. Nephrogenic diabetes insipidus: identification of the genetic defect. *Paediatr Nephrol* 1993; 7: 683.
18. Bichet DG. Nephrogenic diabetes insipidus. In: Cameron JS, Davidson AM, Grunfeld JP et al, eds. *Oxford Textbook of Clinical Nephrology*. Oxford: Oxford University, 1992: 789–800.
19. Canfield MC, Tamarappo BK, Moses AM et al. Identification and characterization of aquaporin-2 water channel mutations causing nephrogenic diabetes insipidus with partial vasopressin response. *Hum Mol Genet* 1997; 6: 865–71.
20. Fujiwara TM, Morgan K, Bichet DG. Molecular biology of diabetes insipidus. *Ann. Rev Med* 1995; 46: 331–43.
21. Boton R, Gaviria M, Battle DC. Prevalence, pathogenesis and treatment of renal dysfunction associated with chronic lithium therapy. *Am J Kidney Dis* 1987; 19: 329–45.
22. Barron WM, et al. Transient vasopressin resistant diabetes insipidus of pregnancy. *N Engl J Med* 1984; 310: 442–4.
23. Dashe AM, Cramm RE, Crist J et al. A water deprivation test for the differential diagnosis of polyuria. *JAMA* 1963; 185: 699–703.
24. Zerbe RE, Robertson GL. A comparison of plasma vasopressin measurement with a standard indirect test in the differential diagnosis of polyuria. *N Engl J Med* 1981; 305: 1539–46.
25. Sato N, Ishizaka H, Yagi H et al. Posterior lobe of the pituitary in diabetes insipidus. Dynamic MR imaging. *Radiology* 1993; 186: 357–60.
26. Crawford JD, Kennedy GC. Animal physiology: chlorothiazide in diabetes insipidus. *Nature* 1959; 183; 891.
27. Usberti M, Deschaux M, Guillot M et al. Renal prostaglandin E2 in nephrogenic diabetes insipidus: effects of inhibition of prostaglandin synthesis by indomethacin. *J Paediatr* 1986; 108: 305.
28. Anderson RJ. Hospital-associated hyponatraemia. *Kidney Int* 1986; 29: 1237.
29. Ladenson JH, Appel FS, Koch DD. Misleading hyponatraemia due to hyperlipidaemia: a method dependent error. *Ann Intern Med* 1981; 95: 707.
30. Halterman R, Berl T. Therapy of dysnatremic disorders. In: Brady H, Wilcox C, eds. *Therapy in Nephrology and Hypertension*. Philadelphia: WB Saunders, 1999: 256.
31. Martin P-Y, Schrier RW. Renal sodium excretion and edematous disorders. *Endocrine Metab Clin North Am* 1993; 24(3): 459–79.
32. Barsoum NR, Levine BS. Current prescriptions for the correction of hyponatraemia and hypernatraemia: are they too simple?. *Nephrol Dial Transplant* 2002; 17: 1176–80.
33. Halperin ML, Bichet DG, Oh MS. Integrative physiology of basal water permeability in the distal nephron: implications for the syndrome of inappropriate secretion of antidiuretic hormone. *Clin Nephrol* 2001; 56: 339–45.
34. Sterns RH. Thomas DJ, Herndon RM. Brain dehydration and neurologic deterioration after rapid correction of hyponatraemia. *Kidney Int* 1989; 35: 69–75.

35. Norenberg MD, Leslie KO. Correction of hyponatraemia and central pontine myelinolysis. *Am J Med* 1982; 73: 882.
36. Pasantes-Morales H, Franco R, Ordaz B, Ochoa LD. Mechanisms counteracting swelling in brain cells during hyponatremia. *Arch Med Res* 2002; 33: 237–44.
37. Omari A, Kormas N, Field M. Delayed onset of central pontine myelinolysis despite appropriate correction of hyponatraemia. *Intern Med J* 2002; 32: 273–4.
38. Arieff AL, Llach F, Massry SG. Neurological manifestations and morbidity of hyponatraemia: correlation with brain water and electrolytes. *Medicine* 1976; 55: 121–9.
39. Lauriat S, Berl T. The hyponatraemic patient. Practical focus on therapy. *J Am Soc Nephrol* 1997; 5: 1599.
40. Reeves WM, Bichet DG, Andreoli TE. Posterior pituitary and water metabolism. In: Wilson JD, Foster DW, Kronenberg, Larsen, eds. *Williams Textbook of Endocrinology*, 9th edn. WB Saunders, 1998: 341–87.
41. Kovacs L, Robertson GL. Disorders of water balance: hyponatraemia and hypernatraemia. *Baillières Clin Endocrinol Metab* 1992; 6: 107.
42. Sterns RH. The management of hyponatraemic emergencies. *Crit Care Clin* 1991; 7: 127–42.
43. Forrest JN Jr, Cox M, Hong C et al. Superiority of demeclocycline over lithium in the treatment of chronic syndrome of inappropriate secretion of antidiuretic hormone. *N Engl J Med* 1978; 298: 173–7.
44. Decaux G, Waterlot Y, Gennette F et al. Inappropriate secretion of antidiuretic hormone treated with furosemide. *BMJ* 1982; 285: 89–90.
45. Riggs JE. Neurologic manifestations of electrolyte disturbances. *Neurol Clin* 2002; 20: 227–39.
46. Decaux G. Treatment of hyponatremic encephalopathy. *J Lab Clin Med* 2001; 138: 403.
47. Gross P. Treatment of severe hyponatremia. *Kidney Int* 2001; 77: 759–64.
48. Lampl C, Yazdi K. Central pontine myelinolysis. *Eur Neurol* 2002; 47: 3–10.
49. Wright FS. Renal potassium handling. *Semin Nephrol* 1987; 7: 174–84.
50. Clark BA, Brown RS. Potassium homeostasis and hyperkalaemic syndromes. *Endocrinol Metab Clin North Am* 1991; 24(3): 573–91.
51. Kamel KS, Halperin ML, Faber MD et al. Disorders of potassium balance. In: Brenner BM, ed. *The Kidney*, 5th edn. Philadelphia: WB Saunders, 1996; 999–1037.
52. Bia MJ, DeFronzo RA. Extrarenal potassium homeostasis. *Am J Physiol* 1981; 240: F257–68.
53. Conlin PR, Dluhy RG, Williams GH. Disorders of the renin–angiotensin–aldosterone system. In: Schrier RW, ed. *Renal and Electrolyte Disorders*, 5th edn. Boston: Little, Brown, 1997: 349–92.
54. DeFronzo RA, Sherwin RS, Dillingham M et al. Influence of basal insulin and glucagon secretion on potassium and sodium metabolism. *J Clin Invest* 1978; 61: 472–9.
55. Clausen T. Adrenergic control of $Na^+ K^+$ homeostasis. *Acta Medica Scand* 1983; 672: 111–15.
56. Ethier JH, Kamel KS, Magner PO et al. The transtubular potassium concentration in patients with hypokalaemia and hyperkalaemia. *Am J Kidney Dis* 1990; 15: 309–15.
57. Kurtz I. Molecular pathogenesis of Bartter's and Gitelman's syndromes. *Kidney Int* 1998; 54: 1396–410.
58. Guay-Woodford LM. Bartter syndrome: unraveling the pathophysiologic enigma. *Am J Med* 1998; 105: 151–61.
59. Winterborn MH, Hewitt GJ, Mitchell MD. The role of prostaglandins in Barrter's syndrome. *Int J Pediatr Nephrol* 1984; 5: 31–8.
60. Knochel JP. Potassium gradients and neuromuscular function. In: Seldin DW, Giebisch G, eds. *The Kidney: Physiology and Pathophysiology*, 2nd edn. New York: Raven Press, 1992: 2191–208.
61. Rastegar A, Soleimani M, Rastegar A. Hypokalaemia and hyperkalaemia. *Postgrad Med J* 2001; 77: 759–64.
62. Davey M, Calidcott D. Calcium salts in management of hyperkalaemia. *Emerg Med J* 2002; 19:92–3.

16

Endocrine hypertension
Jennifer E Lawrence, Robert G Dluhy

Introduction

Hypertension, a major risk factor for cardiovascular disease, is a common disorder and occurs in approximately 20% of the US population. The great majority (90%) carry the diagnosis of essential, or primary, hypertension. It is now clear that essential hypertension is a heritable syndrome reflecting a number of disease processes whereby different mechanisms can lead to an increase in blood pressure. On the other hand, although identifiable secondary causes occur in a smaller percentage (10%) of hypertensive subjects, this small fraction represents a large number of patients.

Broadly speaking, the secondary cause of hypertension can be divided into renal causes (e.g. parenchymal disease, renovascular disease, Liddle's syndrome) and endocrine causes. The latter etiologies are discussed in this chapter. Although endocrine disorders are uncommon, many patients can be diagnosed by the astute clinician, since the signs and symptoms are often distinct. Beyond clinical clues, severity of hypertension or hypertension refractory to conventional antihypertensive agents may prompt the physician to screen for secondary causes. Age and sex of the hypertensive patient may also guide the search for specific secondary etiologies. For example, fibromuscular hyperplasia and Cushing's syndrome are more commonly seen in younger age groups, while primary hypothyroidism most commonly occurs in older female patients. Finally, making a diagnosis of a secondary disorder is gratifying, since it often leads to a cure of the elevated blood pressure.

Primary aldosteronism

Introduction

At the annual meeting for the Central Society for Research in 1954, J. W. Conn reported a syndrome of autonomous production of aldosterone and suppression of renin which resulted in the development of hypertension, hypokalemia and metabolic alkalosis. The aldosterone-producing adenoma, often referred to as Conn's syndrome, was predicted to be the most common form of endocrine hypertension. Subsequently, primary aldosteronism was found to have a variable prevalence, ranging between 0.05% and 14.4% of hypertensive patients.[1–5] Disparity in these percentages is probably due to the use of different hormone screening techniques and the previous reliance on hypokalemia as a screening criterion. Milder normokalemic forms of primary aldosteronism are now being diagnosed with increasing frequency.

Pathophysiology and clinical features

Aldosterone, produced in the zona glomerulosa or the outer zone of the adrenal cortex, is regulated by angiotensin II, potassium and also by adrenocorticotropic hormone (ACTH). Sodium excess and volume expansion normally decreases aldosterone synthesis by suppression of the renin–angiotensin system. Aldosterone binds to the type I mineralocorticoid receptor in the cortical collecting tubule luminal principal cells to increase the number of open sodium channels, resulting in increased reabsorption of sodium. The reabsorption of sodium produces a negative electrical gradient in the tubular lumen, resulting in potassium secretion through potassium channels to maintain electrical neutrality.

Hyperaldosteronism results in volume expansion, suppression of plasma renin activity and hypokalemia. However, one-fifth of patients with primary hyperaldosteronism have normal serum potassium levels, which may reflect a milder form of hyperaldosteronism and/or a decreased delivery of sodium to distal sites for potassium exchange. Metabolic alkalosis occurs secondary to renal tubule urinary hydrogen ion excretion. Mild hypernatremia (serum sodium concentration in the 145 meq/dl range) and resetting of the osmostat occurs so that antidiuretic hormone and thirst occur at a higher sodium concentration.[6] After retention of several liters, an escape from the sodium-retaining actions of aldosterone occurs due to the release of atrial natriuretic peptide. Thus, peripheral edema is not a characteristic feature of primary hyperaldosteronism.

Patients may have neuromuscular symptoms such as cramps, paresthesias or weakness, if hypokalemia is severe.[7] Hypokalemia-induced nephrogenic diabetes insipidus may lead to polyuria and polydipsia. Hypomagnesemia may also be seen. Cardiovascular manifestations include increased systemic vascular resistance, hypertension and cardiac hypertrophy. Hypertension is usually moderate to severe and is often resistant to usual pharmacological interventions. Premature ventricular contractions and electrophysiological disturbances result from hypokalemia. Most of these clinical features arise from the effects of aldosterone on the kidney; however, there is increasing evidence that aldosterone has direct extrarenal actions producing cardiac and vascular smooth muscle hypertrophy and cardiac fibrosis disproportionate to the elevation in blood pressure.[8-10]

Etiologies

The etiologies of primary aldosteronism include aldosterone-producing adenoma (APA), idiopathic hyperaldosteronism (IHA), primary adrenal hyperplasia, glucocorticoid-remediable aldosteronism (GRA), which is also termed familial hyperaldosteronism type I (FH type I), familial hyperaldosteronism type II (FH type II), and adrenal carcinoma. The clinical features of hyperaldosteronism are often most striking in APA. Formerly, it was thought that APA accounted for 65% of cases of primary aldosteronism, with IHA accounting for 30–40%, and GRA accounting for 1–3%.[7] However, as clinical suspicion and screening for primary aldosteronism has increased, milder forms of aldosterone excess, such as IHA and GRA, are being detected and may account for higher percentages.[4]

APA tumors are small tumors, usually measuring less than 2 cm in diameter. Surgical removal of the tumor may result in cure or amelioration of the hypertension—hypokalemia is always reversed. Pathology of such lesions reveals 'hybrid' cells which have histological features of the cells of both the zona glomerulosa and zona fasciculata. APA tumors may be divided into two subtypes: the first is composed predominantly of fasciculata-like cells, where aldosterone secretion is unresponsive to angiotensin II (AII-U-APA); the second is composed predominantly of angiotensin II-responsive glomerulosa-like cells (AII-R-APA). The latter may be misdiagnosed as IHA in which aldosterone production is also responsive to angiotensin II (see below). Aldosterone production is not autonomous in AII-U-APA, since it follows the circadian pattern of ACTH secretion.[11]

Another form of primary aldosteronism, which shares many biochemical features of AII-U-APA, exhibits histological features of unilateral nodular hyperplasia. This form of primary aldosteronism is referred to as primary adrenal hyperplasia (PAH). CT scanning fails to reveal an adenoma. Similar to APA, symptoms associated with PAH may be cured by unilateral adrenalectomy.[12-14]

In idiopathic bilateral hyperplasia (IHA), the adrenal glands appear hypertrophic and have micro/macronodule formation. Microscopically, the zona glomerulosa is hyperplastic. In patients with IHA, the aldosterone response to angiotensin II is exaggerated compared with normal individuals. In contrast to APA, bilateral adrenalectomy usually does not cure or improve hypertension but, similar to APA, does reverse the potassium-wasting state.

Heritable forms of primary aldosteronism

Two types of familial hyperaldosteronism are now recognized. Familial hyperaldosteronism type I (FH type I) is better known as glucocorticoid-remediable aldosteronism (GRA) or glucocorticoid-suppressible hyperaldosteronism (GSH).[15] In this syndrome, which has an autosomal dominant mode of inheritance, aldosterone production is positively, solely and abnormally regulated by ACTH. As a result, glucocorticoid administration profoundly suppresses aldosterone production and reverses this mineralocorticoid excess state.

Because the majority of patients with GRA are not hypokalemic, a potassium level lacks good sensitivity as a screening test for this disorder. Early hemorrhagic stroke and juvenile hypertension are characteristic of GRA pedigrees. Patients with GRA greatly overproduce the hybrid steroid compounds, 18-hydroxycortisol and 18-oxocortisol, which share enzymatic features of both the zona fasciculata and zona glomerulosa. Elevation of these compounds in a 24-h urine collection provides a highly sensitive and specific test to diagnose GRA.[15]

Genetic analysis of GRA kindreds has revealed linkage of GRA to mutations in the aldosterone synthase gene, which is closely related to steroid 11β-hydroxylase, a second gene involved in adrenal steroidogenesis. Both genes are 95% identical in DNA sequence, have identical intron–exon structures, and are located in close proximity on chromosome 8. GRA-affected subjects have two normal copies of genes encoding aldosterone synthase and 11β-hydroxylase, but in addition they have a novel gene duplication: a hybrid, or chimeric, gene.[16] This gene duplication, resulting from an unequal crossing-over between these two homologous genes, contains the 5′ regulatory sequences confirming ACTH responsiveness of 11β-hydroxylase fused to more distal coding sequences of aldosterone synthase. In GRA kindreds, the sites of crossing-over are variable, indicating that, in different pedigrees, these gene duplications arise independently and do not descend from a single ancestral mutation.[16]

Direct genetic screening for the presence of the gene duplication in GRA is 100% sensitive and specific for diagnosing GRA and is recommended for patients with primary aldosteronism without radiographic evidence of tumors, for young hypertensive individuals with suppressed levels of plasma renin activity (especially children), and for at-risk individuals in affected families. Low-dose glucocorticoids, amiloride and spironolactone are effective and directed therapies.[15,17]

Hyperaldosteronism type II (FH type II) is a newly described subset of familial primary aldosteronism with an autosomal dominant mode of inheritance that has been primarily described in Australian hypertensives. In this disorder, the hyperaldosteronism is not reversed with dexamethasone administration, and affected subjects screen negative for the chimeric gene duplication that is characteristic of FH type I or GRA. Affected patients within kindreds exhibit unilateral or bilateral adenomas. The molecular basis for this disorder remains unknown, but mutations in the aldosterone synthase and angiotensin II receptor genes appear to be excluded.[13,18,19]

Screening

Who should be screened for primary aldosteronism? A history of hypertension with 'spontaneous' hypokalemia is suspicious for hyperaldosteronism. However, recent studies suggest that hypokalemia lacks sensitivity as a screening test for primary aldosteronism. Diuretic treatment in patients with primary aldosteronism often precipitates severe hypokalemia (<3 mmol/l). The finding of an incidentally discovered adrenal mass warrants evaluation for hyperaldosteronism in a hypertensive patient. Most aldosterone-producing adenomas are usually less than 2 cm. Since the size of the tumor often correlates with the severity of the clinical presentation, adenomas greater than 2 cm would be expected to be associated with hypertension and hypokalemia. Finally, whenever there is a consideration for secondary hypertension (e.g. recent onset of hypertension in a previously normotensive patient), primary aldosteronism should be considered.

Evaluation of primary aldosteronism begins with hormonal screening for this disorder (Figure 16.1). The initial screening test for primary aldosteronism is usually the plasma aldosterone concentration (PAC) to plasma renin activity (PRA) ratio (PAC/PRA ratio). This ratio is usually less than 270:1 in normotensive subjects when plasma aldosterone concentration (PAC) is measured in pmol/l and plasma renin activity (PRA) is measured in mg/l/h (or ng/ml/h). In primary aldosteronism, the aldosterone levels are usually greater than 555–695 pmol/l in SI units (20–25 ng/dl in conventional units) and the plasma renin activity is suppressed (<0.1 mg/l/h or <0.1 ng/ml/h). A PAC/PRA ratio greater than 810 in SI units (or >30 in conventional units) is 90% sensitive for primary aldosteronism and 91% specific, while PAC/PRA ratios less than 550 in SI units (or <20 in conventional units) are seen in essential hypertension.[20] In secondary hyperaldosteronism, such as from renovascular hypertension, the PAC/PRA should be normal, since aldosterone secretion is increased secondary to activation of the renin–angiotensin system. Measurement of PRA serves to differentiate these forms of hypertension.

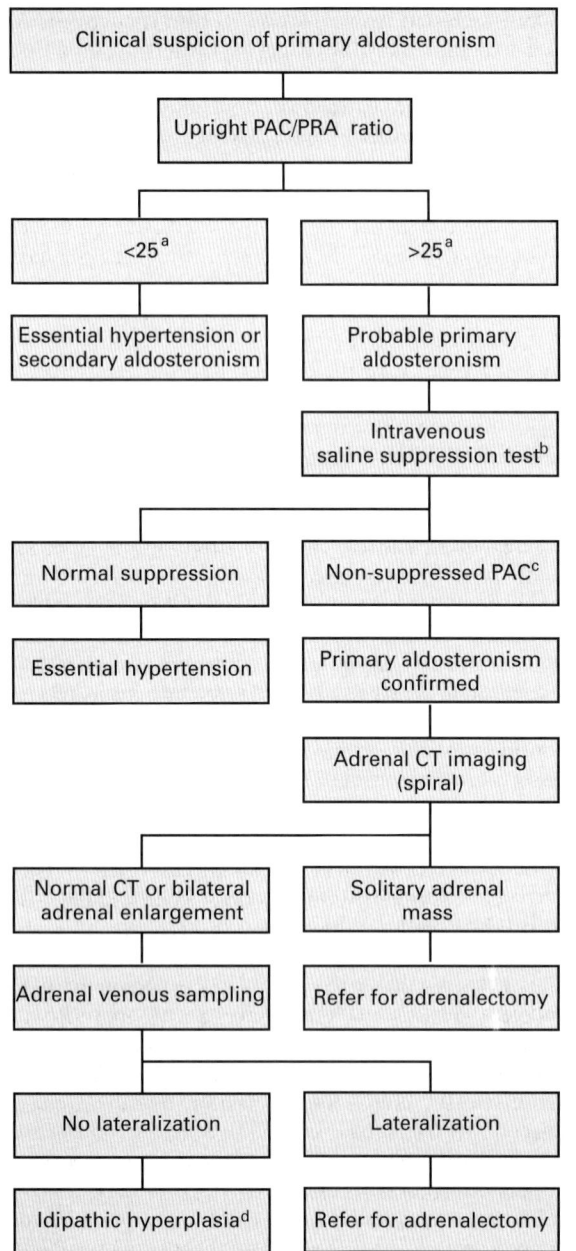

Figure 16.1

Algorithm for diagnosis of primary aldosteronism. [a]PAC/PRA ratio = plasma aldosterone concentration (PAC/plasma renin activity (PRA) ratio. Using conventional units, this ratio is elevated if greater than 25. In SI units, this ratio is considered elevated if greater than 700. [b]Intravenous saline suppression test: administration of 2 or 3 l of isotonic saline over 4 or 6 h respectively. Plasma aldosterone concentrations should decrease to below 166 pmol/L (in SI units) or 6 ng/dl (in conventional units). [c]Non-suppressed plasma aldosterone concentration: >280 pmol/l (in SI units) or > 10 ng/dl (in conventional units). [d]Consider screening for GRA if family history is significant for juvenile onset of hypertension (see text.)

To optimize evaluation for primary aldosteronism, factors that might alter aldosterone secretion should be avoided. Since hypokalemia reduces aldosterone secretion, potassium levels should be repleted before plasma aldosterone is measured. The patient should also be withdrawn from spironolactone, angiotensin converting-enzyme inhibitors (ACEIs), and β-blockers before evaluation, since levels of PRA will be altered by these medications. However, if the screening test is performed on β-blocker or ACEI therapies, and aldosterone levels are frankly elevated, then the likelihood of primary aldosteronism is increased, since ACEIs should increase renin and decrease aldosterone secretion, while β-blockers should decrease both renin and aldosterone secretion.

The captopril test, utilizing 25 mg of this short-acting ACEI, should normally decrease aldosterone levels to less than 416 pmol/l (15 ng/dl).[21,22] Failure to reduce aldosterone levels is consistent with autonomous aldosterone production. Prior captopril administration may also improve the diagnostic sensitivity of the PAC/PRA ratio for diagnosing primary aldosteronism. The cutoff point has been suggested as greater than 550 using SI units (or 20 using conventional units) by some authors versus 1380 using SI units (or 50 using conventional units) by others. Cortisol levels should be obtained to exclude a stress- or ACTH-mediated increase in aldosterone levels that would exaggerate the PAC/PRA ratio.

Establishing a definitive diagnosis

If the screening PAC/PRA ratio is suggestive, but not diagnostic, of primary aldosteronism, confirmation of autonomous aldosterone secretion is necessary. Methods to demonstrate autonomy of aldosterone production focus on volume-expanding maneuvers and include the saline suppression test, the oral salt loading test or the fludrocortisone suppression test (Figure 16.1). Volume expansion should normally suppress the renin–angiotensin system, and as a result the secretion of aldosterone. If suppression is not seen, autonomous secretion is confirmed. The saline suppression test involves intravenous isotonic saline administration over 4–6 h (500 ml/h); plasma aldosterone and plasma cortisol levels are determined at the beginning and end of the infusion. In normal subjects, plasma aldosterone levels will decrease below 166 pmol/l (or 6 ng/dl) following 2 or 3 l of intravenous saline. Values between 166 and 277 pmol/l (6 ng and 10 ng/dl) are indeterminate, while values greater than 277 pmol/l (10 ng/dl) are diagnostic of autonomous aldosterone production. This procedure should be avoided in patients who have compromised cardiac function. Cortisol levels are obtained along with aldosterone levels to exclude a stress- or ACTH-mediated increase in aldosterone levels that would produce a false-positive result.[7]

The oral salt suppression test is an outpatient test. The patient is instructed to eat a high (200 mmol) sodium diet for 3 days, or take two 1-g NaCl tablets (100 mmol) with each meal for 3 days. On the third day of the high-sodium diet, a 24-h urine sample for aldosterone excretion, creatinine and sodium is collected. A urine sodium excretion of greater than 200 mmol per 24 h documents a high sodium intake. The normal aldosterone excretion response is ≤12 μg/24 h.

In the fludrocortisone suppression test, 0.1 mg is given orally every 6 h along with sodium supplementation (20–30 mmol sodium three times daily) for 4 days. Plasma aldosterone concentrations should be suppressed to below 166 pmol/l (6 ng/dl). This test is less popular, as hospitalization is required with frequent potassium measurements to ensure that hypokalemia does not occur.[20]

Features distinguishing APA from IHA

Distinguishing between APA, IHA and the less common forms of primary hyperaldosteronism, such as GRA, is important. Unilateral adrenalectomy of APA cures 69% of patients of their hypertension and invariably reverses hypokalemia. On the other hand, bilateral adrenalectomy in IHA cures hypertension in only 19% of patients, while also reversing hypokalemia in all patients. Therefore, surgical removal of APA is preferred and pharmacological therapy of IHA is the treatment of choice.

Features such as young age (<50 years), severity of hypokalemia ([K] <3.0 mmol/l), severity of hypertension, plasma aldosterone concentration greater than 700 pmol/l (25 ng/dl) or urinary aldosterone >30 μg/24 h favor the diagnosis of APA but lack specificity.[23] Biochemical testing has been used to differentiate APA and IHA. The posture test takes advantage of the fact that aldosterone levels characteristically increase in patients with bilateral hyperplasia secondary to stimulation by angiotensin II. On the other hand, aldosterone levels in APA usually decline, following the circadian release of ACTH; aldosterone production is not regulated by angiotensin II, since the renin–angiotensive system is profoundly suppressed. However, this test lacks specificity and misdiagnoses patients 20% of the time. In addition, it may mislead the physician who is examining a patient with the rare renin-responsive APA to conclude that the patient has idiopathic hyperplasia.

Hormonal testing may help distinguish between these forms of hyperaldosteronism as a result of unique biochemical features. Patients with APA (including the aldosterone-producing renin-responsive tumor subset) typically have serum measurements of 18-hydroxy-corticosterone (18-OH-B), an intermediate in the aldosterone biosynthetic pathway, greater than 100 ng/dl; patients with IHA have values less than 100 ng/dl. However, the diagnostic accuracy is reported to be 82%, since there is significant overlap between the two patient groups.[7]

Adrenal CT with thin-slice (3 mm) spiral technique will often anatomically differentiate between APA and IHA.[12] If a tumor is imaged in a patient with the biochemical features of primary aldosteronism, and, the contralateral adrenal gland is anatomically normal, no further evaluation is usually needed. Since the size of the APA correlates with aldosterone overproduction and the severity of symptoms, an adenoma greater than 2 cm without hypertension and hypokalemia is more likely a non-functioning adrenocortical adenoma (the so-called 'incidentaloma'). On the other hand, APAs <1 cm in size may not be detected by CT scanning, leading to a misdiagnosis of IHA. Of patients who had biochemical features suggestive of APA in a Mayo Clinic series, only 36% had positive CT findings for APA. The remainder had either unilateral limb thickening or normal CT appearance. In the patients who had unilateral limb thickening, 50% were ultimately found to have APA on the normal-appearing contralateral gland. Because structure as seen by imaging often does not correlate with function, adrenal venous sampling is often necessary and is the definitive test to document lateralization in order to distinguish APA from IHA.

Adrenal venous sampling should be considered in patients who are surgical candidates, those who have the hormonal characteristics of an aldosterone-producing adenoma, and those in whom the adrenal CT scan lacks typical anatomical features of either bilateral hyperplasia or a solitary adenoma[24] (Figure 16.1). The technique involves sampling the right and left adrenal venous veins, using catheters placed in the ipsilateral femoral vein. Peripheral samples are also taken from the inferior vena cava. Cortisol and aldosterone levels are drawn peripherally and then simultaneously from each adrenal vein, before and every 10 min for 45 min after 250 μg of synthetic ACTH (cosyntropin) is given. Accessing the right adrenal vein is challenging because it commonly arises from the posterior aspect of the inferior vena cava, is also short (measuring 5–8 mm in length) and connects directly into the vena cava at an almost 90° angle.

In a patient with APA, the adrenal vein aldosterone levels and the aldosterone/cortisol ratio lateralize to the side of the lesion. In the contralateral adrenal vein, the aldosterone to cortisol ratio is less than the ratio measured from the peripheral vein, since aldosterone production is suppressed. The adrenal vein aldosterone/cortisol ratios are usually 4 to 5:1 from the side with the adenoma compared to the contralateral gland. In bilateral hyperplasia, the aldosterone/cortisol ratios are comparable and are usually less than 3.0 but may be as high as 3.5. Ratios between 3.0 and 4.0 are considered indeterminate.

With expertise in adrenal venous sampling accruing, the success rate of successful bilateral adrenal vein catheterization is increasing. Formerly, failure rates were as high as 36%, primarily due to inability to access the right adrenal vein.[24] Currently, with experienced angiographers, the failure rate can be as low as 3%.[23] Risks of the procedure include renal insufficiency and allergic reactions secondary to the radiocontrast injection, as well as direct injuries incurred from the adrenal venous catheterization, such as adrenal ischemia, infarction and injury to the vein.

Treatment

Surgery is usually the treatment of choice for APA unless there are medical contraindications, such as congestive heart failure or severe coronary artery disease. In most centers, surgical resection is accomplished by laparoscopic adrenalectomy, which usually results in shortened length of hospital stay and reduced patient morbidity compared to conventional flank incisions. Resection of APA usually cures or ameliorates the patients of their hypertension (see above) but invariably reverses the hypokalemia. Caution should be exercised in the postoperative management of APA patients, since hypoaldosteronism from the suppressed contralateral gland may result in salt wasting and hyperkalemia.

Spironolactone, a competitive antagonist of the mineralocorticoid receptor, is useful for the treatment of hypokalemia as well as hypertension in patients with primary aldosteronism. Dosages required are between 50 mg and 400 mg daily and are usually administered twice daily. When dosages greater than 100 mg/day are used, long-term side-effects such as gynecomastia and erectile dysfunction often occur in men due to the anti-androgenic actions of spironolactone. In women, spironolactone may lead to menstrual dysfunction and intermenstrual bleeding. Fatigue and gastrointestinal intolerance are other common side-effects. Since spironolactone has a long biological half-life and a slow onset of action, a low dosage should be initiated and clinical response evaluated before increasing the dose.

Potassium levels may require supplementation despite spironolactone in patients with normal renal function. In patients with renal impairment, a potassium-wasting diuretic may be added to reduce the risk of hyperkalemia. The new aldosterone receptor antagonist eplerenone, which should be approved by the FDA in the near future, does not possess the anti-androgenic actions of spironolactone and should be better tolerated, especially in male patients.

When patients are intolerant of the side-effects of spironolactone, other potassium-sparing diuretics, such as triamterene or amiloride, have been used but are usually not as effective as spironolactone.[25] Amiloride inhibits the sodium channel of the distal renal tubule, which is regulated by aldosterone. Sodium and chloride excretion are increased, while potassium excretion is reduced. Amiloride is started at a dosage of 10 mg daily and increased to a maximum of 40 mg daily. Side-effects from amiloride are unusual and mild, such as nausea. As with spironolactone, potassium levels should be monitored in patients with renal dysfunction.

The dihydropyridine calcium channel antagonists have been shown to acutely decrease blood pressure and aldosterone secretion in patients with primary hyperaldosteronism. However, the aldosterone-reducing actions have not been demonstrated with long-term use. In spite of a suppressed renin–angiotensin system, ACEIs and angiotensin II receptor blockers may be helpful in patients who have bilateral adrenal hyperplasia, where there is enhanced sensitivity to the actions of angiotensin II.[8]

Pheochromocytoma

Introduction

Pheochromocytomas are tumors of neuroectodermal origin arising from chromaffin cells and are named for the dark staining reaction which is caused by the oxidation of intracellular catecholamine stores when exposed to dichromate salts. Pheochromocytoma is a rare cause of hypertension, but may be fatal if left undiagnosed and untreated. The incidence is reported to be less than 1% of patients who are evaluated for hypertension, but this may be an underestimate. In one series, the incidence rate was calculated to be 0.8 per 100 000 person-years. In one autopsy series, up to 50% of the pheochromocytomas were diagnosed at postmortem examination, demonstrating that this disorder is frequently undiagnosed.[26,27]

Catecholamine synthesis and metabolism

Catecholamines are formed from the amino acid tyrosine by a process of hydroxylation and decarboxylation. This process of amine precursor uptake and decarboxylation (APUD) is a feature of neuroendocrine tissues which have a common origin. Tyrosine is hydrolyzed to DOPA by the rate-limiting enzyme tyrosine hydroxylase. DOPA is decarboxylated to dopamine. Dopamine is actively transported into granulated vesicles to be hydroxylated to norepinephrine (NE) (noradrenaline) by dopamine β-hydroxylase. These reactions occur in adrenergic neurons in the central nervous system or the peripheral nervous system, or in the chromaffin cells of the adrenal medulla. In adrenal medulla, the cytosolic enzyme, phenylethanolamine-N-methyltransferase (PNMT), converts NE into epinephrine (E) (adrenaline). PNMT activity is regulated by the presence of glucocorticoids by a mechanism still not known. In normal adrenal tissue, in the presence of PNMT, the ratio of E to NE is 4:1. However, in the circulation, the ratio is almost 10:1 NE to E.

Metabolism of catecholamines occurs via two enzyme pathways (Figure 16.2). Catechol-O-methyltransferase (COMT) is found outside of neuronal tissue and converts E to metanephrine and converts NE to normetanephrine. Metanephrine and normetanephrine are oxidized by monoamine oxidase (MAO) to vanillylmandelic acid (VMA). MAO may also oxidize E and NE to dihydroxymandelic acid (DHMA), which is then converted by COMT to VMA.

In pheochromocytoma, the enzymes involved in synthesis are increased and the enzymes involved in catabolism are usually decreased. As storage of the catecholamines is limited, the excess enters into the peripheral circulation. Measurements of these catecholamines and their metabolites are used to confirm the diagnosis of pheochromocytoma (see below).

Clinical manifestations

Hypertension is the most common symptom seen in pheochromocytoma, occurring in 90–100% of patients. Sustained hypertension occurs in approximately half of the patients, paroxysmal hypertension in a third, and normal blood pressure in less than a fifth.[28] In children, hypertension is most often sustained.

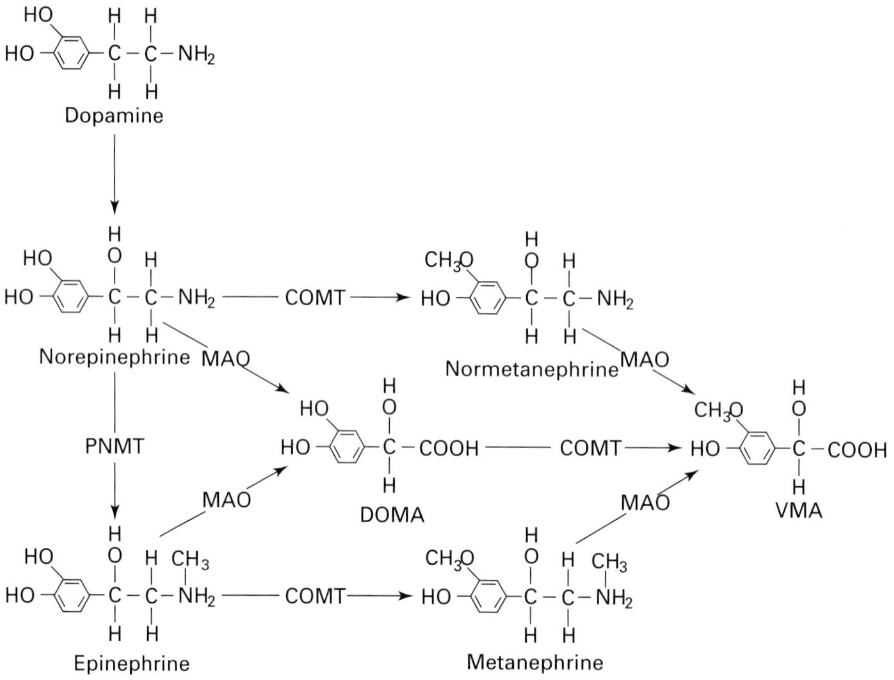

Figure 16.2
Metabolism of catecholamines. Catecholamines are boken down into metanephrines and vanillylmandelic acid (VMA). COMT, catechol-O-methyltransferase; MAO, monoamine oxidase; PNMT, phenylethanolamine-N-methyltransferase.

Patients with pheochromocytoma often present with paroxysmal episodes referred to as spells which include severe headache, palpitations and perspiration (the so-called classic triad).[29] These episodes may occur as frequently as daily, or as infrequently as every few months. More than 90% of patients present with two out of the three symptoms in the classic triad of headache, diaphoresis and palpitations. The headaches are often described as rapid in onset, bursting or throbbing and bilateral in nature, lasting less than an hour. Often, these headaches occur with other symptoms such as pallor or nausea. In most patients, these episodes occur abruptly and diminish over an hour. However, in other patients, the episodes may cease within a minute or continue over a week. Symptoms such as palpitations, anxiety or tremulousness may suggest the predominance of E secretion.[27,30] Less common symptoms include pallor, tremor, Raynaud's phenomenon, livedo reticularis, angina, nausea and mass effect from the tumor.

Orthostatic hypotension may be the presenting symptom in rare cases in which epinephrine, DOPA or dopamine is the predominant hormone secreted.[29] Usually, the drop in blood pressure is to a normal or near-normal range and is accompanied by tachycardia.

Cardiovascular manifestations of pheochromocytoma include dilated cardiomyopathy, which results from years of catecholamine excess. Patients may also present with features of acute myocardial infarction from coronary vasospasm or with arrhythmias.[30]

Diagnosis

The diagnosis of pheochromocytoma may be suspected when a factor such as exertion, trauma, certain drugs, anesthesia, or surgery and/or surgical manipulation of the tumor precipitates a crisis. Tricyclic antidepressants, droperidol, glucagon, metoclopromide, phenothiazines and naloxone have all been reported to precipitate paroxysms.[29,30] Foods or beverages that contain tyramine, such as certain aged cheeses or red wine, may precipitate a crisis. Patients with pheochromocytoma may have a paradoxical rise in blood pressure in response to certain antihypertensives such as β-blockers.

Several disorders may mimic pheochromocytoma and cause elevations in catecholamines. Withdrawal from medications such as clonidine, or withdrawal from alcohol, may mimic pheochromocytoma. Certain cerebral events, including cerebral vasculitis, intracranial lesions with increased intracranial pressure, pre-eclampsia with seizures, subarachnoid hemorrhage, migraine or cluster headache, may give a similar picture. Ingestion of certain drugs should be considered in the differential diagnosis. Examples include: amphetamines, ephedrine, pseudoephedrine, isoproterenol, and phenylpropanolamine. Cocaine, PCP (phencyclidine) and LSD (lysergic acid diethylamide) also lead to excess catecholamine levels. Patients with pheochromocytoma may be mistaken as having panic attacks, hypoglycemic episodes, or accelerated hypertension from other causes of secondary hypertension. Finally, disorders such as mastocytosis and carcinoid in which patients have spells or unusual symptoms, may mimic pheochromocytoma.[31–33]

Most pheochromocytomas are sporadic, but 10% occur within a familial disorder such as multiple endocrine neoplasia type 2A or 2B (MEN 2A or MEN 2B), Von Hippel–Lindau disease, or neurofibromatosis. The MEN syndromes and Von Hippel–Lindau disease have an autosomal dominance pattern of inheritance, with age-related penetrance. When occurring in the setting of a familial disorder, pheochromocytomas are usually intra-adrenal and often bilateral. In one series, up to 83% of the patients with familial pheochromocytoma had bilateral tumors.[34] In MEN 2A, approximately 50% of the patients have pheochromocytoma, usually presenting at a younger age. The mean age of familial pheochromocytoma was 38 ± 11 years, compared to patients with sporadic pheochromocytoma, who were 47 ± 16 years of age.[34] The clinical presentation may vary as well. Sporadic cases usually present with hypertension, whereas most patients with a familial syndrome are often diagnosed by biochemical testing before hypertension is noted.[35] Presumptive treatment of pheochromocytoma in MEN 2 is controversial. At present, prophylactic adrenalectomy is not recommended.

With the relative infrequency of pheochromocytoma, it is important for a physician to know when it is appropriate to screen for the disorder. We feel that the following are reasonable indications for screening:

1. hypertension in association with symptoms suggesting pheochromocytoma.
2. marked lability of blood pressure.
3. refractory hypertension.
4. severe pressor response in anesthesia, surgery, or angiography.
5. unexplained circulatory shock during anesthesia, surgery or pregnancy.
6. family history of pheochromocytoma, or familial disorder such as MEN 2, Von Hippel-Lindau disease neurofibromatosis.
7. all patients with incidentally-discovered adrenal masses.

Biochemical measurement

When clinical suspicion exists, the diagnosis is made with demonstration of elevated circulating or urinary catecholamines or metabolites (Figure 16.3). The methods for screening include: (1) 24-h urine collection for excretion of unmetabolized or free catecholamines—E and NE or catecholamine metabolites metanephrine and normetanephrine, and vanillylmandelic acid; or (2) plasma catecholamines. Of the different metabolites measured in a 24-h urine collection, metanephrines are the most sensitive and specific.[36] When the upper limit of normal for metanephrines is 1.3 mg/24 h, a value greater than 2.3 mg/24 h is usually considered diagnostic for pheochromocytoma (Table 16.1). When collecting 24-h urines, it is important to measure creatinine to verify adequacy of collection, and to add a strong acid (such as 6 M HCl) to a sealed container. When testing for plasma catecholamines, the patient should be fasted overnight and lying comfortably in a supine position with a heparin lock for withdrawing blood, inserted 20–30 min before the collection.

As pheochromocytomas are heterogeneous in their hormone metabolism and secretion, there is no single best test for screening and there is disagreement on the optimum test. For example, with episodic secretion and the short half-life of catecholamines, random plasma assays may miss the peak catecholamine levels. Conversely, plasma levels are useful particularly when collected during an episode. Twenty-four-hour urine collection has the advantage of integrating secretion over time, but is more cumbersome for patients. Urinary metanephrine-to-creatinine ratio can be used as a method to attempt to compensate for overcollection (false-positives) or undercollection (false-negatives).[36] The overnight measurements of urine

Test	Normal levels	Diagnostic levels	Sensitivity	Specificity
Plasma NE	<500 pg/ml	>2000 pg/ml	58–85%	88–99%
Plasma E	<100 pg/ml	>400 pg/ml	33–62%	79–94%
Plasma NE + E			85%	97%
Urine collections:				
NE + E		1.5–2-fold elevated	85–100%	72–99.5%
NMET + MET		>1.8 mg/24 h 1.5–2-fold elevated	97–100%	84–98%
VMA		>11.0 mg/24 h 1.5–2-fold elevated	64–90%	87–98%

NE, norepinephrine; E, epinephrine; MET, metanephrine; NMET, normetanephrine; VMA, vanillylmandelic acid.

From Werbel and Ober with minor modifications (with permission).[32]

Table 16.1
Sensitivity and specificity of biochemical measurements for pheochromocytoma.

catecholamines, especially NE, may also be useful in diagnosing pheochromocytoma.[37]

A plasma catecholamine level greater than 2000 pg/ml is diagnostic for pheochromocytoma (Figure 16.3). Levels between 1000 and 2000 pg/ml fall in a gray zone. In this situation, a clonidine suppression test can be done.[38] Clonidine is a centrally acting α_2 adrenoceptor agonist which normally suppresses the release of catecholamines from neurons. The autonomous release of catecholamines from the tumor is not affected. Plasma catecholamines are checked before and 3 h after oral administration of 0.3 mg of clonidine. In patients without pheochromocytoma, levels drop below 500 pg/ml. To avoid hypotension, the patient should not be on diuretics, to avoid hypovolemia. Tricyclic antidepressants, β-blockers and all antihypertensives should be withheld for 12 h before the test. With these adjustments, the test is considered safe.[30]

If the plasma levels are below 1000 pg/ml and there is a strong clinical suspicion, a glucagon stimulation test can be performed (Figure 16.3).[39] The glucagon stimulation is performed by measurement of baseline plasma catecholamine levels compared to plasma levels determined 2 min after the administration of 1 mg of glucagon intravenously. Patients with pheochromocytoma have a three-fold increase in plasma catecholamine levels or demonstrate values greater than 2000 pg/ml. Pretreatment with α-blockers (such as prazosin) or a calcium channel blocker (such as nifedipine) does not interfere with the assay results.[30] The glucagon test has high specificity (100%) but low sensitivity (81%). The clonidine test has high sensitivity (97%) and low specificity (67%). If both tests are negative, the diagnosis of pheochromocytoma may be excluded.[39]

Plasma metanephrines are considered by some to be more accurate than plasma catecholamines in the diagnosis of pheochromocytoma. This may reflect the fact that pheochromocytomas primarily secrete metabolized catecholamines. Measurement of free metanephrines is probably more useful than measurement of the conjugated form, as that is the compound produced by the chromaffin cells.[40] However, this test is not widely available and experience is limited.

We recommend the use of 24 h collection for catecholamines and metanephrines in the initial evaluation of a patient with suspected pheochromocytoma. If the results are equivocal, plasma catecholamines may be needed to confirm the diagnosis. If the plasma catecholamine levels are increased but not diagnostic (in the gray zone of 1000–2000 pg/ml), a clonidine suppression test is useful. If, on the other hand, plasma catecholamines are low and clinical suspicion is great, a glucagon stimulation test is performed. Plasma metanephrines may also be helpful at this point.

Small adrenal pheochromocytomas often secrete E predominantly, whereas larger tumors tend to secrete predominantly NE.[33] The latter pattern may exist because the larger tumors outgrow the corticomedullary

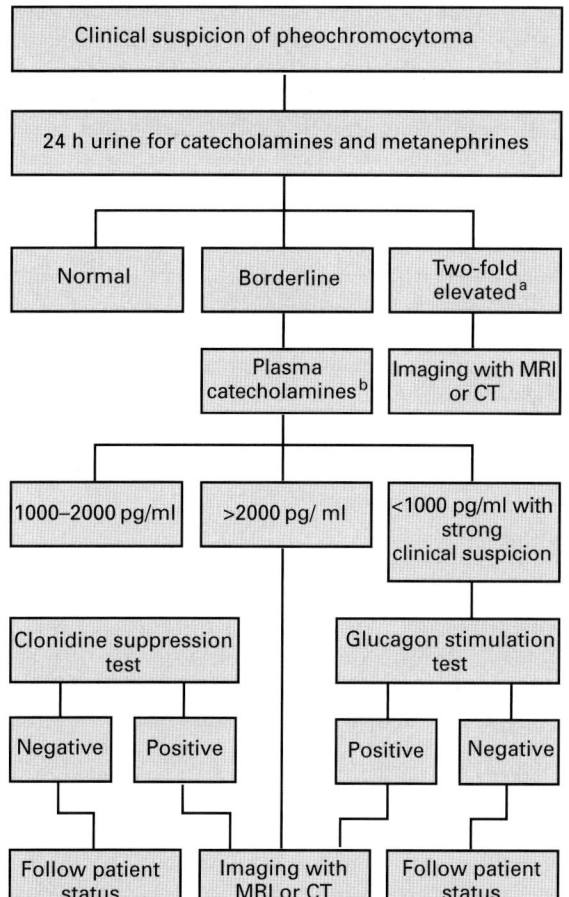

Figure 16.3
Algorithm for diagnosis of pheochromocytoma.
[a]See Table 16.1. [b]Recumbent levels (see text for details).

blood supply and therefore are not exposed to local, high concentrations of glucocorticoids. Glucocorticoids regulate the activity of PNMT, which converts NE to E. Therefore, if there is a predominance of E production, this is probably due to a small intra-adrenal tumor. There is also greater metabolism of catecholamines to metanephrines in large tumors compared to smaller ones.

There are a few areas of caution in interpreting catecholamine or metanephrine values. Radiocontrast dyes, for example, may interfere with some biochemical determinations. Certain drugs, such as labetalol, may cause false-positive results when catecholamines are measured using fluorometric methods of analysis or metanephrines using spectrophotometric methods.[41] Measurements of urinary free catecholamines may also be falsely elevated in labetalol-taking subjects using radioenzymatic assays. Tricyclic antidepressants, compazine, reserpine, clonidine and clofibrate have also been reported to interfere with results of some urinary catecholamine and metabolite measurements.[42,43] In general, such drugs should be discontinued 4–7 days before collection. Blood pressure should be controlled with medications that do not interfere with the assays, such as calcium channel blockers. To better provide resolution against interfering substances, our recommendation is to use the reverse-phase HPLC method and multiple electrochemical detectors. A future direction is to measure these compounds by mass spectroscopy, which should totally eliminate the problem of interfering substances. Stress from myocardial infarction, cerebral vascular accidents or other grave illnesses will cause elevation in catecholamine levels. In renal insufficiency, urinary collections should be expressed in milligrams of creatinine; plasma levels may be falsely elevated in renal failure.[44] In such circumstances, other diagnostic tests, including imaging, are needed for evaluation. It must be kept in mind that catecholamines and metanephrines are not specific markers of pheochromocytoma, but it is the magnitude of the elevation[5] that is diagnostic (see Table 16.1).

Imaging techniques

After a biochemical diagnosis is made, imaging techniques are used to locate the tumor(s). Pheochromocytomas are usually large (2–5 cm in diameter) and may have areas of hemorrhage or necrosis. Patients with MEN syndromes have tumors which tend to be smaller and bilateral.[45] Approximately 98% of pheochromocytomas are located within the abdomen, and 90% are located within adrenal tissue, but pheochromocytomas may occur anywhere within the autonomic nervous system, such as posterior mediastinum, pericardium, or bladder. These tumors may be localized by MRI, CT, MIBG (iodine-labeled meta-iodobenzyl guanidine) or octreotide scintigraphy. Most intra-adrenal tumors are easily imaged by CT or MRI. Although MRI may have greater accuracy, imaging with CT has a sensitivity between 93% and 100%. Contrast agents are not needed to visualize these tumors, due to their size, and, in fact, may precipitate a hypertensive crisis.

MRI is particularly useful for identifying paragangliomas, especially outside of the abdomen, such as intracardiac tumors. On T2–weighted imaging, the tumor is usually three times as intense as liver, and on T1-weighted images, the tumor is usually iso-intense with the liver. With gadolinium-DTPA, the tumors appear hypervascular.[45] However, these general characteristics are not always present, and the pheochromocytomas may appear indistinguishable from other adrenal tumors.

MIBG has chemical similarities to NE and therefore concentrates within intracellular storage granules of catecholamine-secreting tissues.[46] Imaging with MIBG is especially useful for localization of extra-adrenal pheochromocytomas and for postoperative confirmation of tumor resection.[47] Its sensitivity is reported to be greater than 90%, with a specificity of 100%.[46,48] MIBG is labeled with ^{123}I or ^{131}I; the former isotope is considered to provide greater sensitivity. Thyroid uptake should be blocked with iodine prior to administration of the iodine-labeled MIBG. Medicines which might interfere with catecholamine processing should be discontinued 72 h before MIBG evaluation. For example, tricyclic antidepressants or phenylpropanolamine inhibit uptake, and sympathomimetics (cocaine, labetalol or reserpine) deplete the storage vesicle contents. Medications which block adrenergic receptors, such as atypical antidepressants, phenothiazines and butyrophenones, may give false-negative results.[49]

Somatostatin receptors are normally expressed in adrenomedullary and paraganglionic tissues.[50] Somatostatin receptor density is increased on pheochromocytoma tissue, making octreotide, a somatostatin analog, useful in its detection. Octreotide is labeled with ^{111}In-DTPA. Like MIBG, octreotide scanning is most often used for detection of extra-adrenal pheochromocytoma and in the detection of metastases in cases of malignant pheochromocytoma.[51] A positive uptake by octreotide may also be a prognostic indicator as well as offering a therapeutic modality.

Finally, if an adrenal mass is suspicious for pheochromocytoma, and the biochemical tests are not confirmatory, venous sampling may be required. The sampling effluent E/NE ratio is normally 4:1, and higher ratios or reversal of the ratios are suggestive of pheochromocytoma.[52]

Surgical management (Table 16.2)

Although surgery is the therapy of choice, it has a morbidity as high as 40%, with a mortality of 2–4%.[32] Preoperative treatment with α-adrenergic blockers and volume expansion have improved surgical outcomes.[53] Volume expansion should be achieved by a high (150–200 mmol) sodium diet unless contraindicated (e.g. renal insufficiency, congestive heart failure). Traditionally, phenoxybenzamine, a non-competitive α-blocker, is titrated to reduce blood pressure to normal levels and/or to orthostasis. The starting dose is 10 mg daily, and most patients require 80–100 mg in divided doses. Pretreatment with this medication affords intraoperative blood pressure stability by blocking the receptors where catecholamines bind, minimizing the chances

---

5 Days prior to surgery
Initiate high sodium (150–200 mmol) diet; continue phenoxybenzamine administration; check daily weights and vital signs. May need to admit for volume expansion with intravenous saline

1 Day prior to surgery
Transfer to a monitored intensive care unit. Place arterial and Swan-Ganz catheters. Administer isotonic saline to achieve pulmonary capillary wedge pressure (PCWP) greater than 10 mmHg. If SVR (systemic vascular resistance) is greater than 1000 mmHg, start intravenous sodium nitroprusside at 50 mg/min, increasing as needed to 500–1000 mg/min.

Day of surgery
Ensure that patient has two separate intravenous lines: one for possible administration of pressors, and the other for administration of vasodilators. Have available sodium nitroprusside, esmolol, epinephrine and norepinephrine infusions

Table 16.2
Preparation of the patient for surgery.

of hypertensive crisis during intubation, induction with anesthesia, exploration or tumor manipulation. It has been suggested that a non-competitive α-blocker may be better than a competitive inhibitor, because the catecholamine levels, which may be as much as 500 times normal, would overcome a competitive inhibitor.[53] However, phenoxybenzamine's prolonged half-life of 24 h may lead to postoperative hypotension. In addition, complete α-blockade might mask the dramatic fall in blood pressure after tumor resection, which helps the surgeon know that the pheochromocytoma is completely resected.[54] Labetalol, which has an α/β blocking ratio of 1:3 in its oral form, may not be ideal for preparation prior to surgery. The α-blockade is considered weaker than that of phenoxybenzamine and, with the large catecholamine release from manipulation of the tumor, marked hypertension could result. Some have found that additional intraoperative vasodilators were needed to control blood pressure in labetalol-pretreated subjects.[55] The selective α_1 inhibitor, doxazosin, has been shown to be effective in pretreating patients with pheochromocytoma without inducing tachycardia or serious side-effects.[56] Calcium channel blockers, in particular nicardipine from the dihydropyridine group, are increasing in popularity as they seem to stabilize intraoperative systemic vascular resistance (SVR). The proposed benefit comes from their blunting catecholamine-mediated arterial vasoconstriction during tumor manipulation.[57] Improved hemodynamic monitoring during surgery as well as newer intravenous fast-acting vasodilators and β-blockers (such as sodium nitroprusside and esmolol, respectively) and intravenous vasoconstrictors (such as NE or E) have improved surgical outcome.

Tradition and experience have also guided the length of preoperative therapy. Patients are usually treated for 10–14 days, although this length of therapy has not consistently shown improved operative and postoperative outcomes.[53] Unfortunately, there are no consistent features that predict a smooth surgical course, and each patient must be assessed individually when selecting antihypertensive medicines.

The surgical approach depends on the clinical situation. In patients with familial pheochromocytoma, the surgeon may elect to perform a transabdominal incision. When removing a solitary tumor, the flank approach offers reduced blood loss. Although still controversial, some surgeons are gaining experience with laparoscopic adrenalectomy when the tumor is less than 6 cm in size.[58,59] Patients with pheochromocytoma should be referred to a surgeon who has experience with this disorder and who works with anesthesiologists equally experienced in management of pheochromocytoma.

Intraoperative hypotension is treated first with volume expansion, and then with intravenous pressor agents if required. Postoperative hypoglycemia, possibly from reactive hyperinsulinemia, should be anticipated and warrants the routine screening of blood glucose levels in the early postoperative hours.[60]

Once surgery is performed, the catecholamine levels usually return to normal in approximately 2 weeks. If hypertension persists in the setting of normal catecholamine levels, and surgical causes such as inadvertent ligation of the renal artery are excluded, essential hypertension may be the etiology. The Mayo Clinic experience demonstrated that 20% of patients with postoperative hypertension also had essential hypertension.[29]

After surgery, all patients should be followed indefinitely with annual biochemical evaluation and chromogranin A levels. Risk factors for the appearance of another of pheochromocytoma include a familial history of pheochromocytoma, a low ratio of E to total catecholamine, and the presence of large extra-adrenal or bilateral tumors.

Three to thirteen per cent of all pheochromocytomas are malignant, with a 5-year survival rate of 23–44%, compared with a 97% 5-year survival in benign pheochromocytoma.[29,54,61] Tumors metastasize to the lungs or bone, and/or recur locally. Treatment primarily consists of controlling symptoms from excess catecholamines since such the response to chemotherapeutic agents has been disappointing. Although the response rate is suboptimal, the use of I^{131}-MIBG is increasing. Radioactive MIBG is also being used in combination with other chemotherapeutic agents such as vincristine, cyclophosphamide and decarbazine. There is also a palliative role for radiotherapy of bone metastases.

Thyroid hormone function and hypertension

Hypertension is associated with states of thyroid excess as well as deficiency. In hypothyroidism, the hypertension typically is characterized by a rise in diastolic blood pressure. In hyperthyroidism, systolic blood pressure is elevated and diastolic blood pressure is usually lowered, leading to a widened pulse pressure.

The prevalence of isolated systolic hypertension in hyperthyroidism is reported to be between 20% and 30%. This elevation of systolic blood pressure seen in young thyrotoxic patients almost invariably normalizes with treatment. The cardiac manifestations of hyperthyroidism are characterized by an increased heart rate, stroke volume, and cardiac output. There is also an increase in blood volume and a decrease in peripheral vascular resistance. Many of these cardiovascular findings in hyperthyroidism reflect increased activation of the sympathetic system. For example, there is increased heart rate, increased bloodflow to the skin, kidney, heart and muscles, increased body temperature, perspiration, and anxiety. Paradoxically, catecholamine concentrations have been found to be normal or decreased in hyperthyroidism.[62] Instead, there appears to be an increased sensitivity to catecholamines with increased density of β-adrenergic receptors. As a result of enhanced sympathetic activity, β-blockers are effective in decreasing blood pressure, heart rate and some of the neuropsychiatric symptoms that occur with hyperthyroidism. Definitive treatment is reversal of the hyperthyroid state.

It is unclear whether the renin–angiotensin system plays a role in the hypertension of thyroid dysfunction. Hyperthyroid patients have blunted aldosterone secretion and increased renin activity.[63] The total body potassium depletion and heightened adrenergic tone seen in hyperthyroidism may explain some of these findings. Conversely, plasma renin activity is low in hypothyroidism, and increases following thyroxine repletion.[64,65]

The reported prevalence of hypertension in hypothyroid patients is variable, ranging between 0% and 50%.[66] Of 4429 patients screened for secondary causes of hypertension, 3% were incidentally discovered to have primary hypothyroidism.[1] The majority of these subjects were adult women, probably reflecting the increased prevalence of autoimmune thyroiditis in this patient population. In another study, 32% of hypothyroid patients had a reversal of diastolic hypertension with discontinuation of antihypertensive treatment following normalization of thyroid status.[67]

In hypothyroidism, the cardiac manifestations are the converse of those seen in hyperthyroidism. Cardiac output, stroke volume and total blood volume are decreased, while systemic peripheral resistance is increased. Catecholamine levels are either increased or normal after correction for age.[62,68] Treatment for hypertension associated with hypothyroidism is thyroxine replacement, titrating dosage to bring the thyroid-stimulating hormone (TSH) level into the normal range. With advancing age and more longstanding hypertension, the blood pressure response to treatment of hypothyroidism decreases.[69] However, the reversal of hypertension in one-third of hypothyroid patients following treatment underscores the importance of routine screening of hypertensive adults, especially females, for primary hypothyroidism.

Hyperparathyroidism

Primary parathyroidism is a metabolic disorder of increased secretion of parathyroid hormone (PTH) from a parathyroid adenoma, or less commonly parathyroid hyperplasia.

Primary hyperparathyroidism is a common endocrine disorder, with a prevalence of 100 cases per 100 000 population.[70] The disorder usually presents in the fifth and sixth decades of life, with a female preponderance, although it may occur earlier in patients with MEN type 1 and 2A syndromes. Primary hyperparathyroidism occurs secondary to solitary adenoma (80%) or parathyroid hyperplasia (15–20%), or is due to double or multiple gland involvement (5%). The prevalence of hypertension associated with hyperparathyroidism varies from 25% to 70%, but in most studies exceeds the prevalence of essential hypertension in the general population (~20%).

The etiology of hypertension associated with primary hyperparathyroidism has been controversial.[71–74] Hypotheses include hypercalcemia-related renal parenchymal damage, increased vascular tone associated with hypercalcemia, abnormal activation of the renin–angiotensin system, increased activity of the sympathetic system from hypercalcemia, or increased blood pressure from chronically elevated parathyroid levels per se. Although parathyroidectomy typically reverses hypercalcemia, hypertension is not consistently improved. This supports the theory that several factors are likely to be involved in the hypertension associated with primary hyperparathyroidism.

PTH excess may cause hypertension via direct and indirect effects. The syndrome of pseudohypoparathyroidism is associated with an increased prevalence of hypertension (40%–50%).[75,76] In this disorder, PTH resistance is associated with elevated PTH levels, calciuresis, hypocalcemia and hyperphosphatemia, suggesting that PTH per se leads to hypertension. Although acute infusion of PTH leads to vasodilatation, chronic administration may cause vasoconstriction. When

PTH was infused over 12 days in healthy volunteers, reversible hypercalcemia and hypertension occurred.[77] Associated with the development of hypercalcemia and hypertension, there were transient and significant increases in urinary tetrahydroaldosterone excretion and plasma cortisol concentrations. No changes in potassium levels or renin activity were noted in this study. Shorter PTH infusions (1 h) demonstrated increases in plasma renin activity (PRA) without changes in serum ionized calcium, suggesting that PTH has direct effects on the juxtaglomerular apparatus.[78] In patients with essential hypertension, increased levels of PTH have been demonstrated. These elevations have been associated with decreased levels of ionized calcium with increased calciuresis, suggesting that elevated PTH may be compensatory.[79]

Although there is controversy in the literature, PTH has also been hypothesized by some investigators to have direct effects in increasing renin secretion and/or causing a heightened vascular reaction to pressor agents. Elevated levels of PRA and PAC have been observed in hypertensive patients who have primary hyperparathyroidism; following parathyroidectomy, PRA and PAC levels decreased in most of these hypertensive patients.[80]

Some studies demonstrate that in hypertensive hyperparathyroid patients, aldosterone and blood pressure responses to angiotensin II infusions are greater than in normotensive patients. These heightened responses normalized post-parathyroidectomy.[81] The fact that there were differences between the normotensive and hypertensive hyperparathyroid patients suggests that other factors aside from calcium levels may play a role in modulating vasoconstrictive response to angiotensin II. Other authors have found no abnormalities in the renin–angiotensin system in patients with hyperparathyroidism.[82,83]

NE infusions in hypertensive patients with primary hyperparathyroidism are associated with enhanced pressor responsiveness compared to normotensive hyperparathyroid patients and controls. These abnormal pressor responses corrected after parathyroidectomy.[80] There is experimental evidence that release of catecholamines is calcium-dependent.[84] Calcium infusions in hypertensive hyperparathyroid patients led to more marked pressor changes compared to normotensive patients.[85] These correlations suggest a role of hypercalcemia per se and possibly other factors which enhance sympathetic activation or responsiveness to catecholamines. In these hypertensive patients, levels of NE and E and their metabolites were found to be higher when compared to normotensive patients following calcium infusion.

Dietary calcium has also been shown to correlate with blood pressure. For example, a high-calcium diet has been shown to lower blood pressure in normocalcemic hypertensive subjects.[86] Intracellular calcium levels measured in platelets were found to be higher in normotensive hyperparathyroid patients than in hypertensive hyperparathyroid patients, but lower than in patients with essential hypertension.[71] Hypomagnesemia and hypophosphatemia have also been positively correlated with hypertension in patients with hyperparathyroidism.[73]

In summary, while the prevalence of hypertension in primary hyperthyroidism exceeds that seen in the general population, the pathogenesis of hypertension in primary hyperparathyroidism remains unclear. There is also no consensus on the appropriate recommendations for dietary sodium or calcium intake in such patients. A low-calcium diet might stimulate further secretion of PTH, whereas a high-calcium diet might theoretically increase the hypercalcemia. However, since many patients with primary hyperparathyroidism also have essential hypertension, it is important not to counsel the patient that the hypertension will be reversed after surgical cure. In fact, hypertension is not considered a primary indication for surgery in patients with mild asymptomatic primary hyperparathyroidism.[87]

Acromegaly

Hypertension is present in 25–50% of patients with acromegaly, which is at least a 3–4-fold increase in prevalence over the general population.[88–90] Hypertension is usually mild to moderate, and treatment of acromegaly improves the hypertension. Ambulatory blood pressure monitoring has demonstrated an increased frequency (44%) of diastolic hypertension (>81 mmHg) compared with a 19% frequency of systolic hypertension (>132 mmHg).[91] In addition, a blunted nocturnal fall in blood pressure is a feature of acromegaly.[91]

Cardiovascular events are the leading cause of mortality in acromegaly, and hypertension is one factor contributing to this increased mortality.[92] An association between blood pressure and target-organ damage has not consistently been shown, since some patients with left ventricular hypertrophy had no history of hypertension.[89] Increased left ventricular mass and stroke volume may precede the development of hypertension, and acromegalic cardiomyopathy may lead to hypertension.[93]

However, left ventricular mass index is greater in hypertensive than in normotensive acromegalics.[94]

The etiology of hypertension in acromegaly remains unclear, but a leading possibility is volume expansion, since exchangeable sodium (Na_E) is increased in both normotensive and hypertensive acromegalics after adjusting for body mass index.[95,96] Increased renal sodium reabsorption is considered to be an action of growth hormone. Growth hormone infusions in human subjects cause increased sodium and water retention, and edema is a clearcut complication of treatment of growth hormone-deficient hypopituitary patients.[97] Leukocyte oubain-sensitive sodium pump activity, a model of epithelial sodium transport, is increased in acromegalic subjects compared to normal controls. After treatment, this increased pump activity normalizes.[98] There is also direct in vitro evidence of an effect of growth hormone on the leukocyte sodium pump activity, and indirect evidence that pump activity correlates with fasting plasma insulin levels.[98]

Hyperinsulinemia and insulin resistance are cardinal features of acromegaly and may play a role in volume expansion, as insulin is known to increase renal sodium reabsorption.[99–101] Fasting hyperinsulinemia and a hyperinsulinemic response to glucose loading is the rule in acromegalic patients.[100] Thus, hyperinsulinemia is considered to be a mechanism that contributes to the volume expansion seen in acromegaly. Whether growth hormone per se or insulin or both underlie the well-documented volume expansion, sodium retention is seen both in normotensive and hypertensive acromegalics. It is unclear whether the hypertensive subset reflects a greater degree of volume expansion or whether other factors, such as genetic predisposition to hypertension, contribute to the elevation of blood pressure, or both.

Volume expansion in acromegaly would be expected to be associated with reduced activity of the renin–angiotensin–aldosterone system and increased atrial natriuretic peptide (ANP) levels. Several studies have documented a suppressed plasma renin activity and a blunted aldosterone response to sodium restriction in hypertensive acromegalics,[102,103] while others have not corroborated these findings.[104,105] ANP levels in hypertensive acromegalic patients are either normal or elevated.

There is evidence that the dopaminergic control of aldosterone secretion is altered in hypertensive patients with acromegaly. For example, infusion of metoclopramide, a dopaminergic DA_2 receptor antagonist, induces an increase of plasma aldosterone in normal subjects but does not cause a rise in acromegalic patients. This abnormality in the regulation of aldosterone secretion in acromegaly could reflect an alteration in the natriuretic dopamine axis. Finally, growth hormone-producing pituitary neoplasms are a feature of the MEN 1 syndrome which can also be associated with an increased incidence of adrenal neoplasms, such as adrenocortical tumors and pheochromocytoma.

Treatment of hypertension in acromegaly remains empirical, as no randomized studies have been performed. Logically, diuretics could be considered as first-line agents to treat this volume-expanded condition. The clinician is cautioned to have a high index of suspicion for secondary hypertensive disorders in acromegalics, such as renovascular hypertension and primary aldosteronism, especially in patients with refractory or severe hypertension.

Cushing's syndrome

Cushing's syndrome results from glucocorticoid excess (usually hypercortisolism). The diagnosis is established by the measurement of increased cortisol production or the demonstration of autonomy of secretion (i.e. failure to suppress cortisol levels when exogenous glucocorticoids are given). The etiologies of Cushing's syndrome can be divided into three types: ACTH dependent (pituitary or ectopic), ACTH independent (adrenal adenoma or carcinoma), and iatrogenic.

Regardless of etiology, approximately three-quarters of patients with Cushing's syndrome have arterial hypertension. Typically, hypertension is mild, but in several series 15% of patients with Cushing's syndrome had blood pressures greater than 200/120 mmHg.[106] The prevalence of elevated blood pressure is substantially lower (5–25%) with exogenous glucocorticoid intake versus endogenous glucocorticoid excess. Although essential hypertension is common in the general population, signs of glucocorticoid excess should be sought, especially in young hypertensive subjects.

The cause of hypertension in Cushing's syndrome is multifactorial and may also vary according to etiology. There are two theories regarding the pathogenesis of hypertension in Cushing's syndrome: increased cardiac output and elevated peripheral vascular resistance. One is not mutually exclusive of the other. In ACTH-dependent etiologies and in adrenal carcinoma, mineralocorticoids, such as deoxycorticosterone, may be overproduced, resulting in sodium retention and volume expansion. However, in glucocorticoid-mediated hypertension, elevated blood pressure can result even if sodium intake is restricted.[107] A marked increase in cortisol production, as in ectopic ACTH syndrome and adrenal carcinoma, may exceed the capacity of the 11β-hydroxysteroid dehydrogenase (11β-HSD) enzyme, which converts cortisol to the inactive cortisone. As a result, cortisol binds to mineralocortocoid receptors, causing increased sodium and fluid retention, extracellular fluid volume expansion, increased cardiac output and hypertension. Other studies have found that glucocorticoids produce a fluid shift from the intracellular to the extracellular compartment, resulting in increased plasma volume.[108] Enhanced activation of the sympathetic system secondary to glucocorticoid-mediated increased activity of PNMT could result in excess E production and increased cardiac output. In addition, Ritchie et al have reported increased cardiac sensitivity to infused catecholamines, which they concluded was not related to β-adrenoreceptor density but steroid-induced enhancement of receptor coupling.[109]

Regarding enhanced peripheral vascular resistance, both increased vasoconstrictor and reduced vasodilator activities have been reported. Studies have found normal or reduced levels of plasma renin activity in patients with Cushing's syndrome. Glucocorticoids increase production of angiotensinogen within hepatic cells, which should result in increased angiotensin II levels due to the kinetics of the renin–substrate reaction.[110] Another hypothesis is that the increased tissue production of angiotensin II leads to blood pressure elevation. It has been reported that the production of the protein, macrocortin, which inhibits phospholipase A2 activity, leads to decreased vasodilatory activity by reduction in vasodilator prostaglandins.[111] Finally, enhanced vasoconstrictor responsiveness to vasopressors has been inconsistently noted.

Early detection of Cushing's syndrome has important consequences for the patient, since hypertension is often associated with lipid abnormalities and diabetes mellitus, which synergistically lead to greatly increased cardiovascular risk. Accordingly, the clinician should have a high index of suspicion for this disorder in hypertensive patients. While the treatment of hypertension in Cushing's syndrome is largely empirical, clinicians have usually found good responses to interruption of the renin–angiotensin system in combination with diuretics. In certain situations, such as the ectopic ACTH syndrome, where there is a prominent mineralocorticoid action, mineralocorticoid antagonists have been used with gratifying results.

References

1. Anderson GH Jr, Blakeman N, Streeten DH. The effect of age on prevalence of secondary forms of hypertension in 4429 consecutively referred patients. *J Hypertens* 1994; 12(5): 609–15.
2. Gordon RD. Mineralocorticoid hypertension. *Lancet* 1994; 344(8917): 240–3.
3. Hiramatsu K, Yamada T, Yukimura Y et al. A screening test to identify aldosterone-producing adenoma by measuring plasma renin activity. Results in hypertensive patients. *Arch Intern Med* 1981; 141(12): 1589–93.
4. Young WF Jr, Hogan MJ, Klee GG, Grant CS, van Heerden JA. Primary aldosteronism: diagnosis and treatment. *Mayo Clin Proc* 1990; 65(1): 96–110.
5. Lim PO, Rodgers P, Cardale K, Watson AD, MacDonald TM. Potentially high prevalence of primary aldosteronism in a primary-care population. *Lancet* 1999; 353(9146): 40.
6. Ganguly A. Primary aldosteronism. *N Engl J Med* 1998; 339(25): 1828–34.
7. Litchfield WR, Dluhy RG. Primary aldosteronism. *Endocrinol Metab Clin North Am* 1995; 24(3): 593–612.
8. Young M, Fullerton M, Dilley R, Funder J. Mineralocorticoids, hypertension, and cardiac fibrosis. *J Clin Invest* 1994; 93(6): 2578–83.
9. Brilla CG, Matsubara LS, Weber KT. Antifibrotic effects of spironolactone in preventing myocardial fibrosis in systemic arterial hypertension. *Am J Cardiol* 1993; 71(3): 12A–16A.
10. Rocha R, Chander PN, Zuckerman A, Stier CT Jr. Role of aldosterone in renal vascular injury in stroke-prone hypertensive rats. *Hypertension* 1999; 33(1 Pt 2): 232–7.
11. Melby JC. Primary aldosteronism. *Kidney Int* 1984; 26(5): 769–78.
12. Sheaves R, Goldin J, Reznek RH et al. Relative value of computed tomography scanning and venous sampling in establishing the cause of primary hyperaldosteronism. *Eur J Endocrinol* 1996; 134(3): 308–13.
13. Gordon RD. Primary aldosteronism. *J Endocrinol Invest* 1995; 18(7): 495–511.
14. Biglieri EG, Kater CE. Steroid characteristics of mineralocorticoid adrenocortical hypertension. *Clin Chem* 1991; 37(10 Pt 2): 1843–8.
15. Litchfield WR, Dluhy RG, Lifton RP, Rich GM. Glucocorticoid-remediable aldosteronism. *Comp Ther* 1995; 21(10): 553–8.
16. Lifton RP, Dluhy RG, Powers M et al. Hereditary hypertension caused by chimaeric gene duplications and ectopic expression of aldosterone synthase. *Natural Genet* 1992; 2(1): 66–74.
17. Williams GH, Dluhy RG. Glucocorticoid-remediable aldosteronism. *J Endocrinol Invest* 1995; 18(7): 512–17.
18. Torpy DJ, Gordon RD, Lin JP et al. Familial hyperaldosteronism type II: description of a large kindred

19. and exclusion of the aldosterone synthase (CYP11B2) gene. *J Clin Endocrinol Metab* 1998; **83**(9): 3214–18.
19. Stowasser M, Gordon RD, Tunny TJ, Klemm SA, Finn WL, Krek AL. Familial hyperaldosteronism type II: five families with a new variety of primary aldosteronism. *Clin Exp Pharmacol Physiol* 1992; **19**(5): 319–22.
20. Weinberger MH, Fineberg NS. The diagnosis of primary aldosteronism and separation of two major subtypes. *Arch Intern Med* 1993; **153**(18): 2125–9.
21. Lyons DF, Kem DC, Brown RD, Hanson CS, Carollo ML. Single dose captopril as a diagnostic test for primary aldosteronism. *J Clin Endocrinol Metab* 1983; **57**(5): 892–6.
22. Naomi S, Iwaoka T, Umeda T et al. Clinical evaluation of the captopril screening test for primary aldosteronism. *Japan Health J* 1985; **26**(4): 549–56.
23. Young WF Jr, Stanson AW, Grant CS, Thompson GB, van Heerden JA. Primary aldosteronism: adrenal venous sampling. *Surgery* 1996; **120**(6): 913–19; discussion 919–20.
24. Blumenfeld JD, Sealey JE, Schlussel Y et al. Diagnosis and treatment of primary hyperaldosteronism. *Ann Intern Med* 1994; **121**(11): 877–85.
25. Griffing GT, Cole AG, Aurecchia SA, Sindler BH, Komanicky P, Melby JC. Amiloride in primary hyperaldosteronism. *Clin Pharmacol Ther* 1982; **31**(1): 56–61.
26. Beard CM, Sheps SG, Kurland LT, Carney JA, Lie JT. Occurrence of pheochromocytoma in Rochester, Minnesota, 1950 through 1979. *Mayo Clin Proc* 1983; **58**(12): 802–4.
27. Sutton MG, Sheps SG, Lie JT. Prevalence of clinically unsuspected pheochromocytoma. Review of a 50-year autopsy series. *Mayo Clin Proc* 1981; **56**(6): 354–60.
28. Bravo EL. Evolving concepts in the pathophysiology, diagnosis, and treatment of pheochromocytoma. *Endocrine Rev* 1994; **15**(3): 356–68.
29. Sheps SG, Jiang NS, Klee GG, van Heerden JA. Recent developments in the diagnosis and treatment of pheochromocytoma. *Mayo Clin Proc* 1990; **65**(1): 88–95.
30. Bravo EL. Pheochromocytoma: new concepts and future trends. *Kidney Int* 1991; **40**(3): 544–56.
31. Manger WM, Gifford RW Jr. Pheochromocytoma: current diagnosis and management. *Cleve Clin J Med* 1993; **60**(5): 365–78.
32. Werbel SS, Ober KP. Pheochromocytoma. Update on diagnosis, localization, and management. *Med Clin North Am* 1995; **79**(1): 131–53.
33. Bouloux PG, Fakeeh M. Investigation of phaeochromocytoma. *Clin Endocrinol (Oxf)* 1995; **43**(6): 657–64.
34. Mulligan LM, Ponder BA. Genetic basis of endocrine disease: multiple endocrine neoplasia type 2. *J Clin Endocrinol Metab* 1995; **80**(7): 1989–95.
35. Pomares FJ, Canas R, Rodriguez JM, Hernandez AM, Parrilla P, Tebar FJ. Differences between sporadic and multiple endocrine neoplasia type 2A phaeochromocytoma. *Clin Endocrinol (Oxf)* 1998; **48**(2): 195–200.
36. Heron E, Chatellier G, Billaud E, Foos E, Plouin F. The urinary metanephrine-to-creatinine ratio for the diagnosis of pheochromocytoma. *Ann Intern Med* 1996; **125**(4): 300–3.
37. Peaston RT, Lennard TW, Lai LC. Overnight excretion of urinary catecholamines and metabolites in the detection of pheochromocytoma. *J Clin Endocrinol Metab* 1996; **81**(4): 1378–84.
38. Sjoberg RJ, Simcic KJ, Kidd GS. The clonidine suppression test for pheochromocytoma. A review of its utility and pitfalls. *Arch Intern Med* 1992; **152**(6): 1193–7.
39. Grossman E, Goldstein DS, Hoffman A, Keiser HR. Glucagon and clonidine testing in the diagnosis of pheochromocytoma. *Hypertension* 1991; **17**(6 Pt 1): 733–41.
40. Lenders JW, Keiser HR, Goldstein DS et al. Plasma metanephrines in the diagnosis of pheochromocytoma. *Ann Intern Med* 1995; **123**(2): 101–9.
41. Feldman JM. Falsely elevated urinary excretion of catecholamines and metanephrines in patients receiving labetalol therapy. *J Clin Pharmacol* 1987; **27**(4): 288–92.
42. Young WF Jr. Pheochromocytoma and primary aldosteronism: diagnostic approaches. *Endocrinol Metab Clin North Am* 1997; **26**(4): 801–27.
43. Stein PP, Black HR. A simplified diagnostic approach to pheochromocytoma. A review of the literature and report of one institution's experience. *Medicine (Baltimore)* 1991; **70**(1): 46–66.
44. Juan D. Pheochromocytoma: clinical manifestations and diagnostic tests. *Urology* 1981; **17**(1): 1–12.
45. Korobkin M, Francis IR. Adrenal imaging. *Semin Ultrasound CT MR* 1995; **16**(4): 317–30.
46. Scott BA, Gatenby RA. Imaging advances in the diagnosis of endocrine neoplasia. *Curr Opin Oncol* 1998; **10**(1): 37–42.
47. Hanson MW, Feldman JM, Beam CA, Leight GS, Coleman RE. Iodine 131-labeled metaiodobenzylguanidine scintigraphy and biochemical analyses in suspected pheochromocytoma. *Arch Intern Med* 1991; **151**(7): 1397–402.
48. Lauriero F, Rubini G, D'Addabbo F, Rubini D, Schettini F, D'Addabbo A. I-131 MIBG scintigraphy of neuroectodermal tumors. Comparison between I-131 MIBG and In-111 DTPA-octreotide. *Clin Nucl Med* 1995; **20**(3): 243–9.
49. Bouloux PG, Fakeeh M. Investigation of phaeochromocytoma. *Clin Endocrinol (Oxf)* 1995; **43**(6): 657–64.
50. Kennedy JW, Dluhy RG. The biology and clinical relevance of somatostatin receptor scintigraphy in adrenal tumor management. *Yale J Biol Med* 1997; **70**(5–6): 565–75.

51. Tenenbaum F, Lumbroso J, Schlumberger M et al. Comparison of radiolabeled octreotide and meta-iodobenzylguanidine (MIBG) scintigraphy in malignant pheochromocytoma. *J Nucl Med* 1995; 36(1): 1–6.
52. Fonseca V, Bouloux PM. Phaeochromocytoma and paraganglioma. *Baillières Clin Endocrinol Metab* 1993; 7(2): 509–44.
53. Russell WJ, Metcalfe IR, Tonkin AL, Frewin DB. The preoperative management of phaeochromocytoma. *Anaesth Intensive Care* 1998; 26(2): 196–200.
54. Gifford RW Jr, Manger WM, Bravo EL. Pheochromocytoma. *Endocrinol Metab Clin North Am* 1994; 23(2): 387–404.
55. Russell WJ, Kaines AH, Hooper MJ, Frewin DB. Labetalol in the preoperative management of phaeochromocytoma. *Anaesth Intensive Care* 1982; 10(2): 160–3.
56. Miura Y, Yoshinaga K. Doxazosin: a newly developed, selective alpha 1-inhibitor in the management of patients with pheochromocytoma. *Am Heart J* 1988; 116(6 Pt 2): 1785–9.
57. Colson P, Ryckwaert F, Ribstein J, Mann C, Dareau S. Haemodynamic heterogeneity and treatment with the calcium channel blocker nicardipine during phaeochromocytoma surgery. *Acta Anaesthesiol Scand* 1998; 42(9): 1114–19.
58. Winfield HN, Hamilton BD, Bravo EL, Novick AC. Laparoscopic adrenalectomy: the preferred choice? A comparison to open adrenalectomy. *J Urol* 1998; 160(2): 325–9.
59. Suzuki K, Kageyama S, Ueda D et al. Laparoscopic adrenalectomy: clinical experience with 12 cases. *J Urol* 1993; 150(4): 1099–102.
60. Reynolds C, Wilkins GE, Schmidt N, Doll WA, Blix PM. Hyperinsulinism after removal of a pheochromocytoma. *Can Med Assoc J* 1983; 129(4): 349–53.
61. Plouin PF, Chatellier G, Fofol I, Corvol P. Tumor recurrence and hypertension persistence after successful pheochromocytoma operation. *Hypertension* 1997; 29(5): 1133–9.
62. Coulombe P, Dussault JH, Walker P. Plasma catecholamine concentrations in hyperthyroidism and hypothyroidism. *Metabolism* 1976; 25(9): 973–9.
63. Cain JP, Dluhy RG, Williams GH, Selenkow HA, Milech A, Richmond S. Control of aldosterone secretion in hyperthyroidism. *J Clin Endocrinol Metab* 1973; 36(2): 365–71.
64. Resnick LM, Laragh JH. Plasma renin activity in syndromes of thyroid hormone excess and deficiency. *Life Sci* 1982; 30(7–8): 585–6.
65. Hauger-Klevene JH, Brown H, Zavaleta J. Plasma renin activity in hyper- and hypothyroidism: effect of adrenergic blocking agents. *J Clin Endocrinol Metab* 1972; 34(4): 625–9.
66. Saito I, Saruta T. Hypertension in thyroid disorders. *Endocrinol Metab Clin North Am* 1994; 23(2): 379–86.
67. Streeten DH, Anderson GH Jr, Howland T, Chiang R, Smulyan H. Effects of thyroid function on blood pressure. Recognition of hypothyroid hypertension. *Hypertension* 1988; 11(1): 78–83.
68. Christensen NJ. Increased levels of plasma noradrenaline in hypothyroidism. *J Clin Endocrinol Metab* 1972; 35(3): 359–63.
69. Klein I. Thyroid hormone and the cardiovascular system. *Am J Med* 1990; 88(6): 631–7.
70. al Zahrani A, Levine MA. Primary hyperparathyroidism. *Lancet* 1997; 349(9060): 1233–8.
71. Fardella C, Rodriguez-Portales JA. Intracellular calcium and blood pressure: comparison between primary hyperparathyroidism and essential hypertension. *J Endocrinol Invest* 1995; 18(11): 827–32.
72. Maheswaran R, Beevers DG. Clinical correlates in parathyroid hypertension. *J Hypertens Suppl* 1989; 7(6): S190–1.
73. Sangal AK, Kevwitch M, Rao DS, Rival J. Hypomagnesemia and hypertension in primary hyperparathyroidism. *South Med J* 1989; 82(9): 1116–18.
74. Lind L, Ljunghall S. Parathyroid hormone and blood pressure—is there a relationship? *Nephrol Dial Transplant* 1995; 10(4): 450–1.
75. Sowers JR, Tuck ML. Hypertension associated with diabetes mellitus, hypercalcaemic disorders, acromegaly and thyroid disease. *Clin Endocrinol Metab* 1981; 10(3): 631–56.
76. Sowers JR, Brickman AS. Circadian blood pressure and renin, aldosterone, cortisol, and prolactin levels in hypertensive pseudohypoparathyroid patients. *J Clin Endocrinol Metab* 1982; 55(6): 1202–8.
77. Hulter HN, Melby JC, Peterson JC, Cooke CR. Chronic continuous PTH infusion results in hypertension in normal subjects. *J Clin Hypertens* 1986; 2(4): 360–70.
78. Grant FD, Mandel SJ, Brown EM, Williams GH, Seely EW. Interrelationships between the renin–angiotensin–aldosterone and calcium homeostatic systems. *J Clin Endocrinol Metab* 1992; 75(4): 988–92.
79. Hvarfner A, Bergstrom R, Morlin C, Wide L, Ljunghall S. Relationships between calcium metabolic indices and blood pressure in patients with essential hypertension as compared with a healthy population. *J Hypertens* 1987; 5(4): 451–6.
80. Gennari C, Nami R, Gonnelli S. Hypertension and primary hyperparathyroidism: the role of adrenergic and renin–angiotensin–aldosterone systems. *Miner Electrolyte Metab* 1995; 21(1–3): 77–81.
81. Fallo F, Rocco S, Pagotto U, Zangari M, Luisetto G, Mantero F. Aldosterone and pressor responses to angiotensin II in primary hyperparathyroidism. *J Hypertens Suppl* 1989; 7(6): S192–3.
82. Ganguly A, Weinberger MH, Passmore JM et al. The renin-angiotensin-aldosterone system and hyper-

83. Rodriguez-Portales JA, Fardella C. Primary hyperparathyroidism and hypertension: persistently abnormal pressor sensitivity in normotensive patients after surgical cure. *J Endocrinol Invest* 1994; **17**(5): 307–11.
84. Lane JD, Aprison MH. Calcium-dependent release of endogenous serotonin, dopamine and norepinephrine from nerve endings. *Life Sci* 1977; **20**(4): 665–71.
85. Vlachakis ND, Frederics R, Valasquez M, Alexander N, Singer F, Maronde RF. Sympathetic system function and vascular reactivity in hypercalcemic patients. *Hypertension* 1982; **4**(3): 452–8.
86. McCarron DA, Morris CD. Blood pressure response to oral calcium in persons with mild to moderate hypertension. A randomized, double-blind, placebo-controlled, crossover trial. *Ann Intern Med* 1985; **103**(6 Pt 1): 825–31.
87. NIH Conference. Diagnosis and management of asymptomatic primary hyperparathyroidism: consensus development conference statement. *Ann Intern Med* 1991; **114**(7): 593–7.
88. Balzer R, McCullugh EP. Hypertension in acromegaly. *Am J Med Sci* 1959; **237**: 449.
89. Molitch ME. Clinical manifestations of acromegaly. *Endocrinol Metab Clin North Am* 1992; **21**(3): 597–614.
90. Ezzat S, Forster MJ, Berchtold P, Redelmeier DA, Boerlin V, Harris AG. Acromegaly. Clinical and biochemical features in 500 patients. *Medicine (Baltimore)* 1994; **73**(5): 233–40.
91. Terzolo M, Matrella C, Boccuzzi A et al. Twenty-four hour profile of blood pressure in patients with acromegaly. Correlation with demographic, clinical and hormonal features. *J Endocrinol Invest* 1999; **22**(1): 48–54.
92. Wright AD, Hill DM, Lowy C, Fraser TR. Mortality in acromegaly. *Q J Med* 1970; **39**(153): 1–16.
93. Lopez-Velasco R, Escobar-Morreale HF, Vega B et al. Cardiac involvement in acromegaly: specific myocardiopathy or consequence of systemic hypertension? *J Clin Endocrinol Metab* 1997; **82**(4): 1047–53.
94. Lombardi G, Colao A, Ferone D et al. Cardiovascular aspects in acromegaly: effects of treatment. *Metabolism* 1996; **45**: 57–60.
95. Davies DL, Beastall GH, Connell JM, Fraser R, McCruden D, Teasdale GM. Body composition, blood pressure and the renin–angiotensin system in acromegaly before and after treatment. *J Hypertens Suppl* 1985; **3**(suppl 3): S413–15.
96. Snow MH, Piercy DA, Robson V, Wilkinson R. An investigation into the pathogenesis of hypertension in acromegaly. *Clin Sci Mol Med* 1977; **53**(1): 87–91.
97. Biglieri EG, Watlington CO, Forsham PH. Sodium retention with human growth hormone and its subfraction. *J Clin Endocrinol Metab* 1961; **21**: 361–370.
98. Ng LL, Evans DJ. Leucocyte sodium transport in acromegaly. *Clin Endocrinol (Oxf)* 1987; **26**(4): 471–80.
99. Ikeda T, Terasawa H, Ishimura M et al. Correlation between blood pressure and plasma insulin in acromegaly. *J Intern Med* 1993; **234**(1): 61–3.
100. Slowinska-Srzednicka J, Zgliczynski S, Soszynski P, Zgliczynski W, Jeske W. High blood pressure and hyperinsulinaemia in acromegaly and in obesity. *Clin Exp Hypertens (A)* 1989; **11**(3): 407–25.
101. Muggeo M, Bar RS, Roth J, Kahn CR, Gorden P. The insulin resistance of acromegaly: evidence for two alterations in the insulin receptor on circulating monocytes. *J Clin Endocrinol Metab* 1979; **48**(1): 17–25.
102. Cain JP, Williams GH, Dluhy RG. Plasma renin activity and aldosterone secretion in patients with acromegaly. *J Clin Endocrinol Metab* 1972; **34**(1): 73–81.
103. Karlberg BE, Ottosson AM. Acromegaly and hypertension: role of the renin–angiotensin–aldosterone system. *Acta Endocrinol (Copenh)* 1982; **100**(4): 581–7.
104. Ritchie CM, Sheridan B, Fraser R et al. Studies on the pathogenesis of hypertension in Cushing's disease and acromegaly. *Q J Med* 1990; **76**(280): 855–6.
105. Strauch G, Vallotton MB, Touitou Y, Bricaire H. The renin–angiotensin–aldosterone system in normotensive and hypertensive patients with acromegaly. *N Engl J Med* 1972; **287**(16): 795–9.
106. Ross EJ, Linch DC. Cushing's syndrome—killing disease: discriminatory value of signs and symptoms aiding early diagnosis. *Lancet* 1982; **2**: 646–9.
107. Haak D, Mohring J, Mohring B et al. Comparative study on development of corticosterone and DOCA hypertension in rats. *Am J Physiol* 1977; **233**: F403–11.
108. Connell JMC, Whitworth JA, Daves DL et al. Effects of ACTH and cortisol administration on blood pressure, electrolyte metabolism, atrial natriuretic peptide, and renal function in normal man. *J Hypertens*, 1988; **6**:17–23.
109. Ritchie CM, Sheridan B, Fraser R et al. Studies on the pathogenesis of hypertension in Cushing's disease and acromegaly. *Q J Med* 1990; **280**: 855–67.
110. Krakoss LR. Measurement of plasma renin substrate by radioimmunoassay of angiotensin I: Concentration in syndromes associated with steroid excess. *J Clin Endocrinol Metab* 1973; **37**: 608–15.
111. Axelrod L. Inhibition of prostacyclin production mediates permissive effect of glucocorticoids on vascular tone. Perturbations of this mechanism contribute to pathogenesis of Cushing's syndrome and Addison's disease. *Lancet* 1983; **1**: 904–6.

17

Obesity
Pierre-Marc G Bouloux

Introduction

Obesity refers to an excess of body fat; it has become increasingly prevalent in the Western world, representing a major public health risk with significant morbidity and associated comorbidity, such as diabetes mellitus, hypertension, sleep apnea, osteoarthritis and a number of cancers such as endometrial carcinoma (Table 17.1).[1] Obesity has a genetic component that accounts for a significant percentage of the risk of this disorder. Obese patients are frequently subjected to discrimination and may suffer from low self-esteem. It has been estimated that 25–34% of the adult population of the USA is obese, the percentage being greater in racial minorities and women.[2] In the UK, a recent National Audit Report has concluded that the incidence of obesity has increased three-fold over the past 20 years, and that one-fifth of the population is now overweight; this is projected to increase to 1 in 4 by 2010. The cost to the NHS of treating obesity and its comorbidity is estimated at £500 000 000 per annum. Thus, in addition to a reduction in wellbeing, obesity has repercussions on society as a whole through healthcare costs and reduced productivity.[3] Although obesity is occasionally due to another primary disorder (e.g. Cushing's syndrome, hypothyroidism, hyothalamic obesity, Prader Willi syndrome), most cases occur in the absence of an identified disease process.

Healthcare professionals have in general paid little heed to obesity, not considering it as a disease state per se. This negative approach is reinforced by the perceived poor long-term treatment outcomes, with only 5–10% of patients losing weight and then maintaining their reduced weight. Obesity requires lifelong treatment, which in principle is very simple: reduced calorie intake, coupled with increased energy expenditure until a new steady-state weight is reached. Despite the aforementioned, however, modestly successful treatment—e.g. a 10% weight reduction—can result in significant attenuation of the associated health risk.

There are several obesity phenotypes. In constitutional obesity, there is global fat distribution. Visceral obesity, typical of middle-aged men, tends to have an apple-shaped distribution, whereas the obesity of women has been likened to a pear-shape. The fat distribution in Cushing's syndrome and HIV-related lipodystrophy is centripetal, with a prominent dorsocervical and supraclavicular fat pad.

Physiology of adipocytes

A typical adult human has 10–15 kg of fat tissue, whose function is energy storage, thermal and shock insulation, and hormone production.[4] In the morbidly obese individual, adipose mass can excess 100 kg, as a consequence of lipid accretion, the result of the highly efficient nature of lipogenesis in the adipocyte in response to excess energy intake.

Triglyceride synthesis

The primary function of adipocytes is triglyceride storage. Biosynthesis requires glucose as a glycerol backbone for the phosphatidyl ester bond necessary for the fatty acid binding. The principal regulatory steps in biosynthesis are glucose entry (by facilitated diffusion in response to insulin-induced plasma membrane translocation of GLUT 4) into cells to generate glycerol phosphate (glycerol recycling is limited because of the low levels of adipocyte glycerol kinase), and the uptake of free fatty acids from plasma, the

Cardiovascular
   Coronary artery disease
   Hypertension, stroke
   Deep vein thrombosis
Gastrointestinal
   Hiatus hernia
   Reflux disease
   Gallstones
   Colorectal cancer
   Steatosis
   Hemorrhoids
Respiratory
   Primary alveolar hypoventilation
   Obstructive sleep apnea
   Dyspnea
Metabolic
   Type 2 diabetes mellitus
   Dyslipidemia (low high-density lipoprotein)
   Insulin resistance
   PCOS
Neurologic
   Nerve entrapment
   Sciatica
Musculoskeletal
   Osteoarthritis
   Flattened arches
Genitourinary
   Stress incontinence
   Reduced fertility
   Pregnancy complication
   Stearic hindrance during sexual intercourse
Breasts
   Breast cancer
   Gynecomastia
Psychological
   Low self-esteem
   Depression
   Anxiety
Miscellaneous
   Greater operative risk
   Snoring

Table 17.1
Diseases and comorbidity associated with obesity.

consequence of lipoprotein lipase (LPL) activity. LPL is synthesized by adipocytes and secreted before localization in the capillaries, where it is bound to heparan sulfate proteoglycans. It is activated by apolipoprotein CII (present in very low-density lipoprotein (VLDL), high-density lipoprotein (HDL) and chylomicrons) in the capillary lumen. Insulin also stimulates fatty acid synthase activity, as well as LPL activity. The catabolism of LPL is reduced by glucocorticoids. Inhibitors of LPL activity include catecholamines, growth hormone, free fatty acids, testosterone, tumor necrosis factor (TNF) and related cytokines. In the case of adrenaline and growth hormone, inactivation of LPL occurs post-translationally.[4] Adipose tissue contains elevated LPL activity, which remains even after weight loss, implying a role for LPL in the rapid return of obesity following increased calorie intake in the previously obese individual.

Control of lipolysis

Obesity is characterized by increased turnover of adipose tissue triglycerides. The lipolytic pathway involves the regulated enzyme hormone-sensitive lipase (HSL), a cytosolic, neutral lipase that hydrolyses triglycerides into diglycerides and then monoglycerides. Obesity is characterized by elevated basal lipolytic activity. HSL is activated and inhibited by changes in a single serine phosphorylation state. The predominant lipolytic agents for human adipocytes are catecholamines, and to a lesser extent growth hormone. β-Receptors mediate catecholamine-induced lipolysis, whereas α_2-receptors inhibit lipolysis. Insulin is the dominant antilipolytic agent in humans, although, in vitro, neuropeptide (NPY), peptide YY, prostaglandin E_1 and adenosine are also potent inhibitors of lipolysis.

Body fat measurement

Several methods are employed to quantify the degree of fat excess (Table 17.2). Some are purely research tools, while others are applicable to a clinical setting (e.g. anthropometric measurements).[5–9] The Quentelet (or body mass index: BMI) index is clinically the most useful index of obesity, and is the weight in kilograms divided by the square of the height in meters. Height and weight can be measured accurately, being less susceptible to observer error than waist and hip circumferences (and thereby the waist-to-hip ratio: WHR), and caliper-derived skin thickness. Regional fat distribution can be accurately estimated using CT scanning or MRI scanning.

	Cost	Accuracy	Measures regional fat
Height and weight	–	High	No
Skin fold measurement	–	Low	Yes
Circumference of waist/hip	–	Moderate	Yes
Ultrasound	+	Moderate	Yes
Densitometry	++	High	No
Estimates of total body water	+++	High	No
Measurement of total body potassium	++++	High	No
Neutron activation techniques	++++	High	No
Computed tomography	++++	High	Yes
Magnetic resonance imaging	++++	High	Yes
Impedance and conductivity	++	High	No
DEXA	++	High	No

Table 17.2
Techniques for the estimation of body fat and its distribution.

Underwater weighing (densitometry) is the gold standard, and depends on the assumption that fat-free tissue and fat have different but fixed densities. The density of body fat is assumed to be 0.9, and the density of lean body tissue 1.1, when residual lung volume and intestinal gases are properly accounted for. Hydration of tissues is also assumed to be constant, and bone mineral content fixed. A frequently used formula is then used to generate percentage body fat, e.g.

$$\%\text{fat} = 100\,(5.053/\text{density} - 4.164)$$

Total body water estimates usually employ tritiated or deuterated water, and isotope dilution is allowed to reach a steady state after administration. This takes 2–3 h, and body water is assumed to be limited to fat-free mass. Lean body mass is calculated from the assumption of a fixed water percentage in lean tissue (70–72%). Body fat can then be computed from the difference between weight and calculated lean body mass, with a correction for skeletal weight.

Lean body mass can be estimated from measurement of total body potassium, with the assumption that potassium is essentially limited to the fat-free compartment. Potassium is generally measured by isotope dilution using ^{42}K or by assessing ^{40}K in a whole-body counter.

Indirect techniques for measuring body fat employ skinfold measurements. Calibrated calipers are used to measure skinfold thickness at four sites: biceps, triceps, and subscapular and suprailiac sites. Equations and nomograms are used to convert skinfold thickness to body fat. The main problem with this method is that regional fat distribution can vary from individual to individual, but, notwithstanding this, it can be used to monitor an individual through a treatment program.

Impedance measurement is carried out by applying a pair of electrodes to one arm and one leg and using either a single-frequency (50 kHz) or variable-frequency alternating current of approximately 800 A. It estimates primarily the body water, and, depending on the frequency, may provide an estimate of intracellular versus extracellular fluid, using the cell membrane as a capacitor.

Life insurance tables for ideal body weight

Acceptable weights for adults were originally derived form the Metropolitan Life Insurance Company (Table 17.3), based on mortality experience in age- and sex-ranked weights per height at the time of entry into the life insurance system. This has subsequently been modified in the Fogarty Convention, which has generated tables in which average weight is considered to be the median value for a medium frame at each height, and the acceptable range is bracketed by the lowest weight for a small frame and the highest weight for a large frame. Most authorities define obesity as being present when an individual exceeds 20% of his ideal weight.

	AGE			
	19 to 34 Years		Over 35 Years	
HEIGHT	Target	Range	Target	Range
5'0"	112	97–128	123	108–138
5'1"	116	101–132	127	111–143
5'2"	120	104–137	131	115–148
5'3"	124	107–141	135	119–152
5'4"	128	111–146	140	122–157
5'5"	132	114–150	144	126–162
5'6"	136	118–155	148	130–167
5'7"	140	121–160	153	134–172
5'8"	144	125–164	158	138–178
5'9"	149	129–169	162	142–183
5'10"	153	132–174	167	146–188
5'11"	157	136–179	172	151–194
6'0"	162	140–184	177	155–189
6'1"	166	144–189	182	159–205
6'2"	171	148–195	187	164–210
6'3"	176	152–200	192	168–216
6'4"	180	156–205	197	173–222
6'5"	185	160–211	202	177–228
6'6"	190	164–216	208	182–234
BMI kg/m^2	22	19–25	24	21–27

*Subject's height is measured without shoes; subject is weighed without clothes.
Derived from National Research Council, 1989.

Table 17.3
Optimal height-wieght for adults. Reproduced with permission from DeGroot L, Jameson L. Endocrinology (3rd ed). WB Saunders, 1995.

Origins of obesity and regulation of appetite control

Obesity is multifactorial in origin, with important genetic and environmental components. Recently, several single-gene defects have been characterized as contributing to obesity (e.g. leptin and MC4-R gene defects). Many of these involve potential neurotransmitters and signaling systems involved in energy homeostasis (i.e. controlling feeding and energy expenditure). It is useful to review the physiology of hypothalamic peptides and neurotransmitters known to play a role in such energy homeostasis.[10, 11]

The brain plays a critical role in regulation of energy homeostasis through: (1) control of hunger and satiety; (2) influencing the rate of energy expenditure; and (3) regulating secretion of hormones involved in deposition of energy stores. Brain centers receive short-term inputs from the gut and food cues from the environment, and higher brain centers are involved in cognitive and emotional aspects of food ingestion. These appetite-generating signals influence the timing and size of individual meals. Long-term signals are at least in part integrated by the fat-derived hormone leptin, which, upon entering the brain, acts to ensure that food intake and energy expenditure are coupled to the state of energy stores over the long term.

Energy homeostasis is the result of the balance of ingestion of three macronutrients—carbohydrate, fat and lipids—and energy expenditure. Evidence exists that, in humans, carbohydrate and protein balance are efficiently self-regulated, such that carbohydrate and protein oxidation are promoted by carbohydrate and protein intake. By contrast, fat oxidation is not regulated by fat intake, being significantly dependent upon sympathoadrenal activity, in contrast to carbohydrate and protein utilization. A high-fat diet favors fat gain, in part because of greater palatability of fatty food, and because satiety is less with fatty food, with the result that self-compensation by adjustment of subsequent intake is less likely after a high-fat meal. Moreover, meal-induced thermogenesis is lower after a fatty meal (3% of energy content of fat ingested) than after carbohydrate or protein intake (6–7% and 25% respectively).

Total energy expenditure

Obesity results from the cumulative effects of, over a long period, an excess of calorie intake over expenditure. Energy expenditure comprises three components: resting metabolic rate (RMR: accounting for 55–70% of the total), muscular activity (exercise: 15–20%), and the energy expended during digestion. The RMR correlates most closely with lean body mass (fat-free mass). Muscular energy tends to be greater in obese subjects, since increased work is needed to displace the greater mass. When an obese subject loses weight, the RMR is decreased, reflecting a reduction in lean body mass, and energy expended in exercise decreases for the same level of physical activity. The fall in energy expenditure often discourages the efforts of the obese subject to lose weight. Exercise preserves lean body mass as well as enhancing insulin sensitivity and improving cardiac performance.

Hypothalamic neurotransmitters and neuropeptides involved in energy balance

Many substances are known to determine feeding behavior and energy homeostasis in rodents, and evidence is accruing for their importance in humans also.[12,13] In animals, data have been derived from discrete microinjection techniques, and pharmacologic manipulation using agonists and antagonists.

Central nervous system control mechanisms

Anorexigenic signals

α-Melanocyte stimulating hormone (α-MSH)
This inhibits feeding, acting through the melanocortin-4 receptor (MC4-R) in the hypothalamus.[12,14–16] Agouti-related protein (AGRP) antagonizes the actions of α–MSH on MC4-R, causing hyperphagia and obesity in a genetically obese mouse (A^{vy}). One MSH analog (MTII) under development causes weight loss and darkening of the hair in humans.

Corticotropin-releasing factor (CRF)
This inhibits feeding when injected into the third ventricle of rodents, possibly by inhibiting NPY release. It has an additional action in increasing energy expenditure via stimulation of thermogenic tissues, an effect mediated through CRF-2 receptors.

Cocaine- and amphetamine-regulated transcript (CART)
The potential of CART in energy balance has been suggested following the demonstration that leptin coordinately regulates CART expression, and that CART inhibits the feeding response induced by either fasting or NPY.[17]

Neurotensin
This is a 13 amino acid peptide found throughout the brain and gastrointestinal tract, and has been shown to inhibit noradrenaline-induced feeding.

Peripheral (gastrointestinal) signals

Cholecystokinin (CCK)
This is released from the gut after feeding, and inhibits feeding through both peripheral and central pathways. In rodents, systemic CCKa agonists and CCK injected into the paraventricular nucleus inhibits feeding. In humans, intravenous CCK decreases hunger.

Glucagon-like peptide (GLP-1)
This is the 6–29 acid fragment of glucagon, and is processed in the brain and intestine. It is released from the intestine after eating, and enhances insulin secretion as well as delaying gastric emptying. Gastric emptying delay provokes satiety, so GLP-1 also has a central action in decreasing feeding.[18,19]

Leptin
This is a 16 kDa-single-chain peptide produced by adipose tissue, placenta, stomach and skeletal muscle. Its tertiary structure resembles that of cytokines, and the protein is encoded by the *ob* gene, comprising three exons. Leptin circulates in biological fluids both as a free protein and in a form that is bound to the soluble isoform of its receptor (Ob-Re). Its secretion is pulsatile, and shows a circadian

---

Promoting weight loss
   Serotonin
   Cholecystokinin
   α-Melanocyte stimulating factor
   Glucagon-like peptide 1 (GLP-1)
   Corticotropin-releasing-factor
   Leptin
   Cocaine- and amphetamine-regulated transcript (CART)
   Neurotensin
Promoting weight gain
   Serotonin
   Neuropeptide Y
   GHrelin
   Orexin A/B
   Galanin
   Endogenous cannabinoids

Table 17.4
Neurotransmitters involved in energy homeostasis.

rhythm, with a nocturnal rise peaking at 01.00–02.00. The leptin receptor belongs to the gp130 family of cytokine receptors. It has a single membrane-spanning domain and exists in several isoforms (Ob-Ra, Ob-Rb, Ob-Rc, Ob-Rd and Ob-Re) that derive from alternative mRNA splicing. All isoforms have identical ligand-binding domains but differ at the C-terminus. Leptin receptors are widely dispersed both centrally and in peripheral tissues. Injected centrally into rodents, leptin has marked anti-obesity actions, causing profound hypophagia, and increased thermogenesis and brown adipose tissue (BAT) activity, leading to fat mobilization and weight loss. Leptin deficiency in the *ob/ob* mouse is associated with hyperphagia, early-onset morbid obesity and type 2 diabetes. ICV or intravenous leptin dramatically reduced food intake in this mouse, causing weight loss. Congenital (autosomal recessive) leptin deficiency in humans causes a similar phenotype, including hypogonadotropic hypogonadism.[20,21] Leptin-deficient individuals lose weight dramatically with long-term subcutaneous leptin therapy. Leptin is transported into the brain through an isoform of its receptor. Obesity is associated with increased circulating leptin levels, but the saturable transport system limits its access to critical brain sites regulating food intake.

Orexigenic signals

Serotonin

This is thought to participate in the regulation of food intake and appetite. Direct injection of serotonin into the hypothalamus suppresses food intake, and drugs that release serotonin from nerve endings (e.g. fenfluramine) or block its reuptake decrease food intake and body weight.

Neuropeptide Y

This is believed to play a role in the physiologic response to starvation and the promotion of obesity. It is a 36 amino acid peptide, and its central administration, in addition to stimulating appetite, promotes energy storage by suppressing sympathetic outflow to BAT.[22]

Neuropeptide (NPY) can induce dramatic hyperphagia and obesity when injected into the rodent hypothalamus. In addition, it inhibits the sympathetically mediated stimulation of thermogenic tissues, while stimulating insulin secretion. It therefore shifts energy homeostasis towards positive balance and promotes triglyceride deposition in fat cells. Selective NPY Y5 receptor antagonists inhibit feeding in various models of rodent genetic obesity.

Orexin A and B (hypocretin 1 and 2)

These are hypothalamic peptides regulating food intake, being upregulated with fasting. Central administration of either protein stimulates food intake. Antagonists of these peptides may theoretically reduce food intake.[23,24]

Cannabinoids

These stimulate food intake, and cannabinoid antagonists are capable of causing satiety, and are being developed for clinical use. The major active component of cannabis, Δ^9-tetrahydrocannabinol (THC), has been used clinically to attenuate weight loss—particularly in patients with AIDS—and fatty acid-derived endocannabinoids (such as anandamide) have many of the same properties as THC, and act on the CB1-type cannabinoid receptor. There is evidence that leptin downregulates endocannabinoids in rodents. Cannabinoid antagonists are capable of causing satiety, and are being developed for clinical use.

GHrelin

GHrelin injected ICV induces hyperphagia, possibly through NPY release.

Effector systems in energy homeostasis

The adrenergic system and thyroid hormone axis are the most studied, the latter being concerned with long-term setting of energy dissipation, and the former affecting short-term regulation of energy expenditure. Within the adrenergic system, the effector molecules that dissociate fuel oxidation from ATP synthesis reside within the family of mitochondrial proteins known as uncoupling proteins (UCPs).[25] UCP1 belongs to the family of mitochondrial anion carrier proteins, which also includes the ADP/ATP carrier, phosphate carrier, and oxoglutarate carrier. Its action is stimulated by cAMP and free fatty acids, and suppressed by ATP. UCP1 is acutely upregulated by catecholamines via the β_3-receptor, which also stimulates it during cold exposure.[26] UCP2 and UCP3 have different tissue-specific expression and transcriptional regulation. The adrenergic system regulates energy expenditure at the cellular level by regulating expression of UCPs, and at the whole-animal level by enhancing total and basal oxygen consumption.

Changes in body fat composition throughout life

Body fat proportion changes throughout life, young lean men having 15–18% body fat and young women 20–25%. Obesity may be defined as a body fat content exceeding 25% in men and 30% in women. Mortality appears lowest in the BMI range 20–25. The risks of cardiovascular disease, diabetes mellitus, hypertension and gallbladder disease increase within the BMI range 25–30, and progressively in a curvilinear fashion through moderate (30–35) to severe (35–40) obesity. Thereafter, risk becomes exponential, a state known as 'morbid' obesity. Fat distribution plays an independent role in health risk at any given level of obesity. In particular, accumulation of upper abdominal or visceral obesity correlates strongly with insulin-resistant states such as diabetes and hypertension, WHR >0.95 in men and 0.8 in women conferring increased risk. Visceral fat is an important component of the syndrome X cluster comprising non-insulin-dependent diabetes mellitus, premature coronary artery disease, raised LDL and VLDL, and low HDL, polycystic ovarian disease, and hyperuricemia.

Neuroendocrine obesity

Hypothalamic obesity occurs in patients with inherited or acquired disorders affecting the hypothalamus, such as trauma, the sequelae of surgery to the hypothalamus, malignancy (including craniopharyngioma), and inflammatory diseases (sarcoidosis).[27] Disorders of thirst and temperature control may be present, and there is usually evidence of associated partial or complete hypopituitarism. Recently obesity has been associated with impaired prohormone processing associated with mutations of the human prohormone convertase gene.[28]

Polycystic ovarian syndrome has a pleiotropic phenotype including menstrual dysfunction, hirsutes, hyperandrogenism, polycystic ovaries, insulin resistance and obesity. Obesity is present in 50% of patients, often pre-dating the menstrual disturbance in patients, and may participate in the pathophysiology of the condition, since adipose tissue may convert androstenedione to estrone.

Cushing's syndrome is associated with a centripetal pattern of obesity and fat redistribution in the dorsocervical region and supraclavicular regions but sparing the limbs, giving 'a lemon on toothpicks' appearance. A similar phenotype occurs in HIV-positive patients receiving some reverse transcriptase and protease inhibitors, but in this syndrome, there is accompanying lipodystrophy of the face and limbs.

Hypothyroidism can be associated with obesity, whether primary or secondary in origin. Water retention, occasionally associated with hyponatremia, may explain some of the increased weight.

There are several genetic syndromes associated with obesity (Table 17.5).

Endocrine repercussions of obesity

Several endocrine and metabolic changes accompany obesity, but most are secondary to obesity and can be reversed by weight loss.

Prader Willi
  Sporadic inheritance, associated with a 15q11–13 deletion. Patients are of short stature with moderate to severe obesity by age 3. There is hyperphagia and food-seeking behavior. Associated anomalies include neonatal hypotonia, narrow bifrontal diameter, almond-shaped eyes, narrow nasal bridge, down-turned mouth, small, narrow hands and feet, scoliosis and growth hormone deficiency

Bartlet–Biedel syndrome
  This is transmitted as an autosomal recessive condition, and is also associated with pigmentary retinopathy, postaxial polydactyly and renal anomalies

Cohen syndrome
  This is associated with mild to moderate truncal obesity, infantile hypotonia, a high nasal bridge, short philtrum, and prominent central incisors

Borjeson–Forssman–Lehmann syndrome
  This is associated with early childhood obesity, coarse facies, prominent supraorbital ridges, and deep-set eyes and ptosis and large ears

Table 17.5
Genetic syndromes associated with obesity.

Endocrine pancreas

Hyperinsulinism, both fasting and postprandial, is common, and results from the insulin-resistant state induced by obesity. There is altered β-cell pulsatility in obese individuals.

Thyroid gland

There have been reports of increased triiodothyronine (T3) levels in obese patients, possibly the consequence of carbohydrate overfeeding.

Adrenal gland

Although cortisol production rate may be slightly elevated in obesity, cortisol dynamics tend to be normal.

Testes

Total testosterone tends to be low in the massively obese, but free testosterone levels are normal, and the sex hormone-binding globulin (SHBG) levels tend to be low, the consequence of hyperinsulinism. Concentrations of estradiol and estrone tend to be elevated, estrogen production rate being increased as a result of increased extraglandular conversion of androgen precursors to estrogens. Abnormal gonadal steroid production is reversible upon weight loss.

Ovarian function

Menstrual irregularity is more frequent, as is the incidence of polycystic ovarian syndrome.

Hypothalamus and pituitary gland

Basal plasma growth hormone (GH) levels and the GH response to a variety of stimuli are impaired in obesity. Twenty-four-hour integrated GH values are lower in young obese individuals, even though total IGF-1 levels are within the normal range. Free IGF-1 may be increased, leading to GH suppression by negative feedback. Hyperinsulinism leads to decreased IgFBP$_1$ levels, and therefore an increased free IGF-1 level.

Lipid levels and lipoprotein abnormality in the obese

LDL-C tends to be raised, HDL-C lowered, free fatty acids raised, and hypertriglyceridemia present.

Adipose tissue as an endocrine organ

Apart from the production and secretion of the 16-kDa protein leptin, adipose tissue from obese subjects contains an abundance of TNF-α mRNA and protein, and it has been postulated that this may act as a potential mediator of insulin resistance, via alterations in the phosphorylation status of insulin receptor substrate-1 (IRS-1), thereby altering insulin receptor activity. Recent data suggest that the adipocyte product resistin may be responsible for the insulin resistance of obesity, as well as TNF-α.[29] Aromatase activity in adipose tissue will convert adrenal and ovarian (and testicular) androgens into estrogens.

Evaluation of the obese patient

A baseline history and physical examination (functional baseline assessment) is an essential prerequisite. In particular, the history of the obesity, and previous treatments, should be carefully elicited, as well as other modifiable risk factors, such as cigarette smoking, hypertension and dyslipidemia. Several endocrinopathies may be associated with significant obesity: Cushing's syndrome, hypothyroidism, and various medications (e.g. steroids, cyproheptadine, sodium valproate). Complications of obesity should be assessed, such as impaired glucose tolerance or diabetes mellitus, dyslipidemia, hypertension, the presence of cardiovascular disease, sleep apnea, and arthritis. A subject with mild obesity and a favorable pattern of fat distribution is at much lower risk, and can be reassured accordingly. Cessation of smoking is associated with a modest rise in weight (average 2.8 kg), but it has been estimated that a weight gain five times this would be needed to offset the benefits of stopping smoking.

Treatment of obesity

This can be broken down into four main headings: assessment of the individual patient, dietary modification with calorie intake reduction, behavior (lifestyle) modification, and a strategy for prevention of weight regain. The aim is to reduce both weight and overall risks of morbidity and premature mortality, by dietary advice, encouragement of physical activity, and elimination of other comorbid risk factors. Consideration of drug and (in the case of morbid obesity) surgical treatment may also be indicated.

Treatment targets for weight reduction

To return to an ideal body weight is unrealistic for most patients. Proven and definite benefits can be demonstrated with 10% weight loss, and treatment should aim to achieve this at a reasonable and sustainable rate, the optimal rate being about 0.1–1 lb (0.22–2.2 kg) loss per week. This is equal to an energy deficit of around 500–600 kcal per day.

Dietary treatment of obesity

Calorie restriction is the mainstay of treatment, the type of diet being adapted to the patient and the rate, extent and duration of the weight-reducing program.[30] Broadly, diets may be low calorie or very low calorie.

Low-calorie diets

This is simply a balanced supply of fuel sources at a lower amount than required for weight maintenance. In practice, this is frequently achieved by reducing fat intake to about 30%. Such diets generally result in steady but slow weight reduction, and are inadequate in the treatment of severely and morbidly obese subjects.

Very-low-calorie diets

These require medical supervision, and are usually coupled to a supervised program of exercises and nutritional and behavior modification. They usually come in the form of powdered products that are reconstituted in water or skimmed milk and consumed in three or four portions per day. Compliance may be facilitated by the addition of small quantities of high-fiber or low-calorie fresh fruit drinks and vegetables. The total calorie intake usually ranges between 400 and 800 kcal, consisting of good-quality protein and carbohydrate with minimal fat and full supplements of vitamins and minerals. This protects against the excessive loss of lean body mass, while encouraging mobilization of fat stores. These diets can promote significant weight loss in severely obese subjects within 3–6 months. Such diets should be used with caution in patients suffering from cardiac disease, active hepatic or renal disease and pregnancy. Gallstones may be exacerbated during treatment. Weight should be recorded one or two times per week, frequent physician contact being mandatory. Urine ketone assessment is a simple and inexpensive method of checking dietary compliance, trace to large quantities of ketonuria being present after the first week of diet. Several side-effects are common in the first few weeks of treatment, mostly transient in nature (Table 17.6). Lethargy, fatigue, cold intolerance, dry skin, hair loss and halitosis may occur. Adequate hydration can guard against constipation, but diarrhea can sometimes occur. With calorie restriction, the output of solubilizing bile acids is reduced, and gallstones can develop rapidly in up to 25% of cases. Postural hypotension may require some salt supplementation. Menstrual irregularities and loss of libido may occur. Elevations in uric acid, a mild transaminitis and elevations of creatine phosphokinase may occur.

Modification of eating behavior

The patient should be taught new eating habits and self-monitoring techniques to help sustain the period of dieting. This may require the provision of social support, with measures to enhance self-esteem. This can be conveniently accomplished in small group meetings every 2–3 weeks. The reinforcing impact of such an approach cannot be overestimated. The physiology of weight reduction in the obese subject is to gradually drift up to the original set-point. A sustainable exercise program will help maintain a higher level of energy expenditure. Another adjunct is to wear an inextensible nylon cord around the waist, which fits

Postural hypotension	Fatigue
Constipation/diarrhea	Cold intolerance
Nausea and headache	Cholelithiasis
Myalgia	Menstrual irregularity
Arthralgia	Transaminitis

Table 17.6
Side-effects of rapid weight loss.

comfortably at the desired weight, but becomes tight once weight is gained, thereby providing feedback to the wearer.

Exercise programs in obesity

It is increasingly clear that weight loss is better maintained when exercise is part of a weight-reducing program. Following a period of diet-induced weight loss, participation in regular exercise amounting to 1500–2000 kcal/week will result in more successful maintenance of the lesser weight. Regular physical activity has the potential to reverse insulin resistance, improve cardiovascular function and plasma lipid levels, as well as reduce blood pressure. Patients should choose from a variety of activities, particularly those which are enjoyable and can be continued for life.

Drug treatment of obesity

Historically, the first treatments involved the use of amphetamine derivatives, which were anorectic agents. Given their potential for addiction and for abuse, and uncertainties about efficacy and the high risk/benefit ratio, these fell out of favor in the UK. D-Fenfluramine was withdrawn in 1997 because of fears about carcinoid-like cardiac valvular lesions and primary pulmonary hypertension. Most of these drugs interfere with serotoninergic pathways, in sites such as the arcuate and paraventricular parts of the hypothalamus. Acting on 5-HT_{2c} receptors, 5-HT elicits a hypophagic action, possibly through suppression of NPY release. Drugs blocking serotonin reuptake have anti-obesity actions. D-Fenfluramine has, in clinical studies, caused a 10% weight loss in some 33% of patients.

Orlistat (Xenical)

This acts by inhibiting pancreatic and gastric lipase and is a hydrogenated synthetic derivative of lipstatin, produced by the bacterium *Streptococcus toxytricini*. The compound is highly lipophilic, and its β-lactone ring structure is essential for activity. The effect is to reduce fat absorption from the intestine. Weight reductions similar to that seen with D-fenfluramine have been demonstrated (4 kg more than placebo over a 12-month period). Side-effects are predictable: fat malabsorption, with loose or liquid stool after a fatty meal, may condition patients to consume less fat, adding to the therapeutic effect. Orlistat can be prescribed for patients with a BMI > 30 kg/m^2, or 28 kg/m^2 in patients with comorbid factors. Patients should consume less than 30% fat calorie equivalents, and current guidelines stipulate that a patient must lose 2.5 kg in weight through lifestyle changes over the 4 weeks prior to initiating orlistat therapy, which can currently be prescribed for up to 24 months. About one-third of patients fulfill these criteria and will go on to lose an average 16% body weight and keep it up for 2 years.[31] A decrease in the level of fat-soluble vitamins D and E and carotene has been noted on treatment.

Sibutramine

This is a monoamine reuptake inhibitor about to be licensed for use in the UK. It acts by increasing both 5-HT and noradrenaline levels in specific brain regions, thereby inhibiting appetite. There may also be a centrally mediated thermogenic effect. It acts in a dose-dependent manner, and a mean weight loss of 8% can be maintained for 12 months in responders.[32] Side-effects include a slight rise in blood pressure, tachycardia, dry mouth, and headache. There is no evidence of valvulopathies or pulmonary hypertension, but, clearly, vigilance is indicated.

β3 agonists

In rodents, sympathetic stimulation of BAT through β_3 agonists increases heat production and leads to weight loss. In humans, similar drugs can induce modest weight loss, but the use of such agents has been restricted because of lack of specificity of action.

Other drugs that increase energy expenditure

Thyroid hormone is the prototypic drug in this class, but ephedrine with or without caffeine, and terbulaline, have also been used in clinical studies. Side-effects have been limiting. Other therapeutic approaches to the medical management of obesity can be gained from recent reviews.[33,34]

Surgery

Preoperative assessment of the obese patient

This must include a careful clinical history and physical examination for the various complications of obesity, including diabetes mellitus, cardiac problems, pulmonary problems, including sleep apnea, dyslipidemia, hypertension, evidence of reflux esophageal disease, and gallstones. If gallstones are present, cholecystectomy may be performed during any intestinal bypass procedure. Pneumatic compression stockings and heparin are important for prophylaxis of deep vein thrombosis and pulmonary embolus. Obese individuals have higher right atrial pressure and pulmonary artery pressure, and during surgery, both right and left ventricular stroke work decrease. Obese patients are likely to become more hypoxemic during surgery, due in part to the decrease in expiratory reserve volume. Weight is inversely proportional to expiratory reserve volume and to the apnea time necessary to become desaturated.

Jaw wiring

This is undoubtedly very effective in producing weight loss of up to 64 kg in the first year. It is coupled to a low-calorie diet (e.g. 650 kcal), but must not be undertaken in subjects prone to reflux or asthma. It is reserved for the morbidly obese.[36]

When followed up after removal of jaw wires, almost all patients regain their lost weight. Jaw wiring has been reported to give weight losses comparable to jejuno-ileal or gastric bypasses over 6 months of treatment.

The Garrow belt

Garrow observed that professional models used a gold chain around their waist to act as an external feedback signal to help in weight maintenance, and tried to fix a nylon cord around the waists of patients who had lost weight with jaw wiring. In an early report, seven patients who had lost a mean of 31.8 kg with jaw wiring regained only 5.6 kg in 4–14 months with the use of a waist cord.

Gastric balloons

The insertion of a silicone bubble into the stomach, acting as a bezoar, is associated with weight loss, the size of the balloon playing a crucial role. In a study using 300 ml gastric balloons in humans, the balloon group lost more weight than the control group, but less than a 1000-kcal diet group or a group assigned to the gastric balloon and a 1000-kcal diet together. Patients with a smaller gastric capacity lost more weight, and the success of this procedure depends upon tailoring the gastric balloon volume to the stomach capacity.

Jejuno-ileal bypass

Historically, this has been the most widely used surgical technique. In the Payne procedure, 35 cm of jejunum was anastomosed end to side to 10 cm of ileum. In the Scott procedure, 30 cm of jejunum was anastomosed end to end with 15 cm of ileum, the proximal cut portion of the latter being inserted into the transverse colon. Weight loss after surgery was due to both reduced food intake and malabsorption. Anorexia is caused, in part, by bacterial overgrowth in the bypassed segments. The procedures were complicated by diarrhea, vitamin D, vitamin B_{12}, vitamin A and folic acid deficiencies, arthritis, kidney oxalate stones, magnesium and calcium deficiency, and liver disease, rarely progressing to cirrhosis. Hyperoxaluria occurs with a frequency of 4–29%, and oxalate nephropathy may occur more than one decade after surgery.

Variants such as bilio-pancreatic procedures and bilio-intestinal bypass have also been tried.[37] In the former, drainage from the stomach is divided so that the fundus is isolated from the antrum, which is drained along with the pancreatic and biliary ducts. In the latter, the bypassed loop is attached to the gallbladder, allowing bile salt reabsorption in the ileum.

Gastric reduction procedures

These represent the surgical technique of choice. The vertical banded gastroplasty[38] and the Roux-en Y gastrojejunostomy are currently in use, especially in morbid obesity, including that associated with non-insulin-dependent diabetes mellitus. Vertical banded gastroplasty restricts food intake by limiting gastric volume. A 50-ml gastric reservoir is created by a stapling technique, and the reservoir empties through a narrow channel that is reinforced with prosthetic material into the residual stomach. Gastrointestinal continuity is preserved and malabsorption does not occur. The failure rate is about 50%. Bilio-pancreatic diversion has been used successfully in some centers. Nutritional deficiencies may arise.

Surgery should be performed only by an experienced surgical team, supported by appropriate pre- and postoperative support structures to provide dietary advice and behavior modification.[39]

Lipectomy

This is ineffective in producing lasting reductions in body weight, as compensatory hypertrophy of the remaining adipose tissue has been demonstrated.

Plastic surgery

This does have a role to play in the removal of redundant skin and a remaining abdominal panniculus. It is generally recommended that a delay of 1 year following weight stabilization should occur, so as to allow for maximal skin contraction.

Summary

Obesity is a significant cause of morbidity and mortality. Its successful treatment necessitates the input of a multi-disciplinary team, including a nutritionist, clinical psychologist, and physician/surgeon. In order to lose weight successfully, patients need to be exceptionally well motivated and willing to effect a change in lifestyle. The rewards of weight loss in any one obese individual must be of sufficient magnitude to motivate and sustain the changes of behavior, that, in most situations, need to be lifelong. Recent advances in the understanding of the neurochemical basis of appetite control are likely to lead to the design of novel therapeutic approaches in obesity, but until safe and effective treatments are available, surgical approaches to the treatment of obesity are indicated in morbid obesity where lifestyle changes and medical therapy have been unsuccessful.

Further reading

Agarwal N, Shibutani K, SanFilippo JA et al. Hemodynamic and respiratory changes in surgery of the morbidly obese. *Surgery* 1982; 92: 226–34.

Bray GA. Obesity. *Endocrinol Metab Clin North Am* 1996; 25(4).

Garren L, Garren M, Garren R et al. Gastric balloon implantation for weight loss in the morbidly obese. *Am J Gastroenterol* 1985; 80: 860.

Garrow JS. Morbid obesity: medical or surgical treatment? The case for medical treatment. *Int J Obesity* 1987; 11(suppl 3): 1–4.

Garrow J, Summerbell C. Meta analysis: effect of exercise, with or without dieting, on the body composition of overweight subjects. *Eur J Clin Nutr* 1995; 49: 1.

Hofmann AF, Schmuck G, Scopinaro N et al. Hyperoxaluria associated with intestinal bypass surgery for morbid obesity: occurrence, pathogenesis and 6 approaches to treatment. *Int J Obesity* 1981; 5: 513–18.

Hotamisligil GS, Murray DL, Choy LN et al. Tumour necrosis factor alpha inhibits signalling from the insulin receptor. *Proc Natl Acad Sci USA* 1994; 91: 4854–8.

Schrauwen P, Hesselink M. UCP2 and UCP3 in muscle controlling body metabolism. *J Exp Biol* 2002; 205: 2275–85.

Van Itallie TB. Health implications of overweight and obesity in the United States. *Ann Intern Med* 1985; 103(6 pt 2): 983.

References

1. Wadden TA, Brownell KD, Foster GD. Obesity: responding to the global epidemic. *J Consult Clin Psychol* 2002; 70: 510–25.
2. Kuczmarski RJ., Flegal, KM., Campbell., et al. Increasing prevalence of overweight among US adults: The National Health and Nutrition Examination Surveys, 1960–1991. *JAMA* 272:205, 1994
3. Seidell JC: The impact of obesity on health status: Some implications for health care costs. *Int J Obes Relat Metab Disord* 19(suppl6): 13–16, 1995.
4. Ramsay TG: Fat cells. *Endocrinol Metab Clin N Americ* 25, No4 847–870, 1996.
5. Heymsfield, SB., Waki, M., Kehayias J., et al: Chemical and elemental analysis of humans in vivo using improved body composition models. *Am J Physiol* 261 (2pt1): E190–E198, 1991.
6. Kvist H., Chowhury B., Grangard, U., et al: Total and visceral adipose tissue volumes derived from measurements with computed tomography in adult men and women: Predictive equations. *Am J Clin Nutr* 48: 1351–1361, 1988.
7. Bray GA., Greenway FL., Molitch ME et al: Use of anthropometric measures to assess weight loss. *Am J Clin Nutr* 31: 769–773, 1978.
8. Segal KR., Van Loan M., Fitzgerald PI et al: Lean body mass estimation by bioelectrical impedance analysis: A four site cross validation study. *Am J Clin Nutr* 47: 7–14, 1988.
9. Lohman TG., Skinfolds and body density and their rlation to body fatness: A review. *Hum Biol* 53: 181–225, 1981.
10. Kalra SP., Dube, MG., Pu S et al: Interacting appetite regulating pathways in the hypothalamic regulation of body wieght. *Endoc Rev* 20: 68–100, 1999.
11. Lee IM, Blair SN, Allison DB et al. Epidemiological data on the relationships of caloric intake, energy balance and weight gain over the life span with longevity and morbidity. *J Gerontol A Biol Sci Med Sci* 2001; 56: 7–19
12. Flier, JS., Maratos-Flier E: Obesity and the hypothalamus: Novel peptides for new pathways. *Cell* 92: 437–440, 1998
13. Commuzie AG., Allison DB: The search for human obesity genes. *Science* 280: 1374–1377, 1998.
14. Qu D., Ludwig DS., Gammeltoft S., et al: A role for melanin-concentrating hormone in the central regulation of feeding behaviour. *Nature* 380: 243–247, 1997.
15. Ollmann MM., Wilson BD., Yang YK., et al: Antagonism of central melanocortin receptors in vitro and in vivo by agouti-related proteins. *Science* 278: 135–138, 1997.
16. Yeo GS., Faroqi JS., Amimian S, et al: A frameshift mutation in MC4R associated with dominantly inherited human obesity (letter). *Nat Genet* 20: 111–112, 1998.

REFERENCES

17. Kristensen P., Judge ME., Thim L., et al: Hypothalamic CART is a new anorectic peptide regulated by leptin. *Nature* 393: 72–76, 1998.
18. Fehmann HC., Goke R., Goke B: Cell and molecular biology of the incretin hormones glucagon-like peptide-I and glucose-dependent insulin releasing polypeptide. *Endoc Rev* 16: 390–410, 1995.
19. Turton MD., O'Shea D., Gunn IN., et al: A role for glucagon-like peptide-I in the central regulation of feeding. *Nature* 379: 69–72, 1996.
20. Montague CT., Farooqi IS., Whitehead JP., et al: Congenital leptin deficiency is associated with severe early-onset obesity in adults. *Nature* 387: 903–908, 1997.
21. Clement K, Vaisse C., Lahlous N, et al: a mutation in the human leptin receptor causes obesity and pituitary dysfunction. *Nature* 392: 398–401, 1998.
22. Zarjevski N., Cusin I., Vettor R., et al: Chronic intracerebroventricular neuropeptide-Y administration to normal rats mimics hormonal and metabolic changes of obesity. *Endocrinology* 133: 1753–1758, 1993.
23. de Lecea L., Kilduff TS., Peyron C., et al: The hypocretins: Hypothalamic-specific peptide with neuroexcitatory activity. *Proc Natl Acad Sci* USA 95: 322–327, 1998.
24. Sakurai T., Ameniya A., Ishii M., et al: Orexin and orexin receptors: A family of hypothalamic neutopeptides and G protein-coupled receptors that regulate feeding behaviour. *Cell* 92: 573–585, 1998.
25. Gura T: Uncoupling proteins provide new clues to obesity's causes. *Science* 280: 1369–1370, 1998.
26. Lowell, BB., Flier, JS: Brown adipose tissue, beta 3-adrenergic receptors, and obesity. *Ann Rev Med* 48: 307–316, 1997.
27. Bray GA: Syndromes of hypothalamic obesity in MAN. *Pediatr Ann* 13: 525–536, 1984.
28. Jackson RS., Creemers JW., Ohagi S., et al: Obesity and impaired prohormone processing associated with mutations in the human prohormone convertase gene. *Nat Genet* 16: 303–306, 1997.
29. Shuldiner AR, Yang R, Gong D-W. Resistin, obesity and insulin resistance – the emerging role of the adipoclyte as an endocrine organ. *N Engl J Med* 2001; 345: 11345–1346.
30. Wadden TA: Treatment of obesity by moderate and severe caloric restriction. Research of clinical research trials. *Ann Intern Med*: 119: 688–693, 1993.
31. Sjostrom L., Rissanen A., Andersen T., et al: Randomised placebo-controlled trial of orlistat for weight loss and prevention of weight regain in obese patients. European Multicentre Orlistat Study Group. *Lancet* 352: 167–172, 1998.
32. Hanotin C., Thomas F., Jones SP., et al: Efficacy and tolerability of sibutramine in obese patients: A dose-ranging study. *Int J Obes Relat Disord* 22: 32–38, 1998.
33. Brower V. Fighting fat: New drugs against obesity in the pipeline. *EMBO Rep* 2002; 3: 601–3.
34. Hirsch J. The search for new ways to treat obesity. *Proc Natl Acad Sci USA* 2002; 99: 9096–7.
35. Anonymous: NIH conference: Gastrointestinal surgery for severe obesity. Consensus Development Conference Panel [review]. *Ann Intern Med* 115: 956–961, 1991.
36. Ramsay-Stewart G., Martin L: Jaw wiring in the treatment of morbid obesity. *Aus NZJ Surg* 55: 163–167, 1985.
37. Scopinaro N., Gianetta E., Civalleri D., et al: Partial and total biliopancreatic bypass in the surgical treatment of obesity. *Int J Obes* 5: 421–429, 1981.
38. Westerterp KR, Saris WHM., Soeters PB, et al: Determinants of weight loss after vertical banded gastroplasty. *Int J Obes* 15: 529–534, 1991.
39. Greenway FL. Surgery for Obesity. *Endoc and Metab Clin of N Americ* Vol 25, 4: 1005–1027, 1996.

18

Psychoneuroendocrinology
Salim Janmohamed, Ashley B Grossman

Introduction

It has long been recognized that endocrine disease and its treatment can affect the psyche, as exemplified by disorders such as 'myxedematous madness',[1] the affective changes seen in Cushing's syndrome, and the mania produced by dopamine agonists used to treat hyperprolactinemia. Conversely, psychological factors and psychiatric disorders are well known to induce endocrine disturbances that may produce confounding biochemical alterations, as in the loss of diurnal variation in serum cortisol levels associated with depression, or which may result in clinical dysfunction such as the growth retardation observed in children subjected to emotional deprivation.[2] Psychotropic medication can also interfere with endocrine investigation, as seen in the hyperprolactinemia due to neuroleptics, or may even cause overt endocrine illness, such as hypothyroidism due to lithium therapy.

The complex interrelationships between higher mental and endocrine function, in both health and disease, must clearly reflect, among other things, shared neuroanatomical circuits and neurochemical processes. Traditionally, psychoneuroendocrinology has encompassed the study of changes in hypothalamo–pituitary function in mental disorders. This became a practical possibility with the discovery of peptide neuromodulators in the 1970s and the development of measuring techniques such as radioimmunoassay. However, the modern remit of psychoneuroendocrinology is broader than originally entertained, and this chapter will focus on the following topics:

- Psychiatric disorders and medication
    - Depression
    - Bulimia and anorexia nervosa
    - Drug-induced psychosis
        - Testosterone
        - Dopamine agonists

- Endocrine disorders
    - Cushing's syndrome
    - Addison's disease
    - Primary hypothyroidism
    - Thyrotoxicosis
    - Hypopituitarism

Descriptive psychoendocrine studies have their origins in clinical observations, e.g. myxedema and cretinism in the 19th century, and have progressed in tandem with the development of psychopharmacological agents. The validity of many of the conclusions drawn from such investigations is limited, however, by problems related to study design, cohort size, contradictory results from other trials, and interpreting single-sample data in relation to circadian variation in hormone levels. Methodological problems stem from the inaccessibility of the central nervous system (CNS) to detailed examination in depressed subjects and the lack of good animal models of depression. Moreover, establishing cause and effect, i.e. whether the observations reflect etiology or are merely epiphenomena, has proved problematic. Nevertheless, the practicing clinician needs to be aware of the effects of mental disorders and their treatment on neuroendocrine function, as well as understanding the possible effects of neuroendocrine pathology on mental state.

Psychiatric disorders and medication

Psychiatric disorders

Depression
Endogenous depression is associated with a variety of abnormalities of endocrine function, as summarized in

Axis	Finding	Interpretation	Comment
HPA	ACTH and cortisol Sustained (24-h) hypersecretion in 40–70% of patients, including earlier nadir, shortened quiescent period, and increased pulsatility with preserved circadian rhythm (see below)	Increased CRH drive	Raised urinary and salivary cortisol See Figure 18.1.
	CRH Raised CSF levels (most studies)	Increased CRH drive	Similar finding reported in anorexia nervosa and Alzheimer's disease
	CRH test Normal rise in serum cortisol Blunted ACTH response within normal range	Increased CRH drive	Similar in anorexia nervosa and panic disorder. Quantitatively different in Cushing's disease (of differential diagnostic value) but may also be blunted in ACTH-independent Cushing's syndrome
	DST Non-suppression (0.5–2 mg overnight or over 48 h)	Impaired HPA axis function – feedback abnormal	DST (particularly low dose, overnight) may give a false-positive result during investigation of Cushing's syndrome
	Adrenal and pituitary gland morphology State-dependent enlargement in depression	Consistent with increased CRH drive	See Nieschlag[136]
HPT	TSH/fT4 index Blunted TSH rise in response to TRH Administration in unipolar depression	Increased endogenous TRH-like activity?	State or trait marker?
	High-normal fT4 index		Adjunctive T3 treatment of resistant depression

Axis	Finding	Interpretation	Comment
HPG	LH (basal levels; GnRH-stimulated) No consistent abnormality Possible reduced pulse frequency	Reduced GnRH pulse generator frequency	
GH PRL	GH Increased daytime pulse frequency GH pulse peak before sleep rather than in early sleep Blunted GH response to clonidine	? Decreased α_2 adrenoceptor-mediated GH release	Probably secondary to HPA axis disturbances
	Prolactin No consistent abnormalities	?	Stress may elevate serum prolactin
	Somatostatin Reduced CSF levels	?	State marker. Depression not recognized as a particular feature of SSoma
	Abnormalities in circadian rhythm time keeping i.e. 24-h profiles of circulating hormones: cortisol nadir, nocturnal prolactin rise, major GH nocturnal pulse advanced 2–3 h	?	Inconsistent evidence for this phase advance hypothesis of affective illness
Other: Time	Melatonin Decreased amplitude of rhythm Delayed rhythm	?	Melatonin unhelpful Light twice-daily effective treatment, but not melatonin mediated

Table 18.1
Endocrine abnormalities in major depressive illness.[137]

ACTH, adrenocorticotropic hormone; CRH, corticotropin-releasing hormone (100 μg ovine CRH); DST, dexamethasone suppression test; SSoma, somatostatinoma; HPA, hypothalamo-pituitary-adrenal; HPT, hypothalamo-pituitary-thyroid; HPG, hypothalamo-pituitary-gonadal; GH, growth hormone; PRL, prolactin; T3, triiodothyronine; GnRH, gonadotropin-releasing hormone; TRH, thyrotropin-releasing hormone; LH, luteinizing hormone; CSF, cerebrospinal fluid.

Table 18.1. Some are state-dependent markers of endogenous depression, as opposed to trait phenomena. In other words, they resolve with normalization of affect. None of the markers are entirely sensitive or specific, and they are less likely to be found in mild, atypical or bipolar forms of affective disorder. Nor do they, in general, have an exploitable therapeutic corollary, at least from an endocrine point of view; however, thyroid hormones are still used selectively by occasional psychiatrists as an adjunct to more conventional antidepressants in treatment-resistant cases.

The most notable endocrine abnormality is hyperactivity of the hypothalamo–pituitary-adrenal (HPA) axis. In fact, hypercortisolism in depressive illness is perhaps the most consistent finding in biological psychiatry. Other psychological conditions associated with altered HPA axis function are listed in Table 18.2. Disturbances of the hypothalamo–pituitary–thyroid (HPT) axis and hypothalamo–pituitary–gonadal (HPG) axes are well described, but their significance is even less clear. The psychopathology associated with growth hormone (GH) deficiency is elaborated in the section on hypopituitarism.

A number of mediators, particularly neuropeptides, have been investigated for their possible role in depression, but the evidence for their involvement is not compelling. Monoamines, notably noradrenaline (NA) and serotonin (5-HT), are more clearly implicated in the etiology of depression. Their importance is reflected in the development and use of selective reuptake inhibitors. Melatonin, an indoleamine released by the pineal gland, and a transducer of biological rhythms whose synthesis is controlled by NA and 5-HT, is not clearly involved in depressive illness, even including seasonal affective disorder.

Hypothalamo–pituitary–adrenal axis dysfunction: physiology and pathology

The importance of stress, a concept originally defined by Selye in 1936,[3] in the genesis of depression has evolved such that there is now accumulating evidence as to how psychological events and processes may interact with neuroendocrine circuits in the developing brain, from early childhood, to program an individual's psychological phenotype.[4] To some extent, this type of model provides an organic basis for earlier psychoanalytical or Freudian theories emphasizing the importance of childhood events in the genesis of later affective and anxiety disorders.

In health, a number of excitatory (serotoninergic and cholinergic) and inhibitory (adrenergic,[5] GABAergic, opioidergic) neurotransmitter pathways synapse on hypothalamic neurosecretory neurons, which in turn release potent adrenocorticotropic hormone (ACTH) secretagogues from the median eminence: the two hypothalamic secretagogues are corticotropin-releasing hormone (CRH) and arginine vasopressin (AVP). In addition to endogenous circadian rhythms, and feedback loops involving multiple CNS sites, including the hippocampus, physical and psychological stressors are well known to modify the normal diurnal variation in ACTH and cortisol.

There is a substantial amount of evidence favoring the pivotal importance of CRH overactivity in mediating the neuroendocrine, autonomic and behavioral responses to stress and, by implication, in the development of depression. This includes the finding of increased CRH in the cerebrospinal fluid of depressed patients and subsequent normalization as the depression lifts.[6,7] Early and repeated maternal separation of neonatal rat pups has the same effect, and is associated with increased anxiety and depressive-like behavior and higher basal and stress-induced ACTH rises during adulthood.[8] Increased HPA axis activity has been postulated to result from dysfunction of various tonic inhibitory and excitatory control mechanisms. For example, inhibitory opioid peptides regulate the release of both CRH and AVP, and a reduction in opioidergic tone could contribute to HPA axis overactivity. However, while most clinical studies employing the opioid antagonist naloxone are not consistent

Increased HPA axis activity	Decreased HPA axis activity
Melancholic depression	Atypical depression
Obsessive-compulsive disorder	Seasonal affective disorder
Panic disorder	Chronic fatigue syndrome
Anorexia nervosa	Fibromyalgia

Adapted from Tsigos and Chrousos. Physiology of the HPA axis in health and dysregulation in psychiatric and autoimmune disorders. In: Aron D, Tyrell, JB, eds. *Endocrinology and Metabolism Clinics of North America.* Philadelphia: WB Saunders Company, 1994: 451–66.

Table 18.2
Psychiatric/psychological disorders associated with altered HPA axis function

with the notion of opioidergic overactivity in depression, there are data using opioid agonists showing that the HPA axis is abnormally resistant to opioid inhibition in some depressed patients.[9]

Diagnosis

Although patients with endogenous depression do not usually have the physical signs of Cushing's syndrome, it may be difficult to differentiate true from pseudo-Cushing's syndrome due to depression, because of the high background prevalence of obesity, diabetes and hypertension, the affective disorder which can accompany true Cushing's syndrome, and because many of the hormonal abnormalities are found in both conditions. However, proximal myopathy, bruising and thin skin are relatively specific markers of the hypercortisolism associated with true Cushing's syndrome. Despite the presence of hypercortisolemia in depression, diurnal rhythmicity is preserved, albeit with a phase shift compared to non-depressed subjects (Figure 18.1). A commonly used screen, the overnight 0.5–1 mg dexamethasone suppression test (DST), may be abnormal in depression as well as in a number of other psychiatric disorders, including schizophrenia and obsessive-compulsive neurosis. Despite the non-specific nature of the DST, it is still sometimes used in clinical practice as a state marker of affect. Psychotropic medication may produce a false-positive result by inducing hepatic metabolism of dexamethasone. It is noteworthy that benzodiazepines in high doses can produce a false-negative result.[10] Cyclical activity in true Cushing's syndrome may also further complicate investigation. The interpretation of adrenal imaging studies (following biochemical confirmation) may also prove difficult, since radiological evidence of adrenal gland enlargement has also been found in patients with endogenous depression.[11,12]

A number of tests may be useful in making the differential diagnosis between Cushing's syndrome and pseudo-Cushing's states in general.[13] Midnight plasma cortisol values less than 50 nmol/l obtained in the

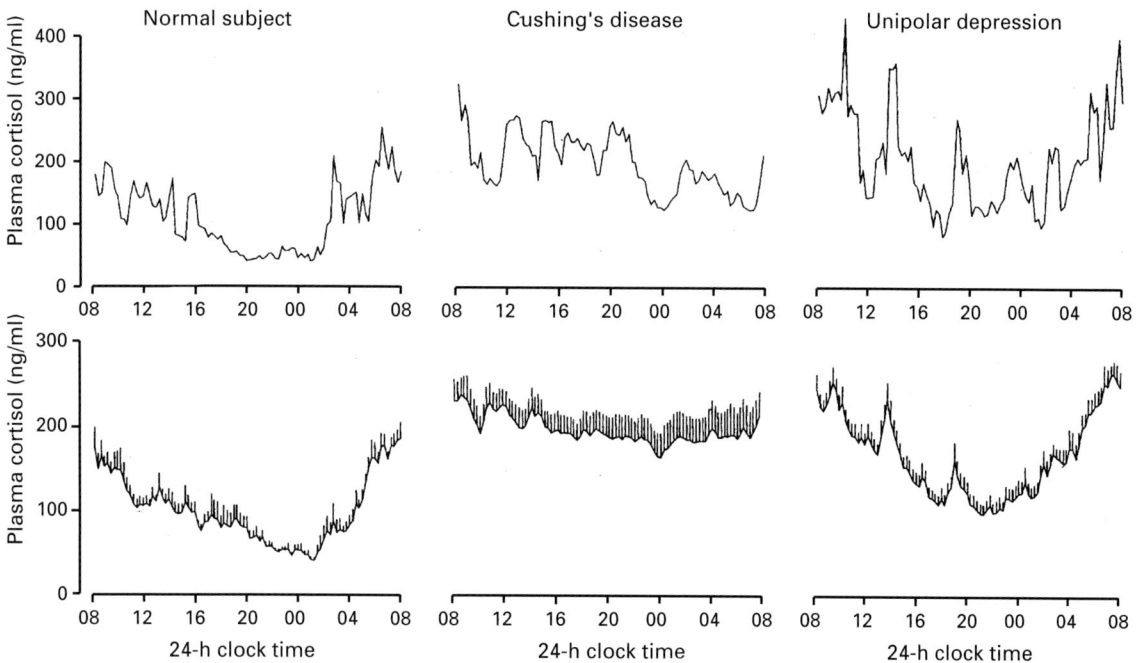

Figure 18.1
Twenty-four-hour profiles of plasma cortisol in normal subjects (left panel), and patients with Cushing's disease (middle panel) and unipolar endogenous depression (right panel). The top three graphs represent individuals. The bottom three graphs represent mean (n = 8–10) and SEM. From Van Cauter E. Physiology and pathology of circadian rhythms. In: Edwards CW, Lincoln DW, eds. Recent Advances in Endocrinology and Metabolism. Edinburgh: Churchill Livingstone, 1989: 109–34.

absence of stress (i.e. while asleep) indicate normality at the time of the test, while values greater than this are a sensitive but non-specific indicator of abnormality.[14] In another study, depressed patients were found to have midnight plasma cortisol values of less than 140 nmol/l, whereas Cushing's syndrome was associated with values greater than 207 nmol/l.[15] Serum cortisol is fully suppressed following the high-dose DST in the majority of depressed patients. It has been claimed that greater diagnostic sensitivity and specificity can be achieved using CRH 2 h after the last dose of dexamethasone in a low-dose dexamethasone suppression test:[16] only in Cushing's disease will cortisol rise in this situation. A blunted ACTH but enhanced cortisol response to CRH alone, presumably signifying downregulation of the pathway including and distal to the CRH receptor in accordance with the paradigm of increased endogenous CRH drive, may be found both in depression and in causes of Cushing's syndrome other than pituitary-dependent disease.

Hypothalamo–pituitary–thyroid axis dysfunction
Psychological symptoms are a well-recognized component of thyroid disease per se (see below), and this should be sought and treated as usual. Most patients with endogenous depression are both clinically and biochemically euthyroid. Nevertheless, a number of observations have been made with respect to the HPT axis. Difficulties arise in dissociating state-dependent changes from effects related to psychotropic therapy. Widely cited findings include a high normal free thyroxine index and a state-dependent elevation of rT3 within the normal range.

Thyrotrophin-releasing hormone (TRH): pathophysiology and diagnostic utility
TRH has a number of behavioral effects in animals, such as anorectic and anti-nociceptive actions and stimulation of movement. In humans, it can increase wellbeing, motivation and coping capacity, not only in physical and psychiatric disease but also in health. Unfortunately, studies of its possible therapeutic value in depression, used both intravenously and by administration of large oral doses, have been disappointing.

A frequently studied neuroendocrine phenomenon in depression is the non-specific finding of a blunted thyroid-stimulating hormone (TSH, i.e. thyrotrophin) response to TRH, despite normal basal levels of thyrotropin and thyroid hormones. Using a 5 mU/l cutoff point, blunting is observed in 25–30% of individuals with major depression, in contrast to 3% of apparently healthy controls with no personal or family history of psychiatric disease.[17] Since the TRH test remains abnormal in up to 50% of patients upon recovery of depression, in those few studies which have attempted individual follow-up, it has also been postulated that TSH blunting is a trait rather than a state marker of depression. Support for this notion has been drawn from the finding that thyrotrophin blunting has been found in patients with a past history of affective illness and apparently normal subjects who have a positive family history. Clearly, one marker cannot represent both a state and a trait marker. Although no association has been found between thyrotrophin blunting and severity or type of depression (unipolar versus bipolar; primary versus secondary), this marker may be associated with duration of illness, inasmuch as it has been found more commonly in chronic than in acute depression.

The putative biological significance of TSH blunting in response to TRH is unclear. Supranormal thyroid hormone levels are not seen in depression and cannot, therefore, underlie this phenomenon. While hypercortisolemia reduces TSH secretion in health and in Cushing's syndrome, such an association has not been found in primary depression. An alternative but unsubstantiated hypothesis is that blunting is a consequence of increased endogenous TRH drive and subsequent downregulation of thyrotroph TSH receptors. It has also been postulated that increased somatostatinergic tone is etiological, but this too has not been robustly demonstrated.

In summary, the TSH response to TRH has been used diagnostically both as a trait marker of depression and to determine the likelihood of a successful treatment outcome and relapse. In both diagnostic and therapeutic terms, TRH has not been of significant clinical value.

Therapeutic use of thyroid hormones in depression
From a clinical endocrinological standpoint, it may seem illogical to use thyroid hormones in the treatment of biochemically euthyroid patients with depression.[18] The basis for doing so originally stemmed from the observation of the greater toxicity of antidepressant drugs in hyperthyroidism. It was subsequently found that tri-iodothyronine (T3), in doses of 20–75 μg daily, can accelerate the therapeutic response to conventional tricyclic antidepressants, such as amitriptyline and imipramine; however, this is an inconsistent effect.[19,20] Moreover, T3 has also been found to convert tricyclic non-responders to therapeutic successes[21,22] in up to 66% of subjects of both sexes. The mechanism for this

interaction is unclear. It does not appear to be related to altered tricyclic pharmacokinetics/blood levels, but may be due to potentiation of central noradrenergic transmission, i.e. a pharmacodynamic effect. Although T3 has been more commonly studied, its therapeutic superiority to T4 has not been established. T3 has been found to be particularly effective in individuals with relatively higher pretreatment levels of T4 and who demonstrate a fall thereafter.[23] Suprahysiological doses of T4 have been used to stabilize patients with rapidly cycling bipolar affective disorder, but this is to be discouraged on endocrine grounds. If thyroid hormones are used adjunctively in affective disorders, it is clearly important to seek and avoid iatrogenic thyrotoxicosis, whatever dose is employed.

Hypothalamo–pituitary–gonadal axis dysfunction

Mood disturbances in the pre-menstrual syndrome (PMS) or late luteal phase dysphoric disorder, adolescence, pregnancy, the puerperium and the climacteric, as well as the much greater incidence of psychiatric disease in women compared to men, are testimony to the possible etiological significance of reproductive hormones[24] in disturbances of affect. The majority of studies of the HPG axis in depression are limited by methodological problems, such as single rather than dynamic measurements of one hormone and failure to control for menstrual phase, menopausal status and gender. Investigations have largely focused on potential abnormalities of feedback by gonadal steroids as well as opioids and CRH, the latter two having inhibitory effects on gonadotropin-releasing hormone (GnRH) release. Essentially, the findings have been inconsistent and inconclusive. While there is no clear evidence that estrogen therapy per se is beneficial in depression, leuprolide (a GnRH analog) has been successfully used to treat PMS, in conjunction with estrogen and progestin to ameliorate the adverse effects of chronic hypoestrogenism.[25]

Prolactin and growth hormone

Prolactin

It is well known that prolactin secretion is under tonic inhibitory control by dopamine released by tuberoinfundibular neurons. Serotonin, acting via 5-HT_{1A} (and possibly also $5\text{-HT}_{2A/C}$) receptors, also causes prolactin release. A number of other hypothalamic neuropeptides also have prolactin-releasing activity, notably TRH, vasopressin and oxytocin. Regulation of prolactin secretion is undoubtedly much more complex than that indicated, but levels may be principally affected by stress (in concert with systemic factors such as hypotension). Psychological/mental stress per se has not unequivocally been shown to affect prolactin release. Even so, it is important to avoid attaching too much significance to a single marginally elevated measurement in the absence of any clinical correlate, since there may have been a (pre-syncopal) stress response to venesection.

No consistent pattern of altered prolactin physiology has been documented in depression. It has proven difficult to control for the effects of associated stress and menstrual phase (for example, luteal levels of prolactin exceed those of the follicular phase in health). Various agents affecting the serotoninergic and dopaminergic pathway have been studied. It was originally held that relatively blunted prolactin responses to serotonin precursors and agonists was a marker of depression, but this is not a robust observation. In contrast, hyperprolactinemia per se, due, for example, to a prolactinoma, has been found to be associated with higher than normal rates of mood disturbance, including depression.[26]

Growth hormone

Reported abnormalities in GH secretion largely point to a blunting of α_2-adrenoceptor-mediated release (probably mediated by an effect on growth hormone-releasing hormone (GHRH)-containing neurons) and by a simultaneous increase in cholinergic responsiveness manifesting as increased somatostatinergic tone. Variable spontaneous GH secretory patterns have been described in depression. The clinical significance of these findings is unknown.

Anorexia and bulimia nervosa

Overview

Anorexia nervosa (AN) is overwhelmingly a disease of adolescent Caucasian females. Like bulimia nervosa (BN), its estimated prevalence in this subpopulation is 1% and may be increasing. The lifetime risk has been estimated to be 3%, and the mortality rate as high as 20%.[27] The approximate overall incidence of AN is up to 2 per 100 000 persons, with individuals from higher social classes and occupations such as ballet dancing being at relatively greater risk.[28]

AN is considered[29] to be a primary psychiatric disorder characterized by the triad of weight loss (>15%; a body mass index of <18 kg/m^2 is considered an alternative), amenorrhea (at least 3 months), and behavioral/perceptual disturbances such as distorted body image and intense fear of weight gain[30] (Table 18.3). Abnormalities of serotoninergic neurotransmission

> A Refusal to maintain body weight at or above a minimally normal weight for age and height (weight loss leading to maintenance of body weight <85% of that expected; or failure to make expected weight gain during period of growth, leading to body weight <85% of that expected)
> B Intense fear of gaining weight or becoming fat, even though underweight
> C Disturbance in the way in which one's body weight, size or shape is experienced (the person claims to feel fat even when obviously underweight), undue influence of body weight or shape on self-evaluation, or denial of seriousness of current body weight
> D Amenorrhea in postmenarchal females: absence of at least three consecutive menstrual cycles (in this classification, a woman is considered to have amenorrhea only if her menses occur solely after hormone administration, e.g. estrogen)
>
> Type
> Restricting (non-binge-eating/non-bulimic) type: During the episode of anorexia nervosa, the person does not regularly engage in binge-eating or purging behavior (i.e. self-induced vomiting or the misuse of laxatives, diuretics, or enemas).
> Non-restricting (binge-eating/bulimic) type: During the episode of anorexia nervosa, the person regularly engages in binge-eating or purging behavior.
> Reprinted from the *Diagnostic and Statistical Manual of Mental Disorders*, 4th edn. (DSM-IV). Washington DC: American Psychiatric Association, 1994: 544–55.

Table 18.3
Diagnostic criteria for anorexia nervosa.

have also been postulated to be etiological.[31] Although binge-eating behavior is commonly associated, it is the principal feature of the related eating disorder BN, in which weight loss is not clinically evident but which may lead to purging behavior. Both disorders are associated with neuroendocrine changes that, in AN at least, are believed to reflect, in part if not entirely, the metabolic adaptation to starvation. Nevertheless, the particular combination of various clinical manifestations such as anorexia, thermoregulatory disturbance and amenorrhea, as well as endocrine abnormalities such as hypogonadotropic hypogonadism, has led to speculation that AN is a primary organic hypothalamic disorder[32] with psychiatric manifestations.

The recent discovery of leptin,[33–36] a peptide produced by adipose tissue and which signals to the hypothalamus, has uncovered an important homeostatic pathway linking peripheral metabolic activity and body weight to reproductive function.[37–39] Leptin levels fall during fasting and leptin 'knockout' mice have neuroendocrine abnormalities similar to those of starvation.[40] It represents an obvious link between two of the cardinal features of AN.[41–43] Other central neuropeptides that may be mechanistically important in the genesis of AN include anorectic agents such as CRH, melanocortin-releasing hormone (MCH) and glucagon-like peptide 1–36 amide (GLP-1), and orectic (stimulating feeding) peptides such as neuropeptide Y (NPY).[44]

Clinical characteristics

The clinical features of AN are protean[45,46] and are summarized in Table 18.4. The psychopathology of AN and BN has been described previously.[29,47–49] The non-psychiatric abnormalities most likely to prompt endocrine assessment are amenorrhea and weight loss; excess facial lanugo hair may also be a presenting complaint. These physical changes tend to improve once critical body mass is re-attained. In contrast, behavioral and perceptual abnormalities may be longer lasting. It is clearly important to exclude structural hypothalamo–pituitary disease masquerading as an eating disorder,[50,51] since there is no single diagnostic clinical or laboratory test for these symptom complexes. Other clinical differential diagnoses worthy of consideration in the context of weight loss include inflammatory bowel disease, infection, particularly tuberculosis and HIV, malignancy and other endocrinopathies such as diabetes mellitus and Addison's disease.

Patients are paradoxically preoccupied with food, spending excessive time in preparing it and exhibiting detailed knowledge of recipes and calorific content. Overconsumption of raw vegetables may contribute to skin yellowing resulting from hypercarotenemia. A period of dieting may pre-date the onset of true AN. Excessive exercise, and gorging and purging, are common accompaniments; pneumomediastinum is a well-recognized complication of AN and particularly

Organ system	Symptoms and signs	Comments
Gastrointestinal	Cachexia	Protein-calorie malnutrition of prime importance
	Abdominal pain and early satiety	Possibly due to slow gastric emptying. Gastric rupture is a well-recognized complication of bingeing subtype of AN and BN. Asymptomatic pancreatitis
	Parotid enlargement	Secondary to malnutrition and vomiting
Metabolic	Cold sensitivity (hypothermia reported)/intolerance. Features similar to Raynaud's phenomenon Reduced basal metabolic rate (often with hyperactivity)	Reduced muscle thermogenesis and subcutaneous fat implicated. Attributed to functional hypothyroidism Related to low body mass
Reproductive	Amenorrhea, hypoestrogenism	Amenorrhea may pre-date or follow obvious weight loss. At risk of osteoporosis.
Cardiorespiratory	Bradycardia and other cardiac arrythmias, bradypnea, hypotension, mitral valve prolapse, peripheral edema	Arrythmias occasionally due to hypokalemia secondary to purging. LV mass may be reduced. Edema *not* related to hypoalbuminemia, but refeeding sometimes an identifiable precipitant
Renal	Polyuria	Impaired renal concentrating ability. Pre-renal uremia
Neurological	Muscle weakness, peripheral neuropathy	
Integumentary	Dryness, increased lanugo hair, hypercarotenemia	Reminiscent of hypothyroidism

NB: Most symptoms are denied.
Endocrine changes are summarized in Table 18.5.

Table 18.4
Non-psychiatric clinical features of anorexia nervosa.

BN. The latter may evolve from a purely restricting form of AN. Denial of symptoms is characteristic, although amenorrhea may be discussed more readily.

Endocrinopathy

A variety of non-specific endocrine abnormalities[52] have been described in AN, whereas the results of endocrine investigations are more usually normal in BN (Table 18.5). These have been considered to be consequences of the metabolic adaptation to starvation. For example, loss of reproductive function has been considered, at least teleologically, to be an appropriate response to excessive weight loss. Awareness of the possible endocrine biochemical findings may be of value in distinguishing AN from primary organic diseases, but these should not be used diagnostically in isolation.

Hypothalamo–pituitary–gonadal axis

Amenorrhea, usually secondary but sometimes primary, precedes significant weight loss in over two-thirds of women with AN. It is postulated to result from reversion of the hypothalamic GnRH pulse generator from an adult towards a typically

	Anorexia nervosa	Bulimia nervosa
LH:	↓ basal (cf. FSH) and LHRH-stimulated release	↓ or → basal (cf. FSH), ↑ LHRH-stimulated release
E2 (cf. T in men)/estrone/P	↓	→ or ↓
ACTH	→ (↓ response to CRH)	→ (↓ response to CRH)
Cortisol	↑ or →	↑ or →
DST	Abnormal (50–90%)	Abnormal (20–60%) See Kaye et al[138]
UFC	↑	→
DHEAS	↓	?
TSH	→ (↓ response to TRH)	→ or ↓ (↓ response to TRH)
T4	↓ or →	→
T3	↓	↓ or →
rT3	↑	?
GH	↑ or → (↓ IGF-1)	↑ or → (↓IGF-1)
Prolactin	↓ or →	↓ or →
Vasopressin:	↓	?

ACTH, adrenocorticotropic hormone (corticotropin); CRH, corticotropin-releasing hormone; UFC, urine free cortisol; DHEAS, dehydroepiandrosterone sulfate; GH, growth hormone; TRH, thyrotropin-releasing hormone; TSH, thyroid-stimulating hormone; T4, thyroxine; T3, triiodothyronine; rT3, reverse T3; LH, luteinizing hormone; LHRH, LH-releasing hormone; FSH, follicle-stimulating hormone; E2, estradiol; P, progesterone; T, testosterone; DST, dexamethatone suppression test; IGF-1, insulin-like growth factor-D; ↑, increased; ↓, decreased; →, unchanged

Table 18.5
Endocrine biochemistry and laboratory features of anorexia nervosa.

pre-pubertal pattern of activity in which gonadotropin levels are constantly low. This is not due to hyperprolactinemia, since both basal and TRH-stimulated serum prolactin levels are either low or normal. Some women have a pubertal pattern characterized by nocturnal sleep-dependent luteinizing hormone (LH) pulses. Recovery from AN is mirrored by progressive normalization of the circadian rhythm of serum gonadotropin levels. Despite restoration of weight, up to one-third of women fail to ovulate in the following year. Consistent with the notion of impaired GnRH release/pulsatility is the attenuation of pituitary responsiveness to acute GnRH stimulation, which itself, as with impaired GnRH release, may result from abnormalities in central noradrenergic (↓), dopaminergic (↓), serotoninergic and opiodergic (↑) neurotransmission. Dopamine and opioid antagonists (e.g. naltrexone) have been reported to stimulate menstruation but, in general, remain research tools and are not diagnostically useful. The response to clomiphene citrate is also typically blunted or absent. Pituitary sensitivity can be restored by continuous low-dose or pulsatile GnRH administration, which, like exogenous gonadotropins, has occasionally been used to induce ovulation.

From an endocrine perspective, the major adverse consequences are those of chronic hypoestrogenism, particularly reduced bone mineral density. Reduced peripheral conversion of estrogen precursors due to diminished subcutaneous fat depots has been hypothesized to contribute to estrogen deficiency, but this is probably of only relatively minor significance. Correspondingly, testosterone deficiency has been described in males. In women, estrogen replacement therapy should be initiated if there is unequivocal osteoporosis and persistent amenorrhea/anovulation associated with hypoestrogenism, since peak bone mass will frequently not have been achieved. The benefit may be limited,[53,54] and confined to maintaining rather than increasing trabecular bone mass in patients who continue to lose weight.[55] Additional therapy with antiresorptive agents such as bisphosphonates should be considered in patients with a particularly high fracture risk. Estrogen deficiency presumably also contributes to mildly elevated LDL-cholesterol, but there are no substantial data to suggest an increased long-term cardiovascular risk as opposed to a lower relative risk as a result of greater physical activity and lipid restriction.

Medication

Testosterone

Sex steroid hormone receptors are widely distributed within the CNS. In men, androgens are pivotal in defining behavioral characteristics such as aggressiveness, personality traits, sexuality and emotions. Contrary to popular belief, exogenous replacement androgen therapy is not clearly associated with adverse psychological sequelae.[56–58] In part, this may relate to the underestimation inherent in the use of self-reported questionnaires. This may seem surprising, given the large body of correlational evidence, albeit contested, demonstrating a relationship between extreme aggressive behavior and endogenous testosterone levels in both men and women.[59] Supraphysiological doses of testosterone used in healthy male volunteers have been shown to increase sexual arousal but not self-reported sexual activity or aggression.[60] One further complexity is the mutual interdependence between testosterone and aggression. Assertive or aggressive behavior followed by a rise in status leads to an increase in testosterone levels.

Increased mental drive and sense of wellbeing, deriving partly from improved physical and sexual performance, are usually achieved as serum testosterone levels are increased in treated hypogonadal men. Compared to the relative passivity of the hypogonadal state, there is no doubt that there is an increase in assertiveness commensurate with normal male behavior during treatment. Some men, however, dislike this and prefer to be under-treated. This may, of course, be suboptimal with respect to bone density.

Supplementing exogenous estrogen with testosterone in (oophorectomized) women has been shown to improve sexuality (arousal, and coital/orgasmic frequency) when compared to estrogen alone,[61] possibly by direct effects on cognitive function or on the peripheral nervous system. It is worth noting, however, that correlational studies have largely failed to provide evidence of a peak in female sexual behavior at the time of the mid-cycle peak in testosterone. Over and above an effect on sexual function, it may also improve mood and wellbeing.[62] Relatively greater hostility may also result from adding testosterone to estrogen therapy.[63] In general, there are few occasions where the addition of testosterone to hormone replacement therapy in women is indicated, unless the woman is also adrenally insufficient and hence lacking in adrenal androgens.

In contrast to the results of prolonged clinical use in hypogonadal patients, there are some limited data demonstrating a dose-dependent relationship between exogenous 'anabolic' androgenic steroids and irritability and aggression in eugonadal men. This has emerged from both field studies and a double-blind trial.[64] Such testosterone analogs used illicitly,[65] e.g. in the sporting world, are not intrinsically different with respect to side-effects, with the exception of 17α-alkylated derivatives, which are known to be hepatotoxic. The significantly higher doses often used, and the secrecy involved as well as their combination with other substances (e.g. GH), mean that it is difficult to firmly attribute causation to any pharmacodynamic effect. The underlying personality type may also be related to the willingness to abuse androgens. In one study employing high-dose 17α-methyltestosterone in normal male volunteers, one episode of mania affected 1 of 20 patients over a period of 2 weeks.[66]

Dopamine receptor agonists

Side-effects such as drowsiness, confusion, psychomotor excitation and hallucinations and other psychotic reactions are well-recognized, but fortunately uncommon, consequences of dopamine analog treatment, an agonist effect presumably mediated by stimulation of (D2) dopamine receptors. They have been reported to occur with doses commonly used[67] in the treatment of hyperprolactinemia and acromegaly,[68] as well as the much higher doses previously used for anti-parkinsonian therapy. Bromocriptine and other ergot alkaloid derivatives such as pergolide and lisuride and the non-ergot quinagolide, may have a greater propensity to cause psychotic reactions than cabergoline (also an ergot derivative), although clinical experience with the latter is relatively limited. Anorexia and weight loss have been documented with quinagolide used in conventional doses; so too have the positive effects of improved motivation, emotional responsiveness and heightened sense of wellbeing, although it is possible that these relate to reduction of serum prolactin and co-normalization of other pituitary hormones.[69]

Psychotic symptoms, including auditory hallucinations, delusions, and significant mood changes, supervened in 1.3% of 600 patients treated with bromocriptine or lisuride, psychiatric diagnoses comprising schizophreniform psychosis (paranoid type), monosymptomatic hypochondriacal psychosis (a type of paranoid illness), and hypomania. These disappeared after treatment was stopped or dosage reduced, thus suggesting that they are dose-dependent.[69,70] Their onset is usually early after initiation of treatment but may be delayed for several months.[68,69] Psychosis may be more likely to occur in patients with a prior history of serious mental disorder, and caution is therefore advised in such circumstances. Obviously, dopamine agonist therapy should be discontinued if psychosis develops. If the endocrine consequences of stopping pose a significant clinical hazard, a trial of dosage reduction might be considered as an alternative, although this may prove both ineffective and hazardous from the psychiatric perspective. Even though some side-effects such as nausea may be mitigated by switching to an alternative dopamine agonist, this should be avoided following a psychotic reaction. It is illogical to continue dopamine agonist treatment and to add antipsychotic therapy, since the latter class of drugs act principally by antagonizing dopamine receptors. Nevertheless, antipsychotic therapy may be required in addition to discontinuing dopamine agonist drugs, albeit temporarily.

Endocrine disorders

Cushing's syndrome

Psychiatric disorders, especially depression, are a common feature of Cushing's syndrome irrespective of its etiology, probably as a direct result of pathological hypercortisolemia. Indeed, one of Harvey Cushing's first patients, reported in the *American Journal of Insanity*, was found in a mental asylum. Psychiatric disorders may result from suppression of the dopaminergic mesocorticolimbic and CRH/locus ceruleus–noradrenergic sympathetic system. There have also been suggestions that ACTH may be more important in the genesis of mental disturbance, since some investigators have found a higher rate in ACTH-dependent compared to ACTH-independent Cushing's syndrome.[72] Peptides co-secreted from the pituitary and the propensity of ACTH-dependent sources of Cushing's syndrome to cycle are interesting in this respect.[73] Against this notion is the observation that therapies aimed at lowering cortisol levels (e.g. metyrapone; bilateral adrenalectomy) are the mainstay in the treatment of Cushingoid mental dysphoria, in spite of causing a rise in ACTH levels.

To varying degrees, mental disturbances may affect 60–80% of patients with Cushing's syndrome.[74] The onset is most commonly recognized after the physical symptoms and signs supervene, but an antecedent psychological disorder may be more common than hitherto recognized;[75] it may precede overt manifestations of endocrine disease by several years.[76] Nevertheless, psychiatric symptoms do not have diagnostic specificity. Conversely, disturbances of HPA activity—reflected in abnormal diagnostic tests—are a frequent finding in primary depression, and this may confound the interpretation of test results (see above). As many as 50% of patients with Cushing's syndrome have been found to meet rigorous criteria for major affective disorder, usually depression.[77,78] Atypical, as opposed to melancholic, depression, itself often associated with a comorbid psychiatric disorder, has been reported to be the commonest variant (17 of 33 patients). It is characterized by hyperphagia, increased fatigue and excessive sleep.[79] Atypical depression has been judged to reflect, in contradistinction to melancholia, hypoactivation of the stress system related to hyposecretion of CRH. The overrepresentation of atypical depression is consonant with the finding of reduced CRH secretion in Cushing's syndrome, secondary to the negative feedback effects of elevated glucocorticoid levels on the hypothalamus and higher centers.[80] Other common symptoms include anxiety and panic.[81]

Interestingly, the depression of Cushing's syndrome has been noted to be intermittent, lasting for periods of a few days, compared to the unremitting dysphoria of endogenous depression.[82] Euphoria or mania may predominate earlier in the course of the illness, and may be commoner in cases of exogenous hypercortisolemia. Symptomatology is not constantly related to drug dosage, but may be more likely with doses of prednisolone exceeding 30 mg (or equivalent). By analogy, no clear association exists between the severity of non-iatrogenic Cushing's syndrome and psychopathological symptoms, although more time-integrated measures of severity and an index of tissue sensitivity to glucocorticoids may be required to assess this.[72,79] Psychiatric symptoms may occur in patients who have previously tolerated the same dose without ill-effect.[83] Although depression, like other psychological disturbances, tends to remit following restoration of normal serum cortisol levels ('cure'), this may be delayed by several months[84] and is not invariable. In one series of 40 patients, improvement in psychiatric symptoms was noted to occur mostly within 2 months of lowering of plasma cortisol, irrespective of the etiology of Cushing's syndrome or mode of treatment.[76] It may be resistant to antidepressant drug therapy and result in suicide. Individual factors, such as personality, and the severity and chronicity of preceding hypercortisolemia, may play a role in determining the psychological response to treatment.

While some symptoms may reflect depression, the symptoms of reduced libido (partly also due to cortisol and androgen excess), sleep disruption (presumably due to night-time hypercortisolemia), cognitive impairment, emotional lability, anxiety, irritability, loss of energy and mild paranoia are also commonly noted (~ 50%) and are worth specific enquiry. As a result, interpersonal problems frequently affect familial and working relationships.

Addison's disease

In Addison's original description, patients were described as having an 'inability to concentrate, drowsiness, restlessness, insomnia, irritability, apprehension, and disturbed sleep'. Psychiatric disturbance is common, manifesting in some fashion in as many as 40–60% of patients. Perceptual abnormalities, often appearing early on, are well recognized and include enhanced sensitivity to but impaired recognition and interpretation of olfactory, gustatory, auditory and tactile stimuli. The apparent absence of more obvious stigmata of adrenocortical failure may cause diagnostic difficulty.

Other presenting symptoms may include apathy, negativism, fatigue, poverty of thought, anhedonia, and social withdrawal, reflecting depression in 20–40% of patients. Organic brain syndrome has a reported incidence of 5–20%.[85] Depending on the acuteness, this may declare itself as psychosis (including paranoid and schizophreniform), delirium, memory impairment, stupor or coma. The role of hyponatremia in the pathogenesis of these psychiatric disturbances is not clear, despite the recognition that a low serum sodium per se is associated with similar psychiatric disturbances and that improvement is sometimes correlated with correction of severe electrolyte imbalance.

In general, symptoms usually remit within a few days of glucocorticoid replacement. Psychosis can take longer to improve, and indeed has been reported to develop as a result of treatment with physiological doses of glucocorticoid, putatively due to upregulation of hippocampal glucocorticoid receptors as a consequence of prolonged hypocortisolemia.[86]

Thyrotoxicosis

Neuropsychiatric problems are very common accompaniments of thyrotoxicosis, irrespective of the underlying etiology, and may lead to a delay in diagnosis or misdiagnosis. It has also been suggested many times that the onset or relapses of the disease may be precipitated by stress, although this has been hard to prove. Increased adrenergic activity may be involved, since β-adrenoceptor blockade ameliorates most of the symptoms. Nervousness, anxiety, restlessness, insomnia and emotional lability and irritability are especially prominent, although, in the elderly, apathy, psychomotor retardation, negativism and social withdrawal may predominate and masquerade as dementia. Depression may affect as many as 14% of patients, usually in the prodromal phase,[75] although in one study 9 of 13 (69%) subjects with thyrotoxic Graves' disease had major depression; additionally, 8 of 13 had generalized anxiety disorder, while 3 of 13 were hypomanic.[87] Cognitive deficits (impaired memory, attention span, planning and productivity) may persist following restoration of euthyroidism.[88]

With the advent of anti-thyroid therapy, more extreme mental disturbance, including confusion, bipolar affective disorder, and paranoid and schizophreniform reactions,[89] has become rarer; it may be more common in patients with underlying psychiatric dysfunction. Only 10 of 8000 cases (0.125%) of overt psychosis were associated with thyrotoxicosis in one early study.[90] Confusion and/or delirium may be apparent in impending or frank thyroid storm. Psychotic reactions[91] have also rarely been described following commencement of anti-thyroid therapy.[92] Anorexia is more likely to complicate severe thyrotoxicosis. In patients with pre-existing epilepsy, the frequency of seizures may increase.

Hypothyroidism

Psychiatric manifestations of hypothyroidism (Table 18.6) have long been recognized, and thyroid function

	Prevalence (%)
Fatigue/lethargy	40
Depression	66–90
Cognitive (e.g. memory) impairment, dementia	
Agitation, irritability, mania	
Delirium	
Psychosis, e.g. paranoid delusions, hallucinations (auditory)	
Affective lability	
Hypersexuality	

Table 18.6
Hypothyroidism: psychiatric features.

testing should be considered in any patient with mental disturbance. As reviewed in Asher's classical paper, the commonest presentations formerly were depression (>50% of patients), or an agitated paranoid state,[7] patients 'admitting rather than complaining of symptoms' because of mental dullness. Other manifestations include chronic insidious personality change, with labile mood, anxiety and emotional withdrawal, psychotic depression and mania. The prevalence of psychosis complicating untreated hypothyroidism, whatever the underlying etiology, was estimated to be 5–15% in 1984,[92] but is presumably falling with increasing routine measurement of thyroid function and earlier initiation of treatment. Symptoms tend to be more severe in the elderly and when hypothyroidism develops rapidly.[85] In the latter situation, there may also be alternating periods of lethargy and restlessness, agitation, and hypersexuality. More subtle neuropsychiatric defects, particularly cognitive impairment and depression, accompany mild hypothyroidism, and so-called subclinical hypothyroidism.

Mental disturbance usually resolves completely within weeks to months following the initiation of thyroid hormone replacement therapy, but often begins to improve within days. Delusions and hallucinations usually disappear in the first week but may return within a short period if treatment is discontinued. This may be as short as 12–18 h in the case of liothyronine (T3). Irreversibility is well recognized in long-standing cases and undetected hypothyroidism affecting the developing brain. Treatment should be started gradually in severe hypothyroidism. In addition to cardiac complications, mania and psychosis may develop, the latter typically in patients with a prior or family history of psychiatric disorder or when high–normal doses of thyroid hormone have been used.[93] The amelioration of psychosis, restlessness and anxiety complicating replacement therapy may be effectively hastened using adjunctive antipsychotic agents or benzodiazepines. Antidepressants used in conjunction with thyroxine may be of value in cases of unresolving severe depression, but such a combination should be employed with caution, because of the potential for increased toxicity of tricyclic agents, as noted above.

Hypopituitarism

The psychopathology of hypopituitarism is likely to result from the combined effects of multiple pituitary hormone deficiencies rather than representing a unique entity, although a distinct apathy syndrome has been described.[94] Hence, a constellation of well-known symptoms may be present, reflecting varying degrees of gonadotroph, corticotroph and thyrotroph failure. Nevertheless, it is common clinical experience that a number of patients remain unwell despite optimal replacement with necessary sex steroids, glucocorticoid, and thyroxine. Other factors, such as the burden of visual impairment and epilepsy, have not been systematically investigated with respect to quality of life (QoL) in hypopituitary patients. Nevertheless, there is increasing evidence[95–98] that at least one important underlying explanation in such cases is untreated adult GH deficiency (GHD).[99] This does not appear to affect all patients equally, and there is wide individual variation.

The psychopathology of growth hormone deficiency

The apparent lack of somatic stigmata of GHD in adults has relatively recently given way to the recognition of physical abnormalities such as an increase in total body fat, mainly intra-abdominal (which may partly relate to the increased cardiovascular mortality), osteoporosis, hyperlipidemia, and decreased muscle strength and exercise tolerance.[96–98,100,101] Further studies have revealed a reduced sense of physical and psychological wellbeing,[102–106] which presumably underlie the observation that patients with hypopituitarism have subnormal socio-economic achievement and poor social interaction, as judged by below-average rates of employment and marriage, particularly if the onset was in childhood.[104,107,108] However, compared to normative data, only limited differences in functioning and QoL were found when GHD adults who had been treated with GH during childhood were compared to their same-sex siblings, suggesting a need for caution in selecting the most appropriate control group; in the same study, adult height and degree of growth over the course of GH therapy were generally found to be unrelated to QoL outcomes.[109] A methodological flaw of this interesting investigation was the failure to reassess the endocrine status of young adults treated for childhood GHD—it is well recognized that the GH status of children with idiopathic GHD frequently normalizes in adulthood. Overall, there is conflicting evidence concerning the possibility that short stature secondary to GHD adversely affects self-esteem, body image and QoL in children.[110,111] Controlling for the effects of chronic disease has been inconsistent, and both a relatively reduced (when compared to diabetic patients) and normal QoL (in relation to 'mastoid surgical' patients) have been found.[99,112] The negative impact of adverse life events, unrelated to hypothalamo–pituitary disease, on QoL has been controlled for by using tools such as the Life Event Inventory.

In adults, the principal psychosocial characteristics of GHD comprise anxiety, depression, irritability, mental fatigue, reduced cognition (especially memory), self-esteem, poor life-fulfilment, and social isolation (Table 18.7). Importantly, the specificity of these abnormalities is confirmed by the repeated observation that the psychiatric morbidity attributed to GHD is significantly improved in patients selected for GH replacement therapy (on the basis of specific criteria), in most,[102,108,113–115] but not all, studies,[112,116–121] as judged by a number of generic psychological health profile assessment tools (usually questionnaires). These include the Nottingham Health Profile, Psychological General Well-Being Schedule, Comprehensive Psychopathological Rating Scale, General Health Questionnaire, Hopkins Symptom Checklist and Short-Form 36. The former, while widely employed, has the disadvantage that it may not be sensitive enough to detect small improvements in QoL. Conflicting results in the literature may also relate to the difficulty in predicting which patients will most benefit from GH, the variable balance between positive effects and side-effects, and the difficulty in measuring QoL.

The appropriateness of self-rating questionnaires to quantify QoL in adult GHD has itself been questioned.[122] It is possible that the conflicting data in the literature are partly related to the type of questionnaire/methodology employed in a particular study.[123,124] A more disease-specific questionnaire, the Assessment of GH Deficiency in Adults (AGHDA),[104] continues to be included in a number of clinical trials and a large international database monitoring the long-term efficacy and safety of GH replacement therapy.[125] It appears to have good reliability, internal consistency and construct validity, and is available in a variety of European languages.[126] It concentrates on body image and fat distribution, low energy level, difficulties with concentration and memory, irritability and temper, lack of strength and stamina, reduced physical and mental drive, dislike of stimulation, and difficulty in coping with stress. A score of >6 is considered to indicate a significantly reduced QoL.[97] Other relatively GHD disease-specific questionnaires are the GHD Questionnaire[127] and a combination of the Modified Impact, Life Fulfilment, and Self-Esteem scales.[128]

Most improvement, predictably, has been found in patients with severe GHD and the greatest deficit in energy and vitality prior to commencing GH.[97,129] The degree of reduction of QoL has been linked to duration of GHD.[108] Improved QoL is frequently evident within the first 3 months of maintenance treatment with GH, but may occasionally be delayed. Since the response to treatment may not be (fully) manifest for 6 months in as many as 30% of patients after the onset of treatment, therapy should be continued for at least this period of time before judgement is made as to its efficacy in improving QoL.[130] Response rates during chronic treatment (20–50 months) have exceeded 80%.[97] Beneficial effects have been documented to last at least as long as 10 years if treatment is continued.[115]

Depression
Anxiety
Irritability/emotional lability
Social isolation
Difficulty with sexual relationships
Reduced sense of wellbeing (mental and physical)
Dissatisfaction with body image
Reduced self-esteem
Poor memory (short and long term)

Table 18.7
Psychological features of adult GH deficiency.

The mechanism by which GH improves QoL is unclear,[118,131] but may involve direct neuroendocrine effects of GH and IGF-1, i.e. within the CNS. There is evidence for GH immunoreactivity in primate cortex, hippocampus and amygdaloid nucleus that persists after hypophysectomy, and GH-binding sites[132] have been found in a variety of human brain areas at autopsy. The high density of binding sites in the choroid plexus may explain the increase in cerebrospinal fluid GH concentration that is observed following GH treatment of GH-deficient adults,[133] and there is evidence that GH affects brain neurotransmitter systems (e.g. reduction in dopamine turnover and increased aspartate and endorphin).[132,134] Other mechanisms, such as changes in body composition, including normalization of total body and extracellular water, and improvement in exercise capacity and muscle strength, have been postulated, and while there is evidence that these changes are induced by GH replacement therapy, there is as yet no evidence to show that they are causally linked to increased QoL. Suboptimal replacement therapy with thyroxine, glucocorticoid and sex hormones has generally been excluded before assessment of GH-specific effects on QoL, but this factor may be relevant in view of the association between QoL and both the likelihood of GH deficiency and the number of pituitary hormone deficiencies.[108,135]

References

1. Asher R. Myxoedematous madness. *BMJ* 1949; 2: 555–62.
2. Powell GF, Brasel JA, Raiti S, Blizzard RM. Emotional deprivation and growth retardation simulating idiopathic hypopituitarism. II. Endocrinologic evaluation of the syndrome. *N Engl J Med* 1967; 276(23): 1279–83.
3. Selye H. A syndrome produced by diverse noxious agents. *Nature* 1936; 138: 32–5.
4. Heim C, Owens MJ, Plotsky PM, Nemeroff CB. Persistent changes in corticotropin-releasing factor systems due to early life stress: relationship to the pathophysiology of major depression and post-traumatic stress disorder. *Psychopharmacol Bull* 1997; 33(2): 185–92.
5. Plotsky PM, Cunningham ETJ, Widmaier EP. Catecholaminergic modulation of corticotropin-releasing factor and adrenocorticotropin secretion. *Endocrine Rev* 1989; 10(4): 437–58.
6. Nemeroff CB, Widerlov E, Bissette G, et al. Elevated concentrations of CSF corticotropin-releasing factor-like immunoreactivity in depressed patients. *Science* 1984; 226: 1342–4.
7. Arborelius L, Owens MJ, Plotsky PM, Nemeroff CB. The role of corticotrophin releasing factor in depression and anxiety disorders. *J Endocrinol* 1999; 160: 1–12.
8. Ladd CO, Owens MJ, Nemeroff CB. Persistent changes in corticotropin-releasing factor neuronal systems induced by maternal deprivation. *Endocrinology* 1996; 137: 1212–18.
9. Garland EJ, Zis AP. Effect of codeine and oxazepam on afternoon cortisol secretion in men. *Psychoneuroendocrinology* 1989; 14: 397–402.
10. Lamberts SW. Neuro-endocrine aspects of the dexamethasone suppression test in psychiatry. *Life Sci* 1986; 39(2): 91–5.
11. Amsterdam JD, Marinelli DL, Arger P, Winokur A. Assessment of adrenal gland volume by computed tomography in depressed patients and healthy volunteers: a pilot study. *Psychiatry Res* 1987; 21(3): 189–97.
12. Nemeroff CB, Krishnan KR, Reed D, Leder R, Beam C, Dunnick NR. Adrenal gland enlargement in major depression. A computed tomographic study. *Arch Gen Psychiatry* 1992; 49(5): 384–7.
13. Newell-Price J, Trainer PJ, Besser GM, Grossman AB. The diagnosis and differential diagnosis of Cushing's syndrome and Pseudo-Cushing's states. *Endocrine Rev* 1998; 19(5): 647–72.
14. Newell-Price J, Trainer PJ, Perry L, Grossman A, Besser M. A single sleeping midnight cortisol has 100% sensitivity for the diagnosis of Cushing's syndrome. *Clin Endocrinol* 1995; 43: 545–50.
15. A single midnight cortisol measurement discriminates Cushing's syndrome from pseudo-Cushing states. 1994.
16. Yanovski JA, Cutler GBJ, Chrousos GP, Nieman LK. Corticotropin-releasing hormone stimulation following low-dose dexamethasone administration. A new test to distinguish Cushing's syndrome from pseudo-Cushing's states. *JAMA* 1993; 269(17): 2232–8.
17. Loosen PT. Thyroid function in affective disorders and alcoholism. *Endocrinol Metab Clin North Am* 1988; 17(1): 55–82.
18. Joffe RT, Sokolov STH, Singer W. Thyroid hormone treatment of depression. *Thyroid* 1995; 5: 235–9.
19. Feighner JP, King LJ, Schuckit MA, Croughan J, Briscoe W. Hormonal potentiation of imipramine and ECT in primary depression. *Am J Psychiatry* 1972; 128: 1230–8.
20. Wilson I, Prange AJ, McClane T, Rabon AM, Lipton MA. Thyroid-hormone enhancement of imipramine in non-retarded depression. *N Engl J Med* 1970; 282: 1063–7.
21. Earle BV. Thyroid hormone and tricyclic antidepressants in resistant depressions. *Am J Psychiatry* 1970; 126: 1667–9.

22. Goodwin FK, Prange AJ, Post RM, Muscettola G, Lipton MA. Potentiation of antidepressant effect by L-triiodothyronine in tricyclic nonresponders. *Am J Psychiatry* 1982; **139**: 34–8.
23. Whybrow P, Coppen A, Prange AJ, Nogeura R, Bailey JE. Thyroid function and the response to liothyronine in depression. *Arch Gen Psychiatry* 1972; **26**: 242–5.
24. Weissman M, Klerman GL. Sex differences and the epidemiology of depression. *Arch Gen Psychiatry* 1977; **34**: 98–111.
25. Mortola JF, Girton L, Fischer U. Successful treatment of severe premenstrual syndrome by combined use of a gonadotropin-releasing hormone agonist and estrogen/progestin. *J Clin Endocrinol Metab* 1991; **72**: 252A–F.
26. Sobrinho LG. In: Neuropsychiatry of Prolactin. Grossman AB, ed. *Psychoneuroendocrinology* 5th edn., vol. 8. Baillière Tindall, 1991; 119–42.
27. Moller-Madsen S, Nystrup J, Nielsen S. Mortality of anorexia nervosa in Denmark during the period 1970–1987. *Acta Psychiatr Scand* 1996; **94**: 454–9.
28. Wakeling A. Epidemiology of anorexia nervosa. *Psychiatry Res* 1996; **62**(1): 3–9.
29. Walsh BT, Devlin MJ. Eating disorders: progress and problems. *Science* 1998; **280**(5368): 1387–90.
30. *Diagnostic and Statistical Manual of Mental Disorders* (DSM-IV), 4th edn. Washington DC: American Psychiatric Association, 1994.
31. Halmi KA. The psychobiology of eating behavior in anorexia nervosa. *Psychiatry Res* 1996; **62**(1): 23–9.
32. Gold PW, Gwirtsman H, Avgerinos PC et al. Abnormal hypothalamic–pituitary–adrenal function in anorexia nervosa. Pathophysiologic mechanisms in underweight and weight-corrected patients. *N Engl J Med* 1986; **314**(21): 1335–42.
33. Rosenbaum M, Leibel RL. The role of leptin in human physiology. *N Engl J Med* 1999; **341**(12): 913–15.
34. Mantzoros CS. The role of leptin in human obesity and disease: a review of current evidence. *Ann Intern Med* 1999; **130**(8): 671–80.
35. Bray GA, York DA. Clinical review 90: Leptin and clinical medicine: a new piece in the puzzle of obesity. *J Clin Endocrinol Metab* 1997; **82**(9): 2771–6.
36. Auwerx J, Staels B. Leptin. *Lancet* 1998; **351**(9104): 737–42.
37. Barash IA, Cheung CC, Weigle DS et al. Leptin is a metabolic signal to the reproductive system. *Endocrinology* 1996; **137**(7): 3144–7.
38. Thong FS, Graham TE. Leptin and reproduction: is it a critical link between adipose tissue, nutrition, and reproduction? *Can J Appl Physiol* 1999; **24**(4): 317–36.
39. Messinis IE, Milingos SD. Leptin in human reproduction. *Human Reprod Update* 1999; **5**(1): 52–63.
40. Ahima RS, Prabakaran D, Mantzoros C et al. Role of leptin in the neuroendocrine response to fasting. *Nature* 1996; **382**(6588): 250–2.
41. Eckert ED, Pomeroy C, Raymond N, Kohler PF, Thuras P, Bowers CY. Leptin in anorexia nervosa. *J Clin Endocrinol Metab* 1998; **83**(3): 791–5.
42. Warren MP, Voussoughian F, Geer EB, Hyle EP, Adberg CL, Ramos RH. Functional hypothalamic amenorrhea: hypoleptinemia and disordered eating. *J Clin Endocrinol Metab* 1999; **84**(3): 873–7.
43. Grinspoon S, Gulick T, Askari H et al. Serum leptin levels in women with anorexia nervosa. *J Clin Endocrinol Metab* 1996; **81**(11): 3861–3.
44. Kalra SP, Dube MG, Pu S, Xu B, Horvath TL, Kalra PS. Interacting appetite-regulating pathways in the hypothalamic regulation of body weight. *Endocrine Rev* 1999; **20**(1): 68–100.
45. Woodside DB. A review of anorexia nervosa and bulimia nervosa. *Curr Problems Pediatrics* 1995; **25**(2): 67–89.
46. Steinhausen HC. Treatment and outcome of adolescent anorexia nervosa. *Hormone Res* 1995; **43**(4): 168–70.
47. Pike KM. Long-term course of anorexia nervosa: response, relapse, remission, and recovery. *Clin Psychol Rev* 1998; **18**(4): 447–75.
48. Powers PS. Initial assessment and early treatment options for anorexia nervosa and bulimia nervosa. *Psychiatr Clin North Am* 1996; **19**(4): 639–55.
49. Hartman D. Anorexia nervosa—diagnosis, aetiology, and treatment. *Postgrad Med J* 1995; **71**(842): 712–16.
50. Heron GB, Johnston DA. Hypothalamic tumor presenting as anorexia nervosa. *Am J Psychiatry* 1976; **133**(5): 580–2.
51. Chipkevitch E. Brain tumors and anorexia nervosa syndrome. *Brain Dev* 1900; **16**(3): 175–9.
52. Bergh C, Sodersten P. Anorexia nervosa, self-starvation and the reward of stress. *Nature Med* 1996; **2**(1): 21–2.
53. Grinspoon S, Herzog D, Klibanski A. Mechanisms and treatment options for bone loss in anorexia nervosa. *Psychopharmacol Bull* 1997; **33**(3): 399–404.
54. Carmichael KA, Carmichael DH. Bone metabolism and osteopenia in eating disorders. *Medicine* 1995; **74**(5): 254–67.
55. Klibanski A, Biller BM, Schoenfeld DA, Herzog DB, Saxe VC. The effects of estrogen administration on trabecular bone loss in young women with anorexia nervosa. *J Clin Endocrinol Metab* 1995; **80**: 898–904.
56. Archer J. The influence of testosterone on human aggression. *Br J Psychol* 1991; **82**: 1–28.
57. Anderson RA. The effects of exogenous testosterone on sexuality and mood of normal men. *J Clin Endocrinol Metab* 1992; **75**: 1503–7.
58. O'Carroll R, Shapiro C, Bancroft J. Androgens, behavior and nocturnal erection in hypogonadal men: the effects of varying the replacement dose. *Clin Endocrinol* 1985; **23**(5): 527–38.
59. Christiansen K. In: Psychotropic effects of androgens. Nieschlag E, Behre HM, eds. *Testosterone: Action, Deficiency, Substitution*, 2nd edn. Berlin: Springer-Verlag; 1998; 107–42.

60. Bagatell CJ, Heiman JR, Matsumoto AM. Metabolic and behavioral effects of high-dose, exogenous testosterone in healthy men. *J Clin Endocrinol Metab* 1994; 79: 561–7.

61. Sherwin BB, Gelfand MM. Differential symptom response to parenteral estrogen and/or androgen administration in the surgical menopause. *Am J Obstet Gynecol* 1985; 151(2): 153–60.

62. Buckler HM, Robertson WR, Wu FC. Which androgen replacement therapy for women? *J Clin Endocrinol Metab* 1998; 83(11): 3920–4.

63. Sherwin BB, Gelfand MM. Sex steroids and affect in the surgical menopause: a double-blind, cross-over study. *Psychoneuroendocrinology* 1985; 10(3): 325–35.

64. Hannan CJJ, Friedl KE, Zold A, Kettler TM, Plymate SR. Psychological and serum homovanillic acid changes in men administered androgenic steroids. *Psychoneuroendocrinology* 1991; 16(4): 335–43.

65. Wilson JD. Androgen abuse by athletes. *Endocrine Rev* 1988; 9(2): 181–99.

66. Su TP, Pagliaro M, Schmidt PJ, Pickar D, Wolkowitz O, Rubinow DR. Neuropsychiatric effects of anabolic steroids in male normal volunteers. *JAMA* 1993; 269(21): 2760–4.

67. Pearson KC. Mental disorders from low-dose bromocriptine. *N Engl J Med* 1981; 305(3): 173.

68. Steinbeck K, Turtle JR. Treatment of acromegaly with bromocriptine. *Aust NZ J Med* 1979; 9: 217–24.

69. Barnett PS, Palazidou E, Miell JP et al Endocrine function, psychiatric and clinical consequences in patients with macroprolactinomas after long-term treatment with the new non-ergot dopamine agonist CV205–502. *Q J Med* 1991; 81(295): 891–906.

70. Turner TH, Cookson JC, Wass JAH, Besser GM. Psychotic reactions during treatment of pituitary tumours with dopamine agonists. *BMJ* 1984; 289: 1101–3.

71. Starkman MN, Schteingart DE. Neuropsychiatric manifestations of patients with Cushing's syndrome. Relationship to cortisol and adrenocorticotropic hormone levels. *Arch Intern Med* 1981; 141(2): 215–19.

72. Cohen SI. Cushing's syndrome: a psychiatric study of 29 patients. *Br J Psychiatry* 1980; 136: 120–4.

73. Ur E. Psychological aspects of hypothalamo–pituitary–adrenal activity. *Psychoneuroendocrinology* 1991; 6: 79–96.

74. Haskett RF. Diagnostic categorization of psychiatric disturbance in Cushing's syndrome. *Am J Psychiatry* 1985; 142(8): 911–16.

75. Sonino N, Fava GA, Belluardo P, Girelli ME, Boscaro M. Course of depression in Cushing's syndrome: response to treatment and comparison with Graves' disease. *Hormone Res* 1993; 39(5–6): 202–6.

76. Jeffcoate WJ, Silverstone JT, Edwards CR, Besser GM. Psychiatric manifestations of Cushing's syndrome: response to lowering of plasma cortisol. *Q J Med* 1979; 48(191): 465–72.

77. Hudson JI, Hudson MS, Griffing GT, Melby JC, Pope HG Jr. Phenomenology and family history of affective disorder in Cushing's disease. *Am J Psychiatry* 1987; 144(7): 951–3.

78. Kelly WF, Kelly MJ, Faragher B. A prospective study of psychiatric and psychological aspects of Cushing's syndrome. *Clin Endocrinol* 1996; 45(6): 715–20.

79. Dorn LD, Burgess ES, Dubbert B et al. Psychopathology in patients with endogenous Cushing's syndrome: 'atypical' or melancholic features. *Clin Endocrinol* 1995; 43(4): 433–42.

80. Kling M, Roy A, Doran AR et al. Cerebrospinal fluid immunoreactive corticotropin-releasing hormone and adrenocorticotropin secretion in Cushing's disease and major depression: potential clinical implications. *J Clin Endocrinol Metab* 1991; 72: 260–71.

81. Loosen PT, Chambliss B, DeBold CR, Shelton R, Orth DN. Psychiatric phenomenology in Cushing's disease. *Pharmacopsychiatry* 1992; 25(4): 192–8.

82. Starkman MN, Schteingart DE, Schork MA. Correlation of bedside cognitive and neuropsychological tests in patients with Cushing's syndrome. *Psychosomatics* 1986; 27(7): 508–11.

83. Smith CK, Barish J, Correa J, Williams RH. Psychiatric disturbance in endocrinologic disease. *Psychosomat Med* 1972; 34(1): 69–86.

84. Kelly WF, Checkley SA, Bender DA, Mashiter K. Cushing's syndrome and depression—a prospective study of 26 patients. *Br J Psychiatry* 1983; 142: 16–19.

85. Leigh H, Kramer SI. The psychiatric manifestations of endocrine disease. *Adv Intern Med* 1984; 29: 413–45.

86. Ur E, Turner TH, Goodwin TJ, Grossman A, Besser GM. Mania in association with hydrocortisone replacement for Addison's disease. *Postgrad Med J* 1992; 68(795): 41–3.

87. Trzepacz PT, McCue M, Klein I, Levey GS, Greenhouse J. A psychiatric and neuropsychological study of patients with untreated Graves' disease. *Gen Hosp Psychiatry* 1988; 10(1): 49–55.

88. Stern RA, Robinson B, Thorner AR, Arruda JE, Prohaska ML, Prange AJ Jr. A survey study of neuropsychiatric complaints in patients with Graves' disease. *J Neuropsychiatry Clin Neurosci* 1996; 8(2): 181–5.

89. Greer S, Parsona V. Schizophrenia-like psychosis in thyroid crisis. *Br J Psychiatry* 1968; 114: 1357–62.

90. Bursten B. Psychoses associated with thyrotoxicosis. *Arch Gen Psychiatry* 1961; 4: 267–73.

91. Caudhill TG, Larinois CK. Severe thyrotoxicosis presenting as acute psychosis. *West J Med* 1991; 155: 292–3.

92. Hall RC. Psychiatric effects of thyroid hormone disturbance. *Psychosomatics* 1983; 24(1): 7–11.

93. Geffken GR, Ward HE, Staab JP, Carmichael SL, Evans DL. Psychiatric morbidity in endocrine disorders. *Psychiatr Clin North Am* 1998; 21(2): 473–89.
94. Weitzner MA. Neuropsychiatry and pituitary disease: an overview. *Psychother Psychosomat* 1998; 67(3): 125–32.
95. McGauley GA. Quality of life assessment before and after growth hormone treatment in adults with growth hormone deficiency. *Acta Paediatr Scand* 1989; 356(suppl): 55–9.
96. de Boer H, Blok GJ, Van der Veen EA. Clinical aspects of growth hormone deficiency in adults. *Endocrine Rev* 1995; 16: 63–86.
97. Monson JP. Adult growth hormone deficiency. *J R Coll Physicians Lond* 1998; 32(1): 19–22.
98. Carroll PV, Christ ER, Bengtsson BA et al. Growth hormone deficiency in adulthood and the effects of growth hormone replacement: a review. *J Clin Endocrinol Metab* 1998; 83: 382–95.
99. Lynch S, Merson S, Beshyah SA et al. Psychiatric morbidity in adults with hypopituitarism. *J R Soc Med* 1994; 87(8): 445–7.
100. Cuneo RC, Salomon F, McGauley GA, Sonksen PH. The growth hormone deficiency syndrome in adults. *Clin Endocrinol* 1992; 37(5): 387–97.
101. Beshyah SA, Freemantle C, Thomas E et al. Abnormal body composition and reduced bone mass in growth hormone deficient hypopituitary adults. *Clin Endocrinol* 1995; 42(2): 179–89.
102. McGauley GA, Cuneo RC, Salomon F, Sonksen PH. Psychological well-being before and after growth hormone treatment in adults with growth hormone deficiency. *Hormone Res* 1990; 33(suppl 4): 52–4.
103. Rosen T, Wiren L, Wilhelmsen L, Wiklund I, Bengtsson BA. Decreased psychological well-being in adult patients with growth hormone deficiency. *Clin Endocrinol* 1994; 40(1): 111–16.
104. Badia X, Lucas A, Sanmarti A, Roset M, Ulied A. One-year follow-up of quality of life in adults with untreated growth hormone deficiency. *Clin Endocrinol* 1998; 49(6): 765–71.
105. Deijen JB, van der Veen EA. The influence of growth hormone (GH) deficiency and GH replacement on quality of life in GH-deficient patients. *J Endocrinol Invest* 1999; 22(5 suppl): 127–36.
106. McGauley G, Cuneo R, Salomon F, Sonksen PH. Growth hormone deficiency and quality of life. *Hormone Res* 1996; 45(1–2): 34–7.
107. Bjork S, Jonsson B, Westphal O, Levin JE. Quality of life of adults with growth hormone deficiency: a controlled study. *Acta Paediatri Scand Suppl* 1989; 356: 55–9.
108. Burman P, Broman JE, Hetta J et al. Quality of life in adults with growth hormone (GH) deficiency: response to treatment with recombinant human GH in a placebo-controlled 21-month trial. *J Clin Endocrinol Metab* 1995; 80(12): 3585–90.
109. Sandberg DE, MacGillivray MH, Clopper RR, Fung C, LeRoux L, Alliger, DE. Quality of life among formerly treated childhood-onset growth hormone-deficient adults: a comparison with unaffected siblings. *J Clin Endocrinol Metab* 1998; 83(4): 1134–42.
110. Stabler B, Clopper RR, Siegel PT, Stoppani C, Compton PG, Underwood LE. Academic achievement and psychological adjustment in short children. The National Cooperative Growth Study. *J Dev Behav Pediatrics* 1994; 15(1): 1–6.
111. Sandberg DE, Brook AE, Campos SP. Short stature: a psychosocial burden requiring growth hormone therapy? *Pediatrics* 1994; 94(6 Pt 1): 832–40.
112. Page RC, Hammersley MS, Burke CW, Wass JA. An account of the quality of life of patients after treatment for non-functioning pituitary tumours. *Clin Endocrinol* 1997; 46(4): 401–6.
113. Bengtsson BA, Eden S, Lonn L et al. Treatment of adults with growth hormone (GH) deficiency with recombinant human GH. *J Clin Endocrinol Metab* 1993; 76(2): 309–17.
114. Almqvist O, Thoren M, Saaf M, Eriksson O. Effects of growth hormone substitution on mental performance in adults with growth hormone deficiency: a pilot study. *Psychoneuroendocrinology* 1986; 11(3): 347–52.
115. Gibney J, Wallace JD, Spinks T et al. The effects of 10 years of recombinant human growth hormone (GH) in adult GH-deficient patients. *J Clin Endocrinol Metab* 1999; 84(8): 2596–602.
116. Florkowski CM, Stevens I, Joyce P, Espiner EA, Donald RA. Growth hormone replacement does not improve psychological well-being in adult hypopituitarism: a randomized crossover trial. *Psychoneuroendocrinology* 1998; 23(1): 57–63.
117. Baum HB, Katznelson L, Sherman JC et al. Effects of physiological growth hormone (GH) therapy on cognition and quality of life in patients with adult-onset GH deficiency. *J Clin Endocrinol Metab* 1998; 83(9): 3184–9.
118. Chrisoulidou A, Kousta E, Beshyah SA, Robinson S, Johnston DG. How much, and by what mechanisms, does growth hormone replacement improve the quality of life in GH-deficient adults? *Baillières Clin Endocrinol Metab* 1998; 12(2): 261–79.
119. Deijen JB, de Boer H, van der Veen EA. Cognitive changes during growth hormone replacement in adult men. *Psychoneuroendocrinology* 1998; 23(1): 45–55.
120. Verhelst J, Abs R, Vandeweghe M et al. Two years of replacement therapy in adults with growth hormone deficiency. *Clin Endocrinol* 1997; 47(4): 485–94.
121. Whitehead HM, Boreham C, McIlrath EM et al. Growth hormone treatment of adults with growth hormone deficiency: results of a 13-month placebo controlled cross-over study. *Clin Endocrinol* 1992; 36(1): 45–52.

122. Murray RD, Shalet SM. The use of self-rating questionnaires as a quantitative measure of quality of life in adult growth hormone deficiency. *J Endocrinol Invest* 1999; 22(5 suppl): 118–26.
123. Wallymahmed ME, Foy P, Shaw D, Hutcheon R, Edwards RH, MacFarlane IA. Quality of life, body composition and muscle strength in adult growth hormone deficiency: the influence of growth hormone replacement therapy for up to 3 years. *Clin Endocrinol* 1997; 47(4): 439–46.
124. Giusti M, Meineri I, Malagamba D et al. Impact of recombinant human growth hormone treatment on psychological profiles in hypopituitary patients with adult-onset growth hormone deficiency. *Eur J Clin Invest* 1998; 28(1): 13–19.
125. Abs R, Bengtsson BA, Hernberg-Stahl E et al. GH replacement in 1034 growth hormone deficient hypopituitary adults: demographic and clinical characteristics, dosing and safety. *Clin Endocrinol* 1999; 50(6): 703–13.
126. McKenna SP, Doward LC, Alonso J et al. The QoL-AGHDA: an instrument for the assessment of quality of life in adults with growth hormone deficiency. *Quality of Life Res* 1999; 8(4): 373–83.
127. Cuneo RC, Judd S, Wallace JD et al. The Australian Multicenter Trial of Growth Hormone (GH) Treatment in GH-Deficient Adults. *J Clin Endocrinol Metab* 1998; 83(1): 107–16.
128. Wallymahmed ME, Baker GA, Humphris G, Dewey M, MacFarlane IA. The development, reliability and validity of a disease specific quality of life model for adults with growth hormone deficiency. *Clin Endocrinol* 1996; 44(4): 403–11.
129. Shalet SM. Growth hormone deficiency and replacement in adults. *BMJ* 1996; 313: 314.
130. Wiren L, Bengtsson BA, Johannsson G. Beneficial effects of long-term GH replacement therapy on quality of life in adults with GH deficiency. *Clin Endocrinol* 1998; 48(5): 613–20.
131. Burman P, Deijen JB. Quality of life and cognitive function in patients with pituitary insufficiency. *Psychother Psychosomat* 1998; 67(3): 154–67.
132. Nyberg F, Burman P. Growth hormone and its receptors in the central nervous system—location and functional significance. *Hormone Res* 1996; 45(1–2): 18–22.
133. Johansson JO, Larson G, Andersson M et al. Treatment of growth hormone-deficient adults with recombinant human growth hormone increases the concentration of growth hormone in the cerebrospinal fluid and affects neurotransmitters. *Neuroendocrinology* 1995; 61(1): 57–66.
134. Burman P, Hetta J, Karlsson A. Effect of growth hormone on brain neurotransmitters. *Lancet* 1993; 342(8885): 1492–3.
135. Toogood AA, Beardwell CG, Shalet SM. The severity of growth hormone deficiency in adults with pituitary disease is related to the degree of hypopituitarism. *Clin Endocrinol* 1994; 41(4): 511–16.
136. Nieschlag E. Testosterone replacement therapy: something old, something new... *Clin Endocrinol* 1996; 45(3): 261–2.
137. De Groot L, ed. *Endocrinology*, 3rd edn. Philadelphia: WB Saunders, 1995.
138. Kaye WH, Gendall K, Kye C. The role of the central nervous system in the psychoneuroendocrine disturbances of anorexia and bulimia nervosa. *Psychiatr Clin North Am* 1998; 21(2): 381–96.

19

Endocrine emergencies
Victor HF Hung, John P Monson

Introduction

The majority of clinical endocrine practice is concerned with the non-acute, elective management of various perturbations of hormonal function and tumors of endocrine glands. However, because of the complex relationships between hormonal systems, salt and water homeostasis, carbohydrate metabolism, immune function and cardiac status, there are specific instances in which endocrine disease may be life-threatening. These situations are relatively uncommon but are particularly important by virtue of their serious nature, the fact that they are generally remediable once the diagnosis has been made, and because, as examples of applied physiology, they have been important in elucidating many of the fundamental principles of hormonal function and homeostasis. In this chapter we will describe the presenting features and emergency management of specific endocrine disorders, with the emphasis on the essential principles of sound clinical practice.

Addisonian crisis

Introduction

Addisonian crisis or acute adrenal insufficiency is a life-threatening condition characterized by fever, nausea, vomiting, postural hypotension and rapid deterioration to cardiovascular collapse and coma. Failure to recognize the diagnosis and initiate appropriate treatment can be fatal. Adrenal insufficiency may develop gradually over months or years, and only becomes clinically obvious in the presence of physical stress, such as infection, surgery or trauma. The term Addisonian crisis, strictly speaking, refers to acute adrenocortical failure. Glucocorticoid deficiency may also be secondary or tertiary depending on whether adrenocorticotropic hormone (ACTH) or corticotropin-releasing hormone (CRH) is primarily deficient. The causes of adrenal insufficiency are listed in Table 19.1.

Clinical assessment[1,2]

Glucocorticoids are important for maintenance of vascular tone and excretion of free water from the body. Deficiency of cortisol will result in dilutional hyponatremia with or without hypotension. On the other hand, mineralocorticoid deficiency will lead to failure of sodium reabsorption and potassium excretion in distal tubules and collecting ducts of the kidney and distal colon. The prominent features of combined glucocorticoid and mineralocorticoid deficiency are thus cardiovascular collapse due to loss of vascular tone and sodium depletion, hyponatremia and hyperkalemia.

If the condition develops gradually, patients with adrenal insufficiency may remain apparently very well, only to decompensate to crisis at times of stress. Common precipitants are trauma, fever, burns, severe exertion, infection, anesthesia, surgery, and salt and volume depletion.

Gastrointestinal symptoms such as nausea, vomiting, diarrhea or steatorrhea and diffuse abdominal pain are common. They can be severe enough to mimic an acute abdominal crisis. If the patient proceeds to surgical exploration without steroid cover, the outcome may be disastrous. Patients may give a history of non-specific fatigue, weakness, weight loss, postural dizziness, anorexia, myalgia and arthralgia. Fever and chills can occur without other signs of infection. Neuropsychiatric manifestations include irritability,

Primary adrenal insufficiency
  Autoimmune
    Addison's disease
    Polyglandular autoimmune syndrome types 1 and 2
  Infection
    Tuberculosis
      Fungal, e.g. histoplasmosis
      Viral: cytomegalovirus, HIV
  Hemorrhage
    Sepsis: *Meningococcus, Pseudomonas,* etc.
    Thromboembolism with anticoagulation
    Bleeding diathesis
    Pregnancy with obstetric stress
    Antiphospholipid syndrome
  Infiltration
    Hemochromatosis
    Amyloidosis
    Sarcoidosis
  Familial
    Congenital adrenal hyperplasia
    Congenital adrenal hypoplasia
    Familial glucocorticoid deficiency
    Adrenoleukodystrophy
    Adrenomyeloneuropathy
  Metastasis
    From lung, breast, melanoma, lymphoma and gastrointestinal tract
  Drugs
    (1) Inhibit cortisol biosynthesis
      Aminoglutethimide
      Ketoconazole
      Metyrapone
      Mitotane (op'DDD)
      Etomidate
    (2) Increase cortisol metabolism[a]
      Rifampicin
      Phenytoin
      Phenobarbitone
      Carbamezepine

Secondary adrenal insufficiency
  Isolated ACTH deficiency
    Autoimmune
    Inherited
  Panhypopituitarism
    Tumor, infection, infarction, Hemorrhage, infiltration, immune, idiopathic, iatrogenic
  Others
    ACTH-blocking antibodies
    ACTH receptor defects

Tertiary adrenal insufficiency
  Sudden withdrawal from long-term steroid therapy
  Cured Cushing's syndrome
    Pituitary
    Adrenal
    Ectopic ACTH
  Hypothalamic
    Tumor
    Infiltration
    Radiotherapy
    Surgery

[a]Steroid deficiency only occurs if ACTH secretion or adrenocortical function is impaired.

Table 19.1
Causes of adrenal insufficiency.

depression, psychosis, apathy, confusion and occasional enhancement of sensory modalities such as taste, olfaction and hearing. If left untreated, coma may ensue.

Attention to the clinical signs of patients with adrenal crisis may give a clue to the diagnosis and usually the cause of adrenal insufficiency. Hyperpigmentation due to increased ACTH secretion, either generalized or localized to buccal mucosa, gingival margins, knuckles, elbows, palmar creases and new scars, is present in 92–96% of patients with primary adrenal insufficiency. Coexisting vitiligo indicates an underlying autoimmune origin. Fine pale wrinkled skin, scanty body hair and other signs of hypopituitarism point to secondary or tertiary adrenal insufficiency. However, decreased axillary and pubic hair can also occur in women with deficient adrenal androgens in primary adrenal failure. Calcification of auricular cartilages has been found exclusively in men with chronic adrenal insufficiency, irrespective of the cause.[2] Clinical features of Cushing's syndrome will alert clinicians to sudden withdrawal of steroids as the cause of the crisis.

In real-life situations, the clinical presentation of adrenal insufficiency can be so non-specific or atypical that the diagnosis is not suspected even at times of crisis. This is particularly true for acute adrenal crisis in adrenal hemorrhage, pituitary apoplexy and sepsis. The full-blown clinical picture simply cannot develop because of the fulminating course. It is, however, worth identifying patients at risk of adrenal insufficiency so that speedy diagnosis and immediate treatment can be possible without delay.

Adrenal hemorrhage may complicate sepsis, thromboembolic disease on anticoagulation, pre-eclampsia, traumatic delivery and bleeding diathesis.[3] Bilateral adrenal hemorrhage resulting from meningococcemia (Waterhouse–Friderichsen syndrome) is a well-known cause of adrenal crisis. Other bacterial septicemic conditions such as *Pneumococcus* and *Pseudomonas* infection may also give a similar picture. Patients with adrenal hemorrhage can present with a sudden drop in hemoglobin together with other biochemical features of adrenal crisis, including hyponatremia, hyperkalemia, pre-renal uremia and eosinphilia. These features are, however, absent in at least half of the reported cases. A high index of suspicion is crucial.

Patients with acquired immune deficiency syndrome (AIDS) have decreased adrenal reserve.[4] Cytomegalovirus and other opportunistic infections can cause necrotizing adrenalitis. Metastatic Kaposi's sarcoma may also involve the adrenals. It is likely that 90% of the adrenal cortex must be destroyed before adrenal failure develops.

Tuberculous adrenalitis has been a major cause of primary adrenal insufficiency, although the incidence is declining with better prevention and treatment. Treatment with rifampicin will further increase the risk of adrenal crisis along the treatment course as a result of hepatic enzyme induction increasing glucocorticoid metabolism.

Pituitary apoplexy is a rare but important cause of secondary adrenal insufficiency with crisis. Severe headache, visual field loss, ophthalmoplegia and mental confusion are classical features.

Acute adrenal insufficiency
   Fever
   Severe gastrointestinal upset: nausea, vomiting, acute abdomen
   Postural hypotension
   Cardiovascular collapse
   Coma
Chronic adrenal insufficiency
   General
      Fatigue, weakness, weight loss, postural dizziness
      Fever, chills
   Gastrointestinal
      Anorexia, nausea, vomiting, diarrhea
      Abdominal pain
   Neuropsychiatric
      Irritability, depression, psychosis, confusion, coma
   Other
      Calcification of auricular cartilage
Precipitants of crisis
   Trauma
   Fever
   Burns
   Severe exertion
   Infection
   Anesthesia
   Surgery
   Sodium and volume depletion
Clues to diagnosis
   Hyperpigmentation (primary adrenal failure)
   At-risk population:
      AIDS
      Tuberculous infection
      On medications
         Enzyme inducers (rifampicin, etc.)
         Cortisol biosynthesis inhibitors (metyrapone, etc.)
   Septic patients or patients on anticoagulants (adrenal hemorrhage)
   Cushing's syndrome (withdrawal of long-term steroids)
   Features of hypopituitarism
   Laboratory parameters
      Hyponatremia
      Hyperkalemia
      Hypoglycemia
      Pre-renal uremia
      Eosinophilia

Table 19.2
Clinical presentation of Addisonian crisis.

Drugs such as diuretics and angiotensin-converting enzyme (ACE) inhibitors promote renal sodium loss and can precipitate adrenal crisis in patients with impaired adrenal reserve. Phenytoin, rifampicin and phenobarbitone cause the same problem by increasing cortisol metabolism. Aminoglutethimide, ketoconazole, metyrapone, mitotane and etomidate can cause adrenal insufficiency by inhibiting cortisol biosynthesis or exerting an adrenolytic effect.

In conclusion, adrenal crisis should be considered in:

1. unexplained shock
2. unexplained fever
3. hyperpigmentation
4. hyponatremia
5. hyperkalemia
6. hypoglycemia
7. patients on steroid treatment.

A summary of the clinical presentation of Addisonian crisis is given in Table 19.2.

Investigation

Hyponatremia and hyperkalemia, pre-renal uremia and metabolic acidosis are the classical features of acute adrenal insufficiency, particularly primary adrenal failure. Dilutional hyponatremia and high urinary sodium without hyperkalemia are found in secondary adrenal failure, the biochemical features being partly related to increased antidiuretic hormone secretion. Hypoglycemia is more common in children with crisis and also in secondary adrenal insufficiency because of accompanying thyroid and growth hormone deficiency. Hypercalcemia is a recognized feature.

Hematologically, normochromic, normocytic anemia, neutropenia, relative eosinopilia and lymphocytosis may be found. Macrocytic anemia may indicate coexisting pernicious anemia.

The combination of a low serum thyroxine and modest elevation of thyroid-stimulating hormone can be a rare presentation of hypoadrenalism without real hypothyroidism. Steroid therapy will reverse the biochemistry. Thyroxine replacement in this situation will precipitate or worsen the crisis. However, coexisting Addison's disease and primary hypothyroidism (Schmidt's syndrome), secondary hypothyroidism in hypopituitarism and sick-euthyroid syndrome should be borne in mind in the interpretation of thyroid function tests.

Chest X-ray may show features of tuberculosis or bronchial carcinoma. Computerized axial tomography of adrenals is usually not indicated in the acute setting, except for confirming bilateral adrenal hemorrhage. Bilateral large adrenals are found in tuberculous adrenalitis, metastatic deposits, amyloidosis and other infiltrative disorders. Otherwise, adrenal atrophy will be found in most other situations.

Subsequent investigations should be directed at defining the cause of adrenal insufficiency when the patient is stable. Low aldosterone, low cortisol response to short and prolonged ACTH tests and high plasma ACTH are expected in primary adrenal failure, while normal aldosterone, stepwise cortisol response on prolonged ACTH test and low plasma ACTH suggest a secondary or tertiary cause. Magnetic resonance imaging of the pituitary and hypothalamus is necessary for detecting any anatomical lesion.

Treatment

Addisonian crisis is a true endocrine emergency that warrants immediate treatment.[1,2,5] One can usually perform therapeutic and diagnostic procedures at the same time to avoid any delay in therapy. The management of adrenal crisis consists of:

1. general measures
2. specific measures
3. treatment of the precipitating illness
4. monitoring of response
5. subsequent management.

General measures

Hypotension, electrolyte imbalance (especially hyponatremia and hyperkalemia) and hypoglycemia are the main problems. Large volumes, usually 3–4 l daily, of 0.9% normal saline or colloid should be given intravenously to reverse the hypovolemia and to correct the sodium deficit. Five per cent dextrose in saline may be necessary to prevent or treat hypoglycemia, which is more common in secondary adrenal insufficiency. Significant hypoglycemia should be treated with 50 ml of 50% dextrose intravenously. Occasionally, inotropic agents such as dopamine are necessary to maintain the blood pressure and renal perfusion. Hypotonic infusions will worsen the hyponatremia and should be avoided. It is advisable to guide fluid therapy by monitoring the vital signs, central venous pressure, urine output, plasma glucose, electrolytes and electrocardiogram in order to prevent fluid overload and arrhythmias. Oxygen therapy should also be instituted to meet the high metabolic demands.

Specific measures

Glucocorticoid replacement is the definitive and life-saving treatment for Addisonian crisis and stabilizing vascular tone. Once the diagnosis is suspected, a bolus dose of 4–8 mg of dexamethasone should be given intravenously for resuscitation. Its action lasts for 12–24 h and it does not interfere with the measurement of plasma cortisol during subsequent tests. If time allows, a short ACTH stimulation test can be performed by taking blood samples for cortisol and aldosterone at baseline and then 30 min and 60 min after 0.25 mg of tetracosactrin (Synacthen) intramuscularly intravenously. Baseline ACTH assay, if handled properly, will be extremely useful in differentiating primary from secondary adrenal insufficiency.

After the diagnostic test, hydrocortisone (100 mg intravenously stat, followed by 100 mg intramuscularly 6-hourly) can be administered and gradually tapered to oral maintenance therapy within 2–3 days if the patient's condition is stable with the resolution of precipitating or complicating illness. Mineralocorticoid replacement is usually not necessary in the acute setting, because of considerable mineralocorticoid activity from high doses (>100 mg daily) of hydrocortisone. It should be borne in mind that intravenous boluses of hydrocortisone have a very short half-life, so that intravenous hydrocortisone should be given as a continuous infusion of 1–3 mg/h if prolonged therapy by this route is required.

Treatment of precipitating illness

Any precipitating factor should be sought and treated accordingly. Broad-spectrum antibiotics should be given to treat bacterial infection after initial samples for culture have been taken. In cases of adrenal hemorrhage, resuscitation with blood transfusion, inotropic agents in addition to glucocorticoids and general fluid therapy are critical. Pituitary apoplexy may require neurosurgical decompression, depending on the conscious level and visual impairment.

Monitoring of response

The improvement in hypovolemia and shock in adrenal crisis after glucocorticoids and saline infusion is expected to be dramatic. Any complicating illness and other possible causes of shock, e.g. septic shock, should be considered if there is a poor response after 4–6 h.

Subsequent management
Maintenance therapy

After the patient is stabilized, intravenous hydrocortisone should be replaced by oral maintenance therapy. The usual oral dose is 20–30 mg daily in two or three divided portions. The adequacy is mainly guided by general wellbeing, blood pressure, body weight and, ideally, by hydrocortisone day profile. The first dose should be taken immediately on wakening and the evening dose not later than 7 p.m. Fludrocortisone (0.05–0.2 mg daily) can be given to patients with primary adrenal insufficiency and the dose is tailored by monitoring blood pressure, plasma electrolytes and recumbent renin activity.

Diagnostic procedure

The patient should be properly reviewed to determine the type and cause of adrenal insufficiency. The result of a short ACTH stimulation test may be difficult to interpret in seriously ill patients. For patients in stable condition, a peak cortisol of 580 nmol/l or more is regarded as an adequate response. A rise to >1000 nmol/l is expected in critically ill patients. The diagnostic tests should be repeated if there is any doubt.

Prevention and education

Patients on regular steroid replacement must be instructed to increase steroid intake during stress to prevent adrenal crisis. For mild illness with minimal fever, no change in steroid is necessary. However, if the patient feels unwell and is febrile, the oral dose should be doubled for 48–72 h. Those who are ill with vomiting or diarrhea should receive hydrocortisone 100 mg intramuscularly every 6–8 h. An ampoule of hydrocortisone (100 mg) should be given to patients, with full instructions, to be stored in the refrigerator for emergency use. Patients who undergo major surgical procedures require a similar regimen. For minor operations or procedures, one needs only a single dose of 100 mg hydrocortisone by intramuscular injection before the procedure.

Prognosis

The prognosis of adrenal insufficiency depends on the underlying etiology. Early recognition and appropriate intervention will definitely improve the outcome.

A summary of the management of Addisonian crisis is given in Table 19.3.

> General measures
>   Hypotension: 3–4 l IV 0.9% isotonic saline
>   or colloids ± inotropes
>   Hypoglycemia: 50 ml 50% dextrose stat
>   and 5% dextrose in saline
>   Ventilation: O_2 therapy
>   Monitoring
>   Vital signs, fluid balance, central venous
>   pressure, serum electrolytes, plasma
>   glucose, ECG
> Specific measures
>   Measure serum cortisol and ACTH
>   Resuscitation with 4–8 mg IV
>   dexamethasone
>   Perform short ACTH (Synacthen) test:
>   cortisol ± aldosterone at 0, 30, 60 min
>   after 0.25 mg IV/IM Synacthen
>   or
>   hydrocortisone 100 mg IV stat after blood
>   taken for cortisol ± aldosterone, then
>   hydrocortisone 100 mg IM 6-hourly or
>   1–3 mg/h IV infusion
>   Change to oral maintenance steroids after
>   48–72 h if stable
> Treatment of precipitating illness/underlying
> disorder
>   Antibiotics for infection
>   Transfusion ± inotropes for adrenal
>   hemorrhage
> Monitoring of response
>   Expect dramatic response to steroids
>   within 4–6 h
>   Consider other cause(s) of shock if poor
>   response after 4–6 h
> Subsequent measures
>   Maintenance therapy
>   20–30 mg/day oral hydrocortisone
>   ± 0.05–0.2 mg/day oral fludrocortisone
>   (in primary adrenal failure)
>   Repeating diagnostic procedures
>   Short Synacthen test, etc.
>   Prevention and education
>   Increase steroids during stress: febrile
>   illnesses, operations, procedures
>   Patient should:
>   Carry a 'steroid card'
>   Wear a MedicAlert bracelet/necklace
>   Store a vial of hydrocortisone
>   (100 mg) in refrigerator for
>   emergency use

Table 19.3
Management of Addisonian crisis.

Hypopituitarism

Introduction

Hypopituitarism can remain clinically silent for months or years and only becomes apparent at times of stress, such as infection, trauma, surgery, anesthesia, consumption of sedatives or various medical diseases, e.g. acute myocardial infarction. However, rapidly evolving acute hypopituitarism presenting with cardiovascular collapse and coma is a life-threatening condition requiring urgent and appropriate intervention.

The secretion of anterior pituitary hormones (growth hormone (GH), luteinizing hormone (LH), follicle-stimulating hormone (FSH), thyroid-stimulating hormone (TSH), ACTH, prolactin (PRL)) is normally tightly regulated by hypothalamic-releasing or -inhibiting factors through the hypothalamo-hypophyseal portal system and also by the feedback inhibition of hormones from respective target organs. On the other hand, vasopressin (ADH) and oxytocin are synthesized in the hypothalamus and stored in the posterior pituitary for release. Partial or complete anterior and posterior hypopituitarism can result from a variety of disorders which interfere with or disrupt the hypothalamic–pituitary unit. It is most commonly associated with pituitary adenoma, particularly after treatment with surgery and radiotherapy. Other etiologies of hypopituitarism, especially pituitary apoplexy, lymphocytic hypophysitis and Sheehan's syndrome, are less common but definitely require special attention by virtue of their unpredictable occurrence and potentially fatal outcome.

Clinical assessment[6–9]

In the context of emergency presentation, glucocorticoid deficiency may manifest as fatigue, weakness, nausea, vomiting, abdominal pain, weight loss and postural hypotension. The latter, usually accompanied by hyperkalemia, is more common in primary than in secondary adrenal failure because of relative preservation of mineralocorticoid function with secondary causes. The pale and sallow complexion is clearly distinguishable from hyperpigmentation in primary adrenocortical insufficiency. Loss of axillary and pubic hair occur in hypopituitarism but also in women with primary adrenal failure because of deficient adrenal androgens. Hyponatremia and hypoglycemia can be found in ACTH deficiency. In cases of fulminant acute hypopituitarism, hypotension and coma may dominate the whole clinical picture.

TSH deficiency shares the same clinical features of primary hypothyroidism, with fatigue, cold intolerance, constipation, weight gain, poor memory, bradycardia, periorbital edema and delayed relaxation of deep tendon reflexes.

Apart from those features attributable to hormonal deficiencies, clinical features from pressure effects of a mass lesion in the hypothalamic–pituitary region may be present, including headache, visual disturbances and cranial nerve involvement. The manifestations of mass effects will be discussed in greater detail below.

Two specific entities of hypopituitarism are worth mentioning: lymphocytic hypophysitis[8] and Sheehan's syndrome.[9] Lymphocytic hypophysitis is characterized by infiltration of the pituitary by lymphocytes and plasma cells with complete or partial hypopituitarism (including isolated ACTH deficiency) and a pituitary mass. The majority of patients are women during pregnancy or in the postpartum period who present with headache, visual abnormalities, weakness and fatigue. However, it is also described in men. Most cases result in deficiency of pituitary hormones requiring long-term replacement. The condition may be confused with Sheehan's syndrome, which is pituitary ischemic necrosis usually following cardiovascular collapse from postpartum hemorrhage. Clinically, it can present acutely with persistent hypotension, tachycardia, failure to lactate and hypoglycemia. The diagnosis should be considered in resistant hypotension despite replacement of blood products for obstetric hemorrhage. On the other hand, it can manifest months or years later with symptoms of hypopituitarism, including fatigue, cold intolerance, decreased body hair and libido and a history of failure of lactation and resumption of menses after delivery.

Investigation

Investigations of hypopituitarism involve:

1. general blood tests
2. hormonal assays
3. imaging of the hypothalamic–pituitary region
4. visual assessment.

General blood tests
Full blood count, plasma urea, creatinine, electrolytes and glucose should be checked for the detection of complications and monitoring of treatment. Panhypopituitarism can cause normochromic normocytic anemia, eosinophilia, hyponatremia and hypoglycemia. A high serum osmolality with a low urine osmolality is suggestive of ADH deficiency.

Hormonal assays
Patients suspected of having acute hypopituitarism should be immediately treated after blood samples have been saved for baseline hormonal assays. The concentration of target hormones (cortisol, thyroxine (T4), insulin-like growth factor-I (IGF-I), estradiol in women and testosterone in men) may be low, with low or inappropriately normal anterior pituitary hormones (ACTH, TSH, GH, LH and FSH), except PRL, which is either normal or slightly elevated in most situations. In combination with typical clinical features of hypopituitarism, baseline hormonal tests are often adequate to make the diagnosis. However, subsequent dynamic endocrine tests may be necessary to confirm the diagnosis, especially in partial hormonal deficiencies.

Imaging studies
Computerized axial tomography (CT) and magnetic resonance imaging (MRI) are useful in defining the pathology in the hypothalamic–pituitary region. In general, MRI is preferable because it is superior in its spatial resolution. However, it may not be possible in patients with claustrophobia, cardiac pacemaker and intracranial metallic implants. CT is better in detecting acute hemorrhage (e.g. in pituitary apoplexy), calcification (e.g. in craniopharyngioma) and bony erosion (e.g. in invasive tumor). Skull X-ray may show enlarged pituitary fossa, calcification and bony erosion.

Visual assessment
Visual acuity, visual fields and color vision should be checked. Formal visual field assessment with Goldman or automated perimetry is useful for monitoring visual deterioration. Visual evoked potential is a more sensitive and an objective means of showing involvement of the optic apparatus.

Treatment[6,7]

Management of hypopituitarism is directed at acute and maintenance measures which, in turn, depend on the onset and severity of pituitary failure.

Acute measures

Immediate life-saving treatment should be instituted once the diagnosis of acute hypopituitarism or hypopituitary coma is suspected after baseline blood for hormone assays is taken. The acute measures involve:

1. general supportive measures
2. hormonal replacement
3. urgent intervention for the underlying cause.

General measures

Hypotension and hyponatremia should be treated with isotonic saline or colloid infusions and monitored by central venous pressure, urine output, blood pressure and plasma electrolytes. In adults, hypoglycemia requires intravenous glucose injection (50 ml of 50% dextrose), but lower concentrations should be used in children to avoid precipitating hyperosmolality. Extra care should be taken in administering isotonic glucose infusions (e.g. 5% dextrose) because of the risk of precipitating severe dilutional hyponatremia due to impaired free water clearance in ACTH and TSH deficiencies. Hypothermia should be treated with passive rewarming measures with blankets or internal rewarming by warm intravenous infusions or gastric perfusion. External rewarming can cause vascular collapse and should be avoided. Adequate oxygen therapy and assisted ventilation are required if hypoventilation ensues. Associated precipitating illnesses such as infection, trauma or acute myocardial infarction should be sought and treated accordingly.

Hormonal replacement

Acute ACTH deficiency is rapidly fatal with cardiovascular collapse and coma. Glucocorticoids (hydrocortisone 100 mg intravenously followed by 100 mg

---

Acute measures
  General measures
    Hypotension: IV 0.9% isotonic saline or colloids
    Hypoglycemia
      50 ml 50% dextrose in adults
      Lower concentration in children (risk of hyperosmolality)
      Beware of dilutional hyponatremia
    Hypothermia: Passive or internal rewarming
    Hypoventilation: O$_2$ therapy ± assisted ventilation
    Precipitating illness: Treat infection, trauma, acute myocardial infarction
    Monitoring: Vital signs, central venous pressure, urine output, serum electrolytes
  Hormonal replacement
    Hydrocortisone 100 mg IV, then 100 mg IM 6-hourly or 1–3 mg/h IV infusion
    Prolonged therapy in
      Infection
      Lymphocytic hypophysitis
      Hypothalamic edema after pituitary surgery for macroadenoma
    Thyroid hormone replacement *after* adequate corticosteroid replacement
    T4 300–500 µg IV bolus, then 50 µg/day IV
    or T3 25 µg IV 8-hourly for 1–2 days
    Start oral replacement if patient is conscious: T4 25–50 µg/day orally
    Cranial diabetes insipidus may be unmasked by corticosteroid therapy
      Desmopressin 10 µg intranasally or 1 µg SC/IM
      Repeat doses if
      Urine output >200 ml/h with sodium concentration ≥138 mmol and serum osmolality >285 mosm/kg
  Urgent intervention of underlying cause
    Consider transsphenoidal decompression for pituitary apoplexy
  Maintenance measures
    Hormonal therapy
      Hydrocortisone, thyroxine, desmopressin replacement as required
      GH, gonadal hormone based on further evaluation
    Treatment of the underlying cause
      Surgery, radiotherapy, medical
    Monitoring
      Clinical, biochemical, radiological assessment
      Life-long follow-up: compliance, disease activity, adequacy of replacement

Table 19.4
Management of hypopituitarism.

intramuscularly or continuous infusion 1–3 mg/h) should be given immediately to stabilize the vascular tone. Dexamethasone, which does not interfere with the cortisol assay, can also be used for initial resuscitation if a short ACTH test is performed. The dose of glucocorticoid can be gradually tapered over 2–3 days to oral maintenance therapy once the patient is stable without any complications. However, it should be maintained in patients with continuing stress (e.g. in infection), lymphocytic hypophysitis and expanding suprasellar tumor with hypothalamic involvement (particularly after transfrontal surgical removal) to reduce hypothalamic edema.

Early thyroid hormone replacement is indicated in hypopituitary coma, especially when hypothermia, hypoventilation and marked bradycardia are present. Intravenous thyroxine (T4 300–500 μg bolus followed by 50 μg daily) or triiodothyronine (T3 25 μg every 8 h for 1–2 days) should be given after commencement of glucocorticoid replacement, to avoid further aggravating the glucocorticoid insufficiency. More detailed discussion of different regimens of thyroid hormone replacement can be found later in this chapter.

ADH deficiency is uncommon in hypopituitarism from pituitary tumor, except with hypothalamic invasion or after surgery. Cranial diabetes insipidus can be unmasked by glucocorticoid replacement. Profuse diuresis with hypovolemia should be treated with appropriate fluid replacement and desmopressin (DDAVP 10 μg intranasally or 1 μg subcutaneously or intramuscularly). Repeated doses of desmopressin may be required if urine output exceeds 200 ml/h in the presence of serum sodium of ≥138 mmol/l and osmolality >285 mosm/kg.

Urgent intervention of the underlying cause

If the patient does not respond to initial treatment, other causes of coma should be sought. Urgent transsphenoidal or transfrontal decompression may be necessary in patients with rapidly expanding hypothalamic–pituitary lesions manifested as progressive visual impairment and mental obtundation, as in pituitary apoplexy or aneurysm. Adequate steroid and antibiotic cover is crucial. However, high-dose steroids alone may be effective in lymphocytic hypophysitis.

Maintenance measures

Following initial stabilization, the treatment of the underlying cause and management of maintenance hormonal replacement therapy is undertaken along similar lines to those described for the elective treatment of pituitary mass lesions and hypopituitarism. It is important to remember that hypopituitarism may improve following surgery[10] or medical therapy for a pituitary macroadenoma.

A summary of the management of hypopituitarism is given in Table 19.4.

Pituitary apoplexy

Introduction

Pituitary apoplexy is a life-threatening clinical syndrome characterized by sudden onset of headache with the variable presence of visual disturbances, ophthalmoplegia, impaired consciousness and variable degree of hypopituitarism due to pressure effects from infarction or hemorrhage of the pituitary gland. It commonly occurs in patients with pituitary adenomas, either previously recognized or undiagnosed, but pituitary infarction can also occur in patients with otherwise normal pituitary glands. Prompt diagnosis and immediate intervention are crucial in preserving vision and saving life, particularly in its most fulminant form with rapidly evolving visual deficits, cardiovascular collapse, coma and death.[11] The mechanism for pituitary apoplexy is still unclear and may be related to ischemia followed by hemorrhagic degeneration of the pituitary tumor. Fragility of tumoral blood vessels or atherosclerotic embolization may also play a role in the pathogenesis. On the other hand, ischemic infarction of a normal pituitary gland may follow a hypotensive episode, such as postpartum hemorrhage in Sheehan's syndrome. Although most apoplectic episodes are spontaneous (i.e. without obvious precipitant),[12] some have been found to be associated with head trauma, pituitary irradiation, anticoagulant therapy or bleeding diathesis, transient increased intracranial pressure (e.g. cough, sneezing), diabetes mellitus, cardiac surgery, diagnostic procedures (e.g. carotid angiography), medications (e.g. bromocriptine, oral contraceptives) or even pituitary function tests, such as triple stimulaton tests, LHRH tests and TRH tests.[11,13]

Clinical assessment[11,14]

While pituitary infarction or hemorrhage can be silent, apoplexy implies the presence of symptoms. The clinical presentation is variable, depending on the size of the pre-existing tumor and the extent of infarction with the expanding hemorrhage and edema. The acute fulminant form of pituitary apoplexy can lead to severe headache, sudden blindness, hemodynamic instability and rapid lapse into coma, with fatal outcome. In its subacute form, however, mild headache and visual disturbance may develop gradually over days or weeks. The mass effects from the expanding lesion, acute hypopituitarism and features of preceding pituitary tumor constitute the cardinal manifestations of the clinical syndrome.

Mass effect

Headache is usually the major and initial symptom. It can be retro-orbital, frontal or diffuse and often severe and sudden in onset. It may be due to dural traction or blood leakage into the subarachnoid space, the latter commonly accompanied by nausea, vomiting, meningeal signs and occasionally fever.

Superior extension of the hemorrhagic lesion will compress the optic chiasm and/or optic nerve with visual field defects (commonly bitemporal hemianopia) and/or loss of visual acuity. Rarely, hypothalamic involvement results in disturbances in sympathetic autoregulation of respiration, temperature, blood pressure and cardiac rhythm.

Lateral expansion causes different combinations of ophthalmoplegia, ptosis and pupillary defects from entrapment of cranial nerves, including oculomotor (III), trochlear (IV) and abducens (VI) nerves in the cavernous sinus. Unilateral III nerve palsy is the most common dysfunction. Unilateral facial pain with corneal anesthesia indicate ophthalmic branch of trigeminal nerve (V) encroachment. Obliteration of the cavernous sinus with eyelid edema and ptosis is an uncommon presentation.

Anterior extension may cause anosmia from olfactory nerve compression or epistaxis and cerebrospinal fluid rhinorrhea from sphenoid bone erosion.

Altered mental state, ranging from mild lethargy to confusion, stupor and coma, may indicate progressive and extensive involvement with increased intracranial pressure and warrant urgent surgical intervention if it is severe. Focal neurological deficits with hemiparesis, hemispheric dysfunction, pyramidal signs or even seizures are unusual and can be the consequences of carotid siphon entrapment or vasospasm from meningeal irritation by the subarachnoid blood or necrotic tissues.

Acute hypopituitarism

Complete or partial hypopituitarism can result from necrosis of the pituitary gland or stalk compression with altered hypothalamic regulation, the latter being potentially reversible with possible recovery of pituitary hormone secretion once the pressure effect is released. The majority of patients with pituitary apoplexy become GH and gonadotropin deficient. Approximately two-thirds of patients have ACTH deficiencies and are at risk of hemodynamic compromise and hypotensive crises. Secondary hypothyroidism occurs in 42–53% of patients.[15] High serum PRL concentration, which frequently accompanies apoplexy, can be due to disconnection hyperprolactinemia or pre-existing prolactinoma. Hypoprolactinemia may also be found in Sheehan's syndrome from pituitary infarction. Cranial diabetes insipidus, however, is relatively rare (2–3%) and may not be clinically obvious in the presence of untreated ACTH deficiency.[15]

Features of the preceding pituitary tumor

Pituitary apoplexy can be the first presentation of pituitary functioning or non-functioning tumors. Hypersecretory states, e.g. in patients with acromegaly, Cushing's diseases and prolactinomas, may resolve or improve after the apoplectic episode. Frequent evaluation of the hormonal status is mandatory to avoid overtreatment.

In conclusion, careful evaluation of the neurological signs, notably the conscious state and visual deficits (by fundoscopy, visual acuity and visual field assessment), and the cardiovascular status is crucial in diagnosis and monitoring the clinical course so as to intervene promptly with neurosurgical decompression in case of deterioration.

Differential diagnosis[11,13]

Pituitary apoplexy can mimic a number of more common intracranial diseases closely. These include migraine, optic neuritis, subarachnoid hemorrhage, meningitis, stroke (particularly midbrain infarction from basilar artery occlusion), and cavernous sinus thrombosis. The differentiation between pituitary apoplexy and subarachnoid hemorrhage is particularly difficult, due to their similar presenting features with headache, alteration of mental state and meningeal signs. Sentinel headache, oculomotor palsy and the subsequent chance of rebleeding may occur in both conditions, although bilateral oculomotor palsies point to pituitary apoplexy. On the other hand, pituitary apoplexy can be clinically indistinguishable from meningitis if there is no visual deficit or focal neurological sign such as hemiparesis and hemispheric dysfunction. Lumbar puncture may not be helpful, as will be discussed later.

A summary of the clinical presentation and differential diagnosis of pituitary apoplexy is given in Table 19.5.

Investigation

Imaging
CT of the hypothalamic–pituitary region and orbits is the most important diagnostic work-up for pituitary apoplexy, especially in the first 24–48 h of presentation. Thin sections (1.5 mm) in the coronal plane are useful in demonstrating acute hemorrhage at the sellar region in the form of a high-density or inhomogeneous lesion. Blood in the subarachnoid space may also be found. After intravenous contrast enhancement, the extent of the underlying pituitary tumor can be delineated. Although CT is the preferred imaging modality in the detection of fresh bleeding in the acute stage, MRI is more sensitive in following the hemorrhage in the subacute setting (4 days to 1 month).[16] On the other hand, carotid or MR angiography can differentiate pituitary apoplexy from cerebral aneurysm with subarachnoid hemorrhage. However, co-occurrence of pituitary tumor and cerebral aneurysm is not uncommon.[11] Lateral skull X-ray may show sellar enlargement, bony erosion or occasionally fracture of the dorsum dellae in pituitary apoplexy.

Endocrine evaluation
Various degrees of hypopituitarism or hypersecretory states can be found, as described previously. Baseline samples for anterior pituitary hormones (TSH, ACTH, GH, LH, FSH and PRL) and their respective target hormones (T4, cortisol, IGF-I, testosterone in men and estradiol in women) should be saved, although detailed assessment can be deferred until the patient becomes stable. Treatment of hormonal deficiency, particularly corticosteroid replacement, should not await laboratory confirmation.

Visual assessment
Careful visual assessment with Goldman or automated perimetry for visual field deficits and Snellen's chart for visual acuity are essential for accurate diagnosis and decision on intervention, as well as for monitoring progress after either conservative treatment or surgical decompression.

Lumbar puncture
Lumbar puncture is frequently performed in patients with headache, meningeal signs and altered mentation,

---

Clinical course
  Acute
    Headache, cardiovascular collapse, ophthalmoplegia, blindness, coma over hours
  Subacute
    Mild headache, visual disturbances over days or weeks
Clinical features
  Mass effect
    Headache
    Visual field deficits
    Visual loss
    Ocular palsy
    Meningism
    Altered mental state
    Stroke-like syndrome
    Seizures
  Acute hypopituitarism
    GH > LH/FSH > ACTH > TSH > ADH in descending order of frequency of deficiency
    Hyperprolactinemia in about two-thirds of patients
  Symptoms of preceding tumor
    Resolution of hypersecretory state
    Apoplexy as first presentation of pituitary tumor
  Precipitating factors
    No precipitant: most common
    Head trauma
    Pituitary irradiation
    Anticoagulant therapy/ bleeding disorder
    Diabetes mellitus
    Cardiac surgery
    Diagnostic procedures (e.g. carotid angiography)
    Medications (bromocriptine, oral contraceptives)
    Pituitary function tests (triple stimulation test, TRH test or LHRH test)
Differential diagnosis
  Migraine
  Optic neuritis
  Subarachnoid hemorrhage
  Meningitis
  Stroke (midbrain infarction from basilar artery occlusion)
  Cavernous sinus thrombosis

Table 19.5
Clinical presentation and differential diagnosis of pituitary apoplexy.

particularly in the presence of fever, but can be misleading in making the distinction between subarachnoid hemorrhage and meningitis from pituitary apoplexy. Xanthochromia and high red blood cell counts, which are the classical cerebrospinal fluid findings in subarachnoid hemorrhage, may also be present in pituitary apoplexy. Similarly, pleocytosis with raised protein concentration in the cerebrospinal fluid can be found both in meningitis and in pituitary apoplexy. The differentiation therefore relies mainly on pituitary imaging. Moreover, lumbar puncture may actually be hazardous in pituitary apoplexy, due to the risk of causing uncal herniation.

Treatment[11,14]

The management of pituitary apoplexy includes:

1. hormonal replacement
2. surgical intervention
3. monitoring of progress.

Hormonal replacement

Once the diagnosis of pituitary apoplexy is suspected, high-dose hydrocortisone (100 mg intravenous bolus followed by 100 mg intramuscularly 6-hourly) or dexamethasone (2 mg intravenously 6-hourly) should be given after blood samples have been saved for hormonal assay, because there is a high incidence of adrenal insufficiency. This is also beneficial in cases of cerebral edema from an enlarging hemorrhagic lesion. As steroid replacement may unmask coexisting cranial diabetes insipidus, careful monitoring of the urine output, electrolytes, serum and urine osmolality is mandatory. Other hormonal replacements are generally not required in the acute setting but may be necessary if hormonal deficiencies persist after the acute episode and are confirmed by subsequent endocrine evaluation after recovery.

Surgical intervention

Urgent transsphenoidal neurosurgical decompression should be performed in patients with altered mental state and visual deficits, as well as in those with a rapidly progressive clinical course. Early intervention frequently improves mental state and preserves vision, probably through relief of the raised intracranial pressure and mass effect from the expanding hemorrhagic lesion. Ophthalmoplegia generally remits spontaneously without surgery, although recovery may be partial. The optimal treatment for patients without neurological deficits is controversial. Some advocate conservative management, particularly for those with mild and subacute presentation. However, there is some evidence that early surgical decompression may partially

---

Hormonal replacement
   Corticosteroid replacement
      Also helpful in relief of cerebral edema
      Hydrocortisone 100 mg IV bolus, then 100 mg IM 6-hourly *or*
      Dexamethasone 2 mg IV 6-hourly
   ADH deficiency
      May be unmasked by corticosteroid therapy
      Desmopressin 10 μg intranasally or 1 μg SC/IM
      Monitor urine output, serum electrolytes, paired serum and urine osmolality
   Other pituitary hormonal deficiencies
      Acute stage: Replacement not needed
      Convalescence: Replacement according to requirement
Surgical intervention
   Indications for urgent transsphenoidal surgical decompression
      Impaired conscious state
      Visual deficits
      Rapidly progressive course
   Normal consciousness and vision
      Optimal time for surgery is controversial
      Ophthalmoplegia usually resolves partially or completely without surgery
      Pituitary hormonal function may improve with early surgery
Monitoring of progress
   Acute stage
      Neurological signs
      Visual acuity and visual fields
      Cardiovascular status
   Recovery
      Full endocrine evaluation
      Visual assessment

Table 19.6
Management of pituitary apoplexy.

or completely restore the pituitary hormonal function by relieving the mass effect at the pituitary stalk.[17]

Monitoring of progress

Patients with pituitary apoplexy should be closely monitored with frequent assessment of neurological signs, visual acuity and fields and cardiovascular status to determine the urgency and the type of treatment. After recovery from the acute event, a full endocrine evaluation and visual assessment are necessary to define the need for long-term hormonal replacement and treatment of any preceding hypersecretory status.

A summary of the management of pituitary apoplexy is given in Table 19.6.

Pituitary macroadenoma with visual loss

Introduction

Pituitary tumors account for approximately 10–15% of all intracranial tumors.[18,19] They can be classified, according to their size, as macroadenomas (>1 cm in diameter) or microadenomas (<1 cm in diameter), and, according to their secretory pattern, as functioning or clinically non-functioning adenomas. The latter can either be non-secretory or secrete inactive hormones or hormonal fragments. Pituitary tumors usually manifest as hypersecretion or hyposecretion of hormones, or their mass effect on adjacent structures, notably the optic chiasm, hypothalamus, cavernous sinus and cranial nerves and sphenoid sinus. A macroadenoma with visual deficit, particularly if it develops acutely, poses a potential emergency in which delay in the diagnosis and intervention can lead to irreversible blindness. Transsphenoidal surgical decompression of a macroadenoma provides rapid relief of the pressure effect of the tumor and frequently improves vision, with a very low mortality risk (<1%). However, effective medical therapies, either acting as first-line treatment or adjunctive measures before surgery, are also available for some types of tumors. Macroprolactinoma and thyrotroph hyperplasia from long-standing untreated primary hypothyroidism can cause visual loss that is readily reversible with dopamine agonists and thyroid hormone replacement, respectively, without surgical intervention. On the other hand, patients with severe Cushing's disease from corticotroph macroadenoma or the very rare situation of thyrotoxicosis from thyrotroph macroadenoma should receive adequate medical preparation before surgery to minimize perioperative complications. This section will therefore focus on important considerations in the management of patients with macroadenoma complicated by visual loss.

Clinical assessment[20]

Patients with pituitary macroadenoma can present with any combination of mass effect of the tumor, hormonal hypersecretion or hormonal hyposecretion. A careful clinical assessment is crucial in selecting appropriate therapy for each individual patient.

Mass effect

While microadenomas rarely cause appreciable pressure effects, macroadenomas commonly displace or invade adjacent neural, vascular or bony structures or even brain parenchyma, depending on the invasiveness and direction of spread of the tumor. The peculiar anatomical position of the pituitary gland accounts for the characteristic clinical presentation of an enlarging macroadenoma. Superior extension can give rise to frontal, temporal, retro-orbital or diffuse headache due to stretching of the diaphragma sellae. The headache may improve once the diaphragm is ruptured. Suprasellar spread of macroadenoma can lead to various visual field defects, such as bitemporal hemianopia, unilateral or bilateral upper temporal quadrantopia from optic chiasm compression or reduced visual acuity with progression to optic atrophy from optic nerve involvement. The pattern of visual loss is governed by the position of the optic chiasm, e.g. pre-fixed or post-fixed, and the direction of tumor invasion. As abrupt or prolonged compression of the optic pathway can result in irreversible visual deficit, the acuteness and the degree of visual impairment actually dictate the urgency and choice of therapeutic intervention. Assessment with a red-headed pin is a sensitive means of detecting visual field abnormalities. Fundoscopic examination and visual acuity measurement with a standard Snellen's chart are mandatory as a baseline for subsequent monitoring of progress and treatment response. Further suprasellar extension to the hypothalamus can cause disturbances in thermoregulation, behavior, sleep pattern, appetite, thirst and water balance. Rarely, obstructive hydrocephalus may occur from involvement of the foramen of Munro or the aqueduct of Sylvius. Lateral extension to the cavernous sinus leads to cranial nerve palsies with ptosis, pupillary defects, diplopia and ophthalmoplegia from oculomotor, abducens and trochlear nerve dysfunction. If the ophthalmic or maxillary branch of the trigeminal nerve is affected, facial pain or paresthesia may ensue. An invasive macroadenoma can also involve the temporal lobe and causes seizures. Anterior or inferior tumor growth results in sellar floor erosion and cerebrospinal fluid rhinorrhea with potential risk of meningitis.

Hormonal hypersecretion and hypopituitarism
The features of functioning pituitary tumors should be borne in mind and appropriate investigations undertaken if indicated. Similarly, clinical features of hypopituitarism should be sought and confirmatory investigations arranged.

Some important considerations
Patients with a macroadenoma should be asked about pregnancy, desire for fertility, and medications, particularly those which may elevate blood PRL concentration, such as antipsychotics, antiemetics and antihypertensives. This information has important implications for subsequent management. Some non-adenomatous pituitary lesions, such as pituitary metastasis, tuberculoma and germinoma, can mimic macroadenomas closely and should be borne in mind with appropriate search for other peripheral lesions, especially if atypical clinical presentation or imaging is present. Lymphocytic hypophysitis can also present with an expanding pituitary mass lesion, headache and visual deficit and should be considered in the differential diagnosis.

Investigation

Investigations of patients suspected to have pituitary macroadenoma should include:

1. endocrine evaluation
2. imaging of the hypothalamic–pituitary region
3. visual assessment.

In all patients presenting with a pituitary mass lesion, an urgent serum PRL measurement is mandatory, as a macroprolactinoma can be effectively treated medically; serum PRL concentration correlates approximately with the size of a prolactinoma, and a serum value of >5000 mU/l (>250 µg/l) in a patient with a pituitary mass lesion is highly suggestive of a macroprolactinoma. A serum level of 3000–5000 mU/l (150–250 µg/l) is borderline. If the serum PRL concentration is <3000 mU/l (<150 µg/l), disconnection hyperprolactinemia is very possible.

Imaging of the hypothalamic–pituitary region
MRI is generally preferable to CT, because of better spatial resolution in the hypothalamic–pituitary region, particularly the optic apparatus, cavernous sinus and pituitary stalk. This is important in defining the extent of the pituitary macroadenoma and in excluding non-pituitary lesions or sometimes a non-adenomatous pituitary mass. With thin sections through the pituitary region in the coronal plane, CT is superior in demonstrating acute hemorrhage as in pituitary apoplexy, bony erosion as in invasive adenoma or carcinoma, and also calcification. Skull X-ray may show sellar enlargement, bony erosion and calcification. Carotid or MRI angiography may be necessary to rule out vascular aneurysms in the vicinity of the pituitary fossa.[6]

Visual assessment
Accurate documentation of the visual acuity, visual fields and color vision is mandatory for diagnosis and monitoring of treatment response in patients with macroadenoma with visual loss. Formal Goldman or computerized perimetry is particularly useful in monitoring progress in visual field deficits. Measurement of the visual evoked potential provides an objective and sensitive means of detecting optic pathway compression. It may also be useful in differentiating simple compression from more severe demyelination lesions of the optic pathway.[21]

Treatment

The choice, either medical or surgical, and the urgency of intervention depends on the acuteness of the visual loss, as well as the nature of the pituitary tumor. The objectives of management should include:

1. decompression of the optic pathway
2. correction of the hypersecretory state
3. treatment of pituitary hormone deficiencies.

Decompression of the optic pathway
Except in the context of a macroprolactinoma, acute visual loss, due to a pituitary mass lesion, requires

urgent transsphenoidal neurosurgical decompression to prevent permanent blindness. Treatment with dopamine agonists (e.g. bromocriptive or cabergoline) has been successful in at least 75% of macroprolactinomas in terms of tumor shrinkage with visual improvement (usually evident within 24 h of commencement of treatment), restoration of serum PRL concentration and other pituitary functions to normal, and prevention of tumor regrowth, in contrast with approximately 30% short-term and 25% long-term surgical cure rates.[22–24] The treatment regimen for dopamine agonist therapy in the acute situation is as described for the elective initiation of treatment. Conversely, the tumor shrinkage effect of bromocriptine in other secretory or non-secretory macroadenomas is inconsistent and only effective in a small proportion (<10%) of cases. Therefore, transsphenoidal surgery remains the treatment of choice to relieve mass effect and improve vision in patients with macroadenomas other than prolactinomas.

In the relatively rare but important situation of expansion of a macroprolactinoma in pregnancy, commencement of bromocriptine is highly effective in achieving tumor shrinkage.

Anti-thyroid medications and β-blockers are indicated to render patients with TSH-secreting macroadenomas euthyroid. Octreotide effectively reduces TSH hypersecretion with tumor shrinkage and acts as an adjunctive therapy.[19,25] Primary hypothyroidism with thyrotroph hyperplasia should be treated with thyroid hormones after adequate hydrocortisone replacement if hypopituitarism is also present. Lymphocytic hypophysitis with mass effects may respond to steroid therapy.

Patients undergoing decompressive pituitary surgery require perioperative steroid cover; hydrocortisone 100 mg 6-hourly intramuscularly, continuing for 7 days to avoid hypothalamic edema, and antibiotic prophylaxis are indicated. Common postoperative complications, including transient or prolonged cranial diabetes insipidus, cerebrospinal fluid rhinorrhea and variable degrees of hypopituitarism, should be treated. Follow-up visual and hormonal assessment should be obtained soon after the operation and 6 weeks afterwards to assess the adequacy of surgery and inform decisions on further treatment. Pituitary imaging is repeated 3–6 months postoperatively to detect any residual tumor. The histology, preferably with immunocytochemical staining, should be reviewed to confirm the pituitary adenoma.

A summary of the acute management of macroadenoma with visual loss is given in Table 19.7

Table 19.7

Acute management of macroadenoma with visual loss.

Decompression of the optic pathway
  Acute visual loss (e.g. pituitary apoplexy)
    Urgent transsphenoidal surgical decompression
  Gradual visual loss (more common)
    Prolactinoma: Dopamine agonists (DA; 75% success in tumor shrinkage)
    Non-prolactinoma: Transsphenoidal surgery to relieve mass effect and improve vision
Correction of the hypersecretory state
  Decision on dopamine agonist trial depends on the prolactin level
  [PRL] > 5000 mU/l (>250 µg/l): Suggests macroprolactinoma
    Start bromocriptine 1.25 mg with meal
    Rapid dose escalation to 7.5 mg/day if no side-effect; more gradual if side-effect ensues
    Clinical improvement may be dramatic within days to weeks
    Monitor: visual fields, visual acuity, [PRL] every 1–2 weeks until stable
    Cabergoline (0.5–3.0 mg/week) if intolerant or resistant to bromocriptine
    Consider surgery if
      Intolerant or resistant to dopamine agonists
      Invasive tumor without immediate response to DA
  [PRL] between 3000–5000 mU/l (150–250 µg/l): Borderline for macroprolactinoma
    Therapeutic trial of DA with careful monitoring of visual fields
    Proceed to surgery if poor response
    Fall in [PRL] to <100 mU/l after DA indicates disconnection hyperprolactinemia
  [PRL] <3000 mU/l (<150 µg/l): Macroprolactinoma unlikely
    Plan transsphenoidal surgical decompression to improve vision
    Medical preparation for other hypersecretory state (see text)
    Perioperative steroid cover: hydrocortisone 100 mg 6-hourly IM up to 7 days
    Antibiotic cover
    Postoperative visual and hormonal assessment
Replacement of pituitary hormone deficiencies
  Hydrocortisone 20–30 mg/day or more in stress
  Thyroid replacement after adequate steroid therapy to avoid adrenal crisis

Thyroid storm

Introduction

Thyroid storm or thyrotoxic crisis is a life-threatening condition characterized by fulminating manifestations of thyrotoxicosis. It implies a grave prognosis requiring urgent treatment. There are no clear or widely accepted diagnostic criteria to differentiate between severe thyrotoxicosis and thyroid storm, the latter indicating a decompensated state. Thyroid function tests serve to support the diagnosis but provide no discrimination between the two.

Thyroid storm usually occurs in patients who have either unrecognized or inadequately treated thyrotoxicosis and is almost invariably precipitated by a stress event such as surgery, infection, trauma or consumption of iodine-rich agents. Hyperthermia, tachyarrhythmias with or without heart failure and altered mental state are the cardinal features. Rarely, patients may present with atypical apathetic thyroid storm with apathy, stupor, cardiac failure, coma and minimal signs of thyrotoxicosis. The detailed pathophysiology of thyroid storm is not well established. However, increased free thyroid hormones secondary to displacement from the binding proteins by circulating inhibitors in systemic illness, increased production rate of hormones or increased stress-induced circulatory catecholamines may each play a part in the whole picture.

Clinical assessment[26,27]

The diagnosis should be based on high clinical suspicion and be confirmed by elevated thyroid hormones. It is crucial to initiate appropriate treatment once the diagnosis of thyroid storm is likely while awaiting the results of investigations. Fever, tachyarrhythmias, and agitation with altered mentation are the cardinal features. Other clinical manifestations are mainly an exaggeration of the sympathetic overactivity and accelerated metabolic rate characteristic of thyrotoxicosis. Usually, at least one provocative factor can be identified. The fever is frequently above 38°C and may be progressive up to 41°C or more. Associated profuse sweating contributes to excessive insensible water loss, resulting in dehydration.

Sinus tachycardia and atrial tachyarrhythmias are common and may lead to rate-dependent heart failure with tachypnea and edema. The blood pressure is variable. Chest pain may indicate exacerbation of underlying ischemic heart disease, pneumonia and pleurisy which has precipitated the thyroid storm or pulmonary embolism, complicating the crisis. Altered mental states with marked agitation, restlessness and tremor are frequent. This may progress to psychosis, seizure and coma. The apathetic variant of thyroid storm is rare and clearly creates a diagnostic difficulty. Gastrointestinal manifestations are common and include nausea, vomiting, diarrhea, abdominal pain and even jaundice. The symptoms may be severe enough to simulate an acute abdominal crisis. There may be a profound myopathy.

However, none of the above clinical features is specific. The diagnosis may be confused with sepsis, pheochromocytoma, malignant hyperthermia, drug or transfusion reactions and many others. It is therefore very important to take a good history, including previous thyroid problems with associated treatment modalities and consumption of any iodine-containing agent such as amiodarone or radiographic contrast medium. Particular attention should be drawn to the presence of goiter, exophthalmos, thyroid thrill or bruit and neck scar during clinical examination. Thyroid storm is more commonly associated with Graves' disease than toxic multinodular goiter or toxic adenoma.

Common precipitating factors of a thyroid storm include surgery, infection, diabetic ketoacidosis, parturition, radioiodine, iodine-rich drugs such as amiodarone, radiocontrast dyes, withdrawal of antithyroid medication, and physical or emotional stress. The crisis typically presents several hours after surgery or delivery, with fever, tachycardia and confusion. Radioiodine and amiodarone can rarely cause destructive thyroiditis, which is resistant to treatment.

The mechanisms of precipitating a thyroid storm are largely unknown but may involve various immunological disturbances with release of cytokines. These will in turn induce an acute rise in the free thyroid hormones by interfering with the binding affinity of the serum thyroid-binding proteins.

A summary of the clinical presentation of thyroid storm is given in Table 19.8.

Investigation

Immediate intervention should be initiated once the diagnosis is suspected before laboratory confirmation. Elevated T4, T3, free T4 (FT4) and free T3 (FT3) with an undetectable TSH confirm the thyrotoxic state

Table 19.8
Clinical presentation of thyroid storm.

Clinical features
- General
  - Fever
  - Sweating
  - Presence of goiter, exophthalmos (Graves')
  - Neck scar
- Neurological
  - Tremor
  - Agitation
  - Restlessness
  - Psychosis
  - Seizure
  - Altered mental state
  - Apathetic thyroid storm: stupor apathy
- Gastrointestinal
  - Nausea
  - Vomiting
  - Diarrhea
  - Abdominal pain
  - Acute abdomen
  - Jaundice
- Cardiovascular
  - Sinus tachycardia
  - Tachyarrhythmias
  - Heart failure
  - Peripheral edema
  - Hypertension or hypotension
  - Chest pain

Precipitating factors
- Surgery
- Infection
- Diabetic ketoacidosis
- Parturition
- Radioiodine
- Iodine-rich agents: amiodarone, radiocontrast
- Withdrawal of anti-thyroid medication
- Physical stress

Differential diagnosis
- Sepsis
- Pheochromocytoma
- Malignant hyperthermia
- Drug or transfusion reactions

which, together with the classical symptoms and signs, will establish the diagnosis of thyroid storm. Increased uptake on a technetium thyroid scan may also help in rapid diagnosis. Associated laboratory features include normochromic, normocytic anemia, leukocytosis, thrombocytosis, pre-renal uremia due to dehydration, hypercalcemia, hypoglycemia or hyperglycemia and deranged liver function tests with decreased albumin, increased alkaline phosphatase, transaminases and even bilirubin. Thyroid antiperoxidase antibodies are usually detectable in patients with Graves' disease. Blood for cortisol should be also taken to exclude coexisting adrenocortical insufficiency.

Further investigations are aimed at detecting precipitating causes and complications. Blood, urine and sputum cultures, chest X-ray and other appropriate screening tests for sepsis should be taken. A chest X-ray may show evidence of cardiac failure or infection. Electrocardiography is essential to diagnose and monitor any tachyarrhythmias and myocardial ischemia. Brain imaging and lumbar puncture may be necessary to rule out meningitis, central nervous system infection, stroke or other causes of altered mental state with fever.

Treatment

The management of thyroid storm[26–29] is directed at:

1. general supportive measures
2. specific measures for reduction of the thyroid hormones and their tissue effects

3. treatment of the precipitating illness
4. prevention and treatment of associated complications
5. monitoring of clinical response.

General measures
Patients with thyroid storm should be admitted to the intensive care unit for meticulous monitoring and therapy. Particular attention to the following problems is crucial.

Fluid balance
Patients may require large quantities of intravenous fluid and electrolytes to compensate for any gastrointestinal loss and insensible fluid losses from profuse sweating, hyperventilation and fever. Central venous pressure monitoring is necessary to monitor the fluid replacement to avoid worsening of any coexisting cardiac arrhythmias and cardiac failure.

Ventilation
Patients may have ventilatory failure secondary to thyrotoxic myopathy or hypokalemic periodic paralysis. Careful monitoring of arterial blood gases and electrolytes is mandatory.

Nutrition
Marked protein breakdown, high oxygen requirement and hepatic glycogen depletion can be seen in thyroid storm. High caloric intake in terms of intravenous dextrose with supplemental insulin may be necessary to counteract the hypercatabolic state. Adequate oxygen therapy is essential even in the absence of clinically obvious cardiac failure or chest infection. Water-soluble vitamins, e.g. vitamin B complex and vitamin C, are beneficial because subclinical deficiencies can occur. Intravenous thiamine, 1–2 mg/kg, should be administered to patients with chronic alcohol abuse or malnourishment to prevent neurological damage.

Hyperthermia
Fever can be as high as 41°C or more, necessitating external cooling measures such as ice packs or cooling blankets. Paracetamol is useful in lowering the body temperature. Salicylates can displace thyroid hormones from their thyroxine-binding globulin and worsen the crisis. They will also increase the metabolic rate and should be avoided. Chlorpromazine has both sedative and central sympathoadrenolytic effects that can be used to control the hyperthermia. It is recommended to give 50 mg orally, intramuscularly or intravenously and repeat every 6 h if necessary. Dantrolene is reserved for severe hyperthermia resistant to the above measures.

Sedation
Patients are frequently agitated and may benefit from sedation. Benzodiazepines and barbiturates are the drugs of choice. The latter have the additional effect of decreasing the levels of thyroid hormones by increasing their metabolism. One should, however, bear in mind that they may mask the signs of underlying stroke, or central nervous system infection.

Specific measures
Various specific therapies control the thyrotoxic crisis at different sites of action. Each drug can have more than one of the following effects:

1. inhibition of hormone synthesis
2. inhibition of hormone release
3. increase in hormone clearance
4. decrease in conversion of T4 to T3
5. antagonizing the adrenergic tissue effects.

Anti-thyroid drugs
High doses of thionamides should be given to block the synthesis of thyroid hormones by inhibiting the organification. Propylthiouracil, 200–300 mg orally, carbimazole, 20–30 mg orally, or methimazole, 20–30 mg orally or rectally, should be given immediately and every 4–6 h to reduce further thyroid hormone production. Propylthiouracil is preferable because of an additional effect on inhibiting conversion of T4 to T3. The drugs can be administered through nasogastric tube if the patient cannot swallow. Rectal and intravenous preparations are available for methimazole if the enteral route is not possible, as in postoperative ileus.

Iodides
Large doses of iodides inhibit thyroid hormone synthesis and release of the stored hormones; this is collectively known as the acute Wolff–Chaikoff effect. Iodides should be administered at least 1 h after antithyroid drugs that block the organification of the given iodine load. Various preparations can be used, including: (1) Lugol's iodine (5% iodine/10% potassium iodide in water) 1 ml orally every 6 h; (2) saturated solution of potassium iodide (SSKI) 2–5 drops orally

every 6 h; (3) sodium iodide (NaI, 10 ml of 10% solution) intravenously; (4) potassium iodide (KI) 120 mg orally every 6 h. The effects of iodides are immediate but may cease after 2 or 3 weeks. They should therefore not be continued beyond 2 weeks, to avoid potential severe relapse of thyrotoxicosis. Iodides are contraindicated in pregnancy because they cross the placenta quite readily and cause fetal hypothyroidism, large goiters and respiratory embarrassment in the fetus. Lithium has been used in iodine-allergic individuals with thyrotoxicosis. It inhibits thyroid hormone secretion and does not interfere with iodine uptake; an escape phenomenon also occurs. Cardiotoxicity and narrow therapeutic index limit its widespread use and its role in thyroid storm is not established.

Sodium ipodate (Oragrafin) and iopanoate

These agents were originally used as oral cholecystographic contrast media and are potent inhibitors of secretion of thyroid hormones and conversion of T4 to T3. They are more effective than inorganic iodides in reducing biologically active T3 by near complete inhibition of peripheral thyroxine deiodinases. The recommended dosage is 1–3 g daily orally. Prolonged use beyond 2 weeks is associated with severe and resistant relapse of thyrotoxicosis and should be avoided.

β-blockers

Propranolol 40–80 mg orally every 6–8 h or 1–2 mg intravenously every 15 min if necessary to a total dose of 10 mg is useful in the control of the peripheral sympathetic effects of thyroid hormones and to inhibit the conversion of T4 to T3 (at daily doses >200 mg). Fever, tremor and tachyarrhythmias and rate-dependent heart failure will respond well to β-blockade. Continuous cardiac monitoring is mandatory. One should, however, be careful if there is a history of cardiac failure. A cardioselective β-blocker may be used cautiously in asthmatic patients. If β-blockade is contraindicated, then reserpine 1–5 mg intramuscularly every 4–6 h, guanethidine 1 mg/kg orally every 12 h or diltiazem 60 mg orally every 4–6 h can be given.

Steroids

Hydrocortisone 200 mg intravenously and then 100 mg every 6 h or dexamethasone 2 mg every 6 h can be used to reduce the peripheral conversion of T4 to T3 and to inhibit the release of thyroid hormones. Glucocorticoid replacement will clearly be indicated in the event of coexisting adrenal insufficiency.

Perchlorate

This agent blocks the active uptake of iodides by the thyroid gland. The recommended dose is 0.5 g twice daily. It is reserved for resistant cases with high intrathyroidal iodine, e.g. in amiodarone-treated patients. A relatively high incidence of bone marrow aplasia limits its use.

Plasmapheresis

Physical removal of circulatory thyroid hormones and thyroid-stimulating immunoglobulins can be useful. However, it is reserved for resistant cases. It should be repeated many times, because only 20% of the T4 pool and even less of the T3 pool can be removed during each session.

Treatment of the precipitating illness

Sepsis is a common precipitant of thyroid storm. Chest and urinary tract infections are particularly common. Biliary tract infection should be excluded, especially if there is liver impairment. Altered mental state and fever may point to encephalitis or meningitis. Broad-spectrum high-dose antibiotics will be needed for infection, because of increased drug metabolism. Prophylactic antibiotic remains controversial, but empirical antibiotic therapy is indicated if occult sepsis is strongly suspected.

Prevention and treatment of complications

Arrhythmias and cardiac failure

Sinus tachycardia and atrial fibrillation are frequent in thyrotoxic crisis. Propranolol and digoxin can be used, but higher than usual doses are needed, due to rapid drug metabolism and clearance. This also applies to diuretics in the treatment of congestive cardiac failure. Continuous cardiac monitoring, frequent clinical assessment and attention to fluid and electrolyte balance are crucial.

Thromboembolism

Anticoagulation with warfarin should be initiated for patients in atrial fibrillation, to prevent embolic stroke. An increased incidence of venous thrombosis and pulmonary embolism is noted in thyroid storm and should be treated accordingly. The effect of warfarin is paradoxically enhanced in thyrotoxicosis, and careful monitoring of coagulation profiles is warranted.

Rhabdomyolysis

Rarely, this may complicate thyrotoxic crisis. Adequate hydration and treatment of associated hyperkalemia, hypocalcemia and renal impairment are essential.

Monitoring of clinical response

Clinical improvement is to be expected within 48–72 h after initiation of anti-thyroid drugs, iodides or sodium ipodate, β-blockers and steroid therapy. Response to treatment is monitored by frequent clinical assessment and serial serum FT3 or T3 levels. Untreated thyroid crisis is invariably fatal. Prompt treatment decreases mortality to approximately 20%.

A summary of the management of thyroid storm is given in Table 19.9.

Myxedema coma

Introduction

Myxedema coma is a decompensated state of untreated or inadequately treated long-standing hypothyroidism. Disturbed mental state, hypothermia, bradycardia and the presence of a precipitating event are the cardinal features. Common precipitants of myxedema coma include infection, prolonged cold exposure as in winter,

---

General measures
    Fluid
        Intravenous fluids and electrolytes; central venous pressure monitoring
    Ventilation
        Ventilatory support if necessary
    Nutrition
        O_2, vitamin B complex and vitamin C, thiamine
        Calories: IV glucose ± SC insulin
    Hyperthermia
        Ice pack, cooling blankets
        Paracetamol, chlorpromazine (50 mg orally/IM/IV)
        Dantrolene in resistant cases
    Sedation
        Benzodiazepines or barbiturates
Specific measures
    Anti-thyroid drugs
        Propylthiouracil 200–300 mg orally 4–6 hourly
        Carbimazole 20–30 mg orally 4–6 hourly
        Methimazole 20 mg orally per rectum 4–6 hourly
    Iodides
        Start >1 h after antithyroid drugs to block iodine organification
        Lugol's iodine 1 ml orally 6-hourly
        SSKI 2–5 drops orally 6-hourly
        NaI 10 ml 10% IV
        KI 120 mg orally 6-hourly
        Lithium for iodine-allergic patients; role in thyroid storm not established
    Sodium ipodate/iopanoate
        Potent inhibitor of hormone release; inhibition of T4 to T3 conversion
        1–3 g orally daily
    β-blockers
        Propranolol 40–80 mg orally 6–8-hourly or 1–2 mg IV every 15 min to a maximum of 10 mg
        Asthmatic: Reserpine 1–5 mg IM 4–6-hourly; guanethidine or diltiazem (see text)
    Steroids
        Hydrocortisone 200 mg IV stat, then 100 mg 6-hourly *or*
        Dexamethasone 2 mg 6-hourly
    Perchlorate
        0.5 g orally 12-hourly in resistant cases due to high intrathyroidal iodine
    Plasmapheresis
        Reserved for resistant cases
Treatment of precipitating illness
    Infection: High-dose broad-spectrum antibiotics
Prevention and treatment of associated complications
    Arrhythmias (e.g. atrial fibrillation): Digoxin and propranolol
    Consider anticoagulation if in atrial fibrillation
    Heart failure: Diuretics and digoxin
    Thromboembolism: Warfarin
    Rhabdomyolysis: Hydration, treatment of electrolyte imbalances
Monitoring of clinical response
    Monitor vital signs, FT3 or T3 levels
    Clinical response is expected within 48–72 h

Table 19.9
Management of thyroid storm.

medications (especially diuretics and sedatives), trauma, surgery, stroke, cardiorespiratory diseases and gastrointestinal bleeding. Impaired thermoregulation and response to infection, progressive cognitive deterioration and polypharmacy make the elderly population particularly vulnerable to the disorder. Given the insidious onset and vague presentation of myxedema coma, it is imperative to exercise a high index of suspicion in diagnosing and treating this rare but fatal disease.

Clinical assessment[30]

The diagnosis of myxedema coma should be made on clinical grounds and supported by laboratory parameters. However, resuscitative measures must not await confirmatory tests. Most patients with myxedema coma have primary hypothyroidism, although secondary hypothyroidism due to hypopituitarism may be the cause. There may be a history of thyroidectomy, radioiodine therapy for thyrotoxicosis or autoimmune thyroiditis. The main manifestations include a variable degree of altered mentation, hypothermia, hypoventilation, bradycardia, pericardial effusion and metabolic and electrolyte disturbances. Classic edematous facies with periorbital swelling and a large tongue may provide clues to the diagnosis.

Family members may notice that the patient suffers from gradual cognitive deterioration, confusion, self-neglect or apathy while at home. Disorientation, poor responsiveness and frank psychosis may be noted clinically. Seizures and coma may ensue and are usually compounded by hypoxia, hypercapnia, hypoglycemia, hyponatremia, infection, sedatives or other concurrent diseases. Hypothermia can pass unnoticed if a low-reading rectal thermometer is not used. On the other hand, the temperature may also be inappropriately normal in a septic patient. Patients with myxedema coma usually have reduced ventilatory drive to hypoxia and hypercapnia. Hypoventilation with carbon dioxide retention is common. It is frequently exacerbated by sedatives, respiratory infection, respiratory muscle weakness due to myopathy, macroglossia and sleep apnea syndrome.

The cardiovascular manifestations can be explained by a decrease in β-adrenergic receptor number and responsiveness with an intact α-adrenergic sensitivity to circulatory catecholamines. This results in a diminished stroke volume, bradycardia and reduced cardiac output due to β-adrenergic refractoriness, together with marked vasoconstriction, intravascular volume contraction, cold extremities and diastolic hypertension attributable to the unopposed α-adrenergic effects.[31] With decreased contractility and increasing afterload from systemic hypertension, cardiac failure may ensue. Cardiomegaly detected on chest X-ray implies long-standing hypertension, congestive heart failure or pericardial effusion. Hypotension is an ominous sign and can suggest occult blood loss, inappropriate diuretic therapy, peripheral vasodilatation secondary to overzealous rewarming, silent myocardial infarction or overwhelming sepsis.

Paralytic ileus and toxic megacolon can complicate myxedema coma, making enteral feeding difficult. Delayed tendon reflexes, thought to be specific for hypothyroidism, can actually be found in hypothermia of whatever cause. Furthermore, the reflexes may be depressed or, if there is concomitant stroke, increased. Brainstem stroke and any cause of hypothermia mimic myxedema coma closely and may at times create diagnostic difficulties.

A summary of the clinical presentation of myxedema coma is given in Table 19.10.

General
    Hypothermia
        Inappropriate normal temperature in sepsis
        Classic edematous facies
            Periorbital swelling and large tongue
Neurological
    Disturbed conscious state
        Disorientation
        Poor responsiveness
        Frank psychosis
        Seizure
        Coma
        Delayed or depressed tendon reflexes
Respiratory
    Hypoventilation
Cardiovascular
    Bradycardia
    Cardiomegaly
        Pericardial effusion
        Diastolic hypertension
    Hypotension
    Search for: Occult blood loss
        Silent myocardial infarction, etc. (see text)
Gastrointestinal
    Paralytic ileus
    Toxic megacolon

Table 19.10
Clinical presentation of myxedema coma.

Investigation

While a markedly elevated TSH and a low T4 or FT4 confirm the diagnosis of hypothyroidism beyond doubt, a normal or low TSH and a low T4 or FT4 can occur in central hypothyroidism or, more commonly, sick-euthyroid syndrome. Clinical and laboratory features of hypothyroidism and associated hypopituitarism may help in making this distinction but can sometimes be difficult.

Various metabolic derangements are found in myxedema coma. Hyponatremia can be partly explained by the elevated ADH and reduced glomerular filtration rate resulting from contracted plasma volume. The exact mechanisms are, however, not fully known. Hypoglycemia is occasionally seen, due to decreased gluconeogenesis and insulin clearance. Serum muscle enzymes, e.g. creatine phosphokinase (mainly the MM fraction), are elevated due to leakage from skeletal muscles and reduced renal clearance. Increased creatine phosphokinase of MB fraction may rarely be found without other evidence of myocardial infarction. Hypercholesterolemia is typical in hypothyroidism. Normochromic, normocytic anemia is common, indicating decreased red cell production and erythropoietin secretion or occult gastrointestinal bleeding. On the other hand, macrocytic anemia, although sometimes present in hypothyroidism alone, suggests the possibility of associated pernicious anemia.

The electrocardiogram typically shows sinus bradycardia, prolonged QT interval, and low voltage with flattening or inversion of T waves. A 'J' wave is seen in severe hypothermia. Evidence of myocardial ischemia may be present. Cardiomegaly, pleural effusions, pulmonary congestion or pulmonary infiltrates may be found on chest X-ray. Abdominal X-ray is useful in detecting dilated bowel loops in ileus or toxic megacolon. Further investigations are necessary to monitor the progress and treatment response, including arterial blood gases, serum urea, creatinine, electrolytes, hemoglobin and white cell counts with differential.

Treatment

Empirical treatment should be initiated once the diagnosis of myxedema coma is clinically suspected to reduce mortality. The management[32,33] should be directed at:

1. general supportive measures
2. specific measures
3. treatment of precipitant(s)
4. prevention and treatment of complications
5. monitoring of clinical response.

General measures
Patients should ideally be admitted to the intensive care unit for close monitoring and aggressive treatment.

Ventilation
Hypoventilation is probably the commonest cause of death in patients with myxedema coma. The multiple aforementioned adverse factors worsen the hypoventilation, with consequent increasing hypercapnia and hypoxemia. A high percentage of oxygen, which may be required due to anemia and intrapulmonary arteriovenous shunting from concomitant pneumonia, will further aggravate the hypercapnia. Early initiation of assisted or mechanical ventilatory support is crucial.

Circulation
As patients are in a state of severe vasoconstriction with reduced intravascular volume, mild diastolic hypertension is expected. If hypotension ensues, careful volume expansion with blood products or crystalloid solutions will improve the circulation and oxygen-carrying capacity. Occult blood loss, silent myocardial infarction or sepsis should be sought and treated accordingly. Inotropic agents should be used cautiously because they can precipitate life-threatening arrhythmias. Digoxin therapy for congestive cardiac failure should be monitored carefully, due to reduced drug clearance in myxedema coma.

Nutrition and electrolytes
Adequate calorie intake is essential for the conversion of T4 to T3, and extra glucose is needed to prevent and treat hypoglycemia. One should beware of excess water load and hyponatremia from intravenous glucose administration. Hyponatremia is usually treated with fluid restriction, but may require hypertonic saline with central venous pressure or pulmonary capillary wedge pressure monitoring if severe. Parenteral feeding may be necessary if paralytic ileus is persistent.

Hypothermia
Passive rewarming measures with blankets and increasing the ambient room temperature are preferred unless

hypothermia is severe (<30°C), when internal warming by infusions or gastric perfusion can be life-saving. External rewarming can precipitate shock and should be avoided.

Specific measures

Thyroid hormone replacement
It is generally recommended that intravenous (IV) thyroid hormone therapy should be given as the initial treatment, because of the sluggish circulation, hypometabolism and poor intestinal absorption in patients with myxedema coma. Various regimens have been suggested:

1) T4 alone: 300–500 μg IV bolus followed by 500 μg IV daily;
2) T3 alone: 25 μg IV 8-hourly for the first 24–48 h *or* 25 μg IV 8-hourly for 1 day and then 12.5 μg 8-hourly via nasogastric tube
3) T4 and T3: T4 200–300 μg IV bolus, then 100 μg IV daily *and* T3 25 μg IV 8-hourly for the first day

Each intravenous regimen should be followed by oral T4 25–50 μg daily when the patient can take oral medication. Those who advocate T4 alone suggest that large doses of T4 will replenish the thyroxine pool and saturate the binding sites for serum proteins. T4 also has a longer half-life (7 days) and smoother action and is thus less likely than T3 to precipitate underlying myocardial ischemia. On the other hand, some prefer T3 as the initial agent, because conversion of T4 to T3 is impaired in critically ill patients, and T3 is active with more rapid onset of action and, therefore, any adverse effects can be reversed quickly by drug withdrawal, due to the short half-life (1 day). Controversy still exists as to the best approach, as no convincing large-scale and comparative data are available in this rare disorder. Most experts, however, recommend intravenous thyroxine alone, because anecdotal evidence suggests a slightly more favorable outcome.

Steroids
Hydrocortisone injection (100 mg every 6-h intramuscularly) should be administered, after blood for cortisol has been taken, until coexisting adrenal insufficiency is excluded. This is to prevent adrenal crisis during thyroid replacement if the underlying diagnosis is hypopituitarism or Schmidt's syndrome (Addison's disease and primary hypothroidism). Stress-induced cortisol secretion may also be impaired in severe hypothyroidism.

Treatment of precipitant(s)
Infection is a common precipitant of myxedema coma. Empirical broad-spectrum antibiotics should be started after sepsis work-up. Classical signs of sepsis, e.g. fever, tachycardia and leukocytosis, may be absent. However, inappropriate normal temperature and a left shift of neutrophils are clues to occult infection. Central nervous system depressants should be stopped. Stroke can precipitate the myxedema coma and should be seriously considered. Computerized axial tomography may be indicated if localizing neurological signs are found.

Prevention and treatment of complications
Thromboembolism can complicate myxedema coma because of sluggish bloodflow and immobilization. The effect of anticoagulants may be prolonged due to slow metabolism. Pericardial effusion should be monitored clinically and followed by echocardiogram. Drainage may be necessary if there is cardiovascular compromise, but this is usually not necessary. Other possible complications are congestive cardiac failure, aspiration pneumonia, arrhythmias and other hypothermia-related complications (disseminated intravascular coagulopathy, rhabdomyolysis, acute renal failure and adult respiratory distress syndrome).

Monitoring of clinical response
With the initiation of appropriate therapy, heart rate, temperature and blood pressure should show some improvement within 12–24 h. Serum T4 and T3 levels may remain low even after 1 week of therapy, but progressive improvement in clinical status with decline in TSH will indicate a good treatment response. Poor prognostic factors include advanced age, slow response to therapy, hypotension and sepsis. Early diagnosis and intervention with cardiorespiratory support and aggressive treatment of infections should reduce the mortality rate to approximately 20%.

A summary of the management of myxedema coma is given in Table 19.11.

Initiate treatment if diagnosis suspected
General measures
    Intensive care unit preferred
    Ventilation
        Early assisted or mechanical ventilation
    Circulation
        Careful volume expansion with blood products/crystalloids ± inotropes, digoxin
    Nutrition
        Adequate calories (enteral or parenteral)
        Treat hyponatremia by fluid restriction
    Hypothermia
        Passive rewarming: Blankets, increased ambient temperature
        Internal rewarming: If <30°C, warm IV infusions and/or gastric perfusions
Specific measures
    Initial intravenous thyroid hormone replacement followed by oral T4 25–50 µg/day if conscious
        T4 alone: 300–500 µg IV bolus, then 50 µg IV daily *or*
        T3 alone: 25 µg IV 8-hourly for 1–2 days or
                  25 µg IV 8-hourly for 1 day, then 12.5 µg 8-hourly via nasogastric tube *or*
        T4 and T3: T4 200–300 µg IV bolus, then 100 µg IV daily
                T3 25 µg IV 8-hourly day 1
Treatment of precipitants
    Infection: Broad-spectrum antibiotics
    Withdraw central nervous system depressants
    CT brain to look for stroke if focal neurological sign
Prevention and treatment of complications
    Thromboembolism: Anticoagulants
    Pericardial effusion: Conservative unless cardiovascular compromise (rare)
    Congestive heart failure, aspiration pneumonia, etc.: Treat accordingly
Monitoring of clinical response
    Monitor heart rate, temperature, blood pressure, and later TSH level
    Clinical improvement usually within 12–24 h

Table 19.11
Management of myxedema coma.

Acute hypercalcemia

Introduction

Hypercalcemia affects about 0.5% of hospitalized patients. In contrast to the predominance of primary hyperparathyroidism in the outpatient setting, hypercalcemia associated with malignancy accounts for at least 50% of hypercalcemia found in hospital. Acute hypercalcemia or hypercalcemic crisis is a life-threatening condition characterized by disturbed mental state, dehydration, marked gastrointestinal symptoms, and variable cardiovascular, renal and neuromuscular involvement in association with profound hypercalcemia (usually serum calcium >3.5 mmol/l). Volume depletion results from vomiting compounded by secondary nephrogenic diabetes insipidus. The majority of cases are related to malignancy, mostly disseminated, but acute hyperparathyroidism, vitamin D excess states, milk alkali syndrome or, rarely, adrenal insufficiency can also present with severe crisis.

Serum calcium concentration is normally tightly regulated by parathyroid hormone (PTH), vitamin D and its metabolites, and calcitonin. However, the protective mechanisms which can be mounted to prevent hypercalcemia are generally less efficient than those guarding against hypocalcemia. Despite the large renal excretory capacity for calcium, it can be compromised by volume depletion and overwhelmed by the escalating calcium load from bone resorption and/or increased intestinal absorption.

The causes of hypercalcemia and their respective main mechanisms are listed in Table 19.12. At least one of the following mechanisms is involved in the pathogenesis of hypercalcemia:

1. increased intestinal calcium absorption
2. increased bone resorption
3. increased renal calcium reabsorption or decreased calcium excretion.

Immediate treatment for hypercalcemic crisis should be directed at rehydration and promoting calcium

Causes	Mechanism(s)[a]
Malignancy	
Local osteolytic hypercalcemia (LOH)	
Multiple myeloma	B
Osteolytic metastases	B
Humoral hypercalcemia of malignancy (HHM)	B, R
Lymphoma (some)[b]	A
Ectopic PTH secretion (rare)	B, R
Hyperparathyroidism	
Primary	B, R
Tertiary	B, R
Granulomatous disorders[b]	
Sarcoidosis	A
Histoplasmosis	A
Tuberculosis	A
Familial hypocalciuric hypercalcemia	R
Endocrine disorders	
Thyrotoxicosis	B
Adrenal insufficiency	?B, R
Pheochromocytoma	B, R
Drugs	
Thiazide	R
Vitamin A	B
Vitamin D	A, B
Lithium	?B, R
Milk alkali syndrome	A, R
Congenital syndromes	
Williams syndrome	A
Jansen's metaphyseal chondrodysplasia	B, R
Others	
Immobilization (especially in Paget's disease)	B
Acute renal failure	R
Rhabdomyolysis	R

[a]A: Increased absorption of calcium; B: increased bone resorption; R: increased renal calcium reabsorption or decreased renal calcium excretion.
[b]Increased local 1 α-hydroxylase activity.

Table 19.12
The causes and respective main mechanisms of hypercalcemia.

excretion, followed by antiresorptive agents and other adjunctive measures. After initial stabilization, etiology-oriented therapy by medical or surgical means (e.g. parathyroidectomy for primary hyperparathyroidism) should be undertaken.

Clinical assessment

The clinical manifestations of hypercalcemia are protean and depend on the severity of hypercalcemia, the rapidity of development, the age of the patient, intercurrent diseases and the underlying etiology.[34,35] The features are non-specific and are listed below:

1. Gastrointestinal—anorexia, nausea, vomiting, constipation, abdominal pain
2. Cardiovascular—dehydration, hypotension/hypertension, bradycardia, arrhythmia, sudden cardiac arrest
3. Renal—polyuria, polydipsia, nocturia, nephrolithiasis, renal insufficiency
4. Neuropsychiatric—depression, irritability, confusion, delirium, coma
5. Musculoskeletal—muscle weakness, myalgia, arthralgia
6. General—weight loss, malaise, fatigue.

Hypercalcemic crisis is more commonly associated with malignancy, in which multiple adverse factors may come into play. The patient may already be debilitated, anorexic, nauseated, constipated, weak or confused from the underlying malignancy and can be made worse by concurrent medications (e.g. narcotics), complications of chemotherapy or radiotherapy, as well as by coexisting medical diseases. Therefore, the diagnosis can sometimes be difficult to make clinically. In most circumstances, however, signs of dehydration, renal insufficiency and altered mentation dominate the clinical picture of hypercalcemic crisis. The clinical course is generally rapidly deteriorating, because hypercalcemia is accelerated by volume depletion, reduced glomerular filtration rate, and enhanced renal calcium reabsorption. The concomitant poor fluid intake, vomiting and disturbed thirst sensation from altered mental state will further aggravate the dehydration and hypercalcemia. Immobilization due to weakness also promotes hypercalcemia by increasing bone resorption. The elderly and the debilitated tend to experience symptoms earlier and deteriorate more rapidly. Clinical vigilance is crucial in preventing unnecessary morbidity and mortality in hypercalcemic patients with malignancy.

Hypercalcemic crisis complicating primary hyperparathyroidism is uncommon. If it occurs, it is usually associated with long-standing hypercalcemia with nephrolithiasis or bone disease. The patient may also harbor an aggressive adenoma or even a carcinoma. On the other hand, a careful drug history may reveal precipitating medications such as thiazide diuretics, lithium, calcium supplements or excessive vitamin A or D.

Investigation

Initial investigations should aim at establishing the diagnosis of severe hypercalcemia and monitoring of treatment response and complications. Serum total calcium, phosphate, magnesium, urea, creatinine and electrolytes, glucose and liver function should be tested, and measurements should be repeated according to clinical conditions. Serum total calcium must be corrected for albumin, which is usually low in patients with disseminated malignancy. Ionized calcium should be obtained if possible. Spot urine for sodium and calcium concentrations will help to distinguish prerenal from established renal failure and may be useful for monitoring fluid therapy. Electrocardiography may show a prolonged QRS complex, heart block, shortened ST segment and low-voltage T waves.

Parallel investigations are aimed at establishing the underlying cause. Full blood count and serum electrophoresis may suggest multiple myeloma. Chest X-ray and skeletal survey can reveal carcinoma of lung, osteolytic metastases or features of hyperparathyroidism (phalangeal subperiosteal erosions or, rarely, osteitis fibrosa cystica—brown tumors). Primary hyperparathyroidism tends to cause a hyperchloremic metabolic acidosis, but hypochloremic metabolic alkalosis is usually present in PTH-related-peptide (PTHrp)-associated malignancies. As most cases of malignant hypercalcemia are associated with increased PTHrp but suppressed PTH, an intact PTH assay is invaluable in differentiating malignant causes from acute hyperparathyroidism (high PTH). However, coexisting primary hyperparathyroidism and malignancy is not uncommon. PTHrp assay is useful but not widely available. Serum PTH may also be elevated in lithium-induced hypercalcemia and familial hypocalciuric hypercalcemia, but they rarely cause hypercalcemic crisis. Serum 1,25-dihydroxycholecalciferol is elevated in granulomatous disorders and some lymphomas, because of local 1α-hydroxylase activity, but the level is low in other malignancies.

A summary of the clinical presentation of hypercalcemic crisis is given in Table 19.13.

Management

Acute hypercalcemic crisis warrants aggressive treatment except in severely debilitated patients with disseminated malignancy, in whom palliative care may be more appropriate. Urgent intervention is indicated for patients with a high calcium level (total corrected serum calcium >3.5 mmol/l) or severe hypercalcemic manifestations, such as altered mental state, marked gastrointestinal disturbances, hypotension or pre-renal uremia. Therapy is mainly directed at restoring circulatory volume, promoting renal calcium clearance, decreasing bone resorption and removing the underlying or precipitating cause if possible.

The management of hypercalcemic crisis[35–37] consists of:

1. general measures
2. specific measures
3. subsequent treatment.

General measures
Fluid therapy

Hypercalcemia inhibits renal tubular ADH action, thereby causing nephrogenic diabetes insipidus and volume depletion. Rehydration with 2–6 l of isotonic saline daily in the initial 24–48 h can correct the hypovolemia, dilute the high calcium level and decrease renal tubular calcium reabsorption. The rate of saline infusion should be adjusted according to the clinical status, central venous pressure and urine output to prevent volume overload.

Loop diuretics

Frusemide therapy prevents fluid overload and promotes further coupled sodium–calcium diuresis after volume repletion. Although the contribution is relatively minor, loop diuretics also inhibit calcium reabsorption in the ascending limb of Henle's loop. The recommended regimen is 20–80 mg of frusemide given every 2–4 h intravenously. However, inadvertent use of frusemide without adequate saline infusion can actually aggravate the dehydration and hence the hypercalcemia. It also frequently leads to hypokalemia, hypomagnesemia and hypophosphatemia, which are deleterious to the already compromised cardiac status in some patients. Careful monitoring of electrolytes and fluid balance is mandatory.

Other general therapies

Any offending agents causing hypercalcemia should be discontinued as soon as possible. Some vitamin D derivatives, such as ergocalciferol (vitamin D_2) or cholecalciferol (vitamin D_3), have long biological half-lives, and their effects can last for weeks to months at times of toxicity. Immobilization promotes osteoclastic bone resorption. Early ambulation should be encouraged if possible. Associated medical conditions such as infections should be sought and treated. Dietary calcium restriction is only advisable in vitamin D excess, granulomatous disorders and some cases of lymphoma. In most other hypercalcemic states, serum 1,25-dihydroxycholecalciferol levels and intestinal calcium absorption are suppressed. No restriction of calcium-rich milk products is particularly relevant to malnourished patients with advanced malignancy.

High clinical suspicion in patients
    With underlying malignancy
    With long-standing hyperparathyroidism
    On thiazides, lithium, vitamin D, calcium
Prominent clinical features: [Ca] >3.5 mmol/l
    Neurological
        Irritability
        Confusion
        Delirium
        Coma
    Gastrointestinal
        Anorexia
        Nausea
        Vomiting
        Severe abdominal pain
    Cardiovascular
        Dehydration
        Hypotension
        Arrhythmia
        Sudden cardiac arrest
    Renal
        Polyuria
        Polydipsia
        Nocturia
        Pre-renal uremia

Table 19.13
Clinical presentation of hypercalcemic crisis.

Specific measures

Although many manifestations of hypercalcemic crisis can be alleviated by fluid replacement and other general measures, the serum calcium normalizes in less than 10% of patients. More effective but slower-acting specific therapies with mostly antiresorptive agents should be instituted simultaneously to bring the calcium level under control.

Bisphosphonates

Being structurally similar to natural pyrophosphate, bisphosphonates bind avidly to hydroxyapatite crystals and prevent their dissolution. They also inhibit osteoclastic bone resorption. Pamidronate has been shown to be more effective than etidronate or clodronate in terms of faster onset, greater reduction in calcium level and longer duration of normocalcemia. The response rate (normalization of serum calcium) ranges from 70% to 100% and is dose-dependent. An appropriate regimen of intravenous infusion of pamidronate in isotonic saline solutions is as follows:

1. If serum calcium is 3–4 mmol/l, give 60 mg over 8 h;
2. If serum calcium is >4 mmol/l, give 90 mg over 24 h.

The calcium level usually falls within 48 h and normalizes within a week. The duration of normocalcemia varies from one to several weeks, depending on the underlying etiology. Repeated administrations may then be necessary. Doses should be reduced in renal insufficiency. Etidronate (7.5 mg/kg intravenous infusion over 4 h for 3–7 days) or clodronate (60-mg single intravenous infusion) can also be used. Side-effects include febrile reactions, hypophosphatemia, hypomagnesemia, lymphopenia and injection site reactions. Hyperphosphatemia is seen in etidronate therapy because of inhibition of urinary phosphate excretion. Bisphosphonates represent a safe and effective first-line therapy for hypercalcemic crises, especially those associated with malignancy. The efficacy may be reduced in acute hyperparathyroidism and a subset of cancer patients with high PTHrp levels, presumably due to lack of effect of bisphosphonates on renal tubular calcium reabsorption.

Calcitonin

Exogenous calcitonin can lower the serum calcium by inhibiting osteoclastic bone resorption through its binding to cell surface receptors on osteoclasts. Its additional inhibition of renal tubular calcium reabsorption possibly underlies the rapid onset of actions (within hours). An analgesic effect in patients with osteolytic metastases may be observed. Modest decline in serum calcium of about 0.5 mmol/l is noticed within 2–6 h after the usual dose of salmon calcitonin (4–8 U/kg subcutaneously or intramuscularly every 6–12 h). Human calcitonin is also available and should be given as 0.5 mg subcutaneously every 12–24 h. The actions of calcitonin wear off rapidly after 2–3 days, due to downregulation of receptors in bone and kidneys. This escape phenomenon may be possibly attenuated for 1–2 weeks by co-administration of glucocorticoids. Calcitonin is useful when administered with other more effective but slower-acting antiresorptive agents (e.g. bisphosphonates) to achieve faster control of hypercalcemia (within the first 48 h). Side-effects are usually mild and generally transient, and include local skin reactions, nausea, vomiting, cramping abdominal pain and flushing of face and hands.

Mithramycin

This tumoricidal antibiotic inhibits osteoclastic bone resorption by interfering with RNA synthesis and osteoclast differentiation. It is highly effective but, because of actual and potential toxicity, it is rarely used and has been substantially replaced by bisphosphonates.

Glucocorticoids

Despite their ineffectiveness in most solid tumors and primary hyperparathyroidism, high-dose glucocorticoids may be very useful in hypercalcemia associated with vitamin D intoxication, granulomatous diseases, especially sarcoidosis, lymphoma or multiple myeloma. Exact mechanisms are unknown but may involve decreased active 1,25-dihydroxycholecalciferol production by activated macrophages, antagonism of vitamin D and cytolytic effects on tumor cells. Either prednisolone (40–60 mg/day orally) or hydrocortisone (100–300 mg/day intravenously) can be used.

Dialysis

Hemodialysis or peritoneal dialysis is reserved for life-threatening hypercalcemic crisis, particularly in patients with renal failure, fluid overload or heart failure. Hemodialysis is more effective than peritoneal dialysis in lowering the calcium level. A low-calcium or calcium-free dialysate is crucial.

General measures
    IV fluids
        2–6 l of isotonic saline in the first 24–48 h
        Monitor vital signs, central venous pressure, urine output
    Loop diuretics
        20–80 mg IV frusemide 2–4-hourly after adequate rehydration
        Caution: Dehydration, electrolyte imbalance
    Others
        Stop offending agents: calcium, vitamin D, thiazide, etc.
        Early mobilization
        Dietary calcium restriction not necessary
Specific measures
    Bisphosphonates
        Effective first-line therapy, onset within 48 h
        Pamidronate 60–90 mg IV depending on serum Ca concentration [Ca]
            [Ca] 3–4 mmol/l: give 60 mg IV, over 8 h
            [Ca] >4 mmol/l: give 90 mg IV over 24 h
        Etidronate 7.5 mg/kg IV over 4 h for 3–7 days
        Clodronate 60 mg single IV infusion
    Calcitonin
        Rapid onset (4–6 h) but short duration due to tachyphylaxis
        Salmon calcitonin 4–8 U/kg SC/IM 6–12-hourly
        Human calcitonin 0.5 mg SC 12–24-hourly
    Mithramycin
        Onset of 24–48 h; 60% effective; duration variable
        12–25 µg/kg IV infusion over 4–24 h
    Glucocorticoids
        Only for vitamin D intoxication, granulomatous diseases, lymphoma, myeloma
        Prednisolone 40–60 mg/day orally
        Hydrocortisone 100–300 mg/day IV
    Dialysis
        For life-threatening crisis, especially in renal failure, fluid overload, heart failure
        Hemodialysis or peritoneal dialysis with low Ca/Ca-free dialysates
    Phosphate
        Effective within min; risk of metastatic calcification
        Only indicated for life-threatening cardiac arrhythmia or encephalopathy
        1–3 mmol/h IV for 12 h
    Edetate
        Rapid action; risk of renal failure
        IV infusion up to 70 mg/kg daily
    Gallium nitrate
        5-day regimen and risk of nephrotoxicity prevent its widespread use
        200 mg/m^2 body surface area IV infusion daily for 5 days
Subsequent treatment
    Clodronate 800–1600 mg 12-hourly orally
    Treatment of the underlying cause
        Malignancy: Surgery or radiotherapy or chemotherapy
        Primary hyperparathyroidism: Parathyroidectomy

Table 19.14
Emergency management of hypercalcemic crisis.

Phosphate

Intravenous phosphate is highly effective in lowering calcium levels within minutes of administration. A suggested regimen is 1–3 mmol of phosphate per hour for 12 h intravenously. However, it has been virtually abandoned because of the risk of widespread metastatic calcification, cardiac arrhythmia, acute renal failure and even sudden death. The only indications are for life-threatening cardiac arrhythmias and severe encephalopathy when dialysis is not immediately available. It is relatively contraindicated in renal failure and hyperphosphatemia.

Edetate

Trisodium edetate given intravenously over 2–3 h up to 70 mg/kg daily acts as a calcium chelator for desperate hypercalcemic crisis. The calcium–edetate complexes are excreted renally and can precipitate acute renal failure. Hemodialysis may be necessary to remove the complexes if renal failure ensues.

Gallium nitrate

Apart from its anti-tumor activity, gallium nitrate has been used in the treatment of malignant hypercalcemia. It apparently adsorbs to and decreases the solubility of hydroxyapatite crystals, thereby inhibiting bone resorption. After 5 days of continuous application of 200 mg/m^2 body surface area of gallium nitrate, about 75% of patients achieve normocalcemia. The onset of action is within 24–48 h, with a mean duration of 11 days. Nephrotoxicity is a major concern, and less frequent adverse effects include nausea, vomiting, hypotension, hypophosphatemia and anemia. Adequate hydration and regular monitoring of urea, electrolytes and full blood counts are therefore essential. The requirement for a 5-day regimen and potential nephrotoxicity prevent its widespread use, especially when safer bisphosphonates are available.

Subsequent treatment

After the acute treatment of severe hypercalcemia, the underlying cause should be established. Further treatment will be governed by the diagnosis. Patients with primary hyperparathyroidism should be treated surgically after initial stabilization. Surgery, chemotherapy or radiotherapy may be indicated for underlying malignancy. Both intravenous and oral bisphosphonates (pamidronate, alendronate and clodronate) have been used successfully in preventing recurrence of hypercalcemia, and for alleviating bone pain and pathological fractures in patients with breast cancer or multiple myeloma. Predictably, the long-term prognosis of patients with malignant hypercalcemia is grave unless effective treatment of the underlying malignancy is possible.

A summary of the emergency management of hypercalcemic crisis is given in Table 19.14.

Acute hypocalcemia

Introduction

Hypocalcemia commonly encountered in clinical practice is usually chronic and stable, with minimal symptoms. However, acute profound hypocalcemia manifesting as tetany, seizure or arrhythmia can constitute an endocrine emergency requiring immediate intervention. The clinical presentation is determined by the concentration of free ionized calcium, which accounts for 50% of the total calcium. Of the remaining 50%, 40% is bound to plasma proteins (mainly albumin) and 10% is complexed to circulating anions, such as lactate, citrate and sulfate. Enhanced protein-binding affinity of calcium as in alkalosis can decrease free calcium and cause hypocalcemic symptoms without appreciable changes in total calcium concentration. Excess anions, either endogenous or exogenous, may also lead to acute symptomatic hypocalcemia by chelating the ionized calcium.

The protective mechanisms mounted against hypocalcemia are generally efficient and involve mainly PTH, and vitamin D and its active metabolite (1,25-dihydroxycholecalciferol). Other hormonal or non-hormonal factors may also participate but are quantitatively less significant. PTH promotes osteoclastic bone resorption, distal renal tubular calcium reabsorption and phosphate excretion. It also increases the conversion of 25-hydroxycholecalciferol to active 1,25-dihydroxycholecalciferol and thereby stimulates intestinal calcium absorption. This coordinated regulatory system serves to maintain calcium homeostasis. The causes of hypocalcemia are listed in Table 19.15.

Clinical assessment

The clinical manifestations of hypocalcemia depend very much on the degree of hypocalcemia (ionized calcium level) and the rate of its development.[38–40] While marked hypocalcemia may be asymptomatic if

PTH related
    Hypoparathyroidism
        Idiopathic
        Autoimmune
        Sporadic
        Congenital
        Infiltration
        Irradiation
        Postsurgical
            Transient
            Permanent
            Hungry bone syndrome
    Pseudoparathyroidism: Type Ia, b, c and II
Vitamin D related
    Vitamin D deficiency
        Nutritional
            Malabsorption
            Drugs: Cholestyramine
            Genetics: Vitamin D-dependent rickets type I
        Renal diseases
        Liver diseases
    Abnormal vitamin D metabolism
        Phenobarbitone
    Vitamin D resistance
        Vitamin D dependent rickets type II
Magnesium related
    Hypermagnesemia
    Hypomagnesemia
        Gastrointestinal loss
        Alcoholism
        Acute pancreatitis
Drugs
    Loop diuretics
    Aminoglycosides
    Cisplatin
Chelator related
    Phosphate
    Iatrogenic
        Chronic renal failure
        Rhabdomyolysis
        Tumor lysis syndrome
    Citrate
        Massive transfusion
        Radiocontrast
    Edetate
Radiocontrast
    Bicarbonate
    Sodium bicarbonate
    Others
    Fluoride
    Foscarnet
Drug related
    Antiresorptive agents
        Bisphosphonates
        Gallium nitrate
        Mithramycin
    Ketoconazole
    Pentamidine
Others
    Acute pancreatitis
    Toxic shock syndrome
    Alkalosis of all causes
    Prematurity
    Osteoblastic metastases
    Critical illness

Table 19.15
Causes of hypocalcemia.

it develops slowly, an acute dramatic fall in serum calcium may be life-threatening. The symptoms will be further modified by coexisting acid–base imbalance, hypomagnesemia, hypokalemia and other metabolic disturbances. Calcium is involved in neurotransmission, smooth and skeletal muscle contractions, exocrine and endocrine secretory processes, and a wide range of metabolic pathways. Clinically, neuromuscular and cardiovascular complications predominate in acute hypocalcemia. Patients may present with symptoms of enhanced neuromuscular excitability with paresthesiae of extremities and circumoral regions, muscle cramps, fasciculation, hyperreflexia, carpopedal spasm and tetany. Chvostek's sign and Trousseau's sign are classic maneuvers for demonstrating latent tetany. Chvostek's sign can be elicited by tapping the facial nerve at the anterior edge of masseter muscle where the parotid duct crosses. Ipsilateral twitching of the facial muscles constitutes a positive test signifying a recent drop in calcium level. Trousseau's sign is carpal spasm induced by inflating the sphygmomanometer on the upper arm 10–20 mmHg above the systolic blood pressure for at least 3 min. However, both signs may be absent in hypocalcemia, and Chvostek's sign, in particular, can occur in normal individuals. In acute hypocalcemia, seizure can arise de novo or in a predisposed patient due to decreased excitation threshold. A generalized and prolonged form of tetany, called cerebral tetany, may mimic a seizure but without loss of consciousness or postictal drowsiness. Smooth muscle spasms, such as bronchospasm, laryngospasm, dysphagia, abdominal pain and biliary colic, can occur with variable severity. Neuropsychiatric symptoms of anxiety, depression, irritability, delirium and psychosis may be found.

Acute profound hypocalcemia may precipitate hypotension due to generalized vasodilatation and decreased aldosterone secretion. Other cardiovascular complications of hypocalcemia include reduced myocardial contractility, bradycardia, prolongation of QT interval on electrocardiogram (ECG) and progression to arrhythmias and congestive cardiac failure. Arrhythmias may be refractory to standard therapies unless calcium is administered. Long-standing hypocalcemia may be manifested as cataract, intracranial calcification (especially in basal ganglia) with or without extrapyramidal features, optic neuritis with unilateral visual loss, papilledema and benign intracranial hypertension. Patients may also have dry skin, coarse hair and brittle nails. Characteristic features of osteomalacia (proximal weakness and myalgia, pseudofractures), autoimmune polyglandular syndrome (hypoparathyroidism, associated mucocutaneous candidiasis, Addison's disease and vitiligo) and pseudohypoparathyroidism (rounded face, short stature, shortened fourth and fifth metacarpals) should be looked for.

A summary of the clinical presentation of hypocalcemia is given in Table 19.16.

Investigation[39]

As approximately 40% of calcium is bound to albumin

Acute
  Neuromuscular
    Paresthesiae of extremities/circumoral region
    Muscle cramps
    Fasciculations
    Hyperreflexia
    Carpopedal spasm
    Tetany
    Seizure
    Chvostek's and Trousseau's sign (latent tetany)
    Cerebral tetany (prolonged and generalized)
  Cardiovascular
    Decreased myocardial contractility
    Hypotension
    Bradycardia
    Prolonged QT interval in ECG
    Arrhythmia
    Congestive heart failure
  Gastrointestinal
    Abdominal pain
    Dysphagia
    Biliary colic
  Respiratory
    Laryngospasm
    Bronchospasm

Chronic
  Neuropsychiatric
    Irritability
    Anxiety
    Depression
    Delirium
    Psychosis
  Ophthalmic
    Cataract
    Optic neuritis
    Papilledema
  Cutaneous
    Dry skin
    Coarse hair
    Brittle nail
  Others
    Intracranial calcifications
    Autoimmune polyglandular syndrome
    Pseudohypoparathyroidism

Table 19.16
Clinical presentation of hypocalcemia.

and other serum proteins, apparent hypocalcemia may be an artefact of hypoalbuminemia. Therefore, calcium concentration should be corrected for albumin by the following formula:

Corrected calcium (mmol/l) = measured calcium (mmol/l) + [40 − serum albumin (g/l)] × 0.02

The corrected calcium concentration correlates with the ionized calcium concentration, which should be directly measured if facilities exist.

The investigations are directed at elucidating the cause of hypocalcemia and monitoring therapy. Serum phosphate, magnesium, urea and electrolytes, creatinine, and liver function tests, including alkaline phosphatase, should be checked. An increased serum phosphate concentration is found in renal failure, phosphate ingestion, tumor lysis syndrome, rhabdomyolysis, hypoparathyroidism and pseudohypoparathyroidism. A low serum phosphate concentration suggests vitamin D deficiency or resistance, 'hungry bone' syndrome after surgical treatment of hyperparathyroidism and osteoblastic metastases. Serum magnesium concentration should also be measured because:

1. Both hypomagnesemia and hypermagnesemia can cause hypocalcemia.
2. Hypomagnesemia and hypocalcemia can have indistinguishable clinical features.
3. Hypomagnesemia and hypocalcemia can coexist in certain conditions, such as malabsorption, or loop diuretic or cisplatin therapy.
4. Hypocalcemia can be refractory to treatment in uncorrected hypomagnesemia.

Two-site immunoradiometric or immunochemiluminometric assay for intact PTH is useful in distinguishing hypoparathyroidism (PTH is low or inappropriately normal) from other causes of hypocalcemia (PTH is high). It is also useful in the differential diagnosis of severe hypocalcemic crisis after parathyroidectomy. PTH level may be high in 'hungry bone' syndrome but low in permanent post-surgical hypoparathyroidism. Measurement of vitamin D metabolites may be necessary to confirm vitamin D deficiency or resistance.

Electrocardiography may show a prolonged QT interval, ST segment prolongation or T wave abnormalities. Skull X-ray can reveal intracranial calcification in chronic hypocalcemia, especially hypoparathyroidism. Bone changes in osteomalacia, osteoblastic metastases or pseudohypoparathyroidism may be evident on a radiological skeletal survey.

Treatment

The management of hypocalcemia can be divided into two phases: acute and maintenance therapy.[39–42] The urgency of treatment depends on the severity of symptoms, which is in turn determined by the ionized calcium concentration, rate of onset and underlying etiology.

Acute therapy

Emergency treatment is indicated for acute symptomatic hypocalcemia, especially when tetany, seizures, hypotension, cardiac failure or arrhythmias are emerging. The intervention should aim at symptomatic relief and preventing complications. It is usually not necessary to restore the calcium to normal levels.

Hypocalcemia

Intravenous calcium is indicated for acute severe hypocalcemia: 10 ml of 10% calcium gluconate (93 mg or 2.25 mmol of elemental calcium) should be given by slow intravenous infusion over 5–10 min. This can be followed by slow infusion ranging from 0.15 to 1.5 mg of elemental calcium/kg per hour if hypocalcemia is likely to recur. Oral vitamin D analogs and calcium supplements may be started at the same time, because they take several days to work. More rapid calcium injection or infusion may precipitate cardiac arrhythmias, especially in patients taking digoxin. Continuous cardiac monitoring is advisable. The rate of infusion should be adjusted according to hypocalcemia symptoms, and serum calcium level should be monitored every several hours. Electrolytes and renal function should also be monitored.

Hypomagnesemia

Magnesium is an effector of PTH secretion, and untreated hypomagnesemia leads to resistant hypocalcemia. Intravenous magnesium sulfate infusion 3–6 g (24–48 mmol) over 24 h should be administered in addition to calcium replacement. Alternatively, intramuscular magnesium (1–2 g (8–16 mmol) every 8 h) can be given but is painful. It may be necessary to continue oral magnesium supplements (as glycerophosphate) for 3–7 days to replenish the magnesium deficit. Dose reduction is required for patients with renal insufficiency. The magnesium level should be checked daily.

Other metabolic disturbances

Hyperphosphatemia, hypermagnesemia, hyperkalemia or hypokalemia, and acid–base disorders should be treated accordingly. Any offending agents, such as diuretics and aminoglycosides, must be withdrawn.

Maintenance therapy

Oral vitamin D derivatives and calcium supplements remain the mainstay of treatment in chronic hypocalcemia. There are several preparations of vitamin D derivatives available for treatment. The choice will depend on the cause of the hypocalcemia and pharmacokinetic properties. The preparations include:

1. ergocalciferol (calciferol, vitamin D_2)
2. cholecalciferol (vitamin D_3)
3. dihydrotachysterol (synthetic)
4. alfacalcidol (1α-hydroxycholecalciferol)
5. calcitriol (1,25-dihydroxycholecalciferol)

Vitamins D_2 and D_3 are the least expensive but require hepatic and renal metabolism to form active calcitriol. They therefore have slower onsets of action (10–14 days) and longer durations of action (weeks to months). Low-dose ergocalciferol (400 units/day) in combination with calcium is used to treat dietary vitamin D deficiency. Patients with malabsorption require specific therapy for the underlying condition, and those on anticonvulsants require higher doses of ergocalciferol. Alfacalcidol and calcitriol are more potent and effective but are more expensive preparations. Their faster onsets of action (1–2 days) and shorter durations of action (2–3 days) are advantageous in treating acute hypocalcemia and in rapid reversal at times of toxicity. Dihydrotachysterol is an active synthetic analog of vitamin D which does not require further metabolism, with intermediate pharmacokinetics and cost. Large daily pharmacological doses (50 000–100 000 units; 1.25–2.5 mg) of vitamin D_2 and D_3 are required for hypoparathyroidism because of deficient 1α-hydroxylase activity. Either alfacalcidol or calcitriol in doses of 0.5–2 μg/day are more effective and are the treatment of choice in hypoparathyroidism. They are also indicated in vitamin D resistance, severe renal disease, and pseudohypoparathyroidism. The equivalent dose of dihydrotachysterol is 375–750 μg/day.

Oral calcium supplements (1–3 g/day) may be necessary as adjunctive maintenance therapy. Calcium carbonate is commonly chosen, due to its higher percentage (40%) of elemental calcium than that in citrate, lactate, gluconate and glubionate. This can be translated to taking fewer tablets. However, calcium citrate is indicated for patients with achlorhydria or those taking histamine receptor-2 blockers (H_2 blockers) or proton pump inhibitors.

Patients on long-term vitamin D and calcium therapy should be monitored by serum calcium and 24-h urine calcium excretion to assess the response to replacement and prevent complications. Serum alkaline phosphatase and PTH level may also be useful in monitoring osteomalacia. The main therapeutic goal is to keep serum calcium in the low–normal range without hypercalciuria.

A summary of the emergency management of hypocalcemia is given in Table 19.17.

Acute therapy
  Indicated for acute symptomatic hypocalcemia: Tetany, seizure, hypotension, etc.
  Aim at symptomatic relief, preventing complications (*not* return [Ca] to normal)
Hypocalcemia
  Calcium gluconate 10 ml 10% (93 mg elemental Ca) slow IV infusion over 5–10 min
  0.5–1.5 mg elemental Ca/kg/h oral IV infusion if necessary
  Avoid faster infusions: Risk of arrhythmias
  Start oral vitamin D analogs and Ca supplements
  Monitor symptoms, [Ca], serum electrolytes, urea and creatinine 4–6 hourly
Hypomagnesemia
  To overcome PTH resistance
  Magnesium sulfate 3–6 g (24–48 mmol) IV infusion over 24 h *or* 1–2 g (8–16 mmol) IV 8-hourly
  Oral magnesium glycerophosphate for 3–7 days to replenish deficit
  Monitor [Mg] daily
Treat other coexisting electrolyte imbalance and acid–base disorders
Withhold offending agent(s)
  Diuretics, aminoglycosides, etc.

Table 19.17
Emergency management of hypocalcemia.

Hypoglycemia

Introduction

Hypoglycemia is probably the most common endocrine emergency in clinical practice. Most patients at risk of hypoglycemia have diabetes mellitus on maintenance treatment with either insulin or oral hypoglycemic drugs. A three-fold increase of severe hypoglycemia has been observed in insulin-dependent diabetes mellitus (IDDM) patients treated with intensive insulin therapy in the Diabetes Control and Complications Trial.[43] Non-insulin-dependent diabetes mellitus (NIDDM) patients are also at risk, particularly those taking long-acting sulfonylureas (e.g. chlorpropamide or glibenclamide). On the other hand, spontaneous hypoglycemia in the non-diabetic population is relatively uncommon but creates both diagnostic and therapeutic challenges to physicians. Appropriate initial evaluation and therapy of hypoglycemia during the acute setting are not only crucial in preventing morbidity or mortality but also helpful in establishing the underlying cause. A sound knowledge of the causes of hypoglycemia, as listed in Table 19.18, is important in formulating a sensible approach to patients with hypoglycemia.

Clinical assessment[44,45]

Biochemically, hypoglycemia is usually defined as a venous plasma glucose level of less than 2.8 mmol/l. The glucose concentration in plasma is 15% higher than in whole blood. However, pathological hypoglycemia is clinically defined by the Whipple triad:

1. the presence of hypoglycemic symptoms
2. concomitant low plasma glucose
3. reversal of symptoms after restoration of normoglycemia.

All three criteria must be satisfied for a firm diagnosis to be made. The central nervous system relies primarily on glucose as the main substrate for normal function. It takes several days for the brain to shift to using ketones as the major fuel in prolonged starvation. The liver is the main source of glucose from glycogenolysis and gluconeogenesis, and the balance between glycogenesis and hepatic glucose output depends on the interaction between insulin on the one hand and glucagon, catecholamines, cortisol, growth hormone and thyroxine on the other.

Hypoglycemia stimulates sympathetic activity and counterregulatory hormone release. It is clinically manifest as adrenergic symptoms consisting of palpitation, tachycardia, sweating, tremor, anxiety, nausea, hunger, pallor or sometimes flushing or angina. These

Medications
  Insulin[a]
  Sulfonylureas[a]
  Others β-blocker
    Ethanol
    Salicylates
    Pentamidine
    Quinine
Tumors
  Islet cell tumor
    Insulinoma
  Non islet-cell tumor
    Mesodermal
      Retroperitoneal leiomyosarcoma
      Fibrosarcoma
      Mesothelioma
    Epithelial: Hepatoma
      Adrenocortical carcinoma
      Gastric carcinoma
Endocrine diseases
  Hypopituitarism
  Addison's disease
  Myxedema coma
Insulin autoimmune syndrome
  Anti-insulin antibodies
  Insulin receptor antibodies
Inborn errors of carbohydrate metabolism
  Galactosemia
  Hereditary fructose intolerance
  Glucose-6-phosphatase deficiency
  Fructose-1,6-diphosphatase deficiency
Postprandial hypoglycemia
  Postgastric surgery
  Reactive to fructose, leucine or galactose
Others
  Liver failure
  Septic shock
  Congestive cardiac failure
  Prolonged starvation
  Ketotic hypoglycemia of childhood

[a] Iatrogenic/accidental/surreptitious.

Table 19.18
Causes of hypoglycemia.

symptoms are non-specific and are also found in hypovolemia, myocardial infarction or other stressful states. However, they act as useful warning signs to allow glucose administration and thereby prevent more severe hypoglycemia and neuroglycopenia. Neuroglycopenic symptoms are protean and usually occur when the plasma glucose concentration is less than 2.6 mmol/l. These include headache, blurred vision, diplopia, incoordination, ataxia, weakness, atypical behavior as a result of loss of normal inhibitions, aggressiveness, confusion, somnolence, seizures and coma. Atypical presentations include a stroke-like syndrome with focal neurological deficit, frank psychosis, dementia, locked-in syndrome and also sensorimotor peripheral neuropathy (usually from chronic recurrent hypoglycemia).

Neuroglycopenic symptoms are usually preceded by adrenergic symptoms, especially in patients with diabetes mellitus. This does not apply to insulinoma patients, who frequently present with neuroglycopenic symptoms such as diplopia, blurring of vision, abnormal behavior, confusion and coma. Not surprisingly, the diagnosis of insulinoma can pass unnoticed for years or even decades. Some patients with insulinoma may have been on prolonged treatment for epilepsy, psychiatric disorder, dementia or stroke prior to recognition of hypoglycemia as the underlying cause of their symptoms. On the other hand, patients with diabetes can also suffer from neuroglycopenia without preceding warning adrenergic symptoms. This phenomenon is known as hypoglycemia unawareness and has been extensively studied, particularly in insulin-dependent diabetes. While impaired glucagon, catecholamine, growth hormone and cortisol responses to hypoglycemia are observed in IDDM patients,[46] NIDDM patients generally have a reduced glucagon response but increased catecholamine and normal growth hormone and cortisol responses.[47] These altered counterregulatory mechanisms may partly explain the hypoglycemia unawareness, which is associated with duration of diabetes and improved metabolic control in IDDM patients. It is worth mentioning that adrenergic symptoms may not only be reduced in autonomic neuropathy (as a complication of diabetes) and the elderly population, but also may be masked by β-blockers, sedatives and alcohol, which also inhibit gluconeogenesis. In view of the frequent absence of adrenergic symptoms, all patients with confusion, seizure or coma should be assumed to have hypoglycemia until proven otherwise.

After the patient has recovered from a hypoglycemic attack, a detailed history is important both in making a correct diagnosis and in preventing future episodes of hypoglycemia. Repeated hypoglycemia in an otherwise stable diabetic patient should alert the physician of the onset of nephropathy, concomitant Addison's disease, hypothyroidism, hypopituitarism or interfering medications. The symptoms and their relation to meals should be documented. A drug history is clearly important. Previous gastric surgery may point to reactive hypoglycemia.

A summary of the diagnosis of hypoglycemia is given in Table 19.19.

Investigation

The diagnosis of hypoglycemia should not be based solely on non-specific symptoms or bedside capillary blood glucose measurements, which are notoriously inaccurate in the hypoglycemic range or when performed with suboptimal technique. Patients with clinically suspected hypoglycemia should have a capillary blood glucose concentration measurement with a reagent strip, and preferably read with a reliable reflectance meter. A low reading should be confirmed by a laboratory glucose measurement. If no clinically obvious cause of hypoglycemia is evident, a further blood sample (about 20 ml) should be centrifuged and the serum saved for later insulin assay. This may obviate the need for future lengthy investigation (e.g. 72-h prolonged fasting) to reproduce a similar spontaneous hypoglycemia episode. A urine sample should be checked for ketones, and this may be helpful in differentiating a hyperinsulinemic state (low ketones) from counterregulatory hormone failure (high ketones), as in hypopituitarism.

After stabilization, subsequent investigations will be directed at finding the cause of hypoglycemia. Urea, electrolytes and liver function tests should be checked to exclude renal impairment (e.g. diabetic nephropathy) or liver failure as the cause of hypoglycemia. The blood sample previously saved during hypoglycemia should be assayed for insulin, C-peptide, β-hydroxybutyrate (blood ketones) and cortisol if indicated. If the insulin concentration is not suppressed, a concomitant low C-peptide level suggests exogenous insulin, and a high C-peptide level indicates endogenous insulin, either from insulinoma or stimulation by oral hypoglycemic agents. Urine for sulfonylurea screen may be necessary for further investigation. A low insulin concentration will be found with all other causes of hypoglycemia. Serum pro-insulin-like growth factor-II (pro-IGF-II) levels may be high with non-islet

Biochemical definition
    Venous plasma glucose concentration
    [glucose]: <2.8 mmol/l
Clinical definition
    Whipple's triad
        Presence of hypoglycemic symptoms
        Concomitant low plasma glucose
        Reversal of symptoms after normoglycemia
Presentation
    Adrenergic symptoms
        Warning but non-specific
        Palpitation
        Sweating
        Tremor
        Anxiety
        Nausea
        Hunger
    Neuroglycopenic symptoms
        Usually [glucose] <2.6 mmol/l
        Headache
        Diplopia
        Incoordination
        Confusion
        Seizure
        Coma
    Atypical presentation
        Stroke-like syndrome
        Psychosis
        Dementia
        Locked-in syndrome
        Sensorineural peripheral neuropathy
    Hypoglycemia unawareness
        Neuroglycopenia without preceding
        adrenergic symptoms
        At-risk population
            Patients with insulinoma
            Intensive control insulin-dependent
            diabetic patients
            Long-standing diabetics especially
            complicated by autonomic neuropathy
            Elderly
            Patients on drugs: β-blockers, sedatives,
            alcohol
    Search for
        Diabetic nephropathy
        Addison's disease
        Hypopituitarism
        Hypothyroidism
        History of gastric surgery
        Drug history, especially oral hypoglycemic
        agents

Table 19.19
Diagnosis of hypoglycemia.

cell tumor. Blood alcohol level may not be helpful in alcohol-induced hypoglycemia, because of a lag period of 6–24 h between ingestion and hypoglycemia.

Treatment

The management of hypoglycemia can be divided into three phases:

1. Acute measures—to prevent and minimize neurological damage.
2. Maintenance therapy—to prevent recurrence of hypoglycemia.
3. Subsequent measures–to search for and treat the underlying cause.

Acute measures

Prolonged severe hypoglycemia can cause irreversible cerebral dysfunction and must be treated promptly. However, as indicated above, it is important to obtain a blood sample for glucose measurement before glucose administration and to save serum for the subsequent measurement of insulin and C-peptide unless the cause is obvious, e.g. hypoglycemia in a patient known to have diabetes. If the patient has a history of malnutrition or chronic alcohol abuse, intravenous thiamine at a bolus dose of 1–2 mg/kg should be given before initiation of glucose treatment, to avoid precipitating Wernicke's encephalopathy. For conscious and cooperative patients, approximately 50 g of oral glucose in the form of glucose drinks, granulated sugar, dextrose tablets or orange juice will usually reverse the hypoglycemia. Alternatively, sugar gel or lump can be given through the buccal mucosa. For those who are unconscious or unable to take sugar orally, an intravenous bolus of 50 ml of 50% (i.e. 25 g) dextrose is adequate in most situations. It is highly irritant and should thus be administered through a large-gauge needle into a large vein if possible. Larger volumes of less concentrated dextrose in intravenous infusions (e.g. 250 ml of 10% dextrose) may be used to minimize the irritation. In children with hypoglycemia, 10% rather than 50% dextrose is used instead, to avoid the serious complication of hyperosmolality. If intravenous access is not immediately available, intramuscular glucagon (1 mg) can be life-saving. Glucagon promotes hepatic glycogenolysis and gluconeogenesis and thereby raises blood glucose to the normal range in 5–10 min, but its action is short-lived. It is not effective in alcohol-induced hypoglycemia or adrenal insufficiency, because of glycogen depletion. Glucagon in these situations may actually aggravate the hypoglycemia by stimulating insulin secretion. Glucocorticoid replacement, after plasma is saved for cortisol measurement, is required in patients suspected of having adrenal insufficiency.

Maintenance therapy

The clinical response of hypoglycemia to intravenous dextrose administration should be rapid and dramatic. Patients with hypoglycemic coma are expected to regain consciousness and become coherent within 5–10 min. The response to intramuscular or intravenous glucagon is slightly slower, with an average time difference of 2–3 min when compared to intravenous glucose.[49] However, complete cognitive recovery may be delayed for 30–60 min after restoration of normoglycemia. If there is no obvious improvement in symptoms or consciousness within 10–15 min, alternative diagnoses (e.g. stroke, drug overdose) should be reconsidered.[50]

As the effect of intravenous glucose is relatively transient, patients should receive a further 25–50 g of oral glucose after clinical recovery to build up sufficient hepatic glycogen stores for preventing recurrence of hypoglycemia. If the hypoglycemic episode is expected to be prolonged or recurrent (e.g. in patients on long-acting sulfonylureas or with hepatic failure or disseminated malignancy), an intravenous infusion of 10% dextrose should be commenced and continued if necessary. The rate of infusion is adjusted according to bedside and laboratory blood glucose every 2–4 h, with the aim of maintaining plasma glucose levels between 5 and 10 mmol/l. Urea and electrolytes should also be monitored regularly because of the risk of dilutional hyponatremia, particularly in patients with defective free water clearance, as in glucocorticoid deficiency. A fatal case of hyponatremic encephalopathy from inadvertent dextrose infusions for treatment of hypoglycemia in a patient with isolated adrenocorticotropin deficiency has been reported recently.[51] Continuous dextrose infusions are not indicated in known diabetic patients with transient hypoglycemia (e.g. missing meal, excess exercise). Early initiation of oral feeding and resumption of the original insulin regimen with or without adjustment are crucial. In patients with insulin-dependent diabetes who are unable to take oral fluids, intravenous 5–10% dextrose and a variable rate of continuous insulin infusion should be commenced.

Subsequent measures

After initial stabilization, subsequent management should be directed at searching for the underlying cause of hypoglycemia and preventing further attacks. For patients with diabetes, any precipitating factor for the hypoglycemic attack must be identified. The drug regimen should be reviewed with the patients and adjusted according to meal time, activity level and home blood glucose monitoring. Hypoglycemia awareness may be improved by reducing the frequency of hypoglycemic episodes. ACE inhibitors commonly used in patients with diabetic nephropathy and/or hypertension can increase insulin sensitivity and predispose to hypoglycemia. Hypoglycemic therapy may need to be adjusted accordingly. As indicated above, recurrent hypoglycemia in patients with diabetes on stable regimens may indicate the onset of nephropathy, coexisting autoimmune Addison's

---

Acute measures
  Prevent/minimize neurological damage
  Save blood sample for insulin and C-peptide ± cortisol unless cause is obvious
  Give thiamine 1–2 mg/kg IV in malnutrition/alcoholic
  Conscious patient: 50 g oral glucose in glucose drinks, juice, sugar gel, etc.
  Unconscious patient: 50 ml 50% or 250 ml 10% IV dextrose; lower concentration used in children
  No IV access: glucagon 1 mg IM (ineffective in alcohol-induced cause or adrenal insufficiency)
Maintenance therapy
  Prevent recurrence of hypoglycemia
  If no clinical improvement after 10–15 min, consider other causes of coma
  After recovery, 25–50 g oral glucose for hepatic glycogen repletion
  Prolonged hypoglycemia: 10% IV infusions ± insulin infusion in IDDM
  Monitor capillary blood and plasma glucose, electrolytes 2–4-hourly until stable
Subsequent measures
  Search for underlying cause
  Review history and drug intake
  Assay for blood insulin/C-peptide/cortisol level if indicated
  Definitive treatment of underlying cause

Table 19.20
Management of hypoglycemia.

disease, hypothyroidism or hypopituitarism requiring further intervention. Saved serum should be assayed for insulin and C-peptide if no obvious cause can be found after clinical assessment. An inappropriate insulin concentration with respect to hypoglycemia strongly suggests an insulinoma that will require subsequent localization procedures. Diazoxide (200–1200 mg/day orally) and octreotide (100–600 μg/day subcutaneously) are useful for patients with insulinoma awaiting surgery or for those with inoperable tumor. Growth hormone and corticosteroid therapy have been used with success for patients with pro-IGF-II-secreting tumors which cannot be completely resected.[49]

A summary of the management of hypoglycemia is given in Table 19.20.

Hyponatremia

Introduction

Hyponatremia is probably the most common electrolyte disorder encountered in a hospitalized population, with an estimated prevalence of approximately 2.5% if plasma sodium ([Na]) below 130 mmol/l is defined as the criterion for diagnosis.[52] The figure is certainly higher if [Na] below 135 mmol/l is adopted, as in most laboratories. The majority of patients with hyponatremia are asymptomatic. However, acute severe hyponatremia, presenting with headache, lethargy, confusion, coma and seizure from cerebral edema, is a medical emergency and warrants prompt intervention to save life and prevent brain damage. Women of reproductive age and small children are particularly vulnerable, apparently due to less effective brain adaptation as a result of the effects of estrogens and physical factors respectively.[53] On the other hand, too rapid correction of marked chronic hyponatremia is associated with central pontine myelinolysis (CPM) or osmotic demyelination syndrome (ODS), resulting in significant neurological deficits and even death. These factors underscore the importance of careful evaluation and therapy.

Clinical assessment

The clinical presentation of hyponatremia depends on the absolute sodium level, its rate of decline and the underlying etiology. While moderate-to-severe hyponatremia (<120 mmol/l) can be well tolerated or only manifest as non-specific symptoms with headache, nausea, vomiting, muscle weakness, lethargy and irritability from gradual brain swelling, a sudden fall in sodium concentration to a similar degree within hours may lead to rapid neurological deterioration with agitation, disorientation, drowsiness or even seizure and coma. The severity of the neurological symptoms therefore actually dictates the urgency of subsequent treatment. On the other hand, as the cause of hyponatremia may not be immediately obvious, careful assessment of the extracellular volume status is essential in the selection of appropriate initial therapy as well as further elucidation of the underlying diagnosis, as shown in Figure 19.1. Being the major cation in extracellular fluid (ECF), sodium is the main contributor to the ECF or serum osmolality. Hyponatremia is thus usually associated with hypoosmolality, except in two situations: pseudohyponatremia and hyponatremia with hypertonicity. The former is an uncommon condition in which serum sodium concentration ([Na]), when measured by methods other than an ion-sensitive electrode, is artefactually low as a consequence of the volume contribution of severe hypertriglyceridemia or hyperproteinemia. The patient is asymptomatic and requires no treatment. Hyponatremia with hypertonicity is most commonly seen in uncontrolled diabetes mellitus. The osmotic effect of hyperglycemia results in water shift from the intracellular to extracellular compartment, with resulting 'translocational hyponatremia'.[54] It is important to recognize this condition, not only because of its common occurrence but also because of the requirement for completely different treatment modalities from those needed for hyponatremia with hypo-osmolality. Intravenous infusion of mannitol or maltose may also result in hyponatremia by the same mechanism.

Hyponatremia generally reflects an excess of water relative to sodium rather than the total body sodium or water, which can be increased, normal or decreased. The majority of patients with hyponatremia and hypoosmolality have impaired renal water excretion in the presence of continued water intake, which perpetuates the hyponatremia. Fluid overload as in congestive heart failure, nephrotic syndrome, cirrhosis and hypoalbuminemia and renal failure is clinically obvious, with varying degrees of edema, raised jugular venous pressure, pleural effusion or ascites. Renal water excretion is impaired due to either primary impairment in the glomerular filtration rate, as in renal failure, or decreased effective circulatory volume with secondarily increased proximal water reabsorption and non-osmotic release of ADH, as in other edematous states. The latter

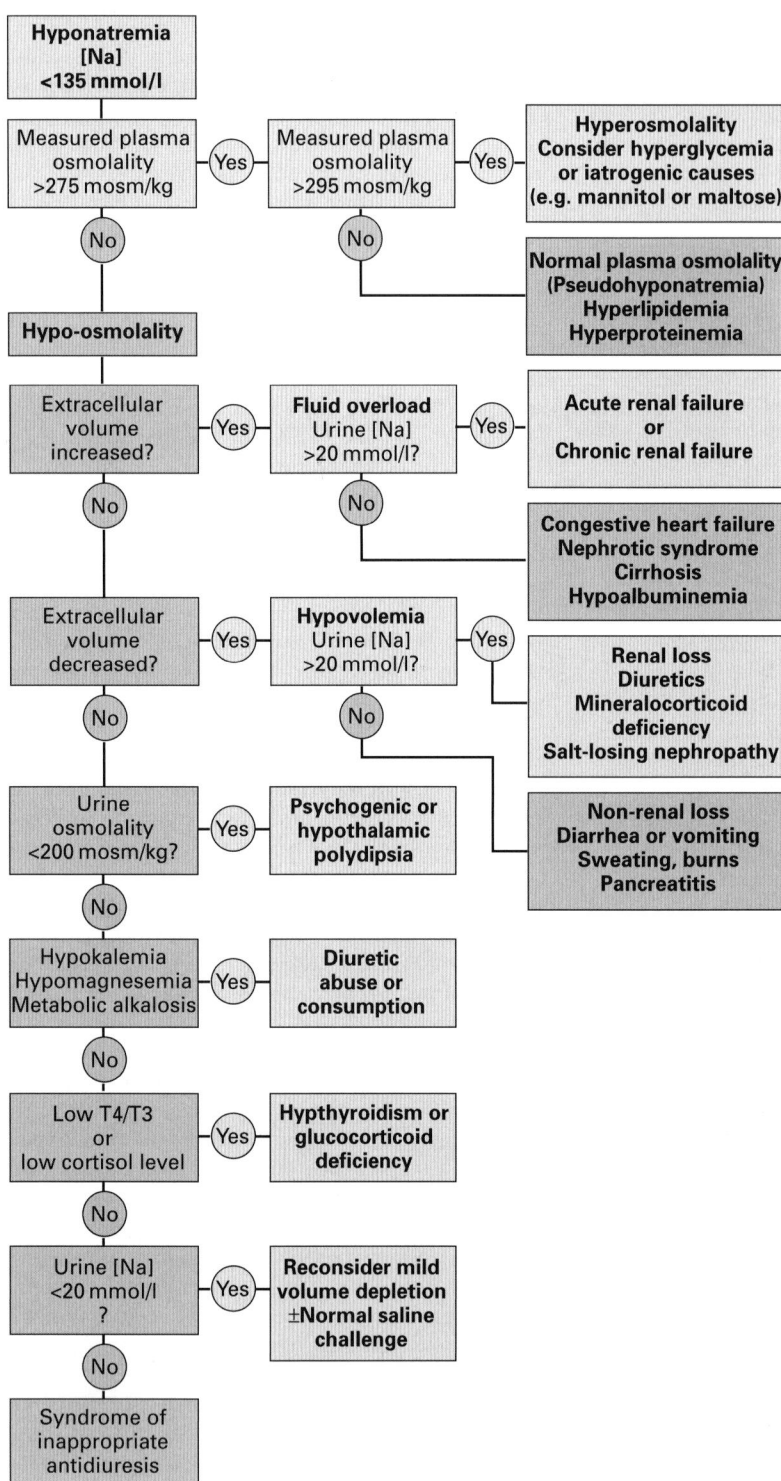

Figure 19.1
Clinical evaluation of hyponatremia.

mechanism also applies in states of volume depletion. The replacement of renal or non-renal solute loss in hypovolemia with water or intravenous hypotonic solutions can precipitate hyponatremia. Clinically, features of dehydration with decreased skin turgor, dry mucosae and postural hypotension can be found.

In the presence of apparent normovolemia, the syndrome of inappropriate antidiuresis (SIAD) contributes a considerable proportion of patients with hyponatremia. However, several important clinical conditions should be ruled out before the diagnosis can be made. Patients with hypothalamic or psychogenic polydipsia ingest enormous amount of water, causing dilutional hyponatremia, which can occasionally be severe enough to cause marked neurological sequelae such as confusion and seizures. A history of psychiatric illness or hypothalamic damage in the presence of a large urine output and low urine osmolality will usually clinch the diagnosis. Thiazide diuretic-related hyponatremia is common and can lead to significant morbidity in the elderly. Impairment of urinary dilution, stimulation of ADH secretion and thirst sensation associated with weight gain are the cardinal features. Associated electrolyte disturbances with a history of diuretic consumption are the clues to this condition. Hypothyroidism and glucocorticoid deficiency are associated with impairment in renal excretion of free water. Both may be resistant to therapy without specific hormonal replacement.

SIAD is frequently associated with a wide range of neoplastic, respiratory and cerebral diseases, as well as various medications. Some of the causes are listed in Table 19.21. Four types of SIAD, according to the relationship between ADH secretion and serum osmolality, have been observed; ADH concentrations are not always elevated, and therefore the term 'SIAD' is used in preference to 'syndrome of inappropriate secretion of ADH'. Postoperative hyponatremia is a clinically important cause of dilutional hyponatremia with increased ADH secretion resulting from stress, pain, nausea and narcotic use during the perioperative period. Postoperative hypotonic fluid replacement tends to aggravate the condition and can be life-threatening, especially in premenopausal women.

Neoplastic
  Bronchogenic carcinoma
  Adenocarcinoma of pancreas and duodenum
  Carcinoma of bladder
  Prostatic carcinoma
  Lymphoma
  Thymoma
Respiratory
  Bacterial or viral pneumonia
  Acute bronchial asthma
  Tuberculosis
  Mechanical ventilation
  Chronic obstructive airway disease
Central nervous system
  Meningitis
  Encephalitis
  Head injury
  Brain tumor
  Brain abscess
  Subarachnoid hemorrhage
  Stroke
  Acute intermittent porphyria
  Guillain–Barré syndrome
Medication
  Cyclophosphamide
  Carbamazepine
  Clofibrate
  Vasopressin
  Desmopressin
  Tricyclic antidepressants
  Narcotics

Table 19.21
Causes of syndrome of inappropriate diuresis.

Investigation

Investigations should be directed at finding the underlying cause of hyponatremia. Measurement of serum osmolality and calculation of the osmolal gap are important in differentiating hyponatremia with hypo-osmolality from pseudohyponatremia and hyponatremia with hypertonicity.

Calculated plasma osmolality (mosm/kg) = $2 \times [Na]$ (mmol/l) + $2 \times [K]$ (mmol/l) + [Glucose] (mmol/l) + [Urea] (mmol/l)

Osmolal gap (mosm/kg) = Measured plasma osmolality (mosm/kg) − calculated plasma osmolality (mosm/kg)

Patients with pseudohyponatremia have normal plasma osmolality and an elevated osmolal gap (>10 mosm/kg). With the widespread use of ion-specific electrodes, this artefact is rarely seen nowadays. In hyponatremia with hypertonicity, the plasma osmolality and the osmolal gap are increased.

When combined with clinical evaluation of volume status, a spot urine sodium concentration (u[Na]) helps in the determination of the underlying etiology (see Figure 19.1). Hypovolemia with u[Na] <20 mmol/l suggests a non-renal cause of sodium loss, while u[Na] >20 mmol/l points to renal loss, such as in diuretic therapy, mineralocorticoid deficiency and salt-losing nephropathy. However, after withdrawal of diuretic therapy, u[Na] can decrease to <20 mmol/l in 1 or 2 days. On the other hand, severe vomiting can result in metabolic alkalosis and some obligate loss of sodium with bicarbonate in the urine; a finding of a low spot urine chloride concentration is helpful.[55] Congestive heart failure, cirrhosis and nephrotic syndrome present with edematous states and u[Na] <20 mmol/l due to abnormal sodium retention. Clinical edema with u[Na] >20 mmol/l is found in acute or chronic renal failure.

Electrolyte disturbances with hypokalemia, hypomagnesemia and metabolic alkalosis are commonly found in cases of diuretic abuse or consumption. High urine output and low urine osmolality (<200 mosm/kg) will suggest psychogenic or hypothalamic polydipsia. Hormonal assays, such as serum cortisol and thyroxine concentration, should be checked, particularly as clinical features may not be obvious. Further dynamic tests may be indicated to confirm the diagnosis of adrenal insufficiency. SIAD is associated with hyponatremia, hypo-osmolality with inappropriately high urine osmolality (>100 mosmol/kg), natriuresis (u[Na] >20 mmol/l) and normal renal, thyroid and adrenal function in the presence of clinical euvolemia. Low serum uric acid and urea concentrations, plasma renin activity and aldosterone are also clues to the diagnosis.

Treatment[54-59]

The urgency and choice of therapy for hyponatremia depend on the degree and rate of development of hyponatremia, as reflected by the presence and severity of the neurological symptoms, and the underlying etiology manifested clinically as change in extracellular volume status. To balance the risk of cerebral edema from untreated hyponatremia and ODS from too rapid correction of low [Na] after brain adaptation, aggressive treatment, such as hypertonic saline, is indicated solely for acute severe symptomatic patients with hyponatremia, to prevent irreversible brain damage, while more conservative therapy (e.g. water restriction) is instituted for asymptomatic patients.

Severe symptomatic hyponatremia

Patients can present with marked neurological symptoms, including disorientation, drowsiness, seizure and even coma. Cautious administration of hypertonic saline serves to relieve cerebral edema and prevent further complications such as tentorial herniation. However, it is important to exclude hyponatremia with hypertonicity, which is aggravated by hypertonic saline. An initial infusion rate of 50–100 ml/h of 3% saline or equivalent is generally safe. Basing the infusion rate on a calculated 'sodium deficit' or 'water excess' is generally unreliable, because the rate of rise in [Na] depends not only on the rate of infusion but also on the urinary sodium excretion. Frequent monitoring (every 1–2 h) of [Na] and u[Na] and clinical status is crucial when aiming at correction of [Na] no faster than 0.5–2 mmol/l/h, depending on the severity of the neurological deficit. The correction rate should not exceed 12 mmol/l in the first 24 h or 25 mmol/l in the first 48 h, to avoid precipitation of ODS. The latter typically manifests several days after a rapid rise in [Na], with dysphasia, spastic quadriparesis, pseudobulbar palsy and swallowing difficulties, and may prove fatal. The risk is increased in cases of alcoholism and hypoxia. Osmotic therapy with hypertonic saline should be stopped once the patient shows clinical improvement or [Na] >12 mmol/l, and conservative therapy with water restriction commenced. Adjunctive loop diuretic therapy (e.g. frusemide) is useful in preventing fluid overload and enhancing free water excretion.

Mild-to-moderate symptomatic hyponatremia

Patients frequently present with non-specific headache, fatigue, nausea, muscle cramps and depression when [Na] has gradually decreased to <120 mmol/l. The treatment aims at preventing further worsening of brain swelling. As the development of hyponatremia usually requires continued water intake, water restriction is the mainstay of therapy unless the patient is hypovolemic. Further management will be directed at the underlying condition and the fluid status. If the hyponatremia persists despite water restriction, as in chronic SIAD, specific pharmacological measures are indicated. Demeclocycline 600–1200 mg orally in divided doses increases free water excretion and [Na] within 3–4 days by inducing nephrogenic diabetes insipidus. It is a

Principles
    Urgency and choice of therapy depend on severity of neurological symptoms and volume status
    Balance the risk of brain swelling from hyponatremia versus osmotic demyelination syndrome

Severe symptomatic hyponatremia
    Rule out hypertonicity
    IV infusion 3% saline at a rate of 50–100 ml/h as initial therapy
    Frequent monitoring of [Na], urinary [Na] and clinical status
    Rate of correction of [Na]
        0.5–2 mmol/l/h, depending on severity
        <12 mmol/l in first 24 h *or*
        <25 mmol/l in first 48 h
    Stop hypertonic saline if clinical improvement or [Na] >125 mmol/l
    Add loop diuretic to prevent fluid overload and enhance free water excretion

Mild-to-moderate symptomatic hyponatremia
    Water restriction except hypovolemia
    Chronic SIAD
        Demeclocycline 600–1200 mg/day orally (side-effect—nephrotoxic in cirrhotic)
        Urea 30 g/day orally (side-effects poor palatability, uremia)
        Lithium: Neurotoxic, cardiotoxic, nephrotoxic, unpredictable efficacy
        IV non-peptide arginine vasopressin antagonist ?role

Asymptomatic hyponatremia
    Hypovolemia
        IV saline 0.9% to restore circulatory volume
        Hydrocortisone 100 mg IV stat, then 100 mg 6-hourly IM in Addison's disease
    Edematous states
        Water and sodium restriction
        Loop diuretic ± inotropes
    Normovolemia
        Thyroid hormone or steroid replacement if necessary
        Water restriction: 500–1000 ml/day, depending on urine output and insensible loss
        Withdraw offending drug, e.g. thiazide
    Borderline volume depletion
        Intravenous isotonic saline challenge; look for fluid overload

Hypertonicity
    Principles
        Restore circulatory volume by rehydration with isotonic saline or 0.45% saline if continuing hypernatremia
        Monitor closely to avoid cerebral edema
        Insulin IV 5–10 u/h initially to control hyperglycemia
        Correction of electrolyte and acid–base disturbances
        Treatment and prevention of complications (e.g. sepsis, thromboembolism)
        Close monitor: clinical status, plasma osmolality, urea, electrolytes, arterial blood gases
        Too rapid correction of hypertonicity: Risk of cerebral edema

Table 19.22
Management of hyponatremia.

relatively safer drug than lithium, which may have cardiotoxic, neurotoxic and nephrotoxic side-effects and also unpredictable efficacy. However, nephrotoxicity has been reported in cirrhotic patients receiving demeclocycline. An oral osmotic diuretic such as urea 30 g/day, can also be used to promote free water clearance, although its use is limited by poor palatability and uremia in high doses.[54] Recently, an intravenous non-peptide arginine vasopressin antagonist has been tried in patients with SIAD, with promising results.[60] Future research is required to define its role.

Asymptomatic hyponatremia

As the risk of ODS from rapid correction of [Na] far outweighs the rate of brain swelling from hyponatremia in this group, the management is directed at the underlying cause and is guided by clinical assessment of fluid status.

In hypovolemia, intravenous infusion of isotonic saline (0.9%) should be instituted to restore the extracellular fluid volume, which will in turn improve cardiac output, renal perfusion and hyponatremia. Patients suspected of having Addison's disease or mineralocorticoid deficiency should receive adequate steroid replacement (100 mg IV stat, then 100 mg IM 6-hourly). Cardiovascular status and plasma urea and electrolytes should be monitored to prevent fluid overload, especially in patients with renal impairment.

In the edematous state, water and sodium restriction are indicated, as the total body sodium is increased. If the response is inadequate, loop diuretics and occasionally inotropes may be useful in promoting water and sodium diuresis.

In clinically normovolemic states, coexisting glucocorticoid or thyroid hormone deficiency should be treated with hormone replacement therapy. Thiazide diuretics should be reduced or discontinued. Further therapy will involve water restriction (500–1000 ml/day, depending on the urine output and insensible loss) and treatment of the underlying neoplastic, respiratory or cerebral disorder, as in SIAD. Demeclocycline is generally not indicated for asymptomatic patients. A trial of isotonic saline may occasionally be indicated if subclinical volume depletion is suspected. Hyponatremia should improve in this situation, but [Na] will remain static in SIAD. Caution should be exercised to prevent fluid overload with saline challenge.

Hypertonicity[61]

As discussed earlier, this is commonly encountered in patients with poorly controlled diabetes, and [Na] can be falsely low due to transcellular water shift. The decrease in [Na] is approximately 1.6 mmol/l for every 5.5 mmol/l increase in plasma glucose. Despite these phenomena, [Na] may, in fact, be high at presentation, due to severe dehydration from vomiting and osmotic diuresis. Clinical features include lethargy, disturbed mental state and coma from cerebral dehydration. Treatment should involve correction of volume depletion, initially by means of intravenous isotonic saline infusion. Initial treatment with isotonic saline is preferred in order to avoid over-rapid correction of hyperosmolality. However, an increase in [Na] during rehydration is common, consequent upon continuing secondary hyperaldosteronism, and a rise in [Na] to >160 mmol/l is an indication for treatment with hypotonic saline (0.45%). A variable-rate continuous insulin infusion is necessary to control hyperglycemia. Treatment and prevention of sepsis and thromboembolism are also important in the management of patients with hypertonicity. Rapid correction of hypertonicity and hyperglycemia can lead to life-threatening cerebral edema and should be avoided by frequent monitoring of neurological and cardiovascular status, plasma osmolality, urea, electrolytes, glucose and arterial blood gases.

A summary of the management of hyponatremia is given in Table 19.22.

References

1. Werbel SS, Ober KP. Endocrine crises: acute adrenal insufficiency. *Endocrinol Metab Clin North Am* 1993; **22**: 303–28.
2. Orth DN, Kovacs WJ. The adrenal cortex: diseases of the adrenal cortex. In: Wilson JD, Foster DW, eds. *Williams Textbook of Endocrinology*, 9th edn. Philadelphia: WB Saunders, 1998; 547–63.
3. Rao RH. Endocrine emergencies: bilateral massive adrenal hemorrhage. *Med Clin North Am* 1995; **79**: 107–30.
4. Donovan DS, Diuhy RG. AIDS and its effect on adrenal gland. *Endocrinologist* 1991; **1**: 227–32.
5. Vallotton MB. Disorders of adrenal cortex. *Baillière's Clin Endocrinol Metab* 1992; **6**: 41–56.
6. Vance ML. Hypopituitarism. *N Engl J Med* 1994; **330**: 1651–62.
7. Abboud CF, Charles F. Anterior pituitary failure. In: Melmed S, ed. *The Pituitary*. Cambridge: Blackwell Science, 1995; 341–412.
8. Thodou E, Asa SL, Kontogeorgos G, Kovacs K, Horvath E, Ezzat S. Lymphocytic hypophysitis: clinicopathological findings. *J Clin Endocrinol Metab* 1995; **80**: 2302–11.

9. Molitch ME. Pituitary disorders. In: Barron WM, Lindheimer MD, eds. *Medical Disorders During Pregnancy*. St Louis: Mosby-Year Book, 1991; 102–47.

10. Arafah BM. Reversible hypopituitarism in patients with large non-functioning pituitary adenomas. *J Clin Endocrinol Metab* 1986; **62**: 1173–9.

11. Rolih CA, Ober KP. Endocrine crises: pituitary apoplexy. *Endocrinol Metab Clin North Am* 1993; **22**: 291–302.

12. Cardoso ER, Peterson EW. Pituitary apoplexy: a review. *Neurosurgery* 1984; **14**: 363–73.

13. Gaillard RC. Endocrine emergencies: pituitary gland emergencies. *Baillière's Clin Endocrinol Metab* 1992; **6**: 57–76.

14. Thorner MO, Vance ML, Laws ER Jr, Horvath E, Kovacs K. The anterior pituitary: pituitary apoplexy. In: Wilson JD, Foster DW, eds. *Williams Textbook of Endocrinology*, 9th edn. Philadelphia: WB Saunders, 1998; 322–3.

15. Veldhius JD, Hammoud JM. Endocrine function after spontaneous infarction of human pituitary: report, review, and reappraisal. *Endocrine Rev* 1980; **1**: 100–7.

16. Glick RP, Tiesi JA, Kyle CA et al. Subacute pituitary apoplexy: clinical and magnetic resonance imaging characteristics. *Neurosurgery* 1990; **27**: 214–18.

17. Arafah BM, Harrington JF, Madhoun ZT, Selman WR. Improvement of pituitary function after surgical decompression for pituitary tumor apoplexy. *J Clin Endocrinol Metab* 1990; **71**: 323–8.

18. Thapar K, Kovacs K, Laws ER et al. Pituitary adenomas: current concepts in classification, histopathology and molecular biology. *Endocrinologist* 1993; **3**: 39–57.

19. Shimon I, Melmed S. Management of pituitary tumors. *Ann Intern Med* 1998; **129**: 472–83.

20. Hennessey JV, Jackson IMD. Clinical features and differential diagnosis of pituitary tumors with emphasis on acromegaly. *Baillière's Clin Endocrinol Metab* 1995; **9**: 271–314.

21. von Werder K. Pituitary enlargement. *Clin Endocrinol (Oxf)* 1996; **44**: 299–303.

22. Molitch ME. Prolactinoma. In: Melmed S, ed. *The Pituitary*. Cambridge: Blackwell Science, 1995: 443–77.

23. Molitch ME, Thorner MO, Wilson C. Therapeutic controversy: management of prolactinomas. *J Clin Endocrinol Metab* 1997; **82**: 996–1000.

24. Molitch ME, Elton RL, Blackwell RE et al. Bromocriptine as primary therapy for prolactin-secreting macroadenomas: results of a prospective multicenter study. *J Clin Endocrinol Metab* 1985; **60**: 698–705.

25. Beck-Peccoz P, Brucker-Davis F, Persani L, Smallridge RC, Weintraub BD. Thyrotrophin-secreting pituitary tumor. *Endocrine Rev* 1996; **17**: 610–38.

26. Burger AG, Philippe J. Endocrine emergencies: thyroid emergencies: thyroid storm. *Baillière's Clin Endocrinol Metab* 1992; **6**: 77–84.

27. Burch HB, Wartofsky L. Endocrine crises: life-threatening thyrotoxicosis: thyroid storm. *Endocrinol Metab Clin North Am* 1993; **22**: 263–78.

28. Tietgens ST, Leinung MC. Endocrine emergencies: thyroid storm. *Med Clin North Am* 1995; **79**: 169–84.

29. Molitch ME. Endocrine emergencies: endocrine emergencies in pregnancy: thyroid. *Baillière's Clin Endocrinol Metab* 1992; **6**: 173–9.

30. Burger AG, Philippe J. Endocrine emergencies: thyroid emergencies: myxedema coma. *Baillière's Clin Endocrinol Metab* 1992; **6**: 84–93.

31. Crowley WF, Ridgway EC, Bough EW et al. Noninvasive evaluation of cardiac function in hypothyroidism: response to gradual thyroxine replacement. *N Engl J Med* 1977; **296**: 1–6.

32. Jordan RM. Endocrine emergencies: myxedema coma: pathophysiology, therapy, and factors affecting prognosis. *Med Clin North Am* 1995; **79**: 185–94.

33. Nicoloff JT, LoPresti JS. Endocrine crises: myxedema coma: a form of decompensated hypothyroidism. *Endocrinol Metab Clin North Am* 1993; **22**: 279–90.

34. Bringhurst FR, Demay MB, Kronenberg HM. Hormones and disorders of mineral metabolism: hypercalcemic disorders. In: Wilson JD, Foster DW, eds. *Williams Textbook of Endocrinology*, 9th edn. Philadelphia: WB Saunders, 1998; 1172–85.

35. Nussbaum SR. Endocrine crises: pathophysiology and management of severe hypercalcemia. *Endocrinol Metab Clin North Am* 1993; **22**: 343–62.

36. Rizzoli P, Bonjour JP. Endocrine emergencies: management of disorders of calcium homeostasis: hypercalcemia. *Baillière's Clin Endocrinol Metab* 1992; **6**: 129–136.

37. Edelson GW, Kleerekoper M. Endocrine emergencies: hypercalcemic crisis. *Med Clin North Am* 1995; **79**: 79–92.

38. Guise TA, Mundy GR. Evaluation of hypocalcemia in children and adults. *J Clin Endocrinol Metab* 1995; **80**: 1473–8.

39. Reber PM, Heath H III. Endocrine emergencies: hypocalcemic emergencies. *Med Clin North Am* 1995; **79**: 93–106.

40. Bringhurst FR, Demay MB, Kronenberg HM. Hormones and disorders of mineral metabolism: hypocalcemic disorders. In: Wilson JD, Foster DW, eds. *Williams Textbook of Endocrinology*, 9th edn. Philadelphia: WB Saunders, 1998: 1185–92.

41. Rizzoli P, Bonjour JP. Endocrine emergencies: management of disorders of calcium homeostasis: hypocalcemia. *Baillière's Clin Endocrinol Metab* 1992; **6**: 136–42.

42. Tohme JF, Bilezikian JP. Endocrine crises: hypocalcemic emergencies. *Endocrinol Metab Clin North Am* 1993; **22**: 363–76.

43. Diabetes Control and Complications Trial Research Group. The effect of intensive treatment of diabetes on the development and progression of long-term complications in insulin-dependent diabetes mellitus. *N Engl J Med* 1993; **329**: 977–86.

44. Service FJ. Endocrine emergencies: hypoglycemia. *Med Clin North Am* 1995; **79**: 1–8.

45. Binder C, Bendtson I. Endocrine emergencies: hypoglycemia. *Baillière's Clin Endocrinol Metab* 1992; **6**: 23–40.
46. Veneman TF, van Haeften TW. Hypoglycemia unawareness in IDDM. *Eur J Clin Invest* 1994; **24**: 785–93.
47. Veneman TF, Erkelens DW. Hypoglycemia unawareness in NIDDM. *J Clin Endocrinol Metab* 1997; **82**: 1682–4.
48. Collier A, Steedman DJ, Patrick AW et al. Comparison of intravenous glucagon and dextrose in treatment of severe hypoglycemia in an accident and emergency department. *Diabetes Care* 1987; **10**: 712–15.
49. Drake WM, Miraki F, Siddiqi A et al. Dose related effects of growth hormone on IGF-I and IGFBP-3 levels in non-islet cell tumour hypoglycemia. *Eur J Endocrinol* 1998; **139**: 532–6.
50. Comi RJ. Endocrine crises: approach to acute hypoglycemia. *Endocrinol Metab Clin North Am* 1993; **22**: 247–62.
51. Liang I, McWilliam L, Owen D, Drayson M, Riley D. Case report: secondary adrenal failure in a young woman presenting as hypoglycemic coma. *Ann Clin Biochem* 1998; **35**: 545–8.
52. Ayus JC, Arieff AL. Brain damage and postoperative hyponatremia: the role of gender. *Neurology* 1996; **46**: 323–8.
53. Anderson RJ, Chung HM, Kluge R et al. Hyponatremia: a prospective analysis of its epidemiology and the pathogenic role of vasopressin. *Ann Intern Med* 1985; **102**: 164–8.
54. Verbalis JG. Hyponatremia. *Baillière's Clin Endocrinol Metab* 1989; **3**: 499–530.
55. Mulloy AL, Caruana RJ. Endocrine emergencies: hyponatremic emergencies. *Med Clin North Am* 1995; **79**: 155–68.
56. Kovacs L, Robertson GL. Disorders of water-balance: hyponatraemia and hypernatraemia. *Baillière's Clin Endocrinol Metab* 1992; **6**: 107–28.
57. Ayus JC, Arieff AI. Endocrine crises: pathogenesis and prevention of hyponatremic encephalopathy. *Endocrinol Metab Clin North Am* 1993; **22**: 425–46.
58. Berl T, Schrier RW. Disorders of water metabolism. In: Schrier RW, ed. *Renal and Electrolyte Disorders*, 5th edn. Philadelphia: Lippincott-Raven, 1997; 1–71.
59. Preston RA. Hyponatremia. In: Preston RA, ed. *Acid–base, Fluids, and Electrolytes Made Ridiculously Simple*. Miami: MedMaster, 1997; 39–64.
60. Saito T, Ishikawa SE, Abe K et al. Acute aquaresis by the nonpeptide arginine vasopressin (AVP) antagonist OPC-31260 improve hyponatraemia in patients with syndrome of inappropriate secretion of antidiuretic hormone (SIADH). *J Clin Endocrinol Metab* 1997; **82**: 1054–7.
61. Lorber D. Nonketotic hypertonicity in diabetes mellitus. *Med Clin North Am* 1995; **79**: 39–52.

Appendix 1

Pituitary function testing
William M Drake, Peter J Trainer

Introduction

Pituitary function testing for hypopituitarism is required in two, quite distinct, clinical situations. The first is in the assessment of a new patient in whom the diagnosis of hypopituitarism has been raised. Patients in this group include: those with target-organ failure (such as hypogonadism or hypoadrenalism) without appropriate elevation of the relevant pituitary trophic hormone; patients with cranial diabetes insipidus; patients with mechanical symptoms consequent upon a pituitary tumor, such as headache and visual failure; and patients in whom a pituitary lesion is documented incidentally during radiological evaluation of an unrelated symptom. The second clinical situation is in the follow-up of patients in whom an evolving endocrinopathy is anticipated. In most such cases, the development of an endocrine deficit will be consequent upon external irradiation as treatment for a pituitary or peri-pituitary tumor, but other examples include sarcoidosis and Langhan's cell histiocytosis, where progressive hypothalamo–pituitary destruction may occur. Hypopituitarism consequent upon a pituitary adenoma and/or its treatment usually develops in a predictable way, with growth hormone (GH) deficiency preceding gonadotropin deficiency, and failure of thyroid-stimulating hormone (TSH) and adrenocorticotropic hormone (ACTH) secretion occurring later. For patients in both groups, pituitary function testing may help identify those patients with hypopituitarism sufficiently severe to threaten their safety, and exclude/provide evidence for hormonal deficiencies as a cause of symptoms such as lethargy and fatigue. A sound knowledge of the physiological basis behind pituitary function tests and their limitations is vital if correct decisions are to be made about patient management. This chapter will discuss various tests of pituitary function and their interpretation, with the aim of producing a rational, reliable and safe strategy for diagnosing hypopituitarism. The clinical features and biochemical diagnosis of the various pituitary syndromes of hypersecretion are discussed elsewhere.

Principles of pituitary assessment

The diagnostic evaluation of pituitary function has several complementary limbs, involving laboratory and radiological investigations. In new patients with suspected hypopituitarism, clinical suspicion arises because of symptoms related to target-organ failure. Hence, it is first necessary to demonstrate target-organ hormonal insufficiency, such as low levels of thyroid hormone or gonadal steroid. Paired testing of both hormones in the pituitary–target-organ feedback loop, sometimes in combination with provocative testing, will prove that target-organ failure is consequent upon lack of stimulation by the relevant pituitary trophic hormone. Additional tests may occasionally be performed in order to determine whether the pituitary itself is at fault, or whether pituitary failure is secondary to understimulation by the hypothalamus: a distinction that has no bearing on the need for hormone replacement therapy. Sophisticated radiological imaging is required to look for possible causes of hypothalamo–pituitary destruction and, together with careful neuro-ophthalmological assessment, helps determine the mechanical effects of any hypothalamo–pituitary mass lesion. Finally, where the cause of pituitary failure is believed to be a systemic illness (such as sarcoidosis), more specific investigations may be needed.

Types of laboratory test

Basal pituitary function tests

Basal blood tests are those taken with the patient resting, unstressed and with no physiological or pharmacological manipulation of the pituitary cell–target cell feedback loop. Such investigations are performed between 7 and 9 a.m., when serum cortisol and testosterone levels are highest, thereby maximizing the chances of basal investigations yielding sufficient information to avoid the need for more complex tests. Paired measurements of both limbs of a pituitary hormone–target hormone loop are required for interpretation of the target hormone level: low levels of target hormone in association with low or normal levels of the relevant pituitary trophic hormone indicate understimulation by the pituitary as the cause of target gland failure.

Stimulation tests

If basal investigations do not yield sufficient diagnostic information about suspected pituitary cell hypofunction, then provocative tests are employed; these are complementary to basal investigations rather than being superior to them. Stimulation tests assess the ability of a given cell type to respond acutely to a stimulus, but do not necessarily provide information about the adequacy of day-to-day hormone production under basal conditions. Two types of provocative tests are used: those that stimulate hormone release indirectly (such as the insulin tolerance and glucagon tests), and direct stimulation tests, in which pharmacological doses of synthetically manufactured peptide are injected and the target cell hormone response measured. Examples include hypothalamic releasing hormone tests and the short synacthen test (see below) The virtue of indirect provocation tests is that the integrity of an entire hypothalamo–pituitary–target cell loop is tested. Hypothalamic releasing hormone tests, with thyrotropin-releasing hormone (TRH), gonadotropin-releasing hormone (GnRH) and growth hormone-releasing hormone (GHRH), discussed below, have no value in the diagnosis of hypopituitarism and cannot predict future pituitary failure. Occasionally, they may help differentiate hypothalamic from pituitary disease, as a normal response to the injection of hypothalamic releasing hormone implies a hypothalamic defect. The major use of releasing hormone tests has been as a tool to increase our understanding of the neuroregulation of pituitary hormone secretion.

Hypothalamo–pituitary–adrenal axis testing

This is probably the most controversial component of pituitary function testing, mainly because assessment of the adequacy of the hypothalamo–pituitary–adrenal (HPA) axis has the most far-reaching consequences for patient health. Biochemical assessment of the HPA axis is performed in two distinct clinical settings, with the aim of establishing adequate cortisol production being common to both. In some patients, symptoms such as tiredness, listlessness and malaise lead to an assessment of ACTH reserve in order to assess whether cortisol deficiency is the cause of those symptoms. The common clinical scenario is that of a patient known to be at risk of developing secondary adrenal insufficiency, due to previous treatment with supraphysiological doses of corticosteroids, or following surgery and/or radiotherapy directed at the pituitary. In asymptomatic 'at-risk' patients it is necessary to assess the patient's ability to mount a response to physiological stress and hence judge the need for emergency steroid cover. Dynamic tests provide an indication of a given patient's ability to respond to physiological stress, but do not assess the appropriateness of basal, unstressed serum cortisol levels and their relationship to symptoms such as lethargy and malaise. An inadequate 'stress response' necessitates steroid cover for surgery, sepsis and accidental trauma, but does not automatically indicate a need for lifelong glucocorticoid replacement. The limitations of the assessment of the basal cortisol production rate must be borne in mind and consideration given to patients' symptoms and wellbeing when instigating lifelong glucocorticoid replacement.

Cortisol production in health

Measurement of the target hormone (cortisol) is common to all tests of the HPA axis. Synthesis and secretion of cortisol is controlled by pituitary-derived ACTH, which, in turn, is regulated by hypothalamic corticotropin-releasing hormone (CRH) and vasopressin. A change in cortisol production rate is the 'final common pathway' for the effect of various neural and humoral inputs that modulate the system at both hypothalamic and pituitary levels: hence the use of serum cortisol levels for the assessment of ACTH reserve. It has the added practical advantage of ease of collection, as ACTH samples require cold centrifugation and flash-freezing, whereas cortisol is measured in serum.

Measurement of cortisol

Cortisol is generally measured by radioimmunoassay (RIA). Administered hydrocortisone, prednisolone and methylprednisolone all interfere with measurements of endogenous cortisol, such that samples for cortisol assay should not be taken within 24 h of exogenous steroid administration. Only 5–10% of cortisol is free, with the remainder bound to cortisol-binding globulin (CBG). Plasma CBG levels therefore significantly alter measurements of serum cortisol. As with sex hormone-binding globulin (SHBG), the rate of hepatic CBG synthesis is increased by oral estrogen preparations that undergo 'first-pass' metabolism by the liver, and in pregnancy. However, CBG is not routinely measured along with cortisol, unlike SHBG with testosterone in the assessment of the pituitary–gonadal axis. Accurate assessment of the HPA axis in pregnancy is extremely difficult, and oral estrogens should be discontinued 6 weeks prior to assessment of the HPA axis.[1] Other circumstances in which CBG levels may complicate assessment of the HPA axis include nephrotic syndrome and hepatic cirrhosis. GH decreases circulating CBG, such that levels are low in acromegaly and fall with initiation of GH therapy in GH-deficient adults.

It is important to note that there is considerable variability in serum cortisol measurements, according to the assay methodology employed.[2] This makes comparisons of cortisol responses between different laboratories extremely difficult, and emphasizes the need for each center to establish its own local reference range, rather than select rigid 'cutoff' values on the basis of population studies, which may have used different methodologies.

Biochemical assessment of the HPA axis relies on several aspects of its physiology. First, cortisol is part of a short (pituitary) and a long (hypothalamic) feedback loop, such that falling cortisol levels stimulate a rise in ACTH and CRH secretion from the pituitary and hypothalamus respectively and vice versa. Second, in the absence of a trophic signal, the adrenal gland undergoes reversible atrophy, with secondary failure of cortisol production. Last, the normal, diurnal pattern of ACTH and cortisol secretion is dramatically modified by pathophysiological stimuli such as trauma and sepsis.

The clinical spectrum of ACTH deficiency varies between hypotension with oliguria and electrolyte abnormalities, and a more subtle dysfunction precipitated only by acute physiological stress such as major surgery or sepsis. A study of the cortisol response to major abdominal surgery in normal and corticosteroid-treated individuals showed that the peak serum cortisol was at least 580 nmol/l (21.6 μg/dL).[3] This study used a fluorimetric method[4] to measure serum cortisol, a technique that, unlike modern RIAs, also detects cortisone. In the same study,[3] serum cortisol responses to hypoglycemia were shown to correlate well with the peak perisurgical serum cortisol measurement. Controlled iatrogenic hypoglycemia is widely accepted as the 'gold standard' by which to judge an individual's ability to mount an adequate cortisol response to physiological stress. The adoption of RIA means that the 'cutoff' serum cortisol level adequate for physiological stress should be lowered from 580 to 500 nmol/l (21 to 18 μg/dL), as modern RIAs measure approximately 15% lower than fluorimetry.[5] This is supported by studies in normal volunteers,[6] although no comparison with cortisol levels during stress has been undertaken.

Having established a minimum serum cortisol level that is adequate for acute physiological stress, which stimulation test best predicts that a patient will be able to achieve such a cortisol response when required? Several tests exist, including measurements of basal serum cortisol, the insulin tolerance test (ITT), glucagon stimulation test, short synacthen test (standard and low dose) and the metyrapone test.

Measurements of basal serum cortisol

Is it possible to infer from measurements of basal serum cortisol whether the HPA axis is capable of responding normally to stress in a given individual? Conversely, below which level does a basal cortisol measurement make dynamic testing unnecessary to confirm ACTH deficiency? Endogenous HPA activity is maximal in the early morning, and samples should be drawn between 7 and 9 a.m. In cases of suspected pituitary insufficiency, a basal morning serum cortisol of <100 nmol/l (<3.6 μg/dL) strongly indicates ACTH deficiency, dynamic testing is not necessary, and glucocorticoid replacement should commence immediately and, in most patients, will be permanent. However, in cases of ACTH deficiency prior to surgery for a pituitary tumor, recovery of ACTH reserve following surgical decompression may occur and the axis should be reassessed postoperatively.

What value of basal serum cortisol indicates an individual's ability to achieve a satisfactory cortisol level during physiological stress? Several studies have documented a close correlation between measurements of basal, unstressed serum cortisol and peak serum cortisol levels during insulin-induced hypoglycemia.[6-8] If it is accepted that a satisfactory peak level is 500 nmol/l (18 μg/dL), then the published evidence suggests that a basal level of 400 nmol/l (14.5 μg/dL) or above is sufficient to avoid the need for an ITT.

In summary, measurements of basal serum cortisol may identify patients for whom a dynamic test of ACTH reserve is unnecessary. Published evidence suggests that dynamic testing of ACTH reserve is required if the basal serum cortisol, measured by modern RIA, lies between 100 (3.6) and 400 nmol/l (14.5 μg/dL) and that values outside this range indicate adrenal insufficiency and a normally functioning HPA axis respectively.

Emergency assessment of the HPA axis

In acutely sick patients with suspected hypoadrenalism, a morning cortisol and/or a dynamic test of ACTH reserve are impractical, and glucocorticoid support must commence immediately. Circadian variation of ACTH release will be absent, and activity of the HPA axis should be maximal. If adrenal insufficiency is suspected, then random serum cortisol and plasma ACTH measurements will suffice for HPA axis assessment. If, subsequently, the random cortisol level is shown to have been appropriate to the clinical situation (>500 nmol/l) (>18 μg/dL), glucocorticoids may be withdrawn. If not, steroid support should continue and dynamic testing must follow resolution of the acute clinical situation. A plasma ACTH will differentiate primary from secondary adrenal insufficiency: a serum cortisol <200 nmol/l (<7.2 μg/dL) with a plasma ACTH >200 μg/l is diagnostic of primary adrenal failure. An elevated plasma renin activity with an inappropriately low serum aldosterone level provides additional evidence of primary adrenal disease.

The insulin tolerance test (ITT) (Table A1.1)

This test[9] seeks to simulate physiological 'stress' in a controlled, supervised environment by inducing hypoglycemia with intravenous short-acting insulin. Hypoglycemia is a powerful stress stimulus that, in the intact pituitary and hypothalamus, induces ACTH and GH release and a rise in serum cortisol levels. It therefore assesses the integrity of the entire HPA axis and has traditionally been regarded as the 'gold standard' for this purpose. Its reproducibility among healthy volunteers is good,[10] but not known among patients with pituitary disease. The assumption that an ability to respond to insulin-induced hypoglycemia will translate into an appropriate cortisol rise during acute illness or major surgery is supported by the observation that the peak cortisol levels of patients undergoing major surgery are comparable to those achieved during an ITT.[2]

Although some physicians are uncomfortable with the use of the ITT, particularly in children, the morbidity of this investigation in experienced hands in a designated metabolic investigation unit is reassuringly low, provided that the exclusion criteria detailed in Table A1.1 are adhered to.[8] The initial dose of insulin used varies in different centers between 0.1 and 0.15 IU/kg, increasing to 0.3 IU/kg for patients with acromegaly, Cushing's syndrome, or other conditions associated with insulin resistance. It is contraindicated in patients with ischemic heart disease or epilepsy and requires careful supervision.

The immediate counterregulatory response to hypoglycemia is characterized by catecholamine release, with consequent hepatic glycogenolysis and correction of hypoglycemia. Glucocorticoids are not part of this phenomenon, although the laying down of hepatic glycogen stores does require glucocorticoid. Hence, in patients with long-standing ACTH deficiency and inadequate glycogen stores, recovery from hypoglycemia may be delayed. It is usual practice to administer oral glucose in the form of a sugary drink, together with a meal, at the conclusion of the test.

A common reason to perform an ITT is to test the ability of the HPA axis to respond to stress following the use of supraphysiological doses of corticosteroids. Such doses may lead to ACTH suppression, with secondary adrenal involution and loss of responsiveness. In this situation, a short synacthen test is mandatory in order to establish that the adrenals are capable of

Indications	Assessment of ACTH and GH reserve
Contraindications	Ischemic heart disease Epilepsy/unexplained syncopal episodes Severe hypoadrenalism (basal serum cortisol <100 nmol/l) Glycogen storage disease Untreated hypothyroidism
Protocol	Must be performed by experienced metabolic nurse and/or physician Resting ECG to be certified normal by attendant physician Ensure that emergency intravenous dextrose and dexamethasone are available Patient must be fasting from 2400 h Insert intravenous cannula approximately 30 min prior to commencement of test Draw sample for basal cortisol Administer 0.15 IU/kg of soluble insulin (e.g. actrapid) as a bolus. Document clinical signs of neuroglycopenia. If not present after 45 min, consider repeating same dose of insulin In cases of severe, prolonged hypoglycemia, syncope or presyncope, termination of the test with intravenous dextrose should be seriously considered. Continue sampling Draw samples for plasma glucose (fluoride bottle), cortisol and GH (both serum) at 30, 45, 60, 90 and 120 min Glucose drink and meal at conclusion of test. NB. Patients with active Cushing's syndrome, acromegaly and other causes of insulin resistance may be insulin resistant and require 0.3 IU/kg (<39.6 mg/dL) of soluble insulin
Interpretation	Plasma glucose <2.2 mmol/l with symptoms and signs of neuroglycopenia necessary for assessment of the adequacy of the stimulus to ACTH/GH release Serum cortisol should rise to >500 nmol/l (>18 μg/dL) Peak GH 9 mU/l (<4.5 μg/L) or less indicates severe GHD

Table A1.1
Protocol for the insulin tolerance (stress) test.

responding to ACTH, prior to an ITT. If the adrenals do not respond to ACTH, an ITT will yield no useful information.

Short synacthen test (SST) (Table A1.2)

This investigation was originally introduced as a test for primary adrenal failure,[11] and involves the injection of a pharmacological dose (250 μg) of synthetic ACTH, with measurement of the serum cortisol response. The basis of its use in the context of hypopituitarism, as an alternative to the ITT, is that chronic underexposure of the adrenal glands to ACTH will result in a blunted cortisol response to exogenously administered ACTH. The test does not distinguish primary from secondary adrenal insufficiency: clinical assessment (pigmentation) and measurement of basal plasma ACTH are usually sufficient for this. The major argument in favor of the SST is its simplicity, as it requires no specialist staff and takes only an hour to complete. The SST does not assess GH reserve. It is universally accepted that the SST cannot be used for the assessment of ACTH reserve in acute hypopituitarism, such as following pituitary infarction (apoplexy) or immediately postoperatively. It takes at least 2 weeks for the adrenal zona fasciculata to involute following withdrawal of ACTH stimulation, during which time the adrenal cortex will remain

Table A1.2
Protocol for short synacthen test.

Indications	Assessment of primary and secondary adrenal failure
Contraindications	History of atopy
Protocol	Non-fasting Insert intravenous cannula approximately 30 min prior to commencement of test Draw sample for basal cortisol Administer 250 mg synacthen intramuscularly Draw samples for cortisol at 30 and 60 min
Interpretation	30-min cortisol should rise to at least 550 nmol/l (19.9 µg/dL) (most useful during longitudinal follow-up of a patient known to be at risk of developing secondary adrenal failure, e.g. following pituitary irradiation

Details of protocols for the other investigations discussed in this Appendix (such as the clomiphene test) are not given here, but can be found elsewhere.[28]

responsive to supraphysiological doses of ACTH. In addition, it should be remembered, in the assessment of new patients with suspected hypothalamic–pituitary disease, that the duration of ACTH deficiency may be unknown and that, as following pituitary surgery or apoplexy, a falsely reassuring SST may result.

The increment in serum cortisol following synacthen has been advocated as a measure of the ability of the HPA axis to respond to stress, but is a poor index of adrenal responsiveness, as there is considerable overlap between normal volunteers and patients with secondary adrenal insufficiency.[12] Further, the cortisol increment is inversely correlated with the basal value, and hence a smaller increment is seen in the early morning, when plasma ACTH and serum cortisol levels are at their highest.[13] The peak serum cortisol response following synacthen shows no diurnal variation and is now the accepted index of adrenal responsiveness.

Serum cortisol levels 30 min after injection of synacthen and the peak cortisol achieved during an ITT are clearly correlated, and it is argued by some that the ITT can be restricted to patients who fail to reach a given threshold 30-min post-synacthen cortisol level (usually between 550 and 600 nmol/l) (19.9 and 21.7 µg/dL), or who require simultaneous assessment of GH reserve. The SST is increasingly being used in preference to the ITT, such that in 1995 50% of UK endocrinologists declared it their investigation of choice in the investigation of the HPA axis, compared to 24% in 1988.[15,16]

Despite its increasing use as a test of ACTH reserve, there is no study showing that a normal SST indicates that the HPA axis is capable of responding normally to major illness or stress. Critics of the use of the SST point to reports of patients with pituitary disease with symptoms and signs of adrenal failure, corrected by glucocorticoid replacement, having recently had a reassuringly 'normal' SST. This problem cannot be corrected by application of a more 'stringent' threshold of serum cortisol, as in two such reported patients the peak serum cortisol value was >950 nmol/l (34.4 µg/dL) 30 min after synacthen. However, it should be stressed that reports exist of patients who have developed acute adrenal crisis following a 'normal' ITT.[17]

Low-dose short synacthen test (LDSST)

In recent years, much interest has arisen in the use of a very low dose of ACTH (typically 1 µg) for the assessment of secondary hypoadrenalism, as the conventional dose of 250 µg produces plasma concentrations that are supraphysiological and beyond the top of the ACTH/cortisol dose–response curve. Proponents of the LDSST argue that chronically understimulated adrenal glands may mount a satisfactory cortisol response to unphysiological concentrations of ACTH, but that only normal glands will respond to 1 µg. Plasma

ACTH levels following injection of 1 μg are comparable to those reached during an ITT in healthy volunteers.[18] The test is quick (a single sample only is drawn 30 min after injection of ACTH) and may be performed at any time of day.

A study of the cortisol responses to the standard and low-dose ACTH tests and to the ITT in patients with suspected or proven pituitary disease[19] showed that, when a serum cortisol of 500 nmol/l (18.1 μg/dL) was used as a 'pass' on the ITT, the LDSST had a sensitivity of 100% and specificity of 80%, with an adequate response defined as a serum cortisol >600 nmol/l (21.7 μg/dL). In other words, there was no patient in whom a serum cortisol level of >600 nmol/l (21.7 μg/dL) provided false reassurance about their ability to 'pass' the ITT. A serum cortisol level <600 nmol/l following 1 μg ACTH indicated the need for an ITT, and the authors advocate the LDSST as a screening procedure for the investigation of secondary ACTH deficiency, reserving the ITT for patients with a borderline response. In a comparison of normal volunteers and patients with pituitary disease, false reassurance was provided in 70% of patients with known secondary adrenal failure using a 30-min serum cortisol value following injection of 5 or 250 μg ACTH, whereas the 1 μg LDSST identified all patients with proven ACTH deficiency.[20] This may partly be accounted for by the use of different protocols for ACTH dilution. No commercial 1-μg preparation of ACTH is available, and concern about the extent to which ACTH may be adsorbed onto the plastic of syringes or saline bags dictates that improved standardization and reproducibility of the LDSST are required prior to its widespread recommendation for the assessment of ACTH deficiency.[21]

Glucagon stimulation test (Table A1.3)

The subcutaneous injection of glucagon, by unknown mechanisms, induces ACTH and GH release, and this has led to its widespread use as a means of assessing the reserve of these two hormones. Glucagon is a less potent stimulus for ACTH release than hypoglycemia, and false-negative results are well recognized. Its injection makes patients feel unwell with nausea and, occasionally, abdominal pain and vomiting. The glucagon test has not been as extensively studied as other investigations, and its interpretation relies upon criteria established for the ITT. However, it remains a useful method of assessing the HPA and GH axes, particularly when the ITT is contraindicated.[22]

Table A1.3
Protocol for glucagon stimulation test.

Indications	Assessment of ACTH and GH deficiency in cases where ITT contraindicated
Contraindications	Glycogen storage disease Severe hypoadrenalism (basal cortisol <100 nmol/l; <3.6 μg/dL) Untreated hypothyroidism
Protocol	Patient must be fasting from 2400 h Insert intravenous cannula approximately 30 min prior to commencement of test Draw sample for basal cortisol Administer 1 mg glucagon SC (1.5 mg if >90 kg) Draw samples for plasma glucose (fluoride bottle), cortisol and GH (both serum) at 90, 120, 150, 180, 210 and 240 min
Interpretation	Plasma glucose should peak at 90 min Serum cortisol should rise to >500 nmol/(718.1 μg/dL)

Metyrapone test

Metyrapone inhibits 11β-hydroxylase, the final enzyme involved in cortisol synthesis. The fall in cortisol levels that follows administration of metyrapone stimulates ACTH release from the intact pituitary. Corticosteroidogenesis increases and serum levels of cortisol precursors such as 11-desoxycortisol rise. This has no effect on ACTH secretion, as 11-desoxycortisol has no glucocorticoid action. In patients with secondary adrenal insufficiency, a fall in cortisol does not stimulate an increase in ACTH secretion, and hence no rise in 11-desoxycortisol level occurs. A typical protocol entails oral administration of 30 mg/kg metyrapone in hospital at midnight. Simultaneous cortisol and 11-desoxycortisol levels are taken between 8 and 9 a.m., and oral glucocorticoids are subsequently administered if the index of suspicion of ACTH deficiency is high. An 11-desoxycortisol level >200 nmol/l (7 µg/dl) indicates normal adrenal function, irrespective of the simultaneous cortisol value, while levels <200 nmol/l, in the presence of a low serum cortisol level, strongly suggest secondary adrenal insufficiency.[23] A low serum cortisol level is required for the interpretation of the test as an indicator of the level of pituitary stimulation. Anticonvulsant therapy such as phenytoin accelerates the metabolism of metyrapone, and an alternative test of the HPA axis should be used in such patients.

A major criticism of this investigation is that it is a test of the ACTH–cortisol feedback mechanism rather than of ACTH reserve. In addition, assays for cortisol precursors are not widely available, and the test is now seldom used in the UK, although it is the investigation of choice for many US physicians in the assessment of ACTH reserve.

Conclusion

It is inevitable that the debate about the optimum method for the assessment of the HPA axis will continue. Practical issues such as cost and staff availability will, to a large extent, affect local policy, but the fundamental clinical issue of patient safety remains the same. Dynamic tests of the integrity of the HPA axis support, rather than substitute for, clinical decisions, and it is important to recognize that the use of sophisticated statistical methods for the comparison of serum cortisol levels in groups of people with or without endocrine disease can never substitute for clinical awareness in the individual patient. Even the ITT cannot provide complete reassurance that an individual will not develop secondary adrenal insufficiency during physiological stress. Changes in methodology and regional variation in the assays used for cortisol measurements hinder comparisons between published experiences of HPA testing and make it difficult to recommend the use of a single protocol. Endocrine physicians should educate their patients about the implications of pituitary disease in terms of the stress response, particularly when an evolving endocrine deficit is anticipated, such as following pituitary irradiation. The ITT is the single most reliable test of the HPA axis but should only be performed under close supervision in specialist centers. If there is any doubt about the adequacy of ACTH reserve, it is sensible to err on the side of caution with respect to the provision of emergency steroid cover, and to consider a trial of oral glucocorticoid replacement therapy in patients with symptoms suggestive of chronic adrenal insufficiency and an equivocal response to dynamic testing.

Pituitary–thyroid axis

Like other pituitary cell types, thyrotrophs interact with their target cells by feedback inhibition, although the marked diurnal and ultradian variations that characterize ACTH and GH release are not present. This means that investigations other than basal blood samples (usually total thyroxine (T4) and TSH; free T4 if female patients are pregnant or taking estrogen) are rarely necessary for the biochemical assessment of thyroid status in the context of pituitary disease. Secondary hypothyroidism is strongly suggested by low levels of circulating T4 (total or free) in the presence of a low or low–normal TSH (TSH is rarely undetectable in hypopituitarism). Illness ('sick euthyroid' syndrome), thyroxine-binding globulin deficiency, supraphysiological doses of glucocorticoids and drugs such as phenytoin may also produce a similar picture. The interpretation of the results is dependent on the overall clinical context and is assisted by measurement of free T4 and tissue markers of thyroid hormone action such as SHBG.

TRH testing

TRH testing is of no value in diagnosing secondary hypothyroidism or predicting imminent TSH deficiency. In normal individuals, intravenous injection of TRH produces a rise in TSH, with levels at 20 min being greater than those at 60 min. Patients with hypothalamic disease classically show a delayed response to TRH, with the 60-min value greater than that at 20 min. Patients with pituitary disease typically have an absent TSH response to TRH, although it is recognized that some patients will respond. This is thought to be due to the fact that some pituitary tumors cause functional disconnection of the hypothalamus from the pituitary, thereby simulating a hypothalamic lesion. Renal failure, depression, malnutrition and extreme illness may all be associated with delayed or absent TRH responses. The uniform adoption of sensitive TSH assays and the risk of syncope or precipitating pituitary apoplexy in patients with pituitary tumors means that the TRH test is now very seldom used in the assessment of pituitary function.

Growth hormone axis

Prior to the recognition of the syndrome of adult GHD, the debate about the optimum method of testing for GH deficiency (GHD) in adults was largely academic, but in the last decade there has been intense interest in establishing diagnostic criteria for adult-onset (AO) GHD.

Normal GH secretion is pulsatile, with, in adults, four to six pulses per 24 h punctuating long periods when GH levels in blood are extremely low. Hence, basal blood samples are unlikely to yield significant diagnostic information, unless they coincide with a GH surge. Measurements of 24-h spontaneous GH profiles have been employed in children, but have proved disappointing in adult practice, as considerable overlap exists between the integrated GH concentration (IGHC) of normal subjects and those of hypopituitary patients.[24] Sleep and exercise are both associated with GH release, but assessing GH secretion by these methods is prohibitively time-consuming for routine clinical use.

Most, if not all, actions of GH are mediated through insulin-like growth factor-I (IGF-I). However, measurement of serum IGF-I is of limited value in the diagnosis of adult-onset GHD, as 30% of patients with proven severe GHD have a serum IGF-I in the lower part of the age-related normal range,[25] but a serum IGF-I below the age-related reference range in the presence of pituitary disease is strongly indicative of GH deficiency. Proof of GHD by two dynamic tests is the current requirement for the prescription of recombinant human GH (rhGH) in many countries.

Pharmacological stimulation of GH release is the most practical and reproducible method of assessing GH reserve, and the ITT has been the most frequently employed test in this regard. ACTH reserve can be assessed simultaneously, and the investigation is safe in experienced hands. Severe GHD is defined as a peak GH response of 9 mU/l (4.5 µg/L) or less,[26] although variability in GH assays between centers must be borne in mind when applying consensus guidelines.

Where the ITT is contraindicated, alternative provocative tests of GH reserve include the glucagon (Figure A1.3), arginine, GH releasing hormone (GHRH) and GH-releasing peptide (GHRP) tests. Arginine stimulates GH release, with a peak occurring between 30 and 120 min, after infusion and is frequently used when a second dynamic test of GH reserve is required and the ITT is contraindicated. It involves the intravenous infusion of 0.5 g/kg (maximum dose 30 g) in 100 ml normal saline over 30 min and sampling for 2 h thereafter. Clonidine testing is of no value for the diagnosis of GHD in adults.

Growth hormone secretagogue testing

Adult-onset GHD is frequently secondary to lack of hypothalamic GHRH consequent upon treatment for a pituitary or peri-pituitary tumor. Injection of GHRH tests the 'readily releasable' pool of pituitary hormone and, indeed, many patients with GHD due to pituitary tumors, hypothalamic disease or radiotherapy have been shown to respond to GHRH administration. With development of new GH releasing peptides (GHRPs), GHRH testing may assume a more significant role in the assessment of the hypopituitary patient. GHRP and combined GHRH/GHRP tests are attracting much interest as convenient and easy-to-perform investigations of GH status. Recent evidence suggests that simultaneous injection of GHRH and hexarelin, a GHRP, is as reliable as the ITT for the diagnosis of GHD in adults.[27]

Assessment of the pituitary–gonadal axis

Regular menstruation in a woman implies normal gonadotrope function, and measurements of gonadotropins and estradiol add little to the clinical assessment. Ovulation is not necessarily implied by regular menstruation: measurement of luteal phase progesterone levels is required for the assessment of subfertility in a patient with pituitary disease and a regular cycle. Unlike with hydrocortisone and thyroxine substitution, social and age-related factors may influence the need to correct any underlying gonadal deficiency in men and women. The benefits of gonadal steroid replacement in terms of avoiding cardiovascular complications and loss of bone mineral density must be set against the temporal relationship of normal physiology. For example, an 80-year-old patient with secondary hypogonadism is likely to feel differently about gonadal steroid replacement therapy than a patient of 30.

Basal measurements of gonadotropin hormones and sex steroid levels are usually sufficient for assessment of the pituitary–gonadal axis. Estradiol and testosterone bind to SHBG: simultaneous measurements of SHBG and gonadal steroid levels are therefore required to assess the 'free' (biologically active) levels of these hormones. Testosterone is measured at 9 a.m., as levels show considerable diurnal variation. Estradiol is best measured in the follicular phase of the menstrual cycle, if patients are menstruating. Ovulation is assessed by measurement of progesterone in the luteal phase (days 18–25) of the cycle.

Dynamic tests may help in the differential diagnosis of secondary gonadal failure but do not significantly alter clinical management. Previously, a combination of clomiphene and luteinizing hormone releasing hormone (LHRH) tests was believed to provide useful evidence in distinguishing hypothalamic from pituitary causes of secondary gonadal failure. Such information has little clinical value, since modern radiological imaging is usually able to distinguish these two groups of causes. Central hypogonadism may be isolated, may occur in the context of a hypothalamo–pituitary tumor or its treatment, or may be the earliest sign of incipient panhypopituitarism. Isolated gonadotropin deficiency is either congenital (e.g. Kallman's syndrome), where it is associated with delayed/absent pubertal development, or acquired and secondary to systemic illness (e.g. AIDS), excessive exercise (e.g. long-distance runners) or psychological disturbance (e.g. anorexia nervosa). In all cases, detailed pituitary function testing is mandatory.

Clomiphene testing

This investigation is essentially a test of gonadotropin-releasing hormone (GnRH) secretory reserve and has been used in the differentiation of gonadotropin deficiency from idiopathic delayed puberty. Clomiphene citrate is a weak estrogen antagonist and competes for hypothalamic and pituitary estrogen receptors, resulting in a rise in hypothalamic GnRH levels over 2–4 days, with consequent release of LH and FSH. Clomiphene acts as a peripheral estrogen agonist, inducing hepatic SHBG synthesis and a rise in measured total testosterone and estradiol levels. Hence, such a rise may be misleading and does not necessarily indicate increased gonadotropin release. Clomiphene should not be given to patients with liver disease, because of its estrogen agonist effects. The test is also contraindicated in depression, because of the risk of mood disturbance, and patients should be warned of the risk of alteration of peripheral vision. Gonadotropin levels double by 10 days, and menstruation usually accompanies a positive clomiphene test in women.

The ability of medroxyprogesterone acetate to induce a menstrual bleed is highly predictive of the response to clomiphene. A normal response to clomiphene in a patient with amenorrhea offers reassurance that the axis is intact and that the problem lies in the hypothalamus, but offers little indication of the etiology. Patients with weight, exercise and stress-induced amenorrhea can have either a normal or absent response to clomiphene, presumably indicative of the severity of the suppression of gonadotropin secretion. The clomiphene test has little role in the modern investigation of amenorrhea.

Gonadotropin-releasing hormone (GnRH) testing

GnRH (LHRH) stimulates LH and FSH release from the pituitary in a dose-dependent manner between 25 and 100 μg. An absent response is characterized by a failure to rise above three times the within-assay coefficient of variation of the basal values. The GnRH test is not used for the diagnosis of hypogonadism, but may assist in establishing its etiology.

In a patient with secondary hypogonadism, a normal response to GnRH implies that hypogonadism is the result of understimulation by the hypothalamus. This may be due to a hypothalamic lesion or disconnection of the pituitary from the hypothalamus by a functional pituitary stalk lesion. Occasionally, the GnRH test may also provide an index of hypothalamic function. GnRH is required for both LH synthesis and release, such that flat or subnormal responses may both be seen in hypothalamic disease with GnRH deficiency.

Prolactin

A clinical syndrome due to prolactin deficiency is not recognized, and its measurement serves only as a guide to the etiology of hypopituitarism. Prolactin physiology differs from that of other anterior pituitary hormones, in that its secretion is principally under tonic inhibition by release of dopamine from the hypothalamus. Levels do not show significant diurnal variation, and so tests other than basal measurements are very rarely required. Physiological stress and various medications that interfere with dopamine action, such as metoclopramide, prochlorperazine and various antipsychotics, raise serum prolactin. TRH stimulates prolactin release, but provides no extra information compared to random serum prolactin measurements, on three separate occasions, to minimize the risk of falsely elevated stress-induced hyperprolactinemia.

Conclusion

Accurate assessment of anterior pituitary function requires a sound knowledge of its normal physiology together with careful integration of clinical and biochemical information. Certain aspects of the optimum method of pituitary function testing, notably the assessment of ACTH reserve, are not universally agreed, such that local circumstances and personal preference may dictate the final choice. Physicians are advised to acquaint themselves with their local laboratory reference ranges and not to allow single hormonal measurements to substitute for clinical awareness, particularly where an evolving endocrine deficit is anticipated, such as following pituitary irradiation. The following protocol is proposed as a reliable and safe strategy for the assessment of suspected hypopituitarism.

New patients

Basal investigations, at 7–9 a.m. (all serum):
  Cortisol
  T4, TSH
  Prolactin
  LH FSH, testosterone/estradiol, SHBG
  IGF-I
Urine/plasma osmolality

If basal serum cortisol <400 nmol/l (<14.4 μg/dL) and/or GHD is suspected, then proceed to ITT. If any abnormality in any of the above tests is found, then proceed to pituitary imaging.

At-risk patients

In such patients (e.g. those who have received pituitary radiotherapy), pituitary function tests should be performed regularly in order to detect asymptomatic hypopituitarism, although there is a paucity of data on the optimum frequency with which this should be done. Our practice is to check basal pituitary function (0700–0900 h) every year, with a dynamic test of ACTH reserve if the basal serum cortisol is <400 nmol/l (<14.4 μg/dL) every 2 years. If patients exhibit the syndrome of GHD, then the dynamic test of choice will be the ITT. GHD occurs early after radiotherapy and, once it has been proven, many physicians use sequential SSTs to document the evolution of ACTH deficiency. Again, data in this regard are scarce, such that accurate, robust local reference ranges are essential.

References

1. Brien TG. Human corticosteroid binding globulin. *Clin Endocrinol* 1981; 14: 193–212.
2. Clark PM, Neylon I, Raggatt PR, Sheppard MC, Stewart PM. Defining the normal cortisol response to the short synacthen test: implications for the investigation of hypothalamic–pituitary disorders. *Clin Endocrinol* 1998; 49: 287–92.
3. Plumpton FS, Besser GM. The adrenocortical response to surgery and insulin-induced hypoglycaemia in corticosteroid-treated and normal subjects. *Br J Surg* 1969; 56: 216–19.
4. Mattingley D. A simple fluorimetric method for the estimation of free 11-hydroxycorticoids in human plasma. *J Clin Pathol* 1962; 15: 374–9.
5. Gashell SJ, Collins CJ, Thorne GC, Groom GV. External quality assessment of assays for cortisol in plasma: use of target data obtained by GC/mass spectrometry. *Clin Chem* 1983; 29: 862–7.
6. Hurel SJ, Thompson CJ, Watson MJ, Baylis PH, Kendall-Taylor P. The short synacthen and insulin stress tests in the assessment of the hypothalamic–pituitary–adrenal axis. *Clin Endocrinol* 1996; 44: 141–6.
7. Pavord SR, Girach A, Price DE et al. A retrospective audit of the combined pituitary function test, using the insulin stress test, TRH and GnRH in a district laboratory. *Clin Endocrinol* 1992; 26: 135–9.
8. Jones SL, Trainer PJ, Perry L, Wass JA, Besser GM, Grossman A. An audit of the insulin tolerance test in

adult subjects in an acute investigation unit over one year. *Clin Endocrinol* 1995; **42**: 101–2.

9. Greenwood FC, Landon J, Stamp TCB. The plasma sugar, free fatty acid, cortisol and growth hormone response to insulin. *J Clin Invest* 1966; **4**: 429–36.

10. Vestergara P, Hoeck HC, Jakobsen PE, Laurber P. Reproducibility of growth hormone and cortisol response to the insulin tolerance test and the short ACTH test in normal adults. *Horm Metab Res* 1997; **29**: 106–10.

11. Wood JB, Frankland AW, James VHT, Landon J. A rapid test of adrenocortical function. *Lancet* 1965; **i**: 243–5.

12. Speckart PF, Nicoloff JT, Bethune JE. Screening for adrenocortical insufficiency with cosyntropin (synthetic ACTH). *Arch Intern Med* 1971; **128**: 761–3.

13. May ME, Carey RM. Rapid adrenocorticotropic hormone test in practice. *Am J Med* 1985; **79**: 679–84.

14. Lindholm J, Kehlet, H. Re-evaluation of the clinical value of the 30 min ACTH test in assessing hypothalamo–pituitary–adrenal function. *Clin Endocrinol* 1987; **26**: 53–9.

15. Clayton RN. Short synacthen test versus insulin stress test for assessment of the hypothalamo–pituitary–adrenal axis: controversy revisited. *Clin Endocrinol* 1996; **44**: 147–9.

16. Stewart PM, Corrie J, Seckl JR, Edwards CR, Padfield PL. A rational approach for assessing the hypothalamo–pituitary-adrenal axis. *Lancet* 1988; **1**: 1208–10.

17. Streeton DHP, Anderson GH, Bonaventura MM. The potential for serious consequences from misinterpreting normal responses to the rapid adrenocorticotropin test. *J Clin Endocrinol Metab* 1996; **81**: 285–90.

18. Darmon P, Dadoun F, Frachebois C et al. On the meaning of the low-dose ACTH (1–24) tests to assess the functionality of the hypothalamic–pituitary–adrenal axis. *Eur J Endocrinol* 1999; **5**: 1–5.

19. Abdu TAM, Elhadd TA, Neary R et al. Comparison of low dose short synacthen test (1 μg), conventional dose short synacthen test (250 μg) and insulin tolerance test for the assessment of the hypothalamo–pituitary–adrenal axis in patients with pituitary disease. *J Clin Endocrinol Metab* 1998; **83**: 8–43.

20. Tjordman K, Jaffe A, Grazas N et al. The role of low dose (1 μg) adrenocorticotropin test in the evaluation of patients with pituitary diseases. *J Clin Endocrinol Metab* 1995; **80**: 1301–5.

21. Streeten DHP. Shortcomings in the low-dose (1 ug) ACTH test for the diagnosis of ACTH deficiency states. *J Clin Endocrinol Metab* 1999; **84**: 835–7.

22. Littley MD, Gibson S, White A, Shalet SM. Comparison of the ACTH and cortisol responses to provocative testing with glucagon and insulin hypoglycaemia in normal subjects. *Clin Endocrinol* 1989; **31**: 527–33.

23. Spiger M, Jubiz W, Meidle W, West CD, Tylor FJ. Single-dose metyrapone test. *Arch Intern Med* 1975; **135**: 698–700.

24. Shalet SM, Toogood A, Rahim A, Brennan BMD. The diagnosis of GH deficiency in children and adults. *Endocrine Rev* 1998; **19**: 203–23.

25. Hoffman DM, O'Sullivan AJ, Baxter RC, Ho KY. Diagnosis of growth hormone deficiency in adults. *Lancet* 1994; **343**: 1064–8.

26. Anonymous. Consensus guidelines for the diagnosis and treatment of adults with growth hormone deficiency: summary statement of the Growth Hormone Research Society Workshop On Adult Growth Hormone Deficiency. *J Clin Endocrinol Metab* 1998; **83**: 379–81.

27. Gasperi M, Aimaretti G, Scarcello G et al. Low dose hexarelin and growth hormone releasing hormone as a diagnostic tool for the diagnosis of GH deficiency in adults: comparison with insulin-induced hypoglycemia test. *J Clin Endocrinol Metab* 1999; **84**: 2633–7.

28. Trainer PJ, Besser GM. *The Bart's Endocrine Protocols*. Churchill Livingstone, 1995.

Appendix 2

Pharmacopoeia

Pierre-Marc G Bouloux and Jessica M Kubie

A
Alendronate sodium
Aminoglutethimide
Anastrozole

B
Bromocriptine

C
Cabergoline
Calcitonin
Carbimazole
Clomiphene citrate
Combined oral contraceptives
Conjugated equine estrogens (Premarin)
Cyproterone acetate

D
dDAVP (Desmopressin)
Dexamethasone
Dydrogesterone

E
Estradiol
Ethinylestradiol
Etidronate (sodium)

F
Finasteride
Fludrocortisone
Flutamide
Follicle-stimulating hormone (FSH)

G
Gonadotropin-releasing hormone–gonadorelin
Gonadotropin-releasing hormone agonists
Growth hormone

H
Human chorionic gonadotropin
Hydrocortisone (cortisol)

K
Ketoconazole

L
Labetalol
Lanreotide
Lithium carbonate

M
Medroxyprogesterone acetate
Menotrophin (hMG)
Metformin
Metyrapone
Mitotane (o'p'-DDD)

N
Norethisterone
Norethisterone enanthate
Norgestimate

O
Octreotide

P
Pamidronate disodium
Pergolide
Phenoxybenzamine
Phentolamine (mesylate)
Prednisolone
Progestogen-only oral contraceptives
Propranolol
Propylthiouracil

Q
Quinagolide

R
Raloxifene
Recombinant human TSH
Risedronate

S
Sildenafil (Viagra)
Sodium ipodate
Spironolactone

T
Testosterone
Thyroxine
Tibolone
Triiodothyronine (T3)

V
Vitamin D and analogues

Alendronate sodium

Mode of action
Alendronate is a bisphosphonate. It inhibits osteoclast activity by being incorporated into the bone matrix, where it is pharmacologically inactive.

Indications
Treatment of postmenopausal osteoporosis.

Dosage
10 mg daily (at least 30 min before breakfast; stand or sit upright for at least 30 min afterwards).

Kinetic data
Preclinical studies show that alendronate transiently distributes to soft tissues following administration but is then rapidly redistributed to bone or excreted in the urine.

Contraindications
Abnormalities of esophageal motility. Hypocalcemia. Renal impairment. Pregnancy and breastfeeding. Inability to stand or sit upright for 30 min. Caution in upper gastrointestinal disorders (dysphagia, symptomatic esophageal disease, gastritis, duodenitis).

Adverse effects
Esophageal reactions (e.g. esophagitis, esophageal ulcers). Gastrointestinal effects (e.g. abdominal pain, diarrhea).

Interactions
Calcium supplements and antacids interfere with the absorption of alendronate.

Aminoglutethimide

Mode of action
This drug inhibits several cytochrome P450-mediated hydroxylation steps in the adrenal cortex, including the initial formation of pregnenolone from cholesterol. Extra-adrenal aromatization of androgens to estrogens is inhibited.

Indications
Adrenal carcinoma. Previously, second-line endocrine therapy for breast cancer but now rarely used in breast cancer. Advanced prostate cancer.

Dosage
250 mg orally three or four times a day. Must be coupled with physiological replacement dosages of hydrocortisone (e.g. hydrocortisone 15 mg twice a day).

Kinetic data
Well absorbed after oral administration. Serum half-life about 7 h.

Contraindications
Pregnancy. Breastfeeding. Porphyria.

Adverse effects
Dizziness, somnolence and lethargy (especially in the elderly). An Addisonian crisis may occur if physiological replacement hydrocortisone is not given, but mineralocorticoid replacement is rarely required. Drug rash and gastrointestinal upsets may occur.

There is a 1% incidence of agranulocytosis.

Interactions
Reduced anticoagulant effect (metabolism of nicoumalone and warfarin accelerated). Increased metabolism of corticosteroids. Reduced plasma concentration of medroxyprogesterone.

Anastrozole

Mode of action
Selective, non-steroidal aromatase inhibitor.

Indications
Advanced breast cancer in postmenopausal women.

Dosage
1 mg daily.

Kinetic data
Absorption is rapid, and maximum plasma concentrations occur within 2 h of dosing. It is eliminated slowly, with a plasma elimination half-life of 40–50 h. It is 40% bound to plasma proteins.

Contraindications
Pregnancy. Breastfeeding. Hepatic disease. Renal impairment. Premenopausal women.

Adverse effects
Hot flashes. Vaginal bleeding. Vaginal dryness. Hair thinning. Gastrointestinal effects.

Interactions
Estrogen-containing therapies should not be co-administered; they would negate its pharmacological action.

Bromocriptine

Mode of action
Bromocriptine is a specific dopamine receptor agonist in the three principal dopaminergic pathways of the central nervous system (CNS): mesolimbic, nigrostriatal and tuberoinfundibular. After interaction of bromocryptine with the D_2 receptor, activation of second messenger systems produces inhibition of adenylate cyclase activity (G_i), potassium efflux (G_k) and inhibition of phosphatidylinositol bisphosphate hydrolysis (G_o).

Since dopamine is the principal restraint on prolactin (PRL) release, the net result is a reduction in PRL gene transcription, mRNA accumulation and ultimately PRL secretion.

The incorporation of bromocriptine into a branched glucose-initiated macromolecular carrier in the long-acting injectable preparation ensures gradual release of the active drug and a prolonged duration of action after intramuscular injection.

Indications
Bromocriptine is mainly used to suppress pathological hyperprolactinemia and galactorrhea. Neoplasmic somatotrophs respond paradoxically to dopamine agonist, with a reduction in growth hormone (GH) concentration to less than 20 mU/l (<10 µg/l) in 54% of acromegalics given bromocriptine. Bromocriptine has also been used as adjunctive therapy in Parkinsonism, allowing a reduction in levadopa dosage by 10–90% in some patients.

Dosage
The initial 1.25-mg oral dose should be taken with a light snack immediately before bedtime, to reduce side-effects. Thereafter, the evening dose can be shifted to the middle of dinner and gradually increased by 1.25 mg every 3 days to a target dose of 5–7.5 mg daily, conventionally taken in two or three divided doses. Should the patient develop side-effects, the dose is temporarily reduced and then gradually increased. Tolerance to adverse effects such as nausea and orthostatic hypotension may develop rapidly. Recent studies have suggested that the drug can be administered as a single dose in the evening in a proportion of patients.

Kinetic data
Bromocriptine is poorly absorbed from the gastrointestinal tract (30–40%) and the bioavailability of the drug is only about 6% because of extensive first-pass hepatic metabolism. The plasma half-life after oral

administration is 15 h, 90–96% of the drug being bound to serum albumin. Metabolism occurs principally in the liver by hydrolysis to lysergic acid and peptides. Excretion is chiefly fecal via the biliary system, with only a minor renal component.

Contraindications

The drug should be avoided in porphyria and in patients with toxemia of pregnancy or hypertension postpartum, and prescribed with caution to patients with hepatic disease, cardiovascular disease, peptic ulceration, or a history of psychotic disorders postpartum, or when hypertensive drugs are prescribed concurrently. Although patients whose hyperprolactinemia has been controlled by bromocriptine are advised to stop the drug when pregnant, there is no evidence of teratogenicity in the offspring of women treated with bromocriptine throughout pregnancy. Indeed, expansion of a prolactinoma during pregnancy is an indication for its administration.

Adverse effects

The prevalence of adverse effects is reduced by gradual introduction of the drug. It is essential to warn all patients starting treatment about the possibility of fainting. Nausea, vomiting and postural hypotension are the most common adverse effects, although headache, nasal congestion, drowsiness, constipation, mouth dryness, digital vasospasm, edema and gastrointestinal bleeding are also reported. Psychosis is a potentially serious problem, and although patients with previous psychiatric disease may be at particular risk, this side-effect has also been encountered in those without a personal or family history of psychiatric disease.

Interactions

Nausea and abdominal pain may be exacerbated by comcomitant ingestion of alcohol, which may also lower tolerance to bromocriptine; patients should be warned of this potential interaction. Erythromycin and possibly other macrolides increase plasma concentration. Octreolide increases plasma concentration. Lack of or decrease in efficacy may occur in patients concomitantly receiving other drugs with dopamine antagonist activity, e.g. phenothiazines, butyrophenone. Metoclopramide and domperidone antagonize the hypoprolactinemic effect.

Cabergoline

Mode of action

Cabergoline is a selective, potent and long-lasting dopamine agonist.

Indications

Hyperprolactinemia, especially if intolerant of bromocriptine. Suppression of lactation. Parkinsonism.

Dosage

The suggested starting dose is 0.25 mg twice weekly, which should be increased to 0.5 mg twice weekly after the first week. Patients not responding should have an increase in dose to 1.0 mg twice weekly.

Kinetic data

The drug is rapidly absorbed, with peak levels reached 0.5–2 h after an oral dose. The evidence suggests biphasic elimination, with an initial rapid half-life of 7.5 h followed by a slow terminal elimination phase with a half-life of 65 h.

Contraindications

Known hypersensitivity to ergot alkaloids and psychotic states.

Adverse effects

Side-effects are generally mild and transient. They include nausea, vomiting, abdominal pain, constipation, drowsiness, depression and headache. There is no evidence of a dose–response relationship for side-effects other than nausea.

Interactions

See bromocriptine.

Calcitonin

The calcitonins are peptide hormones with molecular weights around 8500. The molecule is composed of a chain of 32 amino acid residues with basic features—a disulfide bridge between the cysteine residues in positions 1 and 7, forming a ring of seven amino acid residues at the N-terminus, which carries a free amino group and a proline amide group at the C-terminus—that are identical in all calcitonins and that appear to be essential for biological activity. The central part of the chain, on the other hand, varies considerably from one calcitonin to another, both in the identity of the amino acids present and in their positions in the chain. Currently, three calcitonins—porcine (PCT), human (HCT) and salmon (SCT)—are in general use.

Mode of action

Calcitonin inhibits bone resorption, mainly by a rapid decrease in osteoclast activity. In the kidney it decreases the reabsorption of both calcium and phosphate in the proximal tubules. Overall, it decreases plasma calcium concentration. In addition, the drug has analgesic properties that appear to be distinct from its effect on bone.

Indications

Treatment of osteoporosis where estrogen therapy is contraindicated, especially in patients with high bone turnover, and bone pain. Treatment of Paget's disease of bone, hypercalcemia, metastatic bone pain.

Dosage

Parenteral and nasal preparations are available. The injectable preparation, salcatonin, contains 100 IU/ml in saline of the acetate. Parental calcitonin can be given subcutaneously or intramuscularly; in earlier studies of its effect on osteoporosis, the drug was given subcutaneously. The nasal spray contains 200 units per dose. Paget's disease of bone, 50 units three times weekly to 100 units daily by subcutaneous or intramuscular injection. Post-menopausal osteoporosis, 100 units daily by subcutaneous or intramuscular injection, with dietary calcium and vitamin D supplements.

The recommended dose of intranasal salmon calcitonin is 200 IU daily on alternate days or 5 days a week with adequate calcium supplements; intermittent treatment with 3–6 months on and 1 month off treatment with the nasal spray has been recommended, but further studies are required to establish the optimum daily dose and duration of intranasal calcitonin therapy.

Kinetic data

The drug is rapidly degraded by gastric secretions, which is why it has to be given parenterally or by nasal spray. Peak plasma concentrations are recorded 15–45 min after subcutaneous injection. The plasma half-life is 4–15 min. Animal studies have shown maximal tissue uptake in bone, liver and kidney.

Contraindications

Parenteral calcitonin is not recommended in women of childbearing age, since the drug may cause fetal growth retardation. Similar considerations apply to its administration in lactating mothers. Intranasal calcitonin is not suitable for patients with nasal polypi, epistaxis, sinusitis, empyema antri and nasal obstruction, or for those with otitis media or carcinoma of the middle ear. Intranasal calcitonin is contraindicated in patients with known hypersensitivity to salmon calcitonin, unless they have a negative skin test.

Cautions

Resistance to the effects of calcitonin, and especially to the non-human preparations, has been reported with prolonged use. Whether this resistance is due to the presence of neutralizing antibodies or to downregulation of calcitonin receptors is not clear. Synthetic salmon calcitonin is less immunogenic than porcine calcitonin and is thus preferred for prolonged therapy. In rare cases, parenteral calcitonin therapy has been associated with serious allergic reactions (bronchospasm and anaphylactic shock). Patients with a history of allergy should have an intradermal test using 1:100 dilution of injectable calcitonin in sodium chloride injection. Calcitonin therapy reduces serum calcium concentration, with resultant secondary hyperparathyroidism.

Adverse effects

Parenteral calcitonin may cause side-effects such as nausea, vomiting, facial flushing and unpleasant taste. In rare cases, severe allergic reactions, which should be differentiated from facial flushing, have been reported with parenteral therapy. The intranasal preparation is well tolerated, and preliminary reports suggest a reduction in such adverse effects. The nausea and flushing are usually transient and do not necessitate withdrawal of therapy. Other adverse reactions (noted rarely in patients treated with intranasal calcitonin) include rhinitis, rhinorrhea, hyperemia of nasal mucosa, epistaxis, abdominal discomfort, headache and polyuria. In general, long-term administration of calcitonin is safe, and no serious or long-term effects have been noted in patients.

Carbimazole

Mode of action

Carbimazole reduces thyroid hormone synthesis by inhibiting iodine organification and iodotyrosyl coupling, by inhibiting the enzyme thyroid peroxidase. It also has an immunosuppressive effect and reduces circulating thyroid-stimulating antibody levels. It is completely metabolized to the active metabolite methimazole.

Indications

Hyperthyroidism (Graves' disease). Preparation for thyroidectomy. Sometimes as comcomitant treatment following radio-iodine treatment.

Dosage

Commenced in a dose of 20–60 mg (in divided doses) until patient is euthyroid, and gradually reduced to a maintenance dose of 5–15 mg over a period of usually 18 months.

Kinetic data

Plasma half-life is 4–6 h, and it is metabolized by the liver.

Contraindication

Adverse reaction to the drug previously. Caution in liver disease.

Adverse effects

Agranulocytosis (patient should be warned to stop treatment and seek advice on any sign of infection, such as sore throat, mouth ulcers or fever, and warning noted in notes). Jaundice. Rashes (usually mild papular, occasionally purpuric). Nausea. Headache. Arthralgia. Rarely, alopecia.

Interactions

Increased sensitivity to warfarin has been observed in hyperthyroidism, and careful control of dosage is required as the patient is rendered euthyroid.

Clomiphene citrate

Mode of action

Commercially available preparations of clomiphene are a racemic mixture of the *cis* and *trans* isomers (60:40). The former is a weak estrogen, while the latter has potent antiestrogenic properties. It is thought to act as a partial agonist, binding to the cytoplasmic estradiol receptor. It inhibits or delays replenishment of the receptor, making the target cell insensitive to estrogen; that is, the negative feedback effect of estradiol at the pituitary/hypothalamic level is blocked. Follicle-stimulating hormone (FSH) secretion is thereby increased and follicular growth stimulated. This effect is mediated through an increase in the pulse frequency of gonadotropin-releasing hormone (GnRH) secretion. Clomiphene is thus ineffective in patients with hypothalamic/pituitary dysfunction. The effects of the drug also depend upon the dose used and the estrogen status of the patient.

Indications

Anovulatory and unexplained infertility in women with an intact hypothalamic–pituitary–ovarian axis, including those with polycystic ovaries (PCOs), but excluding those with primary ovarian failure.

Dosage

The usual starting dose is 50 mg orally daily for 5–7 days, starting on day 2, 3 or 5 of the menstrual cycle. The ovarian response should be monitored, preferably by transvaginal ultrasound. Estrogen and progesterone levels in the mid-luteal phase are of value in assessing the ovarian response to clomiphene in retrospect. If ovulation does not occur, the dose may be increased to 100 mg, 150 mg and 200 mg daily, but not beyond. If conception does not occur after four to six courses, the patient should be reassessed and alternative ovarian stimulant therapy given.

Kinetic data

Clomiphene is mainly excreted in the feces, with a small quantity appearing in urine and some returning by the enterohepatic circulation. The half-life of the drug is about 5 days, but the drug remains detectable for up to 30 days.

Contraindications

Pregnancy, liver disease, pituitary tumors and undiagnosed abnormal vaginal bleeding. The drug is ineffective in patients with primary ovarian failure. Its use is not justified in patients with infertility due to bilateral tubal disease or male factors, except in conjunction with in vitro fertilization regimens.

Adverse effects

The incidence of multiple pregnancy during clomiphene therapy is increased to around 8%, the majority being twin pregnancies; high-order multiple pregnancy is rare. There is no evidence of an increase in congenital malformations. Persistent ovarian cysts occur in 5–10% of patients. Ovarian hyperstimulation is rare. There has been concern that ovarian cancer may be a long-term consequence of clomiphene citrate therapy, but there are no definitive prospective studies on that aspect. Nevertheless, the current recommendation is a maximum of six treatment cycles.

Reported side-effects include blurred vision, hot flashes, abdominal discomfort, nausea, vomiting, breast tenderness, weight gain and headache. Objective evidence of ophthalmic disturbance has been reported—scotoma and electroretinographic changes—but these resolve when treatment is discontinued. A variety of symptoms—vertigo, anxiety, depression, insomnia, dermatitis, scalp hair loss—have also been reported in a few patients, but there is no evidence that these are definitively linked with the intake of clomiphene. A small increase (5%) in bromsulphthalein excretion occurs in around 25% of patients treated with the drug; other liver function tests appear unaltered. No long-term effect on hepatic function has been reported.

Interactions

There are no known harmful interactions between clomiphene and other drugs.

Combined oral contraceptives

Composition

The combined oral contraceptive (COC) contains two synthetic steroid hormones: an estrogen and a progestogen. In the majority of UK COCs, the estrogen is ethinylestradiol (EE), but in a few preparations mestranol, structurally very similar to EE, is present. The progestogens used in COCs are all 19-nortestosterone derivatives; they may be norethisterone and levonorgestrel (second generation) and desogestrel, gestodene and norgestimate (third generation). Although many studies have sought to compare the relative selectivity and potency of the different progestogens, there is little agreement regarding the results. In clinical practice it is unlikely that there are significant differences between the progestogens in the doses used in the current COCs.

Table A2.1 lists the various types of combined oral contraception preparations, listed in alphabetical order for progestogen, with the newer third-generation progestogens first.

There are two types of COC: **monophasic**, where the same dose of estrogen and progestogen is given every day for 21 days, after which there is a 7-day gap before the next pack is started; and **phasic** preparations, where the dose of estrogen and progestogen is changed during the cycle. With the **biphasic** pills, the dose changes once in the pill cycle, and in the **triphasic** regimen twice. The **phasic** preparations are designed to lower the total dose of hormone during the

Estrogen	Progestogen	Preparation	Type
	A. Desogestrel (DSG)		
EE 20 µg	DSG 150 µg	Mercilon	Mono
EE 30 µg	DSG 150 µg	Marvelon	Mono
		Graciel	Phasic
	B. Gestodene (GSD)		
EE 30 µg	GSD 75 µg	Femodene	Mono
EE 30 µg	GSD 50 × 6	Triadene	Triphasic
EE 30 × 6	70 × 5	(Tri-Minulet)	
40 × 5	100 × 10		
30 × 10			
	C. Levonergestrel (LNg)		
EE 30 µg	LNg 150 µg	Microgynon 30	Mono
		(Ovranette)	
EE 30 µg	LNg 250 µg	Eugynon 30	Mono
EE 50 µg	LNg 250 µg	Ovran	Mono
EE 30 × 6	LNg 50 µg × 6	Logynon	Triphasic
40 × 5	LNg 75 µg × 5	(Trinordiol)	
30 × 10	LNg 125 µg × 10		
	D. Noresthisterone (NET)		
EE 20 µg	NET-Acetate 1 mg	Loestrin 20	Mono
EE 30 µg	NET-Acetate 1.5 mg	Loestrin 30	Mono
EE 35 µg	NET 500 mg	Brevinor	Mono
		(Norimin)	
EE 35 µg	NET 1 mg	Neocon	Mono
		(Norimin)	
M 50 µg	NET 1 mg	Norinyl-1	Mono
		(Ortho-Novin 1/50)	
EE 35 × 7	NET 500 µg × 7	BiNovum	Biphasic
EE 35 × 14	NET 1 mg × 14		
EE 35 × 7	NET 500 µg × 7	Synphase	Triphasic
EE 35 × 7	NET 1 mg × 9		
EE 35 × 7	NET 500 µg × 5		
	E. Norgestimate (NORG)		
EE 35 µg	NORG 250 µg	Cilest	Mono
	F. Ethynodiol diacetate (ETH-D)		
EE 35 µg	ETH-D 1.5 mg	Conova 30	Mono

EE, ethinylestradiol; M, mestranol; Mono, monophasic.

Table A2.1
Classification of combined oral contraceptive preparations by progestogen used.

pill cycle, the dose being varied in order to maintain endometrial stability and give good cycle control. The two basic regimens for triphasic pills are changes after 7 days, i.e. 7 days, 7 days and 7 days, or after days 6 and 11 (6 days, 5 days, 10 days). Biphasic preparations usually have 7 or 8 days at one dose and then 14 tablets at a different dose.

Mode of action

COCs exert a direct inhibitory action on the hypothalamus and the pituitary, inhibiting the release of follicle-stimulating hormone (FSH), luteinizing hormone (LH) and gonadotropin-releasing hormone (GnRH). The midcycle FSH and LH surges and the preovulatory estradiol peak are either reduced or do not occur. In addition, cervical mucus is thickened, the motility of the fallopian tubes altered and the endometrium desynchronized, so implantation does not occur. Pituitary hormones are suppressed throughout the pill cycle, as are estradiol and progesterone. There is no evidence of ovulation. However, while pituitary suppression and the foregoing effects on the endometrium and cervical mucus occur with the lower-dose pills, follicular activity as evidenced by ultrasound can be seen in up to one-third of patients. These follicles do not appear to be competent; that is, they do not as a rule ovulate and there is no subsequent luteal phase.

The margin of error with low doses, i.e. 20–35 μg EE, is very low. Pill compliance is therefore essential. Missed pills can result in ovulation, which is particularly common if pills are missed either during the first or the last week of pill-taking, which effectively extends the pill-free interval.

Indications

A reversible method of contraception useful for birth spacing or completed families, for those who prefer to take a tablet rather than a delivery system, e.g. injection or implant for contraception.

Dosage

Over the last 30 years, there has been a progressive reduction in the dose of both estrogen and progestogen, in order to minimize side-effects, particularly those related to the estrogen—usually EE. This has been shown to be associated with a reduced incidence of thromboembolic disease. Doses now range from 20 μg to 35 μg per day. The progestogen dosage has also been reduced, but care must be exercised when looking at microgram amounts, as potencies of the various progestogens differ.

Kinetic data

EE is absorbed from the upper gastrointestinal tract and conjugated with sulfates in the bowel wall. A small proportion of the absorbed hormone is found in the free state in the plasma, but the vast majority of EE and its sulfate are bound to albumin. The free EE is metabolized in the liver, EE conjugates and metabolites being excreted through the bile into the large bowel, where they are subsequently hydrolysed by bacterial flora to produce 'free' EE. This is then reabsorbed—the enterohepatic circulation. There is a wide inter-individual variation in the absorption and metabolism of EE, resulting in a 20–30-fold difference in steady-state plasma levels. Peak levels are seen within 1–2 h of oral ingestion in the majority of women.

Norethisterone is well absorbed from the bowel, with peak levels occurring 1–2 h after oral ingestion. It subsequently undergoes first-pass metabolism in the liver, resulting in an average bioavailability of 64%. As with EE, there is a wide inter-individual variation in plasma levels. Levonorgestrel and gestodene are well absorbed from the bowel and do not undergo first-pass liver metabolism, resulting in virtually 100% bioavailability. They are both strongly bound to albumin in the plasma. Desogestrel is a pro-drug and is converted to its active metabolite 3-ketodesogestrel in first-pass metabolism. Norgestimate is active in its parent form, but a small proportion is metabolized to levonorgestrel, 17-deacetylated norgestimate and 3-ketonorgestimate, which all have progestational activity. Oral ingestion of the combined estrogen and progestogen tablet produces peak values which suppress ovulation within 1–2 h. These levels are maintained throughout a 24-h period and do not fall into the non-contraceptive range. Taking one pill a day for 21 days does not cause a depot effect but maintains contraceptive action.

Contraindications

Absolute contraindications
- Pregnancy or suspected pregnancy until the diagnosis rules out pregnancy
- Severe arterial disease risk factors or multiple risk factors (see below for summative effect)
- History of venous thrombosis or arterial thrombosis
- History of valvular heart disease associated with pulmonary hypertension or thrombosis
- Ischemic heart disease
- Hypertension
- Varicose veins when there is a history of thrombosis, familial hyperlipidemia (cholesterol above 6.5 mmol/l) or any prothrombotic coagulation abnormality
- Focal migraine or severe migraine best described as 'crescendo' migraine.
- Active liver disease, porphyria, liver adenoma, gallstones
- Post-hydatidiform mole until plasma β-hCG levels have been normal for 6 months
- History of jaundice during pregnancy
- Breast or genital tract carcinoma

Relative contraindications
- Single risk factor for cardiovascular disease
- Migraine (not focal)
- Homozogous sickle cell disease
- Long-term partial immobilization
- Amenorrhea/oligomenorrhea until after investigation and treatment if indicated
- Hyperprolactinemia until after investigation and treatment if indicated
- Chronic systemic disease such as Crohn's disease, renal disease and diabetes
- Long-term drug therapy which interacts with the COC
- First-degree relative with breast cancer
- During monitoring and after treatment of an abnormal cervical smear

Other risk factors which should be discussed in counseling, particularly with regard to the choice of contraception method, are a family history or personal history of severe depression, long-term immobilization, e.g. in relation to fractured spine or other disease, sickle cell disease and inflammatory bowel disease, including Crohn's disease.

Risk factors for arterial disease include: obesity, hypertension, diabetes mellitus, family history of arterial disease (either cerebrovascular accidents or ischemic heart disease, especially in a first-degree relative under the age of 45 years) and varicose veins if associated with venous thrombosis. The cardiovascular risk factors can be summative, i.e. if more than two are present they may increase the risk significantly and warrant consideration of other methods. The most important risk factor is cigarette smoking, particularly in heavy smokers.

Adverse effects

Nuisance side-effects can occur during the first few cycles of COC use, but these are remarkably few in number with the newer low-dose preparations. They include nausea, headache, breast tenderness, occasional vomiting, change in body weight, and intermenstrual bleeding or spotting, which usually decreases in amount after the third cycle of use.

Changes in mood, depression and loss of libido are more likely to be due to pre-existing situations than to the COC but such symptoms may nevertheless require investigation. Thrombosis is more common in blood groups A, B and AB or when Factor V Leiden is present.

Interactions

Certain clinical interactions are important for COC users.

Diarrhea and vomiting can interfere with absorption and therefore effectiveness of the pill. If severe vomiting occurs, additional contraceptive precautions, e.g. a barrier method, should be used during the episodes of illness and for 7 days after recovery. The pill packet should continue to be taken, but the next pill-free interval should be omitted and the new packet of pills started straight away. This avoids breakthrough ovulation.

COCs should be **discontinued prior to surgery** and alternative contraception provided. It is not, however, necessary to stop the contraceptive pill when undergoing minor surgery (e.g. laparoscopy, sterilization or tooth extraction). Subcutaneous heparin prophylaxis can be given, if indicated, in these circumstances or for emergency surgery.

Drug interaction occurs with certain drugs which induce liver enzymes, enhancing the metabolism of both EE and progestogen so that plasma levels are reduced. The most important are: carbamazepine, phenytoin, phenobarbitone, primidone, griseofulvin and rifampicin. If a short course of any of these drugs, e.g. rifampicin, has to be given, additional contraceptive measures such as a barrier method should be used while the drug is taken and for at least 7 days after ceasing medication. The next packet of pills should then be taken straight away without a pill-free interval.

However, with long-term courses, e.g. an anticonvulsant such as carbamazepine, it is necessary to increase the dose of the oral contraceptive pill in order to compensate for the more prolonged hepatic enzyme induction. This can be achieved with a 50-μg EE pill or by 'tricycling', i.e. taking three packets of pills one after the other so that 12 weeks of continuous pill-taking occurs in order to avoid pill-free intervals. It is important to note that if continuous breakthrough bleeding occurs it will be necessary for the drug levels of the anticonvulsant to be measured and appropriate changes made to the COC dose: in some cases, another method of contraception may be necessary.

COC efficacy may be reduced by some broad-spectrum antibiotics, e.g. ampicillin, when given for short periods of time in high dose. Some antibiotics alter the colonic flora and thus interfere with the recycling of EE. This may result in a reduced plasma concentration, which may be significant in a few women and allow 'breakthrough' ovulation. Additional precautions should be taken while using these drugs for 7 days after the antibiotic course. There is, however, no evidence that long-term low-dose antibiotics for the treatment of acne are a problem for drug interaction. Vitamin C, by contrast, competitively increases plasma EE levels due to competition for sulfate conjugation in the bowel wall. Co-trimoxazole is an enzyme inhibitor and its usage also results in increased hormone levels.

Reasons for stopping oral contraception immediately

COC should be stopped immediately if any of the following symptoms occur. The patient should seek medical advice forthwith or be referred to hospital:

- Sudden breathlessness with blood-stained sputum or productive cough
- Severe pain in the calf or one leg
- Sudden severe chest pain, whether or not radiating to the left arm
- Sudden severe abdominal pain or melena
- Sudden severe headache, especially if prolonged and associated with some loss of vision, vertigo or diplopia. All these conditions require immediate medical advice
- Rise in blood pressure greater than 160/95 mmHg
- Immobilization after an accident or major surgery
- Jaundice

Influence of oral contraceptives on the pharmacotherapeutic effects of other drugs

There are reports suggesting that the use of oral contraceptives may influence the pharmacotherapeutic effects of other drugs. These include: analgesics, antidepressants, antimalarial drugs, benzodiazepine, β-blockers, corticosteroids, hypoglycemic drugs, oral anticoagulants and theophylline. The documentation regarding these interactions varies from 'possible' to 'probable'. So far, however, no evidence has been obtained indicating that clinically significant effects occur which would require adjustment of the COC dose or prescription of an alternative medication.

Conjugated equine estrogens (Premarin)

Composition

A mixture of sodium estrone sulfate (53–61%), sodium equilin sulfate (23–30%) and other estrogenic substances from pregnant mares.

Mode of action

As for estrone, which is the major estrogenic component.

Indications

Treatment of menopausal symptoms and urogenital atrophy. Prevention and treatment of postmenopausal osteoporosis. Treatment of estrogen-responsive prostatic cancer. Palliative treatment of advanced inoperable prostatic cancer. Control of severe dysfunctional uterine bleeding.

Dosage

The recommended initial oral dose for menopausal therapy is 0.625 mg daily. Available as 0.625-, 1.25- and 2.5-mg tablets; 0.625% vaginal cream.

Kinetic data

Oral absorption is good, peak levels being attained within 1–5 h. The preparation is metabolized in the liver to yield estrone in addition to equilin and its metabolites. There is some enterohepatic circulation, but excretion is mainly in urine. Conjugated equine estrogens are well absorbed from the vaginal mucosa.

Contraindications, adverse effects and drug interactions

As discussed under estradiol.

Cyproterone acetate

Mode of action

Cyproterone acetate (CPA) is an anti-androgen which competes with androgens for androgen receptors. It has strong progestogenic properties that result in local action suppressing endometrial formation and at the same time exerting a negative feedback on hypothalamic receptors, leading to a reduction in gonadotropin release. In addition, CPA inhibits adrenal steroidogenesis and has a slight glucocorticoid effect.

Indications

Gonadotropin-independent precocious puberty (alone or in conjunction with gonadotropin-releasing hormone (GnRH) agonists to compensate for the initial stimulatory phase of GnRH agonist therapy). Control of libido in severe hypersexuality and/or sexual deviations in adult men. As palliative therapy of prostatic carcinoma. In conjunction with estrogens in women with the polycystic ovary syndrome (for the control of acne, hirsutism and androgenic alopecia). Idiopathic hirsutism. As the progestogen component of a combined oral contraceptive preparation.

Dosage

In precocious puberty, the recommended dose regimen is 75–100 mg/m^2 in two divided doses, by mouth. In hirsute women, it is given in a dose of 50 or 100 mg daily from days 5 to 15 of the cycle, together with ethinylestradiol (30 μg from days 5 to 26 of the cycle). The low-dose combined pill (2 mg CPA + 35 μg ethinylestradiol) is used for 21 days from day 1 of the cycle.

Kinetic data

CPA is completely absorbed after oral administration, maximal plasma levels after a single dose being achieved at 3–4 h. It is highly lipophilic and hence stored in fat. With daily oral administration, an equilibrium between administration and excretion is established after 8–10 days of therapy. The drug is no longer detectable in plasma 12 days after cessation of oral intake. Elimination from plasma is biphasic; the half-life is prolonged in obese patients, as would be expected. Excretion occurs via bile (70%) and urine (30%). Only small amounts of unchanged drug are found in bile.

Contraindications

The drug should not be used in pregnancy and during lactation. Except for patients with prostatic cancer, CPA is contraindicated in patients with hepatic, malignant or wasting diseases. It is also contraindicated in severe depression and in subjects with a history of thromboembolism.

Cautions

Owing to an initial sedative effect, there may be impaired ability to drive or operate machinery. This effect is dose-dependent. Although, in view of the influence of this drug on adrenal steroidogenesis, it is recommended that patients receiving CPA should carry a 'steroid card' and should receive steroid cover in the event of major stress or illness, signs of adrenal insufficiency are not seen in clinical practice.

Anemia has also been observed; a regular blood count is therefore recommended during treatment. CPA should be used with care in patients with diabetes mellitus, as it may interfere with carbohydrate metabolism.

Adverse effects

In men, CPA inhibits spermatogenesis; abnormal spermatozoa may be produced. The drug reduces the volume of ejaculate and causes infertility. The foregoing effects are reversible. CPA can also cause gynecomastia, changes in weight and hair pattern, skin reactions, fatigue, lassitude and sometimes initial sedation.

Liver abnormalities have been reported in animals. The UK Committee on the Safety of Medicines reported (1995) 91 cases of hepatic reactions—including hepatitis, cholestatic jaundice and hepatic failure—in 91 men treated for prostatic cancer aged between 60 and 90 years. The reactions (32 of which were fatal) typically occurred in men receiving the highest doses of cyproterone acetate for this condition—300 mg daily—over several months. Four cases of hepatic reactions occurred in women taking the oral contraceptive Dianette, which contains only 2 mg cyproterone acetate. The only female fatality was in a woman aged 66 years taking 100 mg cyproterone acetate daily for the treatment of hirsutism. It is therefore recommended that the highest doses of cyproterone acetate for prostatic carcinoma should be given only to cover the testosterone flare associated with GnRH agonist administration, for the treatment of severe hot flashes after orchidectomy or GnHR agonist therapy, or in patients who have not responded to or are intolerant of other forms of therapy for this condition.

Liver function tests should be performed before starting cyproterone acetate treatment and whenever symptoms or signs suggestive of hepatic dysfunction are noted. The drug should be stopped if there is evidence of hepatotoxicity.

Interactions

Alcohol reduces its effects but no potentially hazardous interactions with other drugs are known. Since CPA is metabolized by the liver, the dose of CPA should probably be increased when given in the low-dose contraceptive preparation if enzyme inducers such as antiepileptics are then taken concurrently.

dDAVP (Desmopressin)

Mode of action

Synthetic vasopressin analog. It has 12 times more antidiuretic activity than vasopressin, but less vasoconstrictive activity. It attaches to the specific vasopressin receptor (V2) located at the basal membrane of the collecting tubule. This receptor is coupled to adenylate cyclase, which, when activated, generates cyclic AMP, which in turn stimulates protein kinase A to organize the water channel protein aquaporin 2.

Indications

Diabetes insipidus (treatment and diagnosis). Nocturnal enuresis. Postoperative polydipsia and polyuria.

Preparations

Tablets: 100 µg and 200 µg.
Nasal spray (Desmospray): 10 µg per spray.
Intranasal solution.
Injection: 4 µg/ml.

Dosage

Diabetes insipidus: 300 µg daily in divided doses, with maintenance dose 0.2–1.2 mg. Intranasally: 10–40 µg daily. Injection: 1–4 µg daily.
Nocturnal enuresis: 200 µg at night. Intranasally 20 µg at night.

Kinetic data

Plasma half-life is 75 min.

Contraindications

Caution in cardiac insufficiency, hypertension and renal impairment. Cystic fibrosis.

Adverse effects

Fluid retention. Hyponatremia (can cause convulsions with severe hyponatremia). Nausea. Headache.

Abdominal pains. Epistaxis. When used for nocturnal enuresis, limit fluid intake to minimum and only to satisfy thirst for 8 h after dose.

Interactions

Effect potentiated by indomethacin.

Dexamethasone

Mode of action

Dexamethasone is a highly potent and long-acting glucocorticoid with negligible sodium-retaining properties. Clinical use of the drug is based mainly on its anti-inflammatory and immunosuppressive properties and its effect on the hypothalamo–pituitary–adrenal (HPA) axis.

Indications

Diseases of the connective tissue, liver and gastrointestinal tract. Respiratory distress syndrome. Shock. Raised intracranial pressure. Suppression test of HPA axis function. Congenital adrenal hyperplasia. Glucocorticoid replacement therapy, although hydrocortisone is generally preferred.

Dosage

The dose varies with the indication; overall, the daily oral dose usually varies between 0.5 and 16 mg. It can also be administered by intramuscular or intravenous injection.

Kinetic data

Dexamethasone is well absorbed orally. Peak plasma levels are reached between 1 and 2 h after ingestion and show wide individual variation. The plasma half-life is 3.6 ± 0.9 h and is reduced by simultaneous use of other drugs, e.g. rifampicin, phenobarbitone and phenytoin, and also possibly in chronic renal failure. Dexamethasone metabolism by the liver is slow and limited. Over 60% of the administered dose is excreted in the urine within 24 h, largely as unconjugated steroids.

Contraindications

Systemic infection.

Adverse effects

Patients on prolonged dexamethasone therapy are at risk of collapse and even death if their daily dose is not increased at times of severe physical distress (injury, surgery or infections). They should, therefore, always carry a steroid card and wear a bracelet or necklace indicating that they are taking steroids. Suppression of the HPA axis may persist for up to a year after discontinuation of dexamethasone therapy, so that steroid therapy will be required for a year if the patient is stressed, and the bracelet/necklace should be worn for that length of time.

Severe effects arise from suppression of adrenal function and immune defense mechanisms. The somatic manifestations include growth retardation in children, osteoporosis, thinning of the skin, peptic ulceration, ocular hypertension, subcapsular cataract, pancreatic disturbances and proximal myopathy.

Standard low-dose corticosteroid therapy is generally free from untoward symptoms. On a long-term basis, however, minor gastrointestinal disturbances, such as nausea and vomiting, may occur. Behavioral and personality changes can be caused by corticosteroids, especially at high doses. The more prolonged duration of action of dexamethasone may potentiate adverse effects such as osteoporosis compared with other corticosteroids.

Interactions

Concomitant use of phenytoin, phenobarbitone, ephedrine and rifampicin can reduce the therapeutic efficacy of dexamethasone. The dose of the steroid has therefore to be adjusted during combination therapy and also when these drugs are withdrawn.

Dydrogesterone

Dydrogesterone is a potent, orally active, progestogen similar to endogenous progesterone in its molecular structure and pharmacological effects, but differing from most other synthetic progestogens in its freedom from estrogenic, androgenic and anabolic effects.

Mode of action

The progestational effects of the drug are identical to those of progesterone but with a much greater potency; it causes secretory transformation of the estrogen-primed endometrium.

Indications

Counteraction of the endometrial stimulant effects of estrogen in menopausal therapy. Endometriosis. Dysfunctional uterine bleeding. Dysmenorrhea. Amenorrhea. Irregular cycles. Premenstrual syndrome. Habitual abortion.

Dosage

When estrogen is given continuously (in regimens for menopausal therapy), 10 mg dydrogesterone should be taken twice daily for the first 12–14 days of each calendar month. For endometriosis, 10 mg two to three times daily from days 5 to 25 of the menstrual cycle.

Kinetic data

Dydrogesterone is rapidly absorbed after oral administration. It has a plasma half-life of approximately 6 h and is extensively bound (~97%) to plasma proteins. The metabolites of dydrogesterone are excreted primarily in the urine.

Contraindications

Porphyria.

Adverse effects

Breakthrough bleeding.

Estradiol

Mode of action

All estrogens exert their effects through binding to intracellular receptors. The resulting complex then interacts with nuclear sites, leading to DNA-directed protein synthesis and RNA synthesis. The duration of nuclear binding determines the potency of individual estrogens—estradiol has the longest nuclear binding and estriol the shortest. Estradiol suppresses pituitary gonadotropins, increases calcium absorption from the gut while reducing urinary calcium and bone resorption, and induces endometrial mitosis and proliferation. It promotes growth and maintenance of the female reproductive tract and secondary sexual characteristics.

Indications

Treatment of menopausal symptoms and urogenital atrophy and prevention and treatment of postmenopausal osteoporosis. In treatment of estrogen-responsive prostatic cancer where compliance with conventional therapy is questionable, intramuscular injections of a long-acting estradiol, polyestradiol phosphate, are used. The drug is also given for endometrial stimulation during subfertility treatment, either as a preovulatory supplement to ovulation induction agents, or as part of a combined estradiol/progestogen regimen for enhancing endometrial receptivity during elective embryo transfer cycles.

Dosage

The recommended dose regimens for different conditions are detailed in the relevant chapters. The available doses depend on the route of administration. Oral: 1- and 2-mg tablets. Transdermal gel: 2.5 g per application. Transdermal patch: 25, 50, 100 µg/24 h. Subcutaneous implants: 25, 50, 100 mg. Vaginal application: 25, 100 µg.

Kinetic data

Oral micronized estradiol is very well absorbed, maximum blood levels being reached within 0.5 and 5 h, with a return to baseline levels in 24–30 h. Peak blood levels are achieved more slowly but are maintained for a longer time after transdermal or subcutaneous administrations than after oral ingestion. The drug is bound almost completely (98%) to plasma proteins. It is metabolized in the liver to estrone, estriol and their conjugates (glucuronides, sulfates), excreted in urine (about 80%) and, after some enterohepatic circulation, in feces (7–10%).

Contraindications

Untreated endometrial or breast cancer, undiagnosed vaginal bleeding, acute thrombosis and acute liver disease.

Adverse effects

Endometrial hyperplasia.

Interactions

May interact with hepatic enzyme-inducing drugs (e.g. phenytoin).

Ethinylestradiol

Mode of action

Ethinylestradiol is a potent synthetic estrogen, structurally very similar to the (natural) human estrogen, estradiol. It binds to estrogen receptors present in various tissues. Ethinylestradiol causes proliferation of the vaginal mucosa with subsequent cornification and desquamation of the superficial layer. It produces hyperemia and edema in the uterus, together with proliferation and hypertrophy of the endometrial cells. Cervical secretion is also stimulated. Pituitary follicle-stimulating hormone secretion is suppressed via a hypothalamic mechanism. Ethinylestradiol also induces the synthesis of specific proteins, in particular of sex hormone-binding globulin.

Indications

Excessive growth in adolescent girls. Induction of secondary sex characteristics in hypogonadal young girls. Dysfunctional uterine bleeding. Menopausal symptoms. Prostatic and breast cancer. Oral contraception in combination with a progestogen. Acne and hirsuitism in combination with cyproterone acetate.

Dosage

For induction of breast development: 1–2 µg daily initially, increasing gradually to 5, 10 and 15 µg daily. For oral contraception: 20–35 µg (and in a few preparations 50 µg) daily combined with progestogen.

Kinetic data

The drug is rapidly and completely absorbed after oral administration, with an absorption half-life ranging from 12 to 60 min. In most subjects, peak plasma concentrations are reached in 1 h. Owing to pre-systemic metabolism, only about half of the dose is bioavailable in the systemic circulation, but there is wide (10-fold) individual variation in bioavailability. Only a small proportion (5–15%) of the compound is present in unconjugated form in serum, the remainder being conjugated as sulfate. More than 95% of unconjugated ethinylestradiol and all the ethinylestradiol sulfate present in serum is loosely bound to serum albumin. The half-life of elimination varies from 8 to 24 h. About 60% of the dose is excreted in urine, and 40% in feces. Up to 30% is excreted unoxidized but as glucuronide and sulfate conjugates in urine and bile.

Contraindications

See combined oral contraceptives. Pregnancy. Undiagnosed abnormal bleeding from the genital tract. Untreated endometriosis. Thrombophlebitis or thromboembolic disorders. Past or current, cerebrovascular or coronary artery diseases. Suspected or known estrogen-dependent malignant disease. Impaired liver function. Benign or malignant liver tumors.

Adverse effects

Prolonged and continuous use of ethinylestradiol, without cyclical progestogens, may lead to endometrial hyperplasia and (rarely) to endometrial carcinoma. An overdose may cause nausea and vomiting. Men treated for carcinoma of the prostate with ethinylestradiol develop impotence and gynecomastia.

Interactions

Rifampicin, anticonvulsants and some antibiotics (ampicillin, tetracyline, chloramphenicol) reduce plasma levels of ethinylestradiol. Unwanted pregnancies and intermenstrual bleeding can therefore occur in women on oral contraceptives given any of these drugs.

Women over 40 who smoke cigarettes heavily are at increased risk of myocardial infarction if they take combined oral contraceptives, especially if they take preparations containing 50 µg ethinylestradiol a day.

Hormonal preparation	Doses (mg) in UK	Name in UK	Name (or equivalent) in North America
Oral			
Conjugated Equine Estrogen (CEO)	0.625, 1.25, 2.5	Premarin	Premarin
Estradiol (E2)	2	Zumenon	(Estrace)
E2 valerate	1.0, 2.0	Climaval	(Estrace)
	1.0, 2.0	Progynova	(Estrace)
Piperazine Estrone (E1) sulfate	1.5–3.0	Harmogen	Ogen
Estriol (E3)	0.5–3	Ovestin	(Estrovis)
Mixed estrogens	E3 0.27, E1 1.4, E2 0.6	Hormonin	NA
Estrogen–progestogen preparations	CEO 0.625/1.25 + NG	Prempak-C	NA
	E2 valerate 1 + NET 1	Climagest	NA
	E2 valerate 1, 2 + LNg 0.25, 0.5	Cyclo-Progynova	NA
	E2 2/1 + E3 1/0.5 + NET 1 also E2 4/1 + E3 2/0.5 + NET 1	Trisequens	NA
	E2 valerate 2 + LNg 0.75	Nuvelle	NA
	E2 2 + NET	Kliofem	NA
Tibolone	2.5	Livial	NA
Parenteral			
Transdermal E2 patch	0.025, 0.05, 0.1	Estraderm	Estraderm
	0.05	Evorel	Systen
Transdermal E2 gel	2.5	Estrogel	NA
E2 + progestogen patch	E2 0.05 + NET 0.25	Estracombi	NA
E2 implant	25, 50, 100	Estradiol implant	(Estrapel)
E2 patch + oral progestogen	0.05 + NET 1	Estrapak	NA
	0.05 + NET 1	Evorel-Pak	NA
Vaginal estrogens			
CEO cream	0.625	Premarin	Premarin
E3 cream	0.01%	Ortho-Gynest	NA
	0.1%	Ovestin	(Estragard)
Dienestrol cream	0.01%	Ortho Dienoestrol	NA
E2 pessary	0.025	Vagifem	(Estra vaginal)
E3 pessary	0.5	Ortho-Gynest	NA

NG, norgestrel; NET, norethisterone; LNg, levonorgestrel; NA, not available.

Table A2.2
Hormonal preparations used for menopausal therapy.

Etidronate (sodium)

Mode of action

The bisphosphonates decrease bone resorption by inhibiting osteoclast-mediated bone resorption and by slowing the growth and dissolution of hydroxyapatite crystals in bone.

Indications

Osteoporosis where estrogen therapy is contraindicated. Paget's disease of bone. Hypercalcemia of malignancy.

Dosage

Sodium etidronate 400 mg is given on an empty stomach with water for 14 days every 3 months. It is then interspersed with a calcium supplement such as 500 mg of elemental calcium (calcium carbonate 1.25 g) for 10 weeks to complete a cycle of 12 weeks, repeated if necessary indefinitely. To maximize absorption, food, especially if of high calcium content, such as milk and milk products, vitamins with mineral supplements, laxatives containing magnesium and antacids containing aluminum or calcium, should not be taken within 2 h of bisphosphonate therapy.

Kinetic data

Only 1–6% is absorbed (it is highly water soluble). The drug is not metabolized. Its half-life in plasma is about 6 h, 50% of an intravenous dose being excreted in urine within 24 h. Its half-life in bone exceeds 90 days.

Contraindications

Known hypersensitivity to bisphosphonates. Osteomalacia. Severe renal impairment. Hypercalcemia. Hypercalciuria and renal stones. Pregnancy. Lactation.

Adverse effects

Gastrointestinal side-effects are frequent. These include diarrhea, nausea, dyspepsia, flatulence, abdominal pain, constipation and vomiting. Hyperphosphatemia secondary to increased renal tubular phosphate reabsorption has been noted in some patients with no adverse sequelae. Hyperphosphatemia on its own does not justify withdrawal of therapy, as serum phosphate usually returns to normal in these patients within a few weeks, post-therapy. Hypersensitivity reactions, including angio-edema, urticaria, rash and pruritus, and hematological abnormalities (leucopenia, agranulocytosis, pancytopenia) have been reported but these are rare.

Newer preparations of bisphonsphonates such as disodium pamidronate, alendronate, risedronate and tildronate show encouraging results. Mineralization blockade seems not to be a problem with some of the new bisphosphonates.

Interactions

No potentially hazardous interactions have been reported.

Finasteride

Mode of action

Finasteride is a specific inhibitor of the enzyme 5α-reductase, which metabolizes testosterone into the more potent androgen dihydrotestosterone (DHT) within the prostate. By reducing DHT levels, it may lead to a reduction in prostatic volume and also in obstructive symptoms with long-term use.

Indications

Treatment and control of symptomatic benign prostatic hypertrophy and hirsutism. Androgenic alopecia (male pattern baldness).

Dosage

5 mg daily.

Kinetic data

Maximum plasma levels are reached 2 h after a single dose of finasteride, and absorption is complete after

6–8 h. Minute amounts are excreted unchanged in the feces. The drug is extensively metabolized through oxidative pathways and excreted as metabolites: urine 39%, and feces 57%.

Contraindications

Hypersensitivity to finasteride.

Adverse effects and precautions

Less than 5% of men taking finasteride in clinical trials have experienced decreased libido, impotence and a decreased volume of the ejaculate. As finasteride tends to depress the blood level of prostate-specific antigen, new baseline levels should be established for use as a marker of prostatic malignancy. The use of condoms is recommended if a patient's sexual partner is pregnant or likely to become pregnant, as finasteride is excreted in the semen and could be absorbed systemically into mother and fetus. Women of childbearing potential should also avoid handling crushed or broken tablets, in case of systemic absorption via the skin.

Fludrocortisone

Mode of action

Fludrocortisone is a potent mineralocorticoid drug with relatively little glucocorticoid activity. It is used combined with hydrocortisone in the replacement of adrenal steroids in the treatment of primary adrenal insufficiency. The mineralocorticoid activity of fludrocortisone is very high and its anti-inflammatory activity is of no clinical relevance.

Dosage

50–300 mg given in divided doses.

Adverse effects

These include hypertension, sodium and water retention, potassium loss and are most marked with doses in excess of 2 mg a day. Adequacy of fludrocortisone administration may be assessed by estimating plasma renin activity, which should remain in the low normal range. Adequate replacement of fludrocortisone is generally reflected by a rise in plasma renin activity.

Flutamide

Mode of action

Flutamide is a non-steroidal anti-androgen which reduces prostatic weight in animals. It appears to exert an anti-androgenic effect by inhibiting androgen uptake or by blocking cytoplasmic and nuclear binding of androgen to target tissues.

Indications

Treatment of advanced prostatic carcinoma, especially if refractory to conventional hormonal therapy. Prevention of testosterone 'flare' in the first month of treatment of patients with advanced prostatic carcinoma with gonadotropin-releasing hormone agonists. Hirsutism.

Dosage

250 mg three times daily.

Kinetic data

Rapidly absorbed via the gastrointestinal tract and then rapidly metabolized. Plasma levels of flutamide and/or its metabolites are generally maximal from 4 to 6 h after the dose. Excretion occurs mainly via the kidneys.

Contraindications

Hypersensitivity to flutamide.

Adverse effects

Deaths from severe hepatic injury associated with the use of flutamide have been reported. Apart from its possible effect on liver function, flutamide can produce irreversible gynecomastia and breast tenderness in approximately 40% of patients. Nausea and/or diarrhea have been reported in approximately 10% of patients. Liver function tests should be performed before therapy and at 2 and 4 weeks; the drug should be discontinued if signs of liver damage develop.

Interactions

Adjustment of anticoagulant dose may be necessary when flutamide is administered at the same time as warfarin.

Follicle-stimulating hormone (FSH)

Structure

Purified and highly purified preparations of FSH with no luteinizing activity (urofollitrophin) have been derived from postmenopausal urine. r-hFSH, the product of recombinant DNA technology, is now available for clinical use in both males and females. The biochemical purity of r-hFSH is greater than 99%. Highly purified and recombinant FSH are structurally very similar, having specific activities of 10 000 IU FSH/mg protein compared with 150 IU FSH/mg protein for menotropin (hMG).

Mode of action

FSH binds to specific sites within the gonads and produces its effects via a cAMP-linked second messenger system.

Indications

As discussed under Menotrophin (hMG).

Dosage

Currently, clinical trials use 150 IU thrice weekly for induction of spermatogenesis in men, and 75–150 IU daily for ovulation induction.

Kinetic data

Compared with hMG, highly purified and recombinant FSH preparations have the advantage of more consistent bioactivity and composition and of suitability for subcutaneous administration. Both have 75% bioavailability after intramuscular injection, with elimination half-lives of about 36 h for highly purified FSH and 24 h for recombinant FSH. Renal excretion amounts to 12% of total clearance.

Adverse effects

Mild ovarian enlargement and associated abdominal pain. Nausea and vomiting. Skin irritation at the injection site. The serious complications are the ovarian hyperstimulation syndrome and multiple pregnancy. There is no reported increase in the incidence of congenital malformations.

Gonadotropin-releasing hormone—gonadorelin

Gonadotropin-releasing hormone (GnRH) is a synthetic single-chain decapeptide whose structure is identical in all mammalian species studied to date. The molecular configuration, and hence binding characteristics, are dependent on glycine and the amide group at positions 6 and 10 respectively.

Mode of action

The ability of GnRH to initiate follicle-stimulating hormone (FSH) and luteinizing hormone (LH) synthesis and release is dependent on the second and third amino acids, histidine and tryptophan. These effects are mediated by G proteins, which activate second messenger systems, including the breakdown of polyphosphoinositides, producing diaclyglycerol and inositol triphosphate. These in turn activate protein kinase C, calcium mobilization and hence FSH and LH release. GnRH is normally released in 90-min pulses in the human. Hence, in order to stimulate physiological ovarian follicular development, gonadorelin is administered in 90-min pulses by subcutaneous or intravenous injection to increase pituitary gonadotropin release.

Indications

Hypogonadotropic hypogonadism in both sexes. Investigation of anterior pituitary gonadotropic activity.

Dosage

Gonadorelin should be administered by a special syringe pump designed to deliver one pulse every 90 min. The usual therapeutic dose is 50 µg per pulse if the subcutaneous route is used, and 5 µg per pulse for the intravenous route. The dose for testing anterior pituitary function is 100 µg by intravenous injection.

Kinetic data

The plasma half-life of gonadorelin after intravenous injection is approximately 4 min. Eighty per cent of the drug is metabolized in the liver to the 3–10 GnRH octapeptide, which is further degraded into the fragments and probably to the basic amino acids. Ten per cent is degraded to 2–10 GnRH. The remaining 10% is excreted in the urine.

Contraindications

Hypersensitivity to gonadorelin. Undiagnosed vaginal bleeding.

Adverse effects

Local irritation may occur at the injection site. Rarely, hypersensitivity may occur; this is more likely if injections are repeated after an interval free of therapy.

Gonadotropin-releasing hormone agonists

Structure

The gonadotropin-releasing hormone (GnRH) agonists are derived from the GnRH decapeptide but are 150-fold more potent than the endogenous hormone (Table A2.3). Many agonists have been synthesized, replacing 6-glycine with different amino acids (which makes the molecule superactive) and adding an amide group to the end of the molecule to decrease enzymatic degradation.

Mode of action

The majority of GnRH receptors in the pituitary gland are occupied and internalized by GnRH agonists. This results in an initial short-lived surge in plasma gonadotropins. After the initial stimulation phase, GnRH agonists downregulate pituitary gonadotropin production, leading to suppression of gonadotropin secretion. The marked loss of luteinizing hormone receptors results in inability of the pituitary to react either with the agonist or with endogenous GnRH. The pharmacological gonadectomy induced by prolonged GnRH agonist treatment is reversible.

Indications

Gonadotropin-dependent precocious puberty. Endometriosis. Sex hormone-dependent neoplasms (e.g. prostate, breast). Premenstrual syndrome. Induction of ovulation (prior to gonadotropin therapy), especially in women with polycystic ovaries. Controlled ovarian hyperstimulation in assisted reproduction.

Dosage

The different GnRH agonists are available in appropriate syringes for subcutaneous/intramuscular injection and/or as intranasal spray vials. Depot preparations are all highly viscous and need to be administered by a wide needle. Local anesthetic is usually required.

Buserelin is available for intranasal or subcutaneous administration. The initial dose for subcutaneous injection is 500 µg every 8 h, and the maintenance dose 200 µg daily. The recommended intranasal spray dose is 200 µg to each nostril three times daily.

Goserelin is available in a white to cream-colored cylindrical depot containing 3.6 mg of pure peptide base dispersed in a rigid, biodegradable, polymeric matrix approximately 1.2 mm in diameter and 1 cm in length. The depot is supplied in single doses in preloaded syringe applicators.

Leuprorelin (leuprolide) is available as a subcutaneous injection and an intramuscular depot preparation. The recommended dose is 1 mg by daily subcutaneous injection or 7.5 mg monthly by injection.

Nafarelin is available as a nasal spray. The recommended dose is 200 µg twice daily as one spray to one nostril in the morning and one spray to the other nostril in the evening.

Structure	Name	Form of administration
(D-Trp^6)GnRH	Triptorelin	Monthly microcapsule depot
(D-Nal(2)^6)GnRH	Naferelin	Nasal spray 200 µg/metered spray
(D-Leu^6,Pro^{6}NEt) GnRH	Leuprorelin	Monthly microscapule depot 3.75 mg
(D-His(Bz^l)^6,ProNEt) GnRH	Histrelin	Subcutaneous bolus injections
(D-Ser(Bu^t)^6,Pro^{9}NEt) GnRH	Buserelin	Nasal spray 100 µg/metered spray subcutaneous injections
(D-Ser(Bu^t)^6,AzaGly^{10}) GnRH	Goserelin	Monthly polymer implant 3.6 mg

Table A2.3
Commonly used GnRH agonists.

Kinetic data

GnRH agonists are given as intramuscular, subcutaneous or intranasal preparations, since they are poorly absorbed. GnRH itself has a plasma half-life of only a few minutes after intravenous injection, but its analogs are cleared more slowly. The principal site of clearance is the kidney.

Buserelin is rapidly absorbed after intranasal administration, reaching a peak plasma concentration in 20 min. Approximately 2.5% of the dose delivered intranasally is absorbed into the systemic circulation and is excreted in peptide fragments and also unchanged in urine. The drug has a plasma half-life of 3–6 min.

The release rate of goserelin from the depot governs the shape of the serum profile. In patients with normal renal function, the half-life is 4.2 h, compared with 12 h in those with severely impaired renal function. Continuous release of the drug from the depot formulation produces a near-constant serum concentration throughout the 24-h period. There is a gradual rise to a peak concentration over the 2 weeks after each depot administration, with a gradual decline during the next 2 weeks.

After intramuscular or subcutaneous leuprorelin (leuprolide), the drug is released slowly from its biodegradable copolymer vehicle. With a single dose of 7.5 mg intramuscularly, the plasma level averaged 19.9 ng/ml after 4 h, 0.8 ng/ml after 4 days, remained stable for 2.5 weeks, and was undetectable after 8 weeks. The elimination half-life after intravenous injection is about 3 h.

Nafarelin is rapidly absorbed after intranasal administration, reaching a peak plasma concentration in 20 min. The plasma half-life is approximately 4 h. Bioavailability of the intranasal dose ranges from 1.2% to 5.6%. Degradation of the compound is primarily by action of peptidases.

Contraindications

Pregnancy. Breastfeeding. Undiagnosed vaginal bleeding. Hypersensitivity to the agonist.

Adverse effects

Irritation at the site of administration with skin reactions (urticaria, pruritus, rash). Gastrointestinal adverse effects (constipation, vomiting). Bronchospasm.

The initial flare response may exacerbate signs and symptoms of metastatic prostatic cancer. Other side-effects of GnRH agonists are related to their pharmacological action of pituitary suppression and reduced gonadal steroid secretion. The symptoms include hot flashes, night sweats, decreased libido and impotence. Suppression of libido and erection with breast swelling and tenderness may be reported in males. Hot flashes occur in over 50% of patients. Headache is common in children.

Reduced gonadal steroid secretion also induces progressive bone dimineralization and can result in osteoporosis. Hence GnRH agonists should be administered for a maximum of 6 months when treating non-life-threatening conditions. 'Add-back' therapy is therefore applied.

Sneezing during or immediately after dosing may impair absorption, so the dose should then be repeated. Use of a nasal decongestant impairs absorption if used 30 min before nafarelin.

No serious side-effects have been documented during the decade of their use in clinical practice.

Growth hormone

Structure

The active form of human growth hormone (hGH) consists of a single polypeptide chain of 191 amino acids with disulfide linkages between positions 53 and 175 and between 182 and 189. hGH is now produced by recombinant DNA technology and is synthesized in either bacterial or mammalian cell systems.

Mode of action

hGH stimulates skeletal growth and also promotes the growth of all tissues, an effect mediated by the polypeptide 'insulin-like' growth factor (IGF-1) synthesized in the liver. IGF-1 in turn promotes DNA, RNA and protein synthesis, nitrogen and phosphorus retention, amino acid uptake and cell growth. The hormone also exerts direct metabolic effects—on water and electrolytes, on fat metabolism (stimulating lipolysis), on protein metabolism (stimulating protein anabolism) and a diabetogenic effect by direct antagonism of insulin.

Indications

GH deficiency/insufficiency secondary to pituitary dysfunction, Turner's syndrome, Praeder–Willi syndrome in children, chronic renal insufficiency in children, short for gestational age (SGA).

Dosage

Adult growth hormone deficiency: usually 0.2 mg (0.6 IU) to 0.4 mg (1.2 IU) by subcutaneous injection daily. Adjust dose to keep serum IGF-1 in the upper quartile for the age-related usual range.

Kinetic data

A peak serum concentration of 36.9 ng/ml (range 13–61) occurs 3 h after an intramuscular injection of 41 IU/m^2. Subcutaneous injection of this dose produces a lower concentration, but more prolonged—16.4 and 16.3 ng/ml at 4 and 6 h. The elimination half-life after intravenous injection is 18 min.

Contraindications

Active neoplastic disease and actively growing intracranial tumours.

Adverse effects

Abnormalities in thyroid function may develop during treatment. Adjustment of antidiabetic therapy may be necessary. Fluid retention, carpal tunnel syndrome, arturalgia and myalgia may occur with overdosage. Benign intracranial hypertension has been reported.

Interactions

Glucocorticoid replacement therapy may require adjustment. Oral hypoglycemic therapy or insulin therapy may require adjustment.

Human chorionic gonadotropin

Structure

Human chorionic gonadotropin (hCG) is a 38-kDa dimeric glycoprotein secreted by the placenta and extracted from the urine of pregnant women. It is composed of two subunits, α and β. The α subunit is common to follicle-stimulating hormone, luteinizing hormone (LH) and thyroid-stimulating hormone, while the biological activity depends on the β subunit. The latter is structurally related to the β subunit of LH, with which it shares some biological functions.

Mode of action

hCG simulates the action of pituitary LH, binding to LH receptors on gonadal cells and activating cAMP as a second messenger. Because of its greater availability, hCG is used to stimulate the actions of LH. In the female, it promotes follicular rupture (ovulation), mimicking the midcycle LH surge and increasing progesterone production from the corpus luteum. The longer half-life of hCG compared to LH may, however, contribute to multiple pregnancy and the development of the ovarian hyperstimulation syndrome. In the male, hCG stimulates testosterone production from the interstitial cells of the testis.

Indications

The main indications in the female are anovulatory infertility (when it can also be used in combination with an anti-estrogen or hMG to promote follicular rupture). It has also been used, without good evidence of its efficacy, to treat women with habitual abortion, where this is presumed to be secondary to corpus luteum deficiency. In the male, hCG is used to treat hypogonadotrophic hypogonadism and cryptorchidism in children.

Dosage

hCG is administered by intramuscular or deep subcutaneous injection. The usual dose for ovulation induction is a single injection of 5000 units, but smaller amounts—2500, 2000, 1500, 1000 and even 500 units—can be effective, particularly in patients with multi-follicular development. Regimens for the prevention of habitual abortion include 1000–2000 units daily or 5000 units twice weekly. For hypogonadotropic hypogonadism in the male, 2000 units are administered, initially twice or thrice weekly. The dose is then titrated according to the testosterone response.

Hydrocortisone (cortisol)

Mode of action

Acts by binding to the cytoplasmic glucocorticoid receptor (GR) in glucocorticoid-sensitive cells. Cortisol regulates carbohydrate, lipid and protein metabolism, fluid and electrolyte balance and immune reaction to stress. Production is increased in stress.

Indications

As replacement therapy in adrenocortical insufficiency, hypopituitarism and congenital adrenal hyperplasia. Anaphylactic reaction and shock. Exacerbation of inflammatory bowel disease, asthma and connective tissue disorders when oral or intravenous treatment required.

Preparations

Hydrocortisone tablets 10 and 20 mg. Injection. Topical cream. Rectal forms.

Dosage

15–30 mg as replacement therapy, in divided doses. Doses adjusted according to day curve (hydrocortisone levels obtained at different times of day) and patient's own feeling of wellbeing. Dose is increased during illness.

Kinetic data

Readily absorbed from the gut. Peak concentrations are reached in 60 min and half-life is 100 min. Metabolized in the liver.

Contraindications

Infections. May reactivate latent tuberculosis.

Adverse effects

Adrenal suppression. Osteoporosis. Susceptibility to infection. Diabetes mellitus. Fluid retention. Glaucoma. Psychosis. Dyspepsia. In large doses, florid Cushing's syndrome. See also dexamethasone.

Interactions

Increased risk of gastrointestinal hemorrhage with aspirin and NSAIDs. Rifampicin, aminoglutethimide and antiepileptics accelerate metabolism. Hypokalemia with amphotericin.

Ketoconazole

Mode of action

Ketoconazole is an imidazole antifungal agent which interferes with ergosterol synthesis and therefore alters the permeability of the cell membrane of sensitive fungi. It also inhibits gonadal and adrenal steroid production at several points. In the dosage used in gonadotropin-independent precocious puberty, the drug mainly suppresses the enzyme cytochrome P450C17, which regulates both 17α-hydroxylation and the conversion of 17α-hydroxyprogesterone to androstenedione. It also interferes with binding of testosterone to its binding globulin.

Indications

Systemic mycoses and mucocutaneous candidiasis. Gonadotropin-independent precocious puberty. Malignant neoplasm of the prostate. Cushing's syndrome. Malignant neoplasm of the prostate and adrenal cortex. Hirsutism.

Dosage

In the treatment of gonadotropin-independent precocious puberty and hirsutism, the drug has been used at a dose of 200 mg every 8–12 h, orally.

Kinetic data

The absorption of ketoconazole from the gastrointestinal tract is variable and increases with decreasing stomach pH. Peak serum concentrations of ketoconazole occur within 3 h of administration and are proportional to the dose given. The elimination is biphasic, with a terminal half-life of about 8 h. It is mainly metabolized in the liver to inactive metabolites which are excreted together with unchanged drug, mainly in the feces but partly in the urine.

Contraindications

Hepatic impairment. Pregnancy. Breastfeeding. Hypersensitivity to imidazole drugs.

Cautions

Liver function should be monitored regularly. The risk of developing hepatic complaints is greater in patients taking the drug for more than 14 days.

Adverse effects

The most frequent side-effects are nausea, gastrointestinal disturbances, rashes and, less commonly, headache, somnolence and nervous irritability; gynecomastia and angio-edema occur occasionally. In 0.1–1% of patients, ketoconazole produces hepatic dysfunction, which is usually reversible. A few patients have had a severe hepatotoxic reaction, probably an idiosyncratic reaction to the drug.

Interactions

Antacids and H2 antagonists reduced ketoconazole absorption. The combined administration of ketoconazole with anticoagulants (effect of nicoumalone and warfarin enhanced), antiepileptics (plasma ketoconazole concentration reduced by phenytoin), antihistamines (astemizole and terfenadine metabolism inhibited, with risk of cardiac toxicity), cisapride (metabolism inhibited and risk of cardiotoxicity) and cyclosporin (metabolism inhibited) should be avoided. Concomitant use of rifampicin with ketoconazole may reduce blood levels of both drugs. Acute facial flushing and nausea have been reported after concomitant use of alcohol and ketoconazole.

Labetalol

Mode of action

Labetalol hydrochloride demonstrates both α and ß competitive adrenoreceptor blocking properties. It has been used in hypertension, hypertension with agina and hypertension following acute myocardial infarction, as well as in the hypertensive crises associated wth phaeochromocytoma. Unfortunately, in the latter situation it can interfere with laboratory tests (high performance liquid chromatography with electrochemical detection) estimation of plasma and urinary adrenaline.

Dosage

Initially, 100 mg taken twice daily with food, increasing at intervals of several days to 200 mg twice daily, up to a maximum of 800 mg daily in divided doses. Doses of up to 2.5 g a day have been given without major adverse effects.

By intravenous injection, 50 mg may be given over at least 1 min, repeated after 5 min if necessary to a maximum dose of 200 mg.

Excessive bradycardia can be countered with intravenous injection of atropine sulphate 0.6–2.4 mg.

It can also be given by intravenous infusion, usually at a dose of 2 mg min until satisfactory blood pressure control has been achieved.

Adverse effects

Side-effects include postural hypotension (avoid upright positioning during and for 3h after intravenous administration), tiredness, weakness, headache, rashes, scalp tingling, difficulty in micturition, epigastric pain, nausea, vomiting. Liver damage has also been documented.

Lanreotide

Mode of action
Analog of the hypothalamic release-inhibiting hormone somatostatin.

Indications
Relief of symptoms associated with neuroendocrine (particularly carcinoid) tumors and acromegaly.

Dosage
By intramuscular injection initially 30 mg every 14 days, then every 7–10 days according to response. Lanreotide autogel: by deep subcutaneous injection 60 mg monthly, increasing to 90 mg and 120 mg monthly as required.

Cautions
See Octreotide.

Adverse effects
See Octreotide.

Interactions
Absorption of cyclosporin reduced.

Lithium carbonate

Mode of action
Affects transmembrane sodium fluxes or inhibits the formation of second messenger system linked to the turnover of cellular phosphate diinositides. Inhibits adenylate cyclase and prevents thyroid-stimulating hormone or TSAb activating thyroid cells via the thyroid receptor, resulting in impaired release of thyroid hormones from thyroglobulin.

Indications
Manic depression. Unipolar depression. Mania.

In thyrotoxicosis, it is a second-line drug useful for patients who are intolerant or poorly responsive to other treatment. It is not useful for long-term treatment, but can be used to prepare patients for surgery or radio-iodine treatment.

Preparations
Tablets of 200, 250, 400 and 450 mg. Dose adjusted by measuring lithium levels.

Dosage
Narrow therapeutic window, so concentration should be measured regularly. Maintain adequate fluid intake. Usual dose is 300–450 mg thrice daily.

Kinetic data
Well absorbed. Eliminated unchanged in the urine. Half-life varies with age of patient (range 20–36 h). The concentration should be measured.

Contraindications
Caution in cardiac disease, diseases of salt and water regulation, e.g. Addison's disease, pregnancy and myasthenia gravis.

Adverse effects
Gastrointestinal disturbances and fine tremors. Fluid retention. Weight gain. Polyuria and polydipsia. Hypothyroidism. Nephrogenic diabetes insipidus. Leucocystosis. With toxicity, coarse tremors, ataxia and vomiting leading to circulatory failure, coma and death.

Interactions

With diuretics, ACE inhibitors and NSAIDs, increases lithium levels. With aminophylline and antacids, decreases lithium levels. Lithium toxicity reported with metronidazole. Amiodarone increases chances of hypothyroidism.

Neurotoxicity with phenytoin, carbamazepine, methyldopa, verapamil, diltiazem, metoclopramide without an increase in concentration.

Medroxyprogesterone acetate

Structure

Medroxyprogesterone acetate (MPA) is a synthetic progestogen. The depot preparation is an aqueous suspension of MPA (DMPA) at 150 mg/ml.

Mode of action

The drug induces secretory transformation of estrogenized endometrium, so that the menstrual cycle is disrupted.

The depot preparation blocks cervical mucus, produces a progestogenic endometrium and may affect tubal motility. It is absorbed into the circulation and affects more than 50% of cycles, giving rise to either anovulation or corpus luteum inadequacy.

Indications

Dysfunctional uterine bleeding, especially anovulatory. Endometriosis. Contraception (depot injectable preparation lasting 12 weeks). Amenorrhea/oligomenorrhea. Menopausal therapy (in combination with estrogens). Second-line therapy for breast and endometrial cancer.

Dosage

The dose and duration of therapy depend on the indication—10–20 mg daily for 10 days if given in the second half of the cycle, or 21 days if given from day 5 in dysfunctional uterine bleeding. In combined menopausal regimens, 2.5–5 mg daily is given for 12 days per calendar month. Higher doses can be used with menorrhagia or in endometriosis, e.g. 10 mg three times a day. For contraception, 150 mg/ml is given intramuscularly every 10–12 weeks, the first injection to be given within the first 5 days of the cycle. In breast cancer and in the management of endometrial cancer, 400 mg/day is recommended; the doses range from 100 to 500 mg orally daily, or 0.4–1 g per week intramuscularly.

Kinetic data

The drug is absorbed from the gastrointestinal tract, hydroxylated in the liver and excreted mainly in the feces. MPA and/or its metabolites are reported to be excreted in breast milk, but there is no report of harmful effects to the infant.

Plasma levels rise steeply after injection and become effective for ovulation inhibition within 24 h. Levels gradually fall over the next 12 weeks, maintaining contraceptive efficacy until the next injection is due.

Contraindications

Pregnancy, undiagnosed vaginal bleeding, known sensitivity to MPA, impaired liver function, epilepsy, migraine, porphyria or asthma can be aggravated by fluid retention.

Adverse effects

Acne. Fluid retention. Gastrointestinal disturbances.

Interactions

Aminoglutethimide is an anti-steroidogenic drug which increases metabolism of MPA in liver, so doses may need to be increased.

Menotrophin (hMG)

Structure

Menotrophin (hMG) is a purified preparation of gonadotropins extracted from the urine of postmenopausal women. The preparation is an approximate 50/50 mix of luteinizing hormone (LH) and follicle-stimulating hormone (FSH) molecules (chromatofocusing revealed five immunoreactive FSH isohormones and nine LH isohormones). The relative composition and biological activity of hMG preparations can, however, vary significantly from batch to batch. FSH and LH are related glycoproteins, each comprising an α and β subunit linked by a hydrophobic bond. The α subunit is identical in both hormones, while the β subunit conveys their unique biological properties. The β subunits of FSH and LH have 115 amino-acid residues and a molecular weight of 13 000, but differ in the amino acid sequence and in carbohydrate moieties. The half-lives of LH and FSH have been calculated by bioassay as 1 and 3 h respectively. Similar results were obtained using radioimmunoassay—42 and 193 min for LH and FSH, respectively.

Mode of action

Both LH and FSH bind to specific sites within the gonads and produce their effects via a cAMP-linked second messenger system.

Indications

Induction of spermatogenesis in men with hypothalamic/pituitary failure. Induction of ovulation in women with hypogonadotropic hypogonadism. Ovulation or unexplained infertility. Induction of superovulation for in vitro fertilization (IVF) and gamete intrafallopian tube transfer (GIFT).

Dosage

Ampoules of menotrophin are available in two approximate strengths, namely 75 IU each of FSH and LH or 150 IU each of FSH and LH.

Kinetic data

Peak plasma concentrations of LH and FSH after intramuscular injection are seen at 4 and 6 h respectively. The estimated plasma half-lives of LH and FSH after intravenous injection are 20 min and 2 h respectively. The elimination of hMG after intramuscular injection follows a biexponential curve. The initial rapid phase reflects redistribution from serum to other compartments, while the second slower phase corresponds to metabolism and urinary excretion. The elimination half-life of the FSH component of hMG has been estimated as 48 h.

Contraindications

Untreated hyperprolactinemia. Undiagnosed abnormal vaginal bleeding. Hypersensitivity to menotrophin. The drug is ineffective in ovarian dysgenesis and primary gonadal failure. Its administration is not justified in women with infertility due to bilateral tubal disease or male factors, unless as part of an IVF-GIFT regimen.

Adverse effects

Mild ovarian enlargement. Abdominal pain. Nausea. Vomiting. Headache. Skin irritation at the injection site. The serious complications are the ovarian hyperstimulation syndrome and multiple pregnancy. There is no reported increase in the incidence of congenital malformations. Gynecomastia may occur in males as a result of testicular estradiol synthesis stimulated by the LH-like constituents of hMG.

Metformin

Mode of action

Metformin is a biguanide oral anti-hyperglycemic agent. It exerts its effect mainly by decreasing gluconeogenesis and by increasing peripheral utilization of glucose. It acts only in the presence of endogenous insulin, and so it is effective only in diabetics with some residual functioning pancreatic islet cells.

Indications

Non-insulin-dependent diabetes mellitus when diet has failed and especially if the patient is overweight. It is also used when diabetes is inadequately controlled with sulfonylurea treatment.

In insulin-dependent diabetes, metformin may be given as an adjuvant to patients whose symptoms are poorly controlled.

Dosage

500 mg every 8 h or 850 mg every 12 h with or after food.

Kinetic data

Metformin has a plasma half-life of about 3 h and is not bound to plasma proteins. It is excreted unchanged in the urine.

Contraindications

Hepatic or renal impairment. Predisposition to lactic acidosis. Heart failure. Severe infection or trauma. Dehydration. Alcohol dependence. Pregnancy. Breastfeeding.

Adverse effects

Anorexia. Nausea. Vomiting. Diarrhea. Lactic acidosis (withdraw treatment). Decreased vitamin B_{12} absorption.

Metyrapone

Mode of action

This is a competitive inhibitor of 11-ß hydroxylation in the adrenal cortex, resulting in inhibition of cortisol and to a lesser extent aldosterone production. This leads to an increase in ACTH production, which in turn leads to increased synthesis rate of release of cortisol precursors. Metryapone has been found to be helpful in controlling symptoms of Cushing's syndrome. It may be particularly useful in preparation of the patient for surgery. The dosages used are tailored to cortisol production.

Dosage

For the management of Cushing's syndrome, the range of 250 mg–3 g daily, tailored to cortisol production is suggested.

In resistant edema due to increased aldesterone secretion in cirrhosis, nephrotic syndrome and congestive heart failure, 3 g daily in divided doses.

Adverse effects

Occasional nausea, vomiting, dizziness, headache, hypotension, sedation and rarely abdominal pain, allergic skin reactions, hypoadrenalism and hirsutism. Caution is indicated in patients suffering from hypopituitarism, and patients may develop hypertension on long-term administration. Dosage may have to be adjusted in hypothyroidism or hepatic impairment, where there is a delayed response. Its use may interfere with diagnostic evaluation of steroid related disorders. It should be avoided in porphyria. Drowsiness may affect the performance of skilled tasks, e.g. driving.

Mitotane (o'p'-DDD)

Mode of action

Mitotane is an antineoplastic agent with a selective inhibitory action on adrenal cortex activity.

Indications

Treatment of inoperable adrenocortical tumors. Also used in patients with Cushing's syndrome.

Dosage

Initial dose is 2–6 g daily by mouth in three or four divided doses, adjusted to the maximum tolerated dose, which may range from 2 to 16 g daily.

Kinetic data

Up to 40% of mitotane is absorbed from the gastrointestinal tract. It is metabolized in the liver and other tissues and excreted as metabolites in urine and bile.

Contraindications

Give with care to patients with liver disease.

Adverse effects

Anorexia, nausea, vomiting, diarrhea. About 40% suffer some central toxicity with dizziness, vertigo, sedation, lethargy and mental depression. Permanent brain damage may occur with prolonged use. Ocular side-effects such as blurred vision, diploplia and retinopathy.

Adrenal insufficiency may develop during treatment; concomitant corticosteroid therapy is often required.

Norethisterone

Mode of action

Norethisterone (NET), a synthetic progestogen, exerts its biological activity mainly by interaction with receptors in various tissues, principally those of the reproductive tract, liver and brain. In some tissues, particularly the endometrium, the progesterone receptor to which NET binds is estrogen induced. Its binding affinity to endometrial receptors is similar to that of progesterone itself. Like progesterone, NET will produce secretory changes in estrogen-primed endometrium and affect the activity of many enzymes.

Indications

With an estrogen in some combined oral contraceptives or menopausal preparations. Given alone for contraception (a progestogen-only pill), metropathia hemorrhagica (cystic glandular hyperplasia), postponement of menstruation, endometriosis, menorrhagia, dysfunctional uterine bleeding, hormone replacement therapy and malignant disease.

Dosage

For contraception, see individual preparations (Table A2.1).

For endometriosis, 10–15 mg/day for 4–6 months or longer, starting on day 5 of the cycle.

Kinetic data

NET is absorbed from the gastrointestinal tract and is then rapidly and widely distributed throughout body tissues, with the highest levels accumulating and being metabolized in liver, kidney, intestine and bile. Its effects last for at least 24 h. It is excreted in urine, the elimination half-life varying from 5 to 12 h, with a mean of 7.6 h.

Contraindications

Pregnancy. Severe disturbances of liver function. Porphyria. Current suspicion of thrombosis. Whether a past history of thrombosis is also a contraindication is debatable.

Adverse effects

Breakthrough bleeding. Aggravation of epilepsy. Liver disturbances. Jaundice. Migraine. Nausea. Depression. Bloating. Breast tenderness. Tendency to increase LDL and to lower HDL if used continuously.

Interactions

Many of the drug interactions described with oral contraceptives are considered to be due to the estrogen component; knowledge of the separate effects of progestogens is limited. Important interactions of NET are with rifampicin and penicillins, which reduce its contraceptive effect. Breakthrough bleeding may then occur.

Norethisterone enanthate

Structure

This is a long-acting ester of NET given as an oily solution by injection which provides contraception for 8 weeks.

Mode of action

The drug thickens cervical mucus, suppresses the endometrium and may cause anovulation or corpus luteum inadequacy in up to 50% of cycles.

Dosage

150 mg given by deep intramuscular injection. The vial has to be warmed before being drawn up, due to the viscosity of the oil; otherwise, a significant proportion of the injectable material will be left behind in the phial. Once the injection has been given, either in the gluteal region or upper arm, the injection site should not be massaged, as this will disperse the progestogen.

Kinetic data

Plasma levels, above those required for ovulation inhibition, are seen within a few hours of injection and maintained for at least 8 weeks.

Contraindications

As for MPA.

Adverse effects

The main side-effect is that of irregular bleeding, giving rise to intermenstrual bleeding, spotting, prolonged bleeding or amenorrhea.

Interactions

None known.

Norgestimate

Mode of action

Norgestimate is an orally active progestational steroid which has a strong binding affinity for the progesterone receptor but low androgenicity. A number of its metabolites—principally 17-diacetylnorgestimate, 3-ketonorgestimate and levonorgestrel—have equal binding affinity for the progesterone receptor. Norgestimate has a low binding affinity to sex hormone-binding globulin.

Indications

Oral contraception.

Dosage

250 μg in combination with 35 μg ethinylestradiol.

Kinetic data

Norgestimate is rapidly absorbed after oral ingestion, with peak plasma concentrations occurring by 1 h. It is bound principally to plasma proteins. The drug is metabolized in the gut wall and liver. Its metabolites are excreted by the kidneys and bowel.

Contraindications

As for norethisterone.

Adverse effects

As for norethisterone.

Interactions

As for norethisterone.

Octreotide

Mode of action

Octreotide is an analog of the hypothalamic release-inhibiting hormone somatostatin.

Indications

Symptoms associated with carcinoid tumors with features of carcinoid syndrome. VIPomas. Glucagonomas. Acromegaly. Prevention of complications following pancreatic surgery.

Dosage

Initially, 50 μg by subcutaneous injection once or twice daily, gradually increased according to response to 200 μg three times daily; maintenance dose variable.

For acromegaly, 100–200 μg by subcutaneous injection, three times daily. Octreotide LAR, initially 20 mg by intramuscular injection every 4 weeks for 3 months, increasing to 30 mg every 4 weeks if indicated.

Kinetic data

Octreotide is rapidly absorbed following subcutaneous injection, with a plasma half-life of about 1.5 h.

Cautions

In insulinoma, exacerbation of hypoglycemia may occur. Pregnancy and breastfeeding.

Monitor thyroid function with long-term therapy. Ultrasound examination of the gall bladder before starting treatment and at intervals of 6–12 months.

Adverse effects

Gastrointestinal disturbances. Persistent hyperglycemia may occur with chronic administration, and hypoglycemia has also been reported. Gallstones occur in ~25% of patients. Altered liver function tests, hepatitis, pancreatitis occur rarely. Local reaction at the site of injection.

Interactions

Absorption of cyclosporin reduced. Increased concentration of bromocriptine. Absorption of cimetidine possibly delayed. Possibly reduces insulin and antidiabetic drug requirements in diabetes mellitus.

Pamidronate disodium

Mode of action

This drug is a bisphosphonate, an inhibitor of osteoclastic bone resorption.

Dosage

By slow intravenous infusion. Hypocalemia of malignancy, according to serum calcium level. 15–60 mg in single dose or in divided doses over 2–4 days. Osteolytic lesions and bone pain in bone metastases, 90 mg every 4 weeks. Paget's disease of bone, 30 mg once a week for 6 weeks or 30 mg in the first week, then 60 mg alternate weeks to a maximum total 360 mg - may be repeated every 6 months.

Pergolide

Mode of action

Pergolide is a dopamine agonist with prolonged duration of action, which has been used both in the treatment of hyperprolactinemia and in Parkinson's disease.

Dosage

50 mg at night on day 1, very gradually increasing to a dose of between 100 and 200 mg a day.

Adverse effects

These include hallucinations, confusion, dizziness, dyskinesia, drowsiness, abdominal pain, nausea, vomiting, dyspepsia, diplopia, rhinitis, dyspnea, pleuritis and pleural effusion. Pleural fibrosis, pericarditis, pericardial effusion and retroperitoneal fibrosis have also been documented with this drug. Insomnia, constipation or diarrhea, hypotension, syncope, tachycardia and atrial premature contractions, rash and fever have also been reported, as has the neuroleptic malignant syndrome. The drug should be used with caution in patients who have arrhythmia or underlying cardiac disease or a history of confusion or hallucination. It should not be given in patients with porphyria. Hypotensive reaction may occur, in most patients during the first few days of treatment, and particular care should be exercised when driving or operating machinery. The dosage is titrated according to the prolactin response.

Phenoxybenzamine

Mode of action

Phenoxybenzamine is a non-competitive $\alpha 1/\alpha 2$ adrenoreceptor-blocking drug, useful in the treatment of hypertensive episodes in pheochromocytoma, and also in medical therapy of pheochromocytoma while awaiting surgery or in malignant pheochromocytoma.

Dosage

10 mg daily initially, increasing to 1–2 mg/kg daily in two divided doses.

Phenoxybenzamine may also be given intravenously, preferably through a large vein, the usual dose being 0.5 mg/kg daily in 200 ml of physiological saline over

2h. This may be repeated daily for three consecutive days prior to any surgical or invasive procedure.

Contraindications

Renal impairment. To be avoided in porphyria and to avoid extravasation, as this may be irritant to tissues.

Adverse effects

Postural hypotension with dizziness and marked compensatory tachycardia, lassitude, nasal congestion, miosis, inhibition of ejaculation and rarely gastrointestinal disturbances. There may be decreased sweating and a dry mouth after intravenous infusion and an idiopathic profound hypertension can occur within a few minutes of starting an infusion.

Phentolamine (mesylate)

Mode of action

Phentolamine mesylate is a short-acting, competitive α-adrenoreceptor antagonist. It also has an intrinsic vasodilating action, independent of α-blockade. It induces smooth muscle relaxation, which results in reduced peripheral resistance and increased venous capacitance. Additionally, phentolamine acts as a weak antagonist of 5-hydroxytryptamine and releases histamine from mast cells.

Indications

Hypertensive episodes due to pheochromocytoma.

Dosage

2–5 mg by intravenous injection, repeated as necessary.

Kinetic data

The drug is 54% plasma protein bound and has a plasma half-life of 90 min, although the hemodynamic effect is more prolonged, lasting for up to 12 h.

Contraindications

Hypotension. Ischemic heart disease.

Adverse effects

Flushing and tachycardia, postural hypotension, congestion, prolonged hypotension.

Prednisolone

This has predominantly glucocortical activity and is the corticosteroid most commonly used by mouth for long term disease suppression.

Dosage

This can vary, anything from 2.5 to 80 mg per day orally.

Adverse effects

These include diabetes and osteoporosis, which may be particularly problematic in elderly people, where it may result in osteoporotic fractures, for example of the hip or vertebrae. High doses are also associated with avascular necrosis of the femoral head. Mental disturbance can occur, leading to a paranoid state or indeed depression with risk of suicide. Euphoria may also be observed. Muscle-wasting, particularly proximal myopathy, may also occur and corticosteroid therapy with prednisolone is also weakly linked with peptic ulceration. High doses lead to Cushing's syndrome, with moon-face, striae and acne, usually reversible on withdrawal of treatment, but this must be always tapered gradually to avoid symptoms of acute adrenal insufficiency. In children, administration of corticosteroids may result in suppression of growth. Patients on long-term prednisolone should carry a steroid treatment card. If necessary, a Medicalert bracelet should be used.

Indications

Suppression of inflammation and allergic disorders (e.g. malignant ophthalmic Graves' disease).

Adverse effects

These are minimized by using lowest effective doses for minimum period of time. Gastro-intestinal side-effects include dyspepsia, peptic ulceration, abdominal distension, acute pancreatitis, esophageal ulceration and candidiasis. **Musculoskeletal** effects include proximal myopathy, osteoperosis, vertebral and long bone fractures, avascular osteonecrosis, tendon rupture. **Endocrine** effects include adrenal suppression, menstrual irregularities, hirsutism, weight gain, negative nitrogen and calcium balance, increased appetite, increased susceptibility to and severity of infection. **Neuropsychiatric** effects include euphoria, psychological dependence, depression, insomnia, increased intracranial pressure with papilledema (particularly in children), psychosis and aggravation of schizophrenia. **Ophthalmic** effects include glaucoma, papilledema, posterior subcapsular cataracts, corneal or scleral thinning, exacerbation of ophthalmic viral or fungal disease. Other side-effects include impaired healing, skin atrophy, bruising, striae, telangiectasia, acne, myocardial rupture following recent myocardial infarction, fluid and electrolyte disturbance, leucocytosis. Prednisolone is contraindicated during systemic infection unless specific antimicrobial therapy has been given. Live virus vaccines should be avoided in those receiving immunosuppression. Appropriate monitoring is required if history of tuberculosis is present.

Progestogen-only oral contraceptives

Structure

Four progestogens are available as oral progestogen-only preparations—norethisterone, norgestrel, levonorgestrel and etynodiol diacetate. Of these, levonorgestrel and etynodiol diacetate are metabolized to norethisterone after absorption from the gut, which effectively reduces the choice of preparations to two.

Mode of action

The principal mechanism of action of a progestogen-only pill is on corpus luteum function, where it reduces progesterone secretion. There is also a variable effect on follicle-stimulating hormone and luteinizing hormone production, indicating a degree of pituitary inhibition, but, in contrast to the effects of combined oral contraceptives (COCs), the pituitary still responds to gonadotropin-releasing hormone. The variable suppression of ovarian activity observed in progestogen-only users has led to the suggestion that suppression of progesterone synthesis may be a function of the intrinsic enzyme activity of a particular corpus luteum. A detailed study of hormonal changes in women taking 300 µg norethisterone has shown four main patterns of ovarian response: the changes were similar to those seen in a normal ovulatory cycle in 40%, there was normal follicular but reduced luteal function in 21%, normal or increased follicular activity but with no luteal function in 23%, and no follicular or luteal activity in the remaining 16%.

The progestogen-only pill has additional actions, which contribute to its contraceptive effect. Tubal motility and the rate of ovum transport are altered, fertilization and the capacitation of spermatazoa may be affected, proliferative activity of the endometrium is suppressed, and the number and size of endometrial glands is reduced. The amount of cervical mucus is also less, and it becomes more viscous.

Indications

A progestogen-only oral contraceptive produces reversible contraception, useful for both spacing and completed families. This pill is indicated for any woman who cannot take an estrogen-containing contraceptive, or who prefers tablets to other delivery systems for contraception.

The method is particularly indicated for:

- smokers over the age of 35
- diabetic women
- women with hypertension
- women with migraine
- women with sickle cell disease
- women with a history of thromboembolism
- during lactation.

Although small amounts of progestogen are excreted in breast milk, the concentrations are small and apparently have no significant effect on the infant. Concentrations of progestogen in breast milk are lower after levonorgestrel than after the other preparations. A progestogen-only pill has no effect on the volume or quantity of breast milk.

Progestogen	Name	Dose (mg)	Number of pills per packet
Levonorgestrel	Norgeston/Microval	30	35
Norgestrel	Neogest[a]	75	35
Norethisterone	Micronor/Noriday	350	28
Etynodiol diacetate	Femulen	500	28

[a]Contains 37.5 of active isomer.

Table A2.4
Progestogen-only pills.

Dosage

Table A2.4 indicates the daily dose of the progestogen-only pill and the number of tablets per packet. One tablet is taken every day. Because plasma levels of the progestogen are much lower at the end of the 24-h period after ingestion, it is important to take the pill at the same time each day and to time ingestion of the pill in relation to normal sexual activity, so that the pill is taken 2 h before intercourse or when intercourse is likely to occur.

In menstruating women, the progestogen-only pill should be started on the first day of the cycle, and additional barrier contraception should be used for the first 7 days of the initial cycle. It must be emphasized to the patient that if she forgets to take the pill, even by as little as 3 h, or if its absorption is impaired in any way, as may occur after diarrhea or vomiting, then an additional method, e.g. a barrier method, should be used until unimpaired activity of the progestogen-only pill is possible. Any additional contraceptive measure should be continued for at least 7 days.

Kinetic data

The progestogens used in the progestogen-only contraception formulations have a pharmacokinetic profile which give plasma levels above those required to block cervical mucus and affect endometrial activity within 2 h of ingestion. The resultant impermeability wears off some 22 h later. Provided a daily dose of the progestogen is then taken, blood levels are thus generally adequate to maintain an endometrial and cervical mucus effect over 24 h. There are, however, wide inter-subject variations, which is why timing of ingestion is so critical.

Contraindications

Undiagnosed pregnancy. Undiagnosed abnormal genital tract bleeding. Severe arterial disease. Severe liver disease. Porphyria. After evacuation of hydatidiform mole until gonadotropin levels have returned to normal. History of breast and genital tract carcinoma.

Those with a family history of arterial disease and hypertension have not been found to experience increased vascular problems after progestogen-only oral contraception, presumably due to the low dose of medication. They need not therefore be discouraged from using this method of contraception if they wish to do so.

Adverse effects

The main adverse effect—as with all types of progestogen-only contraceptives—is menstrual irregularity. This irregularity consists of intermenstrual spotting or bleeding and episodes of delayed periods or prolonged bleeding. Provided the patient is adequately counseled, this is seen as a nuisance side-effect rather than a serious problem. If delayed periods occur, pregnancy has to be excluded. Breast discomfort can occur together with some weight changes, but these are minimal, due to the low dose of the progestogen. Skin disorders such as acne have been reported. If depression occurs, it is more likely to be associated with a pre-existing depression rather than to the pill per se. Loss of libido may be a problem, but nausea, vomiting and headache are much less than with a COC.

Interactions

There is no enterohepatic circulation of progestogen. Antibiotics do not therefore interfere with the efficacy of the preparation. Conversely, liver enzyme inducers increase the metabolism of the progestogen-only pill, and women taking an enzyme inducer should use additional precautions, as with the COCs. Although the data sheets recommend caution in regard to drug interaction with anticonvulsant therapy and antibiotics, there is little evidence that severe drug interaction occurs with the low dose in the progestogen-only contraceptives.

Propranolol

Mode of action

Blocks both β_1- and β_2-adrenoreceptors. Decreases conversion of T4 to T3.

Indications

Hypertension. Angina. Post-myocardial infarction. Anxiety. Arthrymias. Migraine. Thyrotoxicosis. Essential tremors.

Preparations

10-, 40- and 80-mg tablets. 80- and 160-mg long-acting capsules. Also available in combination with other drugs.

Dosage

20–160 mg daily in divided doses, although a long-acting modified preparation is available.

Kinetic data

Almost completely absorbed orally. Peak plasma concentration at 2 h with tablets, but longer with modified-release capsules. It is lipid soluble and therefore crosses the blood–brain barrier. Metabolized in the liver and excreted via urine.

Contraindications

Cardiac failure. Asthma and chronic airflow limitation. Peripheral vascular disease. Bradycardia. Hypotension. Sick sinus syndrome. Pheochromacytoma, unless given with α-blocker.

Adverse effects

Exacerbation of asthma. Hypotension. Bradycardia. Heart failure. Conduction disorders. Fatigue. Erectile dysfunction. Worsening of psoriasis. Gastrointestinal disturbances.

Interactions

All drugs causing hypotension and bradycardia. Verapamil and amiodarone important. Vasoconstriction with ergots. Cimetidine and rifampicin increase concentration.

Propylthiouracil

Mode of action

Reduces thyroid hormone synthesis by inhibiting iodine organification and iodotyrosyl coupling, by inhibiting the enzyme thyroid peroxidase. It also has an immunosuppressive effect. Also inhibits peripheral conversion of T4 to T3.

Indications

Hyperthyroidism (especially Graves' disease), to prepare for thyroidectomy. This is the more popular drug in North America.

Preparations

50-mg tablets.

Dosage

Initially 300–600 mg until patient is euthyroid, and gradually reduced to a maintenance dose of 50–150 mg for 18 months.

Kinetic data

Half-life is 75 min.

Contraindications and adverse effects

As for carbimazole, except less excretion in breast milk.

Quinagolide

Mode of action

Quinagolide is a non-ergot selective dopamine D_2 receptor agonist with weak D_1 agonist potency. It exerts a strong inhibitory effect on prolactin secretion. In some patients, the drug may also induce short-lasting small increases in human growth hormone; growth hormone levels may also remain normal or suppressed.

Indications

Hyperprolactinemia.

Dosage

Treatment should be initiated with 25 μg daily for the first 3 days and then 50 μg daily for a further 3 days. From day 7 onwards, the recommended dose is 75 μg daily. The long half-life allows single daily dosing, preferably in the middle of the evening meal. In clinical studies, the dose has ranged from 75 to 1000 μg daily. A definite dose–response relationship has been established for duration, but not for magnitude of prolactin-lowering effect, which, with a single oral dose of 50 μg, was close to maximum.

Kinetic data

Quinagolide is rapidly and well absorbed. It undergoes extensive first-pass metabolism, with more than 95% of the drug excreted as metabolites, with equal amounts in urine and feces. The principal metabolites in blood are N-desethyl and N,N-didesethyl analogs, both compounds possessing biological activity qualitatively similar to that of the parent drug. The elimination half-life of quinagolide is 11.5 h after a single dose and 17 h at a steady state; its protein binding is approximately 90%.

Contraindications

Hypersensitivity to quinagolide. Impaired hepatic and renal function. Caution is required in patients with a history of psychosis, severe cardiovascular disease, peptic ulceration or other gastrointestinal bleeding. Since fertility may be restored with quinagolide therapy, sexually active women who do not wish to conceive should take contraceptive precautions.

Adverse effects

These are those characteristic of dopamine receptor agonists—nausea, vomiting, dizziness, drowsiness, headache and hypotension. They occur predominantly during the first few days of therapy and usually disappear with time. Psychosis may be a particular problem with quinagolide, in view of the potency of its interaction with the D_2 receptor. Significant weight loss has been reported in some patients.

Interactions

Care should be taken when using quinagolide concomitantly with drugs known to have an effect on $5-HT_1$ and $5-HT_2$ receptors. The tolerability of quinagolide may be reduced by alcohol.

Raloxifene

Licensed for the treatment and prevention of post-menopausal osteoperosis. Unlike hormone replacement therapy, raloxifene does not reduce menopausal vasomotor symptoms and in this regard differs from tibolone. It may reduce the incidence of estrogen-receptor positive breast cancer but its role in established breast cancer has not been established as yet. Currently, it is not advised that this drug should be used in breast cancer.

Mode of action

Raloxifene is a selective estrogen-receptor modulator and has been shown to be valuable in the treatment of post-menopausal bone osteoporosis. It has been shown to reduce vertebral fracture risk in elderly post-menopausal women also.

Dosage

61–120 mg daily, reduced significantly the incidence of new vertebral compression fractures. This anti-fracture benefit was seen in groups of women who entered the trial, with or without prevalent vertebral compression fractures. Because an average woman on this trial had T scores ≤2.5 SDs, the raloxifene data suggests that women who have osteoperosis by BMD criteria may benefit more from intervention. The raloxifene trial was not powered for the analysis of hip fracture and the number of hip fractures were small and not significantly different from the placebo group.

Contraindications

History or venous thromboembolism, undiagnosed uterine bleeding, endometrical cancer, hepatic impairment, cholestasis, severe renal impairment, pregnancy and breastfeeding.

Adverse effects

Venous thromboembolism, thrombophlebitis, hot flushes, leg cramps, peripheral edema, influenza-like symptoms, rarely rashes and gastrointestinal disturbances.

Recombinant human thyroid-stimulating hormone (TSH)

Now approved for use in the United Kingdom and United States for use in humans, rTSH facilitates postoperative management of patients with thyroid carcinoma, when therapy doses of ^{131}I are indicated. In clinical trials, the drug has been very effective and in patients with suppressed TSH levels, two daily 0.9 mg injections stimulated thyroidal ^{131}I uptake and thyroglobulin secretion to a degree equal to 2–3 weeks of hormone withdrawal. The results of whole body scanning performed after human rTSH and after thyroxine withdrawal have shown very good, but not perfect, concordance between the two techniques.

Adverse effects

These are minimal, and no anti-TSH antibody formation has been detected, at least in the short term. Treatment therefore allows stimulation of ^{131}I uptake and thyroglobulin secretion without the induction of hypothyroidism which will make ^{131}I whole body scanning and TG testing more acceptable to patients and doctors.

Risedronate
Mode of action

Risedronate is a biphosphonate, which is used in the treatment of osteoporosis. It is absorbed onto hydroxyapatite crystals, so slowing both their rate of growth and dissolution and reducing the increased rate of bone turnover associated with the disease.

Indications and dosage

In Paget's disease of bone, 30 mg daily for 2 months. May be repeated if necessary after at least 2 months.

For treatment and prevention of osteoporosis (including corticosteroid induced osteoporisis) in postmenopausal women, 5 mg daily.

The patient should be counseled to swallow tablets whole, with a full glass of water. On rising, take on an empty stomach at least 30 min before the first food or drink of the day, if taken at any other time of the day, avoid food and drink for at least 2 h before and after risedronate, particularly avoiding calcium-containing products, such as milk and also avoiding iron and mineral supplements and antacids. The patient should sit or stand upright for at least 30 min and not take any tablets at bedtime or before rising.

Contraindications

Hypocalcaemia, pregnancy and breastfeeding.

Adverse effects

Gastro-intestinal effects, including dyspepsia, nausea, diarrhea, constipation, esophageal stricture and duodenitis have been documented. Headache, musculoskeletal pain, rarely glossitis, edema, weight loss, apnea, bronchitis, sinusitis, rash, nocturia, amblyopia, corneal lesions, dry eyes, tinnitis, iritis have been documented.

Sildenafil

Sildenafil citrate is licensed for the treatment of erectile dysfunction and is orally active. Before its prescription, a full assessment should be carried out. Sildenafil has the potential for multiple drug interactions and should not be used on anyone receiving nitrates.

Indications

Erectile dysfunction.

Dosage

Initially 50 mg (in the elderly, 25 mg) taken approximately 1h before sexual activity and subsequent doses adjusted accordingly to the response, from 25 to 100 mg as a single dose. The maximum single dose is 100 mg per 24 hours. The onset of effect may be delayed if it is taken with food.

Adverse effects

Dyspepsia, headache, flushing, dizziness, visual disturbances and increased intraocular pressure and nasal congestion. Hypersensitive to reaction, including rash, priapism and painful red eyes have been reported. Serious cardiovascular events have been reported, particularly in those with severe late cardiac disease and it is strictly contraindicated with nitrates. Caution is advised with cardiovascular disease and in anatomical deformities of the penis (angulation, cavernosal fibrosis and Peyronie's disease). Predisposition to prolonged erection, as in sickle cell anemia, multiple myeloma and leukemia are also relative contraindications.

Sodium ipodate

Mode of action

Inhibits synthesis and release of iodine from the thyroid gland.
 Continued administration for more than a few weeks leads to escape from this block, and therefore it is only useful for short periods.

Indications

To prepare for thyroid surgery. Thyroid storm (thyrotoxic crisis). Originally used as oral cholecystographic agent.

Dosage

500 mg per day orally or single dose of 1 g.

Kinetic data

Following absorption from the gastrointestinal tract, sodium ipodate appears in the bile, where the concentration is such that the biliary tract can be examined radiographically. It is excreted mainly in the urine.

Contraindications

Pregnancy. Breastfeeding. Caution in children. Known allergy.

Adverse effects

Hypersensitivity reaction, including headache and flu-like symptoms. Depression and insomnia on prolonged treatment.

Interactions

Hypersensitivity reactions can be aggravated in patients on β-blockers.

Spironolactone

Mode of action

Aldosterone antagonist, with a steroid-like structure.

Indications

Edema and ascites in cirrhosis of the liver. Congestive cardiac failure. Primary hyperaldosteronism. Hirsutism.

Dosage

100–200 mg daily. Increase to 400 mg if necessary.

Adverse effects

Gastrointestinal disturbances. Gynecomastia. Hyperkalemia. Impotence.

Contraindications and interactions

Concurrent administration of ACE inhibitors, amiloride, triamterene and carbenoxolone should be avoided. Spironolactone synergizes with lithium in manic patients. Patients taking both spironolactone and digoxin show an increase in plasma digoxin, because spironolactone inhibits the tubular secretion of digoxin. Should not be used in Addison's disease, or in severe renal impairment.

Testosterone

Mode of action

Testosterone acts directly on target tissues by binding to specific androgen receptors. The androgen receptor complex is then internalized and binds to chromatin, initiating transcription of specific structural genes. A proportion of its androgenic activity in certain target tissues is mediated by conversion to DHT by 5α-reductase.

Indications

Male hypogonadism, delayed puberty and postmenopausal breast carcinoma. Some esters are being tested as male contraceptives.

Dosage

For adult replacement therapy: testosterone undecanoate 40–80 mg thrice daily orally.

Depot preparations: 250 mg intramuscularly every 3 weeks or 100 mg weekly (Sustanon).

Cutaneous patches. Testoderm—the patch (5 mg) is applied each morning to a clean, dry, shaved area of scrotal skin. Andropatch (2.5, 5 mg) —applied to non-pressure-bearing areas of the skin each night. Viromone (5 mg) applied to non-pressure-bearing areas of the skin each morning. Androgel ia a 100% testosterone gel for skin application, applied once daily.

In delayed puberty: a mixture of testosterone propionate, testosterone phenylpropionate and testosterone isocaproate can be given monthly, by deep intramuscular injection, or oral testosterone undecanoate (40 mg daily) can be given to initiate secondary sexual characteristics, with a gradual increase in dose to mimic the normal timescale of puberty. The usual adult replacement dose is 250 mg intramuscularly every 3 weeks. Subcutaneous implants of testosterone effective for about 4 months (400–600 mg) may also be introduced through a trocar/cannula system. Individual patient dosage requirements vary greatly, and careful monitoring of serum testosterone levels is required, with titration of dosage and frequency accordingly.

Kinetic data

Testosterone is 98% plasma protein bound (to albumin and sex hormone-binding globulin), with the albumin-bound portion readily interchangeable across the capillary membrane. Testosterone is well absorbed orally, but is almost entirely cleared by first-pass metabolism, with 90% of metabolites excreted in the urine. Even intramuscular administration results in a rapid decline of serum levels. For androgen substitution therapy, modifications such as esterification and alkylation have been made to the molecule. These compounds are hydrolysed in the liver, yielding testosterone and, when given by intramuscular injection, they are also released more slowly. The depot injection contains a mixture of propionate, phenylpropionate, isocaproate and decanoate esters. Peak plasma levels occur at 4–5 days and decay to baseline over the next 21 days. Testosterone undecanoate is effective orally due to absorption via the lymphatics, thus avoiding hepatic first-pass metabolism. Peak levels occur 2–6 h after administration, and levels return to baseline at 10–12 h.

Testosterone is well absorbed from genital skin; hence the rationale of using Testoderm. The release is 3.6 mg/24 h: peak levels occur after 2 h, and levels thereafter decline gradually over the next 20 h.

Contraindications

Breast cancer in men. Prostatic cancer. Hypercalcemia. Pregnancy (risk of virilization of a female fetus).

Breast-feeding. Nephrosis. Testosterone should be used cautiously in patients with cardiovascular disorders, renal and hepatic impairment, epilepsy, migraine, diabetes mellitus and other conditions that can be aggravated by possible fluid retention or edema.

Adverse effects

Sodium retention with edema and hypercalcemia. Increased bone maturation. Premature sexual maturation. Early closure of epiphyses in pre-pubertal boys. Priapism. Virilization in women. Suppression of spermatogenesis in men. Raising levels above the physiological range may lead to edema and cause exacerbation of aggressive personality traits.

Thyroxine

Mode of action

Thyroid hormones bind to nuclear thyroid hormone receptors and regulate gene transcription.

Indications

Neonatal hypothyroidism. Deficiency of thyroid hormones, due to disease or iatrogenic causes. To suppress thyroid-stimulating hormone (TSH) secretion after thyroidectomy for thyroid cancer. Thyroxine is *not* indicated for slimming. Its use in shrinking goiter is controversial.

Preparations

25-, 50- and 100-μg tablets. In North America, tablets are available in multiple doses.

Dosage

Usually 100–200 μg daily, adjusted to keep TSH within the lower end of the normal range. However, after thyroid cancer, the dose is maintained to suppress TSH. In the elderly and patients with cardiac disease, treatment should start with very small doses (e.g. 25 μg daily or 50 μg on alternate days), and these should be gradually increased. Increments should be made every 4 weeks.

Kinetic data

50–80% absorbed in the small intestine. Absorption is increased by an empty stomach and decreased by sulcralfate, cholestyramine, iron and aluminum hydroxide. It has an elimination half-life of 6–7 days, and is cleared by the liver. Clearance is increased by thyrotoxicosis.

Contraindications

Thyrotoxicosis (except as block and replacement therapy). In Addison's disease, steroid replacement should be initiated before starting thyroxine.

Adverse effects

Those of overdose.

Interactions

No specific interactions, but may increase clearance of many drugs, including propranolol. Rifampicin, carbamazepine, phenytoin and phenobarbitone accelerate metabolism of thyroxine and may increase requirement. The effect of warfarin is enhanced.

Tibolone

Mode of action

A gonadomimetic steroid with both central and peripheral mechanisms of action. It suppresses serum follicle-stimulating hormone (and to a lesser degree, luteinizing hormone) but stimulates β-endorphin levels, which probably explains it beneficial effects on mood. The drug and its metabolites exhibit varying nuclear binding affinities for estrogen, progesterone and androgen receptors. This accounts for the unique pharmacologic profile of tibolone, such as peripheral estrogenic effects without endometrial stimulation.

Indications

Vasomotor symptoms of the menopause (particularly in older women). Prevention and treatment of menopausal osteoporosis. Prevention of bone demineralization ('add-back' therapy) during treatment of endometriosis or uterine fibroids with gonadotropin-releasing hormone agonists.

Dosage

The recommended dose for climacteric therapy is 2.5 mg nocte; side-effects may be reduced with alternate-day dosing.

Kinetic data

Rapidly absorbed from the gastrointestinal tract within 30 min. Peak levels achieved between 1.5 and 4 h. Metabolized slowly in the liver and intestine to metabolites that also have varying receptor-binding affinities. Elimination half-life is about 45 h. Two-thirds is eliminated in the feces and one-third in the urine.

Contraindications

Severe liver disease. Pregnancy. Breastfeeding. Untreated hormone-dependent tumors. Undiagnosed vaginal bleeding. Cardiovascular or cerebrovascular disease.

Cautions and interactions

Renal impairment. Abnormal liver function tests. Cholestatic jaundice. Rifampicin and antiepileptics accelerate metabolism of tibolone, thereby reducing its plasma concentration.

Adverse effects

Bloating. Weight changes. Nausea. Occasional gastrointestinal disturbances. Seborrheic dermatitis. Dizziness. Ankle edema.

Triiodothyronine (T3)

Mode of action

As for thyroxine. Five times more potent for equivalent dose.

Indications

Limited. In severe myxedema. For imaging after thyroidectomy for cancer (to assess recurrence), T4 is replaced with T3 for a short period before stopping treatment 1 week or so before tracer scanning.

Preparations

20-μg tablets and ampoules.

Dosage

10–20-μg tablets, increased gradually to 60 μg in divided doses. Dose halved in the elderly and those with cardiac disease. In severe myxedema coma, intravenous treatment; 5–20 μg repeated 6–12-hourly.

Kinetic data

Half-life is 12 h. Absorption and elimination is as for thyroxine.

Contraindications

As for thyroxine.

Adverse effects

As for thyroxine. Care is particularly needed in patients with ischemic heart disease. May precipitate adrenal crisis and cardiac rhythm disturbances in patients with coexisting adrenal insufficiency.

Interactions

As for thyroxine.

Vitamin D and analogs

Structure

A wide range of vitamin D preparations suitable for the management of osteoporosis is available. These include:

- ergocalciferol (vitamin D_2)
- cholecalciferol (vitamin D_3)
- alfacalcidol (1α-hydroxycholecalciferol); 1α-OH D_3)
- calcitriol (1,25-dihydroxycholecalciferol).

Mode of action

Vitamin D promotes calcium and phosphate absorption in the gut. It has been suggested that 1,25-dihydroxycholecalciferol, the physiologically active form of vitamin D, may inhibit bone resorption and perhaps even exert a direct effect on osteoblasts, thereby stimulating bone formation.

Indications

Osteomalacia. Prevention of osteoporosis. Treatment of osteoporosis where estrogen therapy is contraindicated. As an adjunct to specific therapy for osteoporosis, especially in postmenopausal women. Prevention of secondary hyperparathyroidism in renal failure. Hypoparathyroidism.

Dosage

An oral supplement of 800 IU (20 µg) cholecalciferol (vitamin D_3) daily. Since there is no commercially plain tablet of this strength available, calcium and vitamin D tablets can be given. Alternatively, 0.5–1 µg/day or an active metabolite of vitamin D (alfacalcidol, calcitrol) is used.

Kinetic data

Vitamin D requires hydroxylation in the kidney to produce the active form. The hydroxylated derivatives (alfacalcidol or calcitrol) should therefore be used in patients with severe renal impairment. Alfacalcidol and calcitrol have a shorter duration of action and hence have the advantage that the problems associated with excessive therapy and hypercalcemia are shorter-lasting and easier to treat.

Contraindications

Hypercalcemia (e.g. hyperparathyroidism). Metastatic calcification. Decalcifying tumors (myeloma). Bone metastasis. Sarcoidosis. Hypercalciuria. Renal stones.

Cautions

All patients receiving vitamin D should be closely monitored and their plasma calcium and albumin checked regularly (initially monthly and later at 6-monthly intervals) and also whenever nausea or vomiting are present. The dose of vitamin D should be titrated against calcium estimation to ensure normocalcemia at all times. Thiazide diuretics reduce urinary calcium excretion and thus increase the risk of hypercalcemia in patients taking vitamin D supplements.

Adverse effects

Mild gastrointestinal disturbances (constipation) can occur, albeit infrequently, if calcium supplements are taken concurrently. Symptoms of overdosage include lassitude, weakness, anorexia, nausea, vomiting, diarrhea, weight loss, headache and vertigo. Patients may present with sweating, polyuria and secondary polydipsia, indicating renal damage. In these circumstances, vitamin D and calcium therapy must be stopped immediately; a high fluid intake and low-calcium diet should be started. Other measures, such as corticosteroid therapy, may be necessary in severe cases. Raised concentrations of calcium and phosphate are found in plasma and urine. Hypercalcemia may cause renal impairment, nephrocalcinosis and renal stones.

Appendix 3

Reference values

Reproduced with permission from Wilson, Foster, Kronenberg and Larsen: Williams Textbook of Endocrinology (4 ed), 2002 © Elsevier Science

Laboratory Parameter	SI	Conventional (C)	Conversion Factor (CF) CF × C = SI
Acetoacetate, plasma	<100 µmol/L	<1 mg/dL	97.95
Adrenal Steroids, plasma			
Aldosterone, supine, saline suppression	<240 pmol/L	<8.5 ng/dL	27.74
Aldosterone, upright, normal diet	140–560 pmol/L	5–20 ng/dL	27.74
Cortisol			
8 AM	140–690 nmol/L	5–25 µg/dL	27.59
4 PM	80–330 nmol/L	3–12 µg/dL	27.59
Overnight dexamethasone suppression	<140 nmol/L	<5 µg/dL	27.59
Dehydroepiandrosterone (DHEA)	7–31 nmol/L	2–9 µg/dL	3.467
Dehydroepiandrosterone Sulfate (DHEAS)	1.3–6.8 µmol/L	200–2500 ng/ml	0.002714
11-Deoxycortisol	<30 nmol/L	<1 µg/gL	28.86
17-Hydroxyprogesterone			
Women, follicular phase	0.6–3 nmol/L	0.2–1 µg/L	3.026
Women, luteal phase	1.5–10.6 nmol/L	0.5–3.5 µg/L	3.026
Men	1.8–9 nmol/L	0.6–3 µg/L	3.026
Adrenal Steroids, urine			
Aldosterone	14–53 nmol/d	5–19 µg/d	2.774
Cortisol, free	55–276 nmol/d	20–100 µg/d	2.759
17-Hydroxycorticosteroids	5.4–27.6 µmol/d	2–10 mg/d	2.759
17-Ketosteroids			
Men	25–88 µmol/d	7–25 mg/d	3.467
Women	14–53 µmol/d	4–16 mg/d	3.467
Ammonia, as **NH3**, plasma	6–47 µmol/L	10–80 µg/dL	0.5872
Angiotensin II, plasma	10–60 ng/L	10–60 pg/mL	–
Arginine Vasopressin (AVP), plasma			
Random fluid intake	0.0–2.8 pmol/L	1–3 pg/ml	9.1
Dehydration 18–24 h	5.5–13 pmol/L	4–14 pg/ml	9.1
Calciferols (as **Cholecaliferol, Vitamin D3**) plasma			
1,25-Dihydroxycholecalciferol [1,25(OH)2D]	36–144 pmol/L	15–60 pg/ml	2.400
25-Hydroxycholecalciferol (25-OH-D)	20–100 nmol/L	8–40 ng/ml	2.496
Calcitonin, plasma			
Normal	<19 ng/L	<19 pg/ml	–
Medullary cancer	>100 ng/L	>100 pg/ml	–

Laboratory Parameter	SI	Conventional (C)	Conversion Factor (CF) CF × C = SI
Calcium			
Ionized serum	1–1.4 mmol/L	4–5.6 mg/dL	0.2495
Total serum	2.2–2.6 mmol/L	9–10.5 mg/dL	0.2595
Catecholamines, urine			
Free Catecholemines	<590 nmol/d	<100 µg/d	5.911
Epinephrine	<275 nmol/d	<50 µg/d	5.458
Metanephrines	<7 µmol/d	<1.3 ng/d	5.485
Norepinephrine	89–473 nmol/d	15–89 µg/d	5.910
Vanillylmandelic acid (VMA)	<40 µmol/d	<8 mg/d	5.046
Chloride, serum	98–106 µmol/L	98–106 mEq/L	–
Cholesterol, total plasma			
Desirable	<5.20 mmol/L	<200 mg/dL	0.02586
Borderline	5.20–8.18 mmol/L	200–239 mg/dL	0.02586
Undesirable	≥6.21 mmol/L	≥240 mg/dL	0.02586
Cholesterol, High-Density Lipoprotein (HDL Cholesterol), plasma			
Desirable	>1.55 mmol/L	>69 mg/dL	0.02586
Borderline	0.9–1.55 mmol/L	35–60 mg/dL	0.02586
Undesirable	<0.9 mmol/L	<35 mg/dL	0.02586
Cholesterol, Low-Density Lipoprotein (LDL Cholesterol), plasma			
Desirable	<3.36 mmol/L	<130 mg/dL	0.02586
Borderline	3.36–4.11 mmol/L	130–159 mg/dL	0.02586
Undesirable	≥4.14 mmol/L	≥160 mg/dL	0.02586
Corticotropin (ACTH), plasma, 8 AM	2–11 pmol/L	9–52 pg/mL	0.2202
Fatty Acids, Free (nonesterified)(FFA), plasma	0.4–0.7 mmol/L	10.6–18 mg/dL	0.03780
Gastrin, plasma	<120 ng/L	<120 pg/mL	–
Glucagon, plasma	50–100 ng/L	50–100 pg/ml	–
Glucose, plasma			
Overnight fast, normal	4.2–6.4 mmol/L	75–115 mg/dL	0.05551
Overnight fast, diabetes mellitus			
National Diabetes Data Group	>7.8 mmol/L	>140 mg/dL	0.05551
American Diabetes Association	>7.0 mmol/L	>126 mg/dL	0.05551
72-h fast, normal men	>2.8 mmol/L	>50 mg/dL	0.05551
72-h fast, normal women	>2.2 mmol/L	>40 mg/dL	0.05551
Glucose Tolerance Test, 2-h postprandial plasma glucose			
Normal	<7.8 mmol/L	<140 mg/dL	0.05551
Impaired glucose tolerance	7.8–11.1 mmol/L	140–200 mg/dL	0.05551
Diabetes mellitus	>11.1 mmol/L	>200 mg/dL	0.05551
Gonadal Steroids, plasma			
Androstenedione			
Women	3.5–7.0 nmol/L	1–2 ng/ml	3.492
Men	3.0–5.0 nmol/L	0.8–1.3 ng/ml	3.492
Dihydrotestosterone			
Women	0.17–1 nmol/L	0.05–3 ng/ml	3.467
Men	0.87–2.6 nmol/L	0.25–0.75 ng/ml	3.467

Laboratory Parameter	SI	Conventional (C)	Conversion Factor (CF) CF × C = SI
Estradiol			
Women, basal	70–220 pmol/L	20–60 pg/ml	3.671
Women, ovulatory surge	>740 pmol/L	>200 pg/ml	3.671
Men	<180 pmol/L	<50 pg/ml	3.671
Progesterone			
Women, luteal phase	6–64 nmol/L	2–20 ng/ml	3.180
Women, follicular phase	<6 nmol/L	<2 ng/ml	3.180
Men	<6 nmol/L	<2 ng/ml	3.180
Testosterone			
Women	<3.5 nmol/L	<1 ng/ml	4.467
Men	10–35 nmol/L	3–10 ng/ml	4.467
Gonadotropins, plasma			
Follicle-Stimulating Hormone (FSH)			
Women, basal	1.4–9.6 IU/L	1.4–9.6 mIU/mL	–
Women, ovulatory surge	2.3–21 IU/L	2.3–21 mIU/mL	–
Women, postmenopausal	34–96 IU/L	34–96 mIU/mL	–
Men	0.9–15 IU/L	0.9–15 mIU/mL	–
Luteinizig Hormone (LH)			
Women, basal	0.8–26 IU/L	0.8–26 mIU/mL	–
Women, ovulatory stage	25–57 IU/L	25–57 mIU/mL	–
Women, postmenopausal	40–104 IU/L	40–104 mIU/mL	–
Men	1.3–13 IU/L	1.3–13 mIU/mL	–
Growth Hormone (GH), plasma			
After 100 g glucose orally	<2 µg/L	<2 ng/mL	–
After insulin-induced hypoglycemia	>9 µg/L	>9 ng/mL	–
Human Chorionic Gonadotropin ß Subunit (ß-hCG), plasma			
Men and nonpregnant women	<3 IU/L	<3 mIU/mL	–
ß-Hydroxybutyrate, plasma	<300 µmol/L	<3 mg/dL	96.05
Insulin, plasma			
Fasting	35–145 pmol/L	5–20 uU/mL	7.175
During hypoglycemia			
(plasma glucose <2.8 nmol/L <50 mg/mL)	<35 pmol/L	<5 uU/mL	7.175
Insulin C Peptide, plasma	0.5–2 µg/L	0.5–2 pg/mL	–
Insulin-Like Growth Factor I (IGF-1, Somatomedin-C)			
Women	0.45–2.2 kU/L	0.45–2.2 U/ml	–
Men	0.34–1.9 kU/L	0.34–1.9 U/ml	–
Lactate, plasma	0.56–2.2 mmol/L	5–20 mg/dL	0.111
Magnesium, serum	0.8–1.30 mmol/L	1.8–3.0 mg/dL	0.4114
Osmolatity, plasma	285–295 mmol/kg	285–295 mOsmol/L	–
Oxytocin, plasma			
Random	1–4 pmol/L	1.25–5 ng/L	0.80
Wome, ovulatory surge	4–8 pmol/L	5–10 ng/L	0.80
Parathyroid Hormone, serum			
(**Intact PTH** using IRMA assay)	10–65 ng/L	10–65 pg/ml	–
Phosphorus, inorganis serum	1–1.5 mmol/L	3.0–4.5 mg/dL	0.3229

Laboratory Parameter	SI	Conventional (C)	Conversion Factor (CF) CF × C = SI
Prolactin, serum			
Nonpregnant women and men	2–15 µg/L	2–15 ng/ml	–
Pyruvate, plasma	39–102 µmol/L	0.3–0.9 mg/dL	0.01129
Renin Activity, plasma, normal-sodium intake			
Supine	3.2 ± 1 µg/L/h	3.2 ± 1 ng/mL/h	–
Standing	9.3 ± 4.3 µg/L/h	9.3 ± 4.3 ng/mL/h	–
Sodium, serum	136–145 mmol/L	136–145 mEq/L	–
Thyroid Function Tests			
Free thyroxine estimate	9–26 pmol/L	0.7–2.0 ng/dL	12.87
Radioactive iodine uptake, 24 h	0.05–0.30	5–30%	–
Resin T_3 uptake, serum	0.25–0.35	25–35%	–
Reverse triiodothyronine (rT_3), serum	0.15–0.61 nmol/L	10–40 ng/dL	0.01536
Thyroid hormone-binding ratio (THBR)	0.85–1.10	85–110%	–
Thyrotropin (TSH), serum	0.5–5 mU/L	0.5–5 µU/mL	–
Thyroxine (T_4), serum	64–154 nmol/L	5–12 µg/dL	12.87
Triiodothyronine (T_3), serum	1.1–2.9 nmol/L	70–190 ng/dL	0.01536
Triglycerides, plasma	<1.80 mmol/L	<160 mg/dL	0.01129
Vitamin D, see **Calciferols**			

Index

Note: Abbreviations: PCOS, polycystic ovary syndrome. 'vs' indicates the differentiation of two or more conditions.

Acid—base disturbances and hyperkalemia, 383
Acromegaly, 51–9, 97, 100, 401–2
    features, 51–3
        hypertension, 401–2
    investigation, 53
ACTH
    in CRH test (in Cushing's syndrome), 67
    deficiency, 489
        diagnosis/assays, 39, 40, 239, 489–90
        treatment, 40, 448–9
    measurement, 490
    in metyrapone test, 494
ACTH-dependent Cushing's syndrome, 60
    causes, 61, 62–3
    diagnosis, 67
ACTH-independent Cushing's syndrome, 60
    causes, 61, 63–6
ACTH-producing tumors
    ectopic, 62, 68
        treatment, 70–1
    pituitary (corticotroph adenomas), 30, 62
        Cushing's syndrome, 62, 68
ACTH stimulation test, short (with tetracosactrin = Synacthen), 39, 491–3
    Addison's disease/Addisonian crisis, 239, 444, 445
    HIV-infected persons, 338
    low-dose, 39, 492–3
Addisonian crisis, 239, 441, 446
    clinical assessment (causes and presentation), 441–4
    investigation, 444
    management, 444–5, 446
        prevention and education, 445
Addison's disease (primary adrenal failure; chronic adrenocortical insufficiency), 235–8, 433, 441–6
    in autoimmune polyglandular disease type 1, 241
    clinical assessment, 237–8
    hyperkalemia, 383
    hypothyroidism and, 444
    management, 239–40, 433
        emergency, 239, 444–6
    psychiatric problems, 433
Adenohypophysis (anterior pituitary), 25
    amenorrhea with disorders of, 133–7
Adenohypophysitis, lymphocytic, see Lymphocytic adenohypophysitis
Adenoma
    adrenal, 63
        aldosterone-producing, see Aldosterone-producing adenoma
    parathyroid
        familial disorders predisposing to, 298
        removal, 298
    pituitary, 44–6, 453–5, see also Macroadenoma; Microadenoma; Pituitary gland, neoplasms
        classification, 30
        corticotroph, see ACTH-producing tumors
        differential diagnosis of sellar and suprasellar lesions from, 42
        gonadotroph, 44–5
        histology, 29
        lactrotroph/prolactin-producing, see Prolactinomas
        MRI, 27
        non-functioning, 44–5
        pituitary apoplexy with, see Pituitary apoplexy
        somatotroph/GH-producing, see Growth hormone-producing adenomas
        thyrotroph, see Thyrotropin-producing adenoma
        with visual loss, 453–5
    thyroid
        toxic, 272
        TSH-R mutations and, 248–50
Adenyl cyclase, G protein for (Gs), see G protein
ADH, see Antidiuretic hormone
Adipose tissue (fat tissue) and adipocytes
    as endocrine organ, 415
    physiology, 407–8, see also Fat, body
    surgical removal (lipectomy), 418
Adolescents, Graves' disease, 227
Adrenal androgens, elevated, women, 209
Adrenal crisis, see Addisonian crisis
Adrenal disease, 235–8, 387–93
    Cushing's syndrome due to, 63–6
    in HIV infection/AIDS, 334
        evaluation for, 337–8
    hyperplastic, see Hyperplasia
    neoplastic, 63–4, 204–5
        aldosterone-producing tumor, see Aldosterone-producing adenoma
        Cushing's syndrome, 63–4, 70, 204–5
        hirsutism with, 204–5
        pheochromocytoma, diagnosis/imaging, 396–7, 397, 398
        secondary (metastases), 345–6
        surgery, 70
Adrenal gland
    disease, see Adrenal disease
    hemorrhage, 443
    in obesity, 414
Adrenal insufficiency/failure (hypoadrenalism)
    acute, see Addisonian crisis
    causes, 442
    chronic/primary, see Addison's disease
Adrenal steroids, reference values, 551-2, see also specific steroids
Adrenergic symptoms, hypoglycemia, 476
Adrenoceptor agonists and antagonists, see Alpha-agonists; Alpha-blockers; Beta-blockers; Beta$_3$-agonists
Adrenocorticotrophic hormone, see ACTH
Adrenoleukodystrophy (ALD), 338–41

INDEX

Adrenoleukodystrophy-related protein (ALDRP), 339
    gene transfer, 341
Adrenomyeloneuropathy, adult-onset, 339
Affective disorder, see Depression
Agenesis
    Müllerian, 142, 143
    parathyroid, 289
AIDS, see HIV disease
Albright's hereditary osteodystrophy, 291
Aldosterone, see also Renin—angiotensin (and aldosterone) system
    assays in aldosteronism diagnosis, 389–91
    physiology, 387–8
Aldosterone antagonist, 392–3, 544
    pharmacology, 544
Aldosterone-producing adenoma (APA), 388
    idiopathic hyperaldosteronism vs, 391–2
    surgery, 392
Aldosteronism (hyperaldosteronism), 387–93
    hypokalemia in, 381, 388
    primary (Conn's syndrome), 387–93
        etiologies, 388
        heritable forms, 388–9
        pathophysiology and clinical features, 387–8
        screening/diagnosis/investigations, 389–93
        treatment, 392–3
Alendronate, osteoporosis, 313
Alfacalcidol, see 1-_-Hydroxyvitamin D
Alimentary tract, see Gastrointestinal tract
Alkali excess, 301
Alkaline phosphate levels, Paget's disease of bone, 318
Alpha-agonists, pharmacology, 532, 538–9
Alpha-blockers (α-adrenergic receptor blockers), 538, 549–50
    erectile dysfunction, 175, 538
    pharmacology, 538, 549–50
    pheochromocytoma, preoperative, 398–9
Alprostadil (PGE$_1$)
    intracavernosal, 173–4
    intraurethral, 173
Amenorrhea, 131–46
    etiology, 131–43
        eating disorders, 132, 429–30
    management, 143–4

primary vs secondary, 131
Aminoglutethimide, 504
    Cushing's syndrome, 69
cAMP, cavernosal smooth muscle and, 167
cAMP-response element modulator gene (CREM) and male infertility, 181, 183–4
Anabolic steroids, osteoporosis, 314
Anastrazole, 505
Androgen(s), see also Antiandrogens
    excess, women (hyperandrogenism), 206–8
        tests, 208–9
    normal production, 205
Androgen deficiency, 147, see also Testosterone
    screening for/diagnosis of, patient groups, 147–8
        erectile dysfunction, 169
    treatment (replacement therapy), 158–65
        contraindications, 161
        in erectile dysfunction, 172–3
        monitoring, 162–5
        psychological effects, 431
Androgen insensitivity syndrome, complete, 142–3
Androgen receptor, infertility and polyglutamine tract length of, 183
Androgen receptor modulators, nonsteroidal selective, 161
Androgen-secreting ovarian tumors, 205
Androstenedione, reference values, 553
Aneurysms, suprasellar, 41
Angiotensin II, see also Renin—angiotensin (and aldosterone) system
    ADH release and, 369
    aldosterone-producing adenomas unresponsive to secretion of, 388
    hyperparathyroidism and, 401
Angiotensin-converting enzyme inhibitors and aldosteronism diagnosis, 390–1
Anorexia nervosa, 427–31
    amenorrhea, 132, 429–30
    clinical characteristics, 428–9
    diagnostic criteria, 428
Anorexigenic drugs, 416, 417
Anorexigenic signals, 411–13, 428
Anovulatory infertility in PCOS, treatment, 139
Antiandrogens, 514–16, 523
    hirsutism, 210–11
    non-steroidal, 523
Antibiotics

interactions with oral contraceptives, 513
    thyroid storm precipitated by sepsis, 459
Antibodies, see also Autoantibodies
    to hCG, 186
    in immunoassays
        in competitive assays, 4–5
        heterophilic, interfering with assay, 11
        'high-dose hook effect', 9
        in non-competitive (immunometric) assays, 5, 9
        specificity and cross-reactivity, 5–6
Antidiabetic drugs, see Hypoglycemics, oral
Antidiuretic hormone (ADH; vasopressin; arginine vasopressin), 368–71
    aquaporins and, 370–1
    deficiency, in hypopituitarism, 449
    diabetes insipidus responsive to, see Cranial diabetes insipidus
    pharmacokinetics, 370
    reference values, 552
    regulation of secretion, 368–9
    renal insensitivity to, see Nephrogenic diabetes insipidus
    syndrome of inappropriate secretion, see Syndrome of inappropriate antidiuresis
Antiestrogens, 544–5
    osteoporosis, 314
    pharmacology, 544–5
Antiphospholipid syndrome, 344
Antiprogestogen, mifepristone as, 533
Antiretroviral drugs, adverse effects, 337
Antithyroid drugs, 508–9, 542
    Graves' disease, 222, 223–4, 226
        in pregnancy, 227, 228
    pharmacology, 508–9, 542
    resistance to thyroid hormone, 261
    thyroid storm, 458, 460
Apomorphine, erectile dysfunction, 175
Appetite
    control, 410, see also Eating
    drugs reducing, 416, 417
    neuropeptides and neurotransmitters affecting, 411–13
Aquaporins, 370–1
    AQP-2 gene mutation, 373
Arginine vasopressin, see Antidiuretic hormone
Aromatase inhibitor, non-steroidal, 505
Arrhythmias

in hypercalcemia, 299
in resistance to thyroid hormone, 255
in thyroid storm, 459
Asherman's syndrome, 143
Assays, see Biochemical investigations and specific tests
Assisted reproduction/conception, male infertility, 188
ATPases, H$^+$/K$^+$, 379
Atrial natriuretic peptide and hypertensive acromegalic patients, 402
Atrophic thyroiditis, presentation with, 232
Attention deficit hyperactivity disorder in resistance to thyroid hormone, 255
Autoantibodies
    21-hydroxylase, 239
    immunoassays and, 10
    insulin, 352
    phospholipids, 344
    thyroglobulin, see Thyroglobulin
    thyroid peroxidase (TPO), 221, 234
    TSH-R, 10, 217, 221, 222, 227
Autoimmune disease, 217–46
    premature ovarian failure, 140
    thyroid, 215–35, 275–9
Autoimmune insulin syndrome, 352
Autoimmune polyglandular syndrome, see Polyglandular syndrome, autoimmune (APS)
Autosomal-dominant non-autoimmune hyperthyroidism, 251
AZF locus, 182–3
Azoospermia
    evaluation, 179–80
    genetic syndromes causing, 181
    treatment, 187–8

Barakat syndrome, 290
Barbiturates and thyroid storm, 458
Bartter's syndrome, 381–2
Basal ganglia calcification, 287, 288
Beckwith–Wiedemann syndrome, 100
Beta$_3$-agonists, obesity, 417
Beta-blockers (β-adrenergic receptor blockers), 541–2
    Graves' disease, 224
    pharmacology, 541–2
    postpartum thyroiditis, 237
    thyroid storm, 459, 460
Biguanide, see Metformin
Binding proteins, assays and, 2–3, 10, see also specific binding proteins
Biochemical investigations (incl. assays), 1–16
    Addison's disease, 239
    aldosteronism, 389–91, 391–2
    Cushing's syndrome (and its differential diagnosis), 66, 67–8
    erectile dysfunction, 167
    failings/limitations, 10–11
        medication and, 2
    hirsutism and PCOS, 208–9
    hyperprolactinemia, 47, 135
    hypogonadism in men, 151
    hypoparathyroidism, 288–9
    hypopituitarism, 447
    hypothalamic—pituitary axis function, 39–41
    interpretation, 12
    lymphocytic and postpartum thyroiditis, 279
    MEN 2, 124–5
    methods, 4–9
    osteoporosis, 309–10
    Paget's disease of bone, 318
    pheochromocytoma, 395–7
    pituitary apoplexy, 451
    pseudohypoparathyroidism, 292
    reference ranges/values, 12, 551–4
    resistance to thyroid hormone, 255–8
    samples, 4
    state of patient, 1–4
Biopsy
    bone, osteoporosis, 310
    testicular, in infertility, 180
    thyroid, in multinodular goiter, 270
Bisphosphonates, 504, 521, 537, 543–4
    hypercalcemia, 302, 468, 469
        of malignancy, 355, 356
    osteoporosis, 313, 504
    Paget's disease of bone, 321–2
    pharmacology, 504, 521, 537, 543–4
    primary hyperparathyroidism, 298
Bleeding, see Hemorrhage
Blood flow in erectile dysfunction, evaluation, 167–9
Blood pressure, raised, 387–406
Blood samples (for assays), 4
Blood tests, hypopituitarism, 447
Blood vessels, see Vasculature
Body composition
    GH deficiency (adult), 90–1
    testosterone replacement and, 163
Body fat and weight, see Fat; Weight
Body mass index, 408

Bone, 287–324
    in acromegaly, 51
    biopsy, osteoporosis, 310
    cancer, see Cancer
    disorders, 287–324
    dysplasia, Paget's disease-like, 316
    fractures, see Fractures
    metabolism, 304–5
    mineral density and mass, 304
        determinants, 304
        GH deficiency (adult), 91–2
        hyperparathyroidism, 296
        osteoporosis, measurement, 307–10
        resistance to thyroid hormone and, 255
        testosterone replacement and, 163
    mineralization, drugs interfering with, 324
    pain, pagetic, 317–18
    turnover (formation/remodelling/resorption)
        drugs inhibiting, 311
        hypercalcemia due to acceleration in, 299
        in osteoporosis, and its assessment, 304–5, 306, 307–10
        in Paget's disease of bone, 316
Bone marrow transplantation, adrenoleukodystrophy, 340
Brachytherapy (interstitial radiotherapy), pituitary tumors, 34
Brain, see also Central nervous system; Neurologic features
    energy homeostasis and, 410, 411–13
    tumors, amenorrhea with, 133
Breast cancer
    drug therapy, 504, 505
    testosterone contraindicated in, 161
Breast enlargement in men (gynecomastia), causes, 151
    testosterone administration, 151, 165
Breastfeeding and prolactinomas, 50
Bromocriptine, 505–6
    hyperprolactinemia, 135–6
    pharmacology, 505–6
    pituitary tumors, 34–5, 50
        GH-producing, 55
    pregnancy and, 50
Bronchial tumors, ectopic hormone production, 62, 70–1

Bulimia nervosa, 427–31
    amenorrhea, 132
    clinical characteristics and psychopathology, 428–9
Buserelin, 525

Cabergoline
    hyperprolactinemia, 136
    pituitary tumors, 35
CAG repeat of androgen receptor gene, infertility and, 183
Calciferol (ergocalciferol; vitamin D_2), 548
    hypocalcemia, 474
    pseudohypoparathyroidism, 293
Calcification, basal ganglia, 287, 288
Calcitonin, 507–8
    hypercalcemia, 303, 468, 469
        of malignancy, 355
    osteoporosis, 312–13, 507
    pharmacology, 507–8
    reference values, 552
Calcitriol (1,25-dihydroxycholecalciferol)
    hypocalcemia, 474
    osteoporosis, 312
    pseudohypoparathyroidism, 293
Calcium
    administration
        in hypocalcemia, 473, 474
        in osteoporosis treatment/prevention, 312
        in pseudohypoparathyroidism, 293
    deficiency, 322–3
    dietary, blood pressure and, 401
    disturbances, 287–324, 464–74, see also Hypercalcemia; Hypocalcemia
        emergencies, 464–74
        in HIV disease/AIDS, 336
    reference values, 552
Calcium channel antagonists
    aldosteronism, 393
    pheochromocytoma, preoperative, 399
Calcium-sensing receptor (CaR; CaSR), mutations, 117, 290
Calorie content in diet, reducing, 415–16
Cancer (malignancy), see also Metastases; Paraneoplastic conditions; Tumors and specific histological types
    bone
        as Paget's disease complication, 319–20

vs Paget's disease, 319–20
    breast, see Breast cancer
    familial/hereditary, clinics, 126
    hypercalcemia in, 300–1, 353–6, 465
        evaluation/investigation, 354–5, 466
        treatment, 355–6
    IGFs and, 88, 97–8
    osteomalacia in, 323–4
    prostate, see Prostate
    thyroid, see Thyroid neoplasms
Cannabinoids and appetite, 413
Captopril tests, aldosteronism, 391
Carbimazole (CBZ) in Graves' disease, 223, 226
    in pregnancy, 227
Carbohydrate metabolism, inborn errors, 475
Carcinoids, ACTH-producing, 62, 70–1
Carcinoma, thyroid,, see also Thyroid neoplasms
Cardiolipin, antibodies to, 344
Cardiovascular system (circulation)
    care, in myxedema coma, 462
    disorders, see also Arrhythmias; Hypertension
        in acromegaly, 51, 401–2
        in anorexia nervosa, 429
        GH deficiency (adult), 92
        in hypocalcemia, 472
        in hypoparathyroidism, 288
        in myxedema coma, 461
        pheochromocytoma, 394
        in resistance to thyroid hormone, 255
        sildenafil and, 171–2
        testosterone replacement and risk of, 164–5
        in thyroid storm, treatment, 459
Cataracts in hypocalcemia, 288
Catecholamines
    assays, pheochromocytoma, 395–7
    reference values, 552
    synthesis/metabolism, 393, 394
Caucasian women, autoimmune endocrinopathies, 215
Cavernosal body, see Corpora cavernosa
CCK, 412
Central nervous system, see also Brain; Neurologic features
    energy homeostasis and, 410, 411–13
    lesions, hyperprolactinemia, 133

in syndrome of inappropriate antidiuresis causation, 376, 481
Central pontine myelinolysis (osmotic demyelination syndrome in hyponatremia correction), 378, 479, 482
Chemotherapy, premature ovarian failure, 140
Chest wall disease, hyperprolactinemia, 134
Children, see also Adolescents; Infants
    Graves' disease, 227
    growth disorders missed in, leading to adult short stature, 98–9
    hypercalcemia in, 301, 302
    nephrogenic diabetes insipidus, 372
Cholecalciferol (vitamin D_3), 548, 549
Cholecystokinin, 412
Chromaffinoma, see Pheochromocytoma
Chromosomes, sex, see Sex chromosome abnormalities
Chronic fatigue syndrome, GH use, 95
Chronic illness, males, androgen/testosterone levels, 147, 152
    screening for deficiency, 147
Chvostek's sign, 288, 471–2
Circulation, see Cardiovascular system
Cirrhosis, 345
Clodronate, 543
    hypercalcemia, 303
        of malignancy, 355
    pharmacology, 543
Clomiphene citrate, 509–10
    in PCOS, 139
    pharmacology, 509–10
Clonidine suppression test
    pheochromocytoma, 396
    pituitary—gonadal axis testing with, 495
CMV adrenalitis, 334
Cocaine- and amphetamine-regulated transcript, 412
Collagen markers and Paget's disease of bone, 318
Coma, myxedema, 460–3, 464
Complement, 11
Computed tomography (CT)
    adrenal (in aldosteronism), 392
    head (incl. hypothalamic—pituitary region)
        craniopharyngioma, 43
        hypopituitarism, 447
        macroadenoma, 454
        pituitary apoplexy, 451

osteoporosis, 308
parathyroid (in hyperparathyroidism), 297
pheochromocytoma (extra-adrenal), 397, 398
Congenital absence of vas deferens, bilateral, 181, 184
Congenital adrenal hyperplasia, 99, 204
diagnosis, 209
hirsutism in, 204, 209
short stature, 99
Congenital disorders (developmental disorders)
amenorrhea, 142–3
GH deficiency due to, 89
parathyroid, 289–90
pituitary, 156–7
Congenital hyperthyroidism, 251
Congenital hypogonadotropic hypogonadism in men, 150–1
Congenital hypothyroidism, 251–3
Conjugated equine estrogen, 514
Conn's syndrome, see Aldosteronism, primary
Contraception
oral, see Oral contraceptive pill
postcoital, 539
Contrast agents, iodinated, see Iodinated contrast agents
Coronary heart disease and sildenafil, 171–2
Corpora cavernosa
anatomy, 165
drug injections in erectile dysfunction, 168, 173–5
physiology, 166
smooth muscle, see Smooth muscle
Corticosteroids, see Glucocorticoids
Corticotroph adenoma, see ACTH-producing tumors
Corticotropin, see ACTH
Corticotropin-releasing hormone (CRH)
anorexigenicity, 412
in Cushing's syndrome diagnosis, 426
ectopic production, 62–3
surgery, 70–1
stress and depression and, 424–5
Corticotropin-releasing hormone test, Cushing's syndrome, 67
Cortisol (hydrocortisone), 527–8
administration, 527–8
ACTH deficiency, 40, 448–9
Addison's disease, 239, 444

myxedema coma, 463
pharmacology, 527–8
pituitary apoplexy, 452
thyroid storm, 459
measurements, 490–1
Addison's disease, 239
basal serum levels, 489–90
Cushing's syndrome, 66
in metyrapone test, 494
reference values, 551–2
in short Synacthen test, 491–2, 492, 493
production in health, 488–489
Cosmesis, hirsutism, 210
Cost-effectiveness, sildenafil, 172
Counselling, erectile dysfunction, 170
CpG islands of *p21*, methylation, pituitary tumors, 21
Cranial diabetes insipidus (central/neurogenic DI), 41
clinical features, 372–3
diagnosis, 374
head trauma-related, 343, 373
investigations of cause, 375
treatment, 375
Craniopharyngioma, 43–4
CREM and male infertility, 181, 183–4
CRH, see Corticotropin–releasing hormone
Critical illness, GH use, 95
Cross-reactivity, immunoassays, 5–6
Cushing's disease, 62
Cushing's syndrome, 59–71, 402–3, 432–3
clinical signs/features, 59–61, 204–5
hirsutism, 204–5
hypertension, 402–3
obesity, 413
diagnosis and differential diagnosis, 67–8, 425–6
investigation, 65, 66
management, 68–71
algorithm, 65
morbidity, 60–1
psychopathology, 61, 425–6, 432–3
Cutaneous disorders, see Skin disorders
Cyclic nucleotide(s), see AMP; GMP
Cyclic nucleotide phosphodiesterase, see Phosphodiesterase
Cyclin-dependent kinases (CDKs) and CDK inhibitors, 21
Cyproterone acetate, 514–16

hirsutism, 210–11
Cyst
ovarian, see Polycystic ovaries; Polycystic ovary syndrome
Rathke's cleft, 43
Cystic fibrosis transmembrane conductance gene (CTFR), infertility and, 180
Cytomegalovirus adrenalitis, 334

Dashe test, 374
DAX-1 and hypogonadotropic hypogonadism, 154–5, 155
DAZ gene family, 183
dDAVP, see Desmopressin
de Quervain's thyroiditis, 273–5
Deafness, resistance to thyroid hormone, 255
Dehydration tests, 374
Dehydroepiandrosterone (DHEA) and DHEA sulfate levels in women
adrenal tumors and, 204–5
assessment, 209
Demecycloline, 378, 482–4, 484
Demyelination syndrome, osmotic (in hyponatremia correction), 378, 479, 482
Dental features, hypoparathyroidism, 288
Depression, 421–7
Cushing's disease, 432–3
Dermatopathies, see Skin disorders
Desmolase deficiencies, premature ovarian failure, 141
Desmopressin (vasopressin analogue; dDAVP), 368, 516
diabetes insipidus, 41, 375
hypopituitarism, 449
pharmacology, 516
Desogestrel (DSG), in oral contraceptive, 511
Developmental disorders, see Congenital disorders
DEXA, osteoporosis, 307, 308
Dexamethasone suppression
in Cushing's syndrome diagnosis, 66, 67, 425, 426
in hirsutism treatment, 211
Dextrose (glucose) in hypoglycemia, 351–2, 477, 478
Diabetes insipidus, 26, 41, 371–6
causes, 41, 372
sarcoidosis, 341
central/cranial/neurogenic, see Cranial diabetes insipidus
diagnosis, 374

gestational, 372, 373
glucose disturbances in, effects, 347
in Langerhans' cell histiocytosis, 342
nephrogenic, see Nephrogenic diabetes insipidus
postoperative, pituitary tumors and, 33
treatment, 375–7
Diabetes mellitus
subfertility, 184
type II, PCOS and, 137
Dialysis, hypercalcemic crisis, 468, 469
Diarrhea with oral contraceptives, 513
Diet and nutrition
calcium in, blood pressure and, 401
energy homeostasis and, 410
management
in adrenoleukodystrophy, 340
in myxedema coma, 472
in obesity, 415
in thyroid storm, 458, 460
DiGeorge syndrome, 289
Digestive tract, see Gastrointestinal tract
Dihydropyridine calcium channel antagonists, aldosteronism, 393
Dihydrotachysterol
hypocalcemia, 474
pseudohypoparathyroidism, 293
Dihydrotestosterone, reference values, 553
1,25-Dihydroxycholecalciferol, see Calcitriol
Disease, pre-existing, assays and, 3–4
Diuretics
in hypercalcemic crisis, 467, 469
hypokalemia with, 380
in osteoporosis, 314
Diurnal secretion, 1
Dopamine agonists, 505–7, 542–3
erectile dysfunction, 175
hyperprolactinemia, 135–6
pharmacology, 505–7, 542–3
pituitary tumors, 34–5, 455
GH-producing, 55, 57–9
pregnancy and, 50
prolactin-producing, 48, 49, 50, 455
psychiatric side-effects, 431–2
Doppler ultrasound, hyperparathyroidism, 297
Doxazocin, erectile dysfunction, 175
Drug(s), 503–50
ADH secretion affected by, 370
adverse effects of/disorders caused by, 504–50

adrenal insufficiency, 442, 444
autoimmune hypothyroidism, 232
in HIV disease, 337
hypercalcemia, 301, 465
hyperkalemia, 383
hyperprolactinemia, 133
hypocalcemia, 471
hypoglycemia, 352, 475
hypogonadism in men, 147–8, 148–9
hypokalemia, 380, 382
osteomalacia, 324
psychiatric effects, 431–2
assay interference by, 2
pharmacopoeia, 503–50
syndrome of inappropriate antidiuresis, 376, 481
Drug therapy (medication), 503–50, see also specific (types of) drugs
Addison's disease, 239–40
Addisonian crisis, 445
aldosteronism, 392–3
anovulatory infertility in PCOS, 139
Cushing's syndrome, 69
erectile dysfunction, 170–2, 172–5, 537–8
Graves' disease, 223–6, 508, 542
ophthalmopathy, 230
in pregnancy, 227, 228
hirsutism, 210
hypercalcemia, 302–3, 467, 468–70
of malignancy, 355, 356
hyperkalemia, 383
hyperparathyroidism, 298
hyperprolactinemia, 135–6
hypocalcemia, 473–4
hyponatremia, 378, 482–4
obesity, 416–17
osteoporosis (incl. prevention), 311–14
Paget's disease of bone, 321–2
pituitary tumors, 34–7, 455
GH-producing (and acromegaly), 54, 55–7
postpartum thyroiditis, 237
resistance to thyroid hormone, 261
subacute granulomatous thyroiditis, 275
thyroid storm, 458–9, 460
Dual-energy X-ray absorptiometry (DEXA), osteoporosis, 307, 308
Dydrogesterone, pharmacology, 517–18

Dyslipidemia, see Lipid disturbances
Dysplasia of bone
fibrous, vs Paget's disease, 319–20
Paget's disease-like, 316
Dysrhythmias, see Arrhythmias

Eating behavior, see also Appetite
disorders of, see Anorexia nervosa; Bulimia nervosa
modifying, in obesity, 416
Ectopic adrenal receptor expression, 65–6
Ectopic hormone production (incl. tumors), 346
ACTH, see ACTH-producing tumors
CRH, see Corticotropin-releasing hormone
GHRH, 51, 56
prolactin, 134
Edetate, hypercalcemia, 469, 470
Elderly, see Older people
Ele-1, 19–20
Electrolytes, see also specific electrolytes
disturbances, 479–84
in HIV disease/AIDS, 336
in intracellular vs extracellular fluids, 367
management, myxedema coma, 462
Embolism, see Thromboembolism
Emergencies, 441–86
Addisonian crisis, 239, 441–6
HPA axis measurement in, 490
thyroid ophthalmopathy, 230
Emesis, see Vomiting
Empty sella (syndrome), 30, 31
hyperprolactinemia, 134
Endometrial curettage and Asherman's syndrome, 143
Endothelin receptor antagonists, erectile dysfunction, 175
Energy
expenditure, 410
drugs increasing, 417–18
homeostasis/balance, 411–13
brain/CNS in, 410, 411–13
regulation, 411–13
Enzymopathies, premature ovarian failure, 141
Erdheim—Chester disease, 342–3
Erection, 165–77
dysfunction (impotence), 165–77
etiology, 168
evaluation, 167–9
prevalence, 165
screening for androgen

deficiency, 147
treatment, 169–75, 537–8
physiology, 165–7
Ergocalciferol, *see* Calciferol
Erythrocytosis, androgens contraindicated in, 161
Estradiol
pharmacology, 518
reference values, 553
Estrogen(s) (used in treatment), *see also* Antiestrogens; Hormone replacement therapy; Oral contraceptive
conjugated equine estrogen, 514
menopausal symptoms, 514, 519
pharmacology, 510–14, 518, 520–1
premenstrual syndrome, 427
primary hyperparathyroidism, 298
Estrogen deficiency in anorexia nervosa, 430
Estrogen receptor modulators, selective, osteoporosis, 313–14
Ethamsylate, 518–20
Ethinylestradiol (EE), 520–1
in oral contraceptive, 511
emergency contraception, 539
pharmacology, 520–1
Etidronate, 521
hypercalcemic crisis, 468
osteoporosis, 313
Paget's disease of bone, 321–2
pharmacology, 521
Etynodiol acetate, 540
Eugonadotropic amenorrhea, 142–3
Euthyroid sick syndrome, *see* Sick euthyroid syndrome
Evidence-based medicine, 13–15
Exercise
amenorrhea with excess of, 132
in obesity, 416
Exercise performance, GH deficiency (adult), 92
Extracellular fluid, solute composition, 367
Eye disease, thyroid, *see* Ophthalmopathy

Familial aldosteronism, 388, 388–9
type I, 388, 388–9
type II, 388, 389
Familial benign hypercalciuric hypercalcemia, 121
Familial cancer clinic, 126
Familial disorders with hypercalcemia predisposition, 117, 121
Familial expansile osteolysis, 316

Familial hypercalcemia and hypercalciuria, 117
Familial hypercalcemic hypercalciuria, 117
Familial hyperparathyroidism—jaw tumor syndrome, 117, 120
Familial isolated hyperparathyroidism, 116, 117, 120–2
Familial medullary thyroid carcinoma (FMTC), 116, 123, 124
Familial non-autoimmune hyperthyroidism, 251
Familial papillary carcinoma of thyroid, 21
Familial prolactinomas, 47
Fat, *see also* Lipid
body, *see also* Adipose tissue
age and, 413
excess, *see* Obesity
in GH deficiency (adult), 90–1
hydrolysis (lipolysis), control, 408
measurement, 408–10
dietary, energy homeostasis and, 410
Fatty acids, very long chain, in adrenoleukodystrophy, 339, 339–40, 340, 341
Feeding, *see* Appetite; Eating behavior
Females, *see* Women
Feminization, testicular, 142–3
Femoral fractures, osteoporotic, 307
Fenfluramine, 416
Ferriman—Gallwey score, 202, 203
Fertile eunuch syndrome, 153
Fertility problems (infertility; subfertility), men, 175–88
pathogenesis/etiology, 177
screening for androgen deficiency, 147
treatment, 184–8
Fertility problems (infertility; subfertility), women, 131–43, 509
in PCOS
management of infertility, 139, 509
presentation with infertility, 138
Fever (hyperthermia), thyroid storm, 458, 460
FGFs, *see* Fibroblast growth factors
Fibroblast growth factors
FGF–2 and MEN 1, 21
FGF–4 and prolactinomas, 20
Fibrosing conditions, 344
Fibrous cystic osteitis, 294

Fibrous dysplasia of bone vs Paget's disease, 319–20
Finasteride, 521–2
hirsutism, 211
pharmacology, 521–2
Fine needle aspiration, multinodular goiter, 270
Fludrocortisone, Addison's disease, 239
Fluid, 367–76
balance
in health, 367–8
treatment addressing, *see* Fluid, restriction; Fluid therapy
imbalance/disturbances, 371–6
in HIV disease/AIDS, 336
in hyponatremia, 479
restriction in hyponatremia, 378
solute composition, intracellular vs extracellular, 367
Fluid therapy
Addisonian crisis, 444
hypercalcemic crisis, 467, 469
thyroid storm, 458, 460
Fluoride salts, 522–3
osteoporosis, 314
Flutamide, 523
hirsutism, 211
pharmacology, 523
Follicle-stimulating hormone (FSH), 523–4, *see also* Gonadotropin
ß-subunit mutation
men, 155–6, 158
women, 140
reference values, 553
testosterone replacement and levels of, 162–3
therapeutic use, 523–4
male infertility, 185, 186
pharmacology of preparations used, 523–4
Follicle-stimulating hormone-producing adenoma, 44
Follicular carcinoma of thyroid, 109–10
Follicular cell, thyroid, TSH and the, 247
Fractures
minimal trauma (in men), screening for androgen deficiency, 147
in osteomalacia, 323–4
osteoporotic, 304, 306–7
Froboese's syndrome (MEN 2B or MEN 3), 116, 123

FSH, *see* Follicle-stimulating hormone

G protein for adenyl cyclase (Gs; Gsp)
    Albright's hereditary osteodystrophy and, 291
    McCune—Albright syndrome and, 64
    neoplasia and, 17–18
    TSH resistance and, 253
Galactorrhea in hyperprolactinemia, 135
Galactosemia, premature ovarian failure, 140–1
Gallium nitrate, hypercalcemia, 303, 469, 470
Garrow belt, 417
Gastric inhibitory polypeptide receptors, ectopic expression, 65–6
Gastric procedures, obesity, 417, 418
Gastrinomas in MEN 1, 118
Gastrointestinal tract
    anorexia nervosa and, 429
    anorexigenic signals, 412
    calcium reabsorption, excessive, 299
    hypercalcemia effects, 299
    in myxedema coma, 461
    potassium loss via, 381
Gene therapy
    adrenoleukodystrophy, 340–1
    pituitary tumors, 38
Genetic factors
    osteoporosis, 306
    Paget's disease of bone, 315–16
    subacute granulomatous thyroiditis, 274
Genetic syndromes and disorders, *see also* Congenital disorders *and specific genes*
    aldosteronism, 388–9
    hypoglycemia, 475
    males
        hypogonadism and, 153–8, 180, 184
        infertility and, 180–4
    nephrogenic diabetes insipidus, 373
Genetic tests, *see* Molecular diagnosis
Genetics (incl. molecular genetics), neoplasia (incl. malignancy), *see also* Familial cancer clinic
    IGFs and, 88, 97
    multiple endocrine neoplasias
        familial isolated hyperparathyroidism, 121
        hyperparathyroidism—jaw tumor syndrome, 120
        MEN 1, 20–1, 116, 117, 118–19
        MEN 2, 123–4
    pituitary and thyroid, 17–24
Genetics (incl. molecular genetics), non-neoplastic conditions
    hypogonadotropic hypogonadism, idiopathic, 153–5
    PCOS, 137
    resistance to thyroid hormone, 257–8
Genital tract abnormalities, amenorrhea, 142–3
Germ cell development, testis, *see* Spermatogenesis
Gestational diabetes insipidus, 372, 373
Gestational hyperthyroidism and TSH-R mutations, 253
Gestodene (GSD), in oral contraceptive, 511
GH, *see* Growth hormone
GHrelin and appetite, 413
GHRH, *see* Growth hormone-releasing hormone
GHRIF, *see* Somatostatin
GHRPs (growth hormone-releasing peptides), 85, 495
GIP receptors, ectopic expression, 65–6
Gitelman's syndrome, 381
GLP-1, 412
Glucagon
    in glucose homeostasis, 347
    therapeutic use, 477–8
Glucagon test, 39, 493
    pheochromocytoma, 396
Glucagon-like peptide-1, 412
Glucocorticoid(s) (corticosteroids)
    administration, 516–17
        ACTH deficiency, 40, 448–9
        Addison's disease, 239–40, 433, 444
        adverse effects/cautions, 335
        Cushing's syndrome, perioperative/postoperative, 69–70, 71
        hirsutism, 211
        in HIV disease/AIDS, 335
        hypercalcemia, 303, 468
        myxedema coma, 463
        non-islet cell tumor hypoglycemia, 352
        pituitary apoplexy, 452
        pituitary tumors, perioperative, 33, 70, 455
        sarcoidosis, 341–2
        subacute granulomatous thyroiditis, 275
        thyroid ophthalmopathy, 230
        thyroid storm, 459, 460
    deficiency, features, 441
    excess (women), screening for, 209
    pharmacology, 335, 516–17
    suppression by dexamethasone, *see* Dexamethasone
Glucocorticoid-remediable aldosteronism, 388, 388–9
Glucose
    administration (dextrose) in hypoglycemia, 351–2, 477, 478
    blood
        abnormal, *see* Hyperglycemia; Hypoglycemia
        homeostasis, 347
        reference values, 553
Glucose tolerance test, oral
    acromegaly, 53
    reference values in, 553
Glycoprotein-producing pituitary tumors, 44–6
cGMP and cavernosal smooth muscle, 167
GNAS1, 291
GnRH, *see* Gonadotropin-releasing hormone
Goiter, 269–85
    multinodular, *see* Multinodular goiter
    non-toxic, 269–85
    in resistance to thyroid hormone, 254
    toxic, *see* Toxic adenoma; Toxic multinodular goiter
Gonad(s)
    dysfunction, *see* Hypogonadism
    dysgenesis, *see* Turner's syndrome
    hypothalamic—pituitary axis and, *see* Hypothalamic—pituitary—gonadal axis
Gonadal steroids, *see* Sex hormones
Gonadorelin, *see* Gonadotropin-releasing hormone, use
Gonadotroph adenoma, 44–5
Gonadotropin, 527, 531–2, *see also* Follicle-stimulating hormone; Luteinizing hormone
    abnormal secretion, *see* Hypergonadotropic disorders *and entries under* Hypogonadotropic

human chorionic, *see* Human chorionic gonadotrophin
pharmacology of various preparations, 527, 531–2
reference values, 553
therapeutic use, 527, 531–2
male infertility, 184–7
Gonadotropin–producing adenoma, 44–5
Gonadotropin-releasing hormone (GnRH; LHRH), 524
anorexia nervosa and, 430
hypogonadotropic amenorrhea and disordered secretion of, 131
mutation in gene for, 155
pulsatile secretion, PCOS and, 206–7
use (gonadorelin), 524
pharmacology, 524
pituitary—gonadal axis testing with, 496
pulsatile administration, males, 186–7
Gonadotropin-releasing hormone (GnRH; LHRH) analogs/agonists, 524–5
in hirsutism, 210
pharmacology, 524–5
Goserelin, 525, 525–6
Grading, pituitary tumors, 28
Granulomatosis, Wegener's, 343
Granulomatous disorders, 341–4
hypercalcemia in, 301, 465
thyroid, 273–5
Graves' disease, 215–29
children/adolescents, 227
clinical assessment, 217–19
familial non-autoimmune hyperthyroidism vs, 251
investigation, 219–20
lymphocytic and postpartum thyroiditis vs, 278–9
management, 222–7, 508, 542
ophthalmopathy, 218, 226–8
pregnancy and, 227–8
Growth, 83–105
disorders of, 83–105
children, missed, leading to adult short stature, 98–9
Growth factors, neoplasia and, 17–20
Growth hormone (GH), 12–13, 495, 526–7
assays, 12–13
interference, 10
in Cushing's syndrome, postoperative assessment, 71
excessive secretion, *see* Acromegaly
neurosecretory dysfunction, 95–6
in obesity, 414
physiology, 83–9
action, 85–9, 495
secretion, 83–5, 495
psychopathology, *see* Psychological dimensions
receptor
agonist, 54, 56–7
deficiency, 96
reference values, 553
replacement therapy (adult), 40–1, 94–5
bone mineral density effects, 91–2
reserve, tests of, 39–40, 495
resistance/insensitivity, 96–7
secretagogs, 83–5
testing, 495
therapeutic use, 95, 526–7
in GH deficiency, *see* replacement therapy *(subheading below)*
in HIV disease/AIDS, 337
in osteoporosis, 314
side-effects, 95, 527
Growth hormone, deficiency, 38, 89–95
adults, 89–95
clinical characteristics, 89–93
diagnosis, 93–4
psychiatric problems, 90, 434–6
replacement therapy, *see* Growth hormone treatment, 94–5
diagnosis, *see* Growth hormone, assays
radiation-induced, 34, 38–9
Growth hormone-binding protein (GHBP), 83
GH assays and, 10
Growth hormone-producing (somatotroph) adenomas, 30
acromegaly, 51, 402
genetics, 18
Growth hormone release-inhibiting hormone, *see* Somatostatin
Growth hormone-releasing hormone (GHRH), 83–4
ectopic production, 51, 56
physiology, 83–4
tests using injection of, 495
Growth hormone-releasing peptides, 85, 495, *see also* GHrelin
Gsp, *see* G protein
Gsx1 mutations, 157
Gut, *see* Gastrointestinal tract
Gynecomastia, *see* Breast enlargement

Hand—Schüller—Christian disease, 342
Hashimoto's (autoimmune) thyroiditis
presentation with, 232
subacute lymphocytic thyroiditis and postpartum thyroiditis as variants of, 275
Head trauma, pituitary dysfunction, *see* Simmonds's disease
Headache in pituitary apoplexy, 450
Hearing loss, resistance to thyroid hormone, 255
Heart, *see also* Cardiovascular system
acromegaly effects, 51, 401–2
arrhythmias, *see* Arrhythmias
coronary disease, sildenafil and, 171–2
failure, in thyroid storm, 459
hypercalcemia effects, 299
in myxedema coma, 461
pheochromocytoma effects, 394
in resistance to thyroid hormone, 255
Height (stature)
in life insurance tables for ideal body weight, 409
measurement, 408
short, missed childhood growth disorders leading to, 98–9
Hemangioma, vertebral, 319
Hemochromatosis, 345
Hemodialysis, hypercalcemic crisis, 468
Hemodynamic effects of sildenafil, 171
Hemodynamic factors influencing ADH secretion, 368, 369
Hemoglobin
hypogonadism and infertility in men and disorders of, 181, 184
testosterone replacement and levels of, 163
Hemorrhage/bleeding
adrenal, 443
uterine, dysfunctional, PCOS and presentation with, 138
Hepatic disease, 345
Heredity, *see entries under* Genetic
Hesx mutations, 157
Heterophilic antibody and immunoassays, 11

Heterozygosity, loss of
    MEN 1 and, 21, 118
    pituitary tumors and, 20–1
Hexarelin, 85, 495
'High-dose hook effect', 9–10
Hip fractures, osteoporotic, 307
Hirsutism, 201–16
    definition, 201
    diagnosis, 208–9
        differential, 203
    evaluation, 208
    idiopathic, PCOS and, 203–4, 206
    management, 209–11
    prevalence, 201–3
Histiocytosis, Langerhans' cell, 342–3
Histomorphometry, osteoporosis, 310
HIV disease/AIDS, 333–8
    adrenal involvement, 443
HLA-B35/B67 and subacute granulomatous thyroiditis, 274
Homeodomain transcription factors, mutations, 156–7
Hormone replacement therapy (HRT; estrogen replacement therapy), 40
    osteoporosis prevention and treatment, 311–12
Human anti-mouse antibodies (HAMA), 11
Human chorionic gonadotrophin (hCG), 527
    antibodies to, 186
    ß-subunit in craniopharyngioma diagnosis, 44
    tumors secreting, 347
    use, 527
        in male infertility treatment, 184, 185, 186, 187
    pharmacology, 527
Human menopausal gonadotrophin (hMG; menotropin), 531–2
    male infertility treatment, 184, 185, 186, 187
    pharmacology, 531–2
Hydrocortisone, *see* Cortisol
Hydrogen ion/potassium ion ATPases, 379
11ß-Hydroxylase inhibition by metyrapone, 69, 494
17_-Hydroxylase deficiency
    diagnosis, 209
    hirsutism, 204
    premature ovarian failure, 141
21-Hydroxylase
    autoantibodies, 239
    deficiency, 99

17-Hydroxyprogesterone, women
    measurement, 209
    PCOS and, 207
5-Hydroxytryptamine (serotonin), orexigenicity, 412
1-_-Hydroxyvitamin D (alfacalcidol), 548, 549
    hypocalcemia, 474
    osteoporosis, 312
    pseudohypoparathyroidism, 293
Hyperaldosteronism, *see* Aldosteronism
Hyperandrogenism, *see* Androgens, excess
Hypercalcemia, 298–303, 464–70
    acute (hypercalcemic crisis), 464–70
    assessment and investigations, 466–7
    causes (other than hyperparathyroidism), 298–303, 465
        HIV disease/AIDS, 336
        malignancy, *see* Cancer
    clinical features, 299, 466
    differential diagnosis, 299–300
    familial predisposition, 117, 121
    therapy, 301–3, 355, 356, 467–70
        emergency, 467–70
Hypercalcemic hypercalciuria, familial, 117
Hypercalciuria
    familial hypercalcemia and, 117
    familial hypercalcemic, 117
Hypercalciuric hypercalcemia, familial benign, 121
Hyperglycemia
    drugs preventing, *see* Hypoglycemics, oral
    effects, 347
Hypergonadotropic disorders
    men, 157–8
    women, amenorrhea, 139–42
Hyperinsulinism/hyperinsulinemia, 100
    in acromegaly, 402
Hyperkalemia, 382–3
    causes, 382–3
        HIV disease/AIDS, 336
    treatment, 383
Hypermagnesemia, hypocalcemia in, 473
Hypernatremia, HIV disease/AIDS, 336
Hyperosmolality (hypertonicity), 484
    hyperkalemia and, 383
    hyponatremia and, 479, 481, 484
Hyperparathyroidism, 293–8, 400–1
    familial, and jaw tumor (syndrome), 117, 120
    familial isolated, 116, 117, 120–2

    hypertension in, 400–1
    in MEN 1, treatment, 116
    primary, 293–8
        asymptomatic, clinical presentation, 294–5
        clinical classification, 294
        diagnosis, 295
        imaging, 296–7
        pathophysiology, 294
        treatment, 294, 297–8
Hyperplasia
    adrenal, 64, 388
        congenital, *see* Congenital adrenal hyperplasia
        idiopathic bilateral, 388
        nodular/macronodular/primary, 64, 388
    parathyroid, 294
    thecal cell (hyperthecosis ovarii), 205
Hyperprolactinemia, 46–50
    amenorrhea in, 133–6
    clinical features, 46–7
    hypothalamic disease causing, 46, 133
    investigation, 47
    treatment, 135–6
Hypertension, 387–406
Hyperthecosis ovarii, 205
Hyperthermia, thyroid storm, 458, 460
Hyperthyroidism, *see also* Graves' disease; Thyrotoxicosis
    congenital/sporadic/autosomal-dominant, TSH-R mutations and, 251
    gestational, TSH-R mutations and, 253
    hypertension in, 399, 400
    males, testosterone assays, 152
    tumors causing, 273
Hypertonic saline, hyponatremia, 378, 482
Hypertonicity, *see* Hyperosmolality
Hypervolemic hyponatremia, 376
Hypoadrenalism, *see* Adrenal insufficiency/failure
Hypocalcemia, 287, 470–4
    clinical features and assessment/investigation, 287–9, 470–3
    emergency treatment, 473–4
    in HIV disease/AIDS, 336
    in hypoparathyroidism, 287
Hypoglycemia, 347–53, 475–9, 490

ADH release, 369
assessment and investigation, 349–50, 466–7, 475–7
causes, 350–3
non-islet cell tumors, 350–2, 475
diagnosis, 348
physiological effects, 347–8, 490
treatment, 351–2, 477–9
unawareness, 476
Hypoglycemics, oral (insulin-sensitizing agents; antidiabetic drugs; antihyperglycemics), 532–3
in PCOS, 139, 210
pharmacology, 532–3
Hypogonadism (gonadal dysfunction)
with anosmia, see Kallmann's syndrome
in HIV disease/AIDS, 335
hypogonadotropic, see Hypogonadotropic hypogonadism
men (testicular dysfunction), 147–65
in adrenoleukodystrophy, 339
evaluation, 148–52
genetic syndromes associated with, 153–8, 180, 184
in hemoglobin disorders, 181, 184
testosterone replacement and sexual aspects of, 162
women, 133
Hypogonadotropic amenorrhea, 131–7
Hypogonadotropic hypogonadism in men, 153–5
congenital, 150–1
evaluation, 151, 179
idiopathic, 151, 153–5
infertility, 177
treatment, 184–7
testicular volume and, 150–1
testosterone replacement and LH and FSH levels, 162–3
Hypogonadotropic hypogonadism in women, idiopathic, 133
Hypokalemia, 380–2
causes, 381
aldosteronism, 381, 388
drugs, 380
HIV disease/AIDS, 336
clinical features, 380
investigation, 381
treatment, 381
Hypomagnesemia, 471
HIV disease/AIDS, 336

hypocalcemia in, 473
treatment, 473, 474
Hyponatremia, 376–8, 479–84
assessment/investigations/, 479–82
asymptomatic, 483, 484
clinical manifestations, 377, 479
HIV disease/AIDS, 336
mild-to-moderate symptomatic, 482–4
severe symptomatic, 482, 483
treatment, 377–8, 482–4
complications of, 378, 479, 482, 484
Hypo-osmolality (hypotonicity), hyponatremia and pseudohyponatremia with, 479, 481
Hypoparathyroidism, 287–90, 471, see also Pseudohypoparathyroidism
acute, 450
causes, 289, 471
clinical features, 287–9
tetany, 287–8, 471–2
Hypophysis, see Pituitary gland
Hypophysitis, lymphocytic, see Lymphocytic adenohypophysitis
Hypopituitarism (pituitary dysfunction/insufficiency), 434–6, 446–9, 487–494
clinical assessment and investigation, 446–7, 487–494
emergencies, 446–9
macroadenoma causing, 454
psychiatric problems, 434–6
radiation-related, 34
traumatic and vascular causes, see Sheehan's syndrome; Simmond's disease
treatment, 447–9
Hypoplasia
Leydig cell, 157
parathyroid, 289
Hypothalamic—pituitary—adrenal (HPA) axis
in AIDS/HIV disease, 334
in hemochromatosis, 345
psychopathology and, 422, 424, 424–6
testing, 488–4
emergency, 490
Hypothalamic—pituitary axis, 28–32, 38–9
classification of diseases, 28–32
erectile dysfunction and lesions of, 169

functional assessment, 39–41
normal, 25–6
radiation damage, 34, 38–9
Hypothalamic—pituitary—gonadal (HPG) axis
in AIDS/HIV disease, 335
evaluation, 337–8
assessment, 495–497
in AIDS/HIV disease, 337–8
psychopathology and, 422, 424, 427
anorexia nervosa, 429–30
Hypothalamic—pituitary—thyroid (HPT) axis, 494–5
psychopathology and, 422, 424, 426–7
testing, 494–5
Hypothalamus
diseases
amenorrhea due to, 131–3
erectile dysfunction and, 169
hyperprolactinemia with, 46, 133
hypopituitarism with, 38
non-endocrine manifestations, 27
obesity due to, 413
sarcoidosis, 341
types, 26
energy balance and, 411–13
imaging, see Imaging
in obesity, 414
Hypothermia, myxedema coma, 462–3
Hypothyroidism, 231–6, 433–4
Addison's disease and (Schmidt's syndrome), 444
autoimmune, 231–6
assessment and investigations, 232, 234–5
clinical features, 232
management, 235–6
childhood, short stature due to, 99
coma in severe hypothyroidism, 460–3, 464
congenital, 251–3
diagnosis/investigations, 234–5, 462
edema in, see Myxedema
hyperprolactinemia in, 134
hypertension in, 399, 400
lymphocytic thyroiditis followed by, 279
obesity in, 414
primary, diagnosis, 232, 233, 234
psychiatric problems, 433–4

radioiodine-induced, 226
Hypotonicity, hyponatremia and pseudo-hyponatremia with, 479, 481
Hypoventilation in myxedema coma, 461, 462
Hypovolemic hyponatremia, 376

Iatrogenic causes of premature ovarian failure, 139–40
IGF, *see* Insulin-like growth factors
IGFBP, *see* Insulin-like growth factor-binding proteins
Imaging
    adrenal, in aldosteronism, 392
    Cushing's syndrome, 68
    erectile dysfunction, 168–9
    head (incl. pituitary—hypothalamic region)
        hypopituitarism, 447
        macroadenomas, 454
        pituitary apoplexy, 451
    hyperparathyroidism, 296–7
    Paget's disease of bone, 318–19
    pheochromocytoma (extra-adrenal), 397–8
Immune system, GH deficiency (adult) and, 93
Immunoassays, 4–9
    accuracy, 8
    automation, 9
    competitive, 4–5
    consensus of methods, 8
    cross-reactivity, 5–6
    design, 4–5
    failings (incl. interference), 9–11
    non-competitive, *see* Immunometric assays
    precision/reproducibility, 7–8
    specificity, 5–6
    standardization/calibration, 6–7
    thyroid hormone and sick euthyroid syndrome, 3–4, 356–7
Immunodepression in AIDS/HIV disease, 334
Immunometric assays, 5
    failings/limitations, 9
Impedance measurement (body fat estimation), 409
Implants, testosterone, 161, *see also* Prostheses
Impotence, *see* Erection, dysfunction
Incidentaloma (adrenal), 392
Infants
    hypercalcemia in, 301, 302

newborn, adrenoleukodystrophy, 338, 340
Infarction, pituitary, *see* Sheehan's syndrome; Simmond's disease
Infections (and sepsis), 345
    adrenal, 443
    myxedema coma precipitated by, 463
    in Paget's disease of bone etiology, 315
    in premature ovarian failure etiology, 140
    thyroid, 279–80
        subacute granulomatous thyroiditis and, 273–4
    thyroid storm precipitated by, 459
Infertility, *see* Fertility problems
Inflammatory disorders, 341–5
Inheritance, *see entries under* Genetic
Injury, head, *see* Simmond's disease
Insulin, *see also* Hyperinsulinism
    acromegaly and, 402
    autoantibodies to, 352
    glucose homeostasis, 347
    hypoglycemia induced by surreptitious administration, 352
    IGFs and, comparisons, 87
    reference values, 554
Insulin hypoglycemia test, 348
Insulin resistance
    in acromegaly, 402
    women (and virilization/PCOS/hyperandrogenism), 205, 207–8
        assessment for, 209
Insulin sensitizing agents, *see* Hypoglycemics, oral
Insulin tolerance or stress test, 39, 490–1
    GH deficiency/reserve and, 93
Insulin-like growth factor(s), 86–9
    comparisons between insulin/IGF-1/IGF-2, 87
    IGF-1, 87
        actions, 87
        in GH resistance/insensitivity, administration, 97
        receptor(s), 86–7
        regulation of expression and action, 86
    IGF-2, 87–8
        overexpression in Beckwith—Wiedemann disease, 100
        tumors secreting, 350–2
    measurement, 39–40, 89
        acromegaly, 53

physiology, 86–8
reference values, 554
resistance syndromes, 100
tumorigenesis and, 88, 97–8
Insulin-like growth factor-binding proteins (IGFBPs), 88–9
    IGF-independent actions, 88–9
    IGFBP-3, 88
        cancer and, 97
        deficiency, 97
    proteases, 88
Insulinoma, 476
Intercurrent illness, assays and, 3
International Standards, immunoassays, 6–7
Internist, male infertility and, 184
Intracellular fluid, solute composition, 367
Intracytoplasmic sperm injection, 188
Intraurethral alprostadil, 173
Iodinated contrast agents, 544
    in thyroid storm, 459
Iodine (and iodide)
    excess, in autoimmune-prone individuals, 278
    radioactive, *see* Radioiodine
    treatment with
        Graves' disease, 224
        thyroid storm, 458–9, 460
Ion channels, potassium, 379
Ionizing radiation,, *see also* Radiation; Radiotherapy
Irradiation, *see* Radiotherapy
Islet cell tumors (insulinoma), 476
Isotonic saline, hyponatremia, 484

Jaw tumor, hyperparathyroidism and, 117, 120
Jaw wiring, 417
Jejunoileal bypass, 417–18
Jensen's syndrome, 302
JunD and menin, 118–19

KALIG-1, 154, 155
Kallmann's syndrome
    men, 154
    women, 133
Kallmann's syndrome interval-1 gene (*KALIG-1*), 154, 155
Kearns—Sayre syndrome, 290
Kenney—Caffey syndrome, 290
Ketoconazole, 528–9
    Cushing's syndrome, 69
    pharmacology, 528–9
        adverse effects, 337, 529

Kidney
  ADH insensitivity/resistance, see Nephrogenic diabetes insipidus
  disease/lesions
    hypercalcemia, 299
    hyperparathyroidism and, 296
    hyperparathyroidism—jaw tumor syndrome, 120
    potassium handling, 380, 382
    vasopressin actions, 370–1
Klinefelter's syndrome, infertility, 180–2

Laboratory evaluation, see Biochemical investigations and specific conditions
Lactotroph adenomas, see Prolactinomas
Langerhans' cell histiocytosis, 342–3
Lanreotide, 529
  pharmacology, 529
  pituitary tumors, 36–7
Laron syndrome, 96–7
Lean body mass, estimation, 409
Lens cataracts in hypocalcemia, 288
Leptin, 27, 412, 428
  deficiency, 412
Letterer—Siwe disease, 342
Leukocytes in semen, 178
Leuprorelin, 525, 526
Levonorgestrel (LNg) in oral contraceptive
  in combined pill, 511
  in emergency contraception, 539
  in progestogen-only pill, 540
Leydig cell hypoplasia, 157
LH, see Luteinizing hormone
Lhx3 mutations, 157
Life insurance tables, ideal body weight, 409
Lifestyle
  female hypogonadotropic amenorrhea and, 132
  male hypogonadism and, 148
Lipase, lipoprotein, 408
Lipectomy, 418
Lipid disturbances (dyslipidemia)
  HIV infection, 336–7
  obesity, 415
Lipolysis, control, 408
Liponecrosis, subcutaneous, 302
Lipoprotein(s), in obesity, 415
Lipoprotein lipase, 408
Lithium, 529–30
  with iodide treatment, 459
  pharmacology, 529–30
Liver disease, 345

Loop diuretics
  in hypercalcemic crisis, 467, 469
  hypokalemia with, 380
Loss of heterozygosity, see Heterozygosity
Lumbar puncture, pituitary apoplexy, 451–2
Lupus erythematosus, systemic, 344
Luteinizing hormone (LH), see also Gonadotropin
  administration (human LH) in male infertility, 185, 186
  assays in male hypogonadism, 151
  testosterone replacement and, 162–3
  PCOS and, 206–7
  reference values, 553
Luteinizing hormone-producing adenoma, 44
Luteinizing hormone receptor, mutations
  men, 155–6, 157–8
    activating, 156, 158
    inactivating, 156, 157
  women, 140
Luteinizing hormone-releasing hormone, see Gonadotropin-releasing hormone
Lymphocytic (adeno)hypophysitis, 41–3, 133, 240, 343–4, 447
  hyperprolactinemia, 134
Lymphocytic thyroiditis, 275–9
Lymphomas, hypercalcemia, 301

McCune—Albright syndrome, 64–5
Macroadenoma, pituitary, 453–5
  MRI, 27, 28
  prolactin-producing, 47, 48
    management, 48–50
  visual loss, 453–5
    assessment and investigation, 453–4
    treatment, 454–5
Macronodular adrenal hyperplasia, 64, 388
Macroprolactin(emia), 10–11, 47
Magnesium disturbances, see Hypermagnesemia; Hypomagnesemia
Magnesium sulfate administration, 473, 474
Magnetic resonance imaging (MRI)
  hypothalamic—pituitary region
    Cushing's syndrome, 68
    hypopituitarism, 447
    lymphocytic hypophysitis, 42
    pituitary apoplexy, 451
    posterior, bright spot, and cranial diabetes insipidus, 375

    sarcoidosis, 43
    tumors, 27, 28, 30, 45, 47, 48, 454
  parathyroid, 297
  pheochromocytoma (extra-adrenal), 397, 398
Males, see Men
Malignancy, see Cancer; Metastases
Marine—Lenhart disease, 219
Masculinization, see Virilization
Mayer—Rokitansky—Küster—Hauser syndrome, 142
MDP (^{99m}Tc) scan, osteoporosis, 309
Measurements, see Biochemical investigations and specific tests
Medical disorders
  chronic, screening males for androgen deficiency, 147
  pre-existing, assays and, 3–4
Medical management, see also Drug therapy
  Cushing's syndrome, 68–9
  Graves' disease, 223–6
  hyperparathyroidism, 298
  Paget's disease of bone, 320–2
  pituitary tumors, 34–7
    GH-producing (and acromegaly), 54
    perioperative, 33
Medication, see Drugs
Medroxyprogesterone acetate, 530–1
  pharmacology, 530–1
  test using, in amenorrhea, 144
Medullary thyroid carcinoma
  familial (FMTC), 116, 123, 124
  MEN 2A and, 122–3
Megestrol acetate in AIDS patients, 337
α-Melanocyte stimulating hormone, 411
Melatonin and seasonal affective disorder, 424
Men, 147–200
  hypogonadism, see Hypogonadism
  osteoporosis, 314
  sexual development, see Sexual development
  sexual function, see Fertility problems; Sexual function
MEN 1 and MEN 1 gene, see Menin (MEN 1); Multiple endocrine neoplasia
Menarche, idiopathic delay, 143
Menin (MEN 1), 118–19
  gene (*MEN 1*), 20–1, 118–19
    in familial isolated hyperparathyroidism and its

diagnosis, 121
    in MEN 1 diagnosis, 119–20
    mutations, 20–1, 118–19
Meningioma, suprasellar, 43
Menopausal gonadotrophin, human, see Human menopausal gonadotrophin
Menopause
    premature, see Ovarian failure
    symptoms, drug therapy, 514, 519
Menotropin, see Human menopausal gonadotrophin
Menstrual abnormalities, see Amenorrhea; Oligomenorrhea
Menstrual cycle, reproductive hormone tests and, 2, see also Premenstrual syndrome
Mental disturbances, see Psychological dimensions
Metabolic acidosis and hyperkalemia, 383
Metabolic disorders/disease, 345–7
    in anorexia nervosa, 429
    bone, 303–14
    inborn errors of carbohydrate metabolism, 475
Metabolism
    bone, 304–5
    GH deficiency (adult) effects, 92
Metanephrine, 393
    assays, pheochromocytoma, 395, 396, 397
Metaraminol, 532
Metastases, 345–6
    in adrenal, 346–7
    from pituitary, 346
    from thyroid, 109, 110
Metformin (a biguanide), 532–3
    PCOS, 139
    pharmacology, 532–3
Methylation of CpG islands of $p21$, pituitary tumors, 21
7-_-Methyl-19-nortestosterone, 161
17-_-Methyltestosterone use, 158, 159
Metyrapone, Cushing's syndrome treatment, 69
Metyrapone test, 494
MIBG scan, pheochromocytoma, 398
MIBI (^{99m}Tc) scan, parathyroid, 297
Microadenoma, pituitary
    MRI, 27, 45
    prolactin-producing, 45, 46–7, 48
        management, 47–8, 50
        pregnancy and, 50
Mifepristone, pharmacology, 533
Milk—alkali syndrome, 301

Milrinone, erectile dysfunction, 175
Mineralocorticoid deficiency, 383, see also Aldosterone
    features, 441
    replacement therapy in Addisonian crisis, 445
Mithramicin, hypercalcemia, 303, 468, 469
Mitotane, 533–4
    Cushing's syndrome, 69
Molecular diagnosis (incl. genetic tests)
    aldosteronism (heritable forms), 389
    familial isolated hyperparathyroidism, 121
    hyperparathyroidism—jaw tumor syndrome, 120
    infertility (males), 180
    MEN 1, 119–20, 122
    MEN 2, 124
        case study, 125, 125–6
    thyroid nodular disease, 270
Molecular genetics, see Genetics
Monoclonal antibody in immunoassays, specificity/hyperspecificity, 6
Mood disorder, see Depression
_-MSH, 411
Müllerian system anomalies, amenorrhea, 142–3
Multinodular goiter, 269–85
    clinical presentation, 269
    diagnosis, 269–71
    pathology, 269
    prevalence, 269
    toxic, see Toxic multinodular goiter
    treatment, 271–2
Multiple endocrine neoplasia (MEN), 115–30
    MEN 1, 115–21
        acromegaly and, 51, 402
        case study, 121–2
        clinical manifestations, 115–16
        diagnosis, 119–20, 120–1
        FGF-2 and, 21
        genetics, 20–1, 116, 117, 118–19
        treatment, 116–18
    MEN 2, 122–6
        case study, 125–6
        clinical manifestations, 122–3
        management, 124–5
        MEN 2A (Sipple's syndrome), 116, 122–3, 123
        MEN 2B (=MEN 3), 116, 123
        pheochromocytoma, see Pheochromocytoma

Muscle strength, GH deficiency (adult), 92
Myalgic encephalomyelitis (chronic fatigue syndrome), GH use, 95
Myelinolysis, central pontine (=osmotic demyelination syndrome in hyponatremia correction), 378, 479, 482
Myeloma, hypercalcemia, 300–1, 353
Myotonic dystrophy, testicular dysfunction, 184
Myxedema, pretibial, 230
Myxedema coma, 460–3, 464

Nafarelin, 525, 526
Nandrolone, osteoporosis, 314
National External Quality Assessment Schemes (NEQAS), 7, 8
Nausea, vasopressin release, 369
Necrosis, tissue, hyperkalemia in, 383
Negative predictive value, 14
Nelson's syndrome, 61, 62
Neonates, adrenoleukodystrophy, 338, 340
Neoplasms, see Tumors
Nephrogenic diabetes insipidus (NPI), 41, 372, 373
    diagnosis, 374
Nephron, vasopressin actions, 370–1
Neuroendocrine disease, 25–81, 95–6
    obesity and, 26–7, 413
Neurohypophysis (posterior pituitary), 25–6
    hormones, 368
    MRI bright spot, and cranial diabetes insipidus, 375
Neurologic features, see also Brain; Central nervous system
    adrenoleukodystrophy, 338, 339
    Graves' disease, 218
    hypercalcemia, 299
    hypoglycemia, 348, 476, 477
    hyponatremia, 378, 481
    hyponatremia correction, 378, 479, 482, 484
    myxedema coma, 461
    pituitary apoplexy, 450
Neuromuscular signs, hypoparathyroidism/hypocalcemia, 287–8, 471–2
Neuropeptide(s)
    depression and, 424
    hypothalamic, in energy balance and eating, 411–13, 428
Neuropeptide Y and appetite, 412
Neuropsychiatric problems, see Psychological dimensions

Neurotensin, 412
Neurotransmitters
　　GH secretion and, 84
　　hypothalamic, in energy balance, 411–13
Newborns, adrenoleukodystrophy, 338, 340
Nitrates and sildenafil, interactions, 172
Nitric oxide, cavernosal smooth muscle and, 166
Nm23 and endocrine neoplasia, 21
Nodular adrenal disease, 63–6, 388
Nodular thyroid disease, 269–85
　　in Grave's disease, 218–19
Non-steroidal antiandrogen, 523
Non-steroidal antiinflammatory drugs, subacute granulomatous thyroiditis, 275
Non-steroidal aromatase inhibitor, 505
Non-steroidal selective androgen receptor modulators, 161
Non-thyroidal illness, thyroid function testing and, 3–4
Noonan's syndrome, 99, 182
Norethisterone (NET), 534
　　in menopausal treatment, 519
　　in oral contraceptive
　　　　combined pill, 511
　　　　progestogen-only pill, 540
　　pharmacology, 534
Norethisterone enanthate, 534–5
Norgestimate, 535
Norgestrel, progestogen-only pill, 540
19-Nortestosterone, osteoporosis, 314
NPS R568, 298
Nutrition, *see* Diet

Obesity, 26–7, 407–20, *see also* Weight
　　disease and comorbidity in, 408
　　endocrine repercussions, 414–15
　　evaluation, 415
　　male, testosterone levels and, 152
　　origins, 410
　　treatment, 415–18
Obstetrics,, *see also* Pregnancy
Octreotide, 535–6
　　hypercalcemia of malignancy, 355
　　pharmacology, 535–6
　　pheochromocytoma imaging, 398
　　pituitary tumors, 36–7
　　　　GH-producing (and acromegaly), 55–6
Older people/elderly, males, androgen/testosterone levels, 147, 152
　　screening for deficiency, 148

Oligomenorrhea, 131
　　definition, 131
　　in PCOS
　　　　management, 138
　　　　presentation, 137
Oncogenes, 17–20
Oophorectomy (ovariectomy), 139–40
Ophthalmopathy, thyroid-associated, 216–18, *see also* Cataracts
　　clinical assessment, 229
　　Graves', 218, 226–8
　　management, 229–30
Optic disk swelling, 288
Optic nerve/chiasm/tract involvement, pituitary tumors, 31, 32
　　management, 454–5
Oral contraceptive pill, 510–14, 539–40
　　amenorrhea following use, 132
　　combined, 510–14
　　dopamine agonists and, 50
　　emergency (postcoital) use, 539
　　in hirsutism, 210
　　immediate stopping, reasons, 513–14
　　pharmacology, 510–14, 539–41
Oral glucose tolerance test, *see* Glucose tolerance test
Orexigenic signals, 411, 412–13
Orexin A and B, 413
Orlistat, 416–17
Osmolality, plasma and urine, *see also* Hyperosmolality; Hypotonicity
　　estimation, 374
Osmoreceptors and ADH secretion, 369
Osmotic demyelination syndrome (in hyponatremia correction), 378, 479, 482
Osteitis fibrosa cystica, 294
Osteoclast differentiation factor, receptor for (ODFR; RANK), 315, 316
Osteodystrophy, Albright's hereditary, 291
Osteolysis, familial expansile, 316
Osteomalacia, 322–4
Osteoporosis, 303–14
　　clinical manifestations, 306–7
　　　　vertebra, 306–7, 319
　　diagnosis, 306–10
　　men, 314
　　pathophysiology, 304–5
　　prevention and management, 310–14, 504, 507
　　primary vs secondary, 305–6
Osteoprotegerin use, 356
Osteosarcomas in Paget's disease, 320
Ovarian failure, premature, 139–42, 240

　　autoimmune aspects, 240
Ovariectomy, 139–40
Ovaries (disorders), 137–42
　　amenorrhea, 137–42
　　androgen production, excess, 207
　　cysts, *see* Polycystic ovaries; Polycystic ovary syndrome
　　hyperthecosis ovarii, 205
　　in obesity, 414
　　in PCOS pathogenesis, 207
　　tumors
　　　　androgen-secreting, 205
　　　　diagnosis, 209
Overgrowth syndromes, 100
Ovulatory failure in PCOS, treatment, 139
Oxandrolone, 536
Oxytocin, 368
　　reference values, 554

p16 and pituitary tumors, 21
p21 and thyroid carcinoma, 21
p27 and pituitary tumors, 21
p53, pituitary tumors and, 21
Paget's disease of bone, 314–22
　　complications, 320
　　diagnosis, 317–20
　　etiopathogenesis, 315–16
　　pathophysiology, 316
　　treatment, 320
Pain, bone, pagetic, 317–18
Pamidronate, 537
　　hypercalcemia, 302, 303, 468
　　　　of malignancy, 355, 356
　　Paget's disease of bone, 322
　　pharmacology, 537
Pancreas
　　endocrine, in obesity, 414
　　in HIV disease/AIDS, 335–6
　　MEN 1-related tumors, 118
Papaverine, 537–8
　　erectile dysfunction, 174–5, 537–8
　　pharmacology, 537–8
Papillary thyroid carcinoma (PTC), 107–9
　　genetics, 19–20
　　　　familial PTC, 21
　　subtypes, 107
Papilledema, 288
Paraganglioma, MRI, 398, *see also* Pheochromocytoma
Paralysis, hypokalemic periodic, 382
Parathyroid gland
　　destruction, 289, 290
　　development failure, 289–90
　　dysfunction due to altered

regulation, 289, 290
imaging, 296–7
neoplasms, *see* Tumors
Parathyroid hormone (PTH)
　abnormal levels, *see* Hyperparathyroidism; Hypoparathyroidism
　actions, 470
　　impaired/resistance to, 290, 290–1
　gene, mutations, 290
　in hypercalcemia differential diagnosis, assay, 466
　in osteoporosis treatment, 314
　synthetic PTH fragment infusion test in pseudohypoparathyroidism, 292
Parathyroid hormone-related protein, 354
　hypercalcemia of malignancy and, 354, 466
Parathyroidectomy
　effects, 290
　in hyperparathyroidism, 294, 297–8
　　guidelines, 294
　in MEN 1, 116
Patches (transdermal), testosterone
　evaluation of local application site, 164
　non-genital, 159, 160
　scrotal, 159, 160
Pediatrics, *see* Children
Pegvisomant, 54, 56–7
Penis
　erection, *see* Erection
　nocturnal tumescence, recording, 169
Perchlorate, thyroid storm, 459, 460
Pergolide, hyperprolactinemia, 136
Periodic paralysis, hypokalemic, 382
Peripheral vasculature resistance and hypertension in Cushing's syndrome, 402, 403
Peritoneal dialysis, hypercalcemic crisis, 468
Peroxisomes
　biogenesis in neonatal adrenoleukodystrophy, 340
　function (membrane transport) in X-linked adrenoleukodystrophy and, 339
　　gene therapy restoring, 341
Petrosal sinus sampling, Cushing's syndrome, 67, 68
PEX1/PEX6, 340

Phenoxybenzamine, preoperative, pheochromocytoma, 398–9
Phentolamine, 538
　erectile dysfunction, 175
　pharmacology, 538
Phenylephrine, 538–9
Pheochromocytoma, 393–9
　clinical manifestations, 393–4
　　Cushing's syndrome, 63
　diagnosis, 394–8
　MEN 2-related, 123, 395
　　treatment, 125
　surgery, 398–9
Phosphate homeostasis, drugs interfering with, 324
Phosphodiesterase (cyclic nucleotide), type 5 (in penile erection), 167
Phosphodiesterase inhibitors (in erectile dysfunction)
　type 4, 175
　type 5, 167, 170–3
Phosphodiesterase type 5, cyclic nucleotide (in penile erection), inhibitors, 167, 170–3
Phospholipids, antibodies to, 344
Photodynamic therapy, pituitary tumors, 37–8
Pigmented nodular adrenal disease, primary, 63–4
Pit-1 mutations, 156
Pituitary apoplexy (with tumors etc.), 28–31, 449–53
　adrenal insufficiency in, 443
　clinical assessment, 449–51
　investigation, 451–2
　treatment, 452–3
Pituitary gland, 27–59, 446–55, 487–494, *see also* Hypothalamic—pituitary—adrenal axis; Hypothalamic—pituitary axis; Hypothalamic—pituitary—gonadal axis
　anterior, *see* Adenohypophysis
　developmental disorders, 156–7
　disorders (in general), 27–59, 446–55
　　amenorrhea in, 133–7
　　emergencies, 446–55
　　erectile dysfunction in, 169
　　in obesity, 414
　　fibrosing pseudotumor, 344
　functional assessment, 487–494
　　principles, 487
　　types of test, 488
　functional impairment (insufficiency/dysfunction), *see* Hypopituitarism
　imaging, *see* Imaging
　lymphocytic hypophysitis, *see* Lymphocytic adenohypophysitis
　neoplasms (incl. cancer), 17–24, 27–38, 133–4, *see also* Adenoma
　　acromegaly and, 51, 402
　　amenorrhea, 133–4
　　classification, 27, 28, 30
　　Cushing's syndrome and, 62, 68
　　genetics, 17–24
　　glycoprotein-producing, 44–6
　　local effects, 28–32
　　in MEN 1, 118
　　metastases from, 346
　　pituitary apoplexy with, *see* Pituitary apoplexy
　　resistance to thyroid hormone vs, 256, 257
　　treatment, 32–8, 136, 452–3
　　visual loss, 31–2, 453–5
　posterior, *see* Neurohypophysis
　postpartum infarction (Sheehan's syndrome), 343, 447
　sarcoidosis, 43, 341
Pituitary resistance to thyroid hormone, 254, 257–8, 260
Pituitary stalk and cranial diabetes insipidus, 375
Plasma osmolality, estimation, 374
Plasmapheresis, thyroid storm, 459
Plastic surgery, obesity, 418
Plicamicin (mithramycin), hypercalcemia, 303, 468, 469
POEMS syndrome, 347
Polyclonal antibody in immunoassays, specificity, 6
Polycystic ovaries, definition, 137
Polycystic ovary syndrome (PCOS), 137–9, 206–8
　clinical presentation and assessment, 137–8
　definition, 137
　genetics, 137
　hirsutism (idiopathic) and, 203–4, 206
　hyperprolactinemia, 134
　obesity in, 413
　pathophysiology, 206–8
Polydipsia, 371–2
　primary, 372, 373
Polyglandular syndrome, autoimmune (APS)

Addison's disease and, 238
　type 1, 238, 240–1
　　clinical features, 241, 290
　type 2, 238, 242
　　clinical features, 241
Polyglutamine tract length of androgen receptor, infertility and, 183
Polyuria, 371–2
　diagnosis in, 374
Pontine myelinolysis, central (=osmotic demyelination syndrome in hyponatremia correction), 378, 479, 482
Positive predictive value, 14
Postcoital contraception, 539
Postpartum pituitary infarction (Sheehan's syndrome), 343, 446
Postpartum thyroiditis, 236–7, 275–9
Potassium, 378–83
　excessive intake or release, 382
　imbalance/disturbances, 380–3
　　HIV disease/AIDS, 336
　normal balance and its regulation, 379–80
　renal handling, 380, 382
　transporters and ion channels, 379
Prader–Willi syndrome, 156
Predictive values, 14
Pre-existing disease, assays and, 3
Pregnancy
　diabetes insipidus, 372, 373
　Graves' disease, 227–8
　hyperthyroidism in, and TSH-R mutations, 253
　pituitary infarction after (Sheehan's syndrome), 343, 446
　pituitary prolactinomas, 50
　thyroiditis following, 236–7, 275–9
　thyrotoxicosis in, 273
Premarin, 514
Premature ovarian failure, *see* Ovarian failure
Premenstrual syndrome, 427
Pretibial myxedema, 230
Progesterone, reference values, 553
Progesterone receptor antagonist, pharmacology, 533
Progestogens (progestagens), 517–18, 530–1, 534–5, 539–41, *see also* Antiprogestogen
　AIDS patients, 337
　in amenorrhea, challenge test, 144
　menopausal symptoms, 519
　in oral contraceptive, pharmacology, 510–14, 539–41

　in combined oral contraceptive, 510–14
　in progestogen-only pill, 539–41
　pharmacology, 517–18, 530–1, 534–5
Prolactin, 427, 497
　autoantibodies to, 10–11
　depression and, 429
　hypersecretion, *see* Hyperprolactinemia
　status, assessment, 501
　　in acromegaly, 53
　　in amenorrhea and hyperprolactinemia, 135
Prolactinomas (lactotroph adenomas), 30, 46–7, 47–50, 133–4
　amenorrhea, 133–4
　familial, 47
　growth factors and genetics, 20
　management, 47–50, 136, 455
　MRI, 45, 47
　in pregnancy, 50
Prop1 mutations, 157
Propranolol, 541–2
　Graves' disease, 224
　postpartum thyroiditis, 237
　thyroid storm, 459, 460
Propylthiouracil (PTU), 542
　Graves' disease, 223, 226
　in pregnancy, 227
　pharmacology, 542
　thyroid storm, 458
Prostaglandin E$_1$, *see* Alprostadil
Prostate
　benign hypertrophy, androgens contraindicated in, 161
　cancer
　　androgens contraindicated in, 161
　　risk with androgen therapy, 163
　follow-up in testosterone replacement therapy, 163–4
Prostate-specific antigen levels, testosterone replacement therapy and, 163–4
Prostheses, penile, 175, *see also* Implants
Protein(s), binding, assays and, 2–3, 10, *see also specific binding proteins*
Protein kinase C and neoplasia, 18
Pseudo-Cushing's syndrome, 60, 61
　Cushing's syndrome vs, 61, 425–6
Pseudohyperkalemia, 382
Pseudohyponatremia, 479, 481–2
　HIV disease/AIDS, 336

Pseudohypoparathyroidism, 290–7
　basal ganglia calcification, 287, 288
　diagnosis, 292
　therapy, 293
　types, 290–2
Pseudotumor, fibrosing pituitary, 344
Psychological dimensions (incl. psychiatric and neuropsychiatric problems), 421–40, *see also specific psychiatric disorders*
　Cushing's syndrome, 61, 425–6, 432–3
　GH and, 427
　　deficiency, 90, 434–6
　hypocalcemia, 472
　resistance to thyroid hormone, 255
Psychosexual counselling, erectile dysfunction, 170
Psychosis, dopamine agonist-induced, 432
PTC/*ret* gene rearrangements, 19–20
PTH, *see* Parathyroid hormone
Pttg, 20
Ptx2a/*Ptx2b* mutations, 157
Pulsatile administration of GnRH, males, 186–7
Pulsatile secretion, 1
　gonadotropin (incl. LH)
　　and idiopathic hypogonadotropic hypogonadism, 153
　　and PCOS, 206
Pyrexia/hyperthermia, thyroid storm, 458, 460

Quality of life and GH deficiency, 435–6
Quentelet index, 408
Quervain's thyroiditis, 273–5
Quinagolide, 542–3

Radiation-related disorders
　pituitary, 34
　　hypopituitarism, 34, 38–9
　premature ovarian failure, 140
　thyroid cancers, 108
Radiography (in assessment)
　osteoporosis, 308
　Paget's disease of bone, 318
Radioiodine
　scans using, pheochromocytoma, 398
　treatment, 112, 225–6
　　cautions and complications, 225, 226
　　Graves' disease (and ophthalmopathy), 225–6, 230

multinodular goiter, 272
toxic adenoma, 272
uptake measurement in subacute granulomatous thyroiditis, 275
Radiolabels in immunoassays, 5
Radiology, see Imaging *and specific methods*
Radionuclide imaging, see Scintigraphy
Radiotherapy, see also Radioiodine
adverse effects, see Radiation-related disorders
pituitary tumors, 33–4, 136
adjuvant, 44–5, 49, 55, 57, 70
complications, 34, 38–9
thyroid cancer, 112, 113
Raloxifene, osteoporosis, 313–14
RANK (receptor activator of nuclear factor [kappa]B), 315, 316
Ras, 18
Rathke's pouch/cleft
cyst, 43
tumor, 43–4
Rb, pituitary tumors and, 21
RBM gene family, 182–3, 183
Receiver operator characteristic curves, 14
Receptor activator of nuclear factor [kappa]B (RANK), 315, 316
5_-Reductase inhibitor, 521–2
hirsutism, 211
pharmacology, 521–2
Reference ranges/values, 12, 551–4
Renal physiology/problems etc., see Kidney
Renin (in plasma) activity
in aldosteronism diagnosis, 389–91
reference values, 554
Renin—angiotensin (and aldosterone) system
in acromegaly, 402
ADH release and, 369
Reproduction, assisted, male infertility, 188
Reproductive function, see Sexual function
Reproductive hormones, see Sex hormones
Reproductive tract abnormalities, amenorrhea, 142–3
Respiratory disorders causing syndrome of inappropriate antidiuresis causation, 481
RET (*ret*)
MEN 2 and, 123–4, 124, 125
thyroid cancer and
medullary carcinoma, 116, 124

papillary carcinoma, 19–20
Retinoblastoma gene and pituitary tumors, 21
Retinoid X receptor, thyroid hormones and, 253
Rhabdomyolysis
hyperkalemia in, 383
in thyrotoxic crisis, 459
Rheumatoid factor, 11
Riedel's thyroiditis, 279, 344
Rieger syndrome, 157
Risedronate, Paget's disease of bone, 322
Rokitansky syndrome, 142
Rolipram, erectile dysfunction, 175
Rosai—Dorfman disease, 342, 343

Saline infusion
Addisonian crisis, 444
hyponatremia, 378, 482, 484
complications, 378, 479, 482, 484
Sarcoidosis, 341–2
hypercalcemia in, 301
pituitary, 43, 341
Sarcomas, bone, Paget's disease and, 320
Schmidt's syndrome, 444
Scintigraphy (radionuclide imaging)
osteoporosis, 309
Paget's disease of bone, 318–19
parathyroid, 297
pheochromocytoma, 398
Scrotal patches, testosterone, 159, 160
Seasonal affective disorder, 424
Sedation, thyroid storm, 458
Selective androgen receptor modulators, non-steroidal, 161
Selective estrogen receptor modulators, osteoporosis, 313–14
Sella
empty, see Empty sella
lesions (incl. tumors), differentiation from suprasellar lesions, 41–4
Semen analysis, 178
Sensitivity (of test), clinical, 13–15
Sepsis, see Infections
Serotonin, orexigenicity, 412
Sex chromosome abnormalities
females, premature ovarian failure, 140
male infertility, 180–3
Sex chromosome-linked adrenoleukodystrophy, 338, 339, 340, 341
Sex hormone(s) (gonadal steroids; reproductive hormones)

menstrual cycle and tests of, 2
reference values, 553
Sex-hormone binding globulin (SHBG), 205
testosterone assays and, 3, 151, 152, 153
Sexual development, males
delayed, screening for androgen deficiency, 147
precocious, LH/FSH receptor mutations and, 156
Sexual function (reproductive function)
men, see also Fertility problems; Psychosexual counselling
HIV disease/AIDS and, 335
hypogonadism and testosterone replacement and, 162
regulation, 165–7
Sheehan's syndrome, 343, 446
Short stature, adults, missed childhood growth disorders leading to, 98–9
Sibutramine, 417
Sick euthyroid syndrome (non-thyroidal illness), 98–9, 356–7
pathophysiology, 356–7
thyroid function testing and, 3–4, 356–7
Sickle cell disease and male gonadal dysfunction, 181, 184
Sildenafil, 167, 170–3
Simmond's disease (pituitary dysfunction due to head trauma), 343
diabetes insipidus, 343, 373
Simpson—Golabi-Behmel syndrome, 100
Sinus histiocytosis with massive lymphadenopathy (Rosai—Dorfman disease), 342, 343
Sipple's syndrome (MEN 2A), 116, 122–3, 123
Skin disorders (dermatopathies)
GH deficiency (adult), 92
in hypoparathyroidism, 288
in thyroid disease, 230–1
Skin patches, see Patches
Skinfold thickness, measurement, 409
Sleep apnea, testosterone replacement therapy and, 161, 164
Smoking and Graves' ophthalmopathy, 228
Smooth muscle, cavernosal, 166
drugs acting on, 173–5
Sodium, see also Saline infusion
disturbances, 376–8, 479–84
in HIV disease/AIDS, 336

urine, measurement, 376, 482
Sodium fluoride, 522–3
  osteoporosis, 314
  pharmacology, 522–3
Sodium iopanate, thyroid storm, 459, 460
Sodium ipodate, 544
  pharmacology, 544
  in thyroid storm, 459, 460
Sodium pump in acromegaly, 402
Soft tissues in acromegaly, 51
Somatostatin (GHRIF), 84–5
  receptors, in pheochromocytoma imaging, 398
Somatostatin analogs, 529, 535–6, *see also* Lanreotide; Octreotide
  ectopic GHRH-producing tumors, 56
  pharmacology, 529
  pituitary tumors, 35–7
    GH-producing (and acromegaly), 55–6, 57–9
Somatotroph (GH-producing) adenoma, genetics, 18
Somatotroph adenomas, *see* Growth hormone-producing adenomas
Spanish Collaborative Group on Male hypogonadotropic hypogonadism, 186
Specificity of assays
  clinical specificity, 13–15
  immunoassays, 5–6
Sperm, *see also* Azoospermia
  evaluation (count/morphology/function etc.), 178, 180
    computer-aided, 180
    intracytoplasmic injection, 188
Spermatogenesis, 175–7
  causes of failure, 176–7
  primary defects, 180–4
Sphenoidal sinus, surgery via, *see* Transsphenoidal
Spine, *see* Vertebra
Spironolactone, 544
  aldosteronism, 392–3
  hirsutism, 211
  pharmacology, 544
Staging system, thyroid cancer, 110
Standardization, immunoassays, 6–7
Stature, *see* Height
Steady state of patient, 1
Stereotactic radiotherapy, pituitary tumors, 34
Steroid(s), *see* Anabolic steroids; Glucocorticoids; Mineralocorticoids; Sex steroids
Steroid receptor coactivator 1 gene, disruption, 258
Stomach, balloons and reduction procedures, 417, 418
Stress and depression, 424
Subcutaneous liponecrosis, 302
Suprasellar lesions (incl. tumors), differentiation from sellar lesions/tumors, 41–4
Surgery
  aldosterone-producing adenoma, 392
  craniopharyngioma, 44
  Cushing's syndrome, 69–71
  IGF-II-producing tumors, 352
  in MEN 2, 124–5
  multinodular goiter, 272
  obesity, 417–18
  parathyroid excision, *see* Parathyroidectomy
  pheochromocytoma, 398–9
  pituitary apoplexy, 452–3
  pituitary tumors, 32, 452–3
    ACTH-producing, 70
    GH-producing, 53–4, 54–5, 57
    prolactin-producing, 48, 48–9, 136
  premature ovarian failure due to, 139
  thyroid excision (e.g. for cancer), *see* Thyroidectomy
  varicocele, in infertile men, 187–8
Synacthen test, *see* ACTH stimulation test
Syndromes of inappropriate antidiuresis (SIAD), 376, 377, 481, 482, 484
  causes/associated conditions, 476, 481
Systemic disease, 333–66
Systemic lupus erythematosus, 344

T3, *see* Triiodothyronine
T4, *see* Thyroxine
Tamoxifen, 544–5
  osteoporosis, 314
  pharmacology, 544–5
Technetium-99m scan
  osteoporosis, 309
  parathyroid, 297
Teeth in hypoparathyroidism, 288
Test(s), *see* Biochemical investigations *and specific tests*
Testicles (testes)
  biopsy, in infertility, 180
  dysfunction, *see* Hypogonadism, men
  germ cell development, *see* Spermatogenesis
  in obesity, 414
  primary failure, 177
  volume measurement (in hypogonadism), 150–1
Testicular feminization, 142–3
Testolactone, pharmacology, 545
Testosterone, 431, 546
  assays, 151–3
    females, in hirsutism and PCOS, 208–9
    male hypogonadism, 151, 151–3
    methods, 152–3
    replacement therapy, target levels and, 162
    sex-hormone binding globulin and, 3, 151, 152, 153
  biosynthesis, 205
  gel preparation, 159, 160
    evaluation of local application site, 164
  implants, 161
  low levels in men, screening for androgen deficiency, 147–8
  reference values, 553
  replacement therapy, 40, 158–65, 546
    contraindications, 161
    in erectile dysfunction, 172–3
    monitoring, 162–5
    in osteoporosis, 314
    preparations used and clinical pharmacology, 158–61
    psychological effects, 431
  sexual function and role of, 165–6
  therapeutic use, 546
    pharmacology, 546
    replacement therapy, *see subheading above*
Testosterone derivatives (incl. esters), 545
  injectable, 158–60
  novel, 161
  oral, 160–1
Tetany, hypoparathyroid, 287–8, 471–2
Tetracosactrin test, *see* ACTH stimulation test
TGF_ and prolactinomas, 20
Thalassemia and male gonadal dysfunction, 181
Thecal cell hyperplasia (hyperthecosis ovarii), 205

565

INDEX

Thiazide diuretics, osteoporosis, 314
Thionamides, see Propylthiouracil
Thirst
    excessive/prolonged, see Polydipsia
    regulation, 370
Thromboembolism
    myxedema coma, 463
    thyroid storm, 459
Thyroglobulin (TG)
    assays
        in postpartum thyroiditis, 279
        in thyroid cancer
        relapse/residual disease, 112
    autoantibodies to, 10, 221, 231, 234
        postpartum, 236
Thyroid gland, see also Hypothalamic—pituitary—thyroid axis; Sick euthyroid syndrome
    function (=hormone function)
        drugs inhibiting,, see also Antithyroid drugs
        HIV disease/AIDS and, 335
        hypertension and, 399–400
        in multinodular goiter, testing, 270–1
        postpartum dysfunction, 236–7, 275–9
        reference values, 554
        in sick euthyroid syndrome, testing, 3–4, 356–7
    in obesity, 414
    size/volume
        assessment, 270
        excessive, see Goiter
Thyroid gland disease, 17–24, 107–14, 215–35, 247–86, 456–63
    autoimmune, 215–35, 275–9
    dermatopathy associated with, 230–1
    neoplastic, see Thyroid neoplasms
    nodular, see Nodular thyroid disease
    ophthalmopathy associated with, see Ophthalmopathy
    psychiatric problems, 433–4
Thyroid hormones, see also Thyroxine; Triiodothyronine
    abnormal production, see Hyperthyroidism; Hypothyroidism
    administration/replacement, 546–7, 548
        autoimmune hypothyroidism, 235, 236
        depression, 427
        hypopituitarism, 449
        myxedema coma, 463, 464
        post-thyroidectomy, 112
    assays
        in Addisonian crisis, 444
        autoantibodies interfering with, 10
        binding proteins and, 3
        in multinodular goiter, 270–1
        in resistance to thyroid hormone, 255
        in sick euthyroid syndrome, 3–4, 356–7
    in depression treatment, 426–7
    function, see Thyroid gland, function
    markers/indices of action, measurement in resistance to thyroid hormone, 256
    pharmacology, 546–7, 548
    receptors (TRs)
        action, 253–4
        resistance to thyroid hormone and, 257, 258–60, 260–1
    resistance to, 253–61
        clinical features, 254–5
        definition, 254
        differential diagnosis, 255–6
        generalized (GRTH), 254
        management, 261
        molecular genetics, 257–8
        pathogenesis of variable tissue resistance, 260
        pituitary (PRTH), 254, 257–8, 260
    suppressive therapy in multinodular goiter, 271–2
    synthesis inhibitors, see Antithyroid drugs
Thyroid neoplasms (incl. cancer/carcinoma), 17–24, 107–14, 272
    exclusion, in nodular disease, 270
    genetics, 17–24, 116
        model of pathogenesis, 22
    MEN and thyroid cancer, 122–3, 123
    prognostic classification, 110
    toxic, 272
    treatment, 110–13
    TSH receptor mutations and, 248–51
        adenomas, 248–50
        cancer, 250–1
Thyroid peroxidase (TOP), autoantibodies, 221, 234
Thyroid-stimulating hormone (TSH; thyrotropin)
    assays
        in Graves' disease, 221
        in multinodular goiter, 270–1
        in resistance to thyroid hormone, 255, 256
    deficiency, features, 447
    resistance, congenital hypothyroidism with, 251–3
    response to TRH, see Thyrotropin-releasing hormone
    suppressive therapy in multinodular goiter, 271
Thyroid-stimulating hormone-producing adenoma, see Thyrotropin-producing adenoma
Thyroid-stimulating hormone receptor, 247–53
    action, 247–8
    autoantibodies, 217, 221, 222, 227
    mutations, 248–53
Thyroid storm (thyrotoxic crisis), 455–60
    clinical assessment and investigation, 456–7
    treatment, 456–60
        of complications, 459–60
Thyroidectomy
    for Graves' disease, 226–7
    for tumors, 111–12
        in MEN 2, therapeutic and prophylactic, 124–5
Thyroiditis, 273–80
    atrophic, presentation with, 232
    granulomatous, subacute, 273–5
    Hashimoto's, see Hashimoto's thyroiditis
    infectious, see Infections
    lymphocytic, 275–9
    postpartum, 236–7, 275–9
    Riedel's, 279, 344
Thyrotoxicosis, 272–3, 433, see also Hyperthyroidism; Toxic adenoma; Toxic multinodular goiter
    psychiatric problems, 433
    severe, thyroid crisis, see Thyroid storm
    tests for, 219–21
    tumors presenting with, 347
Thyrotropin-producing adenoma, 45–6
    resistance to thyroid hormone vs, 256, 257
Thyrotropin-releasing hormone (TRH), 426

pathophysiology/psychopathology, 427
prolactin response to, hyperprolactinemia, 47
TSH response to (TRH testing), 494–5
    depression and, 426
    thyrotroph adenoma, 45
Thyroxine (T4), 546-7, *see also* Thyroid hormones
    administration/replacement, 40, 546-7
        autoimmune hypothyroidism, 235, 236
        depression, 427
        hypopituitarism, 449
        myxedema coma, 463
        post-thyroidectomy, 112
    assays
        autoantibodies interfering with, 10
        binding proteins, 3, 4
        in Graves' disease and its treatment, 221, 223, 224
        in multinodular goiter, 270-1
        replacement therapy, 40
        in sick euthyroid syndrome, 3-4, 357
    causes of raised T4, 256
    pharmacology, 546-7
    reference values, 554
Thyroxine-binding protein, T4 assays and, 3, 4
Tibolone, pharmacology, 547–8
Tiludronate, Paget's disease of bone, 322
Tissue necrosis, hyperkalemia in, 383
TNM system, thyroid cancer, 110
Toxic adenoma, 272
Toxic multinodular goiter, 272
    TSH-R mutations and, 250
Transcription factors, homeodomain, mutations, 156–7
Transdermal patches, *see* Patches
Transforming growth factor-_ and prolactinomas, 20
Transplantation, bone marrow, adrenoleukodystrophy, 340
Transsphenoidal approach
    decompression via, 452–3, 454–5
    pituitary tumors, 32, 53–4, 70, 452–3, 454–5
Transurethral alprostadil, 173
Trauma, head, *see* Simmond's disease
Trazodone, erectile dysfunction, 175

TRH, *see* Thyrotropin-releasing hormone
Triglyceride synthesis/storage, fat tissue, 407–8
3,3,5-Triiodothyroacetic acid use, 261
Triiodothyronine (T3), 548, *see also* Thyroid hormones
    administration, 548
        autoimmune hypothyroidism, 235–6
        depression, 426–7
        hypopituitarism, 449
        myxedema coma, 463
        reference values, 554
    assays
        autoantibodies interfering with, 10
        in Graves' disease, 221
        in multinodular goiter, 270–1
        in sick euthyroid syndrome, 3–4, 356–7
    pharmacology, 548
Trisodium edetate, hypercalcemia, 469, 470
Troglitazone, PCOS, 139
Trousseau's sign, 471–2
TSH, *see* Thyroid-stimulating hormone
Tuberculous adrenalitis, 443
Tubules, renal, ADH actions, 371
Tumor(s), 117, 345–7, *see also* Multiple endocrine neoplasia; Paraneoplastic conditions *and specific types*
    adrenal, *see* Adrenal disease
    brain, amenorrhea with, 133
    ectopic hormone production, *see* Ectopic hormone production
    GH deficiency with, 89
    hyperthyroidism caused by, 273
    hypoglycemia-inducing, 350–2
    hypothalamic, types, 26
    IGFs and tumorigenesis, 88, 97–8
    islet cell (insulinoma), 476
    jaw, familial hyperparathyroidism and, 117, 120
    malignant, *see* Cancer
    osteomalacia with, 323–4
    ovarian, *see* Ovaries
    parathyroid
        familial disorders predisposing to, 298
        removal, 298
    pituitary, *see* Adenoma; Pituitary gland
    sellar and suprasellar, differential diagnosis, 41–4
    syndrome of inappropriate antidi-

uresis caused by, 376, 481
    thyroid, *see* Thyroid neoplasms
Tumor suppressor genes, 20–1
Turner's syndrome (syndrome of gonadal dysgenesis; 45,XO syndrome), 98–9
    male phenotype of (=Noonan's syndrome), 99, 182
    mosaicism (mixed 45,XO/46,XX), 140
        infertility, 182
        premature ovarian failure, 140

Ultrasound
    hyperparathyroidism, 297
    osteoporosis, 308
Urethra, alprostadil administration, 173
Urine
    excessive excretion, *see* Polyuria
    osmolality, estimation, 374
    sodium measurement, 376, 482
Urofollitropin, 523
Uterine bleeding, PCOS and presentation with, 138

Vacuum devices producing erection, 172
Vagina
    congenital absence, 142
    estrogens applied to, 519
Varicocele surgery, infertile men, 187–8
Vas deferens, bilateral congenital absence, 181, 184
Vasculature
    penile, in erection, 166
        in erectile dysfunction, evaluation, 167–9
    peripheral, and hypertension in Cushing's syndrome, 402, 403
Vasoactive amines in erectile dysfunction, 173–5
Vasopressin, *see* Antidiuretic hormone
Vasopressin analogue, *see* Desmopressin
Venous sampling, adrenal, 392
    pheochromocytoma, 398
Ventilatory management, *see also* Hypoventilation
    myxedema coma, 462
    thyroid storm, 458
Vertebra
    osteoporotic, 306–7, 319
    in Paget's disease of bone, differentiation from other conditions, 319
Very long chain fatty acids in adrenoleukodystrophy, 339, 339–40, 340, 341

Viagra (sildenafil), 167, 170–3
Viral origin
    Paget's disease of bone, 315
    subacute granulomatous thyroiditis, 273–4
Virilization, 201–16
    definition, 201
Visual disturbances (with pituitary pathology)
    hypopituitarism, assessment for, 447
    pituitary apoplexy, 450
        assessment for, 451
    tumors, 31–2, 453–5
        assessment, 454
Vitamin D, 471, 548–9
    administration (of preparations and derivatives), 548–9
        hypercalcemia due to, 301, 467
        hypocalcemia, 473, 474
        osteoporosis, 312
        pharmacology, 548–9
        pseudohypoparathyroidism, 293
    deficiency, 322–3, 471
        primary hyperparathyroidism masked by, 298
    drugs interfering with metabolism/absorption, 324
    reference values, 552
Volume expansion in acromegaly, 402
Vomiting
    with oral contraceptives, 513
    vasopressin release, 369

Water, excess, hyponatremia with, 479, see also Fluid; Thirst
Wegener's granulomatosis, 343
Weight (body), see also Obesity
    gain, neuropeptides and neurotransmitters promoting, 411, 412–13
    ideal, life insurance tables, 409
    loss
        amenorrhea with, 132
        neuropeptides and neurotransmitters promoting, 411–12, 428
        in obesity (=weight reduction), 415–18
        PCOS/hirsutism and effects of, 210
    measurement, 408–9
    target, obese patients, 415
Whipple triad, 475, 477
WHO, osteoporosis diagnostic criteria, 308
Williams' syndrome, 302
Women
    Caucasian, autoimmune endocrinopathies, 215
    fertility, see Fertility problems
    hirsutism, see Hirsutism
    virilization, see Virilization
World Health Organization, osteoporosis diagnostic criteria, 308

X-linked adrenoleukodystrophy, 338, 339, 340, 341
X-ray radiograph, see Radiography
Xenical, 416–17
45,XO syndrome, see Turner's syndrome
XX males, 182
47,XXY, infertility, 180–2
47,XYY syndrome, infertility, 182

Y chromosome (and male infertility)
    microdeletion, 181, 182–3
        X chromosome containing portion of, 182
        XYY syndrome, 182
Yohimbine, pharmacology, 549–50

Zollinger—Ellison syndrome in MEN 1, 118